SECOND EDITION

MOTOR SPEECH DISORDERS

Substrates, Differential Diagnosis, and Management

SECOND EDITION

MOTOR SPEECH DISORDERS

Substrates, Differential Diagnosis, and Management

Joseph R. Duffy, PhD, BC-NCD

Head
Section of Speech Pathology
Department of Neurology
Mayo Clinic
Professor
Speech Pathology
Mayo Clinic College of Medicine
Rochester, Minnesota

with 95 illustrations

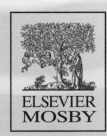

ELSEVIER
MOSBY

ELSEVIER
MOSBY

11830 Westline Industrial Drive
St. Louis, Missouri 63146

NOTICE

Health care is an ever-changing field. Standard safety precautions must be followed, but as new research
and clinical experience broaden our knowledge, changes in treatment and drug therapy may become
necessary or appropriate. Readers are advised to check the most current product information provided by
the manufacturer of each drug to be administered to verify the recommended dose, the method and
duration of administration, and contraindications. It is the responsibility of the licensed health care
provider, relying on experience and knowledge of the patient, to determine dosages and the best treatment
for each individual patient. Neither the publisher nor the author assumes any liability for any injury and/or
damage to persons or property arising from this publication.

The Publisher

ISBN-13: 978-0-323-02452-5
ISBN-10: 0-323-02452-1

Acquisitions Editor: Kathy Falk
Managing Editor: Christie Hart
Publishing Services Manager: Patricia Tannian
Project Manager: Sharon Corell
Designer: Paula Ruckenbrod
Cover Design: Jyotika Shroff

Printed in the United States of America

Last digit is the print number: 9   8   7   6   5

To

my parents, family, and colleagues

for their support and inspiration

Preface

The first edition of this book was published at the midpoint of the "decade of the brain," a time of unprecedented growth in our understanding of the neural bases of cognition and behavior and their disorders. Now, in the early years of the new millennium, the growth curve continues to accelerate. A crude index of the slope of the curve in the arena of motor speech disorders is reflected in a simple MEDLINE inquiry using "dysarthria" and "apraxia of speech" as subject headings or key words. Between 1995 (the year the first edition of this book was published) and September 2004 the search yielded 1075 citations, more than a 50% increase over the number of citations in the preceding decade. Developments in this past decade reflect contributions from speech-language pathology, speech science, neurology, and a number of related disciplines. They have had an impact on what we understand about the neurologic bases of motor speech disorders, their diagnoses, and their management. As is often the case in science and clinical practice, these advances are paradoxically humbling. There is still much to learn.

Readers familiar with the first edition of this book will note that this second edition contains the same number of chapters, only a few changes in chapter titles, and the same basic organization of information within each chapter. The retention of this basic format reflects feedback from many instructors and students who said that it facilitated learning and should not be altered. I have resisted the suggestion from some that the content be simplified because my hope is that the book will be useful to teachers and graduate students committed to a depth of understanding, as well as to professionals in need of a source of information for clinical practice and research. The changes in this edition mostly reflect the integration into the original format of new information and refinements of previous knowledge, rather than any significant paradigm shifts. Some of the changes are based on my own clinical experience, research, and reflection about the topic.

This book addresses the neurologic underpinnings of speech, the speech disorders that can develop when the nervous system goes awry, and the ways in which motor speech disorders can be assessed, diagnosed, and managed. Its contents reflect what we think we know about these things. Within and between the lines of each page, the lacunae will be apparent.

The book is intended primarily for graduate students, practicing clinicians, and researchers in the discipline of speech-language pathology. It will also be of interest to people in related disciplines—such as neurology, neuropsychology, and rehabilitation medicine—who are interested in speech disorders as an index of neurologic disease and its localization, and the differential diagnostic value of speech disorders to medical diagnosis and care.

The book is divided into three major parts that address (1) the neurologic substrates of speech and its disorders, (2) the disorders and their diagnoses, and (3) management. The information included in these three parts is interrelated. Likewise, an understanding of the material presented in all three parts is necessary for one to excel in any of the areas described.

Part One, Chapters 1 through 3, addresses substrates. Chapter 1 provides basic definitions of motor speech disorders (the dysarthrias and apraxia of speech) and discusses their distinction from other speech abnormalities. Data from the Mayo Clinic speech pathology practice—updated from the first edition—are reviewed to provide a sense of the prevalence and distribution of motor speech disorders in multidisciplinary medical practices. The chapter also provides an overview of perceptual, acoustic, and physiologic methods for studying motor speech disorders. Finally, it reviews approaches to characterizing the disorders and introduces the categorization scheme developed by Darley, Aronson, and Brown as the book's vehicle for discussing the dysarthrias.

Chapter 2 reviews the neurologic bases of motor speech and its pathologies. It focuses on structures and functions that are important to speech, the pathologies that may produce motor speech disorders, and some of the physical and behavioral deficits that may accompany motor speech disorders. Its discussion of the relationship of motor speech to the nervous system's final common pathway, direct and indirect activation pathways, and control circuits provides a foundation for understanding the distinctions among the major categories of motor speech disorders that are addressed in subsequent chapters.

Chapter 3 addresses the examination of motor speech disorders. It reviews the purposes and methods of clinical examination, particularly as it relates to differential diagnosis, including history taking, evaluation of each component of the speech mechanism during nonspeech and speech activities, the perceptual analysis of speech, and intelligibility assessment.

Part Two, Chapters 4 through 15, focuses on the disorders and their diagnoses. Chapters 4 through 11 address each major dysarthria type and apraxia of speech. In contrast to the first edition, flaccid dysarthrias (Chapter 4) and hyperkinetic dysarthrias (Chapter 8) are recognized as plural disorders, each with several subtypes that differ in lesion localization and/or underlying neuropathophysiology. Each chapter begins with a brief overview of relevant neurologic and neuropathologic underpinnings and reviews some of the conditions that are commonly or uniquely associated with the disorder under discussion. This is followed by a review of the etiology, localization, associated cognitive problems, and intelligibility for a substantial number of quasi-randomly selected cases with each type of motor speech disorder. Finally, discussion of common patient perceptions and complaints, a review of confirmatory oral mechanism and related findings, and a detailed description of salient perceptual speech characteristics and associated acoustic and physiologic findings are presented. Each chapter ends with four to nine case studies that illustrate some of the major points made in the text. The case studies provide a sense of the clinical reality of the disorders, the ways in which knowledge is applied in clinical practice, and the value and shortcomings of the enterprise.

Chapter 12 addresses forms of neurogenic mutism that reflect severe motor speech disorders, aphasia, or nonaphasic cognitive and affective deficits. Chapter 13 addresses several neurogenic speech disturbances (acquired neurogenic stuttering, palilalia, echolalia, cognitive and affective disturbances, aphasia, pseudoforeign accent, and aprosodia) that have close or distant relationships with motor speech disorders. Both chapters end with illustrative case studies.

One of the most challenging diagnostic problems in medical speech pathology practices involves the distinction between disorders that reflect neuropathology and those that reflect psychopathology or nonorganic influences. Chapter 14 addresses acquired psychogenic and related nonorganic speech disorders. It discusses their common etiologies and describes their most common speech characteristics. The important aspects of history taking and the observations that contribute to diagnosis are reviewed. The variety of speech characteristics associated with psychogenic voice and fluency disorders,

as well as less frequently occurring psychogenic articulation, resonance, and prosodic abnormalities, are described. Case studies at the chapter's end show how people with these disorders sometimes present in clinical practice.

Chapter 15 provides general guidelines for differential diagnosis. It synthesizes and summarizes the information in Chapters 4 through 14 that is most important to differential diagnosis. It emphasizes distinctions among the dysarthrias, between dysarthrias and apraxia of speech, between motor speech disorders and aphasia, among different forms of mutism, between motor speech disorders and other neurogenic speech disorders, and between neurogenic and psychogenic speech disorders.

Part 3, Chapters 16 through 20, addresses management. Chapter 16 provides an overview of principles for managing motor speech disorders. It discusses broad management goals, factors that influence management decisions, and the medical, prosthetic, behavioral, augmentative and alternative communication, counseling, and support aspects of management. It reviews in some detail principles and guidelines for behavioral treatment that can be applied to all motor speech disorders.

Chapter 17 focuses on management of the dysarthrias. It discusses speaker-oriented approaches that include medical, prosthetic, and behavioral interventions. It also examines management in relation to specific types of dysarthria, highlighting the fact that differential diagnoses among the dysarthrias can influence management, and that some approaches are well suited to certain dysarthria types whereas other approaches are not. The chapter also addresses communication-oriented strategies that may be used by dysarthric speakers or their listeners to facilitate communication, independent of dysarthria type and changes in speech production per se. Chapter 18 focuses specifically on the management of apraxia of speech. It makes clear that dysarthrias and apraxia of speech share a number of management attributes but that, because their underlying natures are fundamentally different, their management differs in a number of important ways.

Chapter 19 addresses the management of the other neurogenic speech disturbances discussed in Chapter 13. In keeping with the primary focus of the book, it emphasizes treatment of the speech characteristics associated with them, rather than the affective, cognitive, or linguistic disturbances that may underlie some of them.

Chapter 20 addresses the management of acquired psychogenic speech disorders. This chapter is included because the successful management of psychogenic speech disorders can make a valuable contribution to diagnosis in cases where there is uncertainty about neurogenic versus psychogenic etiology. It is hoped that the chapter contributes to clinicians' differential diagnostic skills as well as their treatment skills.

The impetus for this book grew out of my desire to integrate what is known about the bases of motor speech disorders with the realities of my clinical practice in which differential diagnoses and management are the order of the day. I have learned as much in writing this second edition as I did for the first and have become a wiser and better clinician because of it. I have also become convinced than our ignorance still surpasses our certainty. Some of what I don't know can be found in the minds and daily practices of other clinicians, scientists, and scholars, and some of it represents unanswered or unasked questions. I do hope that the facts and clinical observations reflected in these pages provide a friendly learning vehicle for clinicians and researchers in training, a source of useful information for practicing clinicians and researchers, and some seeds of interest for increasing our understanding of these disorders and our ability to help people who have them.

Joseph R. Duffy

Acknowledgments

Many people deserve recognition and my gratitude for their contributions to the birth of this second edition. They bear no responsibility for any of the book's shortcomings.

I thank the staff at Elsevier for their expert and collegial assistance; John Schrefer, Kellie White, and Jennifer White for helping to get the project off the ground; and especially Kathy Falk and Sharon Corell for guiding it through to completion. The spirit and skill of my secretary, Carie Dittrich, made many things easier.

Several people read drafts of portions of this book and provided valuable feedback. I thank Mick McNeil for his helpful comments on the apraxia of speech chapter, Ray Kent for his review of the unilateral upper motor neuron dysarthria chapter, and Geoff Fredericks for his feedback on many chapters. I am particularly indebted to Jack Thomas for his comments on every chapter of the book.

A special thanks to Ray Kent and his colleagues at the University of Wisconsin for the opportunity to collaborate on motor speech disorders research, work that has influenced the substance of this book. Also, comments about the first edition from many faculty, students, and clinicians have greatly aided my judgments about what did and didn't need fixing for this edition.

A number of people have served as my mentors over the years—the very special influences of Bob Duffy, Fred Darley, and Arnie Aronson float among these pages. The many thousands of patients who have taught me about motor speech disorders, my speech pathology and neurology colleagues in the Department of Neurology at the Mayo Clinic, and my colleagues and very good professional friends have all helped shape this book.

Finally, a special thank you to my wife and colleague Penny Myers for her support, empathy, and patience. She provided the intangibles that helped me finish the race.

Joseph R. Duffy

Contents

Part 1: Substrates

  1. Defining, Understanding, and Categorizing Motor Speech Disorders   3

  2. Neurologic Bases of Motor Speech and Its Pathologies   17

  3. Examination of Motor Speech Disorders   69

Part 2: The Disorders and Their Diagnoses

  4. Flaccid Dysarthrias   109

  5. Spastic Dysarthria   143

  6. Ataxic Dysarthria   163

  7. Hypokinetic Dysarthria   187

  8. Hyperkinetic Dysarthrias   217

  9. Unilateral Upper Motor Neuron Dysarthria   255

10. Mixed Dysarthrias   275

11. Apraxia of Speech   307

12. Neurogenic Mutism   335

13. Other Neurogenic Speech Disturbances   353

14. Acquired Psychogenic and Related Nonorganic Speech Disorders   381

15. Differential Diagnosis   409

Part 3: Management

16. Managing Motor Speech Disorders: General Principles   435

17. Managing the Dysarthrias   465

18. Managing Apraxia of Speech   507

19. Managing Other Neurogenic Speech Disturbances   525

20. Managing Acquired Psychogenic and Related Nonorganic Speech Disorders   535

Substrates

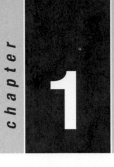

1 Defining, Understanding, and Categorizing Motor Speech Disorders

CHAPTER OUTLINE

    I. The neurology of speech
    II. The neurologic breakdown of speech
   III. Basic definitions
       A. Dysarthria
       B. Apraxia of speech
       C. Motor speech disorders
   IV. Speech disturbances that are distinguishable from motor speech disorders
       A. Other neurologic disorders
       B. Nonneurologic disturbances
       C. Normal variations in speech production
    V. Prevalence and distribution of motor speech disorders
   VI. Methods for studying motor speech disorders
       A. Perceptual methods
       B. Instrumental methods
       C. The clinical salience of the perceptual analysis of motor speech disorders
  VII. Categorizing motor speech disorders
       A. Characterizing motor speech disorders
       B. The perceptual method of classification
VIII. Summary

Speech is a unique, complex, dynamic motor activity through which individuals express thoughts and emotions and respond to and control their environment. It is among the most powerful tools possessed by the human species, and it contributes enormously to the character and quality of life.

Under most circumstances, speech is produced with an ease that belies the complexity of the operations underlying it. The study of normal speech processes helps establish the enormity of the act. Unfortunately, neurologic disease can also unmask the complex underpinnings of speech by disturbing its expression in various predictable ways. These disturbances, the mechanisms that help explain them, the signs and symptoms that define them, and their management are the subjects of this book.

◼ THE NEUROLOGY OF SPEECH

Speech requires the integrity and integration of numerous neurocognitive, neuromuscular, and musculoskeletal activities. These activities can be summarized as follows:

1. When thoughts, feelings, and emotions generate an intent to communicate, they must be organized and converted to verbal symbols in a manner that abides by the rules of language. These activities are referred to as *cognitive-linguistic processes*.

2. The intended verbal message must be organized for neuromuscular execution. This activity includes the selection and sequencing of sensorimotor "programs" that activate the speech muscles at appropriate coarticulated times, durations, and intensities. These activities are referred to as *motor speech planning and programming*.

3. Central and peripheral nervous system activity must combine to regulate and execute speech motor programs by innervating the respiratory, phonatory, resonatory, and articulatory muscles in a manner that generates an acoustic signal that faithfully reflects the goals of the programs. The neuromuscular transmission and subsequent muscle contractions and movements of speech structures are referred to as *neuromuscular execution*.

The combined processes of speech motor planning, programming, and neuromuscular execution are referred to as *motor speech processes*.

◼ THE NEUROLOGIC BREAKDOWN OF SPEECH

When the nervous system becomes disordered, so may the production of speech. In fact, *changes in speech may announce the presence of neurologic disease*. The effects of neurologic disease on speech are often lawful, predictable, and clinically unique and recognizable. Recognizing and understanding predictable patterns of speech disturbance and their underlying neurophysiologic bases are valuable for at least four reasons:

1. *Understanding nervous system organization for speech motor control.* The predictable association of patterns of speech deficit with localizable pathology can contribute to our understanding of the nervous system's anatomic and physiologic organization for speech motor control. Just as the study of aphasia teaches us something about the organization and localization of cognitive-linguistic processes associated with language behavior, the study of motor speech disorders informs us about the physiology and localization of speech production.

2. *Differential diagnosis and localization of neurologic disease.* In 1987 Aronson[3] called the contribution of speech diagnosis to medical diagnosis one of the best-kept secrets of our time by both speech pathology and

medicine. Although this is somewhat less true today, the secret is that speech changes can be the first or only manifestation of both organic and psychiatric disease, and their recognition and diagnosis can contribute to disease localization, diagnosis, and care. This necessitates modification of beliefs that speech diagnosis always follows medical or neurologic diagnosis, and that speech diagnosis and management are separate from medical diagnosis and management. This value becomes evident in many succeeding chapters, especially within the context of the case histories on major motor speech disorders at the end of each chapter.

3. *Prevalence.* Neurologic disorders are common. Few are truly curable, and they are a major cause of disability in the population as a whole.[20,47] Neurologic speech disorders represent a significant proportion of acquired communication disorders (Figure 1-1). An

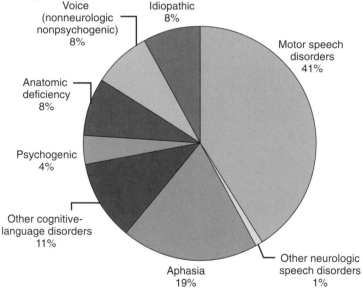

FIGURE 1-1 Distribution of acquired communication disorders, Speech Pathology, Department of Neurology, Mayo Clinic, 1987-1990 plus 1993-2001. Based on 14,269 evaluations of people with a primary speech pathology diagnosis of an acquired communication disorder. Referrals came primarily from neurology, otorhinolaryngology, neurosurgery, physical medicine, internal medicine, and patients themselves. Numbers reflect diagnostic consultations and not the number of patients receiving treatment.

Motor speech disorders include the dysarthrias and apraxia of speech. *Aphasia* includes all types of acquired aphasia. *Other neurologic speech disorders* include stuttering-like behavior, aprosodia, spasmodic dysphonia associated with dystonia or tremor, nonspecific central nervous system mutism or isolated aphonia and reduced loudness, and speech deficits associated with sensory disturbances. *Other cognitive-language disorders* include dementia, confusion, nonaphasic cognitive communication deficits associated with traumatic brain injury, akinetic mutism, alexia with or without agraphia, specific memory loss, ictal speech arrest, neurologic language disorder of undetermined type, and unresponsiveness associated with neurologic disease. *Anatomic deficiency* includes laryngectomy and glossectomy. *Voice (nonneurologic or nonpsychogenic)* disorders include etiologies of vocal abuse, papilloma, intubation and tracheostomy, vocal fold bowing, hormonal imbalance, neoplasm, acromegaly, and surgery. *Psychogenic* includes nonorganic speech disorders characterized by mutism, aphonia or dysphonia, spasmodic dysphonia, dysprosody, stuttering-like behavior, infantile speech, articulation disturbance, foreign accent, high pitch, and abnormal loudness. *Idiopathic* disorders (i.e., of unknown etiology) include dysphonias, stridor, palilalia, monopitch, pseudoforeign accent, and stuttering-like behavior.

increase in their prevalence can be anticipated because of increased survival rates for a number of neurologic conditions and because increasing longevity in the general population gives neurologic disease "more opportunity to introduce itself to us."[16]

4. *Management.* The identification of deviant speech characteristics, their localization to various levels of the speech system, and an understanding of their likely neuropathophysiology can provide important clues for management. For example, knowing that an individual's articulatory distortions are primarily related to incoordination and not to weakness might lead to efforts to assist coordination (e.g., by modifying rate and prosody) rather than attempts to increase strength through exercise.

BASIC DEFINITIONS

It is necessary to define some terms used to refer to certain neurologic speech disturbances. For those learning about these disorders for the first time, the definitions provide a framework for beginning to think about them. For those more familiar with the topic, the definitions establish boundaries of meaning that are sometimes blurred in the medical and speech pathology literature.

Dysarthria

The work of Darley, Aronson, and Brown[11-13] provided the modern definition of dysarthria. Because their pivotal 1969 and 1975 contributions are referenced frequently throughout this book, the abbreviation DAB is used to refer to them. DAB defined dysarthria as the following:

> . . . a collective name for a group of speech disorders resulting from disturbances in muscular control over the speech mechanism due to damage of the central or peripheral nervous system. It designates problems in oral communication due to paralysis, weakness, or incoordination of the speech musculature.[13]

A somewhat modified and expanded definition—although not at odds with the work of DAB—is adopted in this book for two reasons. First, dysarthria can be due to problems other than paralysis, weakness, and incoordination, a fact that was actually established by the work of DAB but not made apparent in their basic definition. Second, adding some detail to the definition helps to better establish the core components and boundaries of the disorder. Thus dysarthria is defined as *a collective name for a group of neurologic speech disorders resulting from*

abnormalities in the strength, speed, range, steadiness, tone, or accuracy of movements required for control of the respiratory, phonatory, resonatory, articulatory, and prosodic aspects of speech production. The responsible pathophysiologic disturbances are due to central or peripheral nervous system abnormalities and most often reflect weakness; spasticity; incoordination; involuntary movements; or excessive, reduced, or variable muscle tone.

This definition explicitly recognizes or implies the following characteristics about the disorder:

1. It is neurologic in origin.
2. It is a disorder of movement or movement control.
3. It can be categorized into different types, each type characterized by distinguishable auditory perceptual characteristics and, presumably, different underlying neuropathophysiology. The ability to categorize the dysarthrias, therefore, has implications for the localization of the causal disorder.

The definition used here is considerably narrower and more specific than that used in many medical dictionaries and texts. For example, some use the term *dysarthria* generically to refer to any disturbance of speech. Others use the term to refer to any neurologic disturbance of speech or language, failing to distinguish it from aphasia, apraxia of speech, and other neurologic communication disorders. Such broad, vague definitions weaken the conceptual and diagnostic value of the term and should be avoided in research and clinical practice.

Apraxia of Speech

Darley[10] was a major force in developing the modern concept and basic definition of apraxia of speech. Many subsequent contributions have led to modifications and refinements in definitions of the disorder and its distinguishing clinical characteristics.

For the purpose of this introductory chapter apraxia of speech is defined as *a neurologic speech disorder reflecting an impaired capacity to plan or program sensorimotor commands necessary for directing movements that result in phonetically and prosodically normal speech. It can occur in the absence of physiologic disturbances associated with the dysarthrias and in the absence of disturbance in any component of language.** A thorough discussion and clinical description of apraxia of speech are provided in Chapter 11.

Unlike dysarthria, the existence of apraxia of speech as a distinct clinical entity is often ignored

---

*This definition is conceptually similar to those used by DAB[11]; Wertz, LaPointe, and Rosenbek[50]; McNeil, Robin, and Schmidt[34]; and McNeil, Doyle, and Wambaugh.[33]

outside the speech pathology literature. Consequently, its clinical manifestations are frequently buried within categories of aphasia or under the generic heading of dysarthria. This is unfortunate for many reasons, especially because the localization of apraxia of speech is different than that for most dysarthria types, and because its management is different from that for dysarthria and aphasia.

Motor Speech Disorders

Motor speech disorders (MSDs) can be defined as *speech disorders resulting from neurologic impairments affecting the motor planning, programming, neuromuscular control, or execution of speech.* They include the dysarthrias and apraxia of speech.

▣ SPEECH DISTURBANCES THAT ARE DISTINGUISHABLE FROM MOTOR SPEECH DISORDERS

Other Neurologic Disorders

Other Neurologic Speech Disturbances

Several disturbances of speech have neither been clearly represented nor defined traditionally as MSDs. They are nonetheless neurologic in origin and distinct in their clinical characteristics. These deficits include, but are not limited to, acquired neurologic stuttering-like behavior, palilalia, echolalia, certain forms of mutism, pseudoforeign dialect, and aprosodia associated with right hemisphere dysfunction. These disorders are discussed in Chapter 13, which focuses on neurologic speech disturbances not typically categorized under the headings of dysarthria or apraxia of speech.

Cognitive, Linguistic, and Cognitive-Linguistic Disturbances

Changes in speech resulting from language and other cognitive deficits (e.g., aphasia, akinetic mutism, other cognitive and affective disturbances that attenuate or inhibit speech) are sometimes difficult to distinguish from MSDs. In addition, because they often co-occur with MSDs, they may make the speech examination and diagnosis of the MSD difficult. Chapter 15 addresses the distinctions among MSDs, aphasia, and other neurologic speech and cognitive-linguistic disturbances that may influence the perceptual characteristics of speech and complicate differential diagnosis.

Sensory Deficits

The emphasis on the motor aspects of speech in this book is not intended to minimize the importance of sensory processes in speech production or the potential impact of sensory disturbances on speech. The effect of congenital deafness, for example, on the development of speech is devastating*; even deafness acquired in adulthood can result in some degradation of speech. The effects of hearing loss on speech production, however, are distinguishable in many ways from MSDs and are not discussed further in this book.

Tactile, kinesthetic, and proprioceptive sensation are also important to the development and maintenance of normal speech, and their malfunction has been implicated in certain MSDs (the role of sensation in motor learning and control is discussed in Chapter 2). Therefore *think of motor speech processes and disorders as sensorimotor and not just motor in character.* Although this book is not intended to discuss speech deficits resulting from primary tactile, kinesthetic, or proprioceptive disturbances, there is a brief discussion of "sensory dysarthria" in Chapters 4 and 6 and the possible influence of sensory disturbances on apraxia of speech in Chapter 11.

Nonneurologic Disturbances

Some influences on speech are not encompassed by cognitive-linguistic or motor speech processes. Some are clearly localized outside the nervous system. Others reside in the "mind" but are neither neuromotor nor specifically cognitive-linguistic in character. These influences are discussed briefly as follows.

Musculoskeletal Defects (e.g., Laryngectomy, Cleft Lip and Palate, Fractures, Abnormal Variants in Cavity Size and Shape)

The integrity of muscle, cartilage, and bone is important to normal speech—injury, disease, congenital absence, loss to aging or poor care (e.g., teeth), or surgical removal of muscle, cartilage, or bone can alter speech. Other physical influences, such as abnormal variations in the size and shape of primary speech structures or the effects of systemic illness, can also alter speech in ways that exceed, mask, or exacerbate the effects of focal neuropathologies on speech. The reader's awareness of these factors is assumed and is not discussed further.

Nonneurologic or Nonpsychogenic Voice Disorders

Certain voice disorders could actually be subsumed under the musculoskeletal defects described in the

---

*See Pratt and Tye-Murray[37] for a comprehensive summary of the speech deficits that may be associated with hearing loss.

preceding section. They are given separate recognition here, however, because they often are more difficult to distinguish from MSDs and sometimes are misinterpreted as reflecting neuropathology. These include, for example, dysphonias associated with hormonal disturbances, head or neck neoplasms, and vocal abuse. The diagnosis may be established by history or during direct laryngeal examination, and experienced clinicians can often hear that the dysphonia is not neurologic. Although these disorders are not addressed in detail in this book, they receive recognition in Chapter 3.*

Psychogenic and Related Nonorganic Disorders

Speech can undergo change as a result of abnormal psychologic states (e.g., schizophrenia, depression, conversion disorder). It can also change as a result of faulty subconscious "learning" or compensation in response to various physical, neurologic, or psychologic influences, sometimes in people who are otherwise psychologically healthy. The speech manifestations of these disorders can be difficult to distinguish from those stemming from neurologic disease. Because these problems reside in the mind, they are arguably fundamentally neurologic (if one believes that the mind and brain are inextricably linked). Because they are not primarily neuromotor in nature, however, they must be distinguished from MSDs.

Psychogenic and related nonorganic voice and speech disorders are not uncommon in neurologic practice and frequently accompany neurologic abnormalities. Their recognition and management are important in medical speech pathology practices. They are discussed in detail in Chapters 14 and 20.

Normal Variations in Speech Production

Age-Related Changes in Speech

Normal aging is associated with changes in speech that are physiologically, acoustically, and perceptually detectable. They include, at the least, changes in pitch, voice quality and stability, loudness, speech breathing patterns, rate, and prosodic variations.†
Because many neurologic disorders are overlaid on an aging nervous system, and because some speech changes associated with aging are similar to those associated with dysarthria, the identification of a speech characteristic as "deviant" and possibly indicative of dysarthria often requires an awareness of the range of normal for the patient's age and general physical condition. Unfortunately, many of these judgments depend on subjective clinical experience, because objective measures are either not easily obtained in clinical settings or are associated with extreme variability of normative data.

Gender

Male and female voice and speech are perceptually different. These differences can influence the detection of abnormalities, at least with some methods of analysis. For example, acoustic indices of laryngeal abnormalities may differ among men and women with the same neurologic disease,[27] and some of the acoustic heterogeneity within specific categories of dysarthria may be explained by gender.[23] Whether gender differences influence clinical perceptual diagnosis is uncertain, but it is nonetheless important to keep them in mind.

Variations in Style

The qualitative character of speech varies as a function of normal differences in personality, emotional state, and speaking roles. Such variations often and justifiably go unnoticed by clinicians and researchers intent upon recognizing abnormality, but they sometimes must be identified explicitly for accurate differential diagnosis.

▪ PREVALENCE AND DISTRIBUTION OF MOTOR SPEECH DISORDERS

The incidence and prevalence of MSDs in the general population are uncertain, but they are undoubtedly common in neurologic practice and probably represent a significant proportion of the communication disorders seen in medical speech-language pathology practices.[53] It has been estimated, for example, that approximately 60% of noncomatose people who have had strokes suffer from some kind of speech or language impairment.[48] More specifically, dysarthria is often present in frequently occurring neurologic conditions. It occurs in 25% of patients with lacunar (small) strokes[1] and about one third of those with traumatic brain injury.[42-54] It is probably present in 60% or more of people with Parkinson's disease (PD), with increased prevalence as the disease progresses.[31,35] It is sometimes a presenting symptom or sign of amyotrophic

---

*Texts such as those by Aronson[2] and Colton and Casper[9] contain comprehensive reviews of a wide variety of voice disorders, including those associated with neurologic disease.

†Useful summaries of age-related speech changes can be found in Baker et al.[4]; Beaseley and Davis[5]; Decoster and Debruyne[14]; Linville[28]; Liss, Weismer, and Rosenbek[30]; Ramig et al.[39]; and Smith, Wasowicz, and Preston.[43]

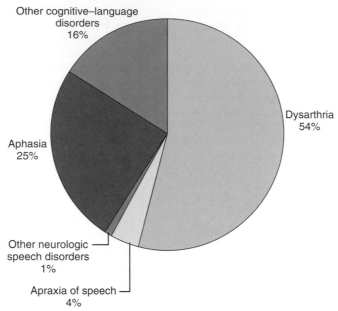

FIGURE 1-2 Distribution of acquired neurologic communication disorders, Speech Pathology, Department of Neurology, Mayo Clinic, 1987-1990 plus 1993-2001. Based on 10,444 evaluations of people whose primary speech pathology diagnosis was an acquired neurologic communication disorder.

Dysarthria includes all dysarthria types, including dysphonia associated with vocal fold paralysis (flaccid) and neurologic spasmodic dysphonia (hyperkinetic). *Apraxia of speech* includes acquired apraxia of speech. *Other neurologic speech disorders* include stuttering-like behavior, aprosodia, nonspecific central nervous system mutism or isolated aphonia and reduced loudness, and speech deficits associated with sensory disturbances. *Aphasia* includes all types of acquired aphasia. *Other cognitive-language disturbances* include dementia, confusion, nonaphasic cognitive communication deficits associated with traumatic brain injury, akinetic mutism, alexia with or without agraphia, specific memory loss, ictal speech arrest, and neurologic language disorder of undetermined type.

lateral sclerosis and often emerges during the disease's course.[19,41]

The representation of MSDs among acquired communication disorders can be appreciated by examining their proportionate distribution in a speech-language pathology practice within a large inpatient and outpatient medical institution. Figure 1-1 summarizes the distribution of acquired communication disorders seen in the Section of Speech Pathology in the Department of Neurology at the Mayo Clinic from 1987-1990 and 1993-2001.* The data indicate that MSDs represent a substantial proportion (41%) of the acquired speech, voice, lan-

guage, and cognitive-communication disturbances that were evaluated. The data might not represent the distribution of these disorders seen in many speech pathology practices. For example, it is possible that the distribution in Figure 1-1 represents a disproportionate number of cases in which a speech-language pathology evaluation was considered necessary for medical diagnosis or clinical management recommendations but not necessarily for ongoing management.

Figure 1-2 isolates from Figure 1-1 the acquired neurologic communication disorders. MSDs (dysarthrias and apraxia of speech) account for 58% of the primary diagnoses and are far more prevalent than any other category, including aphasia. Again, this distribution probably reflects the relative importance or value placed on accurate differential diagnosis of MSDs plus recommendations for management, as opposed to referral for management alone.

These data testify to the prominence of MSDs among acquired communication disorders encountered in comprehensive medical speech pathology practices. They justify ongoing research and the need

*The database is derived from speech pathology diagnostic consultations for outpatients and patients evaluated in two acute care hospitals and a rehabilitation unit. The data reflect patients' primary communication disorder; when more than one disorder was present, primary meant the most severe disorder. The sample is probably fairly representative of the distribution of combined acute, progressive, and chronic acquired communication disorders (with the exception of those related to hearing loss) in large primary and tertiary care inpatient, rehabilitation, and outpatient medical practices.

for clinical diagnostic and management expertise in the area of MSDs.

METHODS FOR STUDYING MOTOR SPEECH DISORDERS

MSDs can be studied in many ways, all of which contribute to their characterization and understanding. The methods can be categorized under two broad headings: perceptual and instrumental. Each method has strengths and shortcomings, each has varying sensitivity to abnormalities in different parts of the speech system, and each has varying relevance to the numerous clinical and theoretical questions that are relevant to understanding MSDs. Therefore progress will likely be greatest if information derived from perceptual and instrumental studies can be integrated into a rich description of the disorders.[24]

Perceptual Methods

Perceptual methods are based primarily on the auditory-perceptual attributes of speech. *They are the "gold standard" for clinical differential diagnosis, judgments of severity, many decisions about management, and the assessment of functional change.* At the same time, they are subject to unreliability of judgments among clinicians, they may be difficult to quantify, and they cannot directly test hypotheses about the pathophysiology underlying perceived speech abnormalities.* In the hands (ears, eyes, and hands, actually) of experienced clinicians, however, the auditory-perceptual classification of MSDs is a valid and essential diagnostic and clinical decision-making tool. It is unlikely that it will be replaced by other methods, however sophisticated, because the evaluation of a speech disorder always begins with a perceptual judgment that speech has changed or is abnormal or different in some way.

DAB[11-13] pioneered the modern use of auditory perceptual assessment to characterize the dysarthrias and to identify the clusters of salient perceptual characteristics that are associated with lesions in different portions of the central and peripheral nervous system. Their approach to classifying the dysarthrias is used by many clinicians charged with differential diagnosis and many researchers investigating the acoustic and physiologic bases of MSDs. In fact, one outcome of the work of DAB was the generation of numerous hypotheses about the physiologic bases of the dysarthrias. These hypotheses grew out of an integration of the perceptual characteristics identified in their studies with what was known or believed

about the general role in movement control played by damaged portions of the nervous system. DAB helped set the direction of acoustic and physiologic studies, the results of which are often interpreted in reference to the clinical hypotheses. With high frequency, acoustic and physiologic studies have confirmed and further refined the perceptually based hypotheses of DAB.

The auditory modality has been the focus of research into the perceptual characteristics of the dysarthrias, but the value of visual and tactile observations in clinical assessment should not be ignored. Although dysarthria is an auditory-perceptual phenomenon and therefore cannot be diagnosed solely on the basis of visual or tactile observation, such observations can provide valuable confirmatory evidence for diagnosis. For example, unilateral upper and lower facial weakness and tongue atrophy and fasciculations are suggestive of lower motor neuron weakness; they help support a diagnosis of flaccid dysarthria when deviant speech characteristics are logically associated with them. Therefore visual and tactile observations of the speech mechanism at rest, during nonspeech movement, and during speech are important and sometimes crucial components of the motor speech examination.

Instrumental Methods

Although "the clinical potential of instrumental analysis of speech and related physiology is now only beginning to be realized,"[44] instrumental analyses—even if only employed within laboratory and clinical research settings—have contributed substantially to the description and understanding of MSDs. In fact, some methods currently have demonstrated clinical value for description and management, and they sometimes contribute to clinical differential diagnosis.

Technology for the instrumental analysis of speech is increasingly user-friendly and affordable, and many techniques are being evaluated for their applicability to questions that can be addressed within clinical settings.[22] The need for systematic research to integrate traditional clinical assessment with instrumental procedures has been recognized.[17,49] These efforts have been evident in numerous venues, to a noteworthy degree since 1982 in the biennial Conference on Motor Speech Disorders and its subsequent publications* that include reports relating "laboratory" research findings to clinical

---

*See Kent[21] for a comprehensive review of the limitations of auditory-perceptual approaches to the assessment of voice and speech disorders, including MSDs.

*These include Berry[6]; Yorkston and Beukelman[52]; Moore, Yorkston, and Beukelman[36]; Till, Yorkston, and Beukelman[45]; Robin, Yorkston and Beukelman[40]; and Cannito, Yorkston, and Beukelman (1998).[8]

practice. Many of the papers employ acoustic and physiologic analyses of MSDs.

With some important exceptions, instrumental methods are not widely used in the clinical evaluation and management of MSDs. One explanation may be a lack of widely accepted standards and normative data for speech tasks and methods and parameters for instrumental measurement.[44] In addition, Gerratt et al.[18] note that: "Clinicians' reluctance to use instrumentation may result from a lack of knowledge and a lack of evidence to support the contribution of instrumentation in dysarthria management. The former requires the attention of training programs; the latter demands the attention of clinical research."

Instrumental methods can be crudely organized under three headings: acoustic, physiologic, and visual imaging. The following discussions emphasize the roles of these methods in clinical practice and our understanding of MSDs.

Acoustic Methods

Acoustic methods can visually display and numerically quantify numerous aspects of the acoustic speech signal. They are tightly bound to auditory-perceptual judgments of speech, because they use the same data, the speech signal. Although they do not always distinguish dysarthric from normal speech,[22] they have contributed substantially to the quantification, description, and understanding of MSDs. They have provided refined, confirmatory, and quantified* support for perceptual judgments that speech rate is slow, voice is breathy or contains tremor or interruptions, pitch and loudness variability are reduced, resonance is hypernasal, articulation is imprecise, speech diadochokinetic rates are irregular, and so on. In addition, qualitative acoustic analyses can make important contributions to theoretical constructs for explaining components of MSDs.[29]

State-of-the-art instrumentation for acoustic analysis has become more affordable, accessible, efficient, and user-friendly to practicing clinicians.[23,25] The capacity of acoustic analysis to make visible and quantify the speech signal can provide baseline data and serve as an index of stability, improvement, or deterioration over time. Acoustic analysis is also a source of feedback during therapy. However, because "only limited progress has been made in identifying acoustic dimensions for certain

types of dysarthria,"[22] its capacity to add to, modify, or refine perceptually based clinical diagnoses has yet to be firmly established.

Physiologic Methods

Auditory-perceptual and acoustic analyses, by definition, are focused on the sound emitted from the vocal tract. Physiologic methods move "upstream" toward the source of activity that generates the speech signal and therefore represent another level of explanation. They focus on the movements of speech structures and air, the muscle contractions that generate movement, the relationships among movements at different levels of the musculoskeletal speech mechanism, the temporal parameters and relationships among central and peripheral neural activity and biomechanical activity, and the temporal relationships among activities in central nervous system structures during the planning and execution of speech. The most commonly employed physiologic methods used to study the movement of air and peripheral structures associated with MSDs include *electromyography, kinematic measures,* and *aerodynamic measures.* The instruments and techniques employed by each method range from simple to elaborate. They also vary as a function of the location under study within the vocal tract.

Physiologic analyses have increased our understanding of speech motor control and how it can break down. They have refined and sometimes challenged perceptually based explanations for the pathophysiology of certain MSDs by clarifying whether various abnormal movements during speech reflect weakness, spasticity, incoordination, reduced range of movement, and so on. They have also helped to identify similarities and differences in the physiologic control of movements among different speech structures. In addition, they have provided insight into whether certain disorders reflect linguistic, motor planning or programming, or neuromuscular deficits, distinctions that can be very difficult or impossible to make on the basis of clinical perceptual assessment alone. Finally, similar to acoustic methods, they can provide feedback during management efforts.

Physiologic analyses of MSDs have much to offer the quantification, description, understanding, and, perhaps, management of MSDs. Similar to acoustic methods, however, their contribution to clinical diagnosis beyond that which can be derived from clinical perceptual assessment is not firmly established.

Visual Imaging Methods

Numerous instruments are available for visually imaging parts of the upper aerodigestive tract during

---

*It is sometimes assumed that because acoustic (and physiologic) analyses can be quantitative, they are more reliable than perceptual measures. In fact, acoustic measures within and among analysis systems have good-to-variable reliability (e.g., Green et al., 1998).[18a] Superior reliability of acoustic over perceptual measures cannot be assumed.[38]

speech, a process that cannot be appreciated simply by watching people talk. These instruments straddle the boundary between perceptual and physiologic measures because, although the instruments can be quantitatively analyzed, the instrumentally-provided visual image is usually interpreted by way of a non-quantified perceptual judgment by the clinician doing the examination. These imaging methods are highlighted here, because, unlike the physiologic methods just discussed, they are widely accepted and used frequently for clinical purposes. The most common clinically used visual imaging methods include videofluoroscopy, nasoendoscopy, laryngoscopy, and videostroboscopy, all of which can be videotaped, saved, and analyzed. They are used most often to evaluate swallowing and velopharyngeal and laryngeal functions for speech. When used to evaluate speech in combination with auditory-perceptual analysis, they frequently influence diagnosis and recommendations for management. Although subject to challenges of reliability similar to those for auditory-perceptual analyses, they are important to both clinical practice and research with MSDs.

It is beyond the scope of this book to review in any depth instrumental methods for studying the dysarthrias.* Gaps in knowledge regarding the reliability, validity, and applicability of a number of instrumental methods to clinical differential diagnosis and management justify a peripheral clinical role for many instrumental methods at this time. It is likely that perceptually based clinical assessment will always be the mainstay of clinical diagnosis. Recognize, however, that instrumental analyses help us understand the underpinnings of MSDs and may someday be widely applicable and important to clinical diagnostic and management efforts. Because they have contributed significantly to the description and understanding of MSDs, clinically relevant findings from acoustic, physiologic, and visual imaging studies are addressed in those chapters dealing with each of the dysarthrias and apraxia of speech.

The Clinical Salience of the Perceptual Analysis of Motor Speech Disorders

The primary emphasis in this book is on clinical perceptual assessment and the auditory perceptual and functional outcomes of management for MSDs. This is not to take issue with Wertz and Rosenbek,[49] who concluded that "the ear may be the final arbiter in detecting apraxia of speech and dysarthria, but combining it with acoustic and physiologic instrumentation will permit us to develop and firm theory and,

more importantly, improve practice." Acoustic and physiologic approaches are clearly an important source of what is known about MSDs,[26] and frequent reference will be made throughout this book to their contributions and relationship to perceptual observations and hypotheses. The emphasis here on perceptual assessment derives from several facts and beliefs:

1. The evaluation of anyone with a suspected motor speech disorder *begins* with a perceptually based assessment of speech. Any acoustic or physiologic assessment that may follow is motivated and directed by the results of the perceptual assessment. If descriptive or diagnostic errors are made at this entry point, whatever follows may be misguided and misleading to both diagnosis and management.

2. The usefulness of perceptually based differential diagnosis, relative to its contribution to localization and diagnosis of neurologic disease, has been established. The degree to which other methods add to, modify, contradict, or contribute equally to that effort is not yet entirely clear. Again, this does not minimize the contribution of acoustic and physiologic methods to the description, understanding, and quantification of MSDs. It does, however, argue for perceptually based methods as the *foundation of clinical practice*. A strong argument also can be made for requiring an adequate description of the salient perceptual characteristics of speech in any research examining the acoustic or physiologic attributes of MSDs; the likelihood that any such research can be replicated, generalized to clinical populations, or meaningfully interpreted by clinicians is greatly diminished or nullified without such description.

3. The standard for judging the functional outcome of management of MSDs is most often based on auditory-perceptual judgments of speech and its understandability and efficiency.

■ CATEGORIZING MOTOR SPEECH DISORDERS

Characterizing Motor Speech Disorders

Because MSDs can be considered in various ways, many different categorization schemes have been developed. DAB[11] and Yorkston et al.[54] identified dimensions that characterize MSDs and are important to both diagnosis and management. Some dimensions reflect a neurologic and etiologic

---

*See McNeil[32] and Kent et al.[25] for comprehensive overviews of acoustic or physiologic methods available for studying MSDs.

approach to classification. Others are tied specifically to the signs and symptoms of the speech disorders themselves.

Variables relevant to neurologic and etiologic perspectives include the following:

1. *Age at onset.* MSDs can be congenital (or developmental) or acquired. This distinction can be reflected in patient behavior and can influence management decisions and prognosis. However, time of onset in acquired disorders is almost always clear, and it rarely challenges clinical diagnosis beyond a careful history and neurologic examination. Clinicians should recognize the distinction, but it is not usually difficult to establish.

   The focus of this book is on acquired rather than congenital or developmental disorders. This reflects (1) an orientation to the contribution of differential diagnosis of MSDs to medical diagnosis and localization, a challenge that is more frequent (and sometimes easier to meet) for acquired than congenital or developmental disorders and (2) the greater wealth of information on differential diagnosis and management in acquired disorders. However, it is likely that many of the principles of classification, diagnosis, and management discussed in this book can be applied or adapted to children with congenital or developmental MSDs.* For example, expert listeners can distinguish the speech of children with athetoid and spastic cerebral palsy,[51] and there are strong parallels between the perceptual attributes and approaches to management for adults with acquired apraxia of speech and developmental apraxia of speech.[15]

2. *Course.* MSDs can be characterized as *congenital* (e.g., as in cerebral palsy or static encephalopathy); *chronic* or *stationary*[†] (e.g., cerebral palsy in adults; after plateauing has occurred in stroke); *improving* (e.g., during spontaneous recovery from stroke or closed head injury); *progressive* or *degenerative* (e.g., amyotrophic lateral sclerosis or PD); or *exacerbating-remitting* (e.g., multiple sclerosis). Monitoring MSDs over time may actually establish the course of disease or help eliminate diagnoses incompatible with a particular course. In many cases, by the time a patient is seen for speech evaluation, the course is already established. Nonetheless, the course of a problem has an important influence on management decisions.

3. *Site of lesion.* Lesions associated with MSDs can include such diverse loci as the neuromuscular junction, the peripheral and cranial nerves, the brainstem, the cerebellum, the basal ganglia, the pyramidal or extrapyramidal pathways, and the cerebral cortex. Establishing a lesion site is a primary goal of neurologic evaluation and one to which differential diagnosis of MSDs can contribute. Conversely, knowledge of a lesion site can predict certain speech deficits. Incompatibility of speech findings with known or postulated lesion sites can raise doubts about presumed localization or suggest the presence of additional lesions or even different diseases. For example, the presence of a mixed hypokinetic-spastic-ataxic dysarthria in someone with a diagnosis of PD should raise questions about the neurologic diagnosis or suggest the presence of neurologic dysfunction beyond that explainable by PD alone.

4. *Neurologic diagnosis.* Broad categories of neurologic disease include degenerative, inflammatory, toxic-metabolic, neoplastic, traumatic, and vascular etiologies. Within each of the broad categories, more specific diagnoses often can be applied. By itself, an MSD usually is not diagnostic of a particular neurologic etiology or specific disease. Because many diseases can affect multiple or variable portions of the nervous system, it is neither particularly useful nor feasible to classify MSDs by disease (e.g., "the dysarthria of multiple sclerosis," or "the dysarthria of stroke"). At the same time, some dysarthria types are found very commonly in some neurologic diseases and rarely or never in others (e.g., when PD causes dysarthria, its type is always hypokinetic; when myasthenia gravis causes dysarthria, its type is always flaccid). Therefore identification of a specific MSD may provide confirmatory (compatible) evidence for disease diagnosis.

---

*van Mourik et al.[46] have argued that dysarthrias acquired in childhood may require a classification scheme different (although as yet unspecified) from that used in this book. In contrast, Cahill, Murdoch, and Theodorus[7] reported that the dysarthria types found in a group of 24 children with traumatic brain injury (TBI) were similar to those in adults with TBI.

[†]Some authors place considerable emphasis on MSDs as chronic conditions.[54] There is no doubt that MSDs are long-term problems in many people. However, it is not unusual for some to have a transient or fluctuating MSD and for others to recover fully (e.g., following a small unilateral stroke or surgical trauma, after resolution of infection, or when it is drug-induced). It is thus important not to *define* MSDs as chronic conditions.

5. *Pathophysiology*. Presumably, it is the underlying pathophysiology (e.g., weakness, spasticity) that determines the unique deviant perceptual features of speech in MSDs. Therefore the presence of certain speech abnormalities suggests one or more pathophysiologic disturbances and vice versa.

Variables relevant to the speech disorders themselves include the following:

1. *Speech components involved*. MSDs can be categorized according to the speech subsystems that are affected. Knowing whether respiration, phonation, resonance, or articulation are impaired can contribute to speech diagnosis and often has an impact on management decisions.

2. *Severity*. Severity, by itself, does not differentiate among MSDs, because each one varies along the severity continuum. It can raise questions about diagnosis, however. For example, speech characteristics suggestive of profound weakness leading to severe reduction in intelligibility are usually accompanied by physical findings that confirm the weakness; if the physical examination is incompatible with underlying weakness, it may be necessary to consider another etiology (e.g., psychogenic, maladaptive speaking strategies).

Severity is always relevant to management decisions. Coupled with information about diagnosis and course of disease, severity helps determine when management is necessary, whether it will be short-term or long-term, whether it should focus on improving speech or developing augmentative forms of communication, and so on.

3. *Perceptual characteristics*. The perceptual characteristics of speech have already been discussed as factors crucial to differential diagnosis and relevant to management. Because it has a firm grounding in clinical research, because it has been heuristically valuable to the acoustic and physiologic study of MSDs, and because it is so salient to daily clinical activity, the perceptually based classification scheme of DAB[11] forms the framework around which MSDs are discussed.

The Perceptual Method of Classification

Table 1-1 summarizes the classification scheme used in this book. It was developed by DAB in their influential studies of the dysarthrias[12,13] and in their classic book, *Motor Speech Disorders*.[11] Their system for classifying the dysarthrias is considered "central to both clinical applications and to ideas of how the neural system regulates the complex processes involved in spoken language."[26]

DAB studied six major types of dysarthria (flaccid, spastic, ataxic, hypokinetic, hyperkinetic, and mixed). The category of mixed dysarthrias includes all possible combinations of the single types, each mix having various predictable or unpredictable relationships with various neurologic diseases. Mixed dysarthrias are discussed in Chapter 10.

Two categories have been added to those studied by DAB. *Unilateral upper motor neuron dysarthria* was alluded to by DAB[11] but not specifically studied by them. It does, however, occur commonly in patients with unilateral cerebral lesions, often occurs with aphasia and apraxia of speech, and is

| table 1-1 | Major types of motor speech disorders and their localization and neuromotor bases |

Type	Localization	Neuromotor Basis
Dysarthria		
Flaccid	Lower motor neuron (final common pathway, motor unit)	Weakness
Spastic	Bilateral upper motor neuron (direct & indirect activation pathways)	Spasticity
Ataxic	Cerebellum (cerebellar control circuit)	Incoordination
Hypokinetic	Basal ganglia control circuit (extrapyramidal)	Rigidity or reduced range of movement
Hyperkinetic	Basal ganglia control circuit (extrapyramidal)	Abnormal movements
Unilateral upper motor neuron	Unilateral upper motor neuron	Weakness, incoordination, or spasticity
Mixed	More than one	More than one
Undetermined	?	?
Apraxia of Speech	Left (dominant) hemisphere	Motor planning or programming

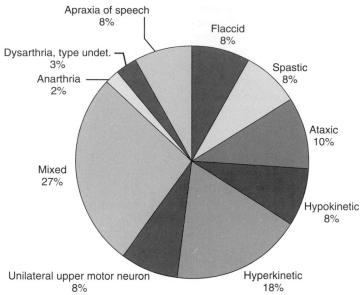

FIGURE 1-3 Distribution of motor speech disorders, Speech Pathology, Department of Neurology, Mayo Clinic, 1987-1990 plus 1993-2001. Based on 6101 evaluations of people whose primary speech pathology diagnosis was a neurologic motor speech disorder.

considered a sign (sometimes the only sign) of unilateral stroke by neurologists. It has therefore been added as a dysarthria type and is discussed as such in Chapter 9. The category of *Type Undetermined* has also been added. It is included to recognize explicitly that perhaps not all perceptually distinct dysarthria types have been recognized and that further subcategorization of already recognized dysarthrias may someday be justified; in fact, it is currently appropriate to subcategorize both flaccid and hyperkinetic dysarthrias. The category also recognizes that although a speech disorder may be recognized as a dysarthria, its manifestations may be sufficiently subtle, complicated, or unusual to lead to a clinical diagnosis of "dysarthria, type undetermined," perhaps with qualifiers that rule out what the clinician is certain the nature of the disorder is not.

Figure 1-3 summarizes the distribution of MSDs seen in the Division of Speech Pathology in the Department of Neurology at the Mayo Clinic from 1987-1990 and from 1993-2001.

SUMMARY

1. Neurologic disease affects speech in a manner that reflects its localization and underlying pathophysiology. These speech disturbances are perceptually distinct, and their recognition can contribute to the localization and diagnosis of neurologic illness. Their recognition can also contribute to our knowledge about the neural organization and control of normal speech and to clinical management decisions.

2. The neurologic breakdown of speech can reflect disturbances in motor planning, programming, control, or neuromuscular execution. These disturbances are called apraxia of speech and dysarthria. They are distinct from one another and from speech abnormalities attributable to primary sensory deficits, other neurologic disturbances that affect communication, musculoskeletal defects, psychopathology, age-related speech changes, and variations attributable to style and personality. Collectively, the dysarthrias and apraxia of speech are known as motor speech disorders (MSDs).

3. MSDs are not unusual in medical practice and are common in neurologic practice. They probably represent a substantial proportion of the communication disorders seen in many medical speech pathology practices, especially practices in which differential diagnosis is valued as an index of the presence and localization of disease.

4. MSDs may be studied perceptually and instrumentally with acoustic, physiologic, and visual imaging methods. Each method contributes to our understanding of the disorders. The perceptual analysis of salient speech characteristics is the first and most important contributor to clinical diagnosis and measures of functional change in response to management.

5. The perceptual method for classifying MSDs developed by Darley, Aronson, and Brown reflects presumed underlying pathophysiology and is related to nervous system localization. It has clinical utility and considerable heuristic value for clinical and laboratory research. It forms the framework for the discussion of diagnosis and management of MSDs in the remainder of this book.

References

1. Arboix A, Marti-Vilata JL: Lacunar infarctions and dysarthria, Arch Neurol 47:127, 1990.
2. Aronson AE: Clinical voice disorders, New York, 1990, Thieme.
3. Aronson AE: The clinical PhD: implication for the survival and liberation of communicative disorders as a health care profession, ASHA Nov:35, 1987.
4. Baker KK et al: Control of vocal loudness in young and old adults, J Speech Lang Hear Res 44:297, 2001.
5. Beaseley DS, Davis GA: Aging: communication processes and disorders, New York, 1981, Grune & Stratton.
6. Berry WR, editor: Clinical dysarthria, San Diego, 1983, College-Hill Press.
7. Cahill LM, Murdoch BE, Theodoros DG: Perceptual analysis of speech following traumatic brain injury in childhood, Brain Inj 16:415, 2002.
8. Cannito MP, Yorkston KM, Beukelman DR, editors: Neuromotor speech disorders, Baltimore, 1998, Paul H Brookes.
9. Colton R, Casper JK: Understanding voice problems, Baltimore, 1996, Williams & Wilkins.
10. Darley FL: Lacunae and research approaches to them. In Milliken C, Darley FL, editors: Brain mechanisms underlying speech and language, New York, 1967, Grune & Stratton.
11. Darley FL, Aronson AE, Brown JR: Motor speech disorders, Philadelphia, 1975, WB Saunders.
12. Darley FL, Aronson AE, Brown JR: Clusters of deviant speech dimensions in the dysarthrias, J Speech Hear Res 12:462, 1969.
13. Darley FL, Aronson AE, Brown JR: Differential diagnostic patterns of dysarthria, J Speech Hear Res 12:246, 1969.
14. Decoster W, Debruyne F: The ageing voice: changes in fundamental frequency, waveform stability and spectrum, Acta Otorhinolaryngol Belg 51:105, 1997.
15. Duffy JR: Apraxia of speech: historical overview and clinical manifestations of the acquired and developmental forms. In Shriberg LD, Campbell TF, editors: Proceedings of the 2002 Childhood Apraxia of Speech Research Symposium, Carlsbad, Calif, 2003, The Hendrix Foundation.
16. Duffy JR: Emerging and future issues in motor speech disorders, Am J Speech Lang Pathol 3:36, 1994.
17. Duffy JR, Kent RD: Darley's contribution to the understanding, differential diagnosis, and scientific study of the dysarthrias, Aphasiology 15:275, 2001.
18. Gerratt BR et al: Use and perceived value of perceptual and instrumental measures in dysarthria management. In Moore CA, Yorkston KM, Beukelman DR, editors: Dysarthria and apraxia of speech: perspectives on management, Baltimore, 1991, Paul H Brookes.
18a. Green JR et al: Reliability of measurements across several acoustic voice analysis systems. In Cannito MP, Yorkston KM, Beukelman DR, editors: Neuromotor speech disorders: nature, assessment, and management, Baltimore, 1998, Brookes Publishing Company.
19. Gubbay SS et al: Amyotrophic lateral sclerosis: a study of its presentation and prognosis, J Neurol 232:295, 1985.
20. Hewer RL: The economic impact of neurologic illness on the health and wealth of the nation and of individuals, J Neurol Neurosurg Psychiatry 63:S19, 1997.
21. Kent RD: Hearing and believing: some limits to the auditory-perceptual assessment of speech and voice disorders, Am J Speech Lang Pathol 5:7, 1996.
22. Kent RD, Vorperian HK, Duffy JR: Reliability of the Multi-Dimensional Voice Program for the analysis of voice samples of subjects with dysarthria, Am J Speech Lang Pathol 8:129, 1999.
23. Kent RD et al: Voice dysfunction in dysarthria: application of the Multi-Dimensional Voice Program, J Commun Dis 36:281, 2003.
24. Kent RD et al: Clinicoanatomic studies in dysarthria: review, critique, and directions for research, J Speech Lang Hear Res 44:535, 2001.
25. Kent RD et al: Acoustic studies of dysarthric speech: methods, progress, and potential, J Commun Dis 32:141, 1999.
26. Kent RD et al: The dysarthrias: speech-voice profiles, related dysfunctions, and neuropathology, J Med Speech Lang Pathol, 6:165, 1998.
27. Kent RD et al: Laryngeal dysfunction in neurological disease: amyotrophic lateral sclerosis, Parkinson's disease, and stroke, J Med Speech Lang Pathol 2:157, 1994.
28. Linville SE: The sound of senescence, J Voice 10:190, 1996.
29. Liss JM, Weismer G: Qualitative acoustic analysis in the study of motor speech disorders [letter], J Acoust Soc Am 92:2984, 1992.
30. Liss JM, Weismer G, Rosenbek JC: Selected acoustic characteristics of speech production in very old males, J Gerontol 45:35, 1990.
31. Logemann JA et al: Frequency and cooccurence of vocal tract dysfunction in the speech of a large sample of Parkinson patients, J Speech Hear Disord 43:47, 1978.
32. McNeil MR, editor: Clinical management of sensorimotor speech disorders, New York, 1997, Thieme.
33. McNeil MR, Doyle PJ, Wambaugh J: Apraxia of speech: a treatable disorder of motor planning and programming. In Nadeau SE, Gonzalez Rothi LJ, Crosson B, editors: Aphasia and language: theory to practice, New York, 2000, Guilford Press.
34. McNeil MR, Robin DA, Schmidt RA: Apraxia of speech: definition, differentiation, and treatment. In McNeil MR, editor: Clinical management of sensorimotor speech disorders, New York, 1997, Thieme.
35. Mlcoch AG: Diagnosis and treatment of parkinsonian dysarthria. In Koller WC, editor: Handbook of Parkinson's disease, New York, 1992, Marcel Decker.
36. Moore CA, Yorkston KM, Beukelman DR, editors: Dysarthria and apraxia of speech: perspectives on management, Baltimore, 1991, Paul H Brookes.

37. Pratt SR, Tye-Murray N: Speech impairment secondary to hearing loss. In McNeil MR, editor: Sensorimotor speech disorders, New York, 1997, Thieme.

38. Rabinov CR et al: Comparing reliability of perceptual ratings of roughness and acoustic measures of jitter, J Speech Hear Res 38:26, 1995.

39. Ramig LO et al: The aging voice: a review, treatment data and familial and genetic perspectives, Folia Phoniatr Logop 53:252, 2001.

40. Robin DR, Yorkston KM, Beukelman DR, editors: Disorders of motor speech: assessment, treatment, and clinical characterization, Baltimore, 1996, Paul H Brookes.

41. Rose FC: Motor neuron disease, New York, 1977, Grune & Stratton.

42. Sarno MT, Buonaguro A, Levita E: Characteristics of verbal impairment in closed head injured patients, Arch Phys Med Rehabil 67:400, 1986.

43. Smith BL, Wasowicz J, Preston J: Temporal characteristics of the speech of normal elderly adults, J Speech Hear Res 30:522, 1987.

44. Till JA: Diagnostic goals and computer-assisted evaluation of speech and related physiology, Special Interest Division 2, neurophysiology and neurogenic speech and language disorders, ASHA 5:3, 1995.

45. Till JA, Yorkston KM, Beukelman DR, editors: Motor speech disorders: advances in assessment and treatment, Baltimore, 1994, Paul H Brookes.

46. Van Mourik M et al: Acquired childhood dysarthria: review of its clinical presentation, Pediatr Neurol 17:299, 1997.

47. Wade DT: Epidemiology of disabling neurologic disease: how and why does disability occur? J Neurol Neurosurg Psychiatry 63:S11, 1997.

48. Weinfeld F: The 1981 national survey of stroke, Stroke 1:1, 1981.

49. Wertz RT, Rosenbek JC: Where the ear fits: a perceptual evaluation of motor speech disorders, Semin Speech Lang 13:39, 1992.

50. Wertz RT, LaPointe LL, Rosenbek JC: Apraxia of speech in adults: the disorder and its management, New York, 1984, Grune & Stratton.

51. Workinger MS, Kent RD: Perceptual analysis of the dysarthrias in children with athetoid and spastic cerebral palsy. In Moore CA, Yorkston KM, Beukelman DR, editors: Dysarthria and apraxia of speech: perspectives on management, Baltimore, 1991, Paul H Brookes.

52. Yorkston KM, Beukelman DR, editors: Recent advances in clinical dysarthria, Boston, 1989, College-Hill Press.

53. Yorkston KM, Beukelman D, Bell K: Clinical management of dysarthric speakers, San Diego, 1988, College-Hill Press.

54. Yorkston KM et al: Management of motor speech disorders in children and adults, Austin, Tex, 1999, Pro-Ed.

2

Neurologic Bases of Motor Speech and Its Pathologies

"We looking at the brain chart of the text-book may never forget the unspeakable complexity of the reactions thus rudely symbolized and spatially indicated."[64]

C.S. Sherrington

CHAPTER OUTLINE

I. Gross neuroanatomy and major neurologic systems
A. Bony boundaries—the skull and spinal column
B. Coverings—the meninges and associated spaces
C. Major anatomic levels of the nervous system
D. Major functional longitudinal systems

II. Primary structural elements of the nervous system
A. The neuron
B. Nerves, tracts, and pathways
C. Supporting (glial) cells
D. Pathologic reactions of structural elements

III. Clinicopathologic correlations
A. Localizing nervous system disease and determining its course
B. Broad etiologic categories

IV. The speech motor system
A. The final common pathway—basic structures and functions
B. The final common pathway and speech
C. The direct activation pathway and speech
D. The indirect activation pathway and speech
E. Control circuits
F. The basal ganglia control circuit and speech
G. The cerebellar control circuit and speech

V. The conceptual-programming level and speech
A. Conceptualization
B. Linguistic planning
C. Motor planning and programming
D. Performance
E. Feedback

VI. Summary

Knowledge of neuroanatomy and neurophysiology is the foundation for differential diagnosis and management of motor speech disorders (MSDs). An examination of that foundation, together with an introduction to broad categories of neurologic disease and their effects, is the purpose of this chapter.

It is not the intent here to review in depth the neuroanatomy, neurophysiology, or neuroscience of speech. Instead, this overview is clinically oriented and applicable to information in subsequent chapters on specific MSDs. The structures and functions that will be emphasized are those that are (1) directly implicated in motor speech activity, (2) relevant to understanding the mechanisms by which MSDs may be produced, and (3) relevant to observable deficits that may accompany MSDs and that are supportive of certain motor speech diagnoses.

Before grappling with the content of this chapter, a caveat and a comfort are in order. The caveat is for readers who are unfamiliar with the neurologic bases of speech or who are just beginning to integrate such information into clinical practice. It is likely that the number of terms and concepts introduced here will be overwhelming and not obviously relevant to MSDs. And, when the facts are grasped, there may be a sense that they are not understood in a way that makes their application easy or automatic. These feelings are natural when learning how to think about problems with which one has little or no experience. The basic reality is that this material will not and perhaps cannot be understood rapidly. The first encounter with it may be somewhat of a struggle.

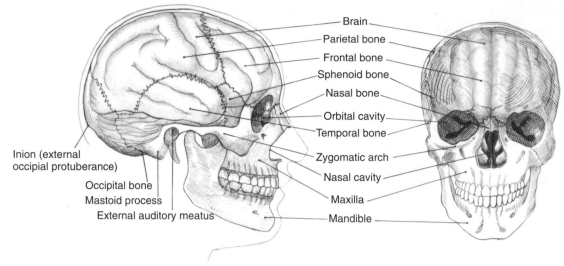

Brain
Parietal bone
Frontal bone
Sphenoid bone
Nasal bone
Orbital cavity
Temporal bone
Zygomatic arch
Nasal cavity
Maxilla
Mandible

Inion (external
occipial protuberance)

Occipital bone
Mastoid process
External auditory meatus

FIGURE 2-1 The major bones of the skull.

The comfort is that, in time, much of this will make sense and be valuable, if not essential, to clinical practice and research with MSDs. An understanding of the material in this chapter may best be achieved by referring back to it when reading chapters on specific MSDs. It may be better still to refer to this chapter in the course of evaluating and working with people with MSDs. The opportunity to integrate this didactic information with patients' medical histories, laboratory and neuroimaging findings, and, most importantly, the sights and sounds of their disordered speech, is probably the best way to understand this material. In fact, it can be argued that this information cannot be integrated as a foundation for clinical practice until clinical practice has actually begun.

◾ GROSS NEUROANATOMY AND MAJOR NEUROLOGIC SYSTEMS*

This section addresses the bony boundaries and coverings of the nervous system; the skull and spinal column represent the bony boundaries, the meninges and their associated spaces the coverings. The major anatomic levels of the nervous system and their relevant structural landmarks are then introduced. This

*The organization and content of major portions of this chapter, including the conceptual approach used to discuss the motor system, rely heavily on the "systems and levels" approach to anatomy, physiology, and pathology used in *Medical Neurosciences,* ed 4, by Bennaroch et al.[8]

is followed by a review of the major functional longitudinal systems of the nervous system. Remember that *clinical localization of disease reflects knowledge of the affected functional system and its location along the length of the nervous system.*

Bony Boundaries—the Skull and Spinal Column

The brain is housed in the skull, the spinal cord within the spinal column. Our primary focus is on the skull, because it contains most of the central nervous system (CNS) structures that subserve speech. It also contains the nuclei (origin) of the cranial nerves that innervate all of the speech muscles except those of respiration.

The bones of the skull (Figure 2-1) form a nonyielding covering for the adult brain. They serve a protective function against trauma. This protection is offset somewhat by the inability of the adult brain to expand in response to pressure from certain internal pathologic conditions (e.g., hemorrhage, hydrocephalus, tumor), a situation that can produce diffuse neurologic abnormalities due to mass effects and increased intracranial pressure.

Viewed from above (Figure 2-2), three distinct shallow cavities are apparent at the base of the skull: the *anterior, middle,* and *posterior fossae.* The posterior and middle fossae contain symmetrically oriented *foramina* (holes) through which the paired cranial nerves exit to innervate peripheral structures, including speech muscles of the head and neck. These fossae help define two of the major levels of the CNS, the *posterior fossa level* and the

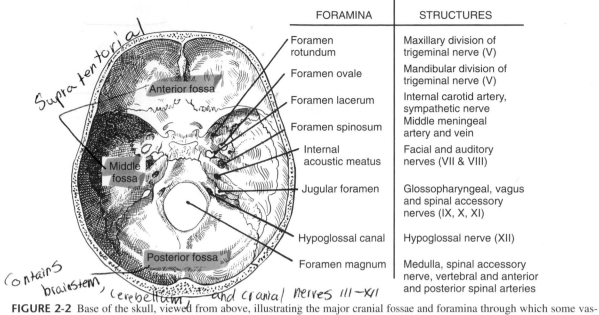

FORAMINA	STRUCTURES
Foramen rotundum	Maxillary division of trigeminal nerve (V)
Foramen ovale	Mandibular division of trigeminal nerve (V)
Foramen lacerum	Internal carotid artery, sympathetic nerve
Foramen spinosum	Middle meningeal artery and vein
Internal acoustic meatus	Facial and auditory nerves (VII & VIII)
Jugular foramen	Glossopharyngeal, vagus and spinal accessory nerves (IX, X, XI)
Hypoglossal canal	Hypoglossal nerve (XII)
Foramen magnum	Medulla, spinal accessory nerve, vertebral and anterior and posterior spinal arteries

[Handwritten annotations: "Supratentorial", "Anterior fossa", "Middle fossa", "Posterior fossa", "Contains brainstem, cerebellum, and cranial nerves III–XII"]

FIGURE 2-2 Base of the skull, viewed from above, illustrating the major cranial fossae and foramina through which some vascular structures and the cranial nerves supplying speech muscles exit.

supratentorial level (anterior and middle fossae). Crude localization of neuropathology often refers to lesions as supratentorial or posterior fossa in origin (Figure 2-3).

Coverings—Meninges and Associated Spaces

The *meninges* (coverings) of the CNS consist of three layers—the dura, arachnoid, and pia mater (see Figure 2-3).

The *dura mater* is the outermost membrane. It consists of two layers of fused tissues that separate in certain regions to form the *intracranial venous sinuses,* areas where venous blood drains from the brain. The folds of the dura in the cranial cavity form two barriers: the *falx cerebri,* which is located between the two hemispheres, and the *tentorium cerebelli,* which separates the cerebellum from the cerebral hemispheres.

The *arachnoid* lies beneath the dura and is applied loosely to the surface of the brain. The *pia mater,* the thin innermost layer, is closely attached to the brain's surface. The pia mater and arachnoid are collectively known as the *leptomeninges.*

The spaces around the meninges are functionally important and relevant to certain pathologies. The *epidural space* is located between the inner bone of the skull and the dura. The *subdural space* is beneath the dura. Blood and pus from injury or infection can accumulate in the epidural and subdural spaces. The *subarachnoid space,* beneath the arachnoid, surrounds the brain and spinal cord and is filled with *cerebrospinal fluid;* it is connected to the interior of the brain through the *ventricular system* (Figure 2-4).

Most diseases capable of producing MSDs that involve the meninges and meningeal spaces stem from infection, venous vascular disorders, hydrocephalus, or trauma with associated hemorrhage and edema.

Major Anatomic Levels of the Nervous System

The major anatomic levels of the nervous system can be related to the boundaries of the skull and spinal column. They are also roughly demarcated by the meninges and portions of the ventricular and vascular systems, which are discussed later. The major anatomic levels and their skeletal, meningeal, ventricular, and vascular characteristics, as well as their relationship to the major types of MSDs, are summarized in Table 2-1.

Supratentorial Level

The supratentorial level is located above the tentorium cerebelli (see Figure 2-3), a nearly horizontal membrane that forms the upper border of the posterior fossa, covers the upper surface of the cerebellum, and separates the anterior and middle fossae

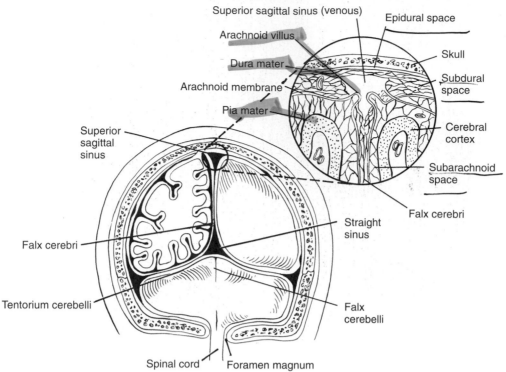

FIGURE 2-3 The supratentorial and posterior fossa levels, and their major boundaries. Also shown *(inset)* are the meninges and their associated spaces.

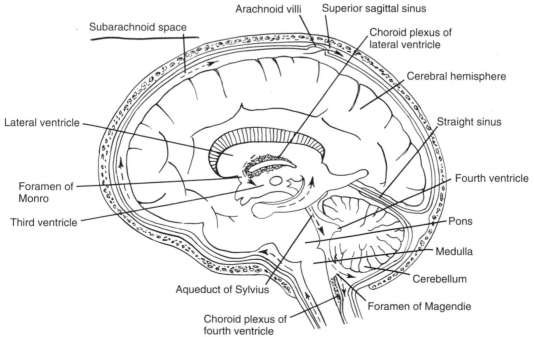

FIGURE 2-4 The subarachnoid space and ventricular system in which cerebrospinal fluid is produced and circulates.

table 2-1	Relationships among the major anatomic levels of the nervous system, skeleton, meninges, ventricular system, vascular system, and major motor speech disorder types				
Anatomic Level	**Skeleton**	**Meninges**	**Ventricular System**	**Vascular System**	**Motor Speech Disorder**
Supratentorial (hemispheres, lobes, basal ganglia, thalamus, cranial nerves I & II)	Skull (anterior & middle fossa)	Above tentorium cerebelli Lateral to falx cerebri	Lateral & third ventricles Subarachnoid space	Carotid arterial system Ophthalmic arteries Middle cerebral arteries Anterior cerebral arteries Vertebrobasilar system Posterior cerebral arteries	Apraxia of speech Dysarthrias Spastic Unilateral UMN Hypokinetic Hyperkinetic
Posterior Fossa Brainstem (pons, medulla, midbrain) & cerebellum	Skull Posterior fossa	Below falx cerebelli	Fourth ventricle Subarachnoid space	Vertebrobasilar system Vertebral arteries Basilar artery	Dysarthrias Spastic Unilateral UMN Hyperkinetic Ataxic Flaccid
Spinal	Vertebral column	Spinal meninges	Spinal Subarachnoid space	Anterior spinal artery Posterior spinal arteries	Dysarthria Flaccid
Peripheral (cranial & spinal nerves)	Face & skull Noncranial & nonspinal bones	None	None	Branches of major extremity vessels	Dysarthria Flaccid

UMN, Upper motor neuron.

from the posterior fossa. The supratentorial level includes the paired *frontal, temporal, parietal,* and *occipital lobes* of the *cerebral hemispheres* (Figure 2-5). It also includes the *basal ganglia, thalamus, hypothalamus,* and *cranial nerves I (olfactory) and II (optic),* which are buried within the depths of the hemispheres.

Posterior Fossa Level

The major structures of the posterior fossa are the *brainstem* (the pons, medulla, and midbrain), the *cerebellum,* and the *origins of cranial nerves III through XII* (see Figure 2-5).

The area of the posterior fossa dorsal to the aqueduct of Sylvius (see Figure 2-4) is known as the *tectum;* it includes the *inferior and superior colliculi* (known collectively as the *corpora quadrigemina),* which are major relay stations for the auditory and

visual systems, respectively. The area ventral to the aqueduct of Sylvius and fourth ventricle is known as the *tegmentum;* it contains white matter pathways and many nuclei, including the *reticular formation.* The large cerebral and cerebellar pathways in the most ventral region below the tegmentum form the base region of the midbrain and pons.

The cerebellum lies dorsal to the fourth ventricle, pons, and medulla. It comprises a *right and left hemisphere* and a midline *vermis.*

Of the 12 paired cranial nerves, 10 (all but I and II) have their origin in and emerge from the brainstem. Several of them represent the last link or *final common pathway* from the nervous system to the speech muscles. Their names, origins, and general functions are summarized in Table 2-2. Although the cranial nerves serving speech have their origin within the skull, they are actually part of the peripheral nervous system (PNS). This distinction is important

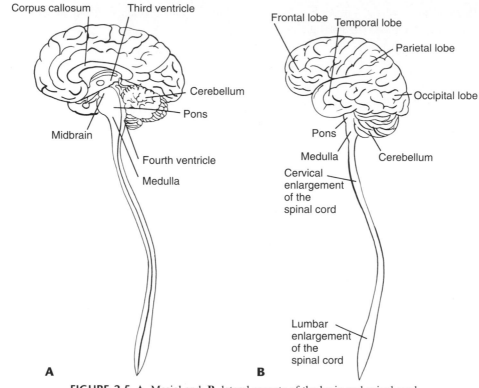

FIGURE 2-5 A, Mesial and, **B,** lateral aspects of the brain and spinal cord.

table 2-2	Location and general functions of the cranial nerves		
	Nerve	**Anatomic Origin**	**Function**
I	Olfactory	Cerebral hemispheres	Smell
II	Optic	Diencephalon	Vision
III	Oculomotor	Midbrain	Eye movement; pupil constriction
IV	Trochlear	Midbrain	Eye movement
V	Trigeminal*	Pons	Jaw movement; face, mouth, jaw sensation
VI	Abducens	Pons	Eye movement
VII	Facial*	Pons	Facial movement; hyoid elevation; stapedius reflex; salivation; lacrimation; taste
VIII	Cochleovestibular	Pons, medulla	Hearing; balance
IX	Glossopharyngeal*	Medulla	Pharyngeal movement; pharynx and tongue sensation; taste
X	Vagus*	Medulla	Pharyngeal, palatal, and laryngeal movement; pharyngeal sensation; control of visceral organs
XI	Accessory*	Medulla, spinal cord	Shoulder and neck movement
XII	Hypoglossal*	Medulla	Tongue movement

*Involved in speech production.

to understanding the pathophysiology of flaccid dysarthria and its differences from other dysarthria types, all of which result from CNS dysfunction.

Spinal Level

The adult *spinal cord* begins at the *foramen magnum,* the large, central opening in the posterior fossa at the lower end of the medulla (see Figures 2-2 and 2-3). The spinal cord is surrounded by the bony *vertebral column,* which includes 7 cervical, 12 thoracic, and 5 lumbar vertebrae. It terminates at the level of the first lumbar vertebra. Thirty-one pairs of spinal nerves are attached to it via *dorsal* (posterior) and *ventral* (anterior) *nerve roots.* The dorsal roots are sensory in function; the ventral roots are motor.

Peripheral Level

The peripheral level, or PNS, consists of the *cranial and spinal nerves.* As already noted, most of the cranial nerves originate in the brainstem, exit from the skull through paired foramina, and travel to and from the muscles they innervate. The spinal nerves, which contain the joined dorsal and ventral roots, enter the peripheral level as they emerge from the vertebral column to travel to and from the muscles they innervate. The course, innervation, and function of the cranial and spinal nerves subserving speech functions are discussed later in this chapter.

Major Functional Longitudinal Systems

Neurologic diagnosis often begins by linking clinical signs and symptoms to one or more of what can be called major longitudinal systems of the nervous system.[8] These systems contain groups of structures that have specific functions. They are called longitudinal because, for the most part, the activities of the system are evident over the length of the nervous system (i.e., from the supratentorial to the peripheral level).

The Cerebrospinal Fluid System (the Ventricular System)

The ventricular system lies within the depths of the brain (see Figure 2-4). The ventricles are cavities that contain *cerebrospinal fluid (CSF),* which is produced by *choroid plexuses* located in each ventricle. Each cerebral hemisphere contains a *lateral ventricle* that is connected by way of the *foramen of Monro* to the midline-located *third ventricle.* The third ventricle narrows into the *aqueduct of Sylvius,* which leads to the *fourth ventricle* between the brainstem and cerebellum. The *foramen of Luschka* and the *foramen of Magendie* in the fourth ventricle link the ventricular system to the subarachnoid space.

The ventricular system and the subarachnoid space comprise the CSF system. CSF circulates throughout the ventricles and subarachnoid space and is absorbed in the *arachnoid villi* in the brain or in the *leptomeninges* within the subarachnoid space in the spinal cord. The CSF system thus can be found within several of the major anatomic levels of the nervous system, including the supratentorial, posterior fossa, and spinal levels. Its primary functions are to *cushion the CNS against physical trauma and to help maintain a stable environment for neural activity.*

The Vascular System (Figures 2-6 to 2-8)

The vascular system is literally the lifeblood of the nervous system. It is found within all major anatomic levels where it provides oxygen and other nutrients to neural structures and removes metabolic wastes from them. It is also a major source of lesions that can lead to MSDs.

All blood vessels that supply the brainstem and cerebral hemispheres arise from the *aortic arch* in the chest. Blood enters the brain by way of the *carotid system* and the *vertebrobasilar system.* These two systems are capable of some communication with each other through connecting channels in the brainstem, known as the *circle of Willis* (see Figure 2-6).

The carotid system originates with the paired *internal carotid arteries* that arise in the neck from the common carotid arteries at the level of the thyroid cartilage (see Figure 2-6). The carotid arteries enter the skull through the carotid canal located in the petrous portion of each temporal bone. They pass through the cavernous sinus lateral to the sphenoid bone and eventually to the circle of Willis.

Each internal carotid artery separates at the circle of Willis into two of the three major cerebral arteries, the *anterior cerebral artery* and the *middle cerebral artery.* The anterior cerebral arteries are connected to each other by the *anterior communicating artery;* they course upward in the midline and supply the medial surface of the cerebral hemispheres and the superior portion of the frontal and parietal lobes. The middle cerebral arteries course laterally, and their branches supply most of the lateral surfaces of the cerebral hemispheres and the deep structures of the frontal and parietal lobes (see Figure 2-8).

Vascular disturbances in the left or right carotid artery and in the left or right anterior and middle cerebral arteries can produce dysarthrias. Left middle cerebral artery disturbances are a common cause of apraxia of speech.

The vertebrobasilar system begins with the paired *vertebral arteries,* which enter the brainstem through the foramen magnum and join at the lower border of the pons to form the *basilar artery.* Branches from these arteries supply the midbrain, pons, medulla, cerebellum, and portions of the cervical spinal cord. The *posterior cerebral arteries*—the third of the major cerebral arteries—are branches of the vertebrobasilar system. They supply the occipital lobe, the thalamus, and the inferior and medial portions of the temporal lobe in each hemisphere (see Figures 2-7 and 2-8). Vascular disturbances in the vertebrobasilar system often lead to MSDs. Table 2-3 summarizes the vascular supply to the brain, the anatomic regions supplied by its components, and some of the neurologic signs associated with vascular disturbances of each component.

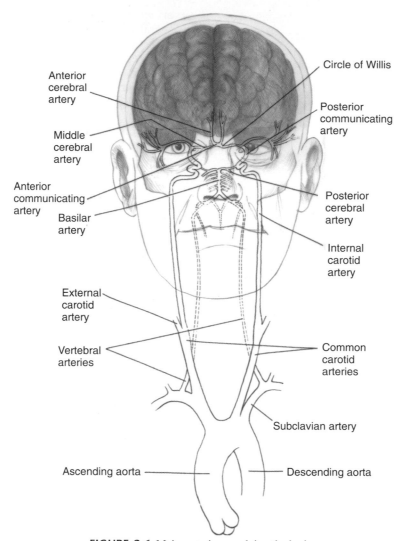

FIGURE 2-6 Major arteries supplying the brain.

The Internal Regulation System (the Visceral System)

The internal regulation system is represented at all major anatomic levels of the nervous system. It includes the hypothalamus and parts of the limbic lobe supratentorially; the reticular formation and portions of some cranial nerves in the posterior fossa; longitudinal pathways in the brainstem and spinal cord; and ganglia, receptors, and effectors at the periphery. It contains afferent and efferent components that interact to *maintain a balanced internal environment (homeostasis) through the regulation of visceral glands and organs.*

The Neurochemical Systems

Neurochemical systems influence all anatomic levels of the nervous system. They include amino acids, acetylcholine, monoamines, neuropeptides, and purines. Some agents are involved in fast neurotransmission, others modulate the responsiveness of neurons to stimuli, and some produce "long-term effects on neuronal activity critical for neural development, learning, and response to injury."[8] The actions of neurochemical agents in the central and peripheral nervous systems have a direct bearing on the planning, programming, control, and execution of speech.

Numerous diseases involving neurochemical systems can lead to motor speech and other neurologic communication disorders. For example, the dopamine system is implicated in Parkinson's disease (hypokinetic dysarthria). The acetylcholine system is implicated in myasthenia gravis (flaccid dysarthrias), movement disorders (hyperkinetic

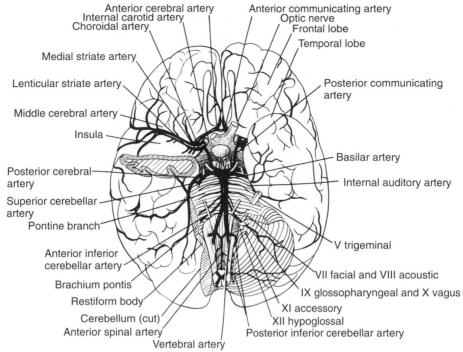

FIGURE 2-7 Inferior view of the carotid, vertebral, and basilar arteries; some of their major branches; and their relationship to major brainstem and cerebral structures.

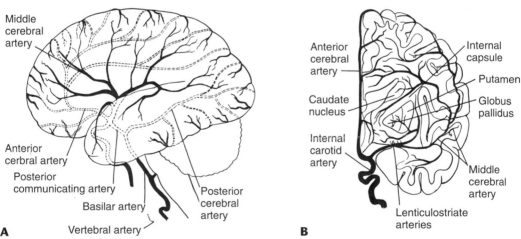

FIGURE 2-8 A Lateral and, **B,** anteroposterior views of the major cerebral arteries and some of their penetrating branches to subcortical structures.

dysarthrias), and Alzheimer's disease (cognitively based communication deficits). In addition, the use of pharmacologic agents to influence neurochemical systems is crucial to the management of many diseases associated with MSDs (e.g., cholinesterase inhibitors to treat myasthenia gravis; dopamine agonists to treat Parkinson's disease).

The Consciousness System

Consciousness system structures are found only at the supratentorial and posterior fossa levels. They include the reticular formation and ascending projection pathways, portions of the thalamus, pathways to widespread areas of the cerebral cortex, and portions of all lobes of the cerebral cortex.

table 2-3	Vascular supply to the brain, some of the major anatomic regions supplied, and some of the primary neurologic and motor speech deficits that result from vascular disturbances. Motor speech disorders and other disorders affecting spoken communication are highlighted in bold.

Main Vessels	Anatomic Region Supplied	Signs
I. Carotid System		
A. Branches of internal carotid artery	Most of cerebral hemispheres	Contralateral hemiplegia
		Contralateral hemianesthesia
		Hemianopsia or ipsilateral blindness
		Aphasia (left)
		Apraxia of speech (left)
		Unilateral UMN dysarthria
		Spastic dysarthria (if bilateral)
		Hypokinetic dysarthria
		Hyperkinetic dysarthria
1. Anterior choroidal	Optic tract; cerebral peduncle; lateral geniculate body; portions of internal capsule	Hemianopsia or upper quadrant defect
		Contralateral hemiplegia
		Thalamic sensory changes
		Unilateral UMN dysarthria?
		Spastic dysarthria (if bilateral)?
2. Ophthalmic	Orbit & surrounding tissue; muscles & bulb of the eye	Unilateral blindness
		Optic atrophy
3. Anterior cerebral	*Cortical branches*	Contralateral lower extremity weakness
	Anterior $\{\frac{3}{4}\}$ of medial surface of cerebral hemispheres; frontal lobe, medial-orbital surface; frontal pole; superior lateral border of hemispheres; anterior $\{\frac{4}{5}\}$ of corpus callosum	Paraplegia (if bilateral)
		Cortical sensory defects, foot & leg
		Contralateral forced grasping & groping
		Sucking reflex
	Deep branches	Incontinence
	Internal capsule, anterior limb; part of head of caudate nucleus	Gait & limb apraxia
		Aphasia?
		Abulia, akinetic mutism, cognitive impairments
		Apraxia of speech (left)?
		Unilateral UMN dysarthria?
		Spastic dysarthria (if bilateral)?
		Hypokinetic dysarthria?
		Hyperkinetic dysarthria?
4. Middle cerebral	*Cortical branches*	Contralateral hemiplegia
	Cortex & white matter of parietal lobe & lateral & inferior frontal lobe; superior parts of temporal lobe & insula	Contralateral cortical sensory deficit
		Homonymous hemianopsia
		Paralysis of conjugate gaze to side opposite lesion
		Aphasia (left)
		Apraxia of speech (left)
		Unilateral UMN dysarthria
		Spastic dysarthria (if bilateral)
		Limb apraxia
	Penetrating branches	Contralateral hemiplegia or hemiparesis
	Putamen; part of head and body of caudate nucleus; outer part of globus pallidus; internal capsule; posterior limb; corona radiata	Contralateral hemisensory deficits
		Contralateral movement disorders
		Aphasia (left)
		Apraxia of speech (left)
		Unilateral UMN dysarthria
II. Vertebrobasilar System		
A. Posterior cerebral	Red nucleus; substantia nigra; cerebral peduncles; reticular formation; oculomotor & trochlear nuclei; superior cerebellar peduncles; hippocampus; portions of thalamus; inferomedial temporal lobe; occipital lobe	Contralateral hemiparesis
		Oculomotor palsy
		Ataxia & tremor
		Memory & attention deficits
		Unilateral sensory loss
		Homonymous hemianopsia
		Movement disorders
		Various visual deficits
		Alexia without agraphia

table 2-3 Vascular supply to the brain, some of the major anatomic regions supplied, and some of the primary neurologic and motor speech deficits that result from vascular disturbances. Motor speech disorders and other disorders affecting spoken communication are highlighted in bold.—cont'd

Main Vessels	Anatomic Region Supplied	Signs
B. Basilar artery	Pons; middle & superior cerebellar peduncles; cerebellar hemispheres; upper midbrain & subthalamus	**Aphasia (left)** **Unilateral UMN dysarthria** **Spastic dysarthria (if bilateral)** **Ataxic dysarthria** **Hyperkinetic dysarthria** Quadriplegia (if bilateral) Hemiplegia Coma (if bilateral) Somnolence Oculomotor deficits Visual defects Nystagmus Ipsilateral cerebellar ataxia Nausea & vomiting Cranial nerve involvement (III-XII) **Spastic dysarthria (if bilateral)** **Anarthria (if bilateral)** **"Locked-in" syndrome (if bilateral)** **Ataxic dysarthria** **Unilateral UMN dysarthria** **Flaccid dysarthria** **Palatal myoclonus**
C. Vertebral artery	Medulla; cerebellum (posterior inferior)	Contralateral hemiplegia & sensory loss Ptosis Ipsilateral weakness of cranial nerves IX, X, XI, XII Nystagmus, vertigo Ipsilateral ataxia Ipsilateral loss of facial sensation (Cranial nerve V) & taste Hiccups Nausea & vomiting **Spastic dysarthria (if bilateral)** **Ataxic dysarthria** **Unilateral UMN dysarthria** **Flaccid dysarthria**

UMN, Upper motor neuron.
*Signs occur with vascular disturbance on the right or left unless otherwise specified in parentheses.

The consciousness system is crucial to maintaining wakefulness, consciousness, awareness of the environment, and, on a higher level, selective and sustained attention. Malfunctions within it can contribute to cognitive deficits, including language and communication, and can also affect the adequacy of motor behavior, including speech.

The Sensory System

The sensory system is found at all major anatomic levels of the nervous system. It includes peripheral receptor organs; afferent fibers in cranial, spinal, and peripheral nerves; dorsal root ganglia (spinal level); ascending pathways in the spinal cord and brainstem; portions of the thalamus; and thalamocortical connections, primarily to sensory cortex in the temporal, parietal, and occipital lobes. Special sensory systems, such as hearing and vision, are also located at the peripheral, posterior fossa, and supratentorial levels.

The Motor System

The motor system is present at all of the major anatomic levels of the nervous system and is directly *responsible for all motor activity involving striated muscle.* It includes efferent connections of the cortex, especially the frontal lobes; the basal ganglia, cerebellum, and related CNS pathways; descending

table 2-4	Structural elements of the nervous system	
Structure	**Locus**	**Function**
Neurons	CNS & PNS	Drive all neurologic functions
Nerves	PNS (brainstem or spinal cord to end organs)	PNS motor & sensory functions
Tracts or pathways	CNS	Communication among groups of neurons
Commissural	Between cerebral hemispheres	
Association	Within cerebral hemispheres	
Projection	To & from higher & lower centers within CNS (e.g., cortex & thalamus)	
Supporting Cells		
Oligodendroglia	Surround CNS axons (myelin)	Insulation: speed transmission
Schwann cells	Surround PNS axons (myelin)	Insulation: speed transmission
Astrocytes	Relate to CNS blood vessels & neurons	Transport substances from blood vessels to neurons
		Blood-brain barrier
Ependymal cells	Lining of ventricles	Separate ventricles from parenchyma
	Choroid plexuses	Produce CSF
Microglia	Scattered in CNS	
	Form microphages	Ingest or remove damaged tissue
Connective tissue	Form meninges	Covering of CNS
	Sheaths on PNS nerve fibers & nerves	Cover & bind fibers together in PNS nerves

CNS, Central nervous system; *CSF*, cerebrospinal fluid; *PNS*, peripheral nervous system.

pathways to motor nuclei of cranial and spinal nerves; efferent fibers within cranial and spinal nerves; and striated muscle. *It is essential to normal reflexes; to maintaining normal muscle tone and posture; and to the planning, initiation, and control of voluntary movement, including speech.*

Lesions in nonmotor areas of the nervous system may produce alterations in speech, but they do so only indirectly through their effects on the motor system. For example, a lesion in the vascular system does not, in and of itself, produce MSDs; any resulting MSD would derive from the effect of that lesion on portions of the motor system involved in speech production.

▨ PRIMARY STRUCTURAL ELEMENTS OF THE NERVOUS SYSTEM

The nervous system is composed of *neurons,* or *nerve cells,* and *supporting cells,* or *glial cells* (Table 2-4). The structure and function of these cells have been studied extensively and are reviewed here only superficially.* An understanding of the physiology of neuronal function is important, because it forms the foundation for understanding the actions of the speech motor system. The cursory summary pro-

---

*Excellent reviews of basic neuronal structure and function can be found in many sources, such as Bhatnagar,[11] Kennedy and Keuhn,[33] Larson,[42] Perkins and Kent,[59] and Stevens.[65]

vided here reflects the more global focus of this book, plus an assumption that the reader already has an understanding of this relatively molecular topic.

The Neuron

The neuron is the most important structural element of the nervous system because its electrochemical activities drive all neurologic functions. Its numbers in humans are astounding, on the order of 100 billion.[56] In the adult, many diseases affecting neurons result in their degeneration and loss.

Neurons in different parts of the nervous system vary in size and shape, but they all contain a *cell body, dendrites,* and an *axon* (Figure 2-9). The cell body is the central processing unit and is responsible for metabolic functions. Dendrites and an axon extend from the cell body into surrounding tissue. Their length and structure vary greatly across different types of neurons. Dendrites are often numerous but short, with many branches; they are responsible for gathering information transmitted from surrounding neurons. Neurons have only one axon that may extend from the cell body for a few millimeters or for several feet, its diameter generally varying with its length. Neurons with axons that travel extended distances are generally specialized for conducting information. Neurons whose axons terminate near their own dendrites and cell body are more involved in complex interactions within pools or net-

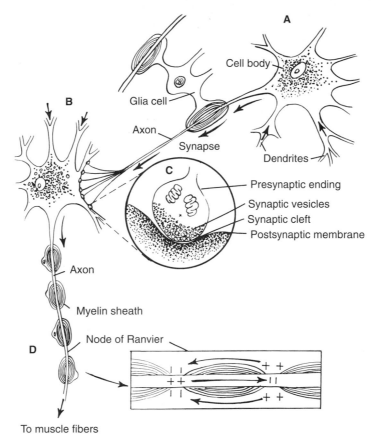

FIGURE 2-9 A, Neuron and, **B** and **C,** *inset,* anatomy of neuron-to-neuron communication. Dendrites receive information while the axon transmits information to other neurons. **D,** *inset,* Action potential is moving through saltatory conduction in the direction of the *arrows* inside the axon.

works of neurons and are involved in "information processing."

The axon conducts electrical energy away from the cell body to the next neuron in a chain or circuit or to muscle or glands. Communication among neurons, or between neurons and muscles, takes place at regions known as *synapses* (see Figures 2-9 and 2-10). In neuronal synapses, the axon usually forms a synapse with the cell body or dendrites of another neuron. In most instances the axon and dendrite (or muscle fibers) are separated by a *synaptic cleft.* At the tip of the axon are tiny *synaptic vesicles* containing a chemical neurotransmitter that carries the axon's signal to a receiving dendrite or to muscle fibers. In neuromuscular synapses, *acetylcholine* is the crucial neurotransmitter substance. If released in sufficient quantity at the neuromuscular junction, it leads to movement through contraction of muscle fibers.

The "message" carried by a single axon to another neuron is simple; it either facilitates or inhibits the neuron receiving it from firing a message of its own. All that varies in the message of a single neuron is the rate at which it is sent. This "go" or "no go" form of communication leads to a limited set of simple, stereotypic outcomes in organisms with few neurons. In the human nervous system, however, axons branch repeatedly, forming anywhere from 1000 to 10,000 synapses, and their cell bodies and dendrites receive information from on the order of 1000 other neurons. (The number of synapses in the brain may be on the order of 100 trillion!) As a result, the "decision" of a neuron to fire or not reflects a summation of the messages it receives from multiple sources.

Nerves, Tracts, and Pathways

The activity of a single neuron is of little consequence to observable human behavior. Only through the activity of many neurons does meaningful sensory, motor, and cognitive activity occur. For example, voluntary movement can result only from the integrated activity of astounding numbers of neurons conducting impulses at many levels of the

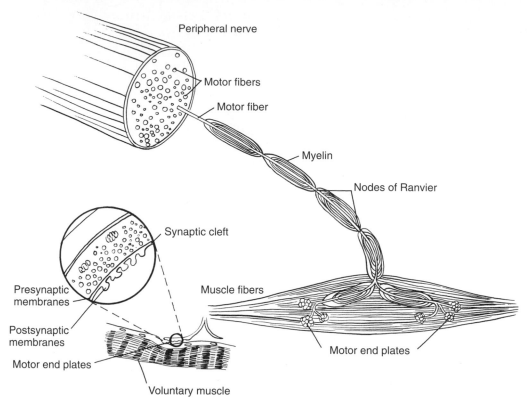

Peripheral nerve

Motor fibers

Motor fiber

Myelin

Nodes of Ranvier

Synaptic cleft

Presynaptic membranes

Muscle fibers

Postsynaptic membranes

Motor end plates

Motor end plates

Voluntary muscle

FIGURE 2-10 Motor unit. A myelinated axon (motor fiber) carries an action potential that results in the release of acetylcholine from synaptic vesicles across the neuromuscular junction *(inset)* to trigger muscle fiber contraction. The final common pathways innervating muscles for speech contain many thousands of such motor units.

CNS motor system, plus the final influence of impulses carried by many axons traveling in nerves to many muscle fibers. Because the focus here is on motor behavior, the greatest interest is in the *combined activities* of groups of neurons that join forces to accomplish particular motor goals.

The major PNS structure is the *nerve* (see Figure 2-10), which is a *collection of nerve fibers (axons)* bound together by connective tissue. Peripheral nerves (cranial and spinal nerves) travel between the CNS (where their cell bodies reside) and peripheral *end organs,* which are the sensory, motor, and visceral structures that they innervate.

A nerve contains up to thousands of nerve fibers of varying sizes. Fibers relevant to speech motor and sensory functions are generally relatively large and *myelinated* (myelin is defined in the next section). They conduct impulses relatively quickly.

The term "nerve" is reserved for groups of fibers that travel together in the PNS. The terms "tracts" or "pathways" refer to groups of fibers that travel together in the CNS. The major distinction between PNS nerves and CNS tracts is that CNS tracts transmit impulses to other neurons, whereas PNS nerves transmit impulses from nerves to end organs such as muscle.

Fiber tracts in the CNS are categorized according to the areas that they connect. *Commissural fiber tracts* connect homologous areas in the two cerebral hemispheres. *Association fiber tracts* connect cortical areas within a hemisphere to one another. *Projection fiber tracts* contain afferent and efferent fibers that connect higher and lower centers in the CNS. Their specific names usually reflect the areas that they connect. For example, afferent projection fibers from the thalamus to the cortex are known as *thalamocortical fibers;* efferent fibers from the cortex to the cranial nerves are known as *corticobulbar fibers;* efferent fibers from the cortex to the red nucleus in the midbrain are known as *corticorubral fibers* ("rubral," meaning red, refers to the red nucleus). Afferent and efferent projection fibers are crucial components of the circuits that direct motor activities.

Supporting (Glial) Cells

Oligodendroglia and Schwann Cells

These cell types form the insulation or *myelin* that surrounds axons in the CNS and PNS. Schwann cells in the PNS form myelin, which can be found wrapped around most peripheral nerves. Small gaps between each myelinated segment of peripheral nerve are known as *nodes of Ranvier.* Electrical signals traveling down axons skip from node to node with a resulting increased speed of transmission, a process known as *saltatory conduction** (see Figures 2-9 and 2-10). *Oligodendroglia cells* are the source of myelin in the CNS.

Astrocytes

Astrocytes are widely distributed in the CNS, lying in proximity to both neurons and capillaries. Evidence suggests that they play a role in CNS metabolism and mechanisms of response to CNS injuries.[56] They are an important part of the *blood-brain barrier,* a mechanism that prevents the passage of many metabolites from the blood into the brain, thereby protecting it from toxic compounds and variations in blood composition.

Ependymal Cells

Ependymal cells line the ventricular system and form a barrier between ventricular fluid and the neuronal substance of the brain *(parenchyma).* They also form the choroid plexuses, which produce ventricular and cerebrospinal fluid.

Microglia

Microglia are small in number and size and are scattered throughout the nervous system. They respond to destructive CNS processes by proliferating and transforming into *macrophages* (scavenger cells) that ingest pathogens and remove damaged tissue.

Connective Tissue

Connective tissues make up the meninges. There is little fibrous connective tissue within the CNS parenchyma. In the PNS, connective tissues form thin layers on myelinated nerve fibers, help bind fibers together within nerves, and can be found covering areas at the trunks of nerves. They are analogous to the meninges that surround the CNS.

---

*In addition to the role of myelin in speeding neural transmission, it also appears to protect axons from injury. For example, in multiple sclerosis (MS), in which demyelination occurs, the loss of myelin seems to predispose axons to subsequent injury, which may contribute to the functional deficits associated with the disease.[61]

Pathologic Reactions of Structural Elements

Nervous system cells respond to neurologic disease. In some disorders, the response is physiologic. In others, there is a structural change that reflects the specific effects of damage or a response to the pathologic process. Some structural responses are nonspecific, whereas others are specific to a particular disease.

Neuronal Reactions

Neuronal loss occurs in response to many disease states. In response to *ischemia* (deprivation of oxygen and cessation of oxidative metabolism, as occurs in stroke) lasting for 2 to 5 minutes, there may be acute swelling of neurons, followed by shrinkage and eventual cell loss.

When axons are severely injured, cell bodies may swell and lose some of their internal components, a process known as *central chromatolysis* or *axonal reaction.* These changes can be seen a few days after injury and peak at 2 to 3 weeks. Unlike ischemic cell change, this process is reversible, with normal appearance reemerging in a few months.

Axons and their myelin sheaths cannot survive when they are separated from their cell bodies by injury or disease. Degeneration of the axon distal to the point of separation is known as *Wallerian degeneration.* In the PNS, however, regeneration of the nerve is possible if the cell body survives. This regeneration happens through sprouting of the portion of the axon still connected to the cell body. If sprouts find their way to the degenerating distal nerve trunk, function eventually may return. This sprouting may occur at a rate of approximately 3 mm per day. *Functionally significant regeneration of nerve tracts does not occur in the CNS.*

Neurofibrillary degeneration is characterized by the formation of clumps of neurofibrils in the cytoplasm of CNS neurons. It is the most common form of degeneration associated with clinical dementia, particularly Alzheimer's disease. *Senile plaques* are a related pathologic change. Deposits of *amyloid* (a fibrous protein) in cell bodies, as well as degenerated nerve processes, characterize them.

Inclusion bodies are abnormal, discrete deposits in nerve cells. Their presence may identify specific diseases (e.g., Parkinson's disease, Pick's disease, certain viral infections).

Abnormal accumulations of metabolic products in nerve cells are known as *storage cells.* Several metabolic diseases can produce such accumulation. Because of the associated degree of swelling that may take place in the cell body, they are referred to as "balloon" cells.

table 2-5	Common localization, development, and evolutionary characteristics for various etiologies of neurologic disease

	Etiology					
	Degenerative	**Inflammatory**	**Toxic or Metabolic**	**Neoplastic**	**Traumatic**	**Vascular**
Localization	Diffuse	Diffuse Focal	Diffuse	Focal	Diffuse Multifocal Focal	Focal Multifocal Diffuse
Development	Chronic	Subacute	Acute Subacute Chronic	Chronic Subacute	Acute	Acute
Evolution	Progressive	Progressive Exacerbate or remit	Progressive Stationary	Progressive	Improving Stationary	Improving Stationary Transient Progressive

When the lower motor neuron innervation of a muscle is destroyed, the muscle will waste away or *atrophy.* In contrast, injury to a CNS axon usually does not result in death of postsynaptic neurons. However, the activities of postsynaptic neurons may be altered by *diaschisis*—a process in which neurons function abnormally because influences necessary to their normal function have been removed by damage to neurons to which they are connected. Diaschisis may explain abnormalities in neuronal function at sites distant from a lesion within the CNS. *Positron emission tomography (PET)* has demonstrated that neuronal cell death in one region of the brain can lead to changes in metabolic functions of adjacent and even distant neuronal regions to which the damaged area has important anatomic connections.* These findings highlight the functional importance of interrelationships among groups of neurons in the CNS, as well as the inadequacies inherent in any attempt to attribute normal or pathologic behavior, including MSDs, solely to activity or pathology in any single structure or pathway.

Supporting Cell Reactions

Myelin may shrink or break down in response to nonspecific injuries, but there are also groups of diseases that specifically affect myelin. In *demyelinating disease,* myelin is attacked by some exogenous agent, broken down, and absorbed. The most common demyelinating disease is *MS,* but demyelinization also occurs in other CNS and PNS diseases, such as *Guillain-Barré syndrome.*

Other diseases that specifically affect myelin are *leukodystrophies,* in which myelin is abnormally formed in response to inborn errors in metabolism. The abnormality leads to the eventual breakdown of myelin.

Astrocytes react to many CNS injuries by forming scars in injured neural tissue. The terms *gliosis, astrocytosis,* and *astrogliosis* refer to this nonspecific process. Astrocytes may also react more specifically to certain diseases, especially metabolic diseases, such as those that may occur in hepatic (liver) failure. They may also form inclusion bodies in cell nuclei in response to certain viral infections.

■ CLINICOPATHOLOGIC CORRELATIONS

It is appropriate at this point to discuss an approach for categorizing the localization, course, and general nature of neurologic disease. Along with the subsequent discussion of the motor system and the neurology of speech, this will set the stage for addressing the assessment of MSDs in the next chapter.

Localizing Nervous System Disease and Determining Its Course

Neurologic signs and symptoms reflect the location of a lesion and not necessarily its specific cause. Disease very often can be localized on the basis of history and clinical examination. Broad categories for describing the localization and history of disease are summarized in Table 2-5.

In broad terms, the *localization* of neurologic disease can be as follows:
  1. *Focal,* involving a single circumscribed area or contiguous group of structures (e.g., left frontal lobe)

---

*For discussions of PET and remote metabolic effects of lesions, see Dobkin et al.,[18] Metter et al.,[50] Mlcoch and Metter,[52] and Powers and Raichle.[60]

2. *Multifocal,* involving more than one area or more than one group of contiguous structures (e.g., cerebellar and cerebral hemisphere plaques associated with MS)
3. *Diffuse,* involving roughly symmetric portions of the nervous system bilaterally (e.g., generalized cerebral atrophy associated with dementia)

Determining specific pathology depends partly on establishing the course or temporal profile of disease. The *development* of symptoms can be as follows:
1. *Acute,* within minutes
2. *Subacute,* within days
3. *Chronic,* within months

The *evolution* or course of disease after symptoms have developed can be as follows:
1. *Transient,* when symptoms resolve completely after onset
2. *Improving,* when severity is reduced but symptoms are not resolved
3. *Progressive,* when symptoms continue to progress or new symptoms appear
4. *Exacerbating-remitting,* when symptoms develop, then resolve or improve, then recur and worsen, and so on
5. *Stationary (or chronic),* when symptoms remain unchanged for an extended period of time

MSDs can appear at any point during the development and evolution of neurologic disease. As a result, their presence may be very informative to localization and diagnosis.

Broad Etiologic Categories

Categorizing types of pathologic changes is useful for understanding neurologic disease. Each category can produce MSDs, but the distribution of MSD types varies across etiologies. Specific diseases associated with each of the following broad etiologic categories are defined and discussed in chapters on the MSDs with which they are most commonly encountered.

Degenerative Diseases

These are characterized by a gradual decline in neuronal function of unknown cause. In some cases, neurons atrophy and disappear, whereas in others neuronal changes may be more specific (e.g., neurofibrillary tangles in Alzheimer's disease).

Many degenerative neurologic diseases are probably genetically determined biochemical disorders that share basic mechanisms that lead to neuronal death. The clinical differences among them are a function of localization, the order in which pathologic changes emerge, and their rate of progression.[8]

Degenerative diseases are most often *chronic, progressive,* and *diffuse,* but they sometimes begin with focal manifestations. When causes for them are found, they are usually shifted to a more specific disease category.

Inflammatory Diseases

These include, but are not limited to, infectious processes. They are characterized by an inflammatory response to microorganisms, toxic chemicals, or immunologic reactions. Their pathologic hallmark is an outpouring of white blood cells. The development of clinical signs and symptoms is usually *subacute.*

Many inflammatory diseases are progressive and diffusely located in the leptomeninges and CSF (as in *meningitis*) or in the brain parenchyma (as in *encephalitis*). Inflammation in the PNS may occur in single nerves *(mononeuritis)* or in multiple nerves *(polyneuritis).*

Some CNS inflammatory diseases are focal. When focal, there may be *abscess formation,* a process in which astrocytes proliferate to form a wall of glial fibers that limits spread of infection, eventually leaving a cavity that reflects loss of the enclosed brain tissue. An abscess can exert mass effects on nearby structures.

Toxic-Metabolic Diseases

Vitamin deficiencies, genetic biochemical disorders, complications of kidney and liver disease, and drug toxicity are examples of toxic and metabolic diseases that can alter neuronal function. Pathologic changes vary but can include edema, ischemia, demyelination, and cell death.[8] Their effects are usually diffuse. Their development and course can be *acute, subacute,* or *chronic.*

Neoplastic Diseases

Any cell type in the nervous system can become neoplastic. However, neurons in the adult nervous system do not normally undergo cell division and, therefore, neuronal neoplasms *(neurocytomas)* are rare. In contrast, astrocytes are very reactive and, consequently, *astrocytomas* are the most common primary CNS tumor. As the terms neurocytoma and astrocytoma suggest, tumors are often named after the cell types from which they arise. Thus cells of the leptomeninges give rise to *meningiomas,* and Schwann cells give rise to *schwannomas.*

Nervous system tumors rarely *metastasize* (spread) outside the CNS, but systemic cancer can metastasize to the CNS. Tumors usually create focal signs and symptoms and are *chronic* or *progressive* in temporal profile.

Not all progressive mass lesions represent neoplasm. Blood clots *(hematomas)* and *edema* are examples of mass lesions that are nonneoplastic in character.

Traumatic Diseases

Traumatic injury usually has an identifiable precipitating event (e.g., automobile accident, fall, gunshot wound). Onset is almost always *acute,* with maximum damage around the time of onset.

PNS traumatic injuries can be focal or multifocal. CNS traumatic injuries are often diffuse initially, as in *concussion* (an immediate and transient loss of consciousness or other neurologic function following head injury). The course is usually one of *resolution or improvement;* residual focal signs and symptoms tend to reflect areas of severe anatomic damage (often associated with contusions, lacerations, and hematomas).

An exception to the general rule of acute onset of signs and symptoms from trauma can occur in *subdural hematoma.* The bleeding in this case is under low pressure, because it occurs in veins crossing from the brain to the dural sinuses, where blood is then drained from the brain. Blood accumulates slowly, and symptoms may not emerge for days or even months.

Traumatic brain injuries (TBIs) can be subdivided into *penetrating* and *closed head injuries (CHIs).* Penetrating head wounds (e.g., bullets, shrapnel) may produce relatively focal neurologic abnormalities, whereas CHIs are often associated with more diffuse abnormalities. Conservative estimates place the incidence in the United States of penetrating head injuries at 12 per 100,000 and the incidence of CHI at 200 per 100,000.[54] CHI is a major cause of death and disability in Americans younger than age 35.[63] Motor vehicle accidents, falls, and sports injuries represent some of the major causes of CHI.

Although cognitive deficits are the most common and perhaps persistent neurologic deficits associated with CHI, motor impairments are not uncommon. Up to 60% of people with CHI in acute rehabilitation settings may be dysarthric.[68]

It is appropriate to discuss briefly the pathogenesis of CHI, because it is complex and applicable to understanding the mechanisms by which it may produce diverse MSDs. Injuries from CHI can create focal lesions, diffuse axonal injury, and superimposed hypoxia or ischemia and microvascular damage.[63] Focal contusions often occur at the site of impact and result in focal neurologic deficits. They are known as *coup injuries.* If the injury is associated with acceleration, the motion of the brain may also cause trauma at sites opposite the point of impact, causing a *contrecoup* lesion. The most common sites of these focal injuries are the orbitofrontal region and the anterior temporal lobes. These are locations where the brain abuts on edges of the skull (see Figures 2-1 and 2-2) and is subject to trauma when the head rapidly decelerates (as in falls or sudden impacts). This often causes rupture (tearing) of veins in the area of trauma, although hemorrhage in CHI can be extradural, subdural, subarachnoid, or intracerebral.

Diffuse axonal injury is viewed as the principal cause of persistent severe neurologic deficit in CHI,[63] but it can occur even after mild concussion. It results from shearing of axons, commonly in the centrum semiovale, corpus callosum, and brainstem. The trauma generates a physiologic response in the affected axons that eventually leads to their being severed. Diffuse axonal injuries occur more frequently when trauma is associated with rotational forces.[26]

Hypoxia and ischemia (see next section on vascular disease) can occur in response to trauma, as can more subtle microvascular damage. These vascular sequelae can result from stretch and strain on blood vessels, from effects on vascular regulatory systems (e.g., decreased vascular system response to changes in carbon dioxide), from transient hypertension, from increased intracranial pressure, and from a transient breakdown in the blood-brain barrier. The most frequent sites of ischemic damage in CHI include the hippocampus, basal ganglia, cortex, and cerebellum.[30]

To summarize, the deficits from CHI result from the direct effects of trauma (coup and contrecoup damage, diffuse axonal injury) and indirectly from biochemical events that occur in response to the trauma. These processes include, but are not limited to, ischemia, altered vascular reactivity, brain swelling, and the creation of conditions that lead to secondary infection. The complex pathophysiology of CHI can obviously lead to a wide variety of focal, multifocal, and diffuse nervous system impairments.

Vascular Diseases

Vascular disease is the most common cause of neurologic disease and, probably, MSDs. The most common type of cerebrovascular disease is *stroke* (or *infarct* or *cerebrovascular accident*), in which neurons are deprived of oxygen and glucose because of an interruption in blood supply. This deprivation is known as *ischemia.*

Stroke is nearly always *sudden in onset* and usually *focal.* Neurons cease to function within seconds of an ischemic event, and pathologic changes occur within minutes. The course of symptoms is usually one of *stabilization and improve-*

ment. When progression of symptoms occurs, it usually reflects the development of *cerebral edema* or continuing infarction of adjacent tissue. Although cerebral edema occurs in response to many pathologic processes, it is common in stroke, because ischemia affects the blood-brain barrier and neuronal and glial cell membranes. Fluid may collect in the extracellular space *(vasogenic edema),* mostly in the white matter of the brain, and cause a significant increase in intracranial pressure. Edema may also be *cytotoxic,* in which there is intracellular accumulation of water, more likely in gray matter, but usually without significant mass effects. Both vasogenic and cytotoxic edema often occur in response to stroke.

Ischemic infarcts account for about 80% of strokes. A common cause of ischemia is *embolism,* in which a fragment of material (an embolus) travels through a blood vessel to a point of arterial narrowing sufficient to block its further passage, with subsequent occlusion of blood flow behind it. Embolic strokes tend to develop suddenly and without warning. Emboli usually come from the heart; the aortic arch and carotid and vertebral arteries are other sources. Embolic material can be a blood clot, atherosclerotic plaque, clump of bacteria, piece of tumor or lining from an artery, or other solid materials that may travel in the bloodstream.

Thrombosis, or the narrowing and occlusion of an artery at a fixed point, can also cause ischemia. Thrombosis frequently reflects a buildup of *atherosclerotic plaque,* made up of lipids (fatty deposits) and fibrous material on the inner wall of a vessel. Thromboses usually occur in the internal carotid, vertebral, or basilar arteries. Thrombotic strokes are sometimes preceded by *transient ischemic attacks (TIAs),* characterized by neurologic symptoms that last for seconds to minutes and are warning signs of cerebrovascular disease and impending stroke. Motor speech and language deficits are among the most common symptoms of TIAs.

Not all thrombotic strokes are associated with atherosclerosis. Some other sources include spontaneous or traumatically induced dissections of the carotid, vertebral, or intracranial arteries at the base of the skull; certain hematologic disorders; and mass effects exerted on arteries by tumors or by *aneurysms.* Aneurysms are *balloonlike malformations in weakened areas of arterial walls.* They are most commonly found in the internal carotid, anterior, or middle cerebral arteries.

Infarcts may also be *hemorrhagic.* In *cerebral hemorrhage,* a vessel ruptures into the brain, with accumulation of blood in neural tissue *(intraparenchymal* or *intracerebral hemorrhage).* These events are often associated with elevated blood pressure and chronic hypertension. Symptoms appear abruptly and are focal, but they may progress because of mass effects from blood accumulation. The thalamus, basal ganglia, brainstem, and cerebellum are common sites of intracerebral hemorrhage.

The most common extracerebral hemorrhage is *subarachnoid hemorrhage,* in which a vessel ruptures on the surface of the brain and blood spreads over its surface and throughout the subarachnoid space. Onset is *abrupt,* but symptoms and pathologic changes are often *diffuse.* Ruptured aneurysms are a common cause of subarachnoid hemorrhage. They may also result from rupture of an *arteriovenous malformation (AVM),* which is a collection of abnormally formed veins and arteries. AVMs can become enlarged by expansion of weak vessel walls and create neurologic symptoms through mass effects. Subarachnoid hemorrhage may eventually occur if the weakened walls rupture. Finally, *subdural* and *extradural hemorrhage* may occur, often from CHIs in which dural blood vessels are torn open.

▧ THE SPEECH MOTOR SYSTEM

The motor system, of which the speech motor system is a part, contains the complex network of structures and pathways that organize, control, and execute movement. It resides at all levels of the nervous system and mediates many activities of striated and visceral muscles. An appreciation of its organization and basic operating principles is necessary to understand normal speech production and MSDs. The remainder of this chapter lays the foundation for that understanding.

The motor system can be subdivided in many ways. Unfortunately, categorizing the components of a complex, integrated, and incompletely understood system inevitably produces some ambiguity, overlap, and confusion. Nonetheless, it would be impossible to develop an understanding of the speech motor system without parsing it in some way.

The motor system can be organized according to its functions, as well as its anatomy. Functional labels contribute to understanding what the components do rather than simply where they are. On this basis, four major functional divisions of the motor system can be delineated (based on Benarroch et al.[8]):

1. The final common pathway
2. The direct activation pathway
3. The indirect activation pathway
4. The control circuits

These divisions have identifiable anatomic correlates, and both anatomic and functional designations are used here in an effort to tie them together in the reader's mind. The four major divisions, their broad functions and primary structures, and some common related designations are summarized in Table 2-6. A fifth division, the conceptual-programming level, is

| table 2-6 | Functional and anatomic divisions of the motor system that are relevant to speech production |

Major Division	Basic Function	Major Structures	Related Designations
Final Common Pathway	Stimulates muscle contraction & movement Other motor divisions must act through it to influence movement	Cranial nerves Spinal nerves	Lower motor neuron system
Direct Activation Pathway	Influences consciously controlled, skilled voluntary movement	Corticobulbar tracts Corticospinal tracts	Upper motor neuron system, direct motor system, pyramidal system or tracts
Indirect Activation Pathway	Mediates subconscious, automatic muscle activities including posture, muscle tone, & movement that support & accompany voluntary movement	Corticorubral tracts Corticoreticular tracts Rubrospinal, reticulospinal vestibulospinal, & related tracts to relevant cranial nerves	Upper motor neuron system, indirect motor system, extrapyramidal system or tracts
Control Circuits	Integration or coordination of sensory information & activities of direct & indirect activation pathways to control movement		
Basal ganglia	Plan & program postural & supportive components of motor activity	Basal ganglia, substantia nigra, subthalamus, cerebral cortex	Extrapyramidal system
Cerebellar	Integrates & coordinates execution of smooth, directed movements	Cerebellum Cerebellar peduncles, reticular formation, red nucleus, pontine nuclei, inferior olive, thalamus, cerebral cortex	Cerebellum

also essential to speech; it includes planning and programming processes. It is discussed under the next major heading in this chapter. The relationships among the four major divisions, planning and programming, sensation, and movement, are illustrated in Figure 2-11.

Although the discussion of the motor system naturally emphasizes *efferent pathways,* the role of sensory or *afferent pathways* cannot be ignored. Sensorimotor integration is necessary for normal movement, and lesions of sensory portions of the sensorimotor system can result in abnormal motor behavior.*

The Final Common Pathway—Basic Structures and Functions

The *final common pathway (FCP)* is often referred to as the *lower motor neuron (LMN) system.*

*Some authors (e.g., McNeil[48]) use the term "sensorimotor speech disorders" to refer to the MSDs discussed in this book.

The words "final common" identify it as the *peripheral mechanism through which all motor activity is mediated;* that is, all other components of the motor system must act through it. It is *the last link in the chain of neural events that lead to movement.*

To understand the role of the FCP in movement requires an appreciation of its interaction with muscle. The FCPs involved in speech generate activity in *skeletal* or *somatic* muscles, which are muscles that can be voluntarily controlled with relative ease. Skeletal muscles move body parts by exerting forces on muscles, tendons, and joints.

A single muscle cannot produce complex movements. It can only relax, stretch, or contract. However, it does contribute to complex movements when integrated with the actions of larger groups of contiguous or distant muscles. The following subsections review some of the basic nerve and muscle functions and the interactions that are involved in skeletal muscle movements.

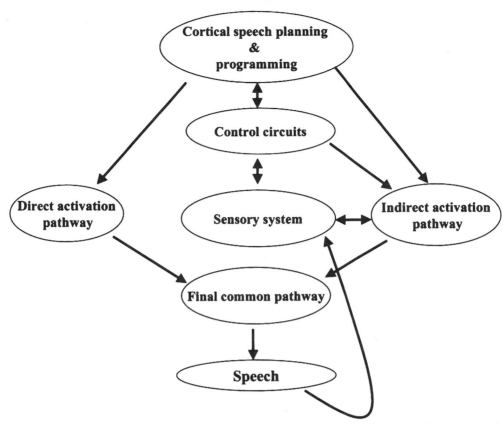

FIGURE 2-11 Relationships among the major divisions of the motor system, the sensory system, the motor speech programmer, and motor speech.

The Motor Unit, Alpha Motor Neurons, and Extrafusal Muscle Fibers

The contractile elements of skeletal muscles are known as *extrafusal muscle fibers.* They are under the direct control of LMNs, or *alpha motor neurons,* whose origins are in the brainstem and in the anterior horns of the spinal cord. LMNs control the activities of groups of muscle fibers. An LMN and the muscle fibers innervated by it are known as a *motor unit* (see Figure 2-10); hundreds of thousands of motor units innervate the muscles of the body. Although this discussion focuses on the activities of single neurons, it must be kept in mind that functional neuromuscular activity requires the combined effects of many neurons acting together in nerves.

The axon of an alpha motor neuron leaves the brainstem or spinal cord as part of a cranial or spinal nerve and travels to a specific muscle. It then subdivides into a number of terminal branches that make contact with muscle fibers. Because they branch, *each axon in a nerve may innervate several muscle fibers.* At the same time, *each muscle fiber may receive input from branches of several different alpha motor neurons.* This redundancy of innervation permits gradations in the force of whole muscle contraction. That is, force can be increased by increasing the rate of firing of individual motor units *(temporal summation)* or by recruiting a greater number of motor units *(spatial summation).*

The number of extrafusal muscle fibers innervated by a single motor neuron determines the size of a motor unit. The number of muscle fibers per axon is known as the *innervation ratio.* Muscles concerned with fine, discrete movements have smaller innervation ratios than those that perform strong-but-cruder movements. For example, proximal limb muscles may have ratios of more than 500:1, whereas one neuron may supply only about 10 to 25 muscle fibers in some facial and laryngeal muscles.[16,28]

In addition to innervating extrafusal muscle fibers, alpha motor neurons also innervate interneurons, or *Renshaw cells,* through collateral fibers from their axons. Renshaw cells are capable of inhibiting alpha motor neurons, in effect producing a negative feedback response, which can immediately turn off the alpha motor neuron after it fires and prepare it to fire again.

Gamma Motor Neurons, Intrafusal Muscle Fibers, the Gamma Motor System, and the Stretch Reflex

In addition to alpha motor neurons, motor nerves contain *gamma motor neurons.* Unlike alpha motor neurons, gamma motor neurons innervate *muscle spindles* or *intrafusal muscle fibers* that are located parallel to extrafusal muscle fibers. Gamma motor neurons are smaller in diameter and slower conducting than alpha motor neurons. Their activity is strongly influenced by the cerebellum, basal ganglia, and indirect activation pathways of the CNS. The activities of alpha motor neurons are more strongly tied to the direct activation pathways.

Gamma motor neurons, their role in a functional unit known as the *gamma loop,* and their relationship to alpha motor neurons and the activities of the direct and indirect activation pathways of the CNS, are important to movement control. They are crucial to maintaining *muscle tone,* a property of normal muscle that establishes its appearance as neither too taut nor too flabby. Muscle tone results from natural tissue elasticity plus a mild degree of resistance that occurs in a muscle in response to its being stretched; it is actually a manifestation of a basic but crucial normal reflex known as the *stretch reflex.*

The stretch reflex represents the "desire" of muscle to maintain its original length whenever it is stretched. Normal muscle tone is a sustained phenomenon, because muscles are never completely relaxed; in a sense they are always maintained in a state of readiness for movement. The sustained nature of muscle tone makes it an ideal support mechanism upon which quick, unsustained, skilled movements may be superimposed. This support is mediated through the *gamma motor system.*

The gamma motor neuron is the efferent component of the gamma motor system. Its firing causes muscle spindles to contract (shorten). This shortening is detected by sensory receptors *(annulospiral endings)* in the spindles that trigger impulses through sensory neurons back to the spinal cord or brainstem, where they synapse with alpha motor neurons. The alpha motor neuron, in turn, directs impulses back to extrafusal muscle fibers, stimulating them to contract until they are the same length as the muscle spindles. Once this equalization has taken place, the sensory receptor no longer detects shortening, and the "loop" is inactivated. During movement this process is, for practical purposes, continuous.

The gamma loop thus consists of the gamma motor neuron, muscle spindle, stretch receptor and sensory neuron, the LMN, and extrafusal muscle fibers. It has been described as a mechanism through which muscle length adjusts reflexively to the relative length of muscle spindles. This mechanism can be used by the indirect activation pathway of the CNS to "preset" the desired length of the muscle spindle for static postures (e.g., extending the arm and holding it stable; possibly for moving the arytenoid cartilages into position for sustained phonation). It can also be used to prepare for the degree of muscle contraction required for intended ongoing movement. The relationships among the alpha and gamma motor neurons, muscle spindles, and the gamma loop are illustrated in Figure 2-12.

Influences upon the FCP

As implied in the preceding discussion, the LMN integrates activity from several sources, including the peripheral sensory system, the direct activation pathway, and the indirect activation pathway. The integrated activity of LMNs results in movement.

The sensory system's *direct* relationship with alpha motor neurons involves synapses at the level of the spinal cord and brainstem. These synapses produce simple, stereotyped, involuntary *reflexes* that are limited to specific muscles and body parts (e.g., the gag reflex). Damage to the peripheral sensory pathways abolishes or reduces reflexes by removing or weakening the trigger for them. Reflexes can also be lost or diminished by damage to the FCP.

Voluntary movement is considerably more complex than the sensory-motor reflexes just described. True volitional or even relatively automatic complex movements depend on the influence of direct and indirect activation pathways and control circuits in the CNS. Nonetheless, such activities can be brought to fruition only through the FCP.

Effects of Damage

Damage to the motor unit prevents the normal activation of muscle fibers. However, because each muscle fiber may be innervated by several alpha motor neurons, damage to a single alpha motor neuron does not eliminate the possibility of muscle fiber contraction. As a result, damage to a nerve may lead only to *weakness* or *paresis* if all of the alpha motor neurons supplying the muscle are not damaged. *Paralysis* results if a muscle is deprived of input from all of its LMNs.

With a loss of innervation, muscles eventually lose bulk and undergo *atrophy.* In addition, excess or spontaneous motor unit activity and a lowered firing threshold may occur in motor unit disease. These spontaneous motor unit discharges may be seen on the surface of the skin as brief localized twitches known as *fasciculations.* Finally, muscles deprived of LMN input also generate slow repetitive action potentials and contract regularly. This process, which cannot be seen, is known as *fibrillation.*

To summarize, the action of the FCP is both simple and profound. On one hand, its role in

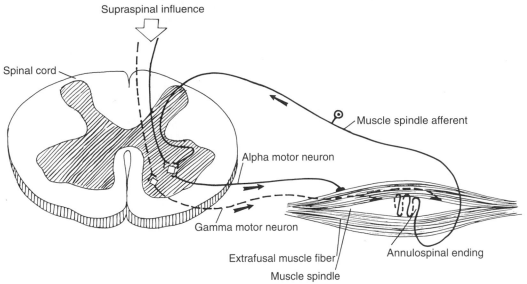

FIGURE 2-12 Motor unit, gamma loop, and stretch reflex. Extrafusal muscle fibers and muscle spindles are stimulated to contract by alpha and gamma motor neurons, respectively. When relaxed, the muscle spindle's sensory receptor (annulospinal ending) is silent. When muscle is stretched by movement, so is the spindle. This is detected by the sensory ending and transmitted to the spinal cord (or brainstem), where the alpha motor neuron is led to fire, producing extrafusal muscle fiber contraction that, in effect, resists the stretch on muscle. The stretch reflex is the basis for normal muscle tone.

Supraspinal (and suprabulbar) influences can use this mechanism to "preset" movement. For example, the indirect activation pathway may stimulate the gamma motor neuron to produce muscle spindle contraction, which is detected by sensory endings and transmitted to alpha motor neurons that then stimulate extrafusal muscle contraction that is sufficient to balance the relationship between the extrafusal muscle and the muscle spindle. The movement "target" is reached when this balance is achieved.

complex and voluntary movement is only as a conduit to muscle of messages "written" and controlled elsewhere. Without it, however, muscle cannot be activated, and movement is impossible. *Damage at this level of the motor system is responsible for the speech characteristics of flaccid dysarthria.*

The Final Common Pathway and Speech

The FCP for speech includes the following:
- The paired cranial nerves that supply muscles involved in phonation, resonance, articulation, and prosody
- The paired spinal nerves involved in respiratory activities and prosody

Following is an overview of the origin, course, and function of the cranial and spinal nerves that are most important for motor speech production.*

Trigeminal Nerve (Cranial Nerve V)

The paired trigeminal nerve is the largest of the cranial nerves. Its sensory functions include the transmission of pain, thermal, and tactile sensation from the face and forehead, mucous membranes of

the nose and mouth, the teeth, and portions of the cranial dura. It also conveys deep pressure and kinesthetic information from the teeth, gums, hard palate, and temporomandibular joint, as well as sensation from stretch receptors in the jaw. Its motor components are responsible for innervating the muscles of mastication and the mylohyoid, anterior belly of the digastric, tensor tympani, and tensor veli palatini muscles.

The nerve emerges on the midlateral surface of the pons as a large sensory and smaller motor root (Figure 2-13). It is divided into *ophthalmic, maxillary,* and *mandibular branches,* all of which arise from the trigeminal ganglion, where most of its sensory nerve cell bodies are located. The ophthalmic branch is concerned with sensation in the upper face and is not discussed further.

The *maxillary branch* is complex in its distribution. Its multiple branches carry sensation from the maxilla and maxillary sinus; the mucous membranes of the mouth; the nasal cavity, palate, and nasopharynx; the teeth; the inferior portion of the auditory meatus; the face; and the meninges of the anterior and middle cranial fossa. Its fibers originate in the *trigeminal ganglion** (also called the *semilunar* or

---

*A more detailed review of the cranial and spinal nerves relevant to speech production can be found in Bhatnager.[11]

*Primary sensory neuron cell bodies of cranial nerves are usually located just outside of the CNS in sensory ganglia.

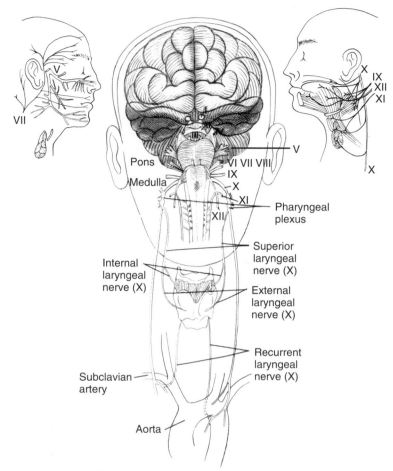

FIGURE 2-13 Primary cranial nerves for speech.

gasserian ganglion), which is located in a depression in the petrous bone on the floor of the middle cranial fossa. They travel outward from the ganglion to the periphery through the *foramen rotundum* in the middle fossa (see Figure 2-2). They travel inward from the ganglion to the brainstem, entering the mid-lateral aspect of the pons. From there, fibers carrying touch sensation from the face synapse with the chief sensory nucleus of the nerve within the pons. Like all peripheral sensory fibers, the primary sensory neurons of the maxillary branch have CNS connections. Some fibers synapse with the adjacent reticular formation. Information is also transmitted in crossed and uncrossed fibers of the *trigeminothalamic tracts* that synapse in the thalamus. Neurons from the thalamus project through the internal capsule to the lower third of the ipsilateral postcentral gyrus in the cortex, where conscious perception of sensation occurs.

Pain and temperature fibers of the maxillary branch descend in the brainstem to various points along the medulla and the upper segment of the cervical spinal cord. These axons synapse with cell bodies in the nucleus of the *spinal tract of the trigeminal nerve;* along the way, small sensory components of cranial nerves IX and X also join the nerve's spinal tract. After these synapses, fibers cross at various levels to the opposite side and ascend in the trigeminothalamic tract to the thalamus. From there, thalamocortical neurons transmit sensory information to the parietal lobe.

The *mandibular branch,* the nerve's largest branch, contains sensory and motor fibers. Its motor nucleus is located in the midpons, close to the nerve's chief sensory nucleus. As it leaves the skull through the *foramen ovale* (see Figure 2-2), it branches repeatedly to send fibers to the tensor veli palatini, tensor tympani, and jaw muscles.

The sensory branches of the mandibular branch carry sensation from the mucous membrane of the mouth, the side of the head and scalp, the lower jaw, and the anterior two thirds of the tongue. They also carry proprioceptive information from muscles involved in jaw movement to the *mesencephalic nucleus* in the midbrain, adjacent to the fourth ventricle. There is evidence for the presence of muscle spindles in the muscles of mastication and evidence of Golgi tendon organs in the temporalis and masseter muscles[43]; these may play an important role in the sensorimotor control of jaw movement during speech.

The central connections of mandibular sensory neurons project to the masticatory nucleus of the nerve to provide reflex control of bite. The motor nucleus also receives sensory input from other cranial nerves (e.g., input from the acoustic nerve influences the part of the motor nerve that innervates the tensor tympani, so that tension on the tympanic membrane can be adjusted for loudness variations).

LMN lesions of the masticatory nucleus or its axons lead to *paresis or paralysis and eventual atrophy of masticatory muscles on the paralyzed side.* Unilateral cranial nerve V lesions do not have major effects on speech. Bilateral lesions can be devastating because the jaw hangs open, cannot be closed, or moves slowly and with limited range, thereby preventing facial, bilabial, and lingual articulatory movements from achieving accurate place and manner of articulation.

Facial Nerve (Cranial Nerve VII)

The paired facial nerve is a mixed motor and sensory nerve. Its motor component supplies the stapedius muscle and muscles of facial expression. Its sensory components provide innervation to the submandibular, sublingual, and lacrimal glands, as well as to taste receptors on the anterior two thirds of the tongue and nasopharynx. Only the motor component has a clear role in speech (see Figure 2-13).

Motor fibers that innervate the muscles of facial expression constitute the largest part of the nerve. They arise in the facial nucleus located in the lower third of the pons. Fibers of the nerve pass medially and arch dorsally, forming a loop around the abducens nucleus, before reaching the lateral surface of the pons and emerging as the facial nerve.

As they leave the pons, motor fibers travel adjacent to nerve's sensory fibers. Accompanied by fibers of cranial (auditory) nerve VIII, motor and sensory divisions of the facial nerve leave the cranial cavity through the *internal auditory meatus* (see Figure 2-2). Motor fibers travel through the facial canal and exit at the stylomastoid foramen below the ear and pass through the parotid gland. From there, the buccal and mandibular branches of the nerve innervate the muscles of facial expression. Motor fibers of the nerve also give off branches to supply the stapedius, the platysma, and other submental muscles.

LMN lesions of the facial nerve can *paralyze muscles on the entire ipsilateral side of the face.* Such lesions affect all voluntary, emotional, and reflex movements. Atrophy occurs, resulting in *facial asymmetry. Fasciculations* may be seen in the perioral area and chin.

Glossopharyngeal Nerve (Cranial Nerve IX)

The paired glossopharyngeal nerve is a mixed motor and sensory nerve. Of relevance for speech are its motor supply to the stylopharyngeus and upper constrictor muscles of the pharynx and its transmission of sensory information from the pharynx, tongue, and eustachian tube (see Figure 2-13).

Motor fibers to the stylopharyngeus muscle originate in the rostral portion of the *nucleus ambiguus,* which is located within the reticular formation in the lateral medulla. The nucleus ambiguus is a complex grouping of cell bodies, containing fibers of cranial nerves IX and X, and portions of cranial nerve XI.

The motor component of the nerve emerges from the medulla just above the rootlets of the vagus nerve. It passes through the *jugular foramen* (see Figure 2-2) with the vagus and accessory nerves to innervate the stylopharyngeus, which elevates the pharynx during swallowing and speech.

The afferent fibers of the nerve, which carry sensation from the pharynx and tongue, arise from cell bodies in the *inferior (petrosal) ganglion* in the jugular foramen. They terminate in the nucleus of the *tractus solitarius,* which lies ventrolateral to the dorsal motor nucleus of the vagus and extends along the length of the medulla. The tractus solitarius also receives visceral afferent fibers from the facial and vagus nerves.

Within the medulla are reflex connections between pharyngeal sensory and motor neurons that mediate the *gag reflex.* CNS neurons carrying pain, temperature, and probably touch and pressure sensation leave the medulla, cross the midline, and ascend to the contralateral thalamus. From there, thalamocortical neurons pass to the postcentral sensory cortex, where sensation reaches conscious awareness.

The effects of glossopharyngeal nerve lesions are difficult to isolate, because such lesions usually also damage the vagus nerve. Damage to the nerve is most predictably associated with *reduced pharyngeal sensation, a decrease in the gag reflex,* and *reduced pharyngeal elevation during swallowing.*[11]

Excessive oral secretions may reflect reduced control of the parotid gland. Lesions of the glossopharyngeal nerve sometime lead to paroxysmal radiating throat pain of unknown etiology known as *glossopharyngeal neuralgia.*

Vagus Nerve (Cranial Nerve X)

The paired vagus nerve is a complex and lengthy mixed motor and sensory nerve (see Figure 2-13) that plays a crucial role in speech production. Its relevant motor functions include the innervation of the striated muscles of the soft palate, pharynx, and larynx. Its relevant sensory role includes transmission of sensation from those same structures. Among its additional functions are parasympathetic innervation to and sensation from the thorax and abdominal viscera, as well as sensory innervation from the external auditory meatus and taste receptors in the posterior pharynx. Only those branches of the vagus nerve relevant to speech production are discussed here.

Motor fibers of the vagus nerve supplying muscles of the soft palate, pharynx, and larynx arise from the posterior two thirds of the *nucleus ambiguus* in the lateral medulla (along with motor fibers of cranial nerve IX and portions of cranial nerve XI). Motor neurons innervating the soft palate and pharynx are located in the most caudal region of the nucleus. Those innervating the larynx are located most rostrally. Sensory fibers from the soft palate, pharynx, and larynx have their cell bodies in the *inferior (nodose) ganglion,* located in or very near the *jugular foramen;* communication with the hypoglossal, accessory, glossopharyngeal, and facial nerves can take place at this level. The central processes of the sensory fibers terminate in the nucleus of the *tractus solitarius.*

The vagus nerve emerges from the lateral aspect of the medulla between the *inferior cerebellar peduncle* and the *inferior olive.* It exits the skull through the jugular foramen with cranial nerves IX and XI (see Figure 2-2). Near its exit from the skull, three branches are identifiable. The *pharyngeal branch* travels down the neck between the internal and external carotid arteries and enters the pharynx at the upper border of the middle pharyngeal constrictor muscle. There it breaks up and joins with branches from the glossopharyngeal and external laryngeal nerves to form the *pharyngeal plexus.* From there it distributes fibers to all the muscles of the pharynx and soft palate except the stylopharyngeus (IX) and the tensor veli palatini (innervated by the mandibular branch of cranial nerve V). It also supplies the palatoglossus muscle of the tongue. The pharyngeal branch is primarily responsible for pharyngeal constriction and for retraction and elevation of the soft palate during velopharyngeal closure for speech and swallowing.

The *superior laryngeal nerve* branch of the vagus descends adjacent to the pharynx, first posterior and then medial to the internal carotid artery. About 2 cm below the inferior ganglion it divides into the internal and external laryngeal nerves.

The *internal laryngeal nerve* is purely sensory. It carries sensation from the mucous membrane lining the larynx down to the level of the vocal folds, the epiglottis, the base of the tongue, aryepiglottic folds, and the dorsum of the arytenoid cartilages. It also transmits information from muscle spindles and other stretch receptors in the larynx.

The *external laryngeal nerve* supplies the inferior pharyngeal constrictor and the cricothyroid muscles. Its innervation of the cricothyroid is especially important for phonation, because the cricothyroid lengthens the vocal folds for pitch adjustments.

The third major branch of the vagus, the *recurrent laryngeal branch,* is so called because it doubles back on itself before reaching the larynx. The right and left recurrent laryngeal nerves take different paths. The right recurrent nerve branches from the vagus nerve anterior to the subclavian artery, then loops below and behind the artery and ascends behind the common carotid artery in the groove between the trachea and the esophagus. It enters the larynx between the inferior horn of the thyroid and cricoid cartilage. The left recurrent nerve is longer than the right, arising from the vagus at the aortic arch. It hooks under the arch near the heart, ascends in the groove between the trachea and esophagus, and enters the larynx between the inferior horn of the thyroid and cricoid cartilage. Both the right and left recurrent laryngeal nerves innervate all of the intrinsic muscles of the larynx except the cricothyroid. General sensation from the vocal folds and larynx lying below them is carried by sensory fibers of the recurrent laryngeal nerves. Thus the superior and recurrent laryngeal nerves are responsible for all laryngeal sensory and motor activities involved in phonation and swallowing.

The effects of vagus nerve lesions depend on the particular branch of the nerve that has been damaged. Damage to all of its branches will produce *weakness of the soft palate, pharynx, and larynx.* Unilateral LMN lesions can affect resonance, voice quality, and swallowing but usually affect phonation more prominently than resonance. Bilateral LMN lesions can have devastating effects on resonance and phonation, with significant secondary effects on prosody and clarity of articulation; swallowing may be significantly impaired. The specific effects of unilateral and bilateral lesions to each of the nerve's branches are discussed in Chapter 4.

Accessory Nerve (Cranial Nerve XI)

The paired accessory nerve (also called the *spinal accessory nerve*) has a cranial and spinal portion (see Figure 2-13). The cranial portion arises from the nucleus ambiguus, emerges from the side of the medulla, and passes through the jugular foramen (see Figure 2-2). Branches from the nerve join the jugular ganglion of the vagus nerve, and the remaining fibers become part of the pharyngeal and superior and recurrent laryngeal branches of the vagus nerve. The cranial portion contributes fibers to the uvula, levator veli palatini, and intrinsic laryngeal muscles but does so while intermingled with fibers of the vagus nerve.

Cell bodies of the spinal portion of the nerve reside in the ventral horn of the first five or six cervical segments of the spinal cord. Its axons ascend in the spinal canal lateral to the spinal cord and enter the posterior fossa through the *foramen magnum.* They then leave the skull through the *jugular foramen* (with the glossopharyngeal, vagus, and cranial portion of the accessory nerve) to innervate the sternocleidomastoid and trapezius muscles.

Lesions in the region of the foramen magnum (where the ascending nerve enters the skull) or in the region of the jugular foramen (where it exits the skull) *can weaken head rotation* toward the side opposite the lesion (sternocleidomastoid weakness). It can also *reduce the ability to elevate or shrug the shoulder* on the side of the lesion.

Hypoglossal Nerve (Cranial Nerve XII)

The paired hypoglossal nerve (see Figure 2-13) is a motor nerve that innervates all intrinsic and all but one of the extrinsic muscles of the tongue (the exception is the palatoglossus, supplied by the vagus nerve). Its long, thin nucleus extends through most of the medulla and lies in the floor of the fourth ventricle. Its fibers travel ventrally to exit from the medulla as a number of rootlets between the medullary pyramids and inferior olive. The rootlets then converge and pass through the *hypoglossal foramen* in the posterior fossa (see Figure 2-2). After leaving the skull, the nerve lies medial to cranial nerves IX, X, and XI and travels in the vicinity of the common carotid artery and internal jugular vein. It eventually loops anteriorly above the greater cornu of the hyoid bone and passes to the intrinsic and extrinsic muscles of the tongue.

The hypoglossal nucleus receives taste and tactile information from the nucleus of the tractus solitarius and the sensory trigeminal nucleus. These sensory processes are important for speech, as well as for chewing, swallowing, and sucking.

Damage to the hypoglossal nucleus or its axons can lead to *atrophy, weakness,* and *fasciculations of the tongue on the side of the lesion.* Unilateral weakness causes the tongue to deviate to the side of the lesion when protruded.

The Spinal Nerves

Upper cervical spinal nerves supply neck and shoulder muscles that are indirectly implicated in voice, resonance, and articulation. For practical purposes, however, the discussion of spinal nerve contributions to speech focuses on respiratory activities.

The discussion of respiratory activity is confined to *external respiration,* or the exchange of air between the lungs and outside atmosphere. *Internal respiration,* or the process of exchanging oxygen and carbon dioxide between the lungs and the blood and cells of the body, is only indirectly relevant to respiratory functions for speech.*

LMNs subserving respiration are spread from the cervical through the thoracic divisions of the spinal cord. Those supplying the diaphragm arise from the third, fourth, and fifth cervical segments of the spinal cord. Those supplying the intercostal and abdominal muscles of respiration are spread throughout the thoracic portion of the spinal cord. Accessory muscles of respiration—certain neck and shoulder girdle muscles (e.g., the sternocleidomastoid)—are spread through the upper and middle cervical cord down to the sixth cervical segment.

Fibers from the third, fourth, and fifth cervical nerves combine in the *cervical plexus* to form the paired *phrenic nerves.* Each phrenic nerve innervates one half of the *diaphragm,* the most important muscle of inhalation and the most important respiratory muscle for speech. The remaining muscles of inhalation (e.g., external and internal intercostal, sternocleidomastoid, scalene, and pectoralis) are innervated by motor neurons from branches of the lower cervical nerves, the intercostal nerves, the phrenic nerve, and the anterior and medial thoracic nerves.

Quiet exhalation occurs primarily through passive forces that bring the rib cage and inhalatory muscles to their resting position. Abdominal muscles are active in forced exhalation, however, and are innervated by the seventh through twelfth intercostal nerves, branches of the iliohypogastric and ilioinguinal nerves, and the lower six thoracic and upper two lumbar nerves.

The CNS is responsible for matching respiratory rate to various metabolic demands that arise from activities including speech. The center for automatic,

---

*Detailed discussion of the neuroanatomy and physiology of respiratory functions for speech can be found in Aronson,[5] Barlow and Farley,[7] Hixon,[29] and Kennedy and Kuehn.[33]

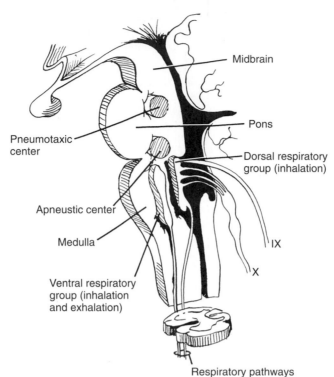

FIGURE 2-14 Respiratory centers and descending respiratory tracts.

rhythmic breathing—as opposed to voluntary or behavioral breathing*—is made up of several widely distributed, bilaterally located groups of neurons in the medulla and pons (Figure 2-14), an area called the *ponto-medullary respiratory oscillator.*[27] Damage to this area can produce respiratory abnormalities and lead to asphyxiation and death.

Dorsal respiratory neurons are located along the length of the medulla in its reticular formation and the nucleus of the tractus solitarius (also the termination point of sensory neurons from the vagus and glossopharyngeal nerves). Stimulation of these neurons produces inhalation and is important to maintaining a smooth rhythm of respiration.

Ventral respiratory neurons are located along the length of the medulla, in its ventrolateral portion. They can stimulate exhalation or inhalation but are primarily responsible for providing force during exhalation.

*Breathing for speech requires temporary overriding by higher brain centers of brainstem-controlled automatic breathing. Although CNS control of respiration for speech is not well understood, it clearly involves the cerebral cortex. Evidence from PET studies has identified contributions from the motor cortex, premotor cortex, supplementary motor area, and cerebellum, bilaterally, during volitional inspiration and expiration.[27]

The *apneustic center* is located in the lower pons. It seems to serve as an additional drive to inspiration. The *pneumotaxic center* is located in the upper pons. It helps regulate inspiratory volume by inhibiting inspiration.

CNS lesions can produce abnormal breathing patterns that may be encountered in people with CNS-based dysarthrias. Perhaps the most common observed by speech-language pathologists is *Cheyne-Stokes respiration* in which the breathing pattern "slowly oscillates between hyperventilation and hypoventilation."[10] It can result from bilateral damage anywhere between the cerebral hemispheres and upper pons. *Apneustic breathing,* caused by lesions of the dorsolateral lower half of the pons, is characterized by a prolonged inspiratory gasp with a pause at the peak of inspiration. *Ataxic breathing,* usually associated with damage to the medulla, is characterized by irregular rate and rhythm of breathing and can be a preterminal respiratory pattern.[10]

Because LMNs supplying the respiratory muscles are distributed widely, diffuse impairment is required to interfere significantly with respiration, especially respiration for speech. The exception to this is damage to the third, fourth, and fifth cervical segment of the spinal cord, where damage can paralyze the diaphragm bilaterally and seriously affect breathing. Significant weakness of respiratory function can affect voice production, loudness, phrase length, and prosody.

The Direct Activation Pathway and Speech

The direct activation pathway has a direct connection and major activating influence on the FCP. It is also known as the *pyramidal tract* or *direct motor system.* It can be divided into the *corticobulbar tract,* which influences the activities of the cranial nerves, and the *corticospinal tract,* which influences the activity of the spinal nerves. Together, they form part of the *upper motor neuron (UMN) system.*

The distinction between the UMN and LMN systems is a basic cornerstone of clinical neurology and is crucial to understanding the distinctive effects of lesions within each system on motor behavior, including speech. The anatomic and physiologic differences between the two systems are fairly straightforward. They are summarized in Table 2-7.

The concept of the UMN system can be confusing, one source of which lies in the degree to which the direct and indirect activation pathways and the control circuits are encompassed by the concept of the UMN. UMNs include neurons that regulate LMNs and that are controlled directly or indirectly by the cortex, cerebellum, or basal ganglia; "in the strictest sense, the neurons in all such pathways should be referred to as upper motoneurons."[25] From this standpoint, the direct and indirect activation pathways, as well as the control circuits, are all part of the UMN system. In practice, however, most clinicians use the term "upper motor neuron" to refer only to the direct and indirect activation pathways.

For our purposes, it is best to think of the UMN system as that part of the motor system that (1) is contained entirely within the CNS and is distinctly different from the location and functions of the LMN system, (2) does not include the basal ganglia and cerebellar control circuits, and (3) does include the direct and indirect activation pathways. These distinctions will be clarified further during discussion of the indirect activation pathway and the control circuits.

The direct activation pathway has a major influence on the cranial and spinal nerves that form the FCP for speech production. It *directly* connects the cortex to the FCP. The effect of the direct activation pathway on the FCP is primarily facilitative. Thus the direct system leads to movement (not inhibition of movement), presumably finely controlled, discrete movement, such as that required for speech.

Cortical Components

The direct activation pathway, including its components that are related to speech production, originates in the cortex of each cerebral hemisphere.

The main launching platform for the direct motor system is the *primary motor cortex* (also called the *precentral gyrus, motor strip,* or *Brodmann's area 4*) (Figure 2-15). It is located just anterior to the *central sulcus,* or *rolandic fissure,* the dividing line between the frontal and parietal lobes. Although the primary motor cortex is the cortical focal point of the pyramidal tracts for speech, only about 30% of the direct

---

table 2-7   Distinctions among the lower motor neuron and upper motor neuron divisions of the nervous system

		Upper Motor Neuron	
	Lower Motor Neuron	*Direct Activation Pathway*	*Indirect Activation Pathway*
Origin	Brainstem & spinal cord	Cerebral cortex	Cerebral cortex
Destination	Muscle	Cranial & spinal nerve nuclei	Cranial & spinal nerve nuclei
Function	Produce muscle actions for reflexes & muscle tone	Direct voluntary, skilled movements	Control posture, tone, & movements supportive of voluntary movement
	Carry out UMN commands for voluntary movements & postural adjustments	*direct spinal cord or brainstem*	
Distinctive Signs of Lesions	Weakness of all movements (voluntary & automatic)	Loss of skilled movement	Spasticity
	Diminished reflexes	Hyporeflexia *reduced reflexes*	Clonus *muscle tension*
	Decreased muscle tone	Babinski sign	Hyperactive stretch reflexes
	Atrophy	Decreased muscle tone	Increased muscle tone
	Fasciculations		Decorticate or decerebrate posture

UMN, Upper motor neuron.

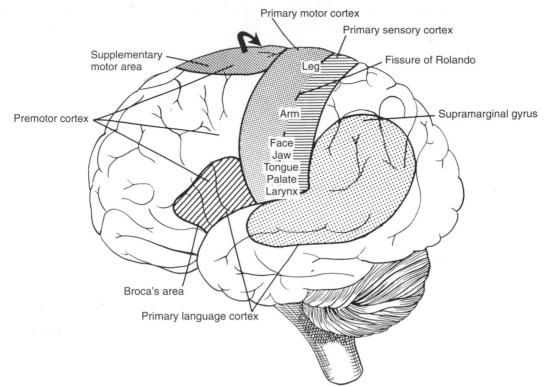

FIGURE 2-15 Major cortical components of the direct and indirect activation pathways and the motor speech planner and programmer.

system originates from it. Its fibers also arise from the *premotor cortex,* located just anterior to the primary motor area in the frontal lobe. The *supplementary motor area,* a portion of the premotor area also of importance for speech, is located on the medial aspect of each hemisphere. Finally, UMN fibers also originate in the postcentral gyrus in the parietal lobe and in adjacent somatosensory association cortex.[11] In addition to sending fibers through the direct activation pathway, these cortical motor areas are also believed to contribute to the indirect activation pathway.

Three characteristics of motor cortex organization further define the cortical anatomic and physiologic organization of the direct activation pathway:

1. Striated muscles are represented in an upside-down fashion along the length of the motor strip. For example, cell bodies sending axons to LMNs that innervate muscles of the face, tongue, and larynx are influenced by neurons in the lowest portion of the strip, whereas the hand, arm, abdomen, leg, and foot, in ascending sequence, are represented at its more upper and superior medial aspects.

2. The number of motor neurons devoted to striated muscle is allocated according to the degree to which fine control of voluntary

movement is required, and not according to muscle size. Therefore the relatively small muscles of the face, tongue, jaw, palate, and larynx are allocated a disproportionately large number of primary motor cortex neurons. This distribution reflects the primary function of the direct activation system for speech—the discrete control of precise movements.

3. The motor cortex is organized in columns of neurons extending vertically from the surface to deeper layers of the cortex. These columns seem to represent functional entities that direct groups of muscles that act on a joint. This organization also presumably includes groups of muscles that work together, even if they do not act on joints, such as the face, tongue, lips, and palate. Therefore it seems that movements, rather than muscles, are represented in the cerebral cortex, because "individual muscles are represented repeatedly, in different combinations, among the columns."[25] This conclusion receives some support from the results of cortical stimulation studies in people undergoing neurosurgery for control of seizures. Stimulation of the motor cortex in such patients leads to

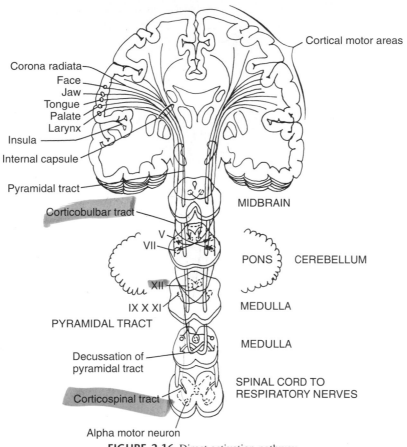

FIGURE 2-16 Direct activation pathway.

movements that include vocalization, tongue protrusion, and palatal elevation, among others.[58] Although not skilled, these behaviors require the activity of groups of muscles, not just single muscles. It is equally important, however, to recognize that stimulation of the motor cortex does not yield words or "meaningful" utterances, suggesting that words or phrases are not stored in discrete areas of the motor cortex (or any other cerebral location, for that matter).

The organization of the *primary sensory cortex* (often called the *sensory strip*), located in the postcentral gyrus, is similar to that of the primary motor cortex. This similarity, particularly the rich allocation of cortical sensory neurons to the relatively small cranial speech muscles, attests to the importance of sensory processes in speech control.

Tracts

Axons of the direct activation pathway for speech travel in the *corticobulbar* and *corticospinal tracts.* Fibers with direct connections to the brainstem nuclei of cranial nerves V, VII, IX, X, XI, and XII travel in the corticobulbar tracts. Fibers with direct connections to the spinal nerves in the anterior horns of the spinal cord that serve respiratory muscles travel in the corticospinal tracts (Figure 2-16).

The corticobulbar and corticospinal tracts in each cerebral hemisphere are arranged in a fanlike mass of fibers that converges from the cortex toward the brainstem. They are collectively known as the *corona radiata.* In the vicinity of the basal ganglia and thalamus, the corona radiata converges into a compact band known as the *internal capsule.* The internal capsule is an important region because it contains all afferent and efferent fibers that project to and from the cortex. Afferent fibers in the internal capsule arise mainly from the thalamus and project as *thalamocortical radiations* to nearly all regions of the cerebral cortex.

A horizontal section of the internal capsule reveals its three major divisions (Figure 2-17). The *anterior limb,* located between the caudate nucleus and putamen, contains anterior thalamic radiations, prefrontal corticopontine fibers, and fibers from the orbital cortex that project to the hypothalamus. The

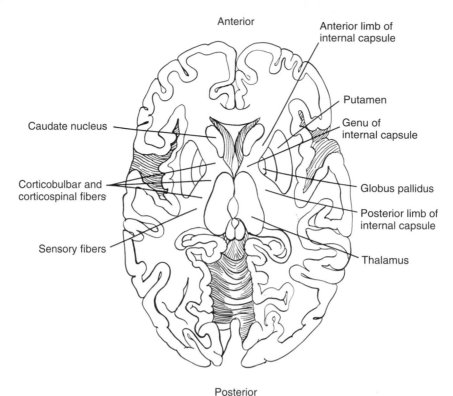

FIGURE 2-17 Internal capsule, thalamus, and basal ganglia *(horizontal section).*

posterior limb, flanked by the thalamus and globus pallidus, contains corticospinal fibers; frontopontine fibers; the superior thalamic radiation (which projects general somatosensory information to the postcentral gyrus); and some corticotectal, corticorubral, and corticoreticular fibers. The *genu,* which lies between the anterior and posterior limbs, contains corticobulbar and corticoreticular fibers. Because thalamocortical, corticobulbar, and corticospinal fibers occupy such a compact area in the internal capsule, *even small capsular lesions can produce widespread motor deficits.* Lesions in the genu and posterior limb produce greater effects on speech than lesions elsewhere in the internal capsule.

Destination

In general, each hemisphere's UMN pathway innervates LMNs predominantly on the opposite side of the body (e.g., the direct activation system originating in the left hemisphere innervates cranial and spinal nerves on the right *[contralateral]* side). However, direct activation pathway innervation of some speech cranial nerves is primarily bilateral, although not necessarily symmetric (Table 2-8). Exceptions include the lower face (cranial nerve VII) and, to a lesser or more variable degree, the

table 2-8	Direct and indirect activation pathway (UMN) innervation of cranial nerves related to speech[57]
Cranial Nerve	**UMN Innervation**
Trigeminal (V)	Bilateral*
Facial (VII)	
Upper face	Bilateral
Lower face	Predominantly contralateral†
Glossopharyngeal (IX)	Bilateral
Vagus (X, all branches)	Bilateral
Accessory (XI)	Bilateral
Hypoglossal (XII)	Contralateral > bilateral‡

UMN, Upper motor neuron.
*Right and left cranial nerves receive input from UMNs coming from both the right and left cerebral hemispheres, although not entirely symmetrically. For example, the excitatory UMN input to the trigeminal nerve is relatively greater from the contralateral hemisphere.[57]
†Right and left cranial nerves receive input mostly from UMN fibers coming from the opposite cerebral hemisphere.
‡UMN supply may be bilateral but with greater input from the contralateral cerebral hemisphere. This may vary among individuals.

tongue (cranial nerve XII),[15] whose innervations are dominated by contralateral corticobulbar fibers.

Corticobulbar pathways to cranial nerve motor nuclei involved in speech do not all project directly from the cortex to motor nuclei of cranial nerves. Many so-called corticobulbar fibers are actually corticoreticular fibers whose influence on cranial nerve nuclei is through synapses in the reticular formation,[14] technically making them part of the indirect rather than the direct activation system. The direct corticobulbar system is a phylogenetically newer system, likely developed for its primary purpose of controlling finely coordinated skilled movements such as speech.

Further increasing the complexity of the direct activation system is the fact that the corticobulbar and corticospinal tracts are not purely motor. They also send fibers to synapse on interneurons that can influence local reflex arcs and nuclei in ascending sensory pathways. In the brainstem, these sensory nuclei include, but are not limited to, the trigeminal sensory nucleus and the nucleus of the tractus solitarius, both of which are relevant to speech and other oromotor activities. These synapses illustrate how descending cortical motor impulses can influence sensory input to the cortex, including that from speech structures.

Function

The direct activation pathway is crucial to voluntary motor activity, especially consciously controlled skilled, discrete-and-often-rapid voluntary movements. Movements generated through the system can be triggered by specific sensory stimuli, but they are not considered reflexes because they are voluntary and not stereotyped. Movements are also generated by cognitive activity that intervenes between sensation and movement and may involve complex planning. Speech clearly falls into the types of movements mediated through the direct activation pathway.

Effects of Damage

Lesions produce a loss or reduction of skilled movements, although weakness is usually not as profound as that associated with LMN lesions. When an UMN lesion is unilateral, weakness is on the opposite side of the body. Because the FCP and peripheral sensation are not part of the direct activation pathways, normal reflexes are preserved.

Because of the predominantly bilateral UMN supply to cranial nerves V, IX, X, and XI, the effects of unilateral UMN lesions on jaw movement and the velopharyngeal, laryngeal, and respiratory functions for speech are usually minor. UMN innervation of the hypoglossal nerve seems to vary in the degree to which it is bilateral, but unilateral UMN lesions will frequently cause some tongue weakness on the side opposite the lesion. Contralateral lower facial weak-ness can be quite prominent after unilateral UMN lesions.

Unilateral UMN lesions can produce a dysarthria that often primarily seems to reflect weakness and loss of skilled movement. It is called *unilateral UMN dysarthria*. Its neuropathologic underpinnings and clinical characteristics are discussed in Chapter 9. Bilateral UMN lesions affecting speech can have mild-to-devastating effects on speech, and they usually reflect the combined effects of direct and indirect activation pathway dysfunction. The resulting speech disorder can reflect bilateral weakness and loss of skilled movement, as well as alterations in muscle tone (spasticity). This dysarthria is known as *spastic dysarthria*. It is discussed in detail in Chapter 5.

The Indirect Activation Pathway and Speech

The indirect activation pathway is complex, and its functions for speech are poorly understood. Its anatomy and activities are difficult to separate completely from those of the basal ganglia and cerebellar control circuits. However, the indirect activation pathway is a source of input to LMNs, whereas the control circuits are not. In addition, separating the control circuits from the indirect activation pathway is clinically valuable, because some dysarthrias are specifically tied to control circuit pathology, whereas others are associated with pathology in portions of the indirect activation pathway that do not include major control circuit structures.

The indirect activation pathway is often referred to as the *extrapyramidal tract* or *indirect motor system*.* The pathway's designation as "indirect" derives from the multiple synapses between its origin in the cerebral cortex and its arrival and activation of the FCP. In a sense, it follows a "local" route, with stops en route to the FCP, in contrast to the "express" or nonstop route followed by the direct activation pathway.

Cortical Components and Tracts

The indirect activation pathway (Figure 2-18) is composed of numerous short pathways and

---

*Benarroche et al.[8] refer to the indirect activation pathways as "brainstem motor pathways," because the regions in which multiple synapses occur before reaching the FCP are located mostly in the brainstem. Because such brainstem motor pathways are influenced by axons projected from the cortex, the indirect activation pathways designation for these pathways will be retained, because it captures their cortical origin and parallel relationship to the direct activation pathways.

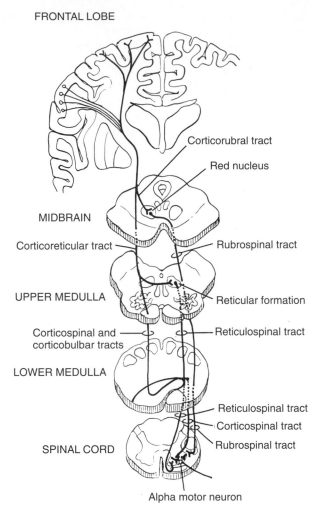

FRONTAL LOBE

Corticorubral tract

Red nucleus

MIDBRAIN

Corticoreticular tract

Rubrospinal tract

UPPER MEDULLA

Reticular formation

Corticospinal and corticobulbar tracts

Reticulospinal tract

LOWER MEDULLA

Reticulospinal tract

Corticospinal tract

Rubrospinal tract

SPINAL CORD

Alpha motor neuron

FIGURE 2-18 Indirect activation pathway. Note that the tracts of this system are intermingled with those of the corticobulbar and corticospinal tracts (the direct activation pathway).

interconnected structures between its origin in the cerebral cortex and its final interaction with cranial nerve nuclei and anterior horn cells of the spinal cord.

Corticoreticular tracts, projecting from the cortex to the reticular formation, arise mostly from the motor, premotor, and sensory cortex. They are intermingled with corticospinal and corticobulbar fibers of the direct activation pathway. They descend to enter the reticular formation in the midbrain, medulla, and pons, where their fibers are distributed bilaterally but with a contralateral predominance. Regions of the reticular formation receiving these fibers have ascending and descending projections, as well as projections to the cerebellum and cranial nerve nuclei. The indirect system also sends fibers from the cortex to the red nucleus through the *corticorubral tracts,* another indirect path from the cortex to the LMNs.

Motor Function Roles of the Reticular Formation and Vestibular and Red Nuclei

The *reticular formation* is a field of scattered cells lying between large nuclei and fiber tracts in the medulla, pons, and midbrain. It is regarded as the neurophysiologic seat of consciousness.[22] It also mediates ascending sensory information, plays an important role in sensorimotor integration, and has complex effects on LMNs. Through its facilitatory and inhibitory influences, it plays a crucial role in the regulation of muscle tone.

Portions of the reticular formation excite extensor motor neurons and inhibit flexor motor neurons, a process that contributes to muscle tone. Fibers in these *reticulospinal tracts* terminate mainly on gamma motor neurons (recall the role of the gamma motor neuron and gamma loop in the stretch reflex and maintenance of normal muscle tone). Other portions of the reticular formation inhibit extensor motor neurons and excite flexors. To exert their influence, these inhibitory reticular fibers must be excited by supratentorial motor pathways. The fibers of these pathways terminate in the spinal cord in the same general areas where corticospinal tracts (direct activation pathway) terminate. The specific influence of the reticular formation on cranial nerve motor function is not well understood. However, collateral fibers from the reticular formation do project to the cranial nerve nuclei, and the lateral zone of the medullary reticular formation is associated with coordinating complex reflexes among multiple cranial nerves involved in swallowing and vomiting.[8,14]

Responses of the reticular formation to stimulation help identify the influence it may have on motor activities that are relevant to speech. Stimulation can facilitate and inhibit reflex activity and cortically induced voluntary movement, influence muscle tone, affect phasic respiratory activities, and facilitate and inhibit ascending sensory information.[14]

The *vestibular nuclei,* located on the floor of the fourth ventricle in the pons and medulla, receive sensory input from the vestibular apparatus of the ear and from the cerebellum. They project to the brainstem, cerebellum, and spinal cord. Ascending and descending brainstem projections of the vestibular nuclei run in the *medial longitudinal fasciculus.* They modulate the activities of the eye and neck muscles.

Vestibular and certain cerebellar influences upon the spinal cord are mediated through the *vestibulospinal tract,* which terminates on both alpha and gamma motor neurons. This tract is thought to facilitate reflex activities and spinal mechanisms that control muscle tone. Although the vestibular system projects to cranial nerve motor nuclei, its specific role in speech is uncertain.

The *red nucleus* is an oval mass of cells in the midbrain. It receives cortical projections through the *corticorubral tracts.* It also serves as a relay station between a pathway from the cerebellum to the ventrolateral nucleus of the thalamus and, ultimately, the cortex. Input from the cerebellum and the basal ganglia can also modify descending activity in the red nucleus. The *rubrospinal tract* assists flexor motor neurons and inhibits extensor alpha and gamma motor neurons, but its major influence is on flexor muscle groups in the limbs. Its specific influence on cranial motor nerves involved in speech is unclear, but a role can be assumed because it is implicated in certain disorders affecting movements of speech structures (e.g., palatopharyngolaryngeal myoclonus).

Destination

The indirect activation pathway influences the activities of both gamma and alpha motor neurons of the FCP. Gamma motor neurons have a lower response threshold than alpha motor neurons, however, so they are more sensitive—respond more readily—to indirect motor system input.

Function

The indirect activation pathway helps regulate reflexes and maintain posture, tone, and associated activities that provide a framework on which the direct activation pathway can accomplish skilled, discrete actions. Its activities are subconscious and typically require the integration of activities of many supporting muscles. It ensures that specific speech movements occur without constant or variable interference with their speed, range, and direction.

Effects of Damage

Diseases affecting the indirect activation pathway are manifest in various ways. In general, lesions affect muscle tone and reflexes and are primarily manifest as spasticity and hyperreflexia, respectively.

The effects of indirect activation pathway lesions are different for flexor and extensor muscles. Lesions damaging corticoreticular fibers above the midbrain and red nucleus produce increased extensor tone in the legs and increased flexor tone in the arms (i.e., the legs tend to be extended and resist bending; the arms tend to flex and resist extension). This occurs because all descending pathways are uninhibited; such a state is known as *decorticate posturing.* Lesions at the level of the midbrain below the red nucleus remove arm flexor excitation and result in excitation of all extensor muscles and a generalized increase in extensor tone; this state is known as *decerebrate posturing.* Lesions below the medulla result in a loss of all descending input and produce generalized flaccidity in muscles supplied by spinal nerves.

Lesions of the brainstem that damage the reticular formation often lead to death. Damage to the indirect activation pathway above that level, however, will produce certain predictable deficits, including decorticate posturing. When cortical controls become nonfunctional, the unchecked reticular system makes extensor muscles hyperexcitable, a condition manifest clinically as increased muscle tone or *spasticity.* The specific muscles that become spastic depend on the level of the lesion, but the effects are usually particularly strong in axial and proximal muscles (toward the center of the body).

Lesions of motor pathways from the cerebral hemispheres are common and are usually referred to as *UMN lesions.* They tend to affect both direct and indirect pathways. Consequently, the clinical picture may include spasticity and increased muscle stretch reflexes as a result of indirect pathway involvement, as well as loss of skilled movements resulting from direct pathway involvement. Weakness can result from damage to direct or indirect pathways. The effects of indirect versus direct activation pathway lesions are summarized in Table 2-7.

Clinical findings in UMN lesions may change over time. When descending CNS pathways to alpha and gamma motor neurons are destroyed, motor activity is initially greatly diminished, as are muscle tone and reflexes. However, because alpha and gamma motor neurons may still be influenced by other input (e.g., peripheral sensory input), they may eventually recover their excitability and even become hyperexcitable. Therefore even though voluntary activity may be absent or diminished, reflexes may become hyperactive, because inhibitory influences from central pathways are lost.

The effects of spasticity on speech, in general, are to slow movement and cause hyperadduction of the vocal folds during phonation. These effects tend to be minimal when UMN lesions are unilateral, but they can range from mild to severe when lesions are bilateral. Bilateral UMN lesions that include the indirect activation pathway are often accompanied by hyperactive reflexes, pathologic reflexes, dysphagia, and disinhibition of the physical expression of emotion.

The dysarthrias resulting from indirect activation pathway involvement are usually encountered in combination with direct pathway involvement. They include *spastic dysarthria* when lesions are bilateral and *unilateral UMN dysarthria* when lesions are unilateral. They are discussed in Chapters 5 and 9, respectively.

Control Circuits

Control circuits are so called because they integrate or help control the diverse activities of the many structures and pathways involved in motor performance. From this standpoint, they can also be considered important contributors to the programming of movements (discussed in more detail later in this chapter). Unlike the direct and indirect activation pathways, the *control circuits do not have direct contact with LMNs.*

Considering the different roles played by the direct and indirect activation pathways in movement, it makes sense that there are mechanisms within the CNS that coordinate or integrate their activities. For example, skilled movements activated through the direct activation pathway need to be planned and controlled with knowledge about the posture, orientation in space, tone, and physical environment in which the movements will occur (aspects of movement mediated through the indirect activation pathway). At the same time, the creation of appropriate posture and tone must be done with some information about the goals to be achieved by voluntary movements that are mediated through the direct activation pathway. This integration and control are accomplished through the activities of the *basal ganglia control circuit* and the *cerebellar control circuit.* These circuits influence movement through their input to the cerebral cortex and, from there, via the direct and indirect activation pathways.

The Basal Ganglia Control Circuit and Speech

Location and Course

The basal ganglia include the caudate nucleus, putamen, and globus pallidus (see Figures 2-17 and 2-19). The term *striatum* refers to the caudate nucleus and putamen, which act together as a functional unit. The putamen and globus pallidus are known collectively as the *lentiform nucleus.* The *substantia nigra* and the *subthalamic nucleus* are anatomically and functionally closely related to the basal ganglia, and, in fact, many clinical neurologists consider them to be part of the basal ganglia.[4] The basal ganglia have important reciprocal connections with diverse areas of the cerebral cortex and strong functional ties to the extrapyramidal pathway or indirect motor system. Because they do not directly influence the FCP, they are more appropriately thought of as a control circuit rather than a major descending pathway for motor activity.

The striatum is the receptive portion of the basal ganglia. It receives major projections from the frontal cortex, as well as input from certain thalamic nuclei and the substantia nigra. The cortical-putamen pathway may be especially important to motor control, because its fibers originate in the premotor cortex; the caudate nucleus receives fibers from the more anterior portions of the frontal lobe.[46] The striatum sends efferent fibers to the substantia nigra and is the major source of input to the globus pallidus.

The major efferent pathways of the basal ganglia originate in the globus pallidus. Most of these efferent fibers go to the ventrolateral nucleus of the thalamus for relay back to the cortex. They also go to the subthalamic nucleus, the nearby red nucleus, and the reticular formation in the brainstem. Basal ganglia pathways are thus made up of several loops: striatum to globus pallidus to thalamus to cortex to

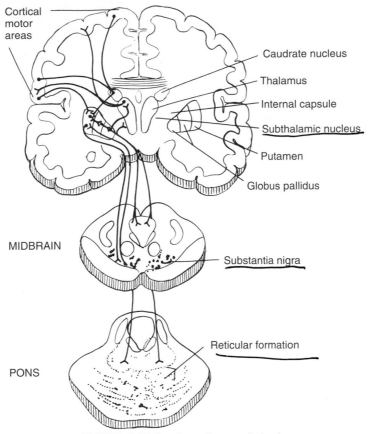

Cortical motor areas

Caudrate nucleus

Thalamus

Internal capsule

Subthalamic nucleus

Putamen

Globus pallidus

MIDBRAIN

Substantia nigra

Reticular formation

PONS

FIGURE 2-19 Basal ganglia control circuit.

striatum, striatum to substantia nigra to striatum, and globus pallidus to subthalamus to globus pallidus.

Basal ganglia functions for motor activity depend on an appropriate balance among several neurotransmitters, the most important of which are *acetylcholine (ACh), dopamine,* and *gamma-aminobutyric acid (GABA).* ACh is the synaptic transmitter for most of the neurons with axonal terminations within the striatum. Dopamine is manufactured in the substantia nigra and transmitted by way of *nigrostriatal tracts* to the striatum, where it also acts as a neurotransmitter; when neurons in the substantia nigra are destroyed, the dopamine content in the striatum is lowered. Finally, most efferent fibers from the striatum to the globus pallidus and from the globus pallidus to the substantia nigra release GABA. The balance among these neurotransmitters is important to motor control, and imbalance among them is implicated in movement disorders associated with several basal ganglia diseases.

Function

The functions of the individual components of the basal ganglia for movement control are not well understood. As a group, however, they seem important for regulating muscle tone and maintaining normal posture and static muscle contraction upon which voluntary, skilled movements are superimposed. They seem important to regulating the amplitude, velocity, and, possibly, the initiation of movement.[3] Recent studies suggest that they play a role in movement selection[32] and motor learning.* It has been suggested that, under conditions of practice, the striatum helps build a repertoire of movements that can be triggered in response to appropriate stimuli.[41]

The basal ganglia control circuit is probably important to generating components of motor programs for speech, particularly those that help maintain a stable musculoskeletal environment in which discrete speech movements can occur. In general, its activities seem to have a damping effect on cortical

---

*For obvious reasons, the emphasis here is on the motor functions of the basal ganglia, but it is noteworthy that the basal ganglia have both motor and cognitive relationships with the cerebral cortex. Activity in basal ganglia–motor cortex circuitry correlates with parameters of movement, whereas activity in basal ganglia–prefrontal cortex circuitry correlates with certain aspects of cognitive function.[51]

discharges. That is, it appears that the cortex initiates impulses for movement that are in excess of those required to accomplish movement goals, and that one role of the basal ganglia is to damp (through inhibition) or modulate (through disinhibition) those impulses to an appropriate degree. The contribution of the basal ganglia to movement may depend on processing of sensory information and perhaps the ability to develop sensory templates that help specify and guide individual movements.[38]

To summarize, the basal ganglia control circuit seems to be an important participant in regulating muscle tone, movements associated with goal-directed activities such as the arm swing during walking, automatic activities such as chewing and walking, postural adjustments during skilled movements such as stabilizing the shoulders and arms during typing, the relationship of movements to the environment such as speaking with restricted jaw movement, and the learning of new movements.[13]

Effects of Damage

The effect of basal ganglia control circuit lesions on movement can be manifest in one of two ways: reduced mobility, or *hypokinesia;* or involuntary movements, or *hyperkinesia.*

Hypokinesia is often associated with disease of the substantia nigra, which results in a deficiency of dopamine supply to the basal ganglia. The effect is an increase in muscle tone, with subsequent increased resistance to passive movements, a condition known as *rigidity.* In rigidity, movements are slow and stiff and may be initiated or stopped with difficulty. This excessive restriction of movement is reflected in the reduced range of movement underlying many of the deviant speech characteristics of *hypokinetic dysarthria.*

It is relevant to note that there seems to be a speech counterpart to the basal ganglia's contribution to some of the automatic aspects of limb movement. For example, in certain basal ganglia diseases (most notably, Parkinson's disease), the face becomes "masked" or expressionless. The hypokinetic dysarthria of such patients can be affectively expressionless as well, even when linguistic content may convey emotionally laden thoughts. These abnormalities highlight the important role of the basal ganglia control circuit in the physical expression of affect. Similarly, its speech pathology demonstrates that dysarthria affects the character of much more than the segmental-phonemic-linguistic messages conveyed in speech; it also affects the suprasegmental-prosodic-emotional components of messages.

Hyperkinesia can result from excessive activity in dopaminergic nerve fibers, thereby reducing the circuit's damping effect on cortical discharges. This results in involuntary movements that can vary considerably in their locus, speed, regularity, and predictability, as well as the conditions that promote or inhibit their occurrence. These excessive and often unpredictable variations in muscle tone and movement underlie many deviant speech characteristics associated with the *hyperkinetic dysarthrias.*

Lesions of the basal ganglia control circuit that involve its subcortical components (i.e., the basal ganglia and their related subcortical nuclei) generally produce more profound speech disturbances than do lesions to its cortical components. This is usually the case for all of the dysarthrias, a fact that underscores the importance of attending to more than the cortical contributions to movement when studying MSDs.

The various movement disorders that may be encountered in disease of the basal ganglia are discussed in Chapters 7 and 8, which deal with hypokinetic dysarthria and hyperkinetic dysarthria, respectively.

The Cerebellar Control Circuit and Speech

Location and Course

The cerebellum and its connections constitute the cerebellar control circuit. The cerebellum can be divided into anterior, posterior, and flocculonodular lobes. From side to side, the midportion of the cerebellum is the *vermis,* which forms the midline of the anterior and posterior lobes. The right and left cerebellar hemispheres are to the side of the vermis (Figure 2-20). Each cerebellar hemisphere is connected to the contralateral thalamus and cerebral hemisphere, and each controls movements on the ipsilateral side of the body.

The *flocculonodular lobe* has primary connections to the vestibular mechanism for modulating equilibrium and the orientation of the head and eyes. The *anterior lobe* is a projection area for spinocerebellar proprioceptive information. It is important for regulating posture, gait, and truncal tone.

The *posterior lobe (neocerebellum)* is a more recent phylogenetic development. Its lateral cerebellar hemispheres are particularly important as a servomechanism for coordinating skilled, sequential voluntary muscle activity. At least for limb movements, for example, there is evidence that these lateral portions of the cerebellum "may compute the muscle activity needed for the braking function of the antagonist muscle, including the onset time and the amplitude, based on the initial position of the limb, the position of the target, and the inertia to be overcome."[23]

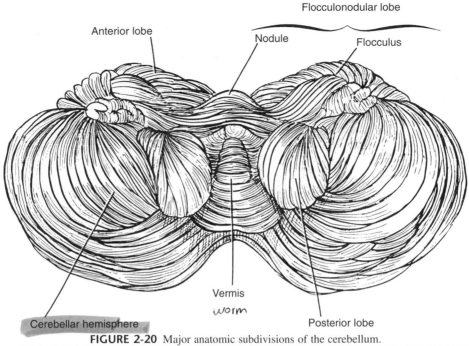

FIGURE 2-20 Major anatomic subdivisions of the cerebellum.

Fiber tracts enter or leave the cerebellum through three structures on each side: the inferior, middle, and superior cerebellar peduncles. The *inferior cerebellar peduncle* contains mostly afferent fibers from the spinal cord and brainstem but also has efferent flow to vestibular mechanisms and to the reticular formation. The *middle cerebellar peduncle* is an afferent pathway from pontine nuclei of the contralateral side. The *superior cerebellar peduncle* contains the major efferent cerebellar pathways. The ratio of afferent to efferent fibers in tracts to and from the cerebellum is about 40:1,[11] testimony to the importance of sensory information in motor control and specifically to the importance of sensation to cerebellar coordination of movement.

The sole output neurons of the cerebellar cortex are *Purkinje cells,* which comprise the middle layer of cells in the cerebellar cortex. The axons of Purkinje cells synapse in the deep cerebellar nuclei, structures from which cerebellar output departs through the superior or inferior cerebellar peduncles. These nuclei include the *dentate, globose, emboliform,* and *fastigial nuclei* (Figure 2-21). The dentate nucleus may be particularly important for speech control, because it seems to be active in initiating movement, executing preplanned motor tasks, and regulating posture.[24]

The areas of the cerebellum that appear most involved in speech control are the vermis and the cerebellar hemispheres. This conclusion is based on the sites of cerebellar damage most frequently encountered in dysarthria resulting from cerebellar lesions. The importance of the cerebellar hemispheres for speech control can also be inferred from their known importance for coordinating skilled, voluntary muscle activity.

The primary and necessary cerebellar pathways for speech production probably include reciprocal connections with the cerebral cortex; auditory feedback and proprioceptive input from speech muscles, tendons, and joints; reciprocal connections with brainstem components of the indirect activation pathway; and cooperative activity with the basal ganglia control circuit through interactions in the thalamus, cortex, and various components of the indirect motor system.

Two cortical-cerebellar pathways appear important for speech control. One is from the primary motor and premotor regions of the cortex to the lateral cerebellar hemispheres via pontine nuclei, with a return pathway to the same cortical areas through deep cerebellar nuclei and ventral thalamic nuclei. This loop seems important to planning and programming learned movements. The second pathway is from descending corticospinal and corticobulbar fibers to the intermediate aspects of the cerebellar hemispheres, with a return pathway to the primary motor cortex through deep cerebellar nuclei and ventral thalamic nuclei. This loop provides the cerebellum with immediate (relatively direct)

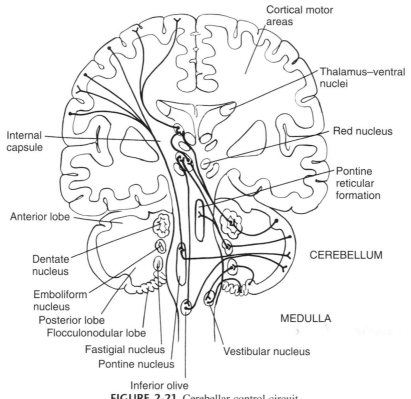

Internal capsule

Anterior lobe

Dentate nucleus

Emboliform nucleus

Posterior lobe

Flocculonodular lobe

Fastigial nucleus

Pontine nucleus

Inferior olive

Cortical motor areas

Thalamus–ventral nuclei

Red nucleus

Pontine reticular formation

CEREBELLUM

MEDULLA

Vestibular nucleus

FIGURE 2-21 Cerebellar control circuit.

information about cortical output,[46] presumably about cortical intentions for skilled movement. The intermediate portions of the cerebellar hemispheres also project to brainstem and spinal motor centers via the red nucleus. The existence of these pathways suggests that the intermediate cerebellum uses sensory input to influence cortical motor output during movement, including speech.

Function

The specific role of the cerebellum in movement control remains a matter of some uncertainty and debate.[23] Nonetheless, the cerebellar control circuit probably influences speech in ways similar to how it is believed to influence movement in general. For example, a basic hypothesis about the cerebellum is that it "helps coordinate the timing between the single components of a movement, scales the size of muscular action, and coordinates the sequence of agonists and antagonists"[17]; it is likely that these timing,* scaling, and coordination roles apply to speech. The apparent role of the cerebellum in maintaining less-than-maximum but constant force

(steadiness) during movement, and the role of the cortico-ponto-neocerebellar component of the circuit in the initiation of fast limb movements,[17] could certainly be adapted for steady-state and phasic aspects of speech. And, in the more general sense, the circuit's participation in motor learning, motor memory, and movement execution by combining movements for skilled motor behavior without conscious awareness[11,41] seems compatible with the needs of motor speech control. Regardless of its specific contributions, however, its involvement in speech motor control is known, because distinctive speech disturbances result from damage to it.*

The cerebellum's role in speech can be conceptualized in the following way[†]:

1. Preliminary information from the cortex about intended speech goals activates the

---

*It also appears that the cerebellum participates in the perceptual processing of durational parameters of speech stimuli.[2]

*It has become apparent in recent years, on the basis of clinical observations and functional neuroimaging studies, that the cerebellum probably makes subtle contributions to a number of cognitive functions, including planning and reasoning, temporal sequencing and timing, attention, visual-spatial processing, learning, memory, and language processing. Its contributions to these functions appears to be independent of motor activity.[46,51]

[†]Relying heavily on discussions by Eccles[20]; Gilman[23]; Kent and Netsell[36]; Kent, Netsell, and Abbs[37]; and Netsell and Kent.[55]

cerebellum's role in long-range movement planning. This role is mostly anticipatory in character and is based on learning, experience, and preliminary sensory information. Input from the cortex also prepares the cerebellum to check the adequacy of speech output as feedback from muscles, tendons, and joints arrives from the periphery.

2. Initial cortical motor speech commands are probably provisional, imprecise, and in excess of those necessary to accomplish movement goals. The exclusive inhibitory output of the cerebellum's Purkinje cells subsequently results in smooth, coordinated, and appropriately timed speech movements, perhaps in a manner analogous to chiseling away from a block of stone to achieve form in a sculpture.[20]

3. The cerebellum can bias or tune muscle spindles to optimize sensory feedback about the state of speech muscles. It interprets this sensory information and integrates it with ongoing input from the cortex about upcoming movement goals. This updating function can influence subsequent cortical motor output and ultimately smooth and time the actions of agonist and antagonist muscles within and among different speech subsystems (phonation, articulation, and so on).

To summarize, the cerebellum receives advance notice about intended speech from the cortex so that it will be prepared to check the adequacy of the outcome when feedback from speech muscles, tendons, and joints arrives from the periphery. With its input to the cortex it can influence subsequent cortical motor speech output based on feedback it has received and ongoing information from the cortex about upcoming speech goals. These corrective modifications help to smooth the coordination of contracting muscles and the opposing activity of antagonistic muscles, resulting in smoothly flowing, well-timed, coordinated speech.

Effects of Damage

Damage to cerebellar control mechanisms produces signs that can be associated with the functions of its lobes. Its effects can be summarized as follows:

- Flocculonodular lesions are associated with *truncal ataxia* (inability to stand or sit without swaying or falling), disturbances in gait, and *nystagmus* (abnormal eye movements).
- Anterior lobe lesions are associated with gait ataxia.
- Posterior lobe lesions, especially in the cerebellar hemispheres, are associated with *limb ataxia* and *hypotonia, intention tremor,* and

incoordination ipsilateral to the side of the lesion. Such lesions can lead to dysarthria.

The effects on speech of cerebellar or cerebellar pathway lesions generally can be attributed to incoordination and possibly hypotonia. They are classified as *ataxic dysarthria.* Damage to the vermis or the cerebellar hemispheres bilaterally generally has more serious consequences for speech than damage to portions of the circuit that lie outside the cerebellum. Ataxic dysarthria is discussed in Chapter 6.

◼ THE CONCEPTUAL-PROGRAMMING LEVEL AND SPEECH

How and where in the nervous system are ideas and the content of speech formulated? How and where is this content transformed into neural impulses that generate muscle contractions and movements that result in meaningful, intelligible speech? What specifies the goals and the sequence of skilled movements for speech that are transmitted through the direct activation pathway? How is the indirect activation pathway informed about motor goals? What is it that the control circuits control? What is the role of sensation in speech production? How can normal speech be produced so quickly? What are the criteria by which the motor system determines that goals have been achieved?

These are only some of many questions relevant to understanding *speech motor control,* or "the systems and strategies that control the production of speech."[34] The answers are, at best, incomplete. Some are to be found within the activities of the direct and indirect activation pathways and the control circuits, but some probably lie within a level of function that Darley, Aronson, and Brown (DAB)[16] called the *conceptual-programming level.* Although the detail they specified for activities that go on at this level was simple and incomplete in comparison to current models of speech control,* the broad stages outlined by them are a useful vehicle for outlining the general processes that precede, include, and follow the planning and programming of speech.

The key components of the conceptual-programming stage represent the highest level of motor organization. The designation "highest" is conferred because neural activity within its key components establishes the meaning or goals of the speech act and the essentials of the plans and programs for achieving them. The designation does not necessarily

---

*Several models of speech formulation and production, as well as their relationship to various motor speech disorders, are discussed or summarized by Kent[34,35]; McNeil, Doyle, and Wambaugh[47]; and Van Der Merwe.[67]

mean that the most severe MSDs always occur with lesions at this level.

The conceptual-programming stage spans the neural and cognitive territory among internal, non-motor, cognitive-linguistic processes that establish an idea or plan that might be expressed and the sensorimotor programming that specifies and controls the movements that result in the plan's realization as speech. It is roughly synonymous with what Van Der Merwe[67] has called "phases in the transformation of the speech code." Where these phases take place is incompletely understood. How they take place is far less certain.

DAB[16] discussed five stages that characterize activities at the conceptual-programming level (summarized in Table 2-9). Taken together, the five stages actually capture what goes on at all levels of the speech sensorimotor system. They include, although with some modifications of the terminology used by DAB, the following:

1. Conceptualization
2. Linguistic planning
3. Motor planning and programming
4. Performance
5. Feedback

The first three stages represent the key, unique components of the conceptual-programming level and are most relevant to this discussion. The performance and feedback stages have already been addressed during discussion of other components of the speech motor system (i.e., the direct and indirect activation pathways, control circuits, and the FCPs).

Conceptualization

This stage includes *an intention or desire to do something and the development of a purpose for action.* These nonlinguistic thoughts, ideas, and feelings, and the desire to act on them, fall into the "sphere of conscious awareness and intentional action."[35] They are cognitive and affective in nature. They precede the specification of the words that could be uttered and the initiation of movement; in fact, conceptualization may remain internal and never emerge as speech.

table 2-9   The conceptual-programming level of speech production

Process	Components	Neural Substrate	Disorders Affecting Speech
Conceptualization	Cognitively and affectively generated thoughts, feelings, and emotions, plus a desire to express them to achieve a goal	Widespread	General cognitive impairment (e.g., dementia) Psychosis Confusion
Linguistic Planning	Highly interactive semantic & syntactic processing, ultimately taking a phonologic form	Left hemisphere perisylvian cortex, with less specific contributions from subcortical structures (thalamus & basal ganglia)	Aphasia
Motor Planning or Programming	Formulation and retrieval of motor commands for production of phonetic segments and syllables at particular rates and with particular patterns of stress and prosody, based on acoustic (and other modality) goals and feedback	1. Dominant hemisphere → somatosensory cortex, premotor cortex (Broca's area), supplementary motor cortex, motor cortex, insula) 2. Control circuits → 3. Limbic system → 4. Right hemisphere → 5. Thalamus and reticular formation →	Apraxia of speech Dysarthrias (? apraxia of speech) Altered affect or prosody ?Aprosodia Dysarthrias
Performance	Motor execution	LMNs (as controlled by direct & indirect activation pathways, control circuits, & feedback)	Dysarthrias
Feedback	Multimodality feedback to the above components	Peripheral & central sensory pathways	Dysarthrias & peripheral sensory-based speech disturbances

LMNs, Lower motor neurons.

Although it can be assumed that conceptualization typically precedes speech, it would be incorrect to assume that any of the conceptual-programming stages operate in a fixed, repetitive sequence during natural speech. *The relationships among the stages reflect parallel and temporally overlapping and interacting phases rather than sequential activities.*

Localization

The neural bases for conceptualization cannot be localized narrowly. Cortical activity is crucial, but it is probably bilateral and widespread. In fact, it is best viewed as a whole brain activity, because alertness, affect, attention, and the sensory and motor processes that frequently acquire the "data" that drive or motivate thought and action are ". . . supported, empowered, and even urged by subcortical systems, including the ascending activating system of the brainstem, the hypothalamus, the limbic system, and various thalamic nuclei."[16]

Effects of Damage

Deficits in conceptualization often reflect anatomically diffuse impairment of cognitive or affective functions. They are commonly associated with dementia or other disturbances of affect, memory, or thought. They are reflected in message content, organization, or affective tone but not in motor planning or execution. Speech associated with such impairments can be motorically normal. Thus, although the conceptual stage is essential to normal, appropriate, and meaningful communication, it is not essential to normal motor speech production.

Linguistic Planning

To accomplish a motor act it is necessary to know the body parts to be used, the space in which the action will take place, and the temporal sequence of its various components. In other words, a plan must be formulated. DAB called this process "spatial-temporal planning,"[16] but, for two reasons, the designation *linguistic planning* will be used instead. First, for speech, *linguistic units* form the content of the plan. Second, the label "spatial-temporal planning" has motor connotations, and it is useful—for both theoretical and clinical reasons—to clearly distinguish language formulation (linguistic planning, including phonologic planning) from the sensorimotor processes necessary for language to be expressed as speech. Like conceptualization, *the linguistic planning phase is nonmotor in nature.*

Once an idea and the intention to express it develop (perhaps even before that), the language system must be activated to formulate the verbal message. Linguistic planning involves cognitive operations on abstract rules. Once semantic and syntactic interactions begin to yield the lexical units and the syntactic and morphologic makeup of an expression, the utterance takes phonologic shape (abstract phonemes are identified and ordered). Linguistic planning requires attention, retrieval, and working memory processes, plus the ability to discard from active processing utterances that have already been formulated and executed.

Localization

Linguistic planning engages the *dominant hemisphere perisylvian cortex,* most importantly the temporoparietal and posterior frontal cortex. In less definitive ways, the dominant hemisphere's thalamus and basal ganglia, and perhaps even the cerebellum, may also be involved. Other cortical areas may be recruited as well, depending on the source of the stimulus to speak (e.g., the occipital lobes when reading). The *left hemisphere* is the dominant hemisphere for linguistic planning (and motor speech planning and programming) in most individuals.

Effects of Damage

Impairment of linguistic planning reflects dominant hemisphere pathology and is called *aphasia* or *dysphasia.* Signs of aphasia include delays and errors in word retrieval, reduced auditory retention span, and other errors and inefficiencies associated with the semantic, syntactic, morphologic, and phonologic aspects of language. These impairments are usually observable in all modalities through which symbols can be conveyed (e.g., speech, verbal comprehension, reading, writing, pantomime, sign language), because the damaged processes are central to, or shared by, all input and output modalities. These problems—particularly phonologic ones—are discussed further in Chapter 15, which focuses on differential diagnosis.

Motor Planning and Programming

Once the phonologic representation of a verbal message is developed, a plan to guide movements for speech must be organized and activated. Although phoneme selection and ordering during linguistic planning are closely related to and difficult to separate from the neural activities required for the emergence of speech, "motor planning of speech is a discernible process aimed at defining motor goals."[67] It is at the heart of the conceptual-programming level for the motor organization of speech. The separation of phonologic processes from motor planning and programming has considerable theoretical, anatomic, and clinical support. This is addressed further in Chapters 11 and 15.

It is appropriate to discuss briefly *motor planning* and *motor programming* (relying heavily on discussions by Brooks[12]; McNeil, Doyle, and Wambaugh[47]; and Van Der Merwe).[67] Planning and programming are intertwined but not synonymous; several features distinguish them neurocognitively and neuroanatomically.

The following points are relevant to notions of motor planning:

1. Motor planning represents the highest level of the motor system and "entails formulating the strategy of action by specifying motor goals."[67] Thus *plans are goal oriented* and reflect general strategies about *what* to do.[12] In a sense, they identify destinations and the steps necessary to reach them but not the details of the specific journey. Plans, as described here, are roughly equivalent to what some have called *preprogramming, central programs,* and *generalized motor programs.*

2. Plans are not formulated anew each time speech takes place. As speech is learned, proprioceptive, tactile, and auditory feedback permit increasingly efficient motor plans to be stored in sensorimotor memory as *engrams*. The stored plans are then accessed and sequenced during subsequent planning in mature speakers.

3. Anatomically, cortical activity is crucial for planning, but planning may also involve other structures (localization is discussed in subsequent sections).

The following points are relevant to notions of motor programming:

1. Programming is at a "lower level" of the motor system hierarchy than planning, because it depends on a plan to guide its substance. Programs are *procedure oriented* and convert strategy into tactics about *how* to accomplish plans.[12] With the destination established by a plan, programs determine and control the specific spatial and temporal details of the journey. In this sense, "motor plans are made up of several programs that, in turn, consist of coordinated, smaller learned subroutines called subprograms."[12]

2. Motor programs for speech probably specify commands for movement that may be modified online as a function of sensory feedback. They "supply specific movement parameterization to specific muscles or muscle groups,"[47] such as details regarding muscle tone, direction, force, range, and rate "according to the requirements of the planned movement as it changes over time."[67]

3. The neural areas that may be crucially involved in motor programming (according to Van Der Merwe[67]) include the basal ganglia, cerebellum, supplementary motor area, motor cortex, and the frontolimbic system (localization is discussed in subsequent sections).

Requirements and Goals

Speech planning and programming involve translation of the abstract, internal linguistic-phonologic representation into a code that can be used by the motor system to generate movements resulting in speech. This is an enormously complex process, one involving more motor fibers than any other human motor activity and capable of speeds that surpass those of any discrete human motor performance. DAB[16] pointed out that about 100 different muscles, each containing about 100 motor units, are involved in speaking. At an average speaking rate of 14 phonemes per second, this translates to about 140,000 neuromuscular events per second. It would be impossible consciously to plan each of these neuromuscular events in such a time frame. Normal adults have little awareness of specific movements during speech unless they are learning how to pronounce a difficult novel word or sequence of words, are trying to correct an inadvertent error of articulation, or are consciously attempting to alter their natural manner of speaking. Most of the time a decision is made about what to say and the process is simply set in motion. It is assumed, therefore, that once speech has been learned, planning and programming usually involve the selection, sequencing, activation, and fine-tuning of *preprogrammed movement sequences* that are considerably more comprehensive than those represented by the contractions of individual muscle fibers, muscles, or even groups of muscles.

What must the motor speech planner and programmer accomplish? Ultimately, and that is what counts, spoken language must meet a condition of perceptual or motor equivalence rather than acoustic or motor invariance, in which *motor equivalence is the capacity to achieve a movement goal in various ways.*[44] In other words, specific linguistic messages can be produced in neuromuscularly variable ways as long as the acoustic result generates an accurate perception in a listener. This flexibility reduces demands on the motor system for perfection, promotes efficiency and speed, and is analogous to what apparently happens during many nonspeech skilled movements. For example, throwing a ball to a target is rarely accomplished in an unvarying way; distance, posture, and requirements for speed vary in nearly infinite ways, and the neural program to accomplish the goal must be modified accordingly.

This goal-oriented or listener-oriented organization of speech highlights a fundamental difference between linguistic and motor mechanisms. An unspoken sentence (language) can be viewed as discrete and context free, separable sequentially into phonemes, morphemes, words, and phrases. In contrast, speech is a continuous and context-dependent activity in which articulators reach targets reliably despite variability in their starting positions. In addition, the acoustic correlates of sequences of abstract phonemes do not reflect a sequence of discrete events. This is because of *coarticulation,* the temporal-spatial overlap of movements associated with the production of more than one sound occurring at a single point in time. In a sense, the speech signal is a partial temporal hologram, in which multiple pieces of information—that is, information about more than one sound—can be found at single points in time. This redundancy greatly increases the speed at which speech can be produced and still be understood. These characteristics suggest that motor commands for successive phonemes are processed simultaneously or that plans for moving the articulators from one position to the next are established in advance. The neural apparatus is apparently organized so that distinctions that can be heard are linked closely to distinctions that can be produced.[59]

Localization of Cortical Components
(See Figure 2-15)

Motor speech planning is, in part, an important function of the *premotor* and *supplementary motor areas* of the dominant hemisphere's frontal lobe. The premotor area (or premotor cortex) receives input from multiple sensory modalities, is linked to the basal ganglia and cerebellum, and has reciprocal connections with the primary motor cortex. It contributes fibers to the corticospinal and corticobulbar pathways, although fewer than does the primary motor cortex. Its influence on the primary motor cortex may be mostly indirect, involving a route through the basal ganglia and their related structures, as well as the thalamus.[3]

The premotor area seems to play a role in motor planning at a relatively abstract point "when choices among competing alternatives need to be made."[49] Its multiple connections with sensory and motor structures suggest that it uses sensory information to organize and guide motor behavior. It also seems to contribute to the planning, initiation, maintenance, inhibition, and perhaps learning of complex move-

ments.[49] Lesions of the premotor cortex are associated with incoordination of lip, tongue, and jaw movements for chewing and swallowing in primates.[66]

Broca's area, a part of the left premotor cortex, appears intimately tied to speech planning and programming. Its role is supported by its connections to portions of the temporal and parietal lobes that are involved in language processes, as well as its proximity to the primary motor cortex. It is located at the foot of the third frontal convolution in the dominant hemisphere, just anterior to the portion of the primary motor area in which the orofacial and neck muscles are richly represented.

It is often assumed that Broca's area is *the* location of the motor speech programmer. This is probably incorrect. On clinical grounds alone, it is clear that damage to other areas of the dominant hemisphere can result in deficits that appear to reflect a disturbance of speech planning or programming. It is noteworthy, however, that these other areas represent loci of interface between Broca's area and language formulation areas, or between Broca's area and other portions of the motor system.

The *supplementary motor area (SMA)* is also associated with planning or programming. Located on the mesial surface of the hemispheres, it receives projections from the primary motor and premotor cortex and from the basal ganglia by way of the thalamus. It projects fibers to the primary motor, premotor, cingulate, and parietal cortex. Its strong connections to the limbic system implicate it in mechanisms that drive or motivate action. It has been shown to be involved in the preparation and execution of sequential and internally driven (as opposed to sensory-guided) movements,[21,40] and it may help to trigger motor activity by releasing inhibition of the primary motor area.[6] It is thought to play a role in the initiation of propositional speech and the control of rhythm, phonation, and articulation.[31] High-frequency repetitive transcranial magnetic stimulation over the SMA interferes with the organization of complex sequences of finger movements.[21] Direct stimulation of the SMA can evoke or arrest vocalization and slow speech or induce dysfluencies and distortions.[58] Surgical lesions in the left SMA can result in mutism or reduced spontaneous speech.[40]

The dominant hemisphere's parietal lobe *somatosensory cortex* and the *supramarginal gyrus* also appear to play a role in speech, especially in the integration of sensory information in preparation for motor activity. Finally, the left hemisphere's *insula,* a mesial area of cortex contiguous with the frontal, temporal, and parietal lobes (see Figure 2-16) and strongly connected with areas of the brain involved in many emotional and purposive behaviors, probably plays an important role in speech and language functions.[9] It recently has been tied to lesions associated with apraxia of speech,[19] suggesting that it may have a specialized role in speech motor planning or programming.

The Role of Sensation

Adequate execution of volitional motor activity may require proprioceptive feedback about muscle activity. Abbs and Kennedy[1] observed that the role of afferent control mechanisms in speech has been underemphasized, even though "speech motor control is almost certainly more than simply transmitting the contents of a predetermined motor tape over existing descending pathways." There is wide agreement that speech motor control is an acquired skill learned through the imitation of acoustic patterns provided by normal speakers. Thus, although by convention we refer to motor speech and MSDs, it is more precise to think of speech as a sensorimotor process and its neurologic aberrations as sensorimotor speech disorders.

There is little doubt that sensation contributes to speech programming and control. However, how this contribution is made is "poorly understood and often neglected in theories and models of speech production."[38] The following points address some characteristics of motor control that seem to require sensory assistance and some facts about the sensory system that permit such assistance.

1. Auditory and sensory input from muscles have diverse input to the speech motor system. They have direct, rapid (i.e., short latency) input to motor neurons supplying speech muscles at the brainstem and spinal levels. These afferent influences also exist in longer latency multisynaptic pathways through the cortex, basal ganglia, and cerebellum.

2. Intelligible speech can be produced by structures that are continuously changing position, in the presence of structural roadblocks (e.g., objects in the mouth), and when structures that normally move are blocked from doing so (e.g., a bite block restricting jaw movement). This means that commands leading to the production of specific sounds cannot be invariant, because the actions depend on the phonetic and physical environment (recall the previous discussion of coarticulation and motor equivalence). Only through knowledge about these states can the system produce a reliable acoustic signal that matches linguistic intent. Because intelligible speech requires relatively reliable achievement of articulatory targets, knowledge about where structures (e.g., the tongue) are coming from and their movement velocity seems essential. Integration of sensory information from peripheral mechanoreceptors may form a primary source of this knowledge.

3. An important concept in motor physiology is that descending pathways from higher brain centers can influence sensory processing at the brainstem and spinal levels. This permits sensory pathways to be pretuned or sensitized by the motor system so optimal use can be made of sensory information. This mechanism is exemplified in the gamma motor neuron system in which muscle spindle sensitivity and readiness to respond can be influenced by UMNs (direct and indirect activation pathways). At the cortical level, primary motor area neurons are most responsive to sensory input from regions to which they provide motor innervation. Finally, the speech system's ability to produce what can be perceived is perhaps the strongest argument for a role of sensory processes in speech motor control.

4. Surgical lesions or surgically placed stimulators in the thalamus and basal ganglia can control certain movement disorders. This is accomplished by interrupting the central afferent component of cortical, basal ganglia, and cerebellar loops that generate and control movement. These observations reflect strong interactions between the sensory and motor systems in movement control.

Reflexes, Learning, and Automaticity of Movement

It is likely that higher levels of the nervous system, such as dominant hemisphere cortical motor areas, determine overall movement goals or plans for speech. It is also likely that noncortical pathways are involved in programming the details and controlling the execution of speech movements. Many aspects of these lower-level, reflexlike processes depend on afferent information from the periphery about movement and the movement environment. These lower-level actions are stereotyped, rapid, and do not require conscious effort. Higher-level regulation of movement by sensorimotor cortex and the control circuits is slower because of increased pathway length and number of synapses; because it is less automatic, more sophisticated and purposeful output geared to accomplishing goal-oriented movement is possible. Motor speech behavior may reflect the cooperation of short-latency, automatic, sensorimotor pathways; longer-latency, relatively more consciously mediated pathways; and intermediate pathways between those extremes.

It is also likely that the allocation of resources for speech motor programming and control among high, low, and intermediate levels of the motor system vary as a function of learning, experience, task complexity, and speaker intentions. It is reasonable to assume that higher levels of the system carry a heavier responsibility when speech is motorically complex or novel; when demands for accuracy and precision are greater than average; or when the speaker intends to be precise, emphatic, intelligible without being ambiguous, or impressive. Conversely, higher-level control may be less vigilant when an utterance is highly overlearned and stereotypic, understood easily in the physical and social context, considered insignificant, or is poorly attended to. It is possible that some aspects of speech are directed by preprogrammed groups of motor commands that are released upon presentation of an appropriate stimulus as long as the relationship between stimulus and response has been established by learning and practice.

Finally, it is quite possible that programming and control requirements differ among various speech structures. For example, the speed, discreteness, and diversity of tongue, lip, and jaw movements during speech appear different and greater than those associated with velopharyngeal and respiratory movements.

Control Circuit Influences

The roles of the basal ganglia and cerebellar control circuits in motor activities, by definition, involve them in speech programming and control. This is because, as already noted, the primary influence of control circuits is through their input to the cortical areas involved in planning and programming speech movements.

It is reasonable to assume that cortical speech areas play an important role in establishing acoustic and motor targets and sequences and in the preliminary movement plan before the initiation of speech. It is also likely that the control circuits are informed of the plan before the initiation of speech, so they may provide a proper tonal and postural environment, as well as information to the cortex about how goals can be achieved. Once speech is initiated, the control circuits probably play an ongoing role in modifying cortical activity and subsequent direct and indirect activation pathway signals to speech muscles.

The basal ganglia control circuit is probably important to the regulation of the slower components of speech, those that provide postural support for rapid speech movements such as those involved in articulation.[1,39] The cerebellar control circuit is probably involved in programming and coordinating more rapid speech movements. Recent studies using PET suggest that the basal ganglia play a role in movement selection or preprogramming, whereas the cerebellum plays a role in optimizing movements by monitoring sensory feedback about movement outcome[32]; it is likely that these specialized contributions also apply to speech.

Limbic System Influences

The limbic system is a supratentorially located group of nuclei and pathways composed of the olfactory areas, hypothalamic and thalamic nuclei, and the limbic lobe of the cortex. The limbic lobe is located on the medial surface of the cortex and includes the orbital frontal region, the cingulate gyrus, and medial portions of the temporal lobe.

The limbic system plays a crucial role in the perception of pain, smell, and taste; visceral and emotional activity; and the mediation of information about internal states such as thirst and hunger, fear, rage, pleasure, and sex. Cortical limbic areas play an important role in regulating memory and learning, modulating drive or motivation, and influencing the affective components of experience.[49]

Nowhere more than in speech are emotions and propositional meaning combined. It is likely that limbic system influences are present before or during the conceptualization stage and that emotional content influences and modifies what happens during linguistic planning, particularly the semantic component. Its influence goes beyond this, however, because speech conveys emotions and meanings beyond those that can be attributed to words. Emotions are conveyed in speech primarily through prosody or suprasegmental variations in pitch, loudness, and duration. The limbic system probably represents a primary drive to the prosodic-emotional character of speech, particularly when the emotion conveyed is involuntary, unintentional, or automatic. Primitive reflex examples are laughter and crying, nonspeech prosodic vocal activities that sometimes cannot be inhibited by voluntary effort. Therefore the emotional components of prosody are mediated less by linguistic activity than by the influence of the limbic system and other cortical areas, most notably in the right hemisphere (see next section).

Cognitive and emotional disorders can affect speech, usually by attenuating or exaggerating prosody in a manner that accurately reflects the individual's general cognitive or emotional state. Conversely, many MSDs result in prosodic disturbances that prevent, exaggerate, or distort the individual's capacity to convey vocally his or her inner emotional state.

Right Hemisphere Influences

It is generally believed that the cortical planning and programming for speech that arises in the left hemisphere is transmitted across the corpus callosum to the right hemisphere, where its motor pathways carry out the program in coordination with the left hemisphere. However, the right hemisphere is not entirely passive regarding speech production, even though its role is not well delineated. Evidence indicates that it contributes to the perception and motor organization of the prosodic components of speech, especially those that express attitudes and emotions.[49]

People with right hemisphere lesions sometimes display "flattened" or reduced prosodic speech variations, a problem that has been called *aprosodia*.[62] There is some dispute about whether the attenuated prosody reflects hypoarousal, depression, or difficulty programming prosodic features for speech.[53] Nonetheless, the deficits are important to recognize and distinguish from the better-understood dysarthrias and apraxia of speech, as well as from prosodic disturbances reflecting other abnormalities of cognition and affect. The role of the right hemisphere in speech production and speech abnormalities associated with right hemisphere damage are discussed in Chapter 13.

Reticular Formation and Thalamic Influences

The role of the reticular formation in activities of the indirect and direct activation pathways, the control circuits, and the sensory system has been discussed. In fact, its multiple functions have led to its significance being buried by discussions of the more "dedicated" portions of the motor system. It is highlighted here simply to emphasize that its multiple roles, connections, and central location give it a significant integrative role in nervous system activities. Its contribution to maintaining alertness, monitoring sensory input, maintaining and helping to focus attention, and refining motor activity influence the emotional and propositional content and neuromuscular adequacy of speech.

The thalamus deserves recognition for the same reasons. Its role in the activities of the control circuits, its importance as a sensory processor, its direct ties to cortical language and motor speech systems, its integrative role in attention and vigilance, and its role within the limbic system make it difficult to assign it a single role. However, its diverse activities include an important role in the circuitry necessary for normal speech production.

Effects of Damage

The motor planning and programming roles of the dominant hemisphere for speech are never more dramatically illustrated than when they become damaged. In fact, such a disturbance helped give birth to behavioral neurology in the mid-1800s as part of attempts to localize diseases affecting "higher-level" motor and cognitive disturbances. The problem, which is distinguishable from aphasia and dysarthria, is known by many labels. For reasons explained later, the disturbance of speech motor planning or programming associated with dominant hemisphere abnormalities is called *apraxia of speech*. Its clinical features and discussion of its nature are addressed in Chapter 11.

Performance

Performance occurs when the FCPs are activated and trigger muscle contractions and movement. Performance is a product of the combined activities of the direct and indirect activation pathways, the control circuits, the final common pathway, feedback from sensory pathways, and ongoing conceptual-programming influences. It has already been discussed within the context of the functions of all other levels of the speech motor system.

Feedback

Feedback provides sensory information about ongoing and completed movements and permits modification of ongoing and future movements based upon that information. This activity may take place at the spinal and brainstem level, in the cerebellum, thalamus, basal ganglia, and cortex. These mechanisms have already been discussed.

SUMMARY

This chapter has presented a broad overview of neuroanatomy and neurophysiology and some basic information about neuropathology. The goal has been to provide a foundation for understanding motor speech activity and its neuropathologies. The major points can be summarized as follows:

1. Most crucial components of the speech motor system have their origins within the skull. They are surrounded by meningeal coverings and spaces for CSF and vascular structures. They are nourished and protected by the ventricular and vascular systems.

2. The major anatomic levels of the nervous system include the supratentorial, posterior fossa, and spinal and peripheral levels, all of which contain components of the motor system.

3. The functional systems of the brain include CSF, vascular, visceral, neurochemical, consciousness, sensory, and motor systems. The cerebrospinal and vascular systems support neurologic functions but have no direct role in speech, because they are not neural in structure. The visceral and consciousness systems have important but indirect influences on speech activities, and damage to them does not necessarily produce specific MSDs. Neurochemical systems drive all neurologic activity and have a direct influence on all aspects of speech production. The sensory system is strongly and rather directly linked to the reflexive and volitional activities of the motor system, including speech. The motor system is directly involved in speech production.

4. The nervous system is made up of neurons and supporting cells. Supporting cells facilitate neuronal function, and pathologic reactions in them can be a cause of, or reaction to, neurologic disease. The neuron is the functional unit of the nervous system. Movement of muscles, tendons, and joints require activity of many neurons that, in the PNS, are grouped together in nerves, and, in the CNS, are grouped together in tracts and pathways. Neuronal death, injury, or degeneration, and other malfunctions of neurons are directly responsible for behavioral disturbances, including MSDs.

5. Neurologic disease can be focal, multifocal, or diffuse in localization, and its development can be acute, subacute, or chronic. Its evolution can be transient, improving, progressive, exacerbating-remitting, or stationary. Causes can be degenerative, inflammatory, toxic-metabolic, neoplastic, traumatic, or vascular. MSDs can be associated with any pattern of localization, temporal course, or etiology.

6. The motor system is present at all anatomic levels of the nervous system. Its major divisions include the final common pathway, the direct activation pathway, the indirect activation pathway, the basal ganglia control circuit, and the cerebellar control circuit. Each division plays a specific role in motor activity, but there is overlap among their anatomy and functions, and they must operate together to produce normal motor behavior. Damage to any of the divisions can produce relatively distinct neurologic deficits whose recognition is helpful to the localization of disease.

7. The motor system for speech is part of the motor system in general. Speech is manifest through movements triggered by cranial and spinal nerves that innervate respiratory, phonatory, resonatory, and articulatory muscles. Cranial nerves V, VII, IX, X, XI, and XII, as well as the phrenic nerves from the cervical level of the spinal cord, are the nerves of the final common pathway that are most important for speech production.

8. The direct activation pathway originates in the cortex and passes directly as corticobulbar and corticospinal tracts to control skilled speech movements carried out through the final common pathway.

9. The indirect activation pathway also originates in the cortex but influences alpha and gamma motor neurons of the LMN system only after synapses at multiple points in the CNS, mostly in the brainstem. It regulates reflex activities of LMNs and maintains posture, tone, and associated activities that provide a stable framework on which skilled actions can be imposed.

10. The basal ganglia control circuit, consisting of the basal ganglia and related structures, affects motor activities primarily through its influence on the cerebral cortex. It assists in generating motor speech programs, especially the components that maintain a stable musculoskeletal environment in which skilled movements can occur. Its ultimate influence on LMNs is primarily through indirect pathways.

11. The cerebellar control circuit, consisting of the cerebellum and related pathways, influences motor activity primarily through its influence on the cortex. It also receives proprioceptive information from the periphery. The circuit's role is to coordinate speech through its knowledge of cortically set goals and its access to results at the periphery.

12. The conceptual-programming level establishes speech goals and the plans and programs for achieving them. Conceptualization—the thoughts and ideas that drive a desire to speak—require cortical activity, but they are not easily localizable and are best thought of as a function of many cortical and subcortical areas of the brain.

13. The language system, with crucial contributions from the left (dominant) hemisphere perisylvian cortex, organizes the linguistic content of spoken language that a speaker intends a listener to perceive.

14. Motor speech planning and programming are at the interface between the language formulation and neuromuscular execution stages of verbal expression. They are responsible for coding linguistic content into neural impulses that are compatible with the operations of the motor system. The goal of motor planning and programming for speech is the generation of movement patterns that result in an acoustic signal

that matches the speaker's intent. Motor speech programs are not and cannot be invariant because of the infinite number of possible utterances, the variability of directions and distances from which articulatory targets must be reached, and because speech gestures overlap in time. The complexity of the movements and the speed at which they are normally accomplished make it probable that many aspects of speech movements in mature speakers are preprogrammed.

15. The left (dominant) hemisphere is crucial to speech planning and programming. The control circuits also play an important role in speech programming and control.

16. Sensory processing at the brainstem and spinal levels, as well as at higher levels of the sensory system, probably plays an important role in the programming and ongoing control of speech movements.

17. It is likely that the responsibilities of various components of the speech planning, programming, and execution system vary as a function of learning, experience, complexity, and speaker intent. This cautions against strict, inflexible localization of speech control to single structures.

18. The limbic system, right hemisphere, reticular formation, and thalamus contribute to the programs that are generated to produce emotional and intended linguistic meanings conveyed in speech.

19. Deficits at the conceptualization and linguistic planning levels can impair the content of speech. Such impairments can exist independently of motor speech disorders.

20. Deficits in the dominant hemisphere's speech planning and programming activities and deficits in the motor system's control and neuromuscular execution of speech are known as apraxia of speech and dysarthria. The assessment of these disorders is the subject of the next chapter.

References

1. Abbs JH, Kennedy JG: Neurophysiological processes of speech movement control. In Lass NJ et al, editors: Speech, language, and hearing, vol. 1, normal processes, Philadelphia, 1982, WB Saunders.

2. Ackermann H et al: Cerebellar contributions to the perception of temporal cues within the speech and nonspeech domain, Brain Lang 67:228, 1999.

3. Adams RD, Victor M: Principles of neurology, New York, 1991, McGraw-Hill.

4. Ahlskog JE: Approach to the patient with a movement disorder: basic principles of neurologic diagnosis. In Adler CH, Ahlskog JE, editors: Parkinson's disease and movement disorders: diagnosis and treatment guidelines for the practicing physician, Totowa, NJ, 2000, Humana Press.

5. Aronson AE: Clinical voice disorders, New York, 1990, Thieme.

6. Ball T et al: The role of higher-order motor areas in voluntary movement as revealed by high-resolution EEG and fMRI, Neuroimage 10:682, 1999.

7. Barlow SM, Farley GR: Neurophysiology of speech. In Kuehn DP, Lemme ML, Baumgartner JM, editors: Neural bases of speech, hearing, and language, Boston, 1989, College-Hill.

8. Benarroch EE et al: Medical neurosciences: an approach to anatomy, pathology, and physiology by systems and levels, Philadelphia, 1999, Lippincott Williams & Wilkins.

9. Bennett S, Netsell RW: Possible roles of the insula in speech and language processing: directions for research, J Med Speech-Lang Pathol 7:253, 1999.

10. Berger JR: Clinical approach to stupor and coma. In Bradley WG et al, editors: Neurology in clinical practice: principles of diagnosis and management, vol 1, ed 3, Boston, 2000, Butterworth-Heinemann.

11. Bhatnager SC: Neuroscience for the study of communicative disorders, Philadelphia, 2002, Lippincott Williams & Wilkins.

12. Brooks VB: The neural basis of motor control, New York, 1986, Oxford University Press.

13. Brown DR: Neurosciences for allied health therapies, St Louis, 1980, Mosby, Inc.

14. Carpenter MB: Core text of neuroanatomy, Baltimore, 1978, Williams & Wilkins.

15. Chen CH, Wu T, Chu NS: Bilateral cortical representation of the intrinsic lingual muscles, Neurology 52:411, 1999.

16. Darley FL, Aronson AE, Brown JR: Motor speech disorders, Philadelphia, 1975, WB Saunders.

17. Diener HC, Dichgans J: Pathophysiology of cerebellar ataxia, Mov Disord 7:95, 1992.

18. Dobkin JA et al: Evidence for transhemispheric diaschisis in unilateral stroke, Arch Neurol 46:1333, 1989.

19. Dronkers NF: A new brain region for coordinating speech articulation, Nature 384:159, 1996.

20. Eccles JC: The understanding of the brain, New York, 1977, McGraw-Hill.

21. Gerloff C et al: Stimulation over the human supplementary motor area interferes with the organization of future elements in complex motor sequences, Brain 120:1587, 1997.

22. Giacino JT: Disorders of consciousness: differential diagnosis and neuropathologic features, Semin Neurol 17:105, 1997.

23. Gilman S: Cerebellar control of movement, Ann Neurol 35:3, 1994.

24. Gilman S, Gloedel JR, Lechtenberg R: Disorders of the cerebellum, Philadelphia, 1981, FA Davis.

25. Gilman W, Winans SS: Manter & Gatz's essentials of clinical neuroanatomy and neurophysiology, Philadelphia, 1982, FA Davis.

26. Gordon B: Postconcussional syndrome. In Johnson RT, editor: Current therapy in neurologic disease, ed 3, Philadelphia, 1990, BC Decker.

27. Gur A: Brain, breathing and breathlessness, Respir Physiol 109:197, 1997.

28. Hageman C: *Flaccid dysarthria. In McNeil MR, editor: Clinical management of sensorimotor speech disorders,* New York, 1997, Thieme.

29. Hixon TJ: *Respiratory functions in speech and song,* Boston, 1987, College-Hill Press.

30. Jennett B, Teasdale G: *Management of head injuries,* Philadelphia, 1981, FA Davis.

31. Jonas S: The supplementary motor region and speech emission, *J Commun Dis* 14:349, 1981.

32. Jueptner M, Weiller C: A review of differences between basal ganglia and cerebellar control of movements as revealed by functional imaging studies, *Brain* 121:1437, 1998.

33. Kennedy JG, Kuehn DP: Neuroanatomy of speech. In Kuehn DP, Lemme ML, Baumgartner J, editors: *Neural bases of speech, hearing, and language,* Boston, 1989, College-Hill.

34. Kent RD: Research on speech motor control and its disorders: a review and perspectives, *J Commun Dis* 33:391, 2000.

35. Kent RD: The acoustic and physiologic characteristics of neurologically impaired speech movements. In Hardcastle WJ, Marchal A, editors: *Speech production and speech modelling,* The Netherlands, 1990, Kluwer Academic Publishers.

36. Kent RD, Netsell R: A case study of an ataxic dysarthric: cineradiographic and spectrographic, *J Speech Hear Disord* 40:115, 1975.

37. Kent RD, Netsell R, Abbs JH: Acoustic characteristics of dysarthria associated with cerebellar disease, *J Speech Hear Res* 22:627, 1979.

38. Kent RD et al: What dysarthrias can tell us about the neural control of speech, *J Phonetics* 28:273, 2000.

39. Kornhuber HH: Cerebral cortex, cerebellum, and basal ganglia: an introduction to their motor function. In Evarts EV, editor: *Central processing of sensory input leading to motor output,* Cambridge, Mass, 1975, MIT Press.

40. Krainik A et al: Role of the supplementary motor area in motor deficit following medial frontal lobe surgery, *Neurology* 57:871, 2001.

41. Laforce R, Doyon J: Distinct contribution of the striatum and cerebellum to motor learning, *Brain Cogn* 45:189, 2001.

42. Larson CR: Basic neurophysiology. In Kuehn DP, Lemme ML, Baumgartner JM, editors: *Neural bases of speech, hearing and language,* Boston, 1989, College-Hill.

43. Larson CR, Pfingst BE: Neuroanatomic bases of hearing and speech. In Lass NJ et al, editors: *Speech, language, and hearing, vol 1, normal processes,* Philadelphia, 1982, WB Saunders.

44. Lindblom B: The interdisciplinary challenge of speech motor control. In Grillner S et al, editors: *Speech motor control,* New York, 1982, Pergamon Press.

45. Marien P, Engelborghs S, DeDeyn P: Cerebellar neurocognition: a new avenue, *Acta Neurol Belg* 101:96, 2001.

46. McClean MD: Neuromotor aspects of speech production and dysarthria. In Yorkston KM, Beukelman DR, Bell KR, editors: *Clinical management of dysarthric speakers,* Boston, 1988, College-Hill Press.

47. McNeil MR, Doyle PJ, Wambaugh J: Apraxia of speech: a treatable disorder of motor planning and programming. In Nadeau SE, Gonzalez Rothi LJ, Crosson B, editors: *Aphasia and language: theory to practice,* New York, 2000, Guilford Press.

48. McNeil MR, editor: *Clinical management of sensorimotor speech disorders,* New York, 1997, Thieme.

49. Mesulam MM: *Principles of behavioral and cognitive neurology,* New York, 2000, Oxford University Press.

50. Metter EJ et al: Local cerebral metabolic rates of glucose in movement and language disorders from positron tomography, *Am J Physiol* 246:R897, 1984.

51. Middleton FA, Strick PL: Basal ganglia and cerebellar loops: motor and cognitive circuits, *Brain Res Brain Res Rev* 31:236, 1998.

52. Mlcoch AG, Metter EJ: Medical aspects of stroke rehabilitation. In Chapey R, editor: *Language intervention strategies in adult aphasia,* Baltimore, 1994, Williams & Wilkins.

53. Myers PS: Communication disorders associated with right hemisphere brain damage. In Chapey R, editor: *Language intervention strategies in adult aphasia,* Baltimore, 1994, Williams & Wilkins.

54. Narayan RK et al: Clinical trials in head injury, *J Neurotrauma* 19:503, 2002.

55. Netsell R, Kent RD: Paroxysmal ataxic dysarthria, *J Speech Hear Disord* 41:93, 1976.

56. Nolte J: *The human brain: an introduction to its functional anatomy,* St Louis, 1999, Mosby.

57. Nordstrom MA et al: Motor cortical control of human masticatory muscles, *Prog Brain Res* 123:203, 1999.

58. Penfield W, Roberts L: *Speech and brain mechanisms,* New York, 1974, Athenium.

59. Perkins WH, Kent RD: *Functional anatomy of speech, language, and hearing,* San Diego, 1986, College-Hill Press.

60. Powers JW, Raichle ME: Positron emission tomography and its application to the study of cerebrovascular disease in man, *Stroke* 16:361, 1985.

61. Rodriguez M: A function of myelin is to protect axons from subsequent injury: implications for deficits in multiple sclerosis (editorial), *Brain* 126:751, 2003.

62. Ross ED: The aprosodias, *Arch Neurol* 38:561, 1981.

63. Salazar AM: Closed head injury. In Johnson RT, editor: *Current therapy in neurologic disease,* Philadelphia, 1990, BC Decker.

64. Sherrington CS: *The integrative action of the nervous system,* London, 1906, Constable & Co.

65. Stevens CF: *The neuron: a Scientific American book,* San Francisco, 1979, WH Freeman & Co.

66. Square PA, Martin RE: The nature and treatment of neuromotor speech disorders in aphasia. In Chapey R, editor: *Language intervention strategies in adult aphasia,* Baltimore, 1994, Williams & Wilkins.

67. Van Der Merwe A: A theoretical framework for the characterization of pathological speech sensorimotor control. In McNeil MR, editor: *Clinical management of sensorimotor speech disorders,* New York, 1997, Thieme.

68. Yorkston KM et al: The relationship between speech and swallowing disorders in head-injured patients, *J Head Trauma Rehabil* 4:1, 1989.

3

Examination of Motor Speech Disorders

"One of the most important parts of a scientist's work is the discovery of patterns in data."[5]

C.E. Brodley, T. Lane, and T.M. Strough

CHAPTER OUTLINE

   I. **Purposes of motor speech examination**
      A. Description
      B. Establishing diagnostic possibilities
      C. Establishing a diagnosis
      D. Establishing implications for localization and disease diagnosis
      E. Specifying severity
  II. **General guidelines for examination**
      A. History
      B. Salient features
      C. Confirmatory signs
      D. Interpretation of findings—diagnosis
 III. **The motor speech examination**
      A. History
      B. Examination of the speech mechanism during nonspeech activities
      C. Assessment of perceptual speech characteristics
      D. Assessment of intelligibility, comprehensibility, and efficiency
  IV. **Summary**

Identifying a speech problem as neurologic and then localizing it within the nervous system is similar to a neurologist's efforts to localize disease and establish a neurologic diagnosis. The differences between the two enterprises are that speech may be only one of a number of neurologic problems, and that speech diagnosis is usually not diagnostic of specific neurologic disease. But these differences sometimes blur. Speech difficulty is sometimes the presenting complaint and the only detectable neurologic abnormality, and its diagnosis may permit localization and a tentative disease diagnosis. Speech examination is thus an important component of many neurologic examinations.

This chapter discusses the examination of speech in people with suspected motor speech disorders (MSDs). It is not the intent here to discuss the interpretation or application of examination findings to diagnosis or management, beyond some illustrative examples. The relationship between examination results and specific speech diagnoses is addressed in each chapter on specific MSDs (Chapters 4 to 14) and in Chapter 15 (Differential Diagnosis). The relationship of examination results to management is addressed in Chapter 16.

■ PURPOSES OF MOTOR SPEECH EXAMINATION

The motor speech examination reflects several goals and activities that are relevant to diagnosis. Different goals are often pursued simultaneously, but they can be isolated and sequenced in a way that helps organize the activities that make up the examination. These goals include description, establishing diagnostic possibilities, establishing a diagnosis, establishing implications for localization and disease diagnosis, and specifying severity.

Description

Description characterizes the features of speech and structures and functions related to speech. It represents the data upon which diagnostic and treatment decisions are made. In some cases the diagnostic process ends with description, because findings

69

cannot establish a diagnosis or even a limited list of diagnostic possibilities. The bases for description derive from the patient's history and description of the problem, the oral mechanism examination, the perceptual characteristics of speech and results of standard clinical tests, and instrumental analyses of speech.

Once speech is described, the clinician asks if the characteristics are normal or abnormal. This is the first step in diagnosis, and an important one. If all aspects of speech are within the range of normal, the diagnosis is normal speech. If some aspects of speech are abnormal, then their meaning must be interpreted. *The process of narrowing diagnostic possibilities and arriving at a specific diagnosis is known as differential diagnosis.*

Establishing Diagnostic Possibilities

If speech is abnormal, then a list of diagnostic possibilities can be generated. Because the emphasis here is on MSDs, the list can grow out of answers to questions such as the following:

1. Is the problem neurologic?
2. If the problem is not neurologic, is it nonetheless organic? For example, is it due to dental or occlusal abnormality, mass lesion of the larynx, or is it psychogenic?
3. If the problem is or is not neurologic, is it recently acquired or longstanding? For example, might it reflect unresolved developmental stuttering, articulation disorder, or language disability?
4. If the problem is neurologic, is it an MSD or another neurologic disorder that is affecting verbal expression (e.g., aphasia, dementia, akinetic mutism)? If an MSD is present, is it a dysarthria or apraxia of speech?
5. If dysarthria is present, what is its type?

Establishing a Diagnosis

Once all reasonable diagnostic possibilities have been recognized, a single diagnosis may emerge or, at the least, the possibilities may be ordered from most to least likely. For example, concluding that speech is not normal, that it is not psychogenic in origin, and that it is a dysarthria but of undetermined type, is of diagnostic value. It implies the existence of an organic process and places the lesion within motor components of the nervous system. If it also can be concluded that the dysarthria is not flaccid, then the lesion is further localized to the central and not the peripheral nervous system, and certain neurologic diagnoses can be eliminated or considered unlikely. If the characteristics of the disorder are unambiguous and compatible with only a single diagnosis, then a single speech diagnosis can be given along with its implications for localization.

Establishing Implications for Localization and Disease Diagnosis

When an MSD is identified, it is appropriate to address explicitly its implications for neurologic localization, especially if the referral source is unfamiliar with the method of classification. For example, if spastic dysarthria is the diagnosis, it is appropriate to state that the disorder is usually associated with bilateral involvement of upper motor neuron (UMN) pathways. If a tentative neurologic diagnosis has already been made, it is appropriate to address the compatibility of the speech diagnosis with it. For example, if the working neurologic diagnosis is Parkinson's disease but the patient has a mixed spastic-ataxic dysarthria, it is important to report that this mixed dysarthria is not compatible with Parkinson's disease. Finally, if neurologic diagnosis is uncertain or if speech is the only sign of disease, it is appropriate to identify possible diagnoses if the MSD is "classically" tied to them. For example, a flaccid dysarthria that emerges only with speech stress testing and recovers with rest has a very strong association with myasthenia gravis.

Specifying Severity

The severity of a MSD should always be estimated. This estimate is important for at least three reasons: (1) subjective or objective measures of severity can be matched against the patient's complaints; gross mismatches between patient and clinician judgment may introduce the possibility of psychogenic contributions, poor insight, or limited concern about speech on the patient's part; (2) it influences prognosis and management decision making; (3) severity estimates at the time of initial examination represent baseline data against which future changes can be compared.

Specifying severity is actually part of the descriptive process. It is highlighted here because of its relevance to estimating functional limitations and disability imposed by the MSD,[50] as opposed to determining the presence of impairment, which is more relevant to diagnosis. Limitations and disability are more relevant to decisions about management than diagnosis.

Once severity is established, it is appropriate to address the implications of the findings for prognosis and management. These are considered in Chapters 16 to 20.

GENERAL GUIDELINES FOR EXAMINATION

The motor speech examination has three essential procedural components: (1) history, (2) identification of salient speech features, and (3) identification of confirmatory signs. With this information, a diagnosis is made, recommendations formulated, and results communicated to the patient, referring professional, and others.

History

An anonymous sage has said that 90% of neurologic diagnosis depends on the patient's history.[38] A wise neurology colleague of the author has said that most clinical neurologic diagnoses are based on speech, either its content or its manner of expression. It would be difficult to argue that the spoken history provided by the patient is less important to motor speech evaluation and diagnosis.

Experienced clinicians often reach a diagnosis by the time greetings and amenities have been exchanged and a history obtained. Subsequent formal examination confirms, documents, refines, and sometimes revises the diagnosis. The history reveals the time course of complaints and the patient's observations about the disorder. It also puts contextual speech on display when anxiety is generally less than during formal examination; when physical effort, task comprehension, and cooperation are not essential; and when the patient may not feel his or her speech is the subject of scrutiny.

Salient Features

Salient features are those that contribute most directly and influentially to diagnosis. They include deviant speech characteristics and their presumed neuromuscular substrates. In 1975 Darley, Aronson, and Brown (DAB) discussed six salient neuromuscular features that influence speech production. They form a useful framework for integrating observations made during examination. They include strength, speed of movement, range of movement, steadiness, tone, and accuracy. Abnormalities associated with these features are summarized in Table 3-1.

Strength

Muscles have sufficient strength to perform their normal functions, plus a reserve of excess strength. Reserve strength permits contraction over time without excessive fatigue, as well as contraction against resistance.

When a muscle is weak, it cannot contract to a desired level, sometimes even for brief periods. It

| | table 3-1 | Salient neuromuscular features of speech and associated abnormalities commonly encountered in motor speech disorders |

Feature	Abnormality Associated with Motor Speech Disorders
Strength	Reduced, usually consistently but sometimes progressively
Speed	Reduced or variable (increased only in hypokinetic dysarthria)
Range	Reduced or variable (predominantly excessive only in hyperkinetic dysarthrias)
Steadiness	Unsteady, either rhythmic or arrhythmic
Tone	Increased, decreased, or variable
Accuracy	Inaccurate, either consistently or inconsistently

may fatigue more rapidly than normal. Sometimes a desired level of contraction can be obtained, but ability to sustain it decreases dramatically after a short time.

Muscle weakness can affect all three of the major speech valves (laryngeal, velopharyngeal, and articulatory), and it can be apparent in all components of speech production (respiration, phonation, resonance, articulation, and prosody). Weakness is most apparent and dramatic in lower motor neuron (LMN) or final common pathway (FCP) lesions and, therefore, in flaccid dysarthrias. Consequences of it can be inferred from perceptual and acoustic analyses, observed visually at rest and during speech, detected during oral mechanism examination, or measured physiologically.

Speed

Movements during speech are rapid, especially the laryngeal, velopharyngeal, and articulatory movements that valve expired air to produce the approximately 14 phonemes per second that characterize conversational speech. These quick, unsustained, and discrete movements are known as *phasic movements*. They can occur as single contractions or repetitively. They begin promptly, reach targets quickly, and relax rapidly. Phasic speech movements are mediated primarily through direct activation UMN pathway input to alpha motor neurons (see Chapter 2).

Excessive speed is uncommon in MSDs, although it may occur in hypokinetic dysarthria. Excessive speech rate in people with dysarthria is nearly always also associated with decreased range of motion.

Slow movements are common in MSDs. Movements may be slow to start, slow in their course, or slow to stop or relax. Single as well as repetitive movements may be slow.

Reduced speed can occur at all major speech valves and during all components of speech production. Slow movement strongly affects the prosodic features of speech because normal prosody is so dependent on quick muscular adjustments that influence rate of syllable production and pitch and loudness variability. The effects of reduced speed are most apparent in spastic dysarthria but also are present in other dysarthria types. The effects of altered speed can be perceived in speech, visibly apparent during speech and oral mechanism examination, and measured physiologically and acoustically.

Range

The distance traveled by speech structures is quite precise for single and repetitive movements. Variation in the range of repetitive movements is normally present but usually small.

Consistent but inappropriately excessive range of motion during voluntary speech is not common in neurologic disease. In contrast, decreased range is common and may occur in the context of slow, normal, or excessively rapid rate. For example, hypokinetic dysarthria is often associated with decreased range of motion and, sometimes, excessively rapid rate. In other instances, range may be variable and unpredictable. Abnormal variability in range is common in ataxic and hyperkinetic dysarthrias.

Abnormalities in range of motion often have a major influence on the prosodic features of speech, sometimes resulting in restricted or excessive prosodic variations. Such abnormalities can occur at all of the major speech valves and during all components of speech production. They can be inferred from acoustic and perceptual analyses of speech, visible during speech and nonspeech movements of the articulators, and measured physiologically.

Steadiness

At rest, there is a measurable 8 to 12 Hz oscillation of the body musculature. During normal movement there are usually no visible interruptions or oscillations of body parts, but oscillation amplitude sometimes increases to visibly detectable levels in healthy people. This visible *physiologic tremor* can occur in extreme fatigue, under emotional stress, or during shivering.

When motor steadiness breaks down in neurologic disease, the results can be broadly categorized as *involuntary movements* or *hyperkinesias*. *Tremor* is the most common involuntary movement. It consists of repetitive, relatively rhythmic oscillations of

a body part, generally ranging in frequency from 3 to 12 Hz. It may occur at rest *(resting tremor),* when a structure is maintained against gravity *(postural tremor),* during movement *(action tremor),* or toward the end of a movement *(terminal tremor).*

Mild tremor may not have any perceptible effect on speech characteristics dependent on respiration, resonance, or articulation. It commonly affects phonation and, when severe, it can affect prosody; its effects are most easily perceived during sustained vowel production. The effects of tremor on speech may be heard or seen during speech, may be seen during oral mechanism examination, and can be measured physiologically and acoustically.

Another major category of involuntary movement consists of random, unpredictable, adventitious movements that may vary in their speed, duration, and amplitude. These abnormal movements include *dystonia, dyskinesia, chorea,* and *athetosis.* They may be severe enough to interrupt or alter the direction of intended movement. They may be present at rest, during sustained postures, or during movement. They can affect movement at all of the major speech valves and all components of speech production. They can affect accuracy and often alter prosody. They are the primary source of abnormal speech in hyperkinetic dysarthrias. The effects of unpredictable hyperkinesias can be perceived during speech, seen during speech and oral mechanism examination, measured physiologically, and inferred from acoustic measurements.

Tone

Muscle tone is discussed in Chapter 2. The gamma loop and indirect activation pathway are crucial for proper maintenance of tone, which creates a stable framework upon which rapid voluntary movements can be superimposed.

In neurologic disease, muscle tone may be excessive or reduced. It may fluctuate slowly or rapidly in a regular or unpredictable fashion. Alterations in tone may occur at all speech valves and during all components of speech production. Abnormal tone is associated with flaccid dysarthrias when consistently reduced, with spastic or hypokinetic dysarthria when consistently increased, and with hyperkinetic dysarthrias when variable. The effects of abnormal tone can be inferred from perceptual speech characteristics, seen during speech and oral mechanism examination, measured physiologically, and inferred from acoustic measurements.

Accuracy

Individual, repetitive, complex sound sequences are normally executed with enough precision to ensure intelligible and efficient transmission of linguistic and emotional meaning. They result from regulation of tone, strength, speed, range, steadiness, and timing of muscle activity. From this standpoint, accuracy is the outcome of well-timed and coordinated activities of all the other neuromuscular features. If strength, speed, range, steadiness, and tone have been properly regulated, speech movements will be accurate. If speech contains inaccuracies and neuromuscular performance is normal, it is possible that the linguistic plan or ideational content is defective, placing the source of the problem outside of the motor system; an alternative explanation is that the problem lies in the planning or programming of movements and not in neuromuscular execution.

Inaccurate movements can result in various speech errors. For example, if force and range of motion are excessive, structures may overshoot targets. If force and range of motion are decreased, target undershooting may occur. If timing is poor, the direction and smoothness of movements may be faulty, and the rhythm of repetitive movements may be maintained poorly.

Inaccurate movements resulting from constantly present defects of strength, speed, range, and tone may result in predictable degrees of articulatory imprecision or other speech abnormalities. If the source of inaccuracy lies in timing or in unpredictable variations in other neuromuscular components, errors may be unpredictable, random, or transient.

Inaccurate movements may occur at all of the major speech valves and at all levels of speech production but are generally perceived most easily in articulation and prosody. Inaccuracy can occur in all dysarthrias, but when it is the result of inadequate timing or coordination, it is usually associated with ataxic dysarthria or apraxia of speech. When associated with random or unpredictable involuntary variations in movement, it often reflects hyperkinetic dysarthria.

It should be apparent that the salient neuromuscular features of movement interact and influence each other. For example, reduced strength is usually associated with reduced tone, range of motion, accuracy, and sometimes steadiness. Increased or variable tone is usually associated with reduced or variable speed, range of motion, steadiness, and accuracy. Reduced range of motion is associated with variations in speed, tone, and accuracy. *It is rare that only a single abnormal neuromuscular feature is present in someone with dysarthria.*

Confirmatory Signs

Confirmatory signs are additional clues about the location of pathology in the nervous system. In the context of speech examination, they are signs other than deviant speech characteristics and the salient neuromuscular features that characterize them that help support the speech diagnosis or increase confidence in it. *MSD diagnosis does not require that confirmatory signs be present.* Therefore observations of a nonspeech nature, even if of the speech muscles, must be considered circumstantial (confirmatory) evidence and not salient. Nonetheless, they can be helpful in establishing a diagnosis.

Confirmatory signs can be manifest in speech or nonspeech muscles. Examples of confirmatory signs within the speech system are atrophy, reduced tone, fasciculations, poorly inhibited laughter or crying, reduced normal reflexes or the presence of pathologic reflexes, and the strength of the cough. It is important to keep in mind that such signs are not diagnostic of MSDs. For example, lingual fasciculations, without any perceivable impairment of lingual articulation, would not warrant a diagnosis of dysarthria. It might reflect a lesion on nerve XII and require further investigation, but a diagnosis of dysarthria would require the presence of a perceptible *speech* deficit.

Confirmatory signs from the nonspeech motor system come from observations of gait, muscle stretch reflexes, superficial and pathologic reflexes, hyperactive limb reflexes, limb atrophy and fasciculations, difficulty initiating limb movements, and so on. They also include observations of strength, speed, accuracy, tone, steadiness, and range of movements in nonspeech muscles.

Confirmatory signs are discussed within each chapter on the specific dysarthrias and apraxia of speech and also briefly during the following overview of the motor speech examination.

Interpretation of Findings—Diagnosis

Once the history and salient speech features and confirmatory signs have been established, they are integrated to formulate an impression about their meaning. This constitutes diagnosis.

No examination is complete without an attempt to establish the meaning of its findings.* It is reasonable to state as principle that *when the results of an examination cannot go beyond description, the reasons why should be stated explicitly.* The absence of a diagnostic interpretation represents an omission of potentially valuable medical information and can

---

*Terms used to introduce diagnostic statements vary in clinical practice, but headings most often include the words *diagnosis, impression,* or *conclusion.* The term *summary* is not an appropriate heading, because the intent is to provide an interpretation of findings, not a brief restatement of them.

convey an impression that although a patient has been assessed, perhaps thoroughly, the results have been neither interpreted nor understood. This can lead to an interpretation by referral sources that speech-language pathology does not contribute to the localization or understanding of speech, language, and communication disorders.

The manner in which diagnostic statements are expressed is influenced by the examination findings plus the intended purposes of the evaluation (e.g., to provide an opinion about the nature of the speech deficit to a neurologist who is uncertain about the neurologic diagnosis; to determine the nature and severity of an MSD for the purpose of management planning). The strength or certainty of diagnostic statements can vary considerably. In some cases, findings may be so ambiguous that they justify only a statement that the diagnosis is uncertain. In others, they may justify a formulation of diagnostic possibilities, perhaps in order from most to least likely. In still others, they may permit a statement about what the disorder is not. And some permit a confidently stated, unambiguous diagnosis. Finally, findings sometimes—perhaps often—lead to a combination of some of the preceding possibilities, such as "the patient has an unambiguous spastic dysarthria, possibly with an accompanying ataxic component. There is no evidence of apraxia of speech." The process of differential diagnosis is discussed in detail in Chapter 15.

■ THE MOTOR SPEECH EXAMINATION

The motor speech examination can be divided into four parts: (1) history; (2) examination of the oral mechanism during nonspeech activities; (3) assessment of perceptual speech characteristics; and (4) assessment of intelligibility, comprehensibility, and efficiency. Instrumental analyses using acoustic, physiologic, or visual imaging methods may also be part of the clinical examination, but in general, they are not essential. Their use during various portions of the examination is noted when appropriate.

History

The history provides basic information about the onset and course of the problem, the patient's awareness of impairment, and the degree to which the problem limits basic activities or reduces participation in various aspects of life. The spoken history also puts on display the salient features, confirmatory signs, and severity of the problem.

No two histories are the same, and the specific questions that elicit histories will vary considerably. Factors affecting how history taking is approached include patients' cognitive ability and personality, whether or not they perceive a problem, what has already been established by other professionals, and the severity of the speech deficit. If patients have cognitive limitations, significantly reduced intelligibility, or an inadequate augmentative means of communication, or if they do not perceive a speech deficit, then the history from them may be limited. If the etiology and time course are already known, they need not be pursued beyond confirmation. The history sometimes must be provided or supplemented by someone who knows the patient well. History taking should usually be controlled by the clinician and not the patient, with questions and their sequence strongly influenced by the facts provided by the patient and by their manner of doing so.

The format of history taking often includes the following.

Introduction and Goal Setting

Once basic amenities have been exchanged, the examination can often begin with a simple but important question, *"Why are you here?"* Some representative responses include "to find out what's wrong with me," "to find out what's wrong with my speech," "to find out if you can help me with my speech," "because my doctor told me to come here," "there's nothing wrong with me," and "I don't know why they brought me here!" The answers are an index of patients' orientation, awareness, and concern about their speech; the priority they place on their speech versus other aspects of their illness; the relative importance to them of diagnosis versus management; their ability to provide a history; the depth and manner in which the history will have to be taken; and the actual severity of the speech disorder. This introduction also allows the clinician to inform the patient about the purposes and procedures of examination and its place in their overall evaluation and management.

Basic Data

Age, education, occupation, and marital and family status should be noted. It is important to establish if there was a history of childhood speech, language or hearing deficit, if treatment for those problems was necessary, and if they had resolved before the current illness began. This is essential when abnormalities are inconsistent with other current medical findings but could be longstanding or developmental in nature. The most common longstanding speech deficits encountered in adults with suspected neurologic disease are persisting developmental articulation errors, articulatory distortions associated with dental or occlusal abnormalities, and developmental stuttering.

Onset and Course

Information about the onset and course of the speech deficit is useful to neurologic diagnosis, prognosis, and management decisions. It also reveals something about the patient's perception of the problem. Relevant questions include the following:

- Do you have any difficulty with your speech? If not, has anyone else commented on a change in your speech?
- When did the speech problem begin? Did it begin suddenly or gradually? Who noticed it first, you or someone else?
- Did you develop any other difficulties when your speech problem began? Were other problems present before the speech problem began? Did other problems develop after the speech problem began?
- Has the speech problem changed? Better, worse, stable, fluctuating?
- Has your speech ever returned to normal? If so, when and for how long?
- Are you taking any medications that affect your speech in a positive or negative way? Are there any other factors that predictably affect your speech (e.g., time of day, stress, fatigue, environment)?

Associated Deficits

Questions about associated deficits that may represent confirmatory symptoms include the following:

- Have you had any difficulty with chewing? Drooling?
- Is it difficult to move food around in your mouth? Why?
- Does food get stuck in your cheeks or on the roof of your mouth? Do you have to remove it with your finger or a utensil?
- Do you have trouble moving food back in your mouth to get a swallow started?
- Do you have trouble with swallowing? Food or liquid? Do you have trouble getting a swallow started? Do you lose food or liquid out of your mouth? Does food or liquid ever go into or out of your nose when you swallow? Does food or liquid go down before you start to swallow and cause coughing or choking? Do you gag or choke when swallowing? Do you choke or cough after completing a swallow? Have you had to modify your diet because of these problems? Have you lost weight?
- Have you had any change in your emotional expression? Do you cry or laugh more easily or less easily than in the past?

Patient's Perception of Deficit

It is important to establish the patient's perception of the problem. This can provide useful confirmatory information.

- What was your speech like when the problem began? Did anything *feel* differently when you spoke?
- Have you noticed any change in the appearance or feeling in your face or mouth?
- Describe your current speech difficulty. How does it sound to you? Is it faster or slower? Louder or quieter? Less precise? Is speaking effortful? If 100% represents your speech before the problem began, where is it now?

Consequences of the Disorder

The following questions address some of the functional consequences of MSDs:

- Do people ever have trouble understanding you? If so, when? What do they or you do if that happens?
- Have you altered any of your work or social activities because of your speech? How? Does your speech prevent you from doing anything? If so, what?

Management

Information about what the patient and others (including professionals) have done to manage the speech disorder is useful for determining prognosis and future management recommendations.

- What have you done to compensate for your speech difficulty? Have you had any help for your speech? If so, when? For how long? What was done? Did it help?
- Do you think you need help with your speech now?

Awareness of Diagnosis and Prognosis

It is important to know what the patient understands about his or her medical diagnosis and prognosis because it influences the manner and depth to which the speech diagnosis and management issues should be discussed. For example, patients who are in the process of evaluation to determine the nature of their disease, or who have just received a diagnosis with a poor prognosis, may be neither interested nor emotionally ready to discuss management of their speech problem.

- What have you been told is the cause of this problem?
- What does the diagnosis mean is going to happen?

Examination of the Speech Mechanism During Nonspeech Activities

Observations of the speech mechanism in the absence of speech can be very informative. In general, it provides information about the size, strength, symmetry, range, tone, steadiness, speed, and accuracy of orofacial movements, particularly of the jaw, face, tongue, and palate. The observations are primarily visual and tactual but also rely on auditory information. The milieu in which the observations are made include (1) at rest, (2) during sustained postures, (3) during movement, and (4) reflexes. Evidence from the examination may help confirm conclusions drawn about speech. Even if not confirmatory of a speech deficit, the observations may nonetheless be salient to neurologic evaluation.

The Face at Rest

At rest, the normal face is grossly symmetric and exhibits normal tone and little spontaneous movement. It is neither droopy nor fixed in a posture associated with strong emotion (e.g., smiling, on the verge of tears).

To observe the face at rest, the patient should be instructed to relax, look forward, let the lips part, and breathe quietly through the mouth. Some people can maintain this relaxed posture more easily with their eyes closed.

The following questions should then be answered:
- Is the face symmetric?
- Are the angles of the mouth symmetric?
- Is asymmetry due to a drooping of the entire face on one side, a droop at the corner of the mouth, or flattening of the nasolabial fold?

Recognize that some asymmetry is the rule rather than the exception; a slight difference in the length and prominence of the nasolabial folds is common. Some asymmetry often can be seen at rest or during voluntary and spontaneous or emotional responses (Figure 3-1).

Additional questions include the following:
- Is the face expressionless, masklike, or unblinking? Is it held in a fixed expression of smiling, astonishment, or perplexity? Does the upper lip appear stiff?
- Are abnormal spontaneous, involuntary movements present? Do the eyes shut tightly and uncontrollably? Is there quick or slow symmetric or asymmetric pursing or retraction of the lips? Are there spontaneous smacking noises of the lips? Can the patient inhibit these movements on request? If so, do they reappear when inhibitory efforts cease?
- Are the lips tremulous or are there tremorlike rhythmic movements of the lips? Are *fascicu-lations* present in the face, especially around the mouth or chin?

The Face During Sustained Postures

Observing the face during sustained postures allows additional observations of symmetry, range of motion, strength and tone, and the ability to maintain a sustained posture.

Useful sustained facial postures include retraction of the lips, rounding or pursing of the lips, puffing the cheeks, and sustained mouth opening. The patient should be asked to sustain each posture after it is demonstrated by the examiner (see Figure 3-1).

The following questions should be answered:
- Are lip retraction, rounding, and puffing symmetric? Is their range of movement normal or restricted? When opening the mouth, is the configuration of the lips symmetric or does one side lag?
- Is the patient able to resist the examiner's attempt to push the upper or lower lip toward the midline when the lips are retracted, or resist the examiner's attempt to spread the lips when they are rounded? Does air escape through the lips when the patient puffs the cheeks or can the seal be broken with less than normal pressure when the examiner pushes in on the cheeks?
- Does *tremulousness* appear or disappear during sustained facial postures? Are additional movements present that distort or alter the ability to maintain the sustained posture?
- Can the patient maintain the posture for several seconds or does he or she stop the effort even when instructed to maintain it?

The Face During Movement

The face should be observed during speech, emotional responses, and volitional nonspeech tasks. During speech and emotional responses, range and symmetry of facial movement and expressiveness should be noted.

There is substantial literature on normal facial asymmetry and its determiners. Evidence suggests that the left side of the face is, on average, more active than the right in the expression of facial emotion, with the implication that the right hemisphere—with its predominant control over innervation of the lower left face—is dominant for emotional facial expression.[2] However, data from neurologically intact people show that asymmetries can be seen in favor of the right or left side of the face and that differences are not necessarily compatible with hypotheses about hemispheric specialization[17,42]; differences in facial morphology,

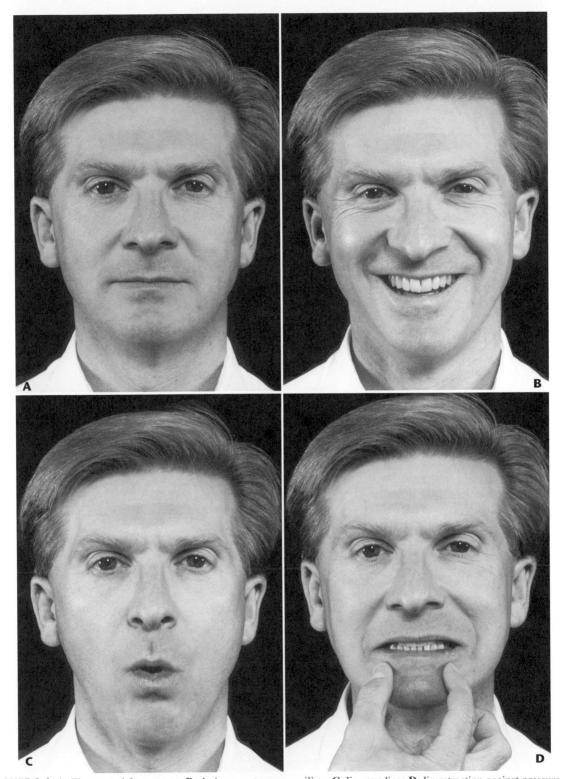

FIGURE 3-1 A, The normal face at rest; **B,** during spontaneous smiling; **C,** lip rounding; **D,** lip retraction against pressure.

Continued

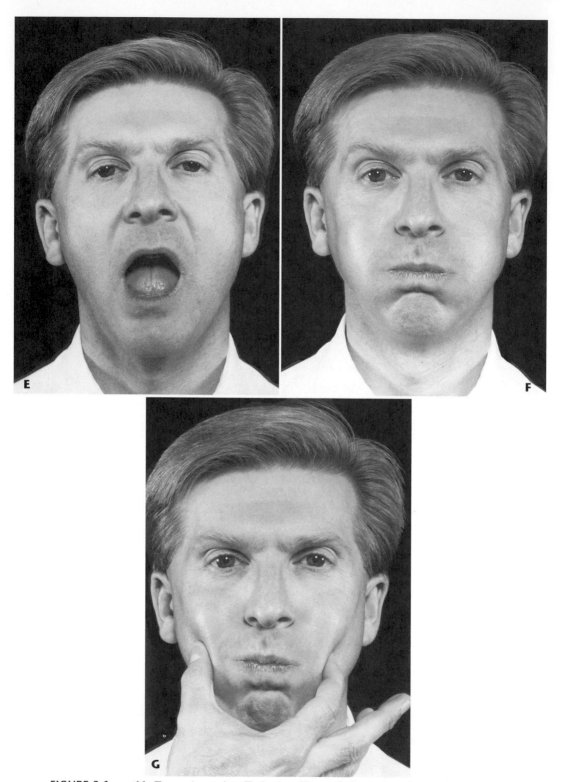

FIGURE 3-1 cont'd. E, mouth opening; **F,** cheek puffing; and, **G,** cheek puffing against pressure.

independent of asymmetric neural innervation, may explain some of the differences among people without neurologic disease. Some studies have found differences in facial asymmetry between the sexes and have argued that they are driven by gender-related differences in cognitive processing by the two cerebral hemispheres.[41] Others have concluded that there are no systematic asymmetry patterns, at least during emotional expression, as a function of gender.[3] Finally, a recent study reported that during repetition of single words the right side of the mouth opened to a greater degree in most people during repetition of single words, presumably reflecting left hemisphere dominance for language or speech programming; this was true for both sexes during single word production, but the asymmetries disappeared in women during word series productions.[18]

In light of these very interesting but probably less than reliably predictable clinical differences, what seems important for basic clinical examination is to remember that *mild facial asymmetries—at rest and during speech and nonspeech emotional expression—are not uncommon, but the direction of the asymmetry is not highly predictable.*

It is also important to remember that *the motor control of voluntary facial movement differs from the control of spontaneous expression.* For example, patients with lower facial paresis resulting from CNS lesions sometimes smile symmetrically in response to a joke, but asymmetry can then be evident when they smile voluntarily; the opposite pattern can be seen in some patients with parkinsonism.[35] Thus it is of value to elicit a spontaneous emotional smile and to compare the extent of facial movement during it to that of a voluntary smile or lip retraction.

Nonspeech tasks can include rapid repetitions of lip pursing, lip retraction, and cheek puffing. The patient should be instructed to repeat the movements as rapidly and steadily as possible. Observations of rate, range, and regularity of movement should be made. Observations of symmetry and the occurrence of regular or irregular involuntary movements should be made during speech and emotional responses.

The patient's emotional responses should be observed. The congenial clinician can usually elicit a spontaneous smile from the patient. When this does not happen naturally, asking "If I told you a joke, would you smile?" while smiling at the patient often is sufficient to trigger a smile. The symmetry of smiling and the degree to which the angles of the mouth elevate to normal height (again, recognizing that some asymmetry is normal) should be noted. More important, the degree of movement asymmetry relative to that observed during voluntary lip retraction should be observed.

Does the patient have difficulty inhibiting laughter or crying? This loss of inhibition can become apparent at any time during examination, but one of the simplest ways to trigger disinhibition is to ask the patient "Do you have any difficulty controlling laughter or crying?" It should be recognized, however, that it can be difficult to distinguish crying that reflects a pathologic loss of motor control from crying that may occur as a result of the psychologic distress, sorrow, and depression that can be expected in people who are coping with disease.

The Jaw at Rest

The jaw is usually lightly closed or slightly open at rest. This can be observed when the face is at rest. The following questions should be answered:

- Does the jaw hang lower than normal?
- Are there spontaneous, apparently involuntary quick or slow movements of the jaw, such as clenching, opening or pulling to one side, or tremorlike up and down movements? Has the patient learned any postural adjustments or tricks that tend to inhibit sustained involuntary movements (e.g., clenching the jaw, holding a pipe in the mouth, touching a hand to the side of the jaw or neck)?

The Jaw During Sustained Posture (Figure 3-2)

The jaw can be observed during sustained facial posture tasks, especially during mouth opening (see Figure 3-1, *E*). The following questions should be answered:

- Does the jaw deviate to one side when the patient attempts to open it as widely as possible? Is the patient able to open the mouth widely or is excursion limited?
- Can the patient resist the examiner's attempt to open the jaw when told to clench the teeth? Can the jaw be closed against resistance from the examiner (either by holding the midline of the jaw with the hand or by placing a tongue blade on the lower teeth and resisting closure)? Do the masseter and temporalis muscles have normal bulk and bulge when the patient bites down?
- Can the patient resist the examiner's attempt to close the jaw when told to hold it open?

The Jaw During Movement

The jaw should be observed for symmetry of opening and closing and for range of motion during speech and spontaneous movements. The patient should be asked to rapidly open and close the mouth;

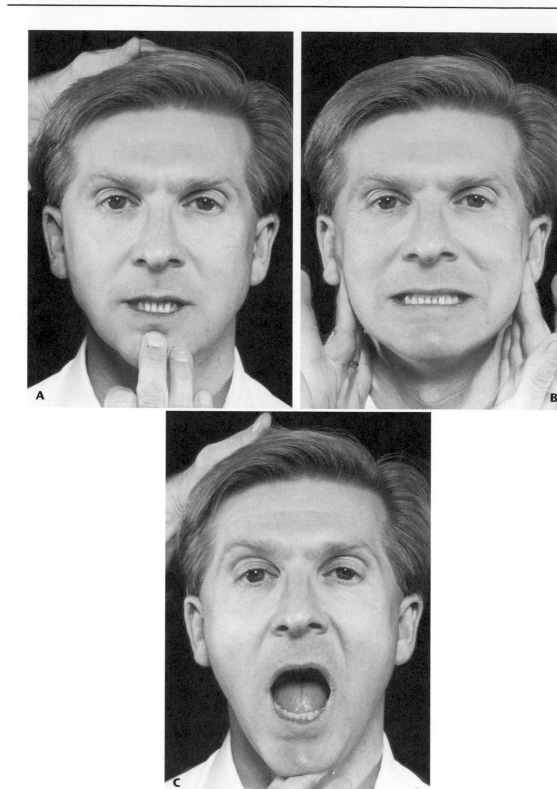

FIGURE 3-2 A, Assessing resistance to jaw opening; **B,** masseter bulk and symmetry during jaw clenching; and, **C,** resistance to jaw closing.

the speed and regularity of movements, as well as involuntary movements that may interrupt the course of jaw alternate motion rates (AMRs), should be noted.

The Tongue at Rest

The tongue should be examined at rest (see Figure 3-1, *E*). The patient should be told to open the mouth, breathe easily, and let the tongue relax on the floor of the mouth. The degree to which the normal tongue lies at rest varies considerably; some low-amplitude spontaneous movement is common. With this in mind, the following questions should be answered:

- Is the tongue full and symmetric? If symmetric, is its size normal? If small, are there symmetric or unilateral grooves or furrowing in the tongue representing atrophy? (Indentations along the tongue's lateral side edges may represent teeth marks and not atrophy.) Are *fasciculations* present (localized twitchlike movements of the tongue)? They are best observed when the tongue is at rest inside the

mouth; with the tongue protruded, normal spontaneous movements can be confused with fasciculations.
- Does the tongue remain quiet on the floor of the mouth? Are quick, slow, or sustained movements of large portions of the tongue apparent in the form of protrusion, retraction, lateralization, or writhing?
- Is the tongue (or oral cavity as a whole) excessively wet or dry? Accumulated saliva may reflect excessive secretions or, more likely in people with neurologic disease, failure to adequately clear secretions. *Xerostomia* (dry mouth) can reflect dehydration, inadequate water intake, autoimmune problems, or the effects of various medications or radiation therapy.

The Tongue During Sustained Postures (Figure 3-3)

The patient should be asked to protrude his or her tongue and sustain the posture. Mild deviation toward one side is not unusual, but the direction of

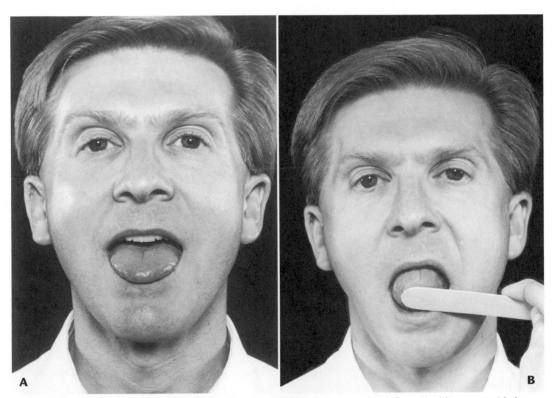

FIGURE 3-3 A, The tongue during protrusion; **B,** resisting pressure to push it inward with a tongue blade.

Continued

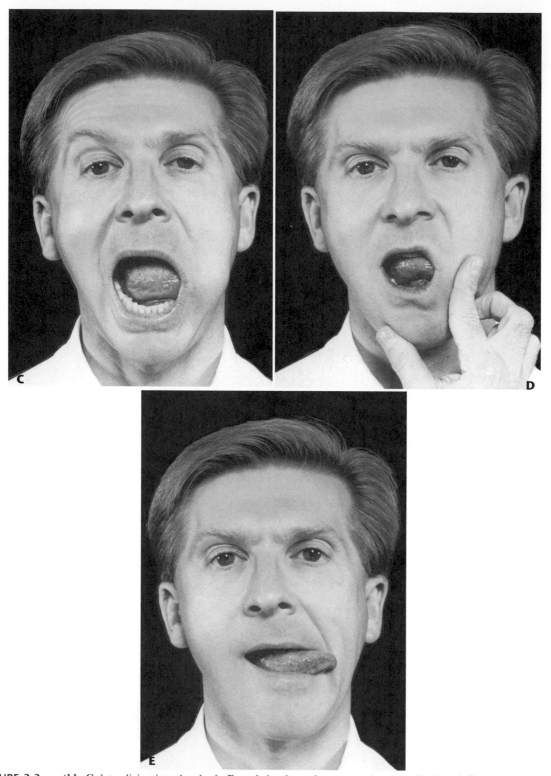

FIGURE 3-3 cont'd. C, lateralizing into the cheek; **D,** resisting inward pressure when lateralized; and, **E,** lateralized outside the mouth, as for lateral lingual alternate motion rates.

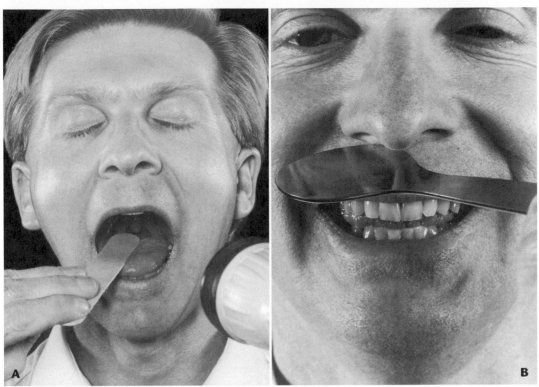

FIGURE 3-4 A, Position for examining the soft palate and pharynx at rest and during phonation and gagging; and, **B,** examining for nasal airflow during prolongation of /i/ or production of pressure consonants.

deviation on repeated trials usually is inconsistent. The meaningfulness of deviation, when subtle, can be determined by having the patient repeat the task several times; consistent deviation to one side may reflect weakness. The following questions should be answered:

- Can the patient protrude the tongue to a normal degree? Does the tongue consistently deviate to one side or the other? Deviation should be judged by the relationship of the tongue to the midline of the chin, especially when unilateral facial weakness is present; an alternative is to hold up the corner of the mouth so that it is roughly symmetric with the unimpaired side, allowing tongue deviation to be judged more validly.
- Can the patient resist the examiner's attempt to push the tongue back into the mouth (a tongue blade placed against the tip of the tongue can be used for this purpose)?

Can the patient push out the cheek on each side with the tongue? If so, can he or she resist pressure from the examiner's finger to push the tongue inward? With the tongue outside the mouth, can the patient resist the examiner's attempt to push the tongue to one side with the tongue blade? Does the

tongue resist pressure at first and then suddenly give way completely?*

The Tongue During Movement

The patient should be asked to move the tongue from side to side as rapidly as possible. Speed, regularity, and range of motion should be noted.

The Velopharynx at Rest

The patient should be asked to open his or her mouth as widely as possible. The tongue should then be depressed gently with a tongue blade (Figure 3-4). The following questions should be answered:

- Does the palate hang low in the mouth? Does it rest on the tongue?

---

*Lingual strength and fatigue can be assessed in a quantifiable way with an instrument known as the Iowa Oral Performance Instrument (IOPI). The IOPI is an air-filled bulb against which the anterior portion of the tongue is pushed, generating a digital readout or analog signal that indexes pressure. It has been used to identify problems of strength or fatigue in children and adults with different neurologic conditions and types of MSDs.[37]

- Are the palatal arches symmetric or does one side hang lower than another? (Normal palates are often mildly asymmetric, especially after tonsillectomy or palatal surgery.)
- Are there spontaneous rhythmic or arrhythmic beating movements of the palate (i.e., myoclonus)?

The Velopharynx During Movement

The patient should be asked to prolong "ah." Important observations relate to the presence, absence, and symmetry of palatal movement. *Inferences about the adequacy of palatal movement for speech on the basis of simple oral inspection should be avoided.* The following questions should be answered:

- Is palatal movement symmetric? If asymmetric, does the palate elevate more strongly to the side opposite that which hung lower at rest?
- Is there evidence of nasal airflow on a mirror held at the nares during vowel prolongation (see Figure 3-4), prolongation or repetition of pressure sounds (/s/, /p/), or words or phrases with nonnasal consonants? Does resonance change during vowel prolongation with the nares occluded versus unoccluded?

The integrity of velopharyngeal closure also can be addressed indirectly by having the patient puff the cheeks and protrude the tongue simultaneously, a procedure known as the *modified tongue-anchor test.*[8,15] The test derives from observations that patients with palatal weakness sometimes impound intraoral pressure by assisting velopharyngeal closure with the back of the tongue. Tongue protrusion during cheek puffing prevents this valving, so the cheeks cannot be puffed, and air will escape nasally if the palate is significantly weak. It sometimes helps if the examiner occludes the nares while the patient puffs and protrudes the tongue, and then releases the nares, observing whether or not air is then emitted nasally. It is important to demonstrate this task to the patient, because some normal individuals have difficulty understanding or coordinating the movements for it. Only the inability to puff the cheeks because of nasal air escape when the tongue is actually protruded is meaningful to the assessment of velopharyngeal weakness. This test may not be valid if there is significant tongue or facial weakness.

To validly observe velopharyngeal activity during speech, videofluoroscopy or nasoendoscopy is necessary. Lateral, frontal, and basal view videofluoroscopy provide good information about palatal, lateral pharyngeal wall, and sphincteric activity of the velopharyngeal mechanism during speech, as does nasoendoscopy. Lateral view videofluoroscopy may be sufficient if documentation of palatal weakness is of primary concern.

The Larynx

The gross integrity of vocal fold adduction can be inferred from two tasks. First, the patient should be asked to cough; the important observation is the *sharpness of the cough,* not its loudness. A weak, "mushy," or breathy cough may reflect vocal fold adductor weakness, poor respiratory support, or both. Second, the patient should be asked to produce a *"coup de glotte" (glottal coup),* which is a sharp glottal stop or grunting sound; this maneuver requires minimal respiratory force and sustained airflow. Again, the *sharpness of the coup* is the important observation. A weak cough but sharp glottal coup may implicate respiratory pathology. A weak coup but normal cough or equally weak cough and coup tends to be associated with laryngeal weakness or combined laryngeal and respiratory weakness.

Weakness of vocal fold abduction can be inferred from the presence of *inhalatory stridor* (noisy or phonated inhalation). This sometimes can be detected during quiet breathing but is more readily detected during rapid inhalation for speech or when the patient takes a deep breath.

Direct visual examination should be pursued whenever structural lesions (e.g., neoplasms, nodules, polyps, inflammation) or LMN lesions of the laryngeal branches of the vagus nerve are a possibility. With regard to CNS lesions, sometimes laryngeal examination identifies vocal fold paresis following UMN stroke[43]; it can also be useful in documenting involuntary laryngeal movements in certain CNS movement disorders. Sophisticated visualization of the larynx can be achieved with an optically precise *rigid oral laryngoscope,* and laryngeal activity during connected speech can be observed with a *flexible fiberoptic laryngoscope. Videostroboscopy* with a rigid or flexible scope provides a simulated slow-motion view of the vocal fold mucosal wave during phonatory vibratory cycles and thus visualization of much more subtle abnormalities of vocal fold function. *Electroglottography* and *acoustic analyses* permit the quantification and analysis of various correlates of vocal fold activity during phonation, but they are rarely necessary to basic clinical diagnosis of MSDs.

Respiration

Hixon and Hoit[20-22] have provided comprehensive, noninstrumental protocols for the clinical examination of the diaphragm, abdominal wall, and rib cage wall in people with known or suspected speech breathing difficulty. They describe observations associated with several tasks that are consistent with normal breathing or with neurologic abnormalities such as weakness, incoordination, and hyperkinesias. They are particularly valuable guides to understanding respiratory movement dynamics and the examination of dysarthric people with prominent or predominant respiratory difficulties. Following is a summary of some useful observations that can be made in the context of a broad-based motor speech examination.

Information about respiratory adequacy for speech can be derived from observations of quiet breathing and a few nonspeech activities. During quiet breathing the following questions should be answered:

- Is posture normal? If not, is the patient slouched in the chair or bent forward or to the side? Does he or she tend to gravitate over time toward abnormal posture, and does it require effort or assistance to resume a more normal posture? Is the head drooped forward? Does it rest on the chest? Is the patient braced in a chair in order to maintain normal posture? Abnormal posture may restrict diaphragm or abdominal or chest wall movements and reduce respiratory support for speech.
- Does the patient complain of shortness of breath at rest, during physical exertion, or during speech? Is breathing rapid, shallow, or labored? (Rate of quiet breathing during wakefulness is about 16 to 18 cycles per minute with each inspiratory and exhalatory cycle taking 2 to 3 seconds.) Are abdominal or chest wall movements asymmetric or limited in range during rest breathing, speech, or maximum inspiration? Is breathing accompanied by shoulder movement, neck extension, retraction of the neck just above the upper sternum on inhalation, or flaring of the nares on inhalation? Rapid, shallow breathing and excessive assistive shoulder or neck movement during breathing may reflect respiratory weakness and predict reduced loudness or phrase length.
- Is breathing rate irregular? Are there any abrupt or slow abdominal or chest wall movements that alter or interrupt normal cyclical breathing during rest breathing, speech, or maximum inspiration? Such irregularities may reflect a movement disorder and predict abnormalities in loudness, prosody, or phrasing.
- Does the patient have *hiccups (singultus)?* Persistent hiccups can be caused by lesions in the medulla and may be an initial manifestation of medullary stroke.[34] They can obviously interfere with respiratory control during speech.
- Sophisticated pulmonary function tests can quantify and often explain sources of abnormal

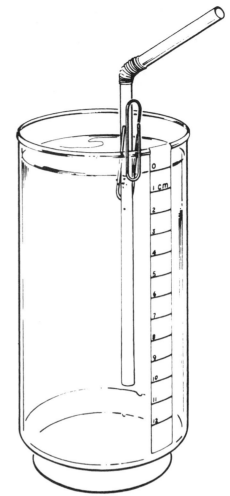

FIGURE 3-5 Water glass manometer for determining ability to generate and sustain respiratory driving pressure sufficient for speech. (From Hixon TJ, Hawley JL, Wilson KJ: An around-the-house device for the clinical determination of respiratory driving pressure: a note on making the simple even simpler, *J Speech Hear Disord* 47:413, 1982, used with permission).

respiratory function. However, in most situations in which respiratory weakness may be present, a few simple tasks can help determine if respiratory support is sufficient for speech.

- As already noted, when weakness is suspected, contrasting the sharpness of the cough versus glottal coup may help separate respiratory from laryngeal contributions to reduced loudness or short phrases. A weak cough with limited abdominal and chest wall excursion may reflect respiratory weakness.
- A simple water glass manometer can be used to estimate the ability to generate respiratory driving pressure sufficient for speech[19] (Figure 3-5). It requires a drinking glass (12 cm or

more in depth) filled with water and calibrated in centimeters and a drinking straw that is affixed by a paper clip to the glass at a given depth. To maintain a stream of bubbles through the straw, a person must sustain breath pressure equal to the depth of the straw in the water. The ability to maintain a stream of bubbles for 5 seconds with the straw at a depth of 5 cm suggests that breath support is sufficient for most speech purposes. For this test to be valid as a measure of respiratory support, the patient must be able to maintain velopharyngeal closure (or have the nares occluded) and a tight lip seal around the straw.

Reflexes

Reflexes can provide confirmatory clues about the gross localization of disease in the CNS or PNS. Those that can be tested in the context of the speech mechanism examination include normal reflexes and primitive or pathologic reflexes. *Normal reflexes are those that reflect normal nervous system function.* Their absence can reflect PNS pathology. *Primitive (or pathologic) reflexes are present during infancy but tend to disappear during maturation;* they may then reappear in the presence of CNS disease, most often in frontal lobe cortical and subcortical regions. Pathologic reflexes represent a *release phenomena,* or reduction of cortical inhibitory influence on lower centers of the brain.

Normal reflexes vary greatly among individuals in the ease with which they are elicited and in the amplitude of the response. Primitive reflexes are present in a certain percentage of normal adults, a percentage that generally increases with age.[23] Therefore the results of oromotor reflex testing can be ambiguous. Cautious interpretation of reflexes as pathologic is required, and not much should be made of them when they are minimally or equivocally present.

1. *Gag reflex*—The gag or pharyngeal reflex is a normal reflex elicited by stroking the back of the tongue, posterior pharyngeal wall, or faucial pillars on both sides with a tongue blade. The afferent pathway for the stimulus is through the glossopharyngeal nerve; the motor response is through the glossopharyngeal and vagus nerves. Elevation of the palate, retraction of the tongue, and sphincteric contraction of the pharyngeal walls characterize the reflex. Normal responses vary greatly, ranging from no response to a vigorous gag elicited merely by touching the tongue.

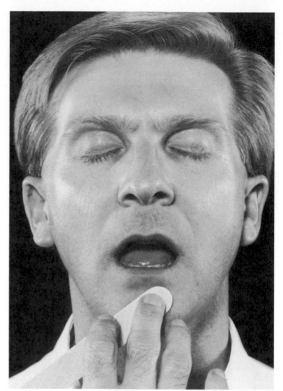

FIGURE 3-6 Position for eliciting the jaw jerk reflex (procedure and response described in text).

In general, the gag reflex is clinically significant only if it is asymmetrically elicited. If absent on one side but not the other, it is probably abnormal on the unresponsive side. When asymmetric it is useful to ask the patient if the stimulus feels different between the two sides; if so, reduced sensation may be responsible for the decreased reflex response. If reported sensation is not different, the motor component of the reflex may be deficient.

2. *Jaw jerk*—The jaw jerk (or maxillary reflex) is a deep muscle stretch reflex that may be pathologic when exaggerated or easily elicited in adults. To test for it, the patient should be relaxed, with the lips parted and the jaw about halfway open. A tongue blade (or fingertip) is placed on the patient's chin, and the blade is then tapped with a reflex hammer or a finger of the other hand (Figure 3-6). The mandibular branch of the trigeminal nerve mediates the afferent and efferent components of the reflex. The reflex is characterized by contraction of the masseter and temporalis muscles, leading to a quick jerk of the jaw toward closing.[4]

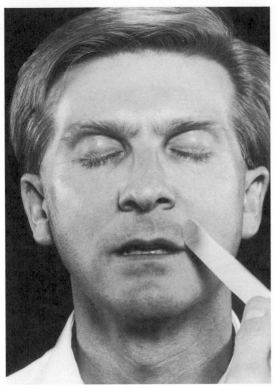

FIGURE 3-7 Position for eliciting the sucking reflex (procedure and response described in text).

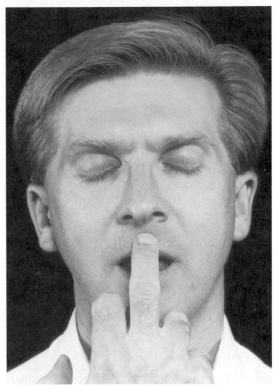

FIGURE 3-8 Position for eliciting the snout reflex (procedure and response described in text).

The jaw jerk is present in about 10% of normal adults.[44] When exaggerated, however, its presence may be confirmatory of bilateral UMN disease above the level of the trigeminal nerve nuclei in the mid pons.

3. *Sucking reflex*—The sucking reflex is a primitive reflex. It is tested by stroking the upper lip with a tongue blade, beginning at the lateral aspect of the upper lip and moving medially toward the philtrum (Figure 3-7). This should be done on both sides. There usually is no response to the stimulus in adults. The positive or pathologic response is a pursing or pouting of the lips. When present, it can be confirmatory of UMN disease above the level of facial nerve nuclei in the pons. It tends to correlate with diffuse involvement of premotor areas of the frontal lobes and is frequently elicited in patients with dementia.[4,44]

When the sucking reflex is very exaggerated, the patient may purse the lips as an object approaches the mouth or may turn the mouth toward a tactile stimulus to the corner of the mouth or cheek. When this occurs, it is called a *rooting reflex.*

4. *Snout reflex*—The primitive snout reflex is similar to the sucking reflex. It can be elicited by a light tap of the finger on the philtrum or tip of the nose[16] (Figure 3-8) or by backward pressure of the examiner's index finger on the midline of the patient's upper lip and philtrum.[23] The reflex is a puckering or protrusion and elevation of the lower lip and depression of the lateral angles of the mouth. Its presence must be interpreted cautiously, because it is present in 17% of normal adults from the third to ninth decades of life, with about double that incidence in people older than age 60.[23]

5. *Palmomental reflex*—The palmomental reflex is a primitive reflex that is elicited by vigorously stroking a blunt object (e.g., a tongue blade) across the palm of the hand. The reflex response is a brief contraction of the mentalis muscle, seen as a slight elevation of muscles in the ipsilateral chin. When pronounced, it may indicate damage to the contralateral paracentral cortex or its projection fibers.[4] Again,

however, about 37% of normal adults from the third to ninth decades have the reflex, with incidence increasing to 60% in the ninth decade.[23] Thus its frequent presence in adults without neurologic disease suggests that it should be interpreted as possibly meaningful only when it is present unilaterally.

Volitional versus "Automatic" Nonspeech Movements of Speech Muscles

Differences can exist between nonspeech volitional movements of speech muscles and movements during relatively automatic or overlearned responses. Differences between movements of the face during emotional responding and voluntary performance have already been discussed.

Just as speech programming ability can be stressed or facilitated, so too can nonspeech programming ability. Whenever supratentorial lesions (particularly dominant hemisphere lesions) or apraxia of speech or aphasia are suspected, the ability to imitate or follow commands for nonspeech movements of the speech muscles should be examined. The goal is to test for *nonverbal oral apraxia*.

The tasks are simple, and several of them are identical to those used in routine oral mechanism examination. They are best elicited by verbal command, but if verbal comprehension is impaired (often the case when aphasia is present), or if the patient comprehends but has difficulty performing a task, imitation should also be used.

The observations are different than those during routine oral mechanism examination. They focus on the ability to perform without off-target approximations, frank errors, or a frustrating awareness that performance is incorrect with accompanying attempts at self-corrections. For example, asked to cough, patients with nonverbal oral apraxia sometimes say "cough, cough" or "huh, huh," then recognize the response's inadequacy and attempt to self-correct. They often improve on imitation but may be inaccurate if tested again a few moments later. Such patients often reflexively perform the acts they cannot do when requested (e.g., unable to cough on command, they may later cough reflexively). These discrepancies reflect a nonverbal oral apraxia and dominant hemisphere pathology. They are frequently but not invariably associated with apraxia of speech and aphasia. Some tasks that are useful for eliciting nonverbal oral apraxia are provided in Box 3-1.[9]

Assessment of Perceptual Speech Characteristics

MSDs can be assessed in many ways. What is important is that the examination elicit behaviors that are

---

box 3-1   Tasks for assessing nonverbal oral movement control and sequencing

Instructions: Ask the patient to perform the following tasks. If he or she fails to respond to a command, use imitation. The following code can be used to score responses:

4. Accurate, immediate, effortless
3. Accurate but awkwardly or slowly produced
2. Accurate after trial and error searching movements
1. Inaccurate or only partially accurate; important component missing or off target

NR = **N**o **r**esponse
V = Accompanying or substituted **v**ocalization or **v**erbalization (e.g., patient says "cough" instead of coughing)
P = **P**erseverative response

Item	Command	Imitation
1. Cough	_____	_____
2. Click your tongue	_____	_____
3. Blow	_____	_____
4. Bite your lower lip	_____	_____
5. Puff out your cheeks	_____	_____
6. Smack your lips	_____	_____
7. Stick out your tongue	_____	_____
8. Lick your lips	_____	_____
9. Bite your lower lip and then click your tongue	_____	_____
10. Smack your lips and then cough	_____	_____

Modified from Darley FL: Differential diagnosis of acquired motor speech disorders. In Darley F, Spriestersbach D, editors: *Diagnostic methods in speech pathology,* ed 2, New York, 1978, Harper & Row.

---

critical to diagnosis and management. It is also important to recognize that *what must be done for diagnostic purposes may not be identical to what is done to establish recommendations for management.* The focus at this point is on methods for identifying the perceptually salient deviant dimensions of speech that lead to diagnosis.

The most useful method for establishing deviant perceptual characteristics of speech derives from the work of DAB. Because their work has been so influential to the understanding of the dysarthrias, and because it remains so clinically relevant, a brief summary of the foundation on which the clinical differential diagnosis of the dysarthrias is based is appropriate.*

---

*See Duffy and Kent[13] for a summary of DAB's contributions to the understanding and scientific study of the dysarthrias, as well as some thoughts about gaps in knowledge and directions for future research.

The Mayo Clinic Dysarthria Studies

The classic text *Motor Speech Disorders*[10] was the outgrowth of extensive clinical research and two important articles that summarized those research efforts.[11,12]

DAB[11,12] analyzed speech samples from 212 patients. A minimum of 30 patients fell into seven groups: (1) bulbar palsy, (2) pseudobulbar palsy, (3) cerebellar lesions, (4) parkinsonism, (5) dystonia, (6) choreoathetosis, and (7) amyotrophic lateral sclerosis (ALS). These groups are equivalent to the categories of flaccid, spastic, ataxic, hypokinetic, hyperkinetic (dystonia and choreoathetosis), and mixed dysarthria, respectively, discussed by DAB in their 1975 book and by many subsequent clinicians and investigators. Each patient had unequivocal neurologic signs and symptoms that placed them into one and only one of the seven groups. Speech was abnormal in all cases. Speech characteristics had not been used to establish neurologic diagnoses.

Audio-recorded samples of reading and, in some cases, conversation and sentence imitation, were reviewed. A list of 38 speech and voice dimensions that seemed pertinent to the range of speech disorders was compiled. The dimensions were related to pitch, loudness, voice and resonance, respiration, prosody, and articulation. Two overall dimensions, intelligibility and bizarreness, were also included.

The authors listened up to 38 times to each sample within each neurologic diagnostic category, each time rating one of the 38 dimensions (certain economies were adopted so that 38 repetitions were not always necessary) on a 7-point, equal-appearing interval scale. Acceptable temporal and interjudge reliability were established.

The deviant speech characteristics for each of the seven groups were analyzed in a manner that allowed comparisons among groups and identification of the most distinctive features within each group. "Clusters" of deviant speech characteristics were also identified. *Clusters represented the tendency for certain deviant speech dimensions to coappear in certain groups of patients.* Each group had a unique pattern of clusters that were logically related to the presumed neuromuscular substrate of the particular neurologic disorder. The analysis also permitted certain inferences about the neuromuscular bases for individual deviant speech characteristics.

DAB expressed hope that their conclusions would serve as hypotheses for "more accurate physiologic and neurophysiologic measurements to further delineate the problems of dysarthria."[12] This was certainly the case, and many subsequent acoustic and physiologic studies have related their findings to the hypotheses of DAB. In addition, numerous subsequent perceptual studies of dysarthria associated with specific neurologic diseases have relied on DAB's methods or the deviant dimensions identified by them. Finally, many clinicians who must differentiate among the dysarthrias rely on their ability to recognize the deviant characteristics and clusters of deviant speech characteristics identified in the work of DAB and subsequent investigators.

Distinctive Speech Characteristics

The distinctive speech characteristics encountered in each of the dysarthrias are addressed in chapters dealing with each dysarthria type. Appendix A lists the 38 dimensions and their definitions, plus several additional characteristics that are relevant to the description of dysarthric speech. The reader should become familiar with all of these terms, because they form the foundation for all subsequent discussion of the dysarthrias.

Box 3-2 is a rating form that may be useful for identifying and rating deviant speech dimensions. It contains all of the characteristics listed in Appendix A. Several features added to the 38 characteristics of DAB are task specific (e.g., AMRs, vowel prolongation).

In our clinic, we rate speech dimensions on a 0 to 4 scale of abnormality (0 = normal, 1 = mild, 2 = moderate, 3 = marked, 4 = severe). This departure from the 7-point scale used by DAB is unimportant, because *the presence of a deviant speech characteristic is generally more important to differential diagnosis than its severity.* The reason for the 0 to 4 scale is its correspondence to commonly used terms for severity (normal, mild, moderate, marked, severe) and its correspondence to the 0 to 4 scale used by many neurologists to rate motor and sensory examination results. It should be noted that the scale can be expanded by 4 points using ratings between categories if necessary (e.g., 0,1 = equivocally present, 2,3 = moderate-marked impairment). Certain dimensions can also be rated plus or minus. For example, rating of reduced loudness can be modified by a minus, increased loudness modified by a plus; when pitch is high it is rated plus, when low minus; when rate is slow it is rated minus, when fast plus. With training and experience, clinicians achieve acceptable reliability when making severity ratings with this scale. The most important challenge to the clinician's ear for diagnostic purposes is learning to detect the presence of deviant dimensions. This is met by experience and the opportunity to check reliability with an experienced clinician.*

---

*A major assumption about the perceptual evaluation of MSDs is that it can be accomplished reliably. Yet such reliability cannot be assumed because perceptual judgments about any behavior can be unreliable. In fact, there are data that document unreliability

| box | 3-2 | Form for rating deviant speech characteristics associated with dysarthria |

Name: _____   Speech diagnosis: _____
Neurologic diagnosis: _____
Age: _____ Date of examination:_____

Dysarthria Rating Scale

Rate speech by assigning a value of 0-4 to each of the dimensions listed below (0 = normal; 1 = mild; 2 = moderate; 3 = marked; 4 = severely deviant). When appropriate, use + to indicate excessive or high and – to indicate reduced or low.

Pitch	Pitch level (+/–) _____	Respiration	Forced inspiration- expiration _____
	Pitch breaks _____		Audible inspiration _____
	Monopitch _____		Inhalatory stridor _____
	Voice tremor _____		Grunt at end of expiration _____
	Myoclonus _____		
	Diplophonia _____ *seen in cp*		
Loudness	Monoloudness _____	**Prosody**	Rate _____
	Excess loudness variation _____		Short phrases _____
	Loudness decay _____		Increased rate in segments ___
	Alternating loudness _____		Increased rate overall _____
	Overall loudness (+/–) ___		Reduced stress _____
			Variable rate _____
			Prolonged intervals _____
			Inappropriate silences _____
			Short rushes of speech _____
			Excess & equal stress _____
Voice quality	Harsh voice _____	**Articulation**	Imprecise consonants _____
	Hoarse (wet) _____		Prolonged phonemes _____
	Breathy voice (continuous) _____		Repeated phonemes _____
	Breathy voice (transient) _____		Irregular articulatory breakdowns _____
	Strained-strangled voice _____		Distorted vowels _____
	Voice stoppages _____		
	Flutter _____		*occurs w/ tourette's*
Resonance (& intraoral pressure)	Hypernasality _____	**Other**	Slow AMRs _____
	Hyponasality _____		Fast AMRs _____
	Nasal emission _____		Irregular AMRs _____
	Weak pressure		*causing* Simple vocal tics _____
	Consonants _____		Palilalia _____
			Coprolalia _____

Modified from dimensions used in Mayo Clinic dysarthria studies,[11,12] plus additional features that may help characterize dysarthria. *AMRs,* Alternating motion rates.

among clinicians and students making perceptual judgments about MSDs.[24,39,40,51,52] However, Kent et al.[29] note that methods used to study reliability probably have not reflected the procedures typically used in clinical practice, and that "the entire examination in either neurology or speech-language pathology may have a robustness that transcends the limitations of individual components of the examination." Duffy and Kent,[13] while stressing the importance of reliability to perceptual descriptions and the diagnosis of dysarthrias, also observed that "it is equally important that studies of reliability, and efforts to train reliability, use methods that represent, approximate, or at least recognize the clinical processes and strategies for arriving at diagnostic conclusions that are used by expert clinicians. If this is ignored, there is a risk that the DAB classification system will be indicted for poor reliability on the basis of evidence derived from studies that have used invalid methods to examine the issue."

Once the ratings have been compiled, they can be used to describe the patient's speech. Experienced clinicians reading an accurate description of deviant speech characteristics often can recognize the important clusters and arrive at an accurate diagnosis without hearing the speech sample. This is not advisable for clinical practice, but it does demonstrate the usefulness of describing speech in this manner.

"Styles" Used for Perceptual Analysis

A symphony can be parsed and its complex underpinnings understood through a careful analysis of its notes, cadence, instruments, and the interactions and temporal relationships among them. Its theme, moods, and message, on the other hand, are best appreciated simply by "taking in" its performance, associating its emotional message with past experience, and appreciating its unique character.

Distinguishing among the dysarthrias can be approached in similar ways. Less experienced clinicians often must be analytic in their approach to diagnosis because they do not yet have an internalized perceptual representation of the dysarthrias for reference. As a result, they carefully identify and list speech characteristics and then match them against the characteristics associated with various dysarthria types. This process is valuable because it trains the ears to recognize salient speech features, and because it is essential to documenting the presence and severity of deviant speech features. What can be missed by this analytic process, however, is the message conveyed by the constant but temporally varying interactions among all of the individual's normal and abnormal speech characteristics. This appreciation of gestalt cannot be obtained by a checklist approach alone.

Experienced clinicians often arrive at a diagnosis by synthesis or complex pattern recognition. They may recognize the speech pattern as a familiar tune, the category of tune represented by a specific dysarthria type. When this occurs, the purpose of listing deviant speech characteristics is to document their presence and severity and summarize some of the reasons for the diagnosis. The risk of this synthesizing approach is that unique and important characteristics may be missed or dismissed, with resultant misdiagnosis. The "taking in" of the pattern of speech, however, can be the most sensitive, reliable, and efficient route to diagnosis.

Tasks for Speech Assessment

A small number of well-selected speech tasks can elicit most of the information necessary for a description and interpretation of abnormal speech. The most important tools for analyzing this information are the ears and eyes of the clinician and an audio or audio-video recorder for repeated analyses when necessary.

The following tasks are designed to isolate as well as possible the respiratory-phonatory, the velopharyngeal, and the articulatory systems for independent assessment and then observe them working together. Because the various tasks differ in their sensitivity to various disorders,[26] their combined use helps ensure detection of deficits that are important to distinguishing among different MSDs.

1. *Vowel prolongation*—Phonation cannot be assessed independent of respiratory function, and disorders at one level can affect function at the other. Fortunately, voice and speech are relatively resistant to respiratory disturbance.

As a result, most neurologic voice abnormalities implicate the laryngeal mechanism rather than the respiratory system.

The simplest task for isolating the respiratory-phonatory system for speech is vowel prolongation. The patient should be instructed to *"take a deep breath and say 'ah' for as long and as steadily as you can, until you run out of air."* This should be followed by a few-second example by the clinician. It is best not to specify pitch or loudness level, because most patients will automatically respond at their habitual pitch and loudness level. If the pitch or loudness produced is noticeably different from conversational levels, the patient should be reinstructed to repeat the task more naturally. It may be necessary to instruct the patient to be higher or lower in pitch, or quieter or louder, and it is often necessary to ask the patient to persist in duration.

The dimensions to be attended to are those categorized under pitch, loudness, and voice quality in Box 3-2. Monopitch and monoloudness should not be rated, because they represent the goal during vowel prolongation. The maximum duration of the vowel should be noted. Maximum vowel duration varies widely among normal speakers; in general, in the absence of other evidence of respiratory or laryngeal abnormality, durations that exceed 8 or 9 seconds can be considered within the normal range for most people (see Table 3-2 for a summary of expected

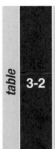

table 3-2 Maximum phonation duration in seconds for the vowel /a/, representing averages across studies of young and elderly (generally older than age 65) male and female adults summarized in Kent, Kent, and Rosenbek's[27] review of maximum performance tests of speech production. Standard deviations are given in parentheses.

	Median*	Minimum†	Maximum‡
Young males	28.5 (8.4)	22.6 (5.5)	34.6 (11.4)
Young females	22.7 (5.7)	15.2 (4.1)	26.5 (11.3)
Elderly males	13.8 (6.3)	13.0 (5.9)	18.1 (6.6)
Elderly females	14.4 (5.7)	10.0 (5.6)	15.4 (5.8)

*Median value of the means and standard deviations reported across studies.
†Lowest mean and lowest standard deviation reported across studies.
‡Highest mean and highest standard deviation reported across studies.
Note: The median of the minimum values in the ranges reported for young males = 15; for young females = 11.8; for elderly males = 8.5; and for elderly females = 6.5.

vowel duration values). Vowel duration can be used as baseline data against which future comparisons can be made, especially when the examiner is convinced that a maximum effort has been made. Acoustic analysis can be used to quantify a number of parameters of voice during vowel prolongation that may be relevant to the description of a dysarthria. For example, it can help disambiguate perceptual uncertainty about whether a tremor is present and can quantify tremor frequency when it is present; measures of variability of fundamental frequency "may be one of the useful indices of phonatory function in relation to neurologic disorder."[30] Direct visualization of the larynx, including videostroboscopy, can identify movement patterns that can confirm or clarify abnormalities associated with paralysis, weakness, tremor, myoclonus, dystonia, and so on.

The jaw, face, tongue, and neck should be observed during vowel prolongation. Patients may display adventitious movements of those structures during what should be a fixed posture task. Quick or slow adventitious movements could represent an underlying movement disorder.

It is appropriate to identify here a disturbance that can compromise the validity of any task designed to assess physiologic support for speech that requires sustained effort or maximum performance. Some patients with damage to the cerebral hemispheres, particularly the right hemisphere, exhibit *motor impersistence,* an inability to maintain simple voluntary acts, such as keeping the eyes closed. When present, motor impersistence may lead to markedly reduced (e.g., <3 seconds) maximum vowel duration, poorly sustained postures during oral mechanism examination—such as keeping the mouth open or protruding the tongue—or poorly sustained speech AMRs or sequential motion rates (SMRs). Motor impersistence probably reflects impairment of mechanisms that permit sustained attention to maintain motor activity.[33] It is not due to reduced physiologic support for motor activity. When present, its possible influence on examination results must be considered.

2. *Alternating motion rates*—AMRs, or *diadochokinetic rates,* are very useful for determining the speed and regularity of reciprocal movements of the jaw, lips, and anterior and posterior tongue. They also permit assessment of articulatory precision, the adequacy of velopharyngeal closure, and respiratory and phonatory support for sustaining the task. These latter observations are usually secondary. *The primary value of AMRs is for assessing speed and regularity of rapid, repetitive articulatory movements.*

The patient should be instructed to *"take a breath and repeat 'puh-puh-puh-puh-puh' for as long and steadily as you can."* This should be followed by a 2- to 3-second example by the clinician. Although the task is to perform for as long as possible, a 3- to 5-second sample usually suffices. Patients can be told to stop when the sample is sufficient for clinical judgments.

When repetitions of /pʌ/ are completed, the patient should be asked to repeat the task for /tʌ/ and /kʌ/. AMRs for other consonant-vowel (CV) syllables can be pursued if other places and manners of articulation are of interest.

Inability to sustain speech AMRs for more than a few seconds often reflects inadequacies at the respiratory-phonatory or velopharyngeal levels. When patients adopt a repetitive rhythm or peculiar cadence, or have difficulty producing regular repetitions, they should be reinstructed or even allowed to practice at a slowed rate before being asked to produce maximum rates. Some patients will produce rapid AMRs at the expense of precision; they should be instructed to go as fast as they can without being imprecise.

Speech AMRs for /pʌ/, /tʌ/, and /kʌ/ usually can be produced precisely at maximum rates of five to seven repetitions per second, with repetition of /kʌ/ usually somewhat slower than /pʌ/ or /tʌ/. Approximate expected values for speech AMRs are summarized in Table 3-3. Acoustic analysis software is now available that will quantify rate and regularity of AMRs automatically, but rates can be adequately estimated with a stopwatch. Experienced clinicians can make judgments of speed and regularity without explicitly computing rate and variability, and the same 0 to 4 scale used for rating perceptual speech characteristics of speech can be employed to do so. For example, mildly slowed AMR rate would be rated −1, severely slowed rate (≈ 1/sec) would be rated −4; markedly rapid rate would be rated +3, and so on. Similarly, mildly irregular AMRs would be rated 1, moderately irregular AMRs rated 2, and so on.

Range of motion of the jaw and lips during speech AMRs should be observed, because it is reduced or variable in some dysarthrias.

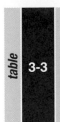

table 3-3	AMR and SMR performance for normal adults across studies of young and elderly adults summarized in Kent, Kent, and Rosenbek's[27] review of maximum performance tests of speech production. Standard deviations are given in parentheses.

Motion Rate Task	Median*	Minimum†	Maximum‡
/pʌ/	6.3 (0.7)	5.0 (0.4)	7.1 (1.2)
/tʌ/	6.2 (0.8)	4.8 (0.4)	7.1 (1.1)
/kʌ/	5.8 (0.8)	4.4 (0.6)	6.4 (1.1)
/pʌtʌkʌ/	5.0 (0.7)	3.6 (0.3)	7.5 (1.3)

AMR, Alternating motion rate; *SMR,* sequential motion rate.
*Median value of the means and standard deviations reported across studies.
†Lowest mean and lowest standard deviation reported across studies.
‡Highest mean and highest standard deviation reported across studies.
Note: The median of the minimum values in the ranges reported for /pʌ/ = 4.8; for /tʌ/ = 4.4; for /kʌ = 4.4; and for /pʌtʌkʌ/ = 4.3.

The rhythmicity of jaw and lip movements should also be observed, because evidence of incoordination can sometimes be seen. Finally, interruptions or extraneous movements of the jaw, lip, and tongue should be noted (e.g., tongue protrusion, lip retraction or pursing, lip smacking), because they may represent an underlying movement disorder.

Speech AMRs are generally slow or normal in rate in people with MSDs, but rapid or accelerated rate can also be pathologic. Irregular AMRs are encountered in some but not all MSDs. Abnormalities of rate and regularity of AMRs are very useful in the identification of several dysarthria types.

3. *Sequential motion rate*—SMR is a measure of ability to move quickly and in proper sequence from one articulatory position to another. Relative to AMRs, sequencing demands for SMRs are heavy; for this reason, *SMRs are particularly useful when apraxia of speech is suspected.*

The patient should be asked to *"take a breath and repeat 'puh-tuh-kuh' over and over again until I tell you to stop."* This should be followed by a 2- to 3-second example by the clinician. Some people need reinstruction in the sequence, and slow or unison practice is sometimes necessary for the task to be grasped. When the sequence cannot be learned, repetition of "buttercup, buttercup, buttercup . . ." is acceptable, but the meaningfulness of the word makes it a simpler task than /pʌtʌkʌ/.

4. *Contextual speech*—The most useful task for evaluating the integrated function of all components of speech, and each of the primary valves, is contextual speech. This includes conversational and narrative speech, as well as reading aloud a standard paragraph containing a representative phonetic sample. The well-known Grandfather Passage is often used for this purpose (see Appendix B).

Conversational speech is elicited during history taking, but the clinician's formal identification of deviant speech characteristics may be deferred so the facts of the history can be attended to. Open-ended questions about the patient's family, work, or hobbies usually elicit a sample sufficient to judge speech characteristics, but sometimes personality traits, depression, anxiety, or cognitive deficits limit responsiveness. Some people respond more readily with narratives about pictured scenes than to more open-ended inquiries.

Reading a standard passage can provide a good sample of connected speech, but adults' ability to read aloud varies widely. Less skilled readers may read slowly, hesitantly, and with pronunciation errors and prosodic features that are inconsistent with their conversational prosody. When such problems are pronounced, reading can be misleading or of little value.

5. *Stress testing*—People with MSDs are susceptible to the effects of fatigue. In fact, regardless of dysarthria type, they often complain of speech deterioration with prolonged conversation or with general physical fatigue over the course of a day. These complaints are obviously important to management issues, but because fatigue is so common it is usually unnecessary to observe its effects on speech for diagnostic purposes. However, whenever LMN weakness of unknown cause is present, or when the patient complains of rapid or dramatic changes in speech with continued speaking or general physical effort, speech stress testing should be pursued. To assess fatigue, the patient should be asked to read aloud naturally or count as precisely as possible at a rate of about two digits per second. This should be continued without rest for 2 to 4 minutes. Significant deterioration of voice quality, resonance, or articulation consistent with perceptual characteristics associated with weakness may reflect the presence of myasthenia gravis, especially if speech then improves significantly after a minute or two of rest. Testing speech muscle

strength before and after stress testing may provide confirmatory evidence of weakness.

6. *Assessing motor speech planning or programming capacity*—Sometimes people produce distorted articulatory substitutions, omissions, repetitions, or additions. They may block, hesitate, or engage in trial-and-error groping for correct articulatory postures during conversation or reading. When this occurs, or when dominant hemisphere pathology is suspected, further assessment of speech motor planning or programming ability should be pursued. An apraxia of speech may be present.

If speech is mildly to moderately impaired, the patient should be asked to perform speech SMRs and to repeat complex multisyllabic words and sentences. Box 3-3[45] provides a list of stimuli that have proven useful for this purpose.

If the patient is mute or barely able to speak, tasks that facilitate speech or place minimal demands on novel motor planning or programming should be used. These tasks include singing a familiar tune, counting, saying the days of the week, completing redundant sentences, and imitating consonant-vowel-consonant (CVC) syllables with identical initial and final consonants. Sometimes, but not invariably, people find it easier to imitate isolated sounds than syllables or words. People with apraxia of speech may respond to these simple tasks with greater ease, making the salient auditory perceptual features of their apraxia more evident. A mismatch between ease of response on complex voluntary tasks versus simpler "automatic" tasks increases the likelihood that apraxia of speech and not dysarthria is the correct diagnosis.

Published Tests for the Diagnosis of Dysarthria

There is only one published test that quantifies distinctions among dysarthria types. A few published measures are available for assessing intelligibility in dysarthria, but they are not intended to establish the presence or type of dysarthria.

The only published diagnostic test is the *Frenchay Dysarthria Assessment (FDA)*.[14] The FDA relies on a rating scale applied to patient-provided information, observations of nonverbal oral structures and functions, and speech. Measures of intelligibility and speaking rate are also made, as well as judgments about hearing, vision, dentition, language, mood, posture, and sensation. The task-oriented portion of the test focuses on reflexes, speech and nonspeech activities of respiration, the lips, jaw, soft palate, tongue and larynx, and the measurement of intelligibility (the intelligibility portion of the test is discussed in the section on intelligibility assessment). The FDA is brief and does not require extensive training to administer and score.

Interjudge reliability coefficients for the test are acceptably high after 3 hours of training. It appears that the test distinguishes among flaccid, spastic, ataxic, hypokinetic, and mixed flaccid-spastic dysarthria with a high degree of accuracy. For example, a discriminant analysis of results for 85 patients with neurologic diagnoses consistent with sites of damage associated with each of the five dysarthria types correctly classified 91% of the patients. Correct classification across dysarthria types ranged from 83% to 100%. The test manual also indicates that an "independent diagnosis" based only on FDA profiles—not direct observation of patients—was in agreement with patients' therapists for 91% of 112 dysarthric patients.

The test manual provides graphs of the means and standard deviations for each of the dysarthria types examined (three of the five groups had fewer than 15 patients). It is clear that there is considerable overlap among the dysarthria types for many of the FDA subtests. Criteria for objectively determining dysarthria type are not provided, nor are the discriminant function formulas that would permit subject placement into a dysarthria category prospectively.

The FDA demonstrates that distinctions among patients with different dysarthria types can be quantified and that the distinctions correlate with neurologic diagnosis. The test relies heavily on patient report and ratings of nonspeech oral activities, and it does not yield a comprehensive description of specific deviant speech characteristics associated with each dysarthria type. For these reasons, it may be viewed most appropriately as a test that distinguishes among patients with different lesion loci on the basis of nonverbal oral findings and certain speech characteristics, rather than a differential diagnostic test of the auditory perceptual features of dysarthria per se. However, with the addition of data for other dysarthria types (e.g., hyperkinetic dysarthrias), an increase in the number of cases per type to the database and discriminant analyses, and provision of discriminant function formulas or other criteria for quantitatively determining dysarthria type for individual patients, the FDA could have increased value as a diagnostic measure of dysarthria.

Published Tests for the Diagnosis of Apraxia of Speech

The only currently available published measure for the assessment of apraxia of speech is the *Apraxia Battery for Adults—Second Edition (ABA-2)*.[7] The

The tasks below require imitation or speaking in response to simple requests. Other tasks that are useful and important for assessing motor programming ability include conversation, narrative picture description, and reading aloud.

Scoring: The following codes may be used to capture response characteristics that may reflect apraxic behaviors.

Distortion (D)
Groping (audible or visible) (G)
Distorted substitution (DS)
Attempts at articulatory self-correction (SC)
Delayed response initiation (DR)

Awareness of errors (AOE)
Slow rate (SR)
Syllable × segregation within multisyllabic words, phrases (S × S)

A numeric code, adapted from the *Porch Index of Communicative Ability,*[36] may also be useful.

15 = correct in all respects
14 = distorted
13 = delayed to respond
10 = self-corrected articulatory
9 = correct after a stimulus response repetition
7 = error clearly related to target

6 = error unrelated to target
5 = rejection or stated inability to respond
4 = unintelligible but differentiated from other responses
3 = unintelligible & relatively undifferentiated from other responses

Broad or narrow transcription of responses can be helpful.

I. "Repeat these sounds after me"

1. /i/ _____   11. /k/ _____
2. /a/ _____   12. /g/ _____
3. /u/ _____   13. /s/ _____
4. /ei/ _____   14. /f/ _____
5. /ai/ _____   15. /tʃ/ _____
6. /au/ _____
7. /m/ _____
8. /p/ _____
9. /t/ _____
10. /n/ _____

II. "Repeat these words after me"

1. mom _____   11. zoos _____
2. Bob _____   12. church _____
3. peep _____   13. shush _____
4. bib _____   14. lull _____
5. tot _____   15. roar _____
6. deed _____
7. kick _____
8. gag _____
9. fife _____
10. sis _____

III. "Repeat these words"

1. cat _____
catnip _____
catapult _____
catastrophe _____
2. please _____
pleasing _____
pleasingly _____
3. thick _____
thicken _____
thickening _____

IV. "Repeat these words three times"

1. animal _____ _____ _____
2. snowman _____ _____ _____
3. artillery _____ _____ _____
4. stethoscope _____ _____ _____
5. rhinoceros _____ _____ _____
6. volcano _____ _____ _____
7. harmonica _____ _____ _____
8. specify _____ _____ _____
9. statistics _____ _____ _____
10. aluminum _____ _____ _____

V. "Repeat these sentences"

1. We saw several wild animals. _____
2. My physician wrote out a prescription. _____
3. The municipal judge sentenced the criminal. _____

VI. "Repeat as fast and as steadily as possible"

1. /pʌpʌpʌpʌ . . ./_____   3. /kʌkʌkʌkʌ . . ./_____
2. /tʌtʌtʌtʌ . . ./_____   4. /pʌtʌkʌpʌtʌkʌ . . ./_____

VII. "Count from 1 to 10"

1. _____   6. _____
2. _____   7. _____
3. _____   8. _____
4. _____   9. _____
5. _____   10. _____

VIII. "Say the days of the week"

1. Sunday ___   5. Thursday ___
2. Monday ___   6. Friday ___
3. Tuesday ___   7. Saturday ___
4. Wednesday ___

IX. "Sing" ("Happy Birthday," "Jingle Bells," or another familiar tune)

1. How well is the tune carried? _____
2. How adequate is articulation? _____

X. Description of conversation and narrative speech. _____

XI. Description of reading aloud. _____

Modified from Wertz RT, LaPointe LL, Rosenbek JC: *Apraxia of speech: the disorder and its treatment,* New York, 1984, Grune & Stratton and unpublished Mayo Clinic tasks for assessing apraxia of speech.

ABA-2 was developed to "verify the presence of apraxia in the adult patient and to estimate the severity of the disorder,"[7] as well as to assist in designing treatment and documenting progress. It contains six subtests, five of which focus on speech or speech-related responses; the sixth subtest assesses limb and nonverbal oral apraxia. The subtests related to speech include (1) diadochokinetic rates for one-, two-, and three-syllable combinations; (2) imitation of words of increasing length; (3) latency and utterance time for naming of pictured multisyllabic words; (4) articulatory adequacy during three consecutive repetitions of polysyllabic words; and (5) an inventory of 15 behaviors or findings based on spontaneous speech, reading, and counting that the author associates with apraxia of speech. It should be noted that not all of the characteristics listed as apraxic in the inventory are unique to the disorder (i.e., some may also occur as manifestations of aphasia), and some may not be characteristic of apraxia of speech at all.

The test was standardized on a sample of 40 persons with apraxia and 49 people with normal speech. Cutoff scores are provided for determining the presence and level of impairment, and guidance is provided for recognizing and interpreting "atypical profiles." Guidance is also provided about treatment planning. The test manual presents data that led to a conclusion that the test is a reliable and valid measure of apraxia, but there are some shortcomings in this regard. For example, test-retest, intrajudge, and interjudge reliability are not reported, and data comparing apraxic to aphasic and dysarthric performance are based on small numbers of aphasic and dysarthric speakers. The latter shortcoming introduces uncertainty about the test's ability to distinguish apraxic from aphasic and dysarthric performance.

The ABA-2 can be administered in a standard fashion to patients with diagnosed or suspected apraxia of speech. Scores can be used to describe patient performance, compare performance over time, and perhaps quantify the diagnosis and severity of the problem. Reliability and validity have not been completely established. Regarding its diagnostic value, the test would benefit from a comparison with some standard for diagnosis. Because there is no other well-established, standardized test for apraxia of speech, judgments by experienced clinicians who agree on clinical criteria for diagnosis should probably represent the "gold standard" for examining this aspect of test validity.

Assessment of Intelligibility, Comprehensibility, and Efficiency

The impact of an MSD on the ability to communicate can be estimated through judgments or measures of intelligibility, comprehensibility, and efficiency. The next few paragraphs rely heavily on the work of Yorkston, Strand, and Kennedy[49] and Yorkston et al.[50] to discuss these concepts. When intelligibility (I), comprehensibility (C), and efficiency (E) are discussed collectively in subsequent paragraphs, they are referred to as *ICE*.

Intelligibility is the degree to which a listener understands the acoustic signal produced by a speaker. In people with MSDs, estimates of intelligibility reflect the acoustic accomplishment of the impaired speech system plus strategies used by the speaker to improve speech production.

Comprehensibility is the degree to which a listener understands speech on the basis of the acoustic signal plus all other information that may contribute to understanding what has been said. The additional information is independent of the acoustic signal and includes knowledge of the topic, semantic and syntactic context, the general physical setting, gestures and signs, orthographic cues, and so on.

Efficiency refers to the rate at which intelligible or comprehensible information is conveyed. It is an important supplement to measures of intelligibility and comprehensibility because it contributes to both the perception of speech normalcy and the normalcy of communication (by whatever means) in social contexts. For example, some people with MSDs are highly intelligible but very inefficient because speech rate is markedly slow; the severity of an MSD is greater in someone with moderately reduced intelligibility and slow rate than someone with comparable intelligibility and normal rate. Some people with MSDs can convey messages using speech and supplemental strategies that are highly comprehensible but so time consuming that their social "success" is limited.

The distinction between intelligibility and comprehensibility is important for at least two practical reasons. First, it tells us that estimates of intelligibility (and its efficiency) are a more valid measure of the functional limitations imposed by MSDs (i.e., the ability to speak normally), whereas estimates of comprehensibility (and its efficiency) are a more valid measure of the disability imposed by MSDs in social, communicative contexts. As a result, intelligibility and comprehensibility (and their efficiency) are distinct ways to describe severity.

The second reason follows from the first. If treatment focuses on reducing impairment or functional limitations imposed by an MSD (i.e., improving the acoustic signal), then intelligibility and its efficiency become the most valid, practical index of change. If treatment focuses on reducing disability (i.e., by also positively manipulating variables independent of the acoustic signal), then comprehensibility and its efficiency become the most valid, practical index of change.

When an MSD is mild, intelligibility and comprehensibility may be unaffected. In fact, MSDs are sometimes so mild that even efficiency, at least from a functional standpoint, also is not compromised. Nevertheless, ICE should always be addressed, because it has great face and ecologic validity as indices of severity. These assessments can range from subjective estimates during interaction with the patient to formal, standardized, quantitative testing.

The degree to which assessment of ICE is pursued depends on the purposes of examination. If the primary purpose is to diagnose or determine the need for treatment, general ratings of ICE can suffice. Such ratings may include judgments by the patient,

significant other, and the clinician. The patient and significant other can be asked if ICE is a problem, how frequently and under what circumstances, and what is generally done to ensure a message is understood (e.g., repetition, yes-no questioning, writing). The clinician may estimate a percentage of intelligible or comprehensible speech based on observations during examination, noting the circumstances under which the judgment is based (e.g., in quiet, with visual contact, when the topic of conversation is known). An estimate of intelligibility or comprehensibility in other (usually less ideal) situations may also be made. Table 3-4 contains a scale that we have found reliable and useful for estimating intelligibil-

table 3-4	Intelligibility rating scale for motor speech disorders

Rating	Dimension	Intelligibility is . . .
10	Environment*	Normal in all environments
	Content[†]	without restrictions on content
	Efficiency[‡]	without need for repairs
9	Environment	Sometimes[§] reduced under adverse conditions
	Content	when content is unrestricted
	Efficiency	but adequate with repairs
8	Environment	Sometimes reduced under ideal conditions
	Content	when content is unrestricted
	Efficiency	but adequate with repairs
7	Environment	Sometimes reduced under adverse conditions
	Content	even when content is restricted
	Efficiency	but adequate with repairs
6	Environment	Sometimes reduced under ideal conditions
	Content	when content is unrestricted
	Efficiency	even when repairs are attempted
5	Environment	Usually[¶] reduced under adverse conditions
	Content	when content is unrestricted
	Efficiency	even when repairs are attempted
4	Environment	Usually reduced under ideal conditions
	Content	even when content is restricted
	Efficiency	but adequate with repairs
3	Environment	Usually reduced under adverse conditions
	Content	even when content is restricted
	Efficiency	even when repairs are attempted
2	Environment	Usually reduced under ideal conditions
	Content	even when content is restricted
	Efficiency	even when repairs are attempted
1	Speech is not a viable means of communication in any environment, regardless of restrictions in content or attempts at repair	

*Environment may be "ideal" (e.g., face-to-face, without visual or auditory deficits in the listener, without competition from noise or visual distractions) or "adverse" (e.g., at a distance, with visual or auditory deficits or distractions).
[†]Content may be "unrestricted" (includes all pragmatically appropriate content, new topics, lengthy narratives, etc.) or "restricted" (e.g., limited to brief responses to questions or statements that permit some prediction of response content).
[‡]Efficiency may be "normal" (rarely in need of repetition or clarification because of poor speech production) or "repairs" may be necessary (repetition, restatement, responses to clarifying questions, modified production such as oral spelling, word-by-word confirmation of listener's repetition, spelling, etc.)
[§]Intelligibility is reduced in 25% or less of utterances.
[¶]Intelligibility is reduced in 50% or more of utterances but not for all utterances.
Note: Not all combinations of deviant dimensions can be captured by a 10-point scale, and there is an obvious gray area between the meaning of "sometimes" and "usually." The point on the scale that most closely approximates the clinician's judgment should be used. Many patients may fit into more than one point on the scale. It is appropriate to assign a range rather than a single point in such cases (e.g., 5-6).

ity that also considers contributions from variables related to comprehensibility, such as speaking environment and message complexity or predictability.

Although comprehensibility of dysarthric speech has been studied, standardized tests for its assessment have not been developed. Measures of intelligibility have received more attention and are therefore emphasized here.

A quantitative estimate of intelligibility can be valuable as a baseline measure when the patient will be treated to improve intelligibility; when an objective, quantified estimate of severity must be made for medical-legal purposes; when treatment may not be pursued but when the patient is to be followed over time to document improvement, stability, or deterioration as a function of medical or surgical intervention, disease progression, and so on; or for research purposes.

Only a few measures have been developed for assessing intelligibility in adult dysarthric speakers. Virtually none have been designed specifically for apraxia of speech, although some of those available for dysarthria can probably be adapted for patients with apraxia of speech if aphasia is not a significant problem.

Assessment of Intelligibility in Dysarthric Speakers (AIDS)[46]

For many years, the AIDS has been the most widely used standardized test for measuring intelligibility, speaking rate, and communicative efficiency in people with dysarthria. It quantifies intelligibility of words and sentences and provides an estimate of communication efficiency by examining the rate of intelligible words per minute in sentences. The single word task requires the patient to read or imitate 50 words randomly selected from among 12 phonetically similar words for each of the 50 items. A judge listens to an audio recording of the responses and identifies the spoken words in a multiple-choice format in which the 12 choices for each word are listed or in a transcription format in which the spoken word is transcribed. The intelligibility score is the percentage of words identified correctly.

In the sentence task, the patient reads or imitates two sentences each, of 5 to 15 words in length, for a total of 220 words. Sentences are selected randomly from a master pool of 100 sentences of each length. The judge transcribes the sentences word by word. The intelligibility score is the percentage of words transcribed correctly.

At least two people must be involved in assessment, one to select the sample for assessment and the other to listen and transcribe or respond in a multiple-choice format to the recorded sample. Repeated assessments for a given patient over time must either use the same judge or groups of judges to control for interjudge variability.

A measure of speaking rate during the sentence task is derived by dividing the number of words (220) by the duration of the sentence sample. Rate of intelligible speech is the number of correctly transcribed words divided by the total duration; a similar measure for rate of unintelligible words can also be computed. The rate of intelligible speech per minute is then divided by 190 (the mean rate of intelligible speech produced by normal speakers on the test, who are nearly 100% intelligible), yielding a *communicative efficiency ratio*. This measure may be particularly useful for mildly impaired speakers whose rate may be slow in spite of good intelligibility.[47]

The AIDS provides an index of severity of impairment, an estimate of the patient's deviation from normal, and a standard for monitoring change over time. Test-retest variability for the word-list test, allowing for differences between stimuli and day-to-day variability, is less than 5%. Variability between sentence lists for the sentence test, however, even within the same day, is higher (approximately 9% to 11%). This latter degree of variability led Yorkston and Beukelman to recommend establishment of stable baseline measures of intelligibility before starting intervention, if the test is to be used to help document treatment effects.

Sentence Intelligibility Test (SIT)[48]

The SIT is an updated Windows version of the sentence portion of the AIDS. It offers a considerable improvement over its predecessor relative to stimulus selection, automaticity and speed of scoring, and data storage.

The SIT is based on the same principles of testing as the AIDS, and it uses the same basic computations to yield measures of intelligibility, rate of intelligible speech, and efficiency. The software package allows for administration, scoring, and storage of results. The program will randomly select 22 or 11 (short version) stimulus sentences from a pool of 1100 sentences ranging from 5 to 15 words in length. The speaker is recorded while reading or imitating the selected sentences. As is the case for the AIDS, the examiner administering the test and the judge transcribing responses must be different people. The computer program computes all relevant scores based on the judge's transcription and marking of timing data.

Several indices of interjudge reliability are provided in the test manual, and they indicate that dispersion of intelligibility and intelligible words per minute scores within a 10% to 20% range fell in the 83% to 100% range, with interjudge correlations all exceeding 0.9. Correlations between scores for different performances by the same speaker also all exceeded 0.9.

Frenchay Dysarthria Assessment (FDA)[14]

The FDA (already discussed) has a component that evaluates the intelligibility of words, sentences, and conversation. In the word task, 10 stimuli are drawn randomly from a set of 50 words. The 10 words, unknown to the examiner, are read by the patient. Performance on the task is rated on a 5-point scale with points on the scale reflecting differences in the number of words correctly recognized or the ease with which they are recognized. Although some of the words on the 50-item list are distinguished by minimal contrasts (park, dark), the 50 stimuli are heterogenous in frequency of occurrence, number of phonemes and syllables, and stress pattern. This word heterogeneity causes problems in selecting equivalent lists, and the intervals between points on the 5-point rating scale may not be equal.[32]

The sentence task is administered and scored like the word task. The sentences actually consist of a standard carrier phrase "the man is" with the final word represented by one of 50 randomly selected words ending with "ing." This task is thus more a measure of single word intelligibility within a sentence context than sentence intelligibility per se.

The conversation task is based on about 5 minutes of conversation that is graded on a 5-point severity scale ranging from "no abnormality" to "totally unintelligible" speech. Although the scale represents a ranking of impaired intelligibility, its quantitative value is limited.

A Word Intelligibility Test

Kent et al.[32] have designed two word intelligibility tests for use with dysarthric speakers. Although not published as standardized tests, they deserve mention because they provide clinically useful information beyond percentage scores for intelligibility and efficiency.

Both tests are single word measures. An intelligibility score representing percentage of intelligible words is generated by judgments of words read by a speaker. The word stimuli and organization of response choices permit examination of 19 phonetic contrasts that may be vulnerable in dysarthria (e.g., front-back vowel contrasts, voicing contrasts for initial and final consonants, fricative-affricate contrasts). The phonetic contrasts have acoustic correlates (e.g., voice onset time and preceding vowel duration for initial and final voicing contrasts, respectively), which permit a more in-depth exploration of features associated with decreased intelli-

gibility. The phonetic feature analysis extends perceptual findings by identifying the effect on articulation or phonetic outcomes of laryngeal and velopharyngeal dysfunction.[32]

In the multiple-choice version, the speaker reads one of four words distinguished by minimal phonetic contrasts (e.g., beat, boot, bit, meat). There are 70 minimal contrast items in the test and any of the four contrasting words for each item can be used (e.g., there are 280 test words). This allows random selection of one of the four words for each of the 70 items, so repeated assessments may be conducted with the same judges.

The paired-word version is designed for use with severely dysarthric patients who cannot reliably produce more complex CVC syllables. Its items consist almost entirely of minimal contrasts within CV or VC syllables (e.g., shoe-chew, eat-it). Sixteen contrasts are tested in three word pairs each.

The test's ability to quantify intelligibility and identify the locus of phonetic difficulties that contribute most to reduced intelligibility has been documented for adults with ataxic, hypokinetic, and various mixed dysarthrias associated with several neurologic diseases (e.g., amyotrophic lateral sclerosis [ALS], cerebral palsy, stroke, parkinsonism, and multiple sclerosis).[1,6,25,28,31,32] The information about the phonetic contributors to reduced intelligibility provided by the test could aid decisions about treatment focus and, possibly, diagnosis. Because the phonetic contrasts examined in the test have measurable acoustic counterparts, test results may also influence the choice of relevant acoustic analyses for individual speakers or specific dysarthria types. These combined attributes have the potential to refine perceptual analyses, direct acoustic and physiologic analyses, document severity, guide emphasis in treatment, and perhaps establish distinctive patterns of phonetic deficits associated with specific dysarthria types.

SUMMARY

1. Diagnosis of MSDs depends on adequate examination of speech and the speech mechanism. Examination includes description, establishing diagnostic possibilities, establishing a diagnosis, establishing implications for localization and disease diagnosis, and specifying severity.

2. The essential components of the motor speech examination include the history; examination of the oral mechanism; assessment of salient features of speech; estimation of intelligibility and severity; and, when appropriate, acoustic and physiologic measures.

3. The history requires goal setting with the patient and acquiring information about relevant events before the onset of speech deficits, the onset and course of the speech problem, the course and nature of associated deficits, the patient's perception of the speech problem and its consequences, current or prior management of the speech problem, and the patient's awareness of the medical diagnosis and prognosis.

4. Speech assessment relies heavily on identification of deviant speech characteristics. Speech tasks include vowel prolongation, AMRs, SMRs, contextual speech, stress testing, and tasks for stressing or facilitating motor speech programming. Accurate diagnosis ideally relies on an analytic approach in which deviant speech characteristics and clusters are identified, plus a synthetic appreciation of the "global" product of all speech characteristics interacting with one another.

5. Examination of the oral mechanism at rest and during nonspeech activities provides confirmatory evidence and information about the size, strength, symmetry, range, tone, steadiness, speed, and accuracy of orofacial structures and their movements. Observations of speech structures are made at rest, during sustained postures and movement, and in response to reflex testing. Assessing volitional versus automatic nonspeech movements of the speech muscles is also important when nonverbal oral apraxia is suspected.

6. Assessments of the intelligibility, comprehensibility, and efficiency of speech serve as indices of the impact of MSDs on the ability to communicate, and as indices of change over time. They can be estimated through clinical judgments or quantitative measures. Estimates of intelligibility reflect the functional impact of MSDs, by themselves, on spoken communication, whereas estimates of comprehensibility reflect the degree of disability imposed by MSDs, allowing for the contribution that information from nonspeech modalities and strategies make to the understanding of speech.

References

1. Ansel BM, Kent RD: Acoustic-phonetic contrasts and intelligibility in the dysarthria associated with mixed cerebral palsy, J Speech Hear Res 35:296, 1992.
2. Borod JC, Haywood CS, Koff E: Neuropsychological aspects of facial asymmetry during emotional expression: a review of the normal adult literature, Neuropsychol Rev 7:41, 1997.
3. Borod JC et al: Facial asymmetry during emotional expression: gender, valence, and measurement, Neuropsychologia 36:1209, 1998.
4. Brazis P, Masdeu JC, Biller J: Localization in clinical neurology, ed 4, Philadelphia, 2001, Lippincott Williams & Wilkins.
5. Brodley CE, Lane T, Stough TM: Knowledge discovery and data mining, Am Sci 87:54, 1999.
6. Bunton K et al: The effects of flattening fundamental frequency contours on sentence intelligibility in speakers with dysarthria, Clin Linguist Phon 15:181, 2001.
7. Dabul B: Apraxia battery for adults, ed 2, Austin, Tex, 2000, Pro-Ed.
8. Dalston R, Warren DW, Dalston ET: The modified tongue-anchor technique as a screening test for velopharyngeal inadequacy: a reassessment, J Speech Hear Disord 55:510, 1990.
9. Darley FL: Differential diagnosis of acquired motor speech disorders. In Darley F and Spriestersbach D, editors: Diagnostic methods in speech pathology, ed 2, New York, 1978, Harper & Row.
10. Darley FL, Aronson AE, Brown JR: Motor speech disorders, Philadelphia, 1975, WB Saunders.
11. Darley FL, Aronson AE, Brown JR: Clusters of deviant speech dimensions in the dysarthrias, J Speech Hear Res 12:462, 1969a.
12. Darley FL, Aronson AE, Brown JR: Differential diagnostic patterns of dysarthria, J Speech Hear Res 12:246, 1969b.
13. Duffy JR, Kent RD: Darley's contribution to the understanding, differential diagnosis, and scientific study of the dysarthrias, Aphasiology 15:275, 2001.
14. Enderby P: Frenchay dysarthria assessment, San Diego, 1983, College-Hill Press.
15. Fox DR, Johns DF: Predicting velopharyngeal closure with a modified tongue-anchor technique, J Speech Hear Disord 35:248, 1970.
16. Gilroy J, Meyer JS: Medical neurology, New York, 1979, Macmillan Publishing.
17. Hager JC, Ekman P: The asymmetry of facial actions is inconsistent with models of hemispheric specialization, Psychophysiology 23:307, 1985.
18. Hausmann M et al: Sex differences in oral asymmetries during word repetition, Neuropsychologia 36:1397, 1998.
19. Hixon TJ, Hawley JL, Wilson KJ: An around-the-house device for the clinical determination of respiratory driving pressure: a note on making the simple even simpler, J Speech Hear Disord 47:413, 1982.
20. Hixon TJ, Hoit JD: Physical examination of the rib cage wall by the speech-language pathologist, Am J Speech-Lang Pathol 9:179, 2000.
21. Hixon TJ, Hoit JD: Physical examination of the abdominal wall by the speech-language pathologist, Am J Speech-Lang Pathol 8:335, 1999.
22. Hixon TJ, Hoit JD: Physical examination of the diaphragm by the speech-language pathologist, Am J Speech-Lang Pathol 7:37, 1998.
23. Jacobs L, Gossman MD: Three primitive reflexes in normal adults, Neurology 30:184, 1980.
24. Kearns KP, Simmons NN: Interobserver reliability and perceptual ratings: more than meets the ear, J Speech Hear Res 31:131, 1988.
25. Kent JF et al: Quantitative description of the dysarthria in women with amyotrophic lateral sclerosis, J Speech Hear Res 35:723, 1992.

26. Kent RD, Kent JF: Task-based profiles of the dysarthrias, Folia Phoniatr Logop 52:48, 2000.

27. Kent RD, Kent JF, Rosenbek JC: Maximum performance tests of speech production, J Speech Hear Disord 52:367, 1987.

28. Kent RD et al: Ataxic dysarthria, J Speech Lang Hear Res 43:1275, 2000.

29. Kent RD et al: The dysarthrias: speech-voice profiles, related dysfunctions, and neuropathology, J Med Speech-Lang Pathol 6:165, 1998.

30. Kent RD et al: A speaking task analysis of the dysarthria in cerebellar disease, Folia Phoniatr Logop 49:63, 1997.

31. Kent RD et al: Impairment of speech intelligibility in men with amyotrophic lateral sclerosis, J Speech Hear Disord 55:721, 1990.

32. Kent RD et al: Toward phonetic intelligibility testing in dysarthria, J Speech Hear Disord 54:482, 1989.

33. Kertesz A et al: Motor impersistence: a right-hemisphere syndrome, Neurology 35:662, 1985.

34. Macken MP et al: Cranial neuropathies. In Bradley WG et al, editors: Neurology in clinical practice: principles of diagnosis and management, vol 2, ed 3, Boston, 2000, Butterworth-Heinemann.

35. Monrad-Krohn GH: On the dissociation of voluntary and emotional innervation in facial paresis of central origin, Brain 47:22, 1924.

36. Porch BE: Porch index of communicative ability, Palo Alto, Calif, 1967, Consulting Psychologists Press.

37. Robin DA et al: Nonspeech assessment of the speech production mechanism. In McNeil MR, editor: Clinical management of sensorimotor speech disorders, New York, 1997, Thieme.

38. Rowland LP: Signs and symptoms in neurologic diagnosis. In Rowland LP, editor: Merritt's textbook of neurology, ed 8, Philadelphia, 1989, Lea & Febiger.

39. Sheard C, Adams RD, Davis PJ: Reliability and agreement of ratings of ataxic dysarthric speech samples with varying intelligibility, J Speech Hear Res 34:285, 1991.

40. Southwood MH, Weismer G: Listener judgments of the bizarreness, acceptability, naturalness, and normalcy of the dysarthria associated with amyotrophic lateral sclerosis, J Med Speech-Lang Pathol 1:151, 1993.

41. Smith WM: Hemispheric and facial asymmetry: gender differences, Laterality 5:251, 2000.

42. Thompson JK: Right brain, left brain: left face, right face: hemisphericity and the expression of facial emotion, Cortex 21:281, 1985.

43. Venketasubramanian N, Seshardi R, Chee N: Vocal cord paresis in acute ischemic stroke, Cerebrovasc Dis 9:157, 1999.

44. Walton J: Essentials of neurology, London, 1982, Pitman.

45. Wertz RT, LaPointe LL, Rosenbek JC: Apraxia of speech: the disorder and its treatment. New York, 1984, Grune & Stratton.

46. Yorkston KM, Beukelman DR: Assessment of intelligibility of dysarthric speech, Tigard, Ore, 1981a, CC Publications.

47. Yorkston KM, Beukelman DR: Communication efficiency of dysarthric speakers as measured by sentence intelligibility and speaking rate, J Speech Hear Disord 46:296, 1981b.

48. Yorkston KM, Beukelman DR: Sentence intelligibility test, Lincoln, Neb, 1996, Tice Technology Services.

49. Yorkston KM, Strand EA, Kennedy MRT: Comprehensibility of dysarthric speech: implications for assessment and treatment planning, Am J Speech-Lang Pathol 5:55, 1996.

50. Yorkston KM et al: Management of motor speech disorders in children and adults, Austin, Tex, 1999, Pro-Ed.

51. Zeplin J, Kent RD: Reliability of auditory-perceptual scaling of dysarthria. In Robin DR, Yorkston K, Beukelman DR, editors: Disorders of motor speech: recent advances in assessment, treatment, and clinical characterization, Baltimore, 1996, Paul H Brookes.

52. Zyski BJ, Weisiger BE: Identification of dysarthria types based on perceptual analysis, J Commun Disord 20:367, 1987.

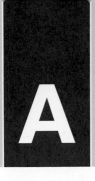

A Deviant Speech Dimensions Encountered in Dysarthrias

LABEL	DESCRIPTION
Mayo Clinic Dysarthria Study Dimensions	
1. Pitch level	Pitch of voice sounds consistently too low or too high for age and sex.
2. Pitch breaks	Pitch of voice shows sudden and uncontrolled variation (falsetto breaks).
3. Monopitch	Voice is characterized by a monopitch or monotone. Voice lacks normal pitch and inflectional changes. It tends to stay at one pitch level.
4. Voice tremor	Voice shows shakiness or tremulousness.
5. Monoloudness	Voice shows monotony of loudness. It lacks normal variations in loudness.
6. Excess loudness variation	Voice shows sudden, uncontrolled alterations in loudness, sometimes becoming too loud, sometimes too weak.
7. Loudness decay	There is progressive diminution or decay of loudness.
8. Alternating loudness	There are alternating changes in loudness.
9. Loudness level (overall)	Voice is insufficiently or excessively loud.
10. Harsh voice	Voice is harsh, rough, and raspy.
11. Hoarse (wet) voice	There is wet, "liquid-sounding" hoarseness.
12. Breathy voice (continuous)	Voice is continuously breathy, weak, and thin.
13. Breathy voice (transient)	Breathiness is transient, periodic, and intermittent.
14. Strained-strangled voice	Voice (phonation) sounds strained or strangled (an apparently effortful squeezing of voice through glottis).
15. Voice stoppages	There are sudden stoppages of voice air stream (as if some obstacle along vocal tract momentarily impedes flow of air).
16. Hypernasality	Voice sounds excessively nasal. Excessive amount of air is resonated by nasal cavities.
17. Hyponasality	Voice is denasal.
18. Nasal emission	There is nasal emission of air stream.
19. Forced inspiration-expiration	Speech is interrupted by sudden, forced inspiration and expiration sighs.
20. Audible inspiration	There is audible, breathy inspiration.
21. Grunt at end of expiration	There is a grunt at the end of expiration.
22. Rate	Rate of actual speech is abnormally slow or rapid.
23. Short phrases	Phrases are short (possibly because inspirations occur more often than normal). Speaker may sound as if he or she has run out of air. Speaker may produce a gasp at the end of a phrase.
24. Increase of rate in segments	Rate increases progressively within given segments of connected speech.
25. Increase of rate overall	Rate increases progressively from beginning to end of sample.
26. Reduced stress	Speech shows reduction of proper stress or emphasis patterns.
27. Variable rate	Rate alternates from slow to fast.
28. Prolonged intervals	There is prolongation of interword or intersyllable intervals.

LABEL	DESCRIPTION
29. Inappropriate silences	There are inappropriate silent intervals.
30. Short rushes of speech	There are short rushes of speech separated by pauses.
31. Excess and equal stress	There is excess stress on usually unstressed parts of speech (e.g., monosyllabic words, unstressed syllables of polysyllabic words).
32. Imprecise consonants	Consonant sounds lack precision. They show slurring, inadequate sharpness, distortions, and lack of crispness. There is clumsiness in going from one consonant sound to another.
33. Prolonged phonemes	There are prolongations of phonemes.
34. Repeated phonemes	There are repetitions of phonemes.
35. Irregular articulatory breakdowns	There is intermittent, nonsystematic breakdown in accuracy of articulation.
36. Distorted vowels	Vowel sounds are distorted throughout their total duration.
37. Intelligibility (overall)	This is a rating of overall intelligibility or understandability of speech.
38. Bizarreness (overall)	This is a rating of degree to which overall speech calls attention to itself because of its unusual, peculiar, or bizarre characteristics.

Other Relevant Dimensions (Not Rated in the Mayo Clinic Dysarthria Studies by Darley, Aronson, and Brown)

39. Diplophonia	Simultaneous perception of two different pitches
40. Flutter	Rapid, relatively low-amplitude voice tremor (perceived as in the 7-12 Hz range), usually most apparent during vowel prolongation.
41. Inhalatory stridor	Similar to audible inspiration (#20) but characterized by actual rough phonation due to vocal fold approximation and oscillation during inhalation.
42. Myoclonus	1-4 Hz rhythmic tremorlike "beats" in the voice, sometimes sufficient to cause brief voice arrests, usually heard only during vowel prolongation.
43. Weak pressure consonants	Pressure consonants lack acoustic distinctiveness or are weak because of excessive nasal airflow during their production.
44. Slow AMRs or fast AMRs	Speech AMRs are slow or fast.
45. Irregular AMRs	Speech AMRs are irregular in duration, pitch, or loudness.
46. Simple vocal tics	Repetitive, rapid, apparently involuntary noises or sounds (e.g., throat clearing, grunting) produced in isolation or during voluntary speech.
47. Palilalia	Compulsive repetition of words or phrases, usually in a context of accelerating rate and decreasing loudness.
48. Coprolalia	Involuntary, compulsive, repetitive obscene language or swearing, uttered loudly, softly, or incompletely.

Permission of Darley FL, Aronson AE, Brown JR: *Motor speech disorders,* Philadelphia, 1975, WB Saunders.
AMRs, Alternating motion rates.

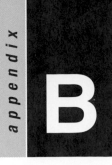
Grandfather Passage

You wish to know all about my grandfather. Well, he is nearly 93 years old, yet he still thinks as swiftly as ever. He dresses himself in an old black frock coat, usually with several buttons missing. A long beard clings to his chin, giving those who observe him a pronounced feeling of the utmost respect. Twice each day he plays skillfully and with zest upon a small organ. Except in the winter when the snow or ice prevents, he slowly takes a short walk in the open air each day. We have often urged him to walk more and smoke less, but he always answers, "Banana oil!" Grandfather likes to be modern in his language.

Number of words = 115

Approximate time to read aloud by normal speakers with normal reading skills = 35 to 45 seconds.

Flaccid Dysarthrias

"The first thing was the tail end of some words were kind of slurred, like I wasn't enunciating properly. Over the last 4 weeks I have had trouble moving food in my mouth and an increase in speech problems."

(37-year-old man with flaccid dysarthria secondary to a skull base tumor in the area of the hypoglossal canals causing bilateral lingual weakness, atrophy, and fasciculations)

CHAPTER OUTLINE

I. Clinical characteristics of flaccid paralysis
   A. Weakness
   B. Hypotonia and reduced reflexes
   C. Atrophy
   D. Fasciculations and fibrillations
   E. Progressive weakness with use

II. Etiologies
   A. Some common terminology
   B. Some associated diseases and conditions

III. Speech pathology
   A. Distribution of etiologies in clinical practice
   B. Patient perceptions and complaints
   C. Trigeminal nerve (V) lesions
   D. Facial nerve (VII) lesions
   E. Glossopharyngeal nerve (IX) lesions
   F. Vagus nerve (X) lesions
   G. Accessory nerve (XI) lesions
   H. Hypoglossal nerve (XII) lesions
   I. Spinal nerve lesions
   J. Multiple cranial nerve lesions
   K. Distribution of speech cranial nerve involvement
      in flaccid dysarthrias
   L. Clusters of deviant speech dimensions

IV. Cases
V. Summary

Flaccid dysarthrias are a perceptually distinctive group of motor speech disorders (MSDs) produced by injury or malfunction of one or more of the cranial or spinal nerves. *They reflect problems in the nuclei, axons, or neuromuscular junctions that make up the* *motor units of the final common pathway (FCP),* and they may be manifest in any or all of the respiratory, phonatory, resonatory, and articulatory components of speech. Their primary deviant speech characteristics can be traced to muscle weakness and reduced muscle tone, and their effects on the speed, range, and accuracy of speech movements. The primacy of weakness as an explanation for the speech characteristics of these disorders leads to their designation as *flaccid* dysarthrias.

Flaccid dysarthrias are encountered in a large medical practice at a frequency comparable to that of the other major single dysarthria types. Based on data for primary communication disorder diagnoses in the Mayo Clinic Speech Pathology practice, they account for 9.1% of all dysarthrias and 8.4% of all MSDs (Figure 1-3).

Unlike most other dysarthria types, flaccid dysarthrias sometimes reflect involvement of only a single muscle group or speech subsystem (e.g., phonatory, articulatory). They can also reflect involvement of several subsystems and muscle groups, in various combinations. Because of these multiple possibilities, it is justifiable to think of *subtypes* of flaccid dysarthria, each characterized by distinct speech abnormalities attributable to unilateral or bilateral damage to a specific cranial or spinal nerve, or combination of cranial or spinal nerves. That is why the plural designation, *flaccid dysarthrias,* is used here. All of its subtypes share a lesion somewhere between the brainstem or spinal cord and the muscles of speech. They also share weakness and reduced muscle tone as their neuromuscular basis. They are perceptually distinguishable from one another on the basis of the specific cranial or spinal nerves that have been damaged.

Close attention to the clinical features of flaccid dysarthrias can help solidify our understanding of peripheral nervous system (PNS) anatomy and physiology. More than any other dysarthria type, flaccid dysarthrias teach us about the course and muscular innervations of the cranial and spinal nerves, the roles of specific muscle groups in speech production, and some of the remarkable and often spontaneous ways by which people adapt and compensate for weakness in order to maintain intelligible speech.

■ CLINICAL CHARACTERISTICS OF FLACCID PARALYSIS

Because flaccid paralysis reflects FCP damage, *reflexive, automatic, and voluntary movements are all affected.* This principle is important in distinguishing lower motor neuron (LMN) lesions from lesions in other parts of the motor system.

Weakness, hypotonia, and diminished reflexes are the primary characteristics of flaccid paralysis. Atrophy, fasciculations, and fibrillations commonly accompany them. Occasionally, rapid weakening with use and recovery with rest are distinguishing features. The presence or absence of these characteristics depends to some extent on the portion of the motor unit that has been damaged. These characteristics are discussed below and summarized in Table 4-1.

Weakness

Weakness in flaccid paralysis stems from damage to any portion of the motor unit, including cranial and spinal nerve cell bodies in the brainstem or spinal cord, the peripheral or cranial nerve leading to muscle, and the neuromuscular junction. It can also result from muscle disease. When damaged, motor units are inactivated and muscles' ability to contract is lost or diminished. When motor unit disease inactivates all of the LMN input to a muscle, *paralysis, the complete inability to contract muscle,* is the result. If some input to muscle remains viable, *paresis, or reduced contraction and weakness,* is the result. The term paralysis, however, is often used generically to refer to weakness, regardless of its severity.

The effects of weakness on muscle can be observed during single (phasic) contractions, during repetitive contractions, and during sustained (tonic) contractions.

Hypotonia and Reduced Reflexes

Flaccid paralysis is also associated with *hypotonia (reduced muscle tone)* and reduced or absent normal reflexes. In flaccid paralysis, the ability of a muscle to contract in response to stretch is compromised, because the motor component of the stretch reflex (discussed in Chapter 2) operates through the FCP. This results in the flabbiness that can be seen or felt in muscles with reduced tone.

Atrophy

Muscle structure can be altered by FCP and muscle diseases. When cranial or spinal nerve nuclei (cell bodies), peripheral nerves, or muscle fibers are involved, muscles eventually *atrophy* or lose bulk. Atrophy is almost always associated with significant weakness.

Fasciculations and Fibrillations

When motor neuron cell bodies are damaged (and, less prominently, when their axons are damaged),

---

table 4-1   Components of the motor unit associated with characteristics of flaccid paralysis

	Damaged Component			
Feature	Cell Body	Axon	Neuromuscular Junction	Muscle
Weakness	+	+	+	+
Hypotonia	+	+	+	+
Diminished reflexes	+	+	+	+
Atrophy	+	+	−	+
Fasciculations	+	+/−	−	−
Fibrillations	+	+/−	−	−
Rapid weakening & recovery with rest	−	−	+	−

+, Present; −, absent; +/−, may or may not be present.

fasciculations and fibrillations may develop. *Fasciculations are visible arrhythmic isolated twitches in resting muscle that result from spontaneous motor unit discharges in response to nerve degeneration or irritation. Fibrillations are invisible, spontaneous, independent contractions of individual muscle fibers that reflect slow repetitive action potentials.* They can be detected electromyographically within approximately 1 to 3 weeks after a muscle is deprived of motor nerve supply. Fasciculations and fibrillations are generally not present in muscle disease.

Progressive Weakness with Use

When disease affects the neuromuscular junction, progressive and rapid weakening of muscle with use and recovery with rest can occur. Even though fatigue is common in people with any type of weakness, *rapid weakening and recovery with rest are prominent in neuromuscular junction disease (e.g., myasthenia gravis [MG]).*

▣ ETIOLOGIES

Flaccid dysarthrias can be caused by any process that damages the motor unit. These include degenerative, inflammatory, toxic, metabolic, neoplastic, traumatic, and vascular diseases.

The distribution of causes of flaccid dysarthrias in the population is unknown and, in fact, it almost certainly varies as a function of the particular cranial or spinal nerves involved, whether or not multiple versus single nerves are involved, and where within the motor unit the pathology actually lies. In general, for example, trauma is the most common cause of peripheral or cranial nerve lesions when a single nerve is injured, whereas toxic and metabolic disorders usually affect many nerves.

Some Common Terminology

Numerous terms are used to describe pathologies of the FCP and muscle. The following definitions may facilitate comprehension of information presented in the remainder of this chapter:

Neuropathy—A general term that refers to any disease of nerve, usually of noninflammatory etiology.

Neuritis—An inflammatory disorder of nerve.

Peripheral neuropathy—Any disorder of nerve in the PNS. Peripheral neuropathies can affect motor, sensory, or autonomic fibers. They may be axonal, demyelinating, or mixed in their effects.

Cranial neuropathies—Peripheral neuropathies involving the cranial nerves.

Mononeuropathy—Neuropathy of a single nerve.

Polyneuropathy—A generalized process producing widespread bilateral and often symmetric effects on the PNS.

Radiculopathy—A PNS disorder involving the root of a spinal nerve, often just proximal to the intervertebral foramen.

Plexopathy—PNS involvement at the point where spinal nerves intermingle (in plexuses) before forming nerves that go to the extremities.

Myelitis—A nonspecific term that indicates inflammation of the spinal cord.

Myelopathy—Any pathologic condition of the spinal cord.

Myopathy—Muscle disease. Myopathies are not associated with sensory disturbances or central nervous system (CNS) pathology. The most common types of myopathy affect proximal rather than distal muscles.

Myositis—Inflammatory muscle disease.

Some Associated Diseases and Conditions

This section summarizes some common conditions that are relatively unique to FCP or muscle diseases whose presence have a strong association with flaccid but not other forms of dysarthria. The conditions discussed here represent only a few of the potential etiologies of flaccid dysarthrias. They are highlighted because of their occurrence within the Mayo Clinic Speech Pathology practice (Box 4-1).

Trauma

Surgery in the brainstem and head, neck, and upper chest can temporarily injure or permanently damage speech cranial nerves. Examples of neurosurgical procedures with known risks for cranial nerve damage include carotid endarterectomy; anterior cervical disk surgery; brainstem vascular procedures; and surgical resection or related procedures for tumors in the posterior fossa, skull base, and cranial nerves (such tumors themselves can lead to cranial nerve palsies). Cardiac, chest, otorhinolaryngologic, and dental procedures directed at the heart, lungs, thyroid gland, neck, jaw, and mouth also hold risks for cranial nerve injuries. Finally, closed head injury, skull fractures, and neck injuries are traumatic events that can lead to flaccid dysarthria through damage to cranial or cervical nerves.

Degenerative Disease

Motor neuron diseases are a group of disorders that involve degeneration of motor neurons. *Amyotrophic*

box 4-1

Etiologies for 154 quasirandomly selected cases with a primary speech pathology diagnosis of flaccid dysarthria at the Mayo Clinic from 1969-1990 and 1999-2001. Percentage of cases for broad etiologic headings is given in parentheses. Specific etiologies under each heading are ordered from most to least frequent.

Traumatic (32%)

Surgical (28%)

1. Neurosurgical (14%)
   Cervical disk
   Carotid endarterectomy
   Carotid aneurysm
   Brainstem vascular
   Carotid artery tumor
   Posterior fossa, pontine, jugular, and acoustic tumors
2. Otorhinolaryngologic or plastic and dental surgery (8%)
   Thyroid
   Parathyroid, maxillectomy for carcinoma, dental surgery, face-lift with liposuction
3. Chest or cardiac surgery (6%)
   Left upper lobectomy for lung carcinoma
   Cardiac

Nonsurgical (4%)

- Closed head injury
- Skull fracture
- Neck injury

Neuropathies of Undetermined Origin (25%)

- Cranial nerve X
- Cranial nerves X and XII
- Cranial nerve VII
- Cranial nerve XII
- Cranial nerves VII and X
- Cranial nerves IX, X, and XI
- Jugular foramen syndrome

Degenerative (13%)

- Amyotrophic lateral sclerosis (motor neuron disease)
- Primary lateral sclerosis

- Multiple systems atrophy
- Undetermined

Muscle Disease (8%)

- Muscular dystrophy
- Myotonic dystrophy
- Myopathy

Myasthenia Gravis (6%)

Tumor (5%)

- Posterior fossa (foramen magnum, jugular foramen, brainstem)
- Tongue or neck, nasopharynx
- Widespread metastases

Vascular (4%)

Brainstem stroke (pons, medulla)

Infectious (2%)

- Polio
- Meningitis

Anatomic Malformation (2%)

- Arnold-Chiari malformation
- Syringobulbia
- Syringomyelia

Demyelinating (1%)

Guillain-Barré syndrome

Other (3%)

- Radiation therapy (palate, nasopharynx)
- Drug toxicity

lateral sclerosis (ALS), the most common motor neuron disease, affects the bulbar, limb, and respiratory muscles. By definition, ALS is a disease of both upper motor neurons (UMNs) and LMNs, but its initial manifestations may be confined to the LMNs of bulbar muscles. Thus progressive bulbar palsy and ALS may produce flaccid dysarthrias secondary to multiple cranial nerve involvement.

Progressive bulbar palsy is a motor neuron disease that primarily affects LMNs supplied by cranial nerves. Although it may also include UMNs that supply the bulbar muscles, it can be limited to LMNs.

Spinal muscle atrophies (sometimes called *progressive muscle atrophy*) form a subgroup of motor neuron diseases that are associated with progressive limb wasting and weakness, with or without cranial nerve weakness. They can be inherited or occur sporadically and may be congenital or present in childhood or adulthood. Bulbar signs and respiratory problems occur less frequently than in typical ALS, but flaccid dysarthria and dysphagia can occur.[42,66]

Kennedy's disease is an uncommon X-linked recessive form of bulbospinal muscle atrophy that can be mistaken for typical ALS. It affects only men, usually after age 30, and is characterized by gynecomastia (excessive breast size), muscle cramps and twitches, limb-girdle muscle weakness, and bulbar involvement. Perioral and facial fasciculations and tongue atrophy are present in most patients, and dysarthria and dysphagia can be significant.[42]

Muscle Disease

Muscular dystrophies are a group of genetic degenerative diseases of skeletal muscle that are associated with degeneration of muscle fibers and proliferation of connective tissue. As a result, affected muscles lose their ability to contract normally. Muscular dystrophies can occur at all ages and vary in severity. Effects are generally diffuse, chronic, and progressive. A *fascioscapulohumeral* form, which may emerge in early adulthood, is partly defined by facial weakness, with potential for effects on speech. Other forms, including *oculopharyngeal muscular dystrophy,* can be associated with dysphagia and dysarthria.[46,65,67] Congenital forms, including *Duchenne's muscular dystrophy,* can be accompanied by cognitive deficits and CNS abnormalities.[25,41]

Myotonic muscular dystrophy is an inherited autosomal dominant disease that affects muscles' normal contractile processes. Myotonia is characterized by the persistence of muscle contraction after stimulation or forcible contraction has ceased. This can be detected clinically as *percussion myotonia*, a persistent myotonic contraction that follows strong percussion. It may be observed after pressure is exerted on the tongue as an obvious depression that persists for several seconds.[39] Muscle atrophy in the disease gives the face a characteristic long and expressionless appearance, with weak voluntary and emotional facial movements. Malocclusion is common.[33] Articulation, phonation, resonance, and swallowing may be affected.[53,36]

Polymyositis is a disease of striated muscle that can be associated with a number of infectious processes. The tongue, jaw, pharyngeal, and laryngeal muscles may be affected, causing dysarthria and dysphagia.[2]

Neuromuscular Junction Disease

Some diseases affect only the neuromuscular junction. MG is the most common of these. MG is an autoimmune disease characterized by rapid weakening of voluntary muscles with use and improvement with rest. It appears that antibodies form against acetylcholine (ACh) receptors in the postsynaptic membrane at the motor end plate. The decreased number of functioning receptors makes muscle less responsive to the ACh that triggers muscle contraction.[6] As a result, muscle contractions progressively diminish with repeated use. Strength may improve with rest as nerves are able to replenish the supply of ACh. A majority of affected people has some

abnormality of the thymus gland. Women are affected more frequently between the ages of 20 and 40, but the sex distribution is approximately equal when onset is after the age of 50.[7,10] Remissions may occur, especially when onset is before age 50. MG is sometimes mistaken for stroke when it emerges in the elderly.[17,35]

Frequent presenting signs of MG include *ptosis* (drooping of the eyelid), weakness of facial muscles, flaccid dysarthria, and dysphagia. Decreased lateral tongue force, reduced bite force, and inspiratory stridor have been documented in patients with MG.[1,54,64] Beyond clinical neurologic examination, MG is commonly diagnosed by single-fiber electromyography (EMG), ACh receptor antibody blood tests, or a Tensilon (edrophonium chloride) test. Injection of Tensilon produces temporary recovery from weakness brought on by prolonged muscular effort. Sometimes speech stress testing is the task used for the Tensilon test. Patients with MG can show rapid development or worsening of flaccid dysarthria during stress testing but rapid improvement after Tensilon injection, even as they continue to speak.

Lambert-Eaton myasthenic syndrome is a rare paraneoplastic* disorder of neuromuscular transmission in which there is inadequate release of ACh from nerve terminals. It is characterized by weakness but with an improved response to repetitive nerve stimulation, a pattern opposite of MG. That is, weakness is greatest at the initiation of muscle use or with slow rates of stimulation; strength increases with repetitive rapid stimulation, apparently because high rates of activation facilitate release of ACh. The syndrome occurs mostly in men with oat cell carcinoma of the lung, less frequently in the absence of primary neoplasm but with evidence of immune system abnormality.[40,45]

Botulism is a serious disease in which botulinum toxin acts on presynaptic membranes for the release of ACh, thus blocking neuromuscular transmission. Contaminated food is the most common cause. Facial, oropharyngeal, and respiratory paralysis can be among presenting signs.[45] Botulism toxin in very small doses is an effective treatment for numerous movement disorders, including certain forms of spasmodic dysphonia. Its therapeutic use is discussed in Chapter 17.

Vascular Disorders

Any brainstem stroke that affects nuclei of speech cranial nerves can lead to flaccid dysarthria. Damage

---

*Paraneoplastic disorders reflect a remote effect of cancer. They are discussed further in Chapter 6.

to lower cranial nerves can also result from dissection of the internal carotid artery.

Some specific vascular syndromes are also associated with flaccid dysarthrias. *Wallenberg's lateral medullary syndrome* is among the more common of these. It is usually caused by occlusion in the intracranial vertebral artery or the posterior inferior cerebellar artery, which affects the lateral portion of the medulla and inferior cerebellum. It leads to ipsilateral facial and contralateral trunk and extremity sensory loss, ipsilateral cerebellar signs, ipsilateral neuro-ophthalmologic abnormalities, and ipsilateral nucleus ambiguus involvement with subsequent palatal, pharyngeal, and laryngeal weakness and associated dysarthria and dysphagia.[8] *Collet-Sicard syndrome* is characterized by unilateral involvement of cranial nerves IX through XII. It can be caused by vascular lesions of the jugular vein and carotid artery below the skull base, as well as by skull base fractures, inflammatory lesions, and tumors. Occlusion of the anterior spinal artery or its source, the vertebral artery, can injure the hypoglossal nerve *(medial medullary syndrome)* and cause lingual weakness.[8]

Anatomic Anomalies

Arnold-Chiari malformation is a congenital anomaly of undetermined etiology characterized by downward elongation of the brainstem and cerebellum into the cervical spinal cord. Signs and symptoms reflect injury to the cerebellum, medulla, and lower cranial nerves. Onset of symptoms is sometimes delayed until adulthood. The damage to the brainstem may lead to flaccid dysarthrias.

Syringomyelia (syrinx = a tube) is an abnormality characterized by elongated cavities lined by glia close to the central canal of the spinal cord. Cavity expansion and compression of anterior horns of the gray matter cause atrophy of the anterior horn cells and axonal degeneration in the spinal cord. The condition may extend upward into the fourth ventricle in the brainstem, where it is called *syringobulbia*. Syringomyelia and syringobulbia can reflect developmental anomalies but can also develop in response to tumor, trauma, or inflammatory conditions. When the brainstem is involved, the ninth through twelfth cranial nerves can be affected.[52,62] Flaccid dysarthrias can result from this.

Demyelinating Disease

Guillain-Barré syndrome is a disorder of unknown cause but is frequently preceded by viral infection. It is characterized by the acute or subacute onset of PNS dysfunction, mainly motor. Focal demyelinization and sometimes axonal degeneration occur in peripheral and cranial nerves. Proximal muscles are affected more severely than distal muscles. Facial, oropharyngeal, and ocular muscles are occasionally affected first, and more than half of affected individuals have facial weakness, dysphagia, and flaccid dysarthria. Recovery is sometimes rapid and complete but may take several months in others. Some individuals are left with permanent weakness.[20]

Chronic demyelinating polyneuritis is similar to Guillain-Barré syndrome but less acute in onset and more prolonged in course. Affected individuals may suffer frequent, recurrent attacks.[48]

Infectious Processes

Polio (poliomyelitis) is a now rare viral disease with an affinity for LMN cell bodies, most often in the lumbar and cervical regions of the spinal cord. Bulbar involvement occurs in 10% to 15% of cases, with cranial nerves IX and X most often affected, but cranial nerve V and VII involvement is not uncommon. The dorsal area of the medulla is generally involved in the bulbar form of the disease; respiratory and circulatory centers in the medulla can also be affected.[2] Survivors often recover function of muscles that are not completely paralyzed, usually within 6 months.

Polio victims occasionally develop the insidious onset of progressive weakness long after the acute attack *(post-polio syndrome)*. This may occur by chance alone, but it may be that previously involved nerves are more susceptible to the effects of aging; it does not appear related to reactivation of the virus.[11]

Herpes zoster is a viral infection that may affect the fifth and seventh nerve ganglia, most often producing pain. When it causes facial paresis, it is known as the *Ramsay-Hunt syndrome*. The herpes virus can also cause superior laryngeal nerve paralysis and dysphonia.[3,24]

Sarcoidosis is a nonviral, chronic granulomatous infection that can occur in all organs and tissues. It occasionally affects the PNS or CNS, most often single or multiple cranial nerves, especially the seventh nerve. Sometimes, cranial neuropathies associated with sarcoidosis result from basilar meningitis.[48]

Individuals with *human immunodeficiency virus (HIV)* who develop *acquired immune deficiency syndrome (AIDS)* may develop neurologic complications as the result of opportunistic infections. *Cryptococcal meningitis* is the most common fungal infection in AIDS. The resulting meningeal inflammation can affect posterior fossa structures and lead to multiple cranial nerve palsies. Other neurologic complications of AIDS that can lead to cranial nerve involvement include *CNS lymphoma* (the most common CNS tumor in AIDS) and *neurosyphilis*.[57] The involvement of cranial nerves for speech may lead to a flaccid dysarthria in such cases.

Other Causes

Skull base tumors can cause cranial neuropathies and flaccid dysarthrias. *Radiation therapy* for the treatment of carcinoma in the neck, oral cavity, and tonsillar area can cause cranial neuropathies and, possibly, associated flaccid dysarthrias. Pathology usually involves axonal degeneration and fibrosis as a result of damaged vascular supply to tissues in the radiated field[37,48]; it may be difficult to separate the effects of axonal degeneration (neurologic weakness) from the effects of necrosis on reduced range of motion of affected structures. The effects of radiation on cranial nerve function may be delayed for years following radiation treatment.[34,56,58]

Cranial mononeuropathies, particularly facial (Bell's palsy) and vocal fold paralyses, are frequently *idiopathic* (of unknown origin). Recovery from such conditions is often quite good.

■ SPEECH PATHOLOGY

Distribution of Etiologies in Clinical Practice

Box 4-1 and Figure 4-1 summarize the etiologies for 154 quasirandomly selected cases seen at the Mayo Clinic with a primary speech pathology diagnosis of flaccid dysarthria. The reader is cautioned that these data may not represent the distribution of etiologies of flaccid dysarthrias in the general population or its distribution in many speech pathology practices. They may approximate the most frequent causes encountered in speech pathology practices within large multidisciplinary primary and tertiary medical settings where patients are referred for diagnosis as well as management of communication disorders.

The data establish that flaccid dysarthrias can result from various medical conditions. Surgical trauma, most often but not always limited to the laryngeal branches of the vagus nerve, was a frequent cause. Surgical trauma to the laryngeal branches of the vagus can occur in cervical disk, thyroid, cardiac, and upper lung surgeries because of the proximity of the vagus nerve to the surgical field. *Carotid endarterectomy*—performed to remove

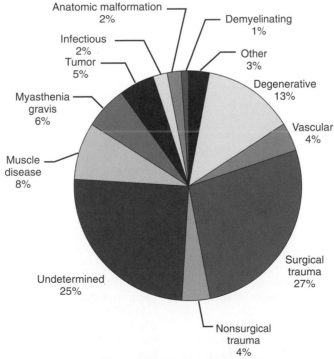

FIGURE 4-1 Distribution of etiologies for 154 quasirandomly selected cases with a primary speech pathology diagnosis of flaccid dysarthria at the Mayo Clinic from 1969-1990 and from 1999-2001 (see Box 4-1 for details).

table 4-2	Neuromuscular deficits associated with flaccid dysarthrias						
Direction	**Rhythm**		**Rate**		**Range**	**Force**	**Tone**
Individual Movements	Repetitive Movements	Individual Movements	Repetitive Movements	Individual Movements	Repetitive Movements	Individual Movements	Muscle Tone
Normal	Regular	Normal or slow	Normal or slow	Reduced	Reduced	Weak	Reduced

Modified from Darley FL, Aronson AE, Brown JR: Differential diagnostic patterns of dysarthria, *J Speech Hear Res* 12:246, 1969.

occlusive or ulcerative plaque from the carotid artery in the neck—injures cranial (especially the tenth and twelfth) and cervical nerves in 12% to 14% of cases.[5,55] Such injuries are usually transient and probably result from retraction or clamping of nerves rather than nerve division and distal degeneration.

Neurosurgical trauma was more likely to result in multiple cranial nerve lesions than was otorhinolaryngologic, plastic, dental, or chest or cardiac surgery. Neck surgery, most often thyroid surgery, was the most frequent cause of isolated laryngeal nerve lesions. Nonsurgical trauma was most often due to closed head injury.

It is noteworthy that 25% of the flaccid dysarthrias were idiopathic, and that the tenth nerve was most often implicated when the idiopathic lesion was confined to a single nerve. The remaining etiologies were less frequent and represented by various conditions, including degenerative disease, muscle disease, MG, tumor, stroke, infectious processes, anatomic malformations, demyelinating disease, and the effects of radiation therapy or drug toxicity.

This retrospective review did not permit a clear delineation of dysarthria severity. However, a judgment about intelligibility was made for 74% of the last 47 patients seen in the sample; 46% were felt to have reduced intelligibility. The degree to which this figure accurately estimates the frequency of intelligibility impairments in the population with flaccid dysarthria is unclear. It is likely that many patients for whom an observation of intelligibility was not made had normal intelligibility, but the sample probably contains a larger number of mildly impaired patients than is encountered in many rehabilitation settings. In general, reduced intelligibility is more common when damage to a cranial or peripheral nerve involved in speech is bilateral or when multiple nerves are involved.

Finally, cognitive impairment is not common in flaccid dysarthria. Among the last 47 patients seen in the sample, cognitive impairment was noted in only 11%. Affected patients had diseases associated with CNS as well as PNS impairments (e.g., muscular dystrophy).

Patient Perceptions and Complaints

People with flaccid dysarthrias sometimes offer complaints or descriptions that differ from those of people with other dysarthria types. Such complaints may provide clues to diagnosis and localization, especially when they can be attributed to muscles supplied by a single cranial nerve. They are noted in the review of deficits associated with each of the cranial nerves because they identify some of the questions that should be asked when weakness is suspected as the primary cause of speech difficulty.

The next several sections address the cranial and spinal nerves that may be involved in flaccid dysarthrias. The anatomic course and function of each nerve is reviewed briefly (greater detail was provided in Chapter 2), as are some of the conditions that can damage each nerve. Nonspeech findings are also discussed. Finally, the salient features of the motor speech examination will be discussed, including the primary auditory perceptual characteristics, accompanying visible deficits, some of the compensatory behaviors that may develop in response to the neuromuscular deficit, and some of the evidence from instrumental studies that further delineate the characteristics and neurologic bases of the speech deficits. The neuromuscular deficits associated with flaccid dysarthrias are summarized in Table 4-2.

Trigeminal Nerve (V) Lesions

Course and Function

The three main branches of cranial nerve V arise in the trigeminal ganglion in the petrous bone of the middle cranial fossa. Central connections from the trigeminal ganglion enter the lateral aspect of the pons and are distributed to various nuclei in the brainstem.

The peripheral distribution of cranial nerve V through its three branches includes the sensory ophthalmic branch, which exits the skull through the superior orbital fissure to innervate the upper face; the sensory maxillary branch, which exits the skull through the foramen rotundum to supply the mid face; and the motor and sensory mandibular branch, which exits the skull through the foramen ovale to supply the jaw muscles, tensor tympani, and tensor veli palatini.

Trigeminal functions for speech are mediated through its maxillary and mandibular branches. Sensory roles are to provide tactile and proprioceptive information about jaw, face, lip, and tongue movements and their relationship to stationary articulatory structures within the mouth (e.g., teeth, alveolus, palate). Motor functions are associated with jaw movements during speech.

Etiologies and Localization of Lesions

Damage to cranial nerve V is usually associated with involvement of other cranial nerves. *It is rarely the only cranial nerve involved in flaccid dysarthrias* (see Table 4-5). Any pathology that can affect the middle cranial fossa can produce weakness or sensory loss in its distribution. Etiologies most often include aneurysm, infection, arteriovenous malformation (AVM), tumors in the middle fossa or cerebellopontine angle, and surgical (e.g., posterior fossa, acoustic neuroma, temporomandibular joint) or nonsurgical trauma to the skull or anywhere along its course to muscle. Peripheral branches are most often damaged in isolation by tumors or fractures of the facial bones or skull. Disease of the neuromuscular junction can cause jaw weakness, as can disease affecting the jaw muscles themselves (myopathies).

Pain of trigeminal origin can indirectly affect speech. *Trigeminal neuralgia* (tic douloureux) is characterized by sudden, brief periods of pain in one or more of the sensory divisions of the trigeminal nerve. It is often idiopathic, but many cases may be due to compression or irritation of the trigeminal sensory roots.[8] Pain can be triggered by sensory input from facial or jaw movements, sometimes leading to restricted lip, face, or jaw movements during speech to avoid triggering pain.

Nonspeech Oral Mechanism

In patients with unilateral mandibular branch lesions, the jaw will deviate to the weak side when opened, and the partly opened jaw may be pushed easily to the weak side by the examiner. The degree of masseter or temporalis contraction felt on palpation when the patient bites down may be decreased on the weak side.

With bilateral weakness, the jaw may hang open at rest. The patient may be unable to close it or may move it slowly or with reduced range. The patient may be unable to resist the examiner's attempts to open or close the jaw and may be unable to clench the teeth strongly enough for normal masseter or temporalis contraction to be felt. Patient complaints may include chewing difficulty, drooling, and recognition that the jaw is difficult to close or move.

If sensory branches to speech structures are affected, the patient may complain of decreased face, cheek, tongue, teeth, or palate sensation. This can be assessed while the patient's eyes are closed by asking him or her to indicate when light touch or pressure applied to the affected areas is detected. Decreased sensation of undetermined origin in one or more of the peripheral branches of the fifth nerve is often referred to as *trigeminal sensory neuropathy*. Viral etiology is common, but association with diabetes, sarcoidosis, and connective tissue disease has also been noted. Facial numbness is occasionally a presenting symptom in multiple sclerosis.[49]

Speech

Effects of cranial nerve V lesions on speech are most apparent during reading, conversation, and alternate motion rates (AMRs). During AMRs, imprecision or slowness for "puh" should be greater than that for "tuh" or "kuh." Vowel prolongation may be normal. In MG, progressive weakening of jaw movements during speech may be observed.

Unilateral damage to the motor division of the fifth nerve generally does not perceptibly affect speech. In contrast, bilateral lesions can have a devastating impact on articulation. The inability to elevate a bilaterally weak jaw can *reduce precision or make impossible bilabial, labiodental, lingual-dental, and lingual-alveolar articulation, as well as lip and tongue adjustments for many vowels, glides, and liquids.* Speech rate may be slowed; this may be either a direct effect of weakness or reflect compensation for weakness. The effects of fifth nerve motor weakness on speech are summarized in Table 4-3.

Lesions to the sensory portion of the mandibular branch, especially if bilateral, can cause loss of face, lip, lingual, and palatal sensation sufficient to result in imprecise articulation of bilabial, labiodental, lingual-alveolar, and lingual-palatal sounds. This can occur without weakness and is presumably due to reduced sensory information about articulatory movements or contacts. Technically, the articulatory distortions resulting from decreased sensation should not be classified as a dysarthria, because the source of the speech deficit is not primarily neuromotor. However, because the source is neurologic and does affect the precision of motor activity, it could be viewed as a *"sensory dysarthria";* the use of such a

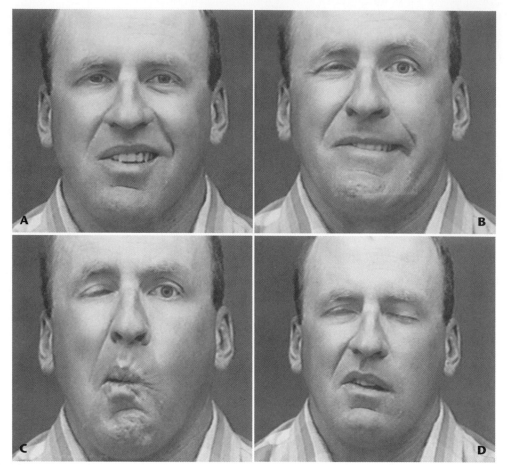

FIGURE 4-2 A, Partially recovered unilateral right facial weakness during spontaneous smile. **B,** Voluntary lip retraction. **C,** Lip pursing, with, **D,** paradoxical, involuntary right lip retraction (synkinesis) when voluntarily closing the eyes. Synkinetic eye closing is also apparent during, **B,** voluntary lip retraction and, **D,** pursing.

term should be accompanied by a statement that the speech deficits are presumed to reflect decreased oral sensation.

Individuals with relatively isolated severe jaw weakness sometimes manually hold the jaw closed to facilitate articulation. Patients with mandibular branch sensory loss sometimes produce exaggerated movements of the jaw, lips, and face during speech, presumably in an attempt to increase sensory feedback. These movements can sometimes be mistaken for, or difficult to distinguish from, hyperkinetic movement disorders. However, sensory loss is usually detectable on touch or pressure sensation testing in patients with trigeminal sensory loss and not in patients with true hyperkinesias.

Finally, as noted previously, patients with trigeminal neuralgia may restrict jaw movement during speech to reduce sensation that might trigger pain. Although apparent visually, this compensatory

restriction of movement may not be apparent auditorily. Mild articulatory distortions and decreased loudness or altered resonance, however, could result from such a strategy.

Facial Nerve (VII) Lesions

Course and Function

Cranial nerve VII is motor and sensory in function, but only its motor component has a clear role in speech. Motor fibers originate in the facial nucleus in the lower third of the pons and exit the cranial cavity, along with fibers of cranial nerve VIII, through the internal auditory meatus. They pass through the facial canal, exit at the stylomastoid foramen below the ear, pass through the parotid gland, and innervate the muscles of facial expression. The facial muscles crucial for speech are those

table 4-3	Effects on speech of unilateral and bilateral cranial nerve and spinal respiratory nerve lesions. The ninth and eleventh nerves are not included because of the negligible or unclear effects of lesions of them on speech.

Cranial Nerves	Respiratory-Phonatory		Resonance		Articulation		Prosody	
	Unilateral	Bilateral	Unilateral	Bilateral	Unilateral	Bilateral	Unilateral	Bilateral
V	None	None	None	None	None	Imprecise • bilabials • labiodentals • lingual-dentals • lingual-alveolars • vowels • glides • liquids	None	Slow rate (compensatory or primary)
VII	None	None	None	None	Mild distortion of bilabials & labiodentals ? Mild distortion of anterior lingual fricatives & affricates	Distortion or inability to produce bilabials & labiodentals ? Vowel distortions ? Anterior lingual fricative & affricate distortions	None	Slow rate (compensatory or primary)
X Above pharyngeal branch	Breathiness Reduced loudness Reduced pitch Short phrases Hoarseness Diplophonia	Breathiness Aphonia Short phrases Inhalatory stridor	Mild hypernasality Nasal emission	Moderate + hypernasality Nasal emission	None (? mildly weak pressure consonants)	Weak pressure consonants	Short phrases	Short phrases

Continued

table 4-3 Effects on speech of unilateral and bilateral cranial nerve and spinal respiratory nerve lesions. The ninth and eleventh nerves are not included because of the negligible or unclear effects of lesions of them on speech.—cont'd

Cranial Nerves	Respiratory-Phonatory		Resonance		Articulation		Prosody	
	Unilateral	Bilateral	Unilateral	Bilateral	Unilateral	Bilateral	Unilateral	Bilateral
X Below pharyngeal branch	Same as above	Same as above	None	None	None	None	Short phrases	Short phrases
X Superior branch only	Breathiness Hoarseness	Breathiness Hoarseness Reduced • loudness • pitch • range	None	None	None	None	Short phrases	Short phrases
X Recurrent branch only	Breathiness Hoarseness Reduced loudness Diplophonia	Breathiness Hoarseness Reduced loudness	None	None	None	None	Short phrases	Short phrases
XII	None	None	None	? Altered	Mildly imprecise lingual consonants	Mild to severe imprecise lingual consonants Vowel distortions	None	Slow rate (compensatory or primary)
Spinal respiratory nerves	None	Reduced • loudness • pitch • variability Strained voice (compensatory)	None	None	None	None	None	Short phrases Reduced pitch & loudness variability

that move the lips and firm the cheeks to permit impounding of intraoral air pressure for bilabial and labiodental articulation.

Etiologies and Localization of Lesions

Cranial nerve VII can be damaged in isolation or along with other cranial nerves. Pathology in the brainstem and posterior fossa can cause seventh nerve damage, but a lesion anywhere along the nerve may affect its functions for speech.

Because cranial (abducens) nerves VI and VII are in close proximity within the pons, especially in the floor of the fourth ventricle, lesions of both the sixth and seventh nerves implicate that part of the brainstem. If cranial nerves VII and VIII are involved, as they frequently are with acoustic neuromas, a lesion is suspected in the area of the internal auditory meatus where both nerves exit the brainstem.

Known infectious causes of facial paralysis include, but are not limited to, infection by herpes zoster, mononucleosis, otitis media, meningitis, Lyme disease, syphilis, sarcoidosis, Guillain-Barré syndrome, and inflammatory polyradiculoneuropathy. Common neoplastic causes include acoustic neuroma, parotid tumor, cerebellopontine angle meningioma, tumor of the facial nerve, and leptomeningeal carcinomatosis.[8,31,38] Vascular lesions and trauma can also cause cranial nerve VII lesions.

Bell's palsy is a relatively common idiopathic condition of undetermined etiology characterized by isolated unilateral cranial nerve VII weakness. Upper and lower facial muscles are affected, and the ability to close the eye on the affected side may be limited. Some patients also have decreased lacrimation, salivation, and taste sensation, as well as hyperacusis (possibly due to involvement of the portion of the nerve that innervates the stapedius). A significant majority reportedly makes full recovery, with better recovery in those younger than age 50.[13] Proposed causes for Bell's palsy include an autoimmune-mediated inflammatory focal neuropathy, herpes simplex viral infection of the nerve, and swelling of the nerve induced by exposure to cold or allergic factors leading to compression by the bony facial canal.[39]

Nonspeech Oral Mechanism

The visible effects of unilateral cranial nerve VII lesions can be striking. At rest, the affected side sags and is hypotonic. The forehead may be unwrinkled, the eyebrow drooped, and the eye open and unblinking. The corner of the mouth may be drawn toward the unaffected side. Drooling on the affected side may occur. The nasolabial fold is often flattened, and the nasal ala may be immobile during respiration. During smiling the face will retract more toward the intact side (see Figure 4-2). Food may squirrel between the teeth and cheek on the weak side because of buccinator weakness. The patient may complain of biting the cheek or lip when chewing or speaking and have difficulty keeping food in the mouth. With milder weakness, asymmetry may be apparent only with use, as in voluntary retraction, pursing, and cheek puffing. Reduced or absent movement is apparent during voluntary, emotional, and reflexive activities. Fasciculations and atrophy may be apparent on the affected side.

Bilateral cranial nerve VII lesions are less common than unilateral lesions. With bilateral lesions, the effects of weakness are on both sides, but they may be less striking visually because of the symmetric appearance. At rest, the mouth may be lax and the space between the upper and lower lips wider than normal. During reflexive smiling the mouth may not pull upward, giving the smile a transverse appearance. The patient may be unable to retract, purse, or puff the cheeks, or the seal on puffing may be overcome easily by the examiner. Fasciculations in the perioral area and chin may be present; patients are usually unaware of them. Patients may complain that their lips do not move well during speech and that they lose food or liquid out of their mouth when eating. Drooling during speech, when concentrating on another activity, or during eating or sleep may be reported or observed.

Abnormal movements of the face sometimes occur with cranial nerve VII lesions. They are noteworthy because they are unexpected in the context of FCP disease and may be confused with hyperkinesias of CNS origin. *Synkinesis* (see Figure 4-2) is the abnormal contraction of muscle adjacent to muscle that is contracting normally (e.g., a normal reflexive or voluntary eye blink may cause a simultaneous movement of lower facial muscles). It reflects aberrant branching or misdirection of regenerating axons of the facial nerve or abnormal activity of residual motor units. It is most commonly seen after recovery from Bell's palsy.[8] *Hemifacial spasm* is characterized by paroxysmal, rapid, irregular, usually unilateral tonic twitching of the facial muscle. It may be due to irritation of the nerve by a pulsating blood vessel in the area of the cerebellopontine angle or facial canal but may also be associated with tumor, vascular abnormalities, or multiple sclerosis.[8] *Facial myokymia* is characterized by rhythmic, undulating movements on an area of the face in which the surface of the skin moves like a "bag of worms." Such movements are more prolonged than fasciculations and reflect alternating brief contractions of adjacent motor units. They are often benign but, if widespread, may be associated with multiple sclerosis, brainstem tumors, syringobulbia, or demyelinating cranial neuropathies.[39,29]

Speech

The speech tasks that are most revealing of cranial nerve VII lesions are conversational speech and reading, speech AMRs, and stress testing.

A *flutter of the cheeks* may be present during conversation because hypotonicity results in less resistance to intraoral air pressure peaks during pressure sound production. Poor bilabial closure on one or both sides may be apparent. There may be a noticeable mismatch between speech AMRs for "puh" versus those for "tuh" and "kuh," with reduced precision and perhaps slowness of "puh" because of lip weakness. In general, precision is reduced more than speed, unless weakness is bilateral and severe. If MG is present, stress testing may generate visible and auditory perceptual deficits attributable to lower face weakness.

The effect of unilateral facial nerve lesions on speech can be more visible than audible. There may be mild, perceptible distortion of bilabial and labiodental consonants and, less frequently, anterior lingual fricatives and affricates. There is usually no perceptible effect on vowels.

Bilateral facial weakness, depending on its degree, can result in distortions or complete inability to produce /p/, /b/, /m/, /w/, /hw/, /f/, and /v/. The distortion of bilabial stops is often in the direction of frication or spirantization. If lip rounding and spreading are markedly reduced, vowels may be distorted. The effects of cranial nerve VII lesions on speech are summarized in Table 4-3.

Patients with unilateral and bilateral facial weakness sometimes spontaneously compensate in an effort to improve speech and physical appearance. In unilateral weakness, they may use a finger to prop up the sagging weak side at rest and during speech or, rarely, actually assist the movement of their lower lip in producing bilabial and labiodental sounds. Some patients exaggerate jaw closure in an effort to approximate the lips. If weakness is bilateral, severe, isolated to the face, and chronic, substitution of lingual articulation for bilabial consonants (e.g., t/p) may occur.[44]

Glossopharyngeal Nerve (IX) Lesions

Course and Function

Motor fibers of cranial nerve IX that are relevant to speech originate in the nucleus ambiguus within the reticular formation in the lateral medulla. The rootlets of cranial nerve IX emerge from the medulla, exit through the jugular foramen in the posterior fossa, and eventually pass into the pharynx to innervate the stylopharyngeus muscle, which elevates the pharynx during swallowing and speech. Afferent fibers originate in the inferior ganglion in the jugular foramen and terminate in the nucleus of the tractus solitarius in the medulla; they carry sensation from the pharynx and posterior tongue and are important to the sensory component of the gag reflex.

Etiologies and Localization of Lesions

Cranial nerve IX is rarely damaged in isolation (at the least; cranial nerve X is also typically involved). It is susceptible to the same pathologic influences that affect the other cranial nerves in the lower brainstem. Intramedullary and extramedullary lesion localization is usually tied to localization of cranial nerve X and XI lesions (discussed later).

Nonspeech Oral Mechanism

Cranial nerve IX is assessed clinically by examining the gag reflex, particularly asymmetry in the ease with which the reflex is elicited. A reduced gag may implicate the sensory or motor components of the reflex, the sensory component if the patient reports decreased sensation in the area. However, a normal gag can be present after intracranial section of the cranial nerve IX, suggesting that cranial nerve X is also involved in pharyngeal function. It is clear, however, that cranial nerve IX may be implicated in dysphagia, with lesions to it presumably affecting pharyngeal elevation during the pharyngeal phase of swallowing.

Some individuals with cranial nerve IX lesions develop brief attacks of severe pain that begin in the throat and radiate down the neck to the back of the lower jaw. Pain can be triggered by swallowing or tongue protrusion. This condition is known as *glossopharyngeal neuralgia*.

Speech

The role of cranial nerve IX in speech cannot be assessed directly. It probably has some influence on resonance and perhaps phonatory functions because of the effects of lesions on pharyngeal elevation. Because cranial nerve IX lesions are usually associated with cranial nerve X lesions, and because cranial nerve X has a crucial and relatively clearly defined role in speech, cranial nerve IX's importance in the assessment of dysarthria can be considered indeterminate for practical purposes.

Vagus Nerve (X) Lesions

Course and Function

Cell bodies of cranial nerve X that are relevant to speech originate in the nucleus ambiguus. Cell bodies of relevant sensory fibers originate in the inferior ganglion located in or near the jugular foramen; central processes of the sensory fibers terminate in the nucleus of the tractus solitarius in the brainstem.

Cranial nerve X exits the skull through the jugular foramen, along with cranial nerves IX and XI. From there it divides into the pharyngeal branch, which enters the pharynx; the superior laryngeal branch, which enters the pharynx and larynx; and the recurrent laryngeal branch, which passes down to upper chest. Cranial nerve X loops around the subclavian artery on the right and around the aorta on the left before traveling back up the neck to enter the larynx.

The pharyngeal branch supplies the muscles of the pharynx except the stylopharyngeus (cranial nerve IX), the muscles of the soft palate except the tensor veli palatini (mandibular branch of cranial nerve V), and the palatoglossus muscle. It is responsible for pharyngeal constriction and palatal elevation and retraction during speech and swallowing.

The internal laryngeal nerve, a component of the superior laryngeal nerve, transmits sensation from mucous membranes of portions of the larynx, epiglottis, base of the tongue, and aryepiglottic folds, and from stretch receptors in the larynx. The external laryngeal nerve—the motor component of the superior laryngeal nerve—supplies the inferior pharyngeal constrictors and the cricothyroid muscles. Its innervation of the cricothyroid muscle is important, because cricothyroid contraction lengthens the vocal folds for pitch adjustments.

The recurrent laryngeal branch of cranial nerve X innervates all of the intrinsic laryngeal muscles except the cricothyroid. Its sensory fibers carry general sensation from the vocal folds and larynx below them.

Etiologies and Localization of Lesions

The localization of cranial nerve X lesions is more complicated than that for other cranial nerves due to its long course and three major branches. The degree of weakness, positioning of paralyzed vocal folds, and degree and type of voice or resonance abnormality depend on the localization of the lesion along the course of the nerve and whether the lesion is unilateral or bilateral. Careful consideration of signs and symptoms stemming from cranial nerve X lesions can often distinguish among lesions that are (1) intramedullary, extramedullary, or above the pharyngeal branch; (2) below the pharyngeal branch but above the superior and recurrent laryngeal branches; or (3) below the superior laryngeal branch.

Vagus nerve lesions can be intramedullary, extramedullary, or extracranial. *Intramedullary lesions* damage the nerve in the brainstem. *Extramedullary lesions* damage the trunk of the nerve as it leaves the body of the brainstem but while it is still within the cranial cavity (i.e., before it exits from the jugular foramen). *Extracranial lesions* damage the nerve after it exits the skull. It is generally the case that as the distance of a lesion from the brainstem increases, the number of muscles, structures, and functions affected by the lesion decreases. Thus intracranial lesions are more likely than extramedullary and extracranial lesions to be bilateral or associated with multiple cranial nerve involvement. Extramedullary lesions are more likely to be unilateral but may still affect several cranial nerves (e.g., cranial nerves IX, X and XI all exit through the jugular foramen on each side of the posterior fossa). Extracranial lesions are more likely to be isolated to cranial nerve X, and perhaps only one of its branches.

The relationships between cranial nerve X lesion loci and impairment of muscle function are summarized in Table 4-4. The most important relationships include the following:

1. Intramedullary, extramedullary, and extracranial lesions above the separation of the pharyngeal, superior laryngeal, and recurrent laryngeal branches affect all muscles supplied by the nerve below the level of the lesion. Therefore pharyngeal and palatal muscles supplied by the pharyngeal branch, the cricothyroid muscle supplied by the superior laryngeal branch, and the remaining intrinsic laryngeal muscles supplied by the recurrent laryngeal branch are weak or paralyzed on the side of the lesion (Figure 4-3).

2. Lesions below the pharyngeal branch, but still high enough in the neck to affect the superior and recurrent branches, spare the upper pharynx and velopharyngeal mechanism but cause paralysis or weakness of the cricothyroid and other intrinsic muscles on the side of the lesion.

3. Lesions of the superior laryngeal branch but not the recurrent laryngeal or pharyngeal branches affect the cricothyroid but not the velopharyngeal mechanism or the remaining intrinsic laryngeal muscles.

4. Lesions affecting only the recurrent laryngeal nerve cause weakness or paralysis of the

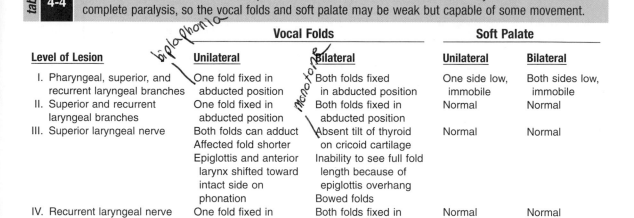

table 4-4 Effects on the vocal folds and soft palate cranial nerve X lesions. Note that many lesions do not cause complete paralysis, so the vocal folds and soft palate may be weak but capable of some movement.

	Vocal Folds		Soft Palate	
Level of Lesion	Unilateral	Bilateral	Unilateral	Bilateral
I. Pharyngeal, superior, and recurrent laryngeal branches	One fold fixed in abducted position	Both folds fixed in abducted position	One side low, immobile	Both sides low, immobile
II. Superior and recurrent laryngeal branches	One fold fixed in abducted position	Both folds fixed in abducted position	Normal	Normal
III. Superior laryngeal nerve	Both folds can adduct Affected fold shorter Epiglottis and anterior larynx shifted toward intact side on phonation	Absent tilt of thyroid on cricoid cartilage Inability to see full fold length because of epiglottis overhang Bowed folds	Normal	Normal
IV. Recurrent laryngeal nerve	One fold fixed in paramedian position	Both folds fixed in paramedian position	Normal	Normal

(handwritten annotations: "biphonia", "Monotone")

Modified from Aronson AE: *Clinical voice disorders*, New York, 1990, Thieme.

intrinsic laryngeal muscles on the side of the lesion, except the cricothyroid.

Intramedullary and extramedullary lesions affecting cranial nerve X can be caused by primary or metastatic tumor, infection, stroke, syringobulbia, Arnold-Chiari malformation, Guillain-Barré syndrome, polio, motor neuron disease, and other inflammatory or demyelinating diseases.[4] Not infrequently, lesions in the posterior fossa affect cranial nerves IX, X, and XI in combination. When this occurs in the area of the jugular foramen, it is called a *jugular foramen syndrome*.

Extracranial cranial nerve X disorders can be caused by myasthenia gravis, tumors in the neck or thorax, aneurysms in the aortic arch or internal carotid or subclavian artery, aortic dissection, and internal carotid artery dissection.[8,19,22] Surgery is a common cause of vocal fold paralysis, most often associated with thyroidectomy; carotid endarterectomy; anterior approach for cervical fusion; and cardiovascular, pulmonary, and skull base procedures.[32] Vagus nerve degeneration and dysphonia have been reported in individuals with severe alcoholic neuropathies.[21]

Nonspeech Oral Mechanism

Unilateral pharyngeal branch lesions are manifest by the following:
1. The soft palate hangs lower on the side of the lesion.
2. It pulls toward the nonparalyzed side on phonation (see Figures 4-3 and 4-4). A palate that hangs low at rest but elevates symmetri-

cally may not be weak. It may be asymmetric as a normal variant or the result of scarring from tonsillectomy. If palatal asymmetry on phonation is ambiguous, the clinician should look for a levator "dimple" representing the point of maximum contraction of the levator veli palatini muscle. If it is centered, the palate may not be weak; if it is displaced to one side, the palate is probably weak on the opposite side.
3. The gag reflex may be diminished on the weak side.

In bilateral lesions:
1. The palate hangs low in the pharynx at rest and moves minimally or not at all during phonation.
2. The gag reflex may be difficult to elicit or absent (recall that this may be normal in some individuals).
3. Nasal regurgitation may occur during swallowing.

Unilateral and bilateral superior laryngeal branch lesions that spare the recurrent laryngeal branch are frequently missed, because the vocal folds can appear normal. However, in unilateral lesions, even though both folds adduct, the affected vocal fold appears shorter than normal, and the epiglottis and anterior larynx are shifted toward the intact side. In bilateral cricothyroid paralysis, both folds appear short and bowed, and the epiglottis overhangs and obscures the anterior portion of the vocal folds.[4]

Unilateral lesions of the recurrent laryngeal nerve but not the pharyngeal or superior laryngeal nerve

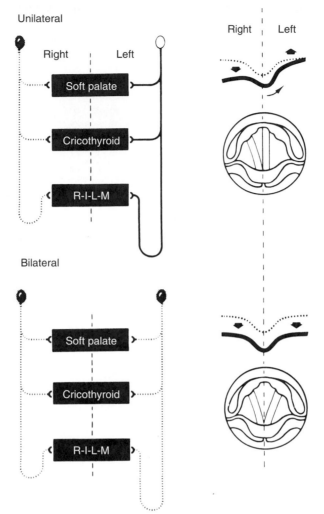

FIGURE 4-3 Effects of unilateral (right) and bilateral cranial (vagus) nerve X lesions above the origin of the pharyngeal, superior laryngeal, and recurrent laryngeal branches of the nerve. When unilateral, the soft palate hangs lower on the right and pulls toward the left on phonation. The right vocal fold is fixed in an abducted position, while the left fold adducts to the midline on phonation. When bilateral, the palate rests low bilaterally and does not move on phonation. Both vocal folds remain in the abducted position on phonation. (From Aronson AE: *Clinical voice disorders,* New York, 1990, Thieme, with permission).

leave the affected vocal fold fixed in the paramedian position. When bilateral, both folds are in the paramedian position. The folds are not completely abducted, because the intact cricothyroid maintains its adductor function and pulls the fold closer to the midline. In unilateral paralysis, dysphagia may be present, the cough and glottal coup can be weak, and there may be airway compromise. In bilateral paralysis, airway compromise and inhalatory stridor often occur, because abductor paralysis prevents widening of the glottis during inhalation. The resulting respiratory distress may require tracheotomy.

Lesions affecting both the recurrent and superior laryngeal branches of the vagus leave the affected vocal folds paralyzed in the abducted position, because all laryngeal adductors are affected. The cough and glottal coup are weak, and dysphagia is common. Signs of weakness are worse with bilateral than unilateral vocal fold lesions.

Speech

Table 4-3 summarizes the effects of unilateral and bilateral cranial nerve X lesions on speech. The effects cross several aspects of speech production, including phonation, resonance, articulation, and prosody, but the effects on resonance and phonation are generally most pronounced.

When the pharyngeal branch is affected unilaterally, there may be little or no perceptible effect or mild-to-moderate hypernasality and nasal emission during pressure consonant production. If weakness is bilateral, *hypernasality* can be marked to severe, *audible nasal emission* may be apparent, and *pressure consonants may be noticeably imprecise* because of inability to impound intraoral pressure. *Loudness may be mildly reduced* because of the damping effects of the nasal cavity on the emitted sound, and *phrase length may be reduced* because of nasal air wastage. *Facial grimacing* may develop in an effort to valve the air stream at the nares. The imprecision of pressure consonants sometimes generates suspicions about tongue, face, or jaw weakness. If consonant imprecision is due solely to velopharyngeal incompetence, occluding the nares during speech facilitates intraoral pressure for articulation and aids assessment of the adequacy of the other articulators.

Unilateral lesions of cranial nerve X below the pharyngeal branch but including the superior and recurrent laryngeal branches can result in *breathiness* or *aphonia, hoarseness, reduced loudness, diplophonia, reduced pitch,* and *pitch breaks.* A *rapid vocal flutter* may be present during vowel prolongation. *Phrases may be short* because of air wastage through the incompletely adducted glottis during phonation; when glottal air wastage is substantial, *speaking on inhalation* is sometimes spontaneously adopted as a compensatory strategy. In bilateral paralysis these characteristics are usually exaggerated.

Lesions of the superior laryngeal nerve that spare the pharyngeal and recurrent laryngeal nerves cause subtle changes in voice. When unilateral, mild breathiness or hoarseness and mild *inability to alter pitch* may be present. Loudness may be normal or mildly reduced. The inability to alter pitch may generate complaints about decreased ability to sing. Bilateral cricothyroid paralysis can cause mild to moderate breathiness and hoarseness, decreased loudness, and markedly reduced ability to alter pitch.

Unilateral recurrent laryngeal nerve lesions that spare the superior laryngeal nerve and pharyngeal branch cause *breathy-hoarse voice quality, decreased loudness,* and sometimes *diplophonia* and *pitch breaks.* Bilateral weakness or paralysis causes *inhalatory stridor,* but the voice may be relatively unaffected because the folds are adducted close to the midline. *Airway compromise,* however, can be a serious problem.

Acoustic and Physiologic Findings

Videofluoroscopy or nasoendoscopy are useful for documenting weakness of the velopharyngeal valve during speech. Bilateral velopharyngeal weakness can be demonstrated by nasoendoscopy and by videofluoroscopy in lateral, frontal, and base views. Laryngoscopic examination is essential in cases with suspected vocal fold weakness, not only for diagnostic purposes but also for management considerations.

The visible characteristics of weak vocal fold activity have been described beyond simple observations of paralysis. Videostroboscopy and high-speed laryngeal photography in patients with unilateral vocal fold paralysis have documented a lack of firm glottal closure during phonation; "light touch" glottic closure, reflecting either less than complete paralysis or assistance to medial fold approximation by the Bernoulli effect; irregular vocal fold vibration; exaggeration of the mucosal wave in the affected fold during phonation; and abnormal frequency and amplitude perturbations in vocal fold activity.[26,63] Greater vibratory amplitude and exaggerated mucosal waves are consistent with hypotonicity. These observations are consistent with the perception of breathiness (lack of firm glottal closure), hoarseness, and perhaps diplophonia associated with vocal fold weakness.

Aerodynamic studies of people with unilateral or bilateral vocal fold weakness have identified increased airflow rates during speech. These findings are consistent with neuromuscular weakness of the vocal folds, with subsequent incomplete vocal fold adduction and excessive air escape through the glottis during phonation.[9,26,60] Relatedly, it has been documented that dysarthric speakers with laryngeal "hypovalving" inspire considerably more volume of air per minute than normal speakers, mostly through increased breaths per minute; have mean speech duration per breath group that is considerably less than normal; expire more air than normal during pauses; and tend to have reduced pause frequency and duration, possibly secondary to poor vocal fold valving or a compensatory effort to increase speaking time.[60] People with inspiratory airway compromise (including unilateral and bilateral vocal fold paralysis) also have increased mean inspiratory duration during speech.[61] Many of these findings are consistent with the perception of breathiness and short phrases in people with laryngeal weakness. They also define some of the efforts that may be made to compensate for vocal fold weakness, such as increased breaths per minute, increased inspiratory volume, and a tendency to reduce pause frequency and duration.

Acoustic studies of people with unilateral vocal fold paralysis or weakness have documented the following characteristics: a breakdown of formant structure, reflected in a long-term average acoustic spectrum characterized by high f_o amplitude with a marked drop-off of harmonics above the first formant; random noise in spectrograms and increased spectral energy levels in high-frequency regions, possibly reflecting turbulent airflow through a partially open glottis; and restricted standard deviation and range of fundamental frequency, suggesting reduced ability to reach upper pitch ranges.[23,43,51] Some studies have noted a relationship between some of these characteristics and perceptual judgments of breathiness and hypofunctional voice.[23,50] Findings of restricted f_o range and variability[43] are consistent with Darley, Aronson, and Brown's (DAB's)[14] finding that monopitch is frequently perceived in flaccid dysarthrias.

Aerodynamic, acoustic, videofluoroscopic, and nasoendoscopic studies have repeatedly shown a relationship among velopharyngeal insufficiency (VPI) and hypernasality, nasal emission, and weak pressure consonants. Although most published studies have examined people with palatal clefts or undefined or mixed dysarthrias, their general findings can probably be generalized to those with velopharyngeal weakness associated with cranial nerve X lesions. In addition to increased nasal airflow with VPI, there are numerous acoustic correlates of listeners' perceptions of hypernasality. These include decreased energy and higher frequency of the first formant, change or shift in center frequencies of formants, increased formant bandwidth, reduced vowel intensity and dynamic intensity range, reduced vocal pitch range, and extra resonances.[12,30] Reduced formant and overall intensity probably reflect the damping characteristics of the nasal cavity. Finally, the connection of the pharyngeal tube to a side branching tube (nasal cavity) leads to the development of antiresonances in the spectrum (i.e., a sharp drop in intensity in a portion of the spectrum where energy is expected). Because these acoustic attributes are correlated with VPI and perceptions stemming from it, they represent quantifiable indices of velopharyngeal weakness that may be useful for documentation of deficits, comparisons over time, and the effects of management.

Accessory Nerve (XI) Lesions

Course and Function

The cranial portion of cranial nerve XI arises from the nucleus ambiguus, emerges from the side of the medulla, and exits the skull through the jugular foramen along with cranial nerves IX and X. It intermingles with fibers of cranial nerve X to help innervate the uvula, levator veli palatini, and intrinsic laryngeal muscles. The spinal portion arises from the first five to six cervical segments of the spinal cord, ascends and enters the posterior fossa through the foramen magnum, and then leaves the skull with fibers of cranial nerves IX and X, and cranial portion of cranial nerve XI, where it innervates the sternocleidomastoid and trapezius muscles.

Etiologies and Localization of Lesions

Etiologies of lesions to the cranial portion of cranial nerve XI are similar to those described for cranial nerve X. The spinal portion can be damaged by lesions in the cervical spinal cord and by compression from lesions in the area of the foramen magnum. Radical neck surgery is another source of eleventh nerve lesions.

Nonspeech Oral Mechanism

Lesions of the spinal portion of cranial nerve XI reduce shoulder elevation on the side of the lesion and weaken head turning to the side opposite the lesion. Such lesions do not generally affect speech. If bilateral weakness causes significant shoulder weakness and head drooping, then respiration, phonation, and resonance may be indirectly and mildly affected by the postural deficit.

Because it is clinically impossible to separate the effects of cranial nerve X lesions from those of lesions to the cranial portion of cranial nerve XI, and because some people argue that the cranial portion of cranial nerve XI is more appropriately considered part of cranial nerve X, it is unnecessary to treat cranial nerve XI as distinctly important to motor speech function.

Hypoglossal Nerve (XII) Lesions

Course and Function

Cranial nerve XII originates in the medulla. Its fibers exit the brainstem as a number of rootlets that converge and pass through the hypoglossal foramen just lateral to the foramen magnum. The nerve travels medial to cranial nerves IX, X, and XI in the vicinity of the common carotid artery and internal jugular vein and passes above the hyoid bone to reach the intrinsic and extrinsic muscles of the tongue.

Cranial nerve XII innervates all of the intrinsic and extrinsic muscles of the tongue, except the palatoglossus (cranial nerve X). It is crucial for lingual articulatory movements, as well as chewing and swallowing.

Etiologies and Localization of Lesions

Hypoglossal nerve lesions can be intramedullary, extramedullary, and extracranial. They can be caused by any condition that can affect the lower cranial nerves. Lesions to it often damage other cranial nerves, especially IX, X, and XI, but it can be damaged in isolation. Common causes of isolated hypoglossal lesions include infection and basilar skull or neck tumor, trauma, or surgery. Approximately 5% of carotid endarterectomies are associated with usually temporary hypoglossal nerve injury.[5] The nerve can also be damaged by carotid and vertebral artery aneurysms; carotid artery dissection; tumors in the neck, salivary glands, or base of the tongue; and radiation therapy.[8,34,47,59]

Nonspeech Oral Mechanism

In unilateral hypoglossal lesions the tongue may be atrophic and shrunken on the weak side (see Figure 4-4). Fasciculations may be apparent. The tongue deviates to the weak side on protrusion, because the action of the unaffected genioglossus muscle is unopposed (Figure 4-5). The ability to curl the tip of the tongue to the weak side inside the mouth is diminished, as is the ability to push the tongue into the cheek against resistance. Voluntary tongue lateralization within the mouth occasionally yields paradoxical results, with the ability to push the tongue into the cheek on the weak side sometimes appearing normal. It may be that some people push the tongue to the weak side with the unaffected side instead of attempting to use the longitudinal fibers on the weak side to turn the tongue to the weak side.

With bilateral lesions the tongue may be atrophic bilaterally, with bilateral fasciculations. It may protrude symmetrically, but with limited range, or not at all. Lateralization and elevation may be impossible. Saliva may accumulate in the mouth, and food may squirrel in the cheeks. Patients may note an inability to move food around in the mouth and may alter their diet to accommodate to this problem. They may complain that the tongue feels "heavy," "thick,"

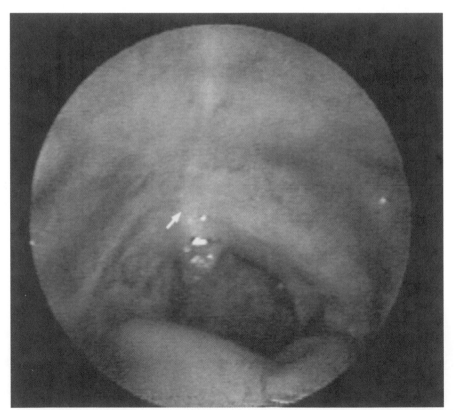

FIGURE 4-4 Palatal movement during phonation in a patient with left palatal weakness. The palate pulls to the right. The *arrow* identifies the levator eminence (dimple), which is also displaced to the right. This patient also has left lingual weakness secondary to a left cranial (hypoglossal) nerve XII lesion; note the smaller left than right side of the tongue because of atrophy on the left.

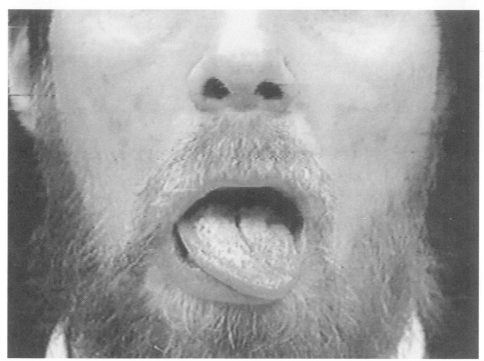

FIGURE 4-5 Deviation of the tongue to the left on protrusion, reflecting a left cranial (hypoglossal) nerve XII lesion.

or "big," or that it does not move well for eating and speaking. Drooling can be related to lingual weakness.

Speech

The overriding speech characteristic in unilateral and bilateral cranial nerve XII lesions is *imprecise articulation* that can be isolated to lingual phonemes. Table 4-3 summarizes the effects of unilateral and bilateral cranial nerve XII lesions on speech.

Isolated unilateral twelfth nerve lesions are often compensated for to a degree that allows perceptually normal speech. Articulatory distortions are generally mild and do not affect intelligibility.

Bilateral lingual weakness causes difficulty with sounds requiring elevation of the tip or back of the tongue. When weakness is mild, anterior lingual consonant distortion is often detected more readily than velar distortions because of their greater number and frequency of occurrence in the language. The movements for the relatively difficult /s/, /ʃ/, /tʃ/ and their voiced cognates, as well as /r/ and /l/, are most susceptible to lingual weakness and may be the "first to go" when weakness develops. When weakness is pronounced, however, velars may be particularly devastated, perhaps because a greater mass must be moved to produce them relative to that for anterior lingual consonants.

Resonance differences are occasionally noted in people with bilateral lingual weakness. The altered resonance is sometimes labeled *hypernasality* or *hyponasality,* but this is probably inaccurate. Although the reason for resonance alterations is unclear, it may be that the weak tongue tends to fall back into the pharynx, altering the shape of the pharynx and, hence, resonance characteristics; reduced tongue movement reduces variability of oral cavity shapes during speech, thus reducing normal resonance variability, leading to a perception of abnormal resonance; or that atrophy alters the size of the oral and pharyngeal cavities, leading to resonance changes.

The most useful tasks for assessing lingual movement for speech are connected speech (including stress testing if MG is suspected) and speech AMRs. Connected speech places heavy demands on rapid, variable movements and may be most useful for identifying lingual distortions. If weakness is limited to the tongue, AMRs for "puh" should be normal, while those for "tuh" and "kuh" may be imprecise or slow. A noticeable mismatch in precision or rate between bilabial and lingual AMRs usually suggests isolated or relatively greater lingual weakness or, if the difference is in favor of lingual AMRs, isolated or relatively greater bilabial weakness. Imprecision and slowness for "kuh" generally exceeds that for "tuh" when the tongue is weak, possibly because elevation of the back of the tongue, with its greater mass, places increased demands on strength (note, however, that AMRs for "kuh" are usually somewhat slower than "tuh" in normal speakers).

Speakers with bilateral lingual weakness often compensate well if other muscles are intact. For example, they may exaggerate jaw movement to facilitate lingual articulation, or they may restrict jaw movement to keep the tongue closer to articulatory targets in the maxilla. Compensatory exaggerated movements occasionally are mistaken for hyperkinetic movement disorders, although the physical mechanism examination usually clarifies the issue.

Acoustic and Physiologic Findings

Studies have demonstrated reduced lingual strength or endurance in individuals with flaccid dysarthria[9,18] and, in some affected individuals, slower than normal lingual AMRs.[18] It is noteworthy, however, that lingual strength in dysarthric individuals may not be related to rate or ratings of intelligibility. It thus appears that tongue strength measures may be useful for quantifying lingual weakness but may not have a strong predictive relationship with speech rate or intelligibility. The lack of relationship between tongue strength and speech rate is consistent with the general perceptual impression that speech rate is noticeably reduced in flaccid dysarthrias only when weakness is quite severe.

Spinal Nerve Lesions

Course, Function, and Localization of Lesions

Upper cervical spinal nerves supplying the neck are indirectly implicated in voice, resonance, and articulation (see discussion of the spinal component of cranial nerve XI). Effects on speech of lesions to these nerves are indirect, usually mild, and poorly understood.

Spinal nerves more directly involved in respiration are spread from the cervical through the thoracic divisions of the spinal cord. Those supplying the diaphragm arise from the third through fifth cervical segments. They combine to form the phrenic nerves, each of which innervates half of the diaphragm, the most important inspiratory respiratory muscle. Remaining inhalatory muscles are supplied by branches of the lower cervical nerves, intercostal nerves, and phrenic nerves. Muscles of forced exhalation, important for control of exhalation during speech, are innervated by motor fibers of the thoracic and intercostal nerves.

Diffuse impairment of spinal nerves supplying respiratory muscles is required to interfere significantly with respiration. The exception is damage to the third through fifth segments of the cervical spinal cord that can paralyze the diaphragm bilaterally and severely compromise breathing.

Etiologies

Spinal cord injuries above C3 can isolate the respiratory muscles from the brainstem respiratory control centers and cause respiratory paralysis. Diseases such as MG, ALS, Guillain-Barré syndrome, and spinal cord injuries affect respiration by weakening muscles or interfering with their innervation.

Nonspeech Oral and Respiratory Mechanisms

Compromised respiratory nerve function can result in rapid, shallow breathing. Flaring of the nasal alae and use of upper chest and shoulder neck muscles to elevate and enlarge the rib cage suggest respiratory compromise. Chest wall and abdominal expansion may be visibly restricted during inhalation, and patients may be unable to hold their breath for more than a few seconds. They may be unable to generate or sustain subglottal air pressure sufficient to support speech as measured by a U-tube or water glass manometer.

Speech

Flaccid dysarthria due to isolated respiratory disturbance is uncommon in many speech pathology practices. It is not clear if this is because the incidence of such disturbances is low, if such patients rarely complain of the effects of such disturbances on speech or spontaneously compensate for them, or if the respiratory compromise for basic life support is so overriding that its effect on speech is of low priority to the patient and his or her medical caregivers. Such speech problems certainly exist and have been described in published reports.[27,28] Patients with respiratory weakness sufficient to affect speech usually also have weakness that interferes with quiet breathing or breathing during other physical activities. These deficits have usually been identified before speech examination. Table 4-3 summarizes the effects of respiratory weakness on speech.

Respiratory weakness reduces the amount and force of expelled air. Reduced vital capacity and control of expiration can result in *short phrases* and *reduced loudness*. Prosodic abnormalities secondary to *altered phrasing* may result, as may *decreased pitch and loudness variability*. Such problems are not universally present, but are not uncommon. For example, in a study of 10 adults with cervical spinal cord injury, three were perceived as normal speakers; three had reduced loudness; two were breathy; two had short phrases; and one had prolonged inspiration, which presumably affected prosody.[28]

Patients with respiratory weakness may inhale with obvious effort, sometimes raising their shoulders and extending their neck in compensation for diaphragmatic weakness. They may attempt to speak on residual air, which may cause the voice to actually sound *strained,* probably secondary to efforts to achieve vocal fold adduction with limited subglottic pressure or to maximize efficient use of the restricted respiratory supply. Many of these characteristics are also evident in people with severe asthma, chronic obstructive pulmonary disease, and other respiratory disturbances of a nonneurologic nature. Finally, inability to extend the duration of exhalation for normal phrase length in speech leads some patients to *speak on inhalation.*

Respiratory weakness in combination with cranial nerve weakness in flaccid dysarthrias is not unusual, and distinguishing between phonatory and prosodic abnormalities due to respiratory versus laryngeal weakness can be difficult. Some clues that help to identify which level is more involved include:

1. Gasping for air, nares flaring, shoulder elevation, and neck retraction on inhalation during speech are rare in isolated laryngeal weakness but not uncommon in respiratory weakness.

2. Patients with isolated laryngeal adductor weakness do not complain of shortness of breath at times other than during speech. Those with respiratory weakness do.

3. Patients with isolated respiratory weakness may have reduced loudness and breathy or strained voice quality but not hoarseness, harshness, or diplophonia. Those with laryngeal weakness are frequently hoarse or harsh and sometimes diplophonic.

4. Patients with greater laryngeal than respiratory weakness may have a glottal coup that is less adequate than their cough (good respiratory force during coughing may overcome vocal fold weakness). The opposite can occur when respiratory weakness exceeds laryngeal weakness (less respiratory force is required for a glottal coup than cough).

Physiologic Findings

Acoustic and physiologic studies of speech in people with isolated respiratory weakness are few. Hixon, Putnam, and Sharp[27] conducted a detailed kinematic analysis of respiratory movements in a man with flaccid paralysis of respiratory muscles. He had considerable capacity for compensatory speech respiratory activities in the form of "neck breathing"

and "glossopharyngeal breathing" (discussed in Chapter 17) The data support contentions that reduced vital capacity need not result in speech difficulty if valving of the air stream can be made more efficient.

Hoit et al.[28] documented abnormal chest wall movement consistent with loss of abdominal muscle function in individuals with cervical spinal injury. They also found speech breathing patterns that reflected compensations for expiratory muscle weakness. Speakers inspired to larger lung and rib cage volumes (they inhaled more deeply) and terminated speech at larger volumes than nonimpaired speakers, presumably to take advantage of higher elastic recoil pressure at those volumes that could drive the upper airway and larynx during phonation. Speakers also used larger lung volumes when asked to increase loudness. These compensatory strategies were developed spontaneously in most cases.

Multiple Cranial Nerve Lesions

When several cranial nerves are damaged, the condition is often referred to as *bulbar palsy.* Damage to more than a single cranial nerve is not unusual. The jaw, face, lips, tongue, palate, pharynx, and larynx can be affected in varying combinations and to varying degrees depending on the particular cranial nerves involved and whether damage is unilateral or bilateral.

Conditions that affect multiple cranial nerves tend to be associated with intracranial pathology. This is because the smallest lesion that can do the most damage is in the brainstem where the cranial nerves are closer together than anywhere else along their course. This is not always the case, however, because multiple cranial nerves may be involved in neuromuscular junction diseases (e.g., myasthenia gravis), and myopathies can affect muscles in the distribution of more than one cranial nerve.

Etiologies

Multiple cranial nerve involvement can be caused by many of the same conditions that affect single cranial nerves. Multiple rather than single cranial nerve involvement is more common in certain diseases, however, including ALS, MG, and brainstem vascular disturbances or tumors.

Nonspeech Oral Mechanism

Clinical examination findings for patients with multiple cranial nerve involvement are no different than those with damage to single cranial nerves. The cumulative effects on function, however, can be much more devastating than the effects of single cranial nerve lesions.

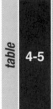

| table 4-5 | Distribution of involvement of cranial nerves V, VII, X, and XII, and spinal respiratory nerves, in 151 quasirandomly selected cases with a primary speech diagnosis of flaccid dysarthria at the Mayo Clinic from 1969-1990 and 1999-2001. Number of instances in which each nerve was the only speech nerve involved, and the number of instances in which each nerve was involved along with other speech nerves, are given. Forty-three percent of the cases had isolated unilateral or bilateral involvement of a single cranial nerve. Fifty-seven percent had more than one cranial nerve involved. As a result, the total number of different nerves reported is 221. |

Nerve	Isolated Unilateral	Isolated Bilateral	Multiple Unilateral	Multiple Bilateral	Percent of Total
V	—	—	2	4	3
VII	—	3	5	22	14
X—Pharyngeal branch only	—	2	—	2	2
Laryngeal branch(es) only	52	7	—	4	29
All branches	10	11	5	35	28
XII	3	6	10	33	24
Respiratory	—	1	—	4	2
Percent of total	29	14	10	47	100

Speech

Deviant speech characteristics associated with multiple cranial nerve lesions are similar to those associated with isolated cranial nerve damage, but the effects are heard in combination. Consequently, they may be more difficult to isolate. In general, the dysarthria is perceived as more severe than in single cranial nerve lesions, but this is not always the case, especially if the measure of severity is intelligibility. For example, a bilateral lesion of the facial nerve could have a greater impact on intelligibility than combined unilateral lesions of cranial nerves V, VII, and X. In general, effective compensatory strategies for maintaining intelligibility are more difficult when multiple cranial nerves are involved than when impairment is to only a single cranial nerve.

Distribution of Speech Cranial Nerve Involvement in Flaccid Dysarthrias

The distribution of cranial nerve involvement in the population of people with flaccid dysarthrias is unknown, but a retrospective review of cases seen in a large medical setting provides clues about the distribution encountered in some practices.

Table 4-5 summarizes the distribution of involvement of cranial nerves V, VII, X, and XII in 151 of 154* of the cases whose etiologies are summarized in Box 4-1. Cautious interpretation should be exercised regarding the representativeness of these

*The three missing cases were insufficiently documented to identify specific cranial nerves.

data for the general population or for all speech pathology practices. In addition, these data represent speech pathologists' judgment about the contribution of cranial nerve weakness to the dysarthria and not necessarily all of the cranial nerves that might have been involved (e.g., unilateral cranial nerve V weakness was not included if it did not appear relevant to the speech deficit).

Several characteristics of the distribution are of interest. First, cranial nerve V and respiratory contributions to flaccid dysarthrias were infrequent. This probably means that they are usually not affected in flaccid dysarthrias or are not often judged to contribute to deviant speech characteristics. Cranial nerves VII and XII were involved much more frequently, and cranial nerve X more often than any other speech cranial nerve. Among the branches of cranial nerve X, the pharyngeal branch was only infrequently implicated without suspected involvement of the superior or recurrent laryngeal branches. In contrast, the laryngeal branches were frequently implicated without pharyngeal branch involvement; this reflects the high frequency of surgery-related or idiopathic vocal fold paralyses below the pharyngeal branch of cranial nerve X. Finally, more than 40% of the sample had unilateral or bilateral involvement of a single cranial nerve (most often cranial nerve X). The majority of the sample had unilateral or bilateral involvement of more than one cranial nerve.

Clusters of Deviant Speech Dimensions

DAB[16] found three clusters of deviant dimensions among 30 patients with bulbar palsy. These clusters are useful in understanding the presumed neuromuscular deficits, the components of the speech system that are most prominently involved, and features of flaccid dysarthrias that distinguish it from other dysarthria types (Table 4-6).

The first cluster was *phonatory incompetence.* It included *breathy voice, audible inspiration,* and *short phrases.* The cluster represents incompetence at the laryngeal valve, including inadequate vocal fold adduction (breathiness due to inadequate vocal fold adduction, as well as short phrases due to air wastage through the glottis) and abduction (audible inspiration due to inadequate vocal fold abduction during inspiration).

The second cluster was *resonatory incompetence.* It included *hypernasality, nasal emission, imprecise consonants,* and *short phrases.* The relationships among these features reflect weakness of the velopharyngeal valve leading to excessive nasal resonance (hypernasality) and nasal air flow during attempts to produce consonants requiring intraoral pressure (nasal emission). Imprecise consonants in this cluster reflect the secondary effect of nasal emission on pressure consonant precision. Short phrases reflect the effect of air wastage through the velopharyngeal port during speech.

The final cluster was *phonatory-prosodic insufficiency.* It consisted of *harsh voice, monopitch,* and *monoloudness.* DAB felt these characteristics reflected hypotonia in laryngeal muscles. This hypothesis receives support from acoustic and physiologic studies and from direct observation of weak or paralyzed vocal folds.

The phonatory and resonatory incompetence clusters are especially important for differential diagnosis, because they were not found in other dysarthria types. Thus the presence of phonatory or resonatory incompetence is suggestive of flaccid dysarthria and implicates LMN weakness at the laryngeal and velopharyngeal valves (cranial nerve X). The third cluster, phonatory-prosodic insufficiency, is of less

value to differential diagnosis, because it is also found in other dysarthria types.

The reader may be struck by the restriction of these clusters to cranial nerve X abnormalities. This does not mean that speech abnormalities attributable to weakness of other cranial nerves do not occur in flaccid dysarthrias, nor does it imply that recognition of other abnormalities is not helpful to diagnosis. The absence of obvious effects of other cranial nerves in the cluster analysis of DAB probably reflects several influences. First, the distribution of cranial nerve involvement in their sample (and those with flaccid dysarthrias in general, as suggested by the findings summarized in Table 4-5) may have been biased toward cranial nerve X lesions. Second, the grouping of all articulatory deficits under the global designation of imprecise consonants and vowel distortions may have masked the specific effects of cranial nerve V, VII, and XII lesions on speech. Third, imprecise consonants can occur in all dysarthria types, so their presence is not likely to be distinctive within clusters that distinguish among types of dysarthria. Finally, the primary purpose of

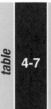

table	4-7	Most deviant speech characteristics encountered in flaccid dysarthrias by Darley, Aronson, and Brown,[15] listed in order from most to least severe. Also listed are the cranial nerves and muscle groups most likely associated with the deviant speech characteristics.

Dimension	Primary Cranial Nerve	Level
Hypernasality*	X	Velopharyngeal
Imprecise		Articulatory
consonants	V	• Jaw
	VII	• Face
	X	• Velopharyngeal
	XII	• Tongue
Breathiness (continuous)*	X	Laryngeal
Monopitch	X	Laryngeal
Nasal emission*	X	Velopharyngeal
Audible inspiration*	X	Laryngeal
Harsh voice quality	X	Laryngeal
Short phrases*	X	Laryngeal or
	Spinal respiratory	respiratory
Monoloudness	X	Laryngeal or
	Spinal respiratory	respiratory

*Tend to be distinctive or more severely impaired in flaccid dysarthrias than any other single dysarthria type.

table	4-6	Clusters of abnormal speech characteristics in flaccid dysarthrias

Cluster Name	Speech Characteristics
Phonatory Incompetence	Breathiness, short phrases, audible inspiration
Resonatory Incompetence	Hypernasality, imprecise consonants, nasal emission, short phrases
Phonatory-prosodic Insufficiency	Harsh voice, monoloudness, monopitch

Modified from Darley FL, Aronson AE, Brown JR: Differential diagnostic patterns of dysarthria, *J Speech Hear Res* 12:246, 1969.

table 4-8 Summary of direct observations and acoustic and physiologic findings in flaccid dysarthrias (based on literature summarized in text). Some findings may reflect efforts to compensate for weakness and not just the primary effects of weakness.

Level	Direct, Acoustic, and Physiologic Observations
Respiratory	Reduced vital capacity
	Termination of speech at larger than normal lung volumes*
	Larger than normal inspiratory and rib cage volumes*
	Abnormal chest wall movements*
	Neck and glossopharyngeal breathing*
Laryngeal or Respiratory	Vocal fold immobility or sluggishness (unilateral or bilateral)
	Incomplete glottal closure (unilateral or bilateral)
	Abnormal vocal fold frequency and amplitude perturbations
	Increased amplitude of vocal fold mucosal wave (unilateral or bilateral)
	Increased airflow rate
	Increased inspiratory volume*
	Increased breaths per minute*
	Reduced pause frequency and duration*
	Reduced speech duration or syllables per breath group*
	Reduced range and variability of f_o
	High amplitude of f_o with reduced energy of harmonics
	Reduced formant intensity and definition
	Increased high-frequency spectral energy (noise)
Velopharyngeal[†]	Reduced or absent palatal movement (unilateral or bilateral)
	Reduced or absent pharyngeal wall movement (unilateral or bilateral)
	Increased nasal airflow
	Decreased energy in f_o
	Increased frequency of f_o
	Reduced pitch range
	Increased formant bandwidth
	Reduced overall intensity and intensity range
	Extra resonances
	Antiresonances
Lingual	Reduced sustained lingual force

*Compensatory or possibly compensatory.
[†]Includes findings from studies of velopharyngeal incompetence associated with cleft palate.

the studies by DAB focused on distinctions among dysarthria types rather than the differential effects on speech of damage to specific cranial nerves within a specific dysarthria type (i.e., flaccid dysarthrias).

The important point here is that investigating the functions of each cranial nerve and the loci of specific speech characteristics is important to examination, description, and diagnosis. Also, because flaccid dysarthrias can be manifest by damage to only a single cranial nerve, and because other dysarthrias are rarely manifest through a single cranial nerve, identification of the offending muscle group is important to differential diagnosis and treatment decisions.

Table 4-7 summarizes the most deviant speech characteristics that were found by DAB in their patients with flaccid dysarthria.[15] The cranial or spinal nerve and the component of the speech mechanism that is most likely implicated in the production of each of the characteristics are also given. Table 4-8 summarizes the acoustic and physiologic correlates of flaccid dysarthrias that were reviewed within the discussion of deficits associated with each of the speech cranial nerves.

Cases

The following cases review the histories, examination findings, and diagnoses for several patients with flaccid dysarthria. As a group, they illustrate some of the similarities and differences that exist among people with this type of dysarthria. Several cases illustrate the prominence of speech deficits in neurologic disease and the importance of speech diagnosis to medical or neurologic diagnosis.

Case 4-1

A 44-year-old woman presented with an 8-month history of speech difficulty that she thought was caused by ongoing stress. The neurologic examination was normal. The neurologist was uncertain but wondered if her complaint was stress related. Speech pathology consultation was requested.

During speech evaluation the patient said that her speech deteriorated when she was tired or under stress, and that it frequently changed while she was coaching a volleyball team. She described it as "slurred, almost like my mouth freezes . . . almost sounds like it goes nasal." She vaguely described an alteration of chewing and swallowing at such times but denied choking or drooling. The speech problem would persist until she rested. Her primary sources of stress were a busy schedule caring for her three school-age children and coaching a high school volleyball team. She described her family life and work as stable and happy but busy.

Speech was initially normal. After 6 minutes of continuous reading aloud, mild sibilant distortions became apparent, along with equivocal hoarseness and intermittent vocal flutter. Speech AMRs were normal, and she did not become hypernasal, but inconsistent nasal airflow was detected on a mirror held at the nares during repetition of nonnasal sounds and phrases. After another 4.5 minutes of reading, she began to interdentalize /s/ and /z/, distort affricates, and mildly distort /r/. AMRs remained normal, and hypernasality was not perceived. The oral mechanism examination immediately following stress testing demonstrated only equivocal lingual weak-

ness. The patient was upset and cried when her speech changed, making it difficult to separate the effects of her emotional response from weakness. Speech returned to normal after 30 seconds of rest.

She was asked to return the following day at 5 PM, following volleyball practice. Although speech was initially normal, it deteriorated quickly and significantly, but its character was the same as that noted the day before. In addition, pitch breaks and some fluttering of the cheeks during speech were apparent.

The speech diagnosis was "flaccid dysarthria characterized by weakness of, at the least, cranial nerves VII, X, and XII, bilaterally, with rapid deterioration with stress testing, consistent with the pattern of breakdown seen in myasthenia gravis." Subsequent EMG and improvement of her symptoms with Mestinon treatment confirmed the diagnosis of MG. She subsequently did well with Mestinon treatment.

Commentary. (1) Speech difficulty can be the first sign of neurologic disease. (2) The presence of psychologic distress at the onset of speech difficulty is insufficient proof of psychogenic etiology. Patients often attribute their physical problem to stress when neurologic disease presents insidiously. In such cases, neurologic and psychologic factors deserve equal attention until a clear cause emerges. (3) Speech diagnosis can localize disease in the motor system. In some cases, speech diagnosis provides strong evidence for a specific neurologic diagnosis.*

*An informative case of a person with MG masking as stroke can be found in Duffy.[17]

Case 4-2

A 37-year-old man presented with a complaint of speech difficulty, problems with "tongue control," and headache and neck pain of 2 months' duration. He described his speech as "slurred" and complained of excess saliva accumulation and difficulty moving food with his tongue.

Oral mechanism examination identified a bilaterally atrophic tongue but no fasciculations. He was barely able to move his tongue in any direction, and tongue strength was rated -4 bilaterally. Saliva pooled in his mouth. Phonation and resonance were normal, as were AMRs for "puh" and "tuh," but those for "kuh" were equivocally slowed and reduced in precision. Lingual sounds were distorted. Nonlingual sounds, rate, and prosody were normal. Jaw and facial movements during speech were exaggerated in apparent compensation for his lingual weakness. Intelligibility was good.

Neurologic examination was otherwise normal except for mild weakness of neck flexor muscles. Skull radiographs showed destruction of the interior portion of the clivus (the bony part of the posterior fossa anterior to the foramen magnum) and an associated nasopharyngeal soft-tissue mass. Magnetic resonance imaging (MRI) and computed tomography (CT) scans identified a destructive tumor mass in the anterior rim of the foramen magnum bilaterally. The patient underwent neurosurgery for radical subtotal removal of a chordoma tumor of the clivus. Postoperatively, articulatory imprecision was mildly worse, but no other speech deficits developed. The patient underwent radiation therapy, and his speech gradually improved, though not to normal. Lingual atrophy and weakness persisted. He did well but 2 years later developed headache, nausea, vomiting, and double vision. There was evidence of tumor recurrence, but further radiation therapy or surgery was not advised because of risks and unlikely benefit. The patient lived outside of the geographic area of treatment and was not seen for further follow-up.

Commentary. (1) Flaccid dysarthrias can be caused by damage to a single cranial nerve, unilaterally or bilaterally. (2) Speech difficulty can be the first sign of neurologic disease. (3) Speech intelligibility can be remarkably preserved in isolated bilateral tongue w eakness.

Case 4-3

A 40-year-old millwright presented with an 8-month history of voice difficulty. His dysphonia began after anterior-approach cervical disk surgery. He had been unable to return to work, because coworkers were unable to hear him in the noisy work environment. He occasionally coughed and choked after swallowing and had to clear his throat frequently.

Speech and oral mechanism examination were normal except for a markedly breathy-hoarse voice quality, moderately decreased loudness, and short phrases secondary to presumed air wastage through the glottis. He could sustain "ah" and "z" for only 2 seconds but sustained "s" for 12 seconds. His cough and glottal coup were markedly weak. There was no evidence of palatal asymmetry, the palate was mobile, and the gag reflex was normal.

The speech pathologist's impression was "suspect vocal cord paralysis secondary to recurrent laryngeal nerve damage caused by surgical trauma." Subsequent laryngeal examination identified a right vocal fold paralysis (paramedian position) and agreed it was probably secondary to surgical trauma. Teflon injection (rarely used currently) of the right vocal fold resulted in normal conversational loudness, ability to sustain "ah" for 14 seconds, /s/ for 12 seconds, and /z/ for 10 seconds. The patient remained unable to produce a loud, shouting voice. He was, however, pleased with his voice improvement and returned to work as a millwright, although with some fatigue in his voice by the end of the workday.

Commentary. (1) Flaccid dysarthrias can result from damage to a single cranial nerve. (2) Flaccid dysarthrias can be caused by surgical trauma. (3) The degree of impairment perceptually does not always predict the impact of the problem on a person's day-to-day functioning (this patient could not work). (4) Some speech deficits can be managed effectively with medical intervention.

Case 4-4

A 76-year-old mildly retarded man presented with a 10- to 11-week history of speech and swallowing difficulty. A swallowing study conducted elsewhere was normal. An ear, nose, and throat (ENT) examination was normal. The physician thought the patient might have amyotrophic lateral sclerosis. He was referred for speech and neurologic examinations.

Speech examination the following day was difficult because of the patient's immature affect, anxiety, and difficulty following directions. He did report that his swallowing problem was present upon awakening one morning and that his speech difficulty followed 1 to 2 days later. He had greater difficulty swallowing food than liquids but he did have nasal regurgitation when swallowing water. He thought all of his problems had worsened since onset.

Oral mechanism examination revealed left ptosis and difficulty closing both eyes completely. His face was moderately weak bilaterally. The tongue was tremulous on protrusion, but there were no fasciculations or atrophy; it was -2,3 weak bilaterally. Palatal movement gradually decreased over repetitions of "ah ah ah . . . ." There was consistent nasal air escape during speech. There was some reduction in speed and range of motion during alternating retraction and pursing of the lips. Cough and glottal coup were weak. Gag reflex was normal.

Speech examination was difficult because of his anxiety and difficulty following directions. However, the following characteristics were apparent: hypernasality (3), weak pressure consonants (3,4), imprecise articulation (2), and reduced rate (0,1). Prolonged "ah" was breathy (0,1), and inhalatory stridor was apparent following maximum vowel prolongation. The patient prolonged "ah" for 20 seconds initially, but over multiple trials this decreased to 12 seconds. It was difficult to get him to persist in speaking for stress testing, but hypernasality and weak pressure consonants appeared to increase over time.

The speech pathologist's impression was "flaccid dysarthria implicating, at the least, cranial nerves X, XII, and VII, bilaterally. There is no evidence of a spastic dysarthria or other CNS-based dysarthria. There is some deterioration of speech during stress testing, raising suspicions about neuromuscular junction disease (does this patient have MG?)."

Subsequent clinical neurologic examination, EMG, and an ACh receptor antibody test confirmed a diagnosis of MG. The patient improved rapidly when treated with Mestinon, but within 3 months his bulbar symptoms worsened and he developed respiratory compromise. He died 1 month later.

Commentary. (1) Speech difficulty can be among the first signs of neurologic disease. (2) Careful speech examination often is more enlightening than anatomic examination of speech structures. (3) The presence of cognitive deficits can make examination difficult. (4) The value of accurate localization and disease diagnosis by speech examination, unfortunately, is not always matched by long-term benefit to the patient.

Case 4-5

A 45-year-old man presented with a 3-month history of dysphagia that began with a choking episode, followed by continuing difficulty swallowing solid foods but not liquids. Speech difficulty, which he described as "slurring" and "difficulty with pronunciation," began approximately 1 month later. The neurologic examination was normal with the exception of possible palatal and tongue weakness. EMG failed to find evidence of neuromuscular junction disease but did find an abnormality of the hypoglossal nerve or its nuclei. MRI scan failed to find evidence of abnormality in the brainstem or posterior fossa. A video swallow study was normal. ENT examination was normal.

During speech evaluation, he complained of some dull, aching pain in his ears, tongue, jaw, and gums that he attributed to increased effort to chew food completely before swallowing. He noted mild difficulty with chewing and a tendency to put food to the left in his mouth. He felt he was able to initiate a swallow but often gagged and had to bring food back up and reinitiate a swallow. He was not aware of drooling during the day but noted that his pillow was frequently wet upon awakening in the morning.

During the examination, he cleared his throat frequently. Jaw strength was normal. There was equivocal weakness of lip rounding. The tongue was moderately weak bilaterally. Tongue protrusion and lateralization were limited (2,3), and there were equivocal fasciculations on the right side of the tongue. The palate elevated more extensively toward the right. There was a trace of nasal emission during pressure sound production. Cough and glottal coup were normal. Speech was characterized

Case 4-5—cont'd

by imprecise articulation, primarily on lingual consonants (0,1) and by hypernasality with occasional audible nasal emission (1). Voice quality was hoarse-breathy (0,1). He was able to sustain a vowel for 25 seconds. Speech AMRs for "puh" and "tuh" were normal, but "kuh" was slow (1). There was no significant deterioration of speech during stress testing.

The clinician's impression was "flaccid dysarthria associated with, at the least, weakness of cranial nerves XII and X, most likely bilateral. There was no significant deterioration of speech during stress testing, as might be encountered in MG. Finally, I hear no evidence to suggest the presence of a spastic component to his dysarthria."

All other laboratory and imaging tests, including tests for MG, were normal. The patient received counseling for management of his dysphagia and was discharged. He returned 3 months later complaining of increased dysphagia and tongue pain. ENT examination revealed a tender, swollen tongue. CT scan of the head and neck identified a mass extending posteriorly from the posterior aspect of the left superior tongue. Subsequent surgery identified extensive squamous cell carcinoma of the tongue with neck metastases. Right and left neck dissection and total glossectomy and laryngectomy were carried out.

Commentary. (1) Speech difficulty can be among the first signs of neurologic and other organic disease. (2) The apparent involvement of more than one cranial nerve does not always place the lesion inside the skull, even when muscle disease and neuromuscular junction disease are not present. (3) Neurologic signs and symptoms do not always mean the patient has primary nervous system disease. Although cranial nerves were affected, the neoplasm in this case was nonneurologic.

Case 4-6

A 24-year-old farmer was hit by a falling piece of heavy farm machinery. He sustained complex skull base, bilateral petrous ridge, and bilateral carotid canal fractures. The accident caused bilateral otorrhea, cranial nerve V palsy, and bilateral cranial nerve VII palsies. EMG and nerve conduction studies demonstrated near-complete paralysis of both cranial nerves VII, with some fibrillation potentials. Surgical management of cranial nerve VII palsies was deferred in the hope that there would be spontaneous regeneration.

The patient initially had significant difficulties with chewing and speech, primarily because he was unable to open his jaw. When seen for speech examination approximately 1 month after onset, his restricted jaw movement had cleared, and he no longer had any chewing or swallowing complaints. He admitted, however, that liquids would sometimes escape his mouth. He recognized that his speech difficulty was related to his facial weakness, but he did not feel that people were having significant difficulty understanding him. He complained that his mouth and lips would get dry easily and that he frequently needed to protrude his tongue to moisten his lips.

Oral mechanism examination was normal with the exception of bilateral facial paralysis. Relative to lower face movements relevant to speech, he was completely unable to make any isolated lip movements toward retraction or rounding. Attempts to puff his cheeks resulted in some flutter of the lips due to air escape. He was able to approximate his lips with his jaw closed. Conversational speech was characterized by distortion of all bilabial and labiodental sounds. He had some mild distortion of anterior lingual fricatives and affricates that the clinician felt was secondary to his facial weakness. There occasionally was mild distortion of /r/ in phonemic environments requiring lip rounding. He did achieve some lip approximation for bilabial sounds, and bilabials and labiodentals were distorted rather than omitted. Speech intelligibility was remarkably adequate in the evaluation setting, although it was felt that it would be mildly reduced in some phonetic environments or under adverse environmental conditions.

It was concluded that the patient had a flaccid dysarthria that was consistent with his bilateral cranial nerve VII paralyses. There was no evidence of speech difficulty that could not be explained by his bilateral facial nerve paralyses. He compensated well, primarily with jaw movement, for his facial weakness.

The patient received training for exercises to help promote lower facial movement and was instructed to do

Case 4-6—cont'd

them twice daily. Speech exercises included materials with consonant-vowel syllables containing /b/, /p/, and /m/ sounds. He was not seen for further follow-up in speech pathology, but his records showed that within 2 months he began to have some recovery of both facial nerves. Approximately 11 months later, he had made further recovery, with mild to moderate persistent weakness. Nearly 2 years after onset, he had made further recovery, but bilateral facial weakness was still evident.

Commentary. (1) Bilateral facial weakness can cause articulatory imprecision for phonemes requiring facial

movement. (2) When a single cranial nerve is damaged, even if bilaterally, considerable compensation is possible if paralysis is not complete and other cranial nerves are functioning normally. (3) The specific speech deficits encountered in flaccid dysarthria depend on the specific cranial nerves that are involved. In this case, all of the patient's speech distortions could be explained by his bilateral facial weakness. (4) Oromotor exercise to improve strength is sometimes justified for people with flaccid dysarthria. In this case, however, it is not possible to conclude that such exercises were responsible for improved strength or speech.

Case 4-7

A 62-year-old woman presented with an 8- to 10-year history of mild swallowing difficulties and a 2- to 3-year history of speech problems. Her history was significant only for radiation treatment to the face for acne at age 13. Clinical neurologic examination was normal with the exception of bilateral weakness in the face, tongue, and sternocleidomastoid muscles.

Speech pathology evaluation revealed normal symmetric jaw movement and strength. The lower face was lacking in tone, but lip retraction and rounding were grossly normal. The tongue was full and symmetric, without atrophy or fasciculations, but it was mild to moderately weak bilaterally. Lateral lingual AMRs were slow. Palatal movement was symmetric, and cough and glottal coup were normal. There were no pathologic oral reflexes. The patient's speech was characterized by equivocally slowed rate and imprecise articulation, particularly for anterior lingual fricatives, liquids, and bilabial sounds. There was some fluttering of the cheeks during production of bilabials. She had some exaggerated lip movements during speech that were judged to be compensatory. Voice quality was normal. Speech AMRs and sequential motion rates were normal. Speech intelligibility was normal.

The speech pathologist concluded that the patient had a "mild flaccid dysarthria whose deviant speech charac-

teristics are consistent with facial and lingual weakness." The clinician stated, "I do not hear anything in her speech to suggest significant weakness in muscles in the distribution of cranial nerves V, IX, X, or XI. I do not hear anything to suggest the presence of a spastic component to her dysarthria, or any other CNS-based dysarthria." It was felt that the patient was compensating adequately for her mild dysarthria. Speech therapy was not recommended.

After a comprehensive neurologic workup, it was concluded that the most likely cause of the patient's cranial and peripheral nerve deficits was her radiation treatment.

Commentary. (1) Flaccid dysarthria can develop in response to radiation-induced cranial nerve weakness. Such effects can be delayed for many years following radiation treatment. (2) Speech evaluation can help rule out certain neurologic diagnostic possibilities. In this case, it was possible to state that there was no evidence of any CNS-based dysarthria and that the speech deficit reflected LMN involvement alone. (3) Speech therapy for dysarthria is not always necessary. In this case, the patient was compensating very well for her impairments and had no difficulty with intelligibility or efficiency of verbal communication. Her need was to establish the etiology of her mild speech and swallowing difficulty.

SUMMARY

1. Flaccid dysarthrias result from damage to the motor units of cranial or spinal nerves that serve the speech muscles. They occur at a frequency comparable to that of other single dysarthria types. They sometimes reflect weakness in only a small number of muscles and can be isolated to lesions of single cranial or spinal nerves. Weakness and hypotonia are the underlying neuromuscular deficits that explain most of the abnormal speech characteristics associated with flaccid dysarthrias.

2. Lesions anywhere within the motor unit can cause flaccid dysarthrias, and various etiologies can produce such lesions. Surgical trauma and

degenerative diseases are common known causes, but etiology is frequently undetermined, particularly when only a single cranial nerve is involved. Muscle disease, MG, tumor, stroke, infection, neuroanatomic malformations, demyelinating diseases, and radiation therapy effects represent other known causes.

3. The speech characteristics and nonspeech examination findings differ among lesions of cranial nerves V, VII, X, and XII, and spinal respiratory nerves. Examination can localize the effects of disease to one or a combination of these nerves.

4. Lesions of the mandibular branch of cranial (trigeminal) nerve V lead to weakness of jaw muscles. When bilateral, jaw weakness can have significant effects on articulation. Lesions of cranial nerve V that affect sensation from the jaw, face, lip, and tongue and stationary points of articulatory contact may also affect speech, primarily articulatory precision.

5. Lesions of cranial (facial) nerve VII can lead to facial weakness and flaccid dysarthria. Unilateral weakness of the face can be associated with mild articulatory distortions. Bilateral lesions may lead to significant distortion of all consonants and vowels requiring facial movement.

6. Lesions of cranial (vagus) nerve X can lead to weakness of velopharyngeal and laryngeal muscles and to some of the most frequently encountered manifestations of flaccid dysarthrias. Lesions of the pharyngeal branch of the nerve can lead to resonatory incompetence, with hypernasality, nasal emission, and weakening of pressure consonant sounds. Lesions of the superior laryngeal and recurrent laryngeal branches can lead to various dysphonias whose perceptual attributes are consistent with weakness and hypotonia of laryngeal muscles. Lesions above the pharyngeal branch of the vagus nerve can lead to both resonatory and laryngeal incompetence, whereas lesions below the pharyngeal branch are associated with laryngeal manifestations only.

7. Lesions of cranial (hypoglossal) nerve XII cause tongue weakness. The resulting flaccid dysarthria is reflected in imprecision of lingual articulation, with severity dependent upon the degree of weakness and whether the lesion is unilateral or bilateral.

8. Lesions affecting spinal respiratory nerves can reduce respiratory support for speech. Weakness at this level can lead to reduced loudness and pitch variability, as well as reduced phrase length per breath group.

9. Phonatory and resonatory incompetence are commonly encountered distinguishing features of flaccid dysarthrias. Although they are tied to involvement of cranial nerve X, it is nonetheless important to attend to speech movements generated through cranial nerves V, VII, and XII. This is important both for a complete description of the speech disorder and because speech deficits isolated to single cranial or spinal nerves are possible in flaccid dysarthrias and unusual in other dysarthria types.

10. Flaccid dysarthrias can be the only, the first, or among the first and most prominent manifestations of neurologic disease. Their recognition and localization to motor units subserving speech can aid the localization and diagnosis of neurologic disease. Their diagnosis and description are important to decision making for medical and behavioral management.

References

1. Abul MM et al: Acute inspiratory stridor: a presentation of myasthenia gravis, J Laryngol Otol 113:1114, 1999.
2. Adams RD, Victor M: Principles of neurology, New York, 1991, McGraw-Hill.
3. Andour KK, Schneider G, Hilsinger RL: Acute superior laryngeal nerve palsy: analysis of 78 cases, Otolaryngol Head Neck Surg 88:418, 1980.
4. Aronson AE: Clinical voice disorders, New York, 1990, Thieme.
5. Ballotta E et al: Cranial and cervical nerve injuries after carotid endarterectomy: a prospective study, Surgery 125:85, 1999.
6. Benarroch EE et al: Medical neurosciences: an approach to anatomy, pathology, and physiology by systems and levels, Philadelphia, 1999, Lippincott Williams & Wilkins.
7. Beekman R, Kuks JB, Oosterhuis HJ: Myasthenia gravis: diagnosis and follow-up of 100 consecutive patients, J Neurol 244:112, 1997.
8. Brazis P, Masdeu JC, Biller J: Localization in clinical neurology, ed 4, Philadelphia, 2001, Lippincott Williams & Wilkins.
9. Cahill LM, Murdoch BE, Theodoros DG: Variability in speech outcome following severe childhood traumatic brain injury: a report of three cases, J Med Speech-Lang Pathol 8:347, 2000.
10. Chitney T, Khoury SJ: Neuroimmunology. In Bradley WG et al, editors: Neurology in clinical practice: principles of diagnosis and management, vol 1, ed 3, Boston, 2000, Butterworth-Heinemann.
11. Corboy JR, Tyler KL: Neurovirology. In Bradley WG et al, editors: Neurology in clinical practice: principles of diagnosis and management, vol 1, ed 3, Boston, 2000, Butterworth-Heinemann.
12. Curtis JF: Acoustics of speech production and nasalization. In Spriestersbach DC, Lerman DS, editors: Cleft palate and communication, New York, 1968, Academic Press.

13. Danielidis V et al: A comparative study of age and degree of facial nerve recovery in patients with Bell's palsy, Eur Arch Otorhinolaryngol 256:520, 1999.

14. Darley FL, Aronson AE, Brown JR: Motor speech disorders, Philadelphia, 1975, WB Saunders.

15. Darley FL, Aronson AE, Brown JR: Clusters of deviant speech dimensions in the dysarthrias. J Speech Hear Res 12:462, 1969a.

16. Darley FL, Aronson AE, Brown JR: Differential diagnostic patterns of dysarthria, J Speech Hear Res 12:246, 1969b.

17. Duffy JR: Stroke with dysarthria: evaluate and treat; garden variety or down the garden path?, Semin Speech Lang 19:93, 1998.

18. Dworkin JP, Aronson AE: Tongue strength and alternate motion rates in normal and dysarthric subjects, J Commun Disord 19:115, 1986.

19. Foster PK et al: Vocal fold paralysis in painless aortic dissection (Ortner's syndrome), Ear Nose Throat J 80:784, 2001.

20. Griffin JW: Diseases of the peripheral nervous system. In Rosenberg RN, editor: The clinical neurosciences, New York, 1983, Churchill Livingstone.

21. Guo YP, McLeod JG, Baverstock J: Pathologic changes in the vagus nerve in diabetes and chronic alcoholism, J Neurol Neurosurg Psychiatry 50:1449, 1987.

22. Guy N et al: Spontaneous internal carotid artery dissection with lower cranial nerve palsy, Can J Neurol Sci 28:265, 2001.

23. Hammarberg B, Fritzell B, Schiratzki H: Teflon injection in 16 patients with paralytic dysphonia: perceptual and acoustic evaluations, J Speech Hear Disord 49:72, 1984.

24. Hartman DE, Daily WW, Morin KN: A case of superior laryngeal nerve paresis and psychogenic dysphonia, J Speech Hear Disord 54:526, 1989.

25. Hinton VJ et al: Selective deficits in verbal working memory associated with a known genetic etiology: the neuropsychological profile of Duchenne muscular dystrophy, J Int Neuropsychol Soc 7:45, 2001.

26. Hirano M, Koike Y, von Leden H: Maximum phonation time and air wastage during phonation, Folia Phoniatr Logop 20:185, 1968.

27. Hixon TJ, Putnam AHB, Sharp JT: Speech production with flaccid paralysis of the rib cage, diaphragm, and abdomen, J Speech Hear Disord 48:315, 1983.

28. Hoit JD et al: Speech breathing in individuals with cervical spinal cord injury, J Speech Hear Res 33:798, 1990.

29. Jacobs L, Kaba S, Pullicino P: The lesion causing continuous facial myokymia in multiple sclerosis, Arch Neurol 51:1115, 1994.

30. Johns DF: Surgical and prosthetic management of neurogenic velopharyngeal incompetency in dysarthria. In Johns DF, editor: Clinical management of neurogenic communication disorders, New York, 1985, Little, Brown.

31. Keane JR: Tongue atrophy from brainstem metastases, Arch Neurol 41:1219, 1984.

32. Kelchner LN et al: Etiology, pathophysiology, treatment choices, and voice results for unilateral adductor vocal fold paralysis: a 3-year retrospective, J Voice 13:592, 1999.

33. Kiliaridis S, Katsaros C: The effects of myotonic dystrophy and Duchenne muscular dystrophy on the orofacial muscles and dentofacial morphology, Acta Odontol Scand 56:369, 1998.

34. King AD et al: Hypoglossal nerve palsy in nasopharyngeal carcinoma, Head Neck 21:614, 1999.

35. Kleiner-Fisman G, Knott HS: Myasthenia gravis mimicking stroke in elderly patients, Mayo Clin Proc 73:1077, 1998.

36. Leonard RJ et al: Swallowing in myotonic muscular dystrophy: a videofluoroscopic study, Arch Phys Med Rehabil 82:979, 2001.

37. Logemann JA et al: Speech and swallowing rehabilitation for head and neck cancer patients, Oncology 11:651, 1997.

38. Matthias C et al: Meningiomas of the cerebellopontine angle, Acta Neurochir Suppl 65:86, 1996.

39. Mayo Clinic Department of Neurology: Mayo Clinic examinations in neurology, ed 7, St Louis, 1998, Mosby.

40. McEvoy KM: Diagnosis and treatment of Lambert-Eaton myasthenic syndrome, Neurol Clin 12:387, 1994.

41. Mercuri E et al: Cognitive abilities in children with congenital muscular dystrophy: correlation with brain MRI and merosin status, Neuromuscul Disord 9:383, 1999.

42. Mitsumoto H: Disorders of upper and lower motor neurons. In Bradley WG et al, editors: Neurology in clinical practice: principles of diagnosis and management, vol 2, ed 3, Boston, 2000, Butterworth-Heinemann.

43. Murry T: Speaking fundamental frequency characteristics associated with voice pathologies, J Speech Hear Disord 43:374, 1978.

44. Nelson MA, Hodge MM: Effects of facial paralysis and audiovisual information on stop place identification, J Speech Lang Hear Res 43:158, 2000.

45. Penn AS: Other disorders of neuromuscular transmission. In Rowland LP, editor: Merritt's textbook of neurology, Philadelphia, 1989, Lea & Febiger.

46. Perie S et al: Dysphagia in oculopharyngeal muscular dystrophy: a series of 22 French cases, Neuromuscul Disord 7:S96, 1997.

47. Pica RA et al: Traumatic internal carotid artery dissection presenting as delayed hemilingual paresis, Am J Neuroradiol 17:86, 1996.

48. Pleasure DE, Schotland DL: Acquired neuropathies. In Rowland LP, editor: Merritt's textbook of neurology, Philadelphia, 1989, Lea & Febiger.

49. Regli F: Symptomatic trigeminal neuralgia. In Samii M, Janetta PJ, editors: The cranial nerves, New York, 1981, Springer-Verlag.

50. Reich AR, Lerman JW: Teflon laryngoplasty: an acoustical and perceptual study, J Speech Hear Disord 43:496, 1978.

51. Rontal E, Rontal M, Rolnick M: The use of spectrograms in the evaluation of voice cord injection, Laryngoscope 85:47, 1975.

52. Rosenbaum RB: Disorders of bones, joints, ligaments, and meninges. In Bradley WG et al, editors: Neurology in clinical practice: principles of diagnosis and management, vol 2, ed 3, Boston, 2000, Butterworth-Heinemann.

53. Salomonson J, Kawamoto H, Wilson L: Velopharyngeal incompetence as the presenting symptoms in myotonic dystrophy, Cleft Palate J 25:296, 1988.

54. Sasakura Y et al: Myasthenia gravis associated with reduced masticatory function, Int J Oral Maxillofac Surg 29:381, 2000.

55. Schauber MD et al: Cranial/cervical nerve dysfunction after carotid endarterectomy, J Vasc Surg 25:481, 1997.

56. Shapiro BE et al: Delayed radiation-induced bulbar palsy, Neurology 46:1604, 1996.

57. Singer EJ: Central nervous system (CNS) complications of HIV disease. Special interest division of publication, Rockville, Md, 1991, American Speech-Language-Hearing Association.

58. Stern Y et al: Vocal cord palsy: possible late complication of radiotherapy for head and neck cancer, Ann Otol Rhinol Laryngol 104:294, 1995.

59. Takimoto T et al: Radiation-induced cranial nerve palsy: hypoglossal nerve and vocal cord palsies, J Laryngol Otol 105:45, 1991.

60. Till JA, Alp LA: Aerodynamic and temporal measures of continuous speech in dysarthric speakers. In Moore CA, Yorkston KM, Beukelman DR, editors: Dysarthria and apraxia of speech: perspectives on management, Baltimore, 1991, Brooks Publishing.

61. Till JA et al: Effects of inspiratory airway impairment on continuous speech. In Robin DA, Yorkston KM, Beukelman DR, editors: Disorders of motor speech: assessment, treatment, and clinical characterization, Baltimore, 1996, Brooks Publishing.

62. Wall M: Brainstem syndromes. In Bradley WG et al, editors: Neurology in clinical practice: principles of diagnosis and management, vol 1, ed 3, Boston, 2000, Butterworth-Heinemann.

63. Watterson T, McFarlane SC, Menicucci AL: Vibratory characteristics of Teflon-injected and noninjected paralyzed vocal folds, J Speech Hear Disord 55:61, 1990.

64. Weijnen FG et al: Tongue force in patients with myasthenia gravis, Acta Neurol Scand 102:303, 2000.

65. Willig TN et al: Swallowing problems in neuromuscular disorders, Arch Phys Med Rehab 75:1175, 1994.

66. Windebank AJ: Motor neuron diseases. In Noseworthy JH, editor: Neurological therapeutics: principles and practice, vol 2, New York, 2003, Martin Dunitz.

67. Young EC, Durant-Jones L: Gradual onset of dysphagia: a study of patients with oculopharyngeal muscular dystrophy, Dysphagia 12:196, 1997.

Symptoms
hyperreflexia
effortful speech
nasal regurgitation
AMRs-slow
but regular

"*It's slower, and sometimes it tires me, and I just don't want to talk anymore . . . the kids don't really say that much about it . . . I think they're in denial.*"

(79-year-old woman with an unambiguous but mild spastic dysarthria of undetermined origin)

CHAPTER OUTLINE

I. Anatomy and basic functions of the direct and indirect activation pathways

II. Clinical characteristics of upper motor neuron lesions and spastic paralysis

III. The relationship of spastic paralysis to spastic dysarthria

IV. Etiologies
   A. Vascular disorders
   B. Degenerative disease
   C. Inflammatory disease

V. Speech pathology
   A. Distribution of etiologies, lesions, and severity in clinical practice
   B. Patient perceptions and complaints
   C. Clinical findings
   D. Acoustic and physiologic findings

VI. Cases

VII. Summary

Spastic dysarthria is a perceptually distinctive motor speech disorder (MSD) produced by bilateral damage to the direct and indirect activation pathways of the central nervous system (CNS). It may be manifest in any or all of the respiratory, phonatory, resonatory, and articulatory components of speech, but it is generally not confined to a single component. Its characteristics reflect the combined effects of weakness and spasticity in a manner that slows movement and reduces its range and force. Spasticity, a hallmark of upper motor neuron (UMN) disease, seems to be the crucial contributor to the distinctive features of the disorder, hence its designation as *spastic* dysarthria. The identification of a dysarthria as spastic can aid the diagnosis of neurologic disease and its localization to CNS motor pathways.

Spastic dysarthria is encountered in a large medical practice at a rate comparable to that of the other major single dysarthria types. Based on data for primary communication disorder diagnoses in the Mayo Clinic Speech Pathology practice, it accounts for 8.2% of all dysarthrias and 7.6% of all MSDs (see Figure 1-3).

The clinical features of spastic dysarthria reflect the effects of excessive muscle tone and weakness on speech. They illustrate well the distinction between speech deficits attributable to weakness alone (as in flaccid dysarthria) from those in which the barriers to normal speech also include neuromuscular resistance to movement.

◼ ANATOMY AND BASIC FUNCTIONS OF THE DIRECT AND INDIRECT ACTIVATION PATHWAYS

The direct activation pathway, also known as the *pyramidal tract* or *direct motor system,* forms part of the UMN system. Its activities lead to movements through the final common pathway (lower motor neurons [LMNs]). The pathway includes the *corticobulbar tracts,* which influence the activities of cranial nerves, and the *corticospinal tracts,* which influence the activities of spinal nerves.

The direct activation pathways are bilateral, one originating in the cortex of the right cerebral hemisphere, the other in the cortex of the left cerebral hemisphere. The pathways from the cortex lead rather directly to the cranial and spinal nerve nuclei in the brainstem and spinal cord. Their fibers primarily innervate muscles on the side of the body opposite the cerebral cortex of origin, but, for the speech muscles, this applies only to the muscles of the lower face, and, to a lesser extent, the tongue. The remaining cranial nerves subserving speech receive bilateral input from the direct (and indirect) activation pathways. This neural redundancy helps to minimize the effects of unilateral UMN lesions on speech and chewing, swallowing, and airway protection functions. Unilateral UMN lesions generally do not have a pronounced effect on jaw, velopharyngeal, laryngeal, or lingual movements for speech.

The direct activation pathway is predominantly *facilitatory.* That is, impulses through it tend to lead to movement, particularly *skilled, discrete movements.*

The indirect activation pathway, also known as the *extrapyramidal tract* or *indirect motor system,* is also part of the UMN system. It originates in the cortex of each cerebral hemisphere, but its course is more complicated than the direct activation pathway's because synapses occur between the cortex and the brainstem and spinal cord. Crucial interneuronal connections include those in the basal ganglia, cerebellum, reticular formation, vestibular nuclei, and red nucleus. The indirect activation pathway is crucial for *regulating reflexes and maintaining posture, tone,* and *associated activities that provide a framework for skilled movements.* Many of its activities are *inhibitory.*

■ CLINICAL CHARACTERISTICS OF UPPER MOTOR NEURON LESIONS AND SPASTIC PARALYSIS

Damage to the direct activation pathway leads to a loss or reduction of fine, discrete movements. Following acute lesions, reduced muscle tone and weakness are evident, but they generally evolve to increased tone and spasticity. Weakness is usually more pronounced in distal than proximal muscles; the distal and speech muscles are those most involved in finely controlled skilled movement. Reflexes tend to be diminished initially but become more pronounced over time.

Direct activation pathway lesions are also associated with a *positive Babinski sign,* a pathologic reflex elicited by applying pressure with a relatively sharp point from the sole of the foot on the side of the heel forward to the little toe and across to the great toe. The normal response is a planting of the toes. A Babinski response is an extension of the great toe and fanning of the other toes. When present in adults, the Babinski sign is associated with CNS disease, reflecting the release of a primitive reflex from CNS inhibition (Babinski's reflex is normal in infants). *Pathologic oral reflexes* are also common

in bilateral UMN disease, including suck, snout, palmomental, and jaw jerk reflexes (defined in Chapter 3).

Damage to the indirect activation pathway affects its predominantly inhibitory role in motor control. As a result, lesions tend to lead to overactivity *(positive signs)* such as increased muscle tone, spasticity, and hyperactive reflexes. These signs are interrelated. Spasticity, for example, is the result of hyperactivity of stretch reflexes, and it goes hand in hand with increased muscle tone. It results in resistance to movement that is generally more pronounced at the beginning of movement or in response to quick movements (i.e., it is velocity dependent). In the limbs, spasticity tends to be biased toward lower extremity extension (i.e., the legs resist bending) and upper extremity flexion (i.e., the arms resist straightening). Physical therapists sometimes hope for spasticity to develop in the legs of patients with UMN lesions, because it facilitates standing.

Patients with UMN lesions and hyperactive reflexes sometimes exhibit *clonus,* a kind of repetitive reflex contraction that occurs when a muscle is kept under tension (stretch) by an examiner (e.g., when the foot is continuously dorsiflexed by the examiner). The reflex response may look like a rhythmic tremor.[30]

Selective damage to only the direct or only the indirect activation pathway is uncommon, because both pathways arise in adjacent and overlapping areas of the cortex and travel in close proximity through much of their course to LMNs. As a result, people with spastic paralysis commonly exhibit decreased skilled movement and weakness from direct activation pathway damage, as well as increased muscle tone and spasticity from indirect activation pathway damage.

Direct and indirect activation pathway signs of UMN lesions are summarized in Table 5-1. The

 table 5-1 Direct and indirect activation pathway signs of upper motor neuron lesions

Damage to	
Direct Activation Pathway (Pyramidal Tracts)	**Indirect Activation Pathway (Extrapyramidal Tracts)**
Loss of fine, skilled movement	Increased muscle tone
Hypotonia	Spasticity
Weakness (distal > proximal)	Clonus
Absent abdominal reflexes	Decorticate or decerebrate posture
Babinski's sign	Hyperactive stretch reflexes
Hyporeflexia	Hyperactive gag reflex

major abnormalities that affect movement in spastic paralysis include *spasticity, weakness, reduced range of movement,* and *slowness of movement.* These abnormalities also appear to represent the most salient features of disordered movement in patients with spastic dysarthria.

◼ THE RELATIONSHIP OF SPASTIC PARALYSIS TO SPASTIC DYSARTHRIA

The neuropathophysiologic underpinnings of spastic dysarthria are more complex and less well understood than those of flaccid dysarthria. This is partly a product of the complexity of the CNS motor pathways and the fact that spastic dysarthria is usually associated with damage to two components of the motor system, the direct and indirect activation pathways. In addition, the degree to which the concept of spasticity can be applied to the cranial nerve innervated portion of the speech system has been questioned.[1,2,7]

Most of what is known about the clinical manifestations of spastic paralysis is based on studies of limb movements that require the movement of joints in agonist and antagonistic relationships with each other.*[1] Many speech movements do not involve the movement of joints, and different speech structures have varying numbers of muscle spindles that are important in the mediation of stretch reflexes. For example, the jaw is well endowed with spindles, the intrinsic muscles of the tongue have some, and the face has none.[7] Furthermore, lip movements do not require the movement of bone, and the tongue is a muscular hydrostat, the movements of which do not involve joints. Relatedly, it seems that different speech structures are affected in somewhat different ways by UMN lesions.[1] Finally, unlike the limbs, speech requires symmetric movements of bilaterally innervated structures. That is, jaw, face, tongue, palate, and laryngeal movements require the synchronous movement of each of their halves so that the structures move as a single unit.

In spite of the differences between bulbar and limb movements, and uncertainty about the degree to which understanding spastic paralysis in the limbs can explain what occurs in the bulbar muscles during speech, it appears that, for practical clinical purposes at least, several of the *general* principles and observations about spastic paralysis discussed in the previous section can be usefully applied to our clinical conceptions of spastic dysarthria.

◼ ETIOLOGIES

Any process that damages the direct and indirect activation pathways bilaterally can cause spastic dysarthria. These include degenerative, inflammatory, toxic, metabolic, traumatic, and vascular diseases. These etiologic categories produce bilateral CNS motor system damage and spastic dysarthria with varying frequency, but the exact distribution of causes of spastic dysarthria is unknown. It does appear, however, that degenerative, vascular, and traumatic disorders are the predominant causes.

Although no general etiologic category is uniquely associated with spastic dysarthria, vascular disorders are more frequently associated with it than with most other dysarthria types. Some of those vascular disorders are discussed as follows. A few other conditions that have a relatively specific association with spastic but not other forms of dysarthria are also addressed. Note that all of the following conditions represent only a few of the potential etiologies of spastic dysarthria. Other diseases associated with spastic dysarthria but that are more frequently associated with other dysarthria types are discussed in the chapters that deal with those specific dysarthria types.

Vascular Disorders

Strokes in the distribution of the internal carotid and middle and posterior cerebral arteries, and less frequently the anterior cerebral artery, can produce spastic dysarthria. However, because these arteries mostly supply structures within the cortex and subcortical structures of the cerebral hemispheres—where the UMN pathways on the left and right are not in close proximity to one another—lesions in both the left and right hemispheres are required to produce the bilateral UMN damage usually associated with spastic dysarthria. In the brainstem, where the right and left UMN pathways are in close proximity to one another, a single infarct in the vertebrobasilar arterial distribution may be sufficient to produce the bilateral UMN damage associated with spastic dysarthria. In general, therefore, *a single brainstem stroke can produce a spastic dysarthria, whereas a single cerebral hemisphere stroke usually does not.**

Some patients with spastic dysarthria have had multiple *lacunes* or *lacunar infarcts*—small, deep infarcts in the small penetrating arteries of the basal ganglia, thalamus, brainstem, and deep cerebral

---

*See Sheean[42] for a concise overview of the pathophysiology of spasticity.

---

*Single cerebral hemisphere stroke sometimes leads to speech characteristics associated with spasticlike dysarthria. This issue is addressed further in Chapter 9.

white matter.* They are usually associated with hypertension. *Lacunar state* is a term applied to patients with numerous lacunar infarcts who frequently have dementia, dysarthria, pseudobulbar affect, dysphagia, hyperreflexia, and incontinence.[8] However, dysarthria (perhaps plus dysphagia) can be the only sign of lacunar strokes. Okuda et al.[35] reported that 11 of their 12 patients with "pure dysarthria" due to stroke had magnetic resonance imaging (MRI) evidence of multiple, bilateral lacunar strokes involving the internal capsule or corona radiata, with 8 of the 11 patients also having evidence (based on single photon emission computed tomography [SPECT]) of frontal hypometabolism.

Relatedly, *Binswanger's disease (subcortical arteriosclerotic encephalopathy)* is a term sometimes applied to patients with vascular dementia. It is characterized by periventricular demyelination of subcortical white matter and is often associated with a history of hypertension.[40] The major lesions are in the subcortical white matter with relative sparing of the cortex and basal ganglia. These bilateral lesions can affect UMN pathways and lead to spastic dysarthria. The association of spastic dysarthria with dementia is an important diagnostic observation, because dysarthria is not commonly associated with common degenerative cortical dementias such as Alzheimer's and Pick's diseases.

Not all occlusive vascular diseases are due to arteriosclerosis or emboli, nor are they solely a disease of the elderly. *Moyamoya disease,* for example, is a chronic, progressive nonatherosclerotic occlusive vascular disease of unknown cause that most frequently affects children, adolescents, or young adults.[9] It can cause stroke and intracranial hemorrhage, with resulting neurologic deficits including speech and language impairments.[21] Because it is associated with bilateral stenosis of the arteries, a resulting dysarthria may be spastic in character. *Cerebral autosomal dominant arteriopathy with subcortical infarcts and leukoencephalopathy (often referred to as CADASIL)* is a hereditary disorder that often presents with stroke manifestations in early adulthood. It is frequently associated with pseudobulbar palsy and cognitive deficits.[15] Because the pathology can be bilateral, an associated dysarthria may be spastic.

Degenerative Disease

Primary lateral sclerosis (PLS) is a rarely occurring subcategory of motor neuron disease (of which amyotrophic lateral sclerosis [ALS] is a major sub-

category). It is manifest by corticospinal and corticobulbar tract signs alone,* with no evidence of LMN involvement. It seems that dysarthria occurs frequently in PLS, and it sometimes is the presenting problem.[39] When dysarthria and dysphagia are the primary manifestations in PLS, the disorder is sometimes referred to as *progressive pseudobulbar palsy.*[†] Because clinical motor findings are limited to descending UMN tracts, it can be assumed that the type of dysarthria is typically spastic. The distinction between PLS and ALS is of more than academic interest because the median disease duration until death for PLS (19 years, as reported by Pringle[39]) is much longer than for ALS (only a few years). Because the dysarthria of PLS is presumably spastic only, the correct distinction between spastic dysarthria and the mixed spastic-flaccid dysarthria often associated with ALS can be of some assistance to neurologic differential diagnosis.

Inflammatory Disease

Leukoencephalitis is an inflammatory demyelinating disease that affects the white matter of the brain or spinal cord. In acute *hemorrhagic leukoencephalitis* the white matter of both hemispheres is destroyed, with similar changes in the brainstem and cerebellar peduncles. This destruction is associated with necrosis of small blood vessels and surrounding brain tissue, with inflammatory reactions in the meninges. There is a tendency for large focal lesions to form in the cerebral hemispheres.[4] The bilateral and multifocal effects of this white matter disease can affect UMN pathways and cause spastic dysarthria (or mixed dysarthrias).

▨ SPEECH PATHOLOGY

Distribution of Etiologies, Lesions, and Severity in Clinical Practice

Box 5-1 and Figure 5-1 summarize the etiologies for 144 quasirandomly selected cases seen at the Mayo Clinic with a primary speech pathology diagnosis of spastic dysarthria. The cautions expressed in Chapter 4 about generalizing these observations to the general population or all speech pathology practices apply here as well.

---

*Mild cognitive impairment has been demonstrated in some patients with PLS.[10]

[†]Windebank[45] uses PLS to refer to a motor neuron disease characterized initially by lower limb spasticity secondary to UMN degeneration. He distinguishes it from progressive pseudobulbar palsy, in which UMN degeneration is characterized primarily by dysarthria and dysphagia.

---

*Lacunar stroke syndromes are discussed in detail in Chapter 9.

box 5-1

Etiologies for 144 quasirandomly selected cases with a primary speech pathology diagnosis of spastic dysarthria at the Mayo Clinic from 1969-1990 and 1999-2001. Percentage of cases for each etiology is given in parentheses. Specific etiologies under each heading are ordered from most to least frequent.

Degenerative (40%)

Unspecified degenerative CNS disease (13%)
ALS (14%)
PSP (5%)
PLS (5%)
CBD (1%)
Spinocerebellar ataxia (1%)
Uncertain (PLS vs. ALS; PSP vs. CBD) (1%)

Vascular (29%)

Nonhemorrhagic stroke (single or multiple) (26%)
Ruptured aneurysm (1%)
Hemorrhagic stroke (1%)
Hypoxic encephalopathy (1%)

Traumatic (10%)

Traumatic brain injury (8%)
Neurosurgical (e.g., tumor resection) (1%)

Undetermined (10%)

Demyelinating (4%)

Multiple sclerosis

Tumor (3%)

CNS tumor (2%)
Paraneoplastic syndrome (1%)

Multiple Causes (2%)

CVA + dementia; tumor + radiation therapy; TBI + alcoholism + PSP

Inflammatory (1%)

Inflammatory brainstem disorder; postencephalitic

Infectious (1%)

Infectious encephalopathy

ALS, Amyotrophic lateral sclerosis; *CBD,* corticobasal degeneration; *CNS,* central nervous system; *CVA,* cerebrovascular accident; *PLS,* primary lateral sclerosis; *PSP,* progressive supranuclear palsy; *TBI,* traumatic brain injury.

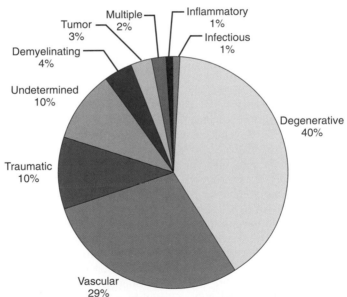

FIGURE 5-1 Distribution of etiologies for 144 quasirandomly selected cases with a primary speech pathology diagnosis of spastic dysarthria at the Mayo Clinic from 1969-1990 and from 1999-2001 (see Box 5-1 for details).

The data establish that spastic dysarthria can result from various medical conditions, the distribution of which are quite different from that associated with flaccid dysarthria. More than 90% of the cases were accounted for by degenerative, vascular, traumatic, demyelinating, and undetermined etiologies. Nearly 70% were accounted for by degenerative and vascular diseases.

Nonhemorrhagic strokes accounted for most of the vascular causes. This is not surprising because such strokes account for the highest proportion of neurovascular disturbances in general. Many of these patients had multiple strokes. Most who had only a single stroke had a brainstem lesion.

Patients with only a single confirmed (by computed tomography [CT] or MRI) stroke in one of the cerebral hemispheres usually had nonspeech clinical signs of bilateral involvement, suggesting the presence of "silent" or undetected infarcts or other pathology in the "intact" hemisphere or brainstem. A few patients with a diagnosis of stroke had no identifiable lesion on CT or MRI, suggesting that *spastic dysarthria may be the only evidence of stroke in some individuals.* It is also possible that characteristics of spastic dysarthria can sometimes result from a unilateral UMN lesion.*

Degenerative diseases associated with spastic dysarthria were often nonspecific. It is not unusual for neurodegenerative disease to defy a more specific diagnosis, especially early in its course. This sometimes remains the case until autopsy. ALS, PLS, and progressive supranuclear palsy (PSP) were the most commonly diagnosed neurodegenerative diseases. It is noteworthy, however, that ALS and PSP can be associated with other dysarthria types and frequently with mixed dysarthrias. ALS, PSP, and other degenerative diseases listed in Box 5-1 are discussed further in Chapter 10.

Traumatic brain injury (TBI) was a fairly frequent cause of spastic dysarthria. Although Yorkston et al.[47] indicate that most TBI-associated dysarthrias are mixed spastic-ataxic or flaccid-spastic, data from the sample reviewed here establish that spastic dysarthria can be the only dysarthria type following TBI. Trauma from intracranial surgery is another possible traumatic cause of spastic dysarthria.

Numerous patients had spastic dysarthria of undetermined etiology. Some of them had several possible diagnoses (e.g., stroke versus degenerative CNS disease) or diagnoses compatible with bilateral UMN involvement. Some had only dysarthria and dysphagia and received only a descriptive diagnosis.

Several patients had multiple sclerosis (MS) (discussed in Chapter 10). Some had tumors. CNS tumors, particularly if localized in the brainstem, can cause spastic dysarthria, as can unilateral hemispheric tumors if they exert mass effects on the brainstem or opposite hemisphere. Only a few patients had inflammatory or infectious disorders.

The data also illustrate that spastic dysarthria can arise from multiple causes or events in the same patient (e.g., TBI plus alcoholism plus PSP). This observation is important, because some patients

---

*In the author's experience, apparent spastic dysarthria in cases of presumed unilateral stroke, with no other clinical evidence of bilateral pathology, is encountered most frequently early after onset of a single unilateral stroke. If true, the reasons for this occurrence are unclear.

being evaluated for a condition that ordinarily might not be associated with spastic dysarthria might develop it because their current illness is added to the effects of a previous or concurrent condition. It is not unusual, for example, to discover in a patient who has developed signs of unilateral stroke and spastic dysarthria that there is a history of prior stroke on the opposite side of the brain (with or without speech disturbance).

The distribution of lesions for the cases summarized in Box 5-1 was spread through the course of the UMN system, including the *cortex, corona radiata, basal ganglia, internal capsule, pons,* and *medulla.* Focal lesions were most obvious when the etiology was vascular. Generalized or diffuse atrophy was frequently the only anatomic abnormality in TBI, degenerative disease, and undetermined etiologies. Approximately one fourth of the patients had no evidence of cerebral pathology on neuroimaging studies. It is important to note that the only clinical sign of bilateral pathology in some patients was their spastic dysarthria and frequently accompanying dysphagia and pathologic oral reflexes.

This retrospective review did not permit a precise delineation of dysarthria severity. However, in a review of the 144 patients reviewed in Box 5-1, intelligibility was specifically commented on in 81%; in those cases, 56% *were judged to have reduced intelligibility.* The degree to which this percentage accurately estimates intelligibility impairments in the population with spastic dysarthria is unclear. It is likely that many patients for whom an observation of intelligibility was not made had normal intelligibility, but the sample probably contains a larger number of mildly impaired patients than is encountered in a typical rehabilitation setting.

Finally, because of its association with bilateral, multifocal, or diffuse CNS disease, it is not uncommon for spastic dysarthria to be accompanied by cognitive disturbances that may include dementia or cognitive-communication deficits associated with right hemisphere impairment, TBI, or aphasia. For the patients in this sample whose cognitive abilities were explicitly judged or formally assessed (83% of the sample), *36% had some impairment of cognitive ability.*

Patient Perceptions and Complaints

People with spastic dysarthria sometimes offer complaints or descriptions that provide clues to the speech diagnosis and its localization. Some of these are only infrequently associated with other dysarthria types.

A frequent complaint is that speech is *slow* or *effortful.* When asked, patients often confirm that it feels as if they are speaking against resistance. The descriptors "slow" and "effortful" are not often heard from patients with other dysarthria types (with the exception of some hyperkinetic dysarthrias). Patients often complain of *fatigue* with speaking, sometimes with accompanying deterioration of speech. With the exception of myasthenia gravis (MG), complaints of fatigue occur more frequently in spastic than flaccid dysarthria, even though deterioration of speech in spastic dysarthria is not usually dramatic and almost never rapid.* Patients also often note that they must speak more slowly to be understood but often admit that they really are unable to speak any faster. Finally, they often complain of *nasal* speech, although this complaint is heard more frequently in people with flaccid dysarthria.

Swallowing complaints are common and often can be associated with both oral and pharyngeal phases of swallowing.† In some patients, a precursor to dysphagia and evidence of a lowered gag reflex threshold is increased gagging when brushing teeth. Patients also complain of *drooling,* more so than for most other single dysarthria types. Finally, many patients complain of or admit to *difficulty controlling their expression of emotion,* especially laughter and crying. This *pseudobulbar affect* is rarely encountered in other single dysarthria types. It is discussed in detail in the next section.

Clinical Findings

Spastic dysarthria is often associated with bilateral motor signs and symptoms in the limbs that make the presence of bilateral CNS involvement obvious.‡ However, it can occur in the absence of bilateral or even unilateral limb findings, and it may, sometimes along with dysphagia and pathologic oral reflexes, be the only sign of neurologic disease. This is not unusual in certain degenerative nervous system diseases.

Bilateral spastic paralysis affecting the bulbar muscles traditionally has been called *pseudobulbar palsy,* and many neurologists use the term to describe the speech of spastic dysarthria. Pseudobulbar palsy is a clinical syndrome that derives its name from its superficial resemblance to bulbar palsy (associated with LMN lesions and flaccid dysarthria). It reflects bilateral lesions of corticobulbar fibers and is most commonly associated with multiple or bilateral strokes, CNS trauma, degenerative CNS disease, encephalopathies, and CNS tumors. Its clinical features include dysarthria, dysphagia, and other oral mechanism abnormalities that are discussed as follows.

Nonspeech Oral Mechanism

Several oral mechanism findings are frequently associated with spastic dysarthria. *Dysphagia* is common and sometimes severe. Although some patients deny chewing or swallowing difficulties, on questioning they may admit that they are careful when swallowing, that chewing meat has become more difficult, or that they chew more slowly or more carefully than before. Nasal regurgitation is unusual in pure spastic dysarthria, but *drooling* is common, and patients often attribute it to excessive saliva production; it is more likely due to decreased frequency of swallowing or poor control of secretions. It may occur when the patient concentrates on some nonspeech activity, particularly if the neck is flexed (e.g., during writing). Patients with or without daytime drooling sometimes note that their pillow is wet upon awakening in the morning, or that saliva has dried around the mouth during the night. Obviously slowed jaw, lip, and facial movement may characterize reflexive swallowing of secretions; the swallow is occasionally audible.

At rest, the nasolabial folds may be smoothed or flattened, or the face may be held in a somewhat fixed, subtle smiling or pouting posture. Reflexive or emotional facial movements frequently emerge slowly but may then overflow and be excessive.

Lability of affect, often called *pseudobulbar affect* or *pathologic laughing and crying,* is frequently apparent. When subtle, patients may have an "on the verge of tears" facial expression. When more obvious, they may cry or laugh in a stereotypic manner for no apparent reason, may fluctuate between laughing and crying, or may have difficulty inhibiting laughter and crying once they begin. The ease with which the response is elicited tends to be

---

*Fatigue is a common complaint in people with neurologic disease. In those with spastic paresis of the limbs, it is usually assumed to be of CNS origin, secondary to impaired recruitment of alpha motor neurons, but it is recognized that mechanisms underlying fatigue can include all elements of the motor system.[18] For example, there is some evidence that biochemical changes in muscles of patients with UMN lesions may contribute to excessive fatigability.[32] The etiology of the muscle changes may be due to disuse, a problem known to reduce muscle volume and weight.[16]

---

†In degenerative or gradually developing neurologic disease, speech and swallowing problems very often emerge concurrently. In the author's experience, which could be subject to referral bias, when one precedes the other, speech difficulty tends to develop first.

---

‡Unilateral UMN lesions produce a syndrome of signs and symptoms that affect movements on the contralateral side of the body. This syndrome sometimes includes unilateral UMN dysarthria, which is addressed in Chapter 9.

table 5-2	Neuromuscular deficits associated with spastic dysarthria						
Direction	**Rhythm**	**Rate**		**Range**		**Force**	**Tone**
Individual Movements	Repetitive Movements	Individual Movements	Repetitive Movements	Individual Movements	Repetitive Movements	Individual Movements	Muscle Tone
Normal	Regular	Slow	Slow	Reduced (weak)	Reduced (biased)	Reduced	Excessive

Modified from Darley FL, Aronson AE, Brown JR: Clusters of deviant speech dimensions in the dysarthria, *J Speech Hear Res* 12:462, 1969.

related to the emotional loading of the interaction, although the emotional response can occur spontaneously or simply in response to being asked if they have difficulty controlling emotional expression. Patients sometimes report that their inner emotional state does not match their physical expression of emotion. These affective responses can occur during speech, sometimes with significant effects on intelligibility or efficiency of communication. Pseudobulbar affect can convey an impression of emotional instability or dementia but can be present without any clear evidence of those disorders and sometimes without other evidence of pseudobulbar palsy,[6] including dysarthria. These uncontrollable emotional responses are often upsetting to patients. Aronson[5] points out that "the reduced threshold for crying and laughter has clinical diagnostic importance and needs to be recognized as one of the great social and psychological burdens borne by patients with pseudobulbar palsy."

Examination of nonspeech oromotor functions usually demonstrates normal jaw strength. The face may be weak bilaterally, and range of lip retraction and pursing may be decreased; however, lower facial weakness is usually not as pronounced as with LMN lesions. The tongue is usually full and symmetric, but range of movement may be reduced and weakness apparent on strength testing. Nonspeech alternate motion rates (AMRs) for jaw, lip retraction and pursing, and lateral or anterior tongue movements are often slow and reduced in range of movement, but they are generally regular in rhythm.

The palate is usually symmetric but may move slowly or minimally on phonation. The gag reflex is often hyperactive.* The cough and glottal coup may be normal in sharpness if respiratory and laryngeal

movements are not too slowed, but they may lack sharpness if slowness is prominent.

Pathologic oral reflexes are common. *Sucking, snout, palmomental,* and *jaw jerk reflexes* are frequently present and are suggestive of bilateral UMN involvement.

Speech

Conversational speech and reading, speech AMRs, and vowel prolongation are the most useful tasks for eliciting the salient and distinguishing characteristics of spastic dysarthria.* Speech stress testing and sequential motion rates (SMRs) are not particularly revealing.

The deviant speech characteristics associated with spastic dysarthria are not easily or usefully described by listing each cranial nerve and the speech characteristics associated with its abnormal function. This is because *spastic dysarthria is associated with impaired movement patterns rather than weakness of individual muscles.* This reflects the organization of CNS motor pathways for the control of movement patterns rather than isolated muscle movements, and it represents an important distinction between LMN and UMN lesions. Therefore *spastic dysarthria is usually associated with deficits at all of the speech valves and for all components of the speech system,* although not always equally. The involvement of multiple speech valves may explain why intelligibility is so frequently affected.

Table 5-2 summarizes the neuromuscular deficits assumed by Darley, Aronson, and Brown (DAB)[12-14]

---

*Some patients with bilateral damage to the lower part of the precentral and postcentral cortex of the cerebral hemispheres may have an absent gag reflex. The constellation of deficits with such lesions is discussed in the section on biopercular syndrome in Chapter 12.

*Speech AMR and vowel prolongation tasks are also sensitive to differences between "developmental" spastic dysarthria and nondysarthric speech. Wit et al.[46] found that performance on such tasks reliably distinguished children with spastic dysarthria associated with cerebral palsy (age 6 to 11 years) from a matched control group. The dysarthric children had reduced maximum sound prolongation and f_o range on vowel prolongation tasks and slower and more variable syllable durations on AMR tasks.

to underlie spastic dysarthria. In general, direction and rhythm or timing of movement are unaffected. The chief disturbances are *slowness and reduced range of individual and repetitive movements, reduced force of movement, and excessive or biased muscle tone or spasticity.* The bias of muscle tone is most apparent at the laryngeal valve, in which the bias is toward hyperadduction during phonation. The relationship between these neuromuscular deficits and the prominent deviant clusters and speech characteristics of spastic dysarthria is apparent in subsequent descriptions of those characteristics. Experimental support for the presumed underlying neuromuscular deficits, especially slowness and reduced range of movement, is reviewed in the section on acoustic and physiologic studies.

Clusters of Deviant Dimensions and Prominent Deviant Speech Characteristics

DAB[13] found four clusters of deviant dimensions in their group of 30 patients with pseudobulbar palsy. These clusters are useful to understanding the neuromuscular deficits presumed to underlie spastic dysarthria, the components of the speech system that are most prominently involved, and the features of spastic dysarthria that distinguish it from other dysarthria types (Table 5-3).

The first cluster is *prosodic excess,* represented by *excess and equal stress* and *slow rate.* These characteristics are probably related to slowness of individual and repetitive movements. Slowness of movement logically reduces speech rate. It probably also contributes to excess and equal stress by reducing the speed of the muscular adjustments necessary for the rapid pitch, loudness, and duration adjustments associated with normal prosody. Slow overall speech rate can also lead to a perception of excess and equalized stress, because longer syllable duration is associated with stressed syllables.

The second cluster is *articulatory-resonatory incompetence,* represented by *imprecise consonants, distorted vowels,* and *hypernasality.* This cluster represents the probable effects of reduced range and force of articulatory movements (presumably including the tongue, jaw, and face) and velopharyngeal movements. The strong interrelationships among velopharyngeal and articulatory features in this cluster implicate the velopharyngeal mechanism's articulatory role, not its resonatory role (i.e., inadequate velopharyngeal closure can result in weak, imprecise pressure consonants).

The third cluster is *prosodic insufficiency,* consisting of *monopitch, monoloudness, reduced stress,* and *short phrases.* For the most part, these characteristics are attributable to reduced vocal variability, with stressed syllables left unstressed or insufficiently different from unstressed syllables, and reduced pitch and loudness variability. Decreased range of movement is a likely explanation for this cluster.

The fourth cluster is *phonatory stenosis,* characterized by *low pitch, harshness, strained-strangled voice, pitch breaks, short phrases,* and *slow rate.* These phonatory characteristics seem to reflect efforts to produce voice through a narrowed glottis with secondary reduction of phrase length and speech rate. The assumption is that laryngeal hypertonus is present with a bias toward excessive adduction or resistance to abduction. The features of slow rate and short phrases may also be related to slowness of movement and inefficient valving at the velopharyngeal and articulatory valves.

DAB noted the presence of *breathiness* in some patients with spastic dysarthria, a characteristic that was not correlated with any of the clusters found for the disorder. This breathiness could reflect a degree of vocal-cord weakness, but it could also represent a compensatory response rather than a primary problem. For example, some patients may actively maintain incomplete adduction to prevent laryngeal stenosis, or, alternatively, may intermittently actively abduct the cords to facilitate exhalation or provide relief from the effort induced by laryngeal stenosis.

Table 5-4 summarizes the most deviant speech dimensions found by DAB.[12] It is noteworthy that the rankings in Table 5-4 represent the order of prominence (severity) of the speech characteristics, not the features that are most distinctive of spastic

table 5-3	Clusters of abnormal speech characteristics in spastic dysarthria
Cluster	**Speech Characteristics**
Prosodic Excess	Excess & equal stress
	Slow rate
Articulatory-Resonatory Incompetence	Imprecise consonants
	Distorted vowels
	Hypernasality
Prosodic Insufficiency	Monopitch
	Monoloudness
	Reduced stress
	Short phrases
Phonatory Stenosis	Low pitch
	Harshness
	Strained-strangled voice
	Pitch breaks
	Short phrases
	Slow rate

Modified from Darley FL, Aronson AE, Brown JR: Clusters of deviant speech dimensions in the dysarthria, *J Speech Hear Res* 12:462, 1969b.

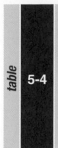

table 5-4

Most deviant speech dimensions encountered in spastic dysarthria by DAB,[13] listed in order from most to least severe. Also listed is the component of the speech system associated with each characteristic. The component "prosodic" is listed when several components of the speech system may contribute to the dimension.

Dimension	Speech Component
Imprecise consonants*	Articulatory
Monopitch	Laryngeal
Reduced stress	Prosodic
Harshness	Laryngeal
Monoloudness	Laryngeal-respiratory
Low pitch*	Laryngeal
Slow rate*	Articulatory-prosodic
Hypernasality	Velopharyngeal
Strained-strangled quality*	Laryngeal
Short phrases	Laryngeal-respiratory-velopharyngeal or articulatory
Distorted vowels	Articulatory
Pitch breaks	Laryngeal
Breathy voice (continuous)	Laryngeal
Excess & equal stress	Prosodic

*Tend to be distinctive or more severely impaired in spastic dysarthria than other single dysarthria types.

table 5-5

Primary distinguishing speech and speech-related findings in spastic dysarthria

Perceptual	
Phonation	Strained-strangled voice quality
Articulation-prosody	Slow rate
	Slow & regular alternating motion rates
Physical	Dysphagia, drooling
	Weak face & tongue
	Pathologic reflexes (suck, snout, palmomental, jaw jerk)
	Pseudobulbar affect
Patient Complaints	Slow speech rate
	Increased effort to speak
	Fatigue when speaking
	Chewing-swallowing difficulty
	Poor control of emotional expression

speech AMRs are the most distinctive clues to the presence of spastic dysarthria.

Table 5-5 summarizes the primary distinguishing speech characteristics and common oral mechanism examination findings and patient complaints encountered in spastic dysarthria.

Acoustic and Physiologic Findings

This section focuses primarily on acoustic and physiologic studies of acquired spastic dysarthria, but a few studies of children and adults with cerebral palsy are also relevant. The results of these studies are summarized in Table 5-6. Figure 5-2 illustrates some acoustic correlates of perceived slow and regular AMRs. Figure 5-3 illustrates some acoustic correlates of perceived slow speech rate and prosodic abnormalities commonly associated with spastic dysarthria.

Respiration

Little is known about speech-related respiratory characteristics in acquired spastic dysarthria. It is quite possible, however, that they bear a resemblance to some of the documented respiratory difficulties of children and adults with spastic cerebral palsy. These abnormalities include reduced inhalatory and exhalatory respiratory volumes leading to shallow breathing; paradoxical breathing in which abdominal muscles fail to relax during inhalation with resultant restriction of respiratory intake; and reduced vital capacity.[5,14]

dysarthria. For example, imprecise consonants, although rated as the most severely impaired characteristic in spastic dysarthria, are found in all major dysarthria types and therefore are not a *distinguishing* characteristic of spastic dysarthria.

Numerous studies support DAB's identification of slow rate as a pervasive and perceptually salient feature of spastic dysarthria. For example, Kammermeier[25] (as summarized by DAB[14]) found a mean reading rate of 104 words per minute in patients with spastic dysarthria, slower than in those with bulbar palsy, Parkinson's disease, cerebellar disease, and dystonia. Slow speech AMRs have been documented in several studies.[17,22,28,38] In studies in which comparisons have been made to other dysarthria types, patients with spastic dysarthria have had the slowest AMRs. Linebaugh and Wolfe[29] documented slow rate of syllable production in spastic dysarthria, as well as a moderate relationship between rate and intelligibility and speech naturalness ratings.

What features of spastic dysarthria help distinguish it from other types of MSDs? Among the many abnormalities that may be detected, *strained-harsh voice quality, slow speech rate, and slow and regular*

table 5-6	Summary of acoustic and physiologic findings in studies of spastic dysarthria*

Speech Component	Acoustic or Physiologic Observation
Respiratory (or respiratory or laryngeal) (based on studies of spastic cerebral palsy)	Reduced: Inhalatory & exhalatory volumes Respiratory intake Vital capacity Maximum vowel prolongation Poor visuomotor tracking with respiratory movements
Laryngeal	Decreased: Harmonic-to-noise ratio Laryngeal airflow Fundamental frequency variability Increased: Shimmer & jitter Standard deviation of f_o Subglottal pressure Glottal resistance Nonsyntactic breaks Hyperadduction of true & false cords during speech Poor visuomotor tracking with pitch variations
Velopharyngeal	Slow velopharyngeal movement Incomplete velopharyngeal closure
Articulatory or Rate or Prosody	Reduced: Overall rate (words per minute, syllables per second, phoneme duration) Alternate motion rates (AMRs) Speed & range of tongue, jaw, & palatal movements Acceleration & deceleration of articulators Maximum speed of lip movements Rate & slope of F2 transitions Rate of amplitude variation Tongue strength Ability to sustain maximum tongue contraction Vowel space Completeness of articulatory contacts Completeness of consonant clusters Sharpness of voiceless stops Spectral tilt for /s/ (imprecision) Oral pressures Sound pressure level contrasts in consonants Amplitude of release bursts for stops Frequency & intensity increases for initial word stress Articulatory effort for final word stress Increased: Duration of nonphonated intervals Variability of noise amplitude or spectrum shape during /s/ Noise before closure for /s/ Duration of phoneme-to-phoneme transitions Intersyllable duration Temporal & amplitude variability for AMRs Centralization of vowel formants Acoustic energy during intersyllable gaps (imprecision) Voicing of voiceless stops Incomplete lingual articulatory contacts Spirantization

*Note that many of these observations are based on studies of only one or a few speakers, and not all speakers with spastic dysarthria exhibit all of these features. Note also that these characteristics may not be unique to spastic dysarthria; many can be observed in other motor speech disorders or nonneurologic conditions.

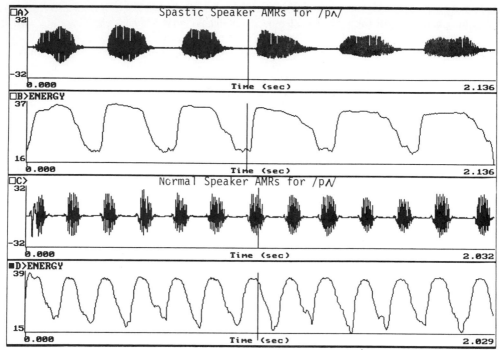

FIGURE 5-2 Raw waveform and energy tracings of speech alternate motion rates (AMRs) for /p⇒/ by a normal speaker *(bottom two panels)* and a speaker with spastic dysarthria. The normal speaker's AMRs are normal in rate (≈6.5 Hz) and relatively regular in duration and amplitude. In contrast, the spastic speaker's AMRs are slow (≈3 Hz) and regular. These attributes represent the acoustic correlates of perceived slow and regular AMRs that are common in spastic dysarthria.

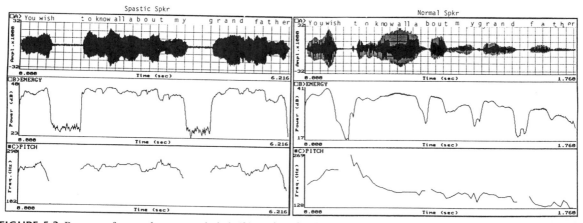

FIGURE 5-3 Raw waveform and energy and pitch (f_o) tracings for the sentence "You wish to know all about my grandfather" by a normal female speaker *(tracings on right)* and a female speaker with spastic dysarthria *(tracings on left)*.

The normal speaker completes the sentence in less than 2 seconds with normal variability in syllable duration and amplitude (energy tracing) and normal variability and declination in f_o across the sentence (pitch tracing).

In contrast, the spastic speaker is slow (≈6.2 seconds for the utterance). The silent breaks evident in all tracings between "wish" and "to" and between "my" and "grandfather" are considerably lengthened and reflect slowness in achieving and releasing stop closure for /t/ and /g/, respectively. Other portions of the utterance in the energy and pitch tracings show little syllable distinctiveness, reflecting continuous voicing and restricted loudness and pitch variability. These acoustic attributes reflect the perceptible slow rate and monopitch and monoloudness that are characteristic of many speakers with spastic dysarthria.

The degree to which respiratory abnormalities affect speech in spastic dysarthria is unclear. Complicating their understanding is the fact that laryngeal valve hyperadduction is usually present, so even normal expiratory capacity must work against laryngeal resistance to airflow. In some cases, efforts to overcome severe glottic constriction during speech are so great that the speaker will seek momentary relief by volitionally releasing a considerable quantity of air. The result is intermittent breathiness and air wastage that can lead to reduced utterance length per breath group. Therefore deviations of respiratory activity may reflect the primary effects of underlying respiratory deficits but also secondary effects from abnormal laryngeal (and possibly resonatory and articulatory) activities as well.

Laryngeal Function

Visual examination of the larynx at rest may reveal normal-appearing vocal folds. However, bilateral hyperadduction of the true and false vocal cords during speech may be apparent.[5,48]

Studies of patients with pseudobulbar palsy or multiple bilateral strokes have examined connected speech and vowel prolongation using various acoustic measures related to laryngeal function. They have found evidence of increased shimmer and jitter,* increased nonsyntactic breaks, increased standard deviation of fundamental frequency (f_o), decreased harmonic-to-noise ratio, decreased pitch variability, decreased words per minute and syllables per second, and decreased maximum vowel prolongation[25] (as reported by DAB[14]; Sherard, Marquardt, and Cannito[43]).

Using electromyography and aerodynamic measures, Murdoch, Thompson, and Stokes[33] reported that approximately half of their 14 subjects with stroke had hyperfunctional features such as increased subglottal air pressure, increased glottal resistance, and decreased laryngeal airflow. Other subjects had hypofunctional activity (including perceived breathiness in some subjects), thought possibly to reflect compensation or laryngeal hypertonus and muscle stiffness. Perceptual results did not concur with instrumental findings in approximately half of the subjects (e.g., some subjects with perceived hyperfunctional features had instrumental findings suggestive of laryngeal hypofunction, and vice versa). The authors questioned if this could be

due to inadequacies of perceptual or instrumental methods, different tasks used for the two methods, or different compensatory strategies.

The findings of these studies generally align well with several of the primary perceptual features of spastic dysarthria, including monopitch, strained-harsh voice quality, and slow rate. Evidence of hypofunction from aerodynamic studies raises the possibility of weakness at the laryngeal level but might also reflect compensatory strategies, variations in the muscular dynamics of laryngeal spasticity, or methodological artifacts. Incongruities between perceptual and instrumental findings could also reflect methodological artifacts but might also reflect the sensitivity of instrumental methods to abnormalities that are dismissed or escape detection perceptually.

Velopharyngeal Function

On oral inspection, the palate may move sluggishly or not at all during vowel prolongation. Palatal immobility, slow movement, and incomplete velopharyngeal closure may be apparent during videofluoroscopy and nasoendoscopy.

Thompson and Murdoch[44] found that 7 of 19 subjects with "UMN dysarthria" had hypernasality based on accelerometric recordings. Ziegler and von Cramon,[48] noting the tendency of some of their spastic subjects to voice voiceless stops, speculated that such distortions might be facilitated by incomplete velopharyngeal and oral cavity contacts that prevent interruption of phonation, even if vocal fold capacity is normal.* This explanation was supported by one of their subject's ability to produce voiceless stops when air wastage through the velopharyngeal port was decreased with the nares occluded. This observation illustrates the interactions at different levels of the speech system that may affect articulatory outcomes.

Articulation, Rate, and Prosody

Numerous acoustic and physiologic studies have contributed to a better understanding of the articulatory dynamics and rate and prosodic impairments in spastic dysarthria. A few of the studies summarized here are detailed to illustrate the logic behind them and how they relate to clinical perceptual findings.

---

*Shimmer and jitter are "short-term" measures of departures from regularity (perturbation) in the voice. Shimmer reflects "cycle-to-cycle variations in the peak amplitude of the laryngeal waveform." Jitter reflects "cycle-to-cycle variation in the fundamental period."[27]

---

*The rapid laryngeal adjustments necessary for producing voiceless consonants are another source of voicing errors.

Acoustic studies support conclusions that rate of movement is slow and that range and precision of movement are reduced. Evidence of slowness comes from findings of reduced overall speech rate, increased word durations, increased syllable durations, prolonged phonemes, slow transitions from one phoneme to another, lengthened intersyllable pauses, reduced rate of amplitude variations, and slow speech AMRs. Evidence of imprecision and reduced range of movement derives from findings of acoustic energy within intersyllable gaps (imprecise articulation, spirantization) and centralization of vowel formants indicating restricted range of movement.[17,22,28,29,36,38,48] Some findings,[28,38] while confirming perceptual judgments of slow AMRs, suggest a degree of variability in timing and amplitude that has not generally been noted in perceptual studies.

Several other acoustic attributes suggest that imprecise articulation may be related to slowness, reduced range of movement, or weakness at the articulatory, velopharyngeal, or laryngeal valves. These include reduced sharpness of voiceless stops with a tendency toward voicing and reduced sound pressure level (SPL) contrasts in consonants (Alajouanine, Sabouraud, and Gremy, 1959, as summarized by DAB[14]; Ziegler and von Cramon[48]). Ziegler and von Cramon[48] attributed reduced SPL differences to inadequate voicing and hypernasality, as well as to the presence of friction noise (spirantization) with decreased amplitude of release bursts during production of stops. They noted that adequate production of stops and vowels was usually accomplished at the expense of articulatory rate. It is also instructive to note that voice onset time (VOT)—an acoustic reflection of timing control between laryngeal and supralaryngeal movements—is measurable less frequently in stop consonants of people with spastic dysarthria (84% measurable) than neurologically normal speakers (95% measurable).[37] This is most often due to lack of a burst signifying release of stop consonants, suggesting imprecision or a lack of firm articulatory contact. This implies that the greater than normal inability to make certain acoustic measurements in dysarthric speakers is an indirect way to document abnormality and, depending on the measure, may permit inferences about abnormal movement dynamics.

Chen and Stevens[11] used spectral analysis and spectrographic observations of /s/ in the initial position of words in a study of two normal and eight dysarthric subjects. Four of the dysarthric speakers had spastic cerebral palsy and can be presumed to have had spastic dysarthria. They had abnormal values on a number of the acoustic measures, but three deserve mention because together they predicted speech intelligibility: (1) spectral tilt, a measure (in dB) of the high-frequency prominence relative to the mid-frequency spectrum amplitude for /s/, served as an indirect measure of the proximity of the tongue blade to the lips and hence an indirect measure of articulatory precision; (2) time variation, a measure of variability of noise amplitude or spectrum shape during the /s/, was an indirect measure of the maintenance of a reasonably fixed tongue blade position and shape, and possibly fixed jaw position and relatively constant intraoral pressure; (3) precursor, a measure of the amount of inadvertent noise or voicing energy before the closure for the /s/, was an indirect measure of coordination among expiratory pressure, vocal fold configuration for the voiceless /s/, and the placement and shaping of the tongue blade for /s/.

A few studies have found different effects across speech structures. Ziegler and von Cramon[48] acoustically analyzed consonant-vowel-consonant (CVC) sequences and found disproportionate impairment of tongue-back movements relative to tongue-blade movements. Some studies have found relative preservation of range and control of jaw movement,[22,31] and Hirose[22] speculated that this might permit the jaw to compensate to some degree for inadequate tongue and lip articulatory movements. In a nonspeech visuomotor tracking study, McClean, Beukelman, and Yorkston[31] required subjects to track a sinusoidal wave with lower-lip and jaw movement (using strain gauge transducers), respiratory activity (by transducing air pressure changes in a face mask), and laryngeal activity (by altering f_o). Their one subject with spastic dysarthria had subnormal levels of respiratory tracking and greatly reduced tracking with the larynx but normal control of the jaw and lip. These observations suggest that spastic dysarthria may be associated with fine motor control difficulties that may vary across levels of the speech system.

In a kinematic study of lower lip trajectories during sentence production, Ackermann et al.[3] found reduced maximum speed of lip opening and closing gestures, as well as reduced peak velocity to maximum amplitude of lip movements, in three speakers with spastic dysarthria. These findings were interpreted as a reflection of "stiffness" and "central paresis due to an impairment of the upper motor neurons." Several other studies, using various physiologic methods, have documented slowness and reduced range of movement of the tongue, jaw, or palate.[22-24,26]

Using a rubber bulb tongue pressure transducer system, Thompson, Murdoch, and Stokes[44] examined tongue strength, rate of repetitive tongue movements, and ability to sustain maximum tongue contraction in 16 adults with stroke-related "UMN type dysarthria." Three of the subjects had bilateral lesions and may have had spastic dysarthria. In comparison to normal speakers, the dysarthric speakers had reduced tongue strength, reduced rate of repetitive tongue movements, and reduced ability to sustain maximum tongue contractions (i.e., reduced endurance or fatigue). Of interest, the transduced measures of tongue function were not significantly related to perceived articulatory adequacy. The authors suggested that the lack of relationship may have been because only some of the subjects had reduced strength beyond a critical level at which speech is affected, or that the relationship is not a linear one. Dworkin and Aronson[17] also found reduced tongue strength in speakers with spastic dysarthria, although not more so than in individuals with other dysarthria types.

Electropalatography has been employed to measure lingual-palatal contact during speech in a small number of people with spastic dysarthria. Detected abnormalities have included incomplete patterns of articulatory contact, smaller areas of contact, and greater numbers of contacts.[19,20] These abnormalities could reflect spatial as well as timing disturbances, and they imply reduced precision and accuracy of lingual speech movements.

Slow speech rate helps explain the presence of prosodic abnormalities in spastic dysarthria, but few investigations have examined vocal-stress patterns. Murry[34] tested the ability of five individuals with spastic dysarthria to vary stress during multiple productions of three-word sentences in which stress was placed on varying words. Peak intraoral pressure, duration of the pressure pulse, f_o, vowel duration, and vowel intensity were measured. In contrast to normal speakers, spastic speakers conveyed phrase final word stress only with frequency and intensity changes. They also generally conveyed stress less adequately than normal and usually by compensation. For example, spastic speakers seemed to use increased articulatory effort for phrase initial word stress. For final word stress, they increased f_o and intensity, but articulatory effort was compromised. Murry[34] concluded that when spastic dysarthric subjects use consonant-related cues to stress an initial word, vowel-related cues are decreased relative to baseline. For final word stress, they switch to a vowel strategy and reduce articulatory effort. They did not generally use vowel duration cues to vary stress in any position.

Finally, Roy et al.[41] examined several perceptual, acoustic, and physiologic parameters in a man with severe spastic dysarthria from a TBI. Before initiation of treatment, acoustic analyses identified slow and shallow F2 format transitions (i.e., slow movement and reduced range of movement) and reduced vowel space (i.e., reduced acoustic distinctiveness among different vowels). Nasometry and aerodynamic measures of velopharyngeal function identified reduced oral pressures, increased nasal airflow, and increased nasalance. All findings are consistent with auditory perceptual features of spastic dysarthria. The study is noteworthy because it illustrates the value of combining perceptual, acoustic, and physiologic measures to understand specific speech subsystem contributors to reduced intelligibility and their contribution to treatment decisions and measurement of change.

To summarize, acoustic and physiologic studies have documented the presence of impairments at all levels of the speech system in spastic dysarthria, and, for the most part, they provide strong support for many of the perceptually recognizable features of the disorder. Within each speech subsystem there is evidence of slowness, reduced range and precision of movements, and sometimes variability of movement control. The studies support and refine perceptual observations of imprecise articulation and indicate that at least some affected people lack precision and control for articulatory placement. Physiologic studies have defined some of the movement dynamics underlying the perception of slow rate, and they support inferences that spastic dysarthria reflects a combination of spasticity and weakness. There is some evidence that the motor control difficulties associated with the disorder can vary across levels of the speech system. Finally, there is evidence that some acoustic correlates of precision, steadiness, and coordination in spastic dysarthria are related to intelligibility. Chen and Stevens[11] concluded that one goal of ongoing acoustic analyses should be "to assemble a set of parameters that, in combination, can predict the intelligibility of a dysarthric speech signal and can be interpreted in terms of deviations in control of the speech production system." If this goal can be met, and if the related analyses can be relatively automated and cost-effective, acoustic analysis will become highly valuable in many clinical settings.

Cases

Case 5-1

A 65-year-old woman presented with a 6-month history of "slurred speech" and dysphagia. Prior history was unremarkable, except for hypertension that did not require medication. Her initial difficulty with swallowing was greater for liquids than solids and had progressed to a point where she had extreme difficulty with liquids. She had not lost weight, nor had she had difficulty with aspiration or nasal regurgitation. A short time after her dysphagia developed, she noted speech difficulty that had also gradually progressed. She had been placed on Mestinon for MG by a neurologist at another institution, without benefit.

The neurologic examination, beyond her speech difficulty and dysphagia, revealed mild bilateral facial weakness and bilaterally increased deep tendon and Babinski reflexes. Arm and leg AMRs were diminished slightly on the left. Laboratory tests were essentially normal, as were screenings for hereditary demyelinating syndromes. Nerve conduction studies and electromyogram (EMG) were normal, including EMG examination of the tongue. MRI of the head was normal.

During speech examination, the patient said she initially attributed her swallowing difficulty to her dentures. At onset, her tongue felt "thick," and she was aware of a "nasal tone" to her voice. Psychologic stress and prolonged speaking made speech worse. She admitted to occasionally biting her cheek when chewing; food sometimes squirreled in her cheeks. She had compensated by chewing more slowly and eating smaller amounts to prevent choking. She admitted to difficulty controlling emotional expression.

She frequently had an "on the verge of crying" facial expression. Jaw strength was normal. The lower face was weak (−1) on voluntary lip retraction. The tongue was full and symmetric, but lateral tongue movements were slow (−2, 3). The tongue was moderately weak bilater-

ally, slightly more so on the left. The palate was symmetric and mobile. Gag reflex, cough, and glottal coup were normal. A sucking reflex was equivocally present.

Conversational speech and reading were characterized by reduced rate (2), monopitch and monoloudness (2), strained-harsh-groaning voice quality (1,2), occasional pitch breaks, hypernasality (0,1), and imprecise articulation (1,2). Prolonged "ah" was sustained for 11 seconds and was equivocally strained. Her speech AMRs were slow (2,3) but regular. Intelligibility was judged normal in the quiet one-to-one setting but probably mildly compromised in noise.

Acoustic analysis showed f_o (242 Hz) and measures of jitter and shimmer to be grossly normal. Speech AMRs for /pʌ/, /tʌ/, and /kʌ/ were 2.8, 2.8, and 2.5 Hz, respectively.

The clinician concluded: "Spastic dysarthria, suggestive of bilateral UMN involvement affecting the bulbar muscles. There are no clear-cut features of flaccid dysarthria, nor do I note characteristics that could be interpreted as ataxic." Speech therapy and management for her dysphagia were recommended.

The neurologist concluded that the patient had progressive UMN dysfunction of undetermined etiology but wondered about primary lateral sclerosis. Reevaluation in 3 to 6 months was recommended. She did not return for follow-up.

Commentary. (1) Degenerative neurologic disease can present as dysarthria or dysphagia. (2) Diagnosis of spastic dysarthria places the lesion in the CNS, bilaterally, and can help to rule out disease isolated to LMNs (e.g., MG). (3) Early during their course it is not unusual for degenerative diseases in which spastic dysarthria and dysphagia are the primary signs to defy more specific neurologic diagnosis, and for neuroimaging studies to be normal.

Case 5-2

[handwritten annotations: @ risk for stroke / high blood pressure]

A 41-year-old right-handed man from Saudi Arabia was hospitalized for management of hypertension and speech and swallowing difficulties. According to his family, he had fairly adequate English language skills.

The patient had a 2-year history of hypertension for which he had refused to take medication. Eleven months previously, over the course of an evening, he developed left hemiplegia. Ten days later he lost consciousness and upon awakening 17 days later was unable to speak or swallow. His left hemiplegia persisted, but he had no motor signs on the right side of the body. With therapy his left-sided weakness improved, but swallowing and speech remained significantly impaired. He had been fed through a nasogastric tube, but more recently he had been eating puréed foods while lying supine.

Neurologic examination revealed a left hemiparesis. Upper limb reflexes were hyperactive bilaterally, left greater than right. He was unable to speak. Questions were raised about whether the patient had an "expressive aphasia," or if a component of his speech difficulty was psychogenic. It was assumed that his lesion was unilateral (right).

On speech examination, he was nearly *anarthric* *[handwritten: or no speak]* (speechless due to severe dysarthria). He could produce a nasally emitted and resonated, quiet but strained-strangled undifferentiated vowel with great effort but little else. With his lips closed he produced a prolonged and strained /m/. Voluntary lip and jaw movements were slow and limited in range but were more extensive during reflexive swallowing; the jaw opened widely during a reflexive yawn. Suck, snout, and jaw jerk reflexes were present. At rest the tongue sat in a relatively retracted position. Tongue movement was minimal and slow; he was unable to extend it beyond the edge of the lower teeth and unable to elevate or move it laterally. The palate hung so low in the pharynx that the uvula could not be seen; a gag reflex could not be elicited. Surprisingly, his cough was sharp.

There was no evidence of language difficulty. He followed two-step commands and communicated effectively through writing, although with occasional spelling errors.

It was concluded that he had a "severe spastic dysarthria without any evidence of aphasia or apraxia of speech, and no clear evidence of a psychogenic contribution to his speechlessness. To produce a dysarthria like this, the lesion should be bilateral."

Subsequent CT scan revealed old infarcts in the centrum semiovale of both hemispheres, as well as an infarction in the right posterior parietal cortex (Figure 5-4).

A brief period of speech therapy was undertaken, but it was soon apparent that intelligible speech would not

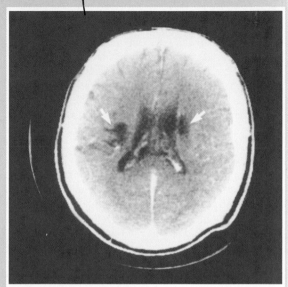

FIGURE 5-4 Computed tomography scan for Case 5-2. Relatively small infarcts in the centrum semiovale bilaterally *(arrows)* were associated with a severe spastic dysarthria.

be achieved. Vocal loudness increased and hypernasality decreased when the palate was elevated from the surface of the tongue with a tongue depressor. A palatal lift prosthesis was made to ease swallowing, but the weight of the velum on the device made it impossible to keep the prosthesis securely fastened. The patient underwent pharyngeal flap surgery and was then able to eat puréed food while sitting in an upright position, although it took 2 hours for him to complete a meal. He could breathe orally. Writing was an effective, portable, but somewhat inefficient means of communication for him. He returned to his home before other means of augmentative communication could be thoroughly investigated.

Commentary. (1) The presence of significant spastic dysarthria should raise questions about bilateral UMN involvement, even when limb findings suggest that the lesion is only unilateral. (2) Lesions do not have to be large to produce devastating consequences for speech. The patient's centrum semiovale lesions were small, but their locus was sufficient to interrupt UMN pathways to the bulbar speech muscles bilaterally. (3) Severe spastic dysarthria is almost always accompanied by significant dysphagia. (4) Accurate diagnosis of the speech deficit helped to rule out aphasia, as well as significant psychogenic influences. This information was useful in counseling the patient and family, particularly their understanding of the nature of the problem and their acceptance of limitations on future recovery of speech.

Case 5-3

A 71-year-old woman presented with a 3-month history of "lost voice." Prior medical history was unremarkable. The only abnormality on ear, nose, and throat (ENT) examination was decreased tongue mobility. "Neurologic dysphonia" and possible "LMN disease" were suspected. Speech pathology and neurology consultations were arranged.

During speech evaluation, the patient recalled that her progressing speech difficulty had been present for approximately 15 months. She complained that her voice was strained, that speech was slow, and that speaking was effortful. She had difficulty swallowing liquids, with occasional choking and infrequent nasal regurgitation. She had not had to modify her diet, nor had she lost weight. She denied change or difficulty controlling emotional expression, drooling, and difficulty with memory or other cognitive skills.

Speech AMRs of the jaw, lower face, and tongue were slow (2) but regular. Jaw and lower face strength were normal; the left side of the tongue was equivocally weak. There was a slight droop at the right corner of the mouth and a subtle "snarl" of the left upper lip at rest. The palate was symmetric and relatively immobile during vowel prolongation but moved normally during gagging. Nasal emission was apparent during pressure sound production. Her cough was normal. Suck, snout, and jaw jerk reflexes were not detected.

A strained-harsh-groaning voice quality (2), reduced rate (1,2), hypernasality (1,2), imprecise articulation (1), and monopitch and monoloudness (1,2) characterized connected speech. Lip and jaw movements were slightly exaggerated during speech, possibly reflecting compensatory efforts to maintain intelligibility. Speech AMRs were slow (2,3). "Ah" was strained (3) and sustained for only 6 seconds.

The clinician concluded, "Spastic dysarthria, moderately severe. No clear evidence of a flaccid (LMN) component. Speech characteristics are strongly suggestive of bilateral UMN dysfunction affecting the bulbar musculature." She was referred for speech therapy and management of her dysphagia, which she pursued closer to home.

Neurologic examination noted brisk muscle stretch reflexes but no pathologic reflexes. No fasciculations were detected. Subsequent EMG failed to identify fibrillations or fasciculation potentials. MRI of the head, with special attention to the brainstem, was normal. The neurologist concluded that the patient had a pseudobulbar palsy with spastic dysarthria plus minimal findings in the upper limbs. ALS was suspected, but a diagnosis could not be confirmed. She was not seen for subsequent follow-up.

Commentary. (1) Speech difficulty can be the presenting complaint in neurologic disease. (2) Spastic dysarthria can occur in the absence of other significant neurologic deficits and can progress without significant clinical findings in the limbs. (3) Spastic dysarthria is frequently accompanied by dysphagia. (4) Dysarthria affecting the bulbar muscles, in the absence of limb findings, is sometimes misinterpreted as LMN disease (frequently MG). Careful speech examination can help establish the presence of bilateral UMN involvement in such cases.

Case 5-4

An 80-year-old woman was admitted to the hospital neurology service following the sudden onset of speech difficulty. She had a 10-year history of hypertension. Approximately a year before the current admission she had the sudden onset of dysarthria, dysphagia, and right-hand clumsiness, all which resolved within 10 days.

Neurologic examination identified significant dysarthria, dysphagia, and left-hand weakness, as well as hyperactive reflexes on the left. A diagnosis of a right internal capsule or pontine infarct was made. Subsequent MRI and CT scans identified moderate generalized atrophy and multiple focal areas of abnormality in the hemispheric white matter bilaterally, consistent with subcortical ischemic disease.

Speech examination revealed both left and right lower facial weakness with reduced range of movement on smiling, lip rounding, and lip puffing. Tongue protrusion and lateralization were limited in range. Gag reflex was hypoactive. A sucking reflex was not present. A hoarse, strained voice quality, reduced loudness, imprecise articulation, hypernasality, and monopitch and monoloudness characterized contextual speech. Speech AMRs were slow (2) but regular. Speech intelligibility was reduced. There was no evidence of aphasic language impairment or apraxia of speech.

The clinician concluded that the patient had a "marked spastic dysarthria with significantly reduced speech intelligibility. The tongue is markedly weak, but this is probably on a bilateral UMN basis."

Speech therapy was recommended, which she pursued closer to home. Neuropsychological assessment identified moderate generalized cognitive dysfunction, most evident in areas of attention and concentration, new learning and memory, and reasoning and problem solving.

Commentary. (1) Although excellent recovery from unilateral UMN lesions causing dysarthria is possible, additional lesions on the other side of the brain can result in spastic dysarthria with significant reduction of speech intelligibility. (2) When spastic dysarthria is present following an apparent unilateral cerebral event, suspicions should be raised about bilateral lesions. In this case, the history and current event helped establish the presence of more than one lesion.

SUMMARY

1. Spastic dysarthria results from damage to the direct and indirect activation pathways (UMNs) bilaterally. It occurs at a frequency comparable to that of other single dysarthria types. Its deviant speech characteristics reflect impaired movements and movement patterns, usually at all levels of speech production. The combined effects of spasticity and weakness on the speed, range, and force of movement seem to account for most deviant speech characteristics of the disorder.

2. Clinical signs that accompany spastic dysarthria usually include weakness, loss of skilled movement, spasticity, hyperactive reflexes, and pathologic reflexes. The salient effects of UMN lesions on speech movements include spasticity, weakness, reduced range of movement, and slowness of movement.

3. Degenerative and vascular etiologies probably account for a majority of cases of spastic dysarthria, but traumatic, demyelinating, neoplastic, and undetermined etiologies are not uncommon. Most patients with spastic dysarthria have other clinical signs or neuroimaging evidence of bilateral UMN dysfunction, but spastic dysarthria can be the only neurologic sign in some cases. The distribution of offending lesions can be widespread in the UMN system, including pathways ranging from the cortex to brainstem.

4. Dysphagia and pseudobulbar affect are common in people with spastic dysarthria. Complaints that speech is slow and effortful and deteriorates with fatigue are also common.

5. The major clusters of deviant speech characteristics in spastic dysarthria include prosodic excess, articulatory-resonatory incompetence, prosodic insufficiency, and phonatory stenosis. Although many deviant speech characteristics can be detected in spastic dysarthria, strained-harsh voice quality, slow speech rate, and slow and regular speech AMRs are the most distinctive clues to the presence of spastic dysarthria.

6. In general, acoustic and physiologic studies of individuals with spastic dysarthria have provided quantitative support for its clinical perceptual characteristics. They have helped to specify more completely the location and dynamics of abnormal movements that lead to the perceived speech abnormalities.

7. Spastic dysarthria can be the only, the first, or among the first or most prominent manifestations of neurologic disease. Its recognition and correlation with bilateral UMN dysfunction can aid the localization and diagnosis of neurologic disease and may influence decision making for medical and behavioral management.

References

1. Abbs JH, Hunker CJ, Barlow SM: Differential speech motor subsystem impairments with suprabulbar lesions: neurophysiological framework and supporting data. In Berry WR, editor: Clinical dysarthria, San Diego, 1983, College-Hill Press.

2. Abbs JH, Kennedy JG: Neurophysiological processes of speech movement control. In Lass NJ et al, editors: Speech, language, and hearing, vol 1, normal processes, Philadelphia, 1982, WB Saunders.

3. Ackermann H et al: Kinematic analysis of articulatory movements in central motor disorders, Mov Disord 6:1019, 1997.

4. Adams RD, Victor M: Principles of neurology, New York, 1991, McGraw-Hill.

5. Aronson AE: Clinical voice disorders, New York, 1990, Thieme.

6. Asfora WT et al: Is the syndrome of pathological laughing and crying a manifestation of pseudobulbar palsy? J Neurol Neurosurg Psychiatry 52:523, 1989.

7. Barlow SM, Abbs JH: Orofacial fine motor control impairments in congenital spasticity: evidence against hypertonus-related performance deficits, Neurology 34:145, 1984.

8. Bayles KA, Kaszniak AW: Communication and cognition in normal aging and dementia, Boston, 1987, College-Hill Press.

9. Biller J, Love BB: Ischemic cerebrovascular disease. In Bradley WG et al, editors: Neurology in clinical practice: principles of diagnosis and management, vol 2, ed 3, Boston, 2000, Butterworth-Heinemann.

10. Caselli RJ, Smith BE, Osborne D: Primary lateral sclerosis: a neuropsychological study, Neurology 45:2005, 1995.

11. Chen H, Stevens KN: An acoustical study of the fricative /s/ in the speech of individuals with dysarthria, J Speech Lang Hear Res 44:1300, 2001.

12. Darley FL, Aronson AE, Brown JR: Differential diagnostic patterns of dysarthria, J Speech Hear Res 12:246, 1969a.

13. Darley FL, Aronson AE, Brown JR: Clusters of deviant speech dimensions in the dysarthria, J Speech Hear Res 12:462, 1969b.

14. Darley FL, Aronson AE, Brown JR: Motor speech disorders, Philadelphia, 1975, WB Saunders.

15. Dichgans M et al: The phenotypic spectrum of CADASIL: clinical findings in 102 cases, Ann Neurol 44:731, 1998.

16. Duchateau J, Hainaut K: Electrical and mechanical change in immobilized human muscle, J Appl Psychol 62:2168, 1987.

17. Dworkin JP, Aronson AE: Tongue strength and alternate motion rates in normal and dysarthria subjects, J Commun Disord 19:115, 1986.

18. Enoka RM, Stuart DG: Neurobiology of muscle fatigue, J Appl Physiol 72:1631, 1992.

19. Goozée JV, Murdoch BE, Theodoros DG: Electropalatographic assessment of tongue-to-palate contacts exhibited in dysarthria following traumatic brain injury: spatial characteristics, J Med Speech-Lang Pathol 11:115, 2003.

20. Hardcastle WJ, Barry RA, Clark CJ: Articulatory and voicing characteristics of adult dysarthric and verbal dyspraxia speakers: an instrumental study, Br J Commun Disord 20:249, 1985.

21. Hartman DE, Vishwanat B, Heun R: Cases of atypical neurovascular disease, stroke, and aphasia, J Med Speech-Lang Pathol 8:53, 2000.

22. Hirose H: Pathophysiology of motor speech disorders (dysarthria), Folia Phoniatr Logop 38:61, 1986.

23. Hirose H, Kiritani S, Sawashima J: Patterns of dysarthric movement in patients with amyotrophic lateral sclerosis and pseudobulbar palsy, Folia Phoniatr Logop 34:106, 1982a.

24. Hirose H, Kiritani S, Sawashima J: Velocity of articulatory movements in normal and dysarthric subjects, Folia Phoniatr Logop 34:210, 1982b.

25. Kammermeier MA: A Comparison of Phonatory Phenomena Among Groups of Neurologically Impaired Speakers [PhD dissertation]. Minneapolis/St Paul; University of Minnesota; 1969.

26. Kent R, Netsell R, Bauer LL: Cineradiographic assessment of articulatory mobility in the dysarthrias, J Speech Hear Disord 40:467, 1975.

27. Kent RD, Read C: The acoustic analysis of speech, San Diego, 1992, Singular Publishing Group.

28. Kent RD et al: Acoustic studies of dysarthric speech: methods, progress, and potential, J Commun Disord 32:141, 1999.

29. Linebaugh CW, Wolfe VE: Relationships between articulation rate, intelligibility, and naturalness in spastic and ataxic speakers. In McNeil M, Rosenbek J, Aronson A, editors: The dysarthrias: physiology acoustics perception management, Austin, Tex, 1984, Pro-Ed.

30. Mayo Clinic Department of Neurology: Mayo Clinic examinations in neurology, ed 7, St Louis, 1998, Mosby.

31. McClean MD, Beukelman DR, Yorkston KM: Speech-muscle visuomotor tracking in dysarthric and nonimpaired speakers, J Speech Hear Res 30:276, 1987.

32. Miller RG et al: Excessive muscular fatigue in patients with spastic paraparesis, Neurology 40:1271, 1990.

33. Murdoch BE, Thompson EC, Stokes PD: Phonatory and laryngeal dysfunction following upper motor neuron vascular lesions, J Med Speech-Lang Pathol 2:177, 1994.

34. Murry T: The production of stress in three types of dysarthric speech. In Berry W, editor: Clinical dysarthria, Boston, 1983, College-Hill Press.

35. Okuda B et al: Cerebral blood flow in pure dysarthria: role of frontal cortical hypoperfusion, Stroke 30:109, 1999.

36. Ozawa Y et al: Symptomatic differences in decreased alternating motion rates between individuals with spastic and with ataxic dysarthria: an acoustic analysis, Folia Phoniatr Logop 53:67, 2001.

37. Ozsancak C et al: Measurement of voice onset time in dysarthric patients: methodological considerations, Folia Phoniatr Logop 53:48, 2001.

38. Portnoy RA, Aronson AE: Diadochokinetic syllable rate and regularity in normal and in spastic ataxic dysarthric subjects, J Speech Hear Disord 47:324, 1982.

39. Pringle CE et al: Primary lateral sclerosis, Brain 115:495, 1992.

40. Rossor MN: The dementias. In Bradley WG et al, editors: Neurology in clinical practice: principles of diagnosis and management, vol 1, ed 3, Boston, 2000, Butterworth-Heinemann.

41. Roy N et al: A description of phonetic, acoustic, and physiological changes associated with improved intelligibility in a speaker with spastic dysarthria, Am J Speech-Lang Pathol 10:274, 2001.

42. Sheean G: The pathophysiology of spasticity, Eur J Neurol 9:3, 2002.

43. Sherrard KC, Marquardt TP, Cannito MP: Phonatory and temporal aspects of spasmodic dysphonia and pseudobulbar dysarthria: an acoustic analysis, J Med Speech-Lang Pathol 8:271, 2000.

44. Thompson EC, Murdoch BE, Stokes PD: Tongue function in subjects with upper motor neuron type dysarthria following cerebrovascular accident, J Med Speech-Lang Pathol 3:27, 1995.

45. Windebank AJ: Motor neuron diseases. In Noseworthy JH, editor: Neurological therapeutics: principles and practice, vol 2, New York, 2003, Martin Dunitz.

46. Wit J et al: Maximum performance tests in children with developmental dysarthria, J Speech Hear Res 36:452, 1994.

47. Yorkston KM et al: Management of motor speech disorders in children and adults, Austin, Tex, 1999, Pro-Ed.

48. Ziegler W, von Cramon D: Spastic dysarthria after acquired brain injury: an acoustic study, Br J Commun Disord 21:173, 1986.

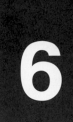

6

Ataxic Dysarthria

"Well, I slur the 'ph' and the 'th' and some of the harsh sounds. And they come real slurred, almost like I was drunk . . . and it's like I can't control my lips and tongue, and they'll occasionally get in my way. I know this could be carelessness, but it very seldom used to happen. Now it happens quite often!"

(62-year-old man with degenerative cerebellar disease and ataxic dysarthria)

CHAPTER OUTLINE

I. Anatomy and basic functions of the cerebellar control circuit
II. Localization of speech within the cerebellum
III. Clinical characteristics of cerebellar lesions and ataxia
IV. Etiologies
    A. Degenerative diseases
    B. Vascular disorders
    C. Neoplastic disorders
    D. Trauma
    E. Toxic or metabolic conditions
    F. Other causes
V. Speech pathology
    A. Distribution of etiologies, lesions, and severity in clinical practice
    B. Patient perceptions and complaints
    C. Clinical findings
    D. Acoustic and physiologic findings
VI. Cases
VII. Summary

Ataxic dysarthria is a perceptually distinctive motor speech disorder (MSD) associated with damage to the cerebellar control circuit. It may be manifest in any or all of the respiratory, phonatory, resonatory, and articulatory levels of speech, but *its characteristics are most evident in articulation and prosody.* The disorder reflects the effects of incoordination and reduced muscle tone, the products of which are slowness and inaccuracy in the force, range, timing, and direction of speech movements. Ataxia is an important contributor to the speech deficits of patients with cerebellar disease, hence the disorder's designation *ataxic* dysarthria. The identification of a dysarthria as ataxic can aid the diagnosis of neurologic disease and its localization to the cerebellum or cerebellar control circuit.

Ataxic dysarthria is encountered as the primary speech pathology in a large medical practice at a rate comparable to that for most other major single dysarthria types. Based on data for primary communication disorder diagnoses within the Mayo Clinic Speech Pathology practice, it accounts for 10.8% of all dysarthrias and 9.9% of all MSDs (see Figure 1-3).

The clinical features of ataxic dysarthria illustrate the important role of the cerebellum and its connections in speech motor control. Of all the individual dysarthria types, it most clearly reflects a breakdown in timing and coordination. When one listens to the speech of a person with ataxic dysarthria, the impression is not one of underlying weakness, resistance to movement, or restriction of movement, but rather one of an activity that is poorly timed and coordinated.

◼ ANATOMY AND BASIC FUNCTIONS OF THE CEREBELLAR CONTROL CIRCUIT

The cerebellar control circuit consists of the cerebellum and its connections. Its components are described in detail in Chapter 2. Here its structures, pathways, and functions that are most relevant to speech are briefly summarized.

The vermis forms the midportion of the anterior and posterior lobes of the cerebellum. To the sides of the vermis are the right and left cerebellar hemispheres, each of which is connected to the opposite thalamus and cerebral hemisphere. Each cerebellar hemisphere is involved in controlling movement on the ipsilateral side of the body. Thus the left cerebral and right cerebellar hemispheres cooperate in coordinating movement on the right side of the body, and the right cerebral and left cerebellar hemispheres cooperate in coordinating movement on the left side of the body. The lateral cerebellar hemispheres are particularly important to the coordination of skilled voluntary muscle activity and tone.

Purkinje cells, whose functions are inhibitory, are the sole output neurons of the cerebellar cortex. They synapse with deep cerebellar nuclei, and their output departs the cerebellum through the superior and inferior cerebellar peduncles.

The cerebellum influences and is informed about activities at several levels of the motor system. The primary and essential connections for its role in speech control include: (1) reciprocal connections with the cerebral cortex; (2) auditory and proprioceptive feedback from speech muscles, tendons, and joints; (3) reciprocal connections with brainstem components of the indirect activation pathway; and (4) cooperation with the basal ganglia control circuit through loops among the thalamus, cerebral cortex, and components of the indirect motor system.

From a functional standpoint, *the cerebellum helps time the components of movement, scale the size of muscle actions, and coordinate sequences of muscle contractions for skilled motor behavior.*[20,31,68] It presumably receives notice of intended movements from the cerebral cortex and monitors the adequacy of movement outcomes based on feedback from muscles, tendons, and joints. It can influence subsequent cortical motor output based on that feedback and on ongoing information from the cortex about upcoming movement goals. This permits it to make modifications that smooth the timing and coordination of movement.

■ LOCALIZATION OF SPEECH WITHIN THE CEREBELLUM

The localization of speech within the cerebellum is uncertain. Brown, Darley, and Aronson,[23] examining disparities in gait, limb, and speech disturbances in people with cerebellar disease, concluded that areas other than the anterior portion of the vermis are probably important or sufficient for motor speech control. They also concluded that ataxic dysarthria usually results from bilateral or generalized cerebellar disease, even though it may sometimes be due to a more focal lesion.

Where are such focal lesions? Chiu, Chen, and Tseng,[25] examining 15 patients with cerebellar disease and dysarthria, concluded that midline structures and the vermis and fastigial nucleus were the primary locus for coordination of speech. Ackermann et al.[8] concluded that ataxic dysarthria is especially associated with damage to paramedian regions of the superior cerebellar hemispheres, that lesions in the dentate nucleus are linked to phonatory disturbances, and that the most severe articulatory deficits are associated with bilateral lesions. Several studies of people with cerebellar tumors or small cerebellar infarcts implicate the paravermal areas and lateral cerebellar hemispheres.[8,12,13,69] Kent et al.,[64] noting that lesions generally include vermal and paravermal areas, as well as the lateral cerebellar hemispheres, concluded, "Possibly, different parts of the cerebellum are involved in motor control of different motor systems within speech production, or they are involved with different functions of motor control." In general, therefore, *ataxic dysarthria is most commonly associated with bilateral or generalized cerebellar disease. When lesions in the cerebellum are focal, the lateral hemispheres and posteromedial or paravermal regions are implicated.*

Lesions causing ataxic speech may not be confined to the cerebellum. Clinical evidence indicates that it also can result from lesions to the superior cerebellar peduncle or anywhere along the frontopontocerebellar pathways.[64,98]

Might speech functions be lateralized within the cerebellum, similar to the lateralization of speech and language within the cerebral hemispheres? Holmes[51] observed that disease affecting only one lateral cerebellar hemisphere could affect speech, but that speech usually improves rapidly when lesions are unilateral. Lechtenberg and Gilman[69] observed that dysarthria in 31 patients with nondegenerative cerebellar dysarthria was much more common when the disease was exclusively or predominantly in the left cerebellar hemisphere than when it was exclusively or predominantly in the right cerebellar hemisphere or vermis. Because prosodic disturbances are prominent in ataxic dysarthria, they felt that the "dominance" of the left cerebellar hemisphere is logically related to its strong ties to the right cerebral hemisphere and its apparently important role in prosodic functions. In contrast, however, Ackermann et al.[8] reported that three of their four patients with dysarthria resulting from unilateral cerebellar strokes had right-sided lesions. Also, Gironell, Arboix, and Marti-Vilalta[44] reported a case with dysarthria from a right-sided paravermal stroke and argued that the superior right paravermal zone might be the "cerebellar speech centre."*

---

*Kent and Rosenbek[60] have discussed the relationship of cerebellar functions to speech prosody, and the relationship of prosodic disturbances in cerebellar disease to the aprosody and dysprosody that may occur with right and left cerebral hemisphere lesions, respectively. They said, "We should not conclude that the cerebellum is normally a generator of prosody. It may instead be part of a larger neuronal circuit that regulates the prosodic base of speech."

The notion of lateralized cerebellar dominance, or different speech roles for the right versus left cerebellar hemispheres, is certainly relevant to our understanding of speech motor control. That there may be an asymmetric distribution of cerebellar lesions that lead to ataxic dysarthria also raises the possibility of different "types" of ataxic dysarthria that are dependent upon the lateralization of cerebellar lesions. It should be noted, however, that ataxic dysarthria is not just a prosodic disturbance (articulation, at the least, is also affected), and that several other dysarthria types (and aprosodia and apraxia of speech) also affect prosody, although in a manner distinguishable from that resulting from cerebellar lesions. In addition, Kent et al.[64] note that a full understanding of cerebellar localization for speech must account for remote effects of lesions as well as local effects. For example, one consequence of cerebellar disease seems to be a diminished facilitatory influence of the cerebellum on the motor cortex of the cerebral hemispheres.[71] Finally, as Gilman, Bloedel, and Lechtenberg[42] state, "It is unlikely that only one cerebellar locus could be responsible for all of the facets of speech disorder occurring with cerebellar disease." Thus at this point, caution should be exercised in drawing conclusions about the lateralization of speech functions within the cerebellum.

■ CLINICAL CHARACTERISTICS OF CEREBELLAR LESIONS AND ATAXIA

Difficulties with standing and walking are the most common signs of cerebellar disease, and gait is often referred to as *ataxic.* Stance and gait are usually broad based, and truncal instability may lead to falls. Steps may be irregularly placed, and the legs lifted too high and slapped to the ground. There may be no difference in steadiness when standing with the feet together with the eyes open versus closed *(Romberg test).*

Titubation is a rhythmic tremor of the body or head that can occur with cerebellar disease. It is usually manifest as rocking of the trunk or head forward or back, side to side, or in a rotary motion, several times per second.

The most common of the abnormal eye movements that can occur in cerebellar disease is *nystagmus,* which is characterized by rapid oscillation or back and forth jerky movements of the eyes at rest or with lateral or upward gaze. Patients may also exhibit *ocular dysmetria,* in which small, rapid eye movements develop as they attempt to fix on a visual target and attempt to correct for inaccurate fixation.

Hypotonia, a decrease in resistance to passive movement, can occur in cerebellar disease. It can be associated with excessive *pendulousness,* in which

an extremity, allowed to swing freely in a pendular manner, has a greater than average number of oscillations before coming to rest; this is a function of decreased muscle tone or decreased resistance to movement. A related phenomenon, known as *impaired check and excessive rebound,* can also occur. For example, when asked to maintain the arm in an outstretched position with the eyes shut, a light tap on the wrist results in a large displacement of the limb followed by overshoot beyond the original position when it returns. The wide excursion reflects impaired check, whereas overshoot reflects excessive rebound.

Dysmetria, a common sign of cerebellar disease, is a disturbance in the trajectory of a body part during movement or an inability to control range of movement. It is often characterized by overshooting or undershooting of targets, as well as by abnormalities in speed, giving movements an irregular appearance. It is frequently detected when patients are asked to repetitively touch the tip of their index finger to their nose and then to fully extend the arm to touch the examiner's finger (nose-finger-nose test).[78]

Dysdiadokokinesis is a manifestation of *decomposition of movement (dyssynergia),* which refers to errors in the sequence and speed of component parts of a movement, with a resultant lack of coordination. It can be elicited by testing alternating repetitive movements. A common task is the *knee-pat test* in which the patient pats the knee alternately with the palm and dorsum of the hand, gradually increasing to a maximum rate; side-to-side tongue wiggling and patting the floor with the ball of the foot are examples of other alternate motion rate (AMR) tasks used to elicit dysdiadokokinesis. Poor performance on such tasks is characterized by abnormalities in rate, rhythm, amplitude, and precision. Speech AMRs are analogous to these tests of coordination and speed.

Ataxia is the product of dysmetria, dysdiadokokinesis, and decomposition of movement. Ataxic movements are halting, imprecise, jerky, poorly coordinated, and lacking in speed and fluidity or smoothness. Ataxia is generally associated with disease of the cerebellar hemispheres.*

Cerebellar disease is sometimes associated with *intention* or *kinetic tremor* that is apparent during movement or sustained postures and is usually most obvious as a target is approximated *(terminal tremor).* This cerebellar tremor usually occurs with disorders of the lateral cerebellar hemispheres.

Some signs that occur in conjunction with cerebellar disease do not reflect cerebellar dysfunction

*The relevance of dysarthria to the diagnosis and quantification of ataxia and cerebellar syndromes is reflected in its inclusion as one of four major symptom categories in the International Cooperative Ataxia Rating Scale.[97]

per se. Mild facial weakness, often limited to the lower face, occurs frequently with focal cerebellar lesions, more often with cerebellar hemisphere than midline lesions.[42] Although pressure effects on cranial nerve VII are a possible explanation, there may be other, as yet undetermined, explanations. Abnormalities of cranial nerves V, VI, and VIII may also be encountered.

Finally, *cognitive disturbances may be present*. Cognitive deficits encountered in people with cerebellar disease traditionally have been discounted as an artifact of accompanying noncerebellar deficits. However, recent clinical observations and functional neuroimaging studies suggest that the cerebellum contributes to a number of cognitive functions, including language processing, that are not necessarily related to motor activities.[38,77,81] In the author's experience, the content, organization, and pragmatics of verbal statements made by some people with ataxic dysarthria and what appear to be isolated cerebellar deficits are not quite normal. These abnormalities seem more akin to nonaphasic cognitive-communication deficits than to aphasic language impairments.

▪ ETIOLOGIES

Any process that damages the cerebellum or cerebellar control circuit can cause ataxic dysarthria. These processes include degenerative, demyelinating, vascular, neoplastic, inflammatory, traumatic, and toxic or metabolic diseases. These etiologic categories are associated with ataxic dysarthria with varying frequency. The exact distribution of causes of ataxic dysarthria is unknown, but degenerative, demyelinating, and vascular diseases seem to be the most frequent known causes (see Figure 6-1 and Box 6-1).

The presence of ataxic dysarthria, by itself, is not diagnostic of any specific neurologic disease. However, several diseases are associated with ataxic dysarthria more frequently than with other dysarthria types. In addition, some diseases specifically affect the cerebellum and are uniquely associated with ataxic dysarthria. Some common neurologic conditions that are associated with ataxic dysarthria more frequently than with other dysarthria types are discussed as follows. Other diseases that can produce it but are more frequently associated with other dysarthria types (especially mixed dysarthrias) are discussed in the chapters that address those specific dysarthrias.

Degenerative Diseases

Degenerative diseases that affect the cerebellum are not uncommon. Their mechanisms are generally poorly understood, but an increasing number seem to have a hereditary basis.

The most common and well-characterized *hereditary ataxias* may be autosomal dominant or autosomal recessive; X-linked forms have been described

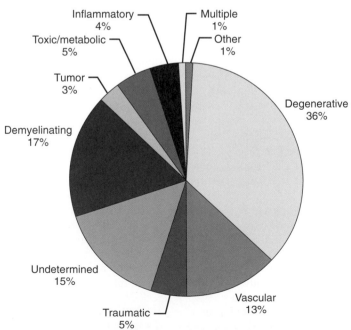

FIGURE 6-1 Distribution of etiologies for 166 quasirandomly selected cases with a primary speech pathology diagnosis of ataxic dysarthria at the Mayo Clinic from 1969-90 and 1999-2001 (see Box 6-1 for details).

Etiologies for 166 quasirandomly selected cases with a primary speech pathology diagnosis of ataxic dysarthria at the Mayo Clinic from 1969-1990 and 1999-2001. Percentage of cases for each etiology is given in parentheses. Specific etiologies under each heading are ordered from most to least frequent.

Degenerative (35%)

Cerebellar degeneration, unspecified etiology (14%)
OPCA (5%)
Shy-Drager syndrome (2%)
Multiple systems atrophy (2%)
Cerebellar atrophy, hereditary (1%)
Other (10%)
   Cerebellar and brainstem degeneration; PSP; Friedreich's ataxia; spinocerebellar degeneration; degenerative CNS disease; corticocerebellar degeneration; hereditary cerebral calcinosis

Demyelinating (17%)

Multiple sclerosis (16%)
Unspecified demyelinating disease (1%)

Undetermined (15%)

Undetermined cerebellar ataxia (4%)
Undetermined cerebellar atrophy (2%)
Other (9%)
   Dysarthria only; paroxysmal periodic ataxia; undetermined cerebellar and brainstem disease; undetermined cerebellar lesion; Wilson's disease vs. liver disease; encephalitis vs. undetermined brainstem disease; tumor vs. AVM; undetermined neurologic problem

Vascular (13%)

Nonhemorrhagic stroke (single or multiple) (9%)
Hemorrhagic stroke (2%)
Other (2%)
   Ruptured aneurysm, lupus, intracranial arteritis, anoxia

Toxic or Metabolic (5%)

Prescribed medication (anticonvulsants, lithium) (3%)
Other (2%)
   Alcohol or drug abuse; anoxic encephalopathy associated with intentional drug overdose

Traumatic (5%)

Closed head injury (3%)
Penetrating head injury (1%)
Postoperative (1%)

Inflammatory (4%)

Encephalitis (2%)
Meningitis (1%)
Multifocal leukoencephalopathy (1%)

Tumor (3%)

Paraneoplastic syndrome, brainstem tumor, cerebellopontine angle tumor

Multiple (1%)

Stroke + ? CNS degenerative disease

Other (1%)

Depression or personality disorder, hypothyroidism

AVM, Arteriovenous malformation; *CNS,* central nervous system; *OPCA,* olivopontocerebellar atrophy; *PSP,* progressive supranuclear palsy.

but are uncommon and not well characterized. Hereditary ataxias can be fatal or nonfatal and can begin in childhood or adulthood. They usually evolve over several decades. Some are largely confined to the cerebellum. When they also affect spinal cord tracts they are called *spinocerebellar,* and when they also affect the inferior olive and pontine nuclei they are called *olivopontocerebellar.*

Various *hereditary spinocerebellar ataxias (SCAs)* have overlapping phenotypes, but molecular genetics has permitted increasingly definitive molecular classification. Many recessively inherited ataxias produce initial symptoms in childhood. *Friedreich's ataxia* is the most common, with a prevalence of 1 in 50,000 persons. It usually begins before age 20 and it evolves to incapacitation and death over a course of approximately 20 years. Its cardinal features include limb and gait ataxia, dysarthria, absent muscle stretch reflexes in the

lower limbs, sensory loss, and signs of corticospinal tract involvement.[36] LMN weakness, as well as dystonia, chorea, and other movement disorders, may also occur. Several studies have examined the dysarthria associated with the disorder,[39,43,54,84] each describing speech characteristics consistent with ataxic dysarthria. Some imply that the dysarthria is mixed in character, with ataxic and spastic components.[54,84] Because the disease can affect portions of the motor system beyond the cerebellum, it is not surprising that its associated dysarthria is not always only ataxic in character.

*Ataxia telangiectasia** is another progressive autosomal recessive disorder in which dysarthria is a frequent neurologic manifestation; truncal

---

*Telangiectasia involves dilatation of capillary vessels and minute arteries.

or appendicular ataxia, choreoathetosis, dystonia, sensory loss, and distal muscle atrophy are among additional neurologic signs. The dysarthria has not been well described, but ataxic and mixed dysarthrias (ataxic, hyperkinetic, or flaccid) are logical possibilities. Dysarthria has also been reported in autosomal recessive *ataxia with isolated vitamin E deficiency,* a treatable disorder that emerges in childhood or adolescence and can resemble the Friedreich's ataxia phenotype.[36]

Dominantly inherited cerebellar ataxias have an estimated incidence in the general population of 5 in 100,000.[36] They tend to begin between 20 and 40 years of age. The terminology used to describe their genotype uses SCA types, such as SCA-1 and SCA-2. A recent review of hereditary ataxias[36] indicates that dysarthria is a characteristic of many SCA types that have been described. Their clinical features suggest that ataxic dysarthria should be a predominant dysarthria type, but, because multiple portions of the motor system can be involved in many SCAs, nearly any type seems logically possible. Finally, *episodic (or paroxysmal) ataxias* are uncommon, usually autosomal dominant conditions in which intermittent, brief attacks (seconds to minutes) of ataxia and dysarthria (presumably ataxic) occur, sometimes with other neurologic signs (e.g., myokymia, diplopia, nystagmus, vertigo). Their recognition is important, because they may be effectively treated pharmacologically, often with acetazolamide.[36]

Olivopontocerebellar atrophy (OPCA) is a degenerative disease that can be hereditary or sporadic. It is a heterogeneous condition associated with neurologic diseases that are broadly grouped under the heading of *multiple systems atrophy (MSA).**[90] OPCA is associated with degeneration of the pontine, arcuate, and olivary nuclei, the middle cerebellar peduncles, and the cerebellum. It can also be associated with degenerative changes in the basal ganglia, cerebral cortex, spinal cord, and even peripheral nerves. The clinical features are variable, but cerebellar findings are the most common. Parkinsonism, movement disorders, pyramidal and ophthalmologic signs, bulbar and pseudobulbar palsy, and dementia can also occur.[47]

Multiple sclerosis (MS), a demyelinating disease, may cause cerebellar lesions and ataxic dysarthria. Discussion of MS is deferred to Chapter 10, because MS lesions often are not confined to the cerebellum. However, a condition associated with MS, known as *paroxysmal ataxic dysarthria (PAD),* deserves mention here, because its occurrence may be suggestive of MS[35] or episodic ataxia, as described previously. In PAD, brief episodes of ataxic dysarthria occur in an individual whose speech may be otherwise normal. Netsell and Kent[85] reviewed 10 cases in the literature and 3 cases of their own with PAD and an established or provisional diagnosis of MS. The group's distinctive characteristics included: (1) a few to several hundred episodes per day, each lasting 5 to 30 seconds; (2) speech characteristics consistent with those of ataxic dysarthria; (3) the possibility of remission and reappearance at a later time, with or without new symptoms; (4) no evidence of associated seizures; (5) overbreathing sometimes evoked the paroxysms; (6) the paroxysms remitted in each case with administration of carbamazepine (Tegretol).

Vascular Disorders

Vascular lesions can affect cerebellar function. Lesions are most commonly caused by aneurysms, arteriovenous malformations (AVMs), cerebellar hemorrhage, or stroke within the vertebrobasilar system. The lateral regions of the vertebrobasilar system, including the posterior inferior cerebellar artery (PICA) at the level of the medulla, the anterior inferior cerebellar artery (AICA) at the level of the pons, and the superior cerebellar artery at the level of the midbrain, are most often implicated in cerebellar and superior cerebellar peduncle lesions that lead to ataxic dysarthria.[21,34,44] Ataxic dysarthria may be more common with superior cerebellar artery than with PICA or AICA distribution lesions.[18]

Von-Hippel Lindau disease is an inherited autosomal dominant condition characterized by hemangioblastomas* of the cerebellum and retina, as well as visceral cysts and tumors. The cerebellar tumors are usually removed surgically, but recurrence is possible. The tumors can also occur in the medulla and spinal cord and infrequently in the cerebral hemispheres. Diagnosis is usually made after the second decade.[93]

Neoplastic Disorders

Tumors within the cerebellum or that exert mass effects on it can lead to cerebellar signs, including ataxic dysarthria. Cerebellopontine angle tumors, which often arise from the meninges (meningiomas) or supporting cells of cranial nerves, can lead to

---

*A hemangioma is a benign, slow-growing tumor made up of newly formed blood vessels. A hemangioblastoma is a capillary hemangioma of the brain that consists of proliferated blood vessels or angioblasts (blood cells and vessels are derived from angioblasts).

early cerebellar signs because of pressure on the middle cerebellar peduncle, dentate nucleus, and posterior cerebellar lobes. There also may be involvement of multiple cranial nerves, including V, VI, VII, VIII, and X, plus other signs of brainstem dysfunction.[21] Such tumors can lead to ataxic dysarthria, as well as to flaccid and spastic dysarthria.

Some posterior fossa tumors, particularly medulloblastomas and astrocytomas, are more common in children and young adults. They often arise in the midline and can displace portions of the cerebellum and sometimes infiltrate the cerebellar hemispheres.[17] Surgical intervention and subsequent radiation therapy can also impair cerebellar functions.

Sixteen percent of metastatic brain tumors develop in the cerebellum.[52] Signs and symptoms of cerebellar disease can be the first evidence that the patient has a tumor, the primary tumor remaining occult.

Neoplasm outside the central nervous system (CNS) is frequently suspected in patients with signs of nonfamilial cerebellar degeneration of late onset. This suspicion is fueled by the existence of *paraneoplastic disorders,* rare and intriguing autoimmune conditions associated with cancer. *Paraneoplastic cerebellar degeneration* is thought to be one of the most common CNS paraneoplastic syndromes. Affected people usually have carcinoma outside the CNS (usually ovarian or lung), but the neurologic disorder does not reflect actual metastatic invasion by tumor and often precedes actual clinical evidence of the primary tumor by weeks to years. The syndrome tends to emerge and progress over weeks to months. Purkinje cells are predominantly affected, and antibodies to Purkinje cells are often present. Along with nystagmus and ataxia of gait and limbs, dysarthria is a common and sometimes first clinical manifestation of paraneoplastic cerebellar disease.[14,26] Its type has been confirmed as ataxic or mixed ataxic-spastic.[87]

Trauma

Traumatic brain injury (TBI) is frequently associated with limb ataxia and dysarthria.[41,101,103] Anoxia secondary to TBI is often invoked as the cause of cerebellar deficits, but damage to the superior cerebellar peduncles, which are vulnerable to the rotational injuries associated with TBI, has also been associated with cerebellar signs, including dysarthria.[24]

"Punch-drunk" encephalopathy or *dementia pugilistica* is often encountered in boxers who have sustained repeated cerebral injuries. The cerebellum is among the areas of the CNS that undergo pathologic changes,[11] and affected individuals can be ataxic and have ataxic dysarthria.

Toxic or Metabolic Conditions

Acute and chronic alcohol abuse can produce cerebellar signs and symptoms, the most common of which are abnormal stance and gait. Cerebellar degeneration associated with alcoholism is well documented.[16] Although ataxic speech frequently occurs with acute alcohol intoxication, permanent dysarthria in chronic alcoholism is not common.[42]

Neurotoxic levels of several drugs can produce cerebellar signs and symptoms. These drugs include anticonvulsants, such as phenytoin (Dilantin), carbamazepine (Tegretol), valproic acid (Depakote), and primidone (Mysoline). Lithium, used to treat manic depressive illness, can produce sometimes-irreversible neurotoxic effects that include postural or intention tremor, ataxia, hyperkinesia, and dysarthria[56,67]; in the author's experience the dysarthria is often ataxic but sometimes spastic or hyperkinetic. Ataxic dysarthria has been reported as the initial sign of acute cerebellar toxicity in response to cytosine arabinoside (ara-C) for treatment of acute leukemia.[33,66] Valium, an antianxiety drug, has also been associated with ataxic dysarthria.[82] Finally, signs of cerebellar dysfunction can develop with severe malnutrition and vitamin deficiencies (e.g., thiamine, vitamin E).[100]

Other Causes

Hypothyroidism is an endocrine disturbance caused by insufficient secretion of thyroxin by the thyroid glands. When severe *(myxedema),* it can lead to ataxic dysarthria.[55] It can be accompanied by a hoarse, gravelly, and excessively low-pitched dysphonia caused by mass loading of the vocal folds with myxomatous material.[15]

Normal pressure hydrocephalus (NPH) is a condition in which the ventricles may be enlarged while normal cerebrospinal fluid (CSF) pressure is maintained. It has been associated with trauma, subarachnoid hemorrhage, and meningitis, but etiology is often unclear. It is recognized by a triad of symptoms that include progressive gait disorder, impaired mental function, and urinary incontinence.[92] Dysarthria can occur in NPH and it can be ataxic in character.

Cerebellar signs and symptoms, including dysarthria, can occur as uncommon manifestations of heat stroke.[76] A number of viral, bacterial, and other infectious processes can lead to CNS disease with prominent cerebellar dysfunction in children and adults (e.g., rubella, Creutzfeldt-Jacob disease, Lyme disease, CNS tuberculosis).[100] Although uncommon, *Guillain-Barré syndrome*—usually associated with flaccid dysarthria—can sometimes be characterized by ataxia and, subsequently, ataxic dysarthria. This variant of the disease is sometimes called *Fisher syndrome*.[91]

Finally, lack of proprioceptive input can lead to *sensory ataxia*, a problem that emerges in certain sensory neuropathies. Dysarthria has been reported in people with severe peripheral axonal loss that disproportionately affects sensory nerves.[37] The author has seen a small number of patients with known sensory neuropathy whose speech characteristics were consistent with those of ataxic dysarthria.

■ SPEECH PATHOLOGY

Distribution of Etiologies, Lesions, and Severity in Clinical Practice

Box 6-1 and Figure 6-1 summarize the etiologies for 166 quasirandomly selected cases seen at the Mayo Clinic with a speech pathology diagnosis of ataxic dysarthria. The cautions expressed in Chapter 4 about generalizing these data to the general population or all speech pathology practices also apply here.

The data establish that ataxic dysarthria can result from a number of medical conditions. Ninety percent of the cases are accounted for by degenerative, demyelinating, vascular, toxic or metabolic, traumatic, and undetermined etiologies. Degenerative, demyelinating, and vascular diseases account for more than 65% of the cases.

Degenerative diseases were the most frequent cause (35%), with approximately 40% of them accounted for by relatively isolated cerebellar degenerative disease of undetermined etiology. The remainder of the degenerative etiologies included more specific entities such as OPCA, Shy-Drager syndrome, multiple systems atrophy, progressive supranuclear palsy (PSP), and cerebellar and brainstem degeneration. Most of these latter conditions are typically associated with degeneration that affects more than the cerebellum; consequently, they are often associated with other or additional dysarthria types. They are described more completely in Chapter 10. The remaining etiologies (Friedreich's ataxia and spinocerebellar degeneration) have already been defined.

MS accounted for nearly all of the demyelinating etiologies. Its 16% representation within the sample suggests that ataxic dysarthria is not uncommon in MS and may occur as the only dysarthria type in MS more frequently than other single dysarthria types (e.g., MS accounted for 4% of the cases of spastic dysarthria that were reviewed in Chapter 5). However, because lesions may be disseminated in many locations of the nervous system in MS, mixed dysarthrias are common. MS is discussed in more detail in Chapter 10.

A substantial number of patients did not receive a definitive etiologic diagnosis. Within this group were patients with several possible diagnoses (e.g., tumor vs. AVM) plus a number whose symptoms and course were too subtle or short-lived to be understood. It is likely that some of these patients had degenerative cerebellar diseases and probable that a clearer diagnostic picture emerged as the disease progressed.

Nonhemorrhagic stroke accounted for most of the vascular causes. A majority of those with stroke had a single event, with the remainder having multiple strokes. Nearly half of the vascular cases had an identifiable lesion in the cerebellum. Most of the remaining cases had lesions in the brainstem or midbrain. It is likely that the ataxic dysarthria in these latter cases resulted from damage to major cerebellar pathways. For example, lesions of the superior cerebellar peduncles can lead to the same abnormalities that occur with cerebellar hemispheric lesions.[98] A few cases had supratentorial lesions (e.g., posterior right frontal lobe, multiple lesions in the periventricular white matter); whether the lesions in these cases were responsible for the ataxic dysarthria is a matter of conjecture, but they do support the notion that ataxic dysarthria can result from lesions anywhere along the corticocerebellar pathways (see Chapter 9 for further discussion of this possibility).

Toxic or metabolic causes for ataxic dysarthria are noteworthy, because they were not evident in the cases of flaccid or spastic dysarthria that were reviewed in Chapters 4 and 5. Most often, the ataxic dysarthria was secondary to anticonvulsant medications prescribed for epilepsy. Medication effects should always be suspected as a possible cause of ataxic dysarthria in individuals with seizure disorders who are on anticonvulsant medications.

The association of ataxic dysarthria with TBI in this sample is in general agreement with the observations of Yorkston et al.[103] TBI accounted for a somewhat smaller proportion of cases of ataxic dysarthria reviewed here than cases of spastic dysarthria reviewed in Chapter 5. This does not necessarily mean that isolated spastic dysarthria occurs more frequently than isolated ataxic dysarthria in the TBI population, because these cases were selected on the basis of dysarthria diagnosis and not on the basis of etiology.

The data also establish that ataxic dysarthria can occur in association with inflammatory disease, such as encephalitis and meningitis, demonstrating that focal deficits can occur in conditions that are often diffuse in nature. Tumors associated with ataxic dysarthria were relatively uncommon but were con-

sistently located in the cerebellum or adjacent to it (cerebellopontine angle) or affected cerebellar function indirectly (paraneoplastic syndrome).

Of those patients who had abnormalities detected by neuroimaging, approximately half had lesions or atrophy that were confined to or included the cerebellum; others had lesions more generally localized to the brainstem or posterior fossa. A significant minority had evidence of generalized, diffuse, or multifocal abnormalities. A few had evidence of cerebral hemisphere lesions without evidence of cerebellar or posterior fossa abnormalities. This latter finding obviously does not rule out cerebellar or brainstem lesions in such patients, but as already discussed, it raises the possibility that ataxic speech characteristics may occur in individuals with supratentorial lesions.

Because many causes of ataxic dysarthria in the sample defied detection by neuroimaging (e.g., degenerative, toxic, undetermined etiologies), clinical findings often had to be relied on for localization. In this regard, the great majority of the sample had nonspeech clinical signs of cerebellar involvement. In general, the clinical neurologic findings and neuroimaging data indicate that most patients with ataxic dysarthria have lesions or clinical signs that are localizable to the cerebellum or to the cerebellar pathways in the brainstem. This is reassuring, because the sample was selected on the basis of speech diagnosis and not localization of disease. Therefore the data generally confirm the localizing value of a diagnosis of ataxic dysarthria.

This retrospective review did not permit a precise description of dysarthria severity. However, in those patients for whom a judgment of intelligibility was stated (69% of the sample), *48% had reduced intelligibility*. The degree to which this figure accurately estimates the frequency of intelligibility impairments in the population with ataxic dysarthria is unclear. It is likely that many patients for whom an observation of intelligibility was not made had normal intelligibility; however, the sample probably contains a larger number of mildly impaired patients than is encountered in a typical rehabilitation setting.

Finally, *cognitive deficits were noted in 15% of the patients* in the sample. The reasons for these deficits are uncertain, but they could reflect incidental problems stemming from abnormalities in noncerebellar structures or direct or indirect effects of the cerebellar abnormalities themselves.

Patient Perceptions and Complaints

People with ataxic dysarthria sometimes describe their speech in ways that provide clues to their speech diagnosis and its localization. Similar to those with other dysarthria types, they often complain that their speech is *slurred*. Unlike most patients with other dysarthria types, however, they also often refer to the *"drunken"* quality of their speech, either as they perceive it ("I sound like I'm drunk") or as others have commented upon it ("People ask me if I've been drinking"). They may also report dramatic deterioration in their speech with limited alcohol intake. They occasionally report an inability to coordinate their breathing with speaking and sometimes note that they bite their cheek or tongue while talking or eating. When the dysarthria is mild, they may comment that speech proceeds normally until they suddenly *stumble over words*. They may complain about the negative effects of fatigue on their speech, but perhaps less so than those with flaccid or spastic dysarthria. They do not often complain of exerting increased physical effort in speaking. They often report that slowing speech rate improves intelligibility.

Drooling is an uncommon complaint. Swallowing complaints are much less frequent than encountered with flaccid or spastic dysarthria, and they usually relate to the oral phase of swallowing. This is consistent with observations that the cerebellum does not play an important role in swallowing.[75]

Clinical Findings

Ataxic dysarthria usually occurs with other signs of cerebellar disease, but sometimes it is the initial or only sign of cerebellar dysfunction.* In such cases, recognition of the dysarthria as ataxic can be valuable to neurologic localization, especially because there may be no other oromotor evidence of neurologic disease.

Nonspeech Oral Mechanism

The oral mechanism examination is often normal. That is, the size, strength, and symmetry of the jaw, face, tongue, and palate may be normal at rest, during emotional expression, and during sustained postures. The gag reflex is usually normal, and pathologic oral reflexes are absent. Drooling is uncommon, and the reflexive swallow is usually normal on casual observation.

Nonspeech AMRs of the jaw, lips, and tongue may be irregular. This is usually most apparent on lateral wiggling of the tongue or retraction and pursing of the lips; judgments that nonspeech AMRs are irregular should be interpreted cautiously, and only after observing many normal individuals, because normal performance is frequently somewhat irregular on these tasks. It is more relevant and

---

*For example, Brown, Darley, and Aronson[23] noted that ataxic dysarthria was the initial symptom in 7 of their 30 patients with cerebellar disease.

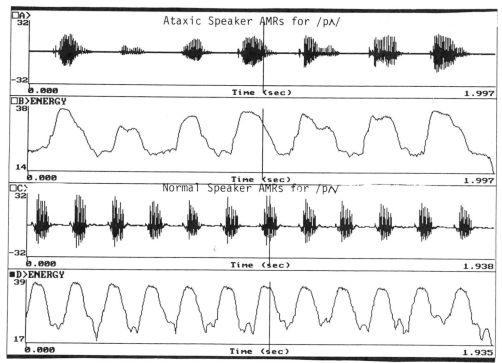

FIGURE 6-2 Raw waveform and energy tracings of speech alternate motion rates (AMRs) for /pʌ/ by a normal speaker *(bottom two panels)* and a speaker with ataxic dysarthria. The normal speaker's AMRs are normal in rate (≈6.5 Hz) and are relatively regular in duration and amplitude. In contrast, the ataxic speaker's are slow (≈3.5 Hz) and irregular in amplitude, syllable duration, and intersyllable interval; these latter attributes represent the acoustic correlates of perceived irregular AMRs.

valuable to observe the direction and smoothness of jaw and lip movements during connected speech and speech AMRs for evidence of dysmetria. Irregular movements during speech are often observable, are not frequently observed in normal speakers, and are more relevant to the speech diagnosis than non-speech AMRs.

Speech

Conversational speech, reading, and speech AMRs are the most useful tasks for observing the salient and distinguishing characteristics of ataxic dysarthria. Repetition of sentences containing multi-syllabic words (e.g., "My physician wrote out a prescription"; "The municipal judge sentenced the criminal") may promote distinctive, irregular articulatory breakdowns and prosodic abnormalities. Speech AMRs can be particularly revealing (see Figure 6-2). *Irregular speech AMRs are a distinguishing characteristic of ataxic dysarthria.*

Similar to spastic dysarthria, the deviant speech characteristics of ataxic dysarthria are not easily described by listing each cranial nerve and the speech characteristics associated with its abnormal function. Ataxic dysarthria is associated with impaired coordination of movement patterns rather

than with deficits in individual muscles, and it is the breakdown in coordination among simultaneous and sequenced movements that gives it its distinctive character. *It is predominantly an articulatory and prosodic disorder.*

Table 6-1 summarizes the neuromuscular deficits presumed by Darley, Aronson, and Brown (DAB)[27-29] to underlie ataxic dysarthria. In general, they include inaccurate movements, slow movements, and hypotonia of affected muscles. As a result, individual and repetitive movements contain errors in timing, force, range, and direction, and they tend to be slow and often irregular. The relationships among these characteristics and the specific deviant characteristics associated with ataxic dysarthria are discussed as follows. Experimental support for the presumed underlying neuromuscular deficits, especially those that reflect the global impression of incoordination, are reviewed in the section on acoustic and physiologic findings.

Clusters of Deviant Dimensions and Prominent Deviant Speech Characteristics

DAB[28] found three distinct clusters of deviant speech dimensions in their group of 30 patients with cerebellar disorders. These clusters are useful to under-

table 6-1	Neuromuscular deficits associated with ataxic dysarthria						
Direction	**Rhythm**	**Rate**		**Range**		**Force**	**Tone**
Individual Movements	**Repetitive Movements**	**Individual Movements**	**Repetitive Movements**	**Individual Movements**	**Repetitive Movements**	**Individual Movements**	**Muscle Tone**
Inaccurate	Irregular	Slow	Slow	Excessive to normal	Excessive to normal	Normal to excessive	Reduced

Modified from Darley FL, Aronson AE, Brown JR: Differential diagnostic patterns of dysarthria, *J Speech Hear Res* 12:246, 1969.

table 6-2	Clusters of abnormal speech characteristics in ataxic dysarthria
Cluster	**Speech Characteristics**
Articulatory Inaccuracy	Imprecise consonants
	Irregular articulatory breakdowns
	Distorted vowels
Prosodic Excess	Excess & equal stress
	Prolonged phonemes
	Prolonged intervals
	Slow rate
Phonatory-Prosodic Insufficiency	Harshness
	Monopitch
	Monoloudness

Modified from Darley FL, Aronson AE, Brown JR: Differential diagnostic patterns of dysarthria, *J Speech Hear Res* 12:246, 1969b.

standing the neuromuscular deficits that underlie ataxic dysarthria, the components of the speech system that are most prominently involved, and the features that distinguish ataxic dysarthria from other dysarthria types. These clusters are summarized in Table 6-2.

The first cluster is *articulatory inaccuracy,* represented by *imprecise consonants, irregular articulatory breakdowns,* and *vowel distortions.* These features reflect inaccuracy in the direction of articulatory movements and dysrhythmia of repetitive movements. They implicate movements of the jaw, face, and tongue primarily but do not exclude poorly controlled movements at the velopharyngeal or laryngeal valves.

The second cluster is *prosodic excess,* composed of *excess and equal stress, prolonged phonemes, prolonged intervals,* and *slow rate.* This cluster seems related to the slowness of individual and repetitive movements that are prominent in ataxia in general. DAB[29] noted that the slowing of repetitive movements seems to include "slowness, even metering of patterns, and excessive vocal emphasis on usually unemphasized words and syllables . . ." This cluster is probably related to descriptions of speech in individuals with cerebellar disease as *scanning* in character, a term defined in slightly different

ways by various authors.[94,99] It refers to slowness, a word-by-word cadence, syllable segregation, and relatively equal and obvious emphasis on each syllable or word whether normally stressed or unstressed (see Figure 6-3).

The third cluster is *phonatory-prosodic insufficiency,* composed of *harshness,* monopitch,* and *monoloudness.* DAB attributed this cluster to insufficient excursion of muscles (presumably laryngeal and, possibly, respiratory) as a result of hypotonia.

Table 6-3 summarizes the most deviant speech dimensions found by DAB.[27] The component of the speech system most prominently associated with each characteristic is also included. The rankings in the table represent the order of prominence (severity) of the speech characteristics and not necessarily the features that best distinguish ataxic dysarthria from other dysarthria types.[†]

A few additional comments are warranted about some of the clusters and prominent speech characteristics, because they are relevant to clinical diagnosis. These are based on some data embedded within those presented by DAB[27,28] or reflect clinical impressions from assessments of many patients with cerebellar disease.

1. The cluster of prosodic excess, particularly features of excess and equal stress and prolonged phonemes and intervals, although quite distinctive of ataxic dysarthria, is not prominent in all patients. For example, only 20 to 24 of DAB's 30 subjects with cerebellar

*Although harshness was among the most deviant characteristics noted by DAB, in the author's experience it does not seem to occur frequently or be more than mildly evident in people with isolated ataxic dysarthria. In general, the presence of significant harshness in someone with ataxic dysarthria should raise questions about an accompanying spastic component.

†Kent et al.[62] point out that descriptions of the salient features of ataxic dysarthria are quite similar across different languages and dialects. In the author's experience, ataxic dysarthria (and other types) often can be recognized without difficulty in languages with which a clinician has little knowledge, simply on the basis of perceptual judgments of speech AMRs, vowel prolongation, and rate and prosodic features of conversational speech.

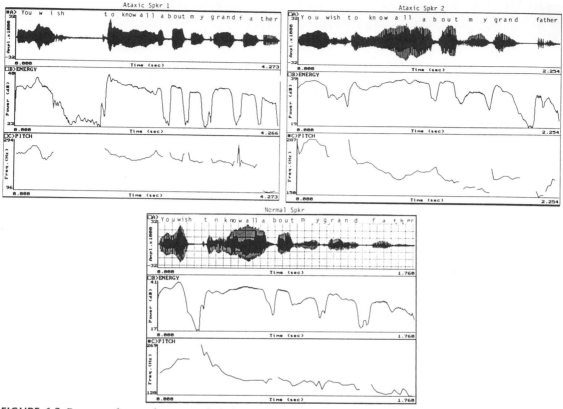

FIGURE 6-3 Raw waveform and energy and pitch *(f_o)* tracings for the sentence "You wish to know all about my grandfather" by a normal female speaker *(bottom tracings)* and two females with ataxic dysarthria *(upper tracings)*. The normal speaker completes the sentence in less than 2 seconds with normal variability in syllable duration and amplitude *(energy tracing)* and normal variability and declination in f_o across the sentence *(pitch tracing)*. Ataxic Speaker 1 is slow ($\approx$4.3 seconds for the utterance). Note also the relatively equal amplitude and duration of syllables for ". . . about my grandfather" in the energy tracing and the relative absence of f_o variability and declination in the pitch tracing. These represent acoustic correlates of the slow rate, excess and equal stress, and monoloudness and monopitch that are often apparent in ataxic dysarthria.

Ataxic Speaker 2 is not dramatically slow, and the energy and pitch tracings are grossly similar to the normal speaker's. Note, however, that the word "grandfather" is produced more rapidly, particularly the syllables for "father"; the stressed syllable "fa" is shorter than the unstressed "ther" *(energy tracing)*. These alterations are associated with perceivable breakdowns in articulation, as well as dysprosody characterized by abnormal stress and syllable durations.

disease exhibited the speech features of this cluster. This lack of pervasiveness is not simply a function of severity because some patients with marked ataxic dysarthria and decreased intelligibility do not have prominent prosodic excess. In such cases it may be the cluster of articulatory inaccuracy that predominates, with irregular articulatory breakdowns giving speech an "intoxicated," irregular character rather than a measured quality.

2. Relatedly, not all patients with ataxic dysarthria have irregular speech AMRs, even though irregular AMRs are a distinctive and fairly pervasive marker of the disorder. It is the author's impression that irregular AMRs occur less frequently in patients with promi-

nent prosodic excess (whose AMRs may be quite slow) and are more prominent in those with significant irregular articulatory breakdowns. Of course, many patients with ataxic dysarthria have both prosodic excess and articulatory inaccuracy.

3. Irregular articulatory breakdowns are sometimes associated with *telescoping,* an occurrence that refers to an inconsistent breakdown of articulation in which a syllable or series of syllables are suddenly or unpredictably run together, giving speech a transient accelerated character.

4. Some ataxic speakers exhibit *explosive loudness* and poorly modulated pitch and loudness variations. These characteristics do not appear within the most deviant characteristics

table 6-3	The most deviant speech dimensions encountered in ataxic dysarthria by Darley, Aronson, and Brown,[27] listed in order from most to least severe. Also listed is the component of the speech system associated with each characteristic. The component "prosodic" is listed when several components of the speech system may contribute to the dimension. Characteristics listed under "Other" include features not among the most deviant but that were judged deviant in a number of subjects and are not typical of most other dysarthria types.

Dimension	Speech Component
Imprecise consonants	Articulatory
Excess & equal stress*	Prosodic
Irregular articulatory breakdowns*	Articulatory
Distorted vowels*	Articulatory-prosodic
Harsh voice quality	Phonatory
Prolonged phonemes*	Articulatory-prosodic
Prolonged intervals	Prosodic
Monopitch	Phonatory-prosodic
Monoloudness	Phonatory-prosodic
Slow rate	Prosodic
Other	
Excess loudness variations*	Respiratory-phonatory-prosodic
Voice tremor	Phonatory

*Tend to be distinctive or more severely impaired than in any other single dysarthria type.

or clusters of ataxic dysarthria, but they are striking when present. DAB observed excess loudness variability in one third of their subjects and noted that this feature is probably a component of what some have described as "explosive speech." Although it may not occur frequently, explosive loudness has traditionally been associated with cerebellar dysfunction.[45]

5. *Voice tremor* is not frequently encountered in ataxic dysarthria and does not emerge among the clusters of deviant speech characteristics or among its most deviant speech characteristics.[27,28] However, cerebellar disease can be associated with tremor of the laryngeal and respiratory muscles that results in a slow voice tremor of approximately 3 Hz.

6. Abnormal resonance is rare in ataxic dysarthria. However, intermittent *hyponasality* is perceived in some speakers. These infrequent occurrences presumably reflect improper timing of velar and articulatory ges-

tures for nasal consonants. Although uncommon, *intermittent hyponasality* is probably more frequently encountered in ataxic dysarthria than any other dysarthria type.

7. If some patients with ataxic dysarthria have predominant prosodic excess while others have predominant articulatory inaccuracy, if the two clusters can occur relatively independently, and if some patients with ataxic dysarthria truly have predominant explosive loudness, this means that *there may be subtypes of ataxic dysarthria.* If true, subtypes might be tied to differences in lesion location within the cerebellar control circuit, differences in the nature of the cerebellar disorder, or differences among speech subsystem impairments (findings relevant to the possibility of subtypes are reviewed in the next section).

What features of ataxic dysarthria help distinguish it from other MSDs? Among all of the abnormal speech characteristics that may be detected, *irregular articulatory breakdowns, irregular speech AMRs, excess and equal stress, excess loudness variations,* and *distorted vowels* are the most common distinctive clues to the presence of the disorder.

Table 6-4 summarizes the primary distinguishing speech characteristics and common oral mechanism examination findings and patient complaints associated with ataxic dysarthria.

Acoustic and Physiologic Findings

Respiratory and Laryngeal Function

The few physiologic investigations of respiration during speech in ataxic dysarthria make it clear that respiratory functions can be disturbed. Some early studies of a single or a few subjects found evidence of reduced vital capacity, incoordination between rib cage and abdominal movements, and incoordination between the timing of onset of respiration and phonation leading to air wastage.[1,23]

In a comprehensive study employing spirometric and kinematic techniques, Murdoch et al.[83] examined respiratory function during speech and nonspeech tasks in 12 people with cerebellar disease and ataxic dysarthria. Several differences were found between normal controls and a significant proportion of the ataxic speakers during vowel prolongation, syllable repetition, and reading and conversational tasks. The most salient findings for the ataxic speakers included: (1) reduced vital capacity, (2) paradoxical movements or abrupt changes in movements of the rib cage and abdomen, (3) irregularities in chest wall movements during sustained vowels and syllable repetition, and (4) a tendency to initiate utterances at

table 6-4	Primary distinguishing speech and speech-related findings in ataxic dysarthria

Perceptual	
Phonation-respiration	Excessive loudness variations
Articulation-prosody	Irregular articulatory breakdowns
	Irregular AMRs
	Distorted vowels
	Excess & equal stress
	Prolonged phonemes
Physical	Dysmetric jaw, face, & tongue AMRs
Patient Complaints	"Drunk" or intoxicated speech
	Stumbling over words
	Biting tongue or cheek when speaking or eating
	Speech deteriorates with alcohol
	Poor coordination of breathing with speech

AMRs, Alternate motion rates.

lower than normal lung volume levels. These abnormalities seemed to reflect poor coordination of chest wall components of respiration, something the authors felt could explain some of the prosodic abnormalities perceived in ataxic speakers.

The existence of respiratory incoordination was confirmed by McClean, Beukelman, and Yorkston,[79] who examined the ability of an ataxic speaker to track a visually presented sinusoidal target by controlling respiratory movements. The subject's control of respiratory movements bore only a limited relationship to target movements, and there was marked variability in performance. The subject was also unable to vary fundamental frequency (f_o) to perform the tracking task (normal speakers and some individuals with other dysarthria types could), suggesting that the task's demands far exceeded the subject's motor control ability.

DAB[29] summarized a number of early acoustic studies that bear on the issue of laryngeal speech control.[46,53,70,94] In general, studies suggest that patients with cerebellar involvement may display "restricted pitch and intensity variability, and individual patterns of aberrant vocal fold vibration that may be related to perceived voice quality deviations or may precede the development of audible changes in voice."[29] DAB pointed out that what might be perceived as phonatory abnormalities could also be the result of dysfunction at the respiratory level.

Subsequent studies support the frequent clinical perception of unsteadiness during vowel prolongation and frequent instability of pitch and loudness within connected speech. That is, acoustic studies of

varying numbers of people with various cerebellar diseases who presumably had ataxic dysarthria often report (in varying proportions of those tested) increased rather than decreased variability on several measures of long-term and short-term phonatory stability.[39,40,61,65] These abnormalities have generally been identified on vowel prolongation tasks but have sometimes been derived from AMR and sentence-level tasks. They include abnormal variability in long-term measures of f_o and intensity,*[39,61,63] increased jitter and shimmer values,[7,63] increased pitch level,[7] harshness,[61] and abnormal voice onset time (VOT) values (see next section for details). These abnormalities have been reported in men and women, but occasional gender differences have been observed; for example, Kent et al.[63] found a high occurrence of abnormal shimmer values for female but not male ataxic speakers.

Although voice tremor is only infrequently evident in ataxic dysarthria, it has been confirmed by acoustic analysis in some speakers.[6,7,20] For example, Ackermann and Ziegler[6] found a 3-Hz voice tremor in a woman with chronic cerebellar atrophy with an ataxic dysarthria and voice tremor; respiratory and articulatory tremor were ruled out, because rhythmic oscillations were not present during sustained voiceless fricatives. This tremor rate is consistent with other forms of cerebellar postural tremor. It is of interest that Kent et al.[63] found that a rate of approximately three syllables per second often occurred during AMR, sentence repetition, and conversation tasks, corresponding to the frequency of cerebellar tremor. The authors speculated that tremor rate may serve "as an attractor for syllable tempo," possibly explaining the tendency toward uniform syllable duration and equal stress in conversation; that is, the tremor may serve as a temporal substrate for voluntary movements, with temporal irregularities arising "because of inaccuracies in muscle activation (e.g., variant contraction times in the musculature) or intersystem incoordination."

Taken together, these abnormalities suggest that ataxic dysarthria, at least in some individuals, is characterized in part by *phonatory instability or phonatory-respiratory instability.* The explanations for this instability most often point to problems of coordination, timing, or control. For example, Ackermann and Ziegler[6,7] speculated that asymmetrically distributed motor deficits at the laryngeal level and altered sensory (e.g., proprioceptive) control of laryngeal or respiratory reflexes could account for impaired control of tension in intrinsic laryngeal muscles, leading to phonatory instability.

*Kent et al.[61] noted that long-term measures of f_o and amplitude variability might be particularly sensitive indices of phonatory dysfunction in ataxic dysarthria, and MSDs in general.

In addition, voicing errors imply poor laryngeal control or laryngeal-supraglottic timing errors.[61]

Articulation, Rate, and Prosody

A number of acoustic and physiologic studies support, quantify, and help explain the clinical perception of slow rate, irregular articulatory breakdowns, and prosodic abnormalities in ataxic dysarthria.

Various acoustic analyses have documented *slow rate* on AMR tasks and during word and sentence production.*[†] Slowness of movement in ataxic speech has also been demonstrated in a cineradiographic study of articulatory movements[58] and in a kinematic study of lower lip movements during speech.[5,9]

Slowness during connected speech in ataxic dysarthria includes longer sentence and syllable durations, longer formant transitions, lengthened consonant clusters and vowel nuclei in words and syllables, and, sometimes, longer VOT.[10,25,49,57,59,61,72] There also is evidence that some ataxic speakers have difficulty changing speech rate or producing faster speech rates,[40,61] suggesting that slow rate is not just, or not always, compensatory.

It is reasonable to ask if slow rate might predict intelligibility or severity in ataxic dysarthria. It appears this may not be the case. Although Ziegler and Wessel[105] found that maximum AMR rate was a good predictor of severity and intelligibility, Kent et al.[63] found that AMR rate was not correlated with perceived overall severity of dysarthria during conversation. In addition, Linebaugh and Wolfe[72] found no relationship between duration and measures of intelligibility or naturalness. These latter findings support general clinical observations that intelligibility can be quite good in some speakers whose rate is slow. They also support the clinical impression that *speech characteristics or speaking tasks that may be sensitive to the presence and type of a disorder do not necessarily predict intelligibility or other ratings of severity.*

What is the basis for slow rate? Hypotonia has been offered as one explanation.[25,40,49,58] That is, the reduced tone and muscular tension that characterize hypotonia may delay the generation of muscle force and reduce the rate of muscle contraction, with resultant slowness of movement and prolongation of sounds.[58] Another explanation is that cerebellar damage—because it may interfere with the cerebellum's role in revising provisional cortical motor commands—may lead to a heavier reliance on basic cortical motor programs for movement control. Because cortical revisions of a motor program presumably take longer than cerebellar revisions, speech segment durations might be increased to allow time for the longer and slower cortical loops to operate.[9,25,59] This explanation is intriguing, and it raises questions about whether imposition of cortical control in response to cerebellar damage occurs "automatically," is dependent on the specific nature of the cerebellar deficit, reflects an intentional compensatory response by the speaker, or represents a combination of these possibilities. The outcome in any case would be a slowing of speech rate.

In addition to slow rate—and more relevant to the truly distinctive perceptual characteristics of ataxic dysarthria—acoustic and physiologic studies have frequently documented and sometimes specified the parameters of *abnormalities in rhythm on speech AMR tasks.* The sensitivity of the AMR task to timing problems confirms its usefulness in the perceptual and acoustic assessment of the disorder (see Figure 6-2). The loci of increased variability in AMRs have included VOT, vowel duration, syllable gaps, and minimum and maximum energy values.[61,63] Irregularities in chest wall movements during speech AMRs have also been documented kinematically in some ataxic speakers.[†83] All of these findings, plus others discussed later, speak to the presence of *timing problems* in the disorder. Kent et al.[61] concluded that *temporal dysregulation* is a primary component of ataxic dysarthria and that its effects "are most evident in the production of longer syllabic strings, even if they take the form of simple syllable repetition," suggesting that the cerebellum may have a major role in regulating precise timing during long or complex sequences of motor activity.

Timing abnormalities are also evident in measures of VOT, which are felt to be a sensitive index of laryngeal control or laryngeal-articulatory coordination. Abnormal VOT values are found frequently in ataxic speakers.[3,25,59,61] They include shorter than normal VOT, longer than normal VOT, and overlapping or more variable than normal VOT across repeated responses,[25,59,61] all which suggest abnormal variability beyond that explainable by general slowness. The

---

*The work of Kent and Netsell[58] is an excellent example of how inferences derived from acoustic and physiologic studies can lead to refinements or modifications of hypotheses generated by perceptual analyses of the dysarthrias.

[†]References 2, 4, 19, 32, 39, 40, 48, 57, 58, 59, 61, 86, 88, 96, 104, 105.

---

*References 4, 19, 39, 40, 50, 59, 61, 63, 88, 96, 104, 105.

[†]These irregularities within the speech system are not necessarily unique to speech. For example, McNeil et al.[80] studied isometric force and static position control of the upper and lower lip, tongue, and jaw during nonspeech tasks in four ataxic speakers. They had greater force and position instability than normal speakers. McClean, Beukelman, and Yorkston's[79] ataxic speaker performed poorly on a nonspeech visuomotor tracking task involving the lower lip and jaw.

finding of Kent et al.[61] that the most frequent intelligibility errors in a group of ataxic speakers were related to voicing contrasts attests to the relevance of poor VOT control to some perceptual errors.

Several acoustic and aerodynamic studies have quantified and determined the loci of problems with stress and prosody at the word and sentence level (see Figure 6-3). They lend further support to conclusions that problems with timing, coordination, and control are common in the disorder. Markedly abnormal fluctuations in f_o and intensity, restriction of f_o variation, excessive interword pauses, irregularity of segment durations, and apparent increased articulatory effort (as reflected in peak intraoral air pressure) have been documented.[24,40,58,84,102] Aberrations in speech segment duration with increased length of utterance were documented by Kent, Netsell, and Abbs,[59] who found that the normal tendency to reduce base word duration as the number of syllables in words increases was inconsistent in ataxic speakers. For example, the duration of the syllable "please" in the sequence "please, pleasing, pleasingly" showed inconsistent reductions, small reductions, and occasional lengthening of the base word as the number of syllables increased. Although lengthened segments (slow rate) seemed characteristic of the ataxic speakers, inconsistent degrees of lengthening altered speech stress and timing patterns. Lax and unstressed vowels were more likely to be disproportionately lengthened, a finding that fits well with the perception of excess and equal stress or *scanning* in some speakers. The authors speculated that ataxic speakers do not decrease syllable duration when it is appropriate, because such reductions require flexibility in sequencing complex motor instructions. The lack of flexibility may lead to a syllable-by-syllable motor control strategy with subsequent abnormal stress patterns.

Problems of stress and prosody identified in instrumental studies clearly have perceptual salience. For example, Liss et al.[74] found that listeners transcribing ataxic speech had difficulty distinguishing strong and weak syllables, even when they had been familiarized with ataxic speech, and even though their intelligibility scores improved with familiarization. Listeners also seem to have difficulty determining lexical boundaries in speakers with ataxic dysarthria, partly as a function of abnormalities in speech rhythm.

The apparent coexistence of the clusters of prosodic excess and phonatory-prosodic insufficiency in ataxic dysarthria (as established by DAB) is curious, because they seem to be mutually exclusive abnormalities. Observations and analysis of this paradoxical relationship seem to confirm the presence of both problems in the disorder, although whether they coexist within the same patient is not quite so clear. Across patients, acoustic studies have

identified both excessive and reduced variability of speech segment durations.[2,39,40,59,61] The existence of scanning (prosodic excess) has been documented in acoustic studies,[48,60,95] with its specific acoustic characteristics represented by limited variation in syllable duration, fairly regular spacing between syllabic nuclei, and a generally flat f_o contour. In general, these features are consistent with "an equalization across syllables with respect to their prosodic content."[60] Thus in the scanning speech of ataxic dysarthria, variability of segment durations and f_o may actually be less than normal, a seeming contradiction to many findings of variability that have already been discussed.

Hartelius et al.[48] offered an explanation for this paradox. Their 14 ataxic speakers had longer than normal syllable durations and less variability (more *isochrony,* or syllable equalization) in their production of consecutive syllables within sentences, a pattern suggestive of *inflexibility.* However, they also had increased variability of syllable duration across repetitions of the same sentence, as well as increased variability of interstress intervals (i.e., the intervals between stressed vowels within sentences); these characteristics suggest *instability.* The authors felt that this cooccurrence of both inflexibility and instability of temporal control could explain the apparently contradictory perceptual characteristics of prosodic excess and phonatory-prosodic insufficiency.

Is prosodic excess more prominent or important than phonatory-prosodic insufficiency or articulatory inaccuracy to the diagnosis and understanding of ataxic dysarthria? Although Ackermann et al.[8] emphasized irregular articulatory breakdowns as the core speech disturbance, as opposed to scanning or prosodic excess, this does not always seem to be the case clinically. It seems possible that the apparent paradoxical cooccurrence of prosodic excess and articulatory inaccuracy (particularly irregular articulatory breakdowns) might reflect individual differences. That is, if subtypes of ataxic dysarthria exist, they could reflect differences in the degree to which inflexibility versus instability of motor control predominate, leaving some affected people with predominant prosodic insufficiency and articulatory inaccuracy, others with predominant problems of excess stress, and others with a more equal combination of the two.

There is some acoustic evidence that suggests subgroups of ataxic dysarthria do exist, although not along the lines just discussed. Subgroups have been identified as a function of variability in the temporal characteristics and intensity of speech AMRs, with differences in variability among subgroups possibly reflecting different subsystem impairments[19] but not necessarily differences in the nature of the cerebellar disorder.[63] Boutsen, Bakker, and Duffy[19] identified three subgroups from among a group of 27 ataxic speakers. One group had similar durational variability among AMRs for "puh," "tuh," and "kuh." For the other two groups durational variability was dependent on the specific syllable. These differences were not related to severity or etiology, and they raised the possibility of different subsystem impairment. The authors concluded, "ataxic dysarthria may not be a unitary disorder in which differences among patients' speech characteristics are simply a function of dysarthria severity." Relatedly, Kent et al.[62] suggested that global effects related to temporal dysregulation and positioning errors may be common to all patients with the disorder, whereas other abnormalities might be variable across patients and reflect specific impairments in different muscle systems.

The general observations derived from acoustic and physiologic studies reviewed in this section are summarized in Table 6-5.

table 6-5	Summary of acoustic and physiologic findings in studies of ataxic dysarthria. Note that many of these observations are based on studies of only one or a few speakers, and that not all speakers with ataxic dysarthria exhibit these features. These characteristics are not necessarily unique to ataxic dysarthria; some may also be characteristic of other motor speech disorders, or nonneurologic conditions.

Speech Component	Acoustic or Physiologic Observation
Respiratory or Laryngeal	Abnormal & paradoxical rib cage & abdominal movements Irregularities in chest wall movements Initiation of utterances at reduced lung volume levels Reduced vital capacity (probably secondary to incoordination) Poor visuomotor tracking with respiratory movements & f_o Increased long-term variability of f_o & peak amplitude during vowel prolongation & AMRs Increased shimmer & jitter Voice tremor (≈ 3 Hz)

Articulation, Rate, and Prosody	Reduced rate:
	  Increased syllable & sentence duration
	  Increased duration of formant transitions
	  Longer VOT (but sometimes shorter)
	  Lengthened consonant clusters & vowel nuclei
	  Slow AMRs
	  Disproportionate lengthening of lax or unstressed vowels
	  Excessive interword pauses
	  Difficulty initiating purposeful movement
	  Slow lip, tongue, & jaw movements
	  Difficulty increasing speech rate
	
	Increased variability, inconsistency, or instability of:
	  Segment durations
	  Rate
	  Intensity (maximum & minimum energy values)
	  AMR rate & intensity
	  f_o
	  VOT
	  Range & velocity of articulatory movements, especially AMRs
	  Inconsistent reduction of base word (first syllable) duration as number of syllables in words increases
	  Inconsistent velopharyngeal closure
	
	Reduced variability or restriction of:
	  Anterior-posterior tongue movements during vowel production
	  Syllable duration
	  Spacing between syllabic nuclei
	  f_o contour in connected speech
	
	Other:
	  Breakdown in rhythmic EMG patterns in articulatory muscles during syllable repetition
	  Poor visuomotor tracking with lower lip & jaw movements on nonspeech tasks
	  Increased instability of force & static position control in lip, tongue, & jaw on nonspeech tasks
	  Occasional failure of articulatory contact for consonants.

AMRs, Alternate motion rates; *EMG,* electromyelogram; f_o, fundamental frequency; *VOT,* voice onset time.

Cases

Case 6-1

A 41-year-old woman presented for speech evaluation before neurologic assessment. She had been aware of a change in her speech for approximately a year, and people frequently asked if she was "on drugs or drinking." Speech deteriorated under conditions of stress or fatigue, but she felt intelligibility remained normal. She denied chewing or swallowing difficulty. She mentioned that her 49-year-old brother also had gait, balance, and speech difficulties.

Oral mechanism examination was normal in size, strength, and symmetry. Gag reflex was hypoactive. Cough and glottal coup were normal. Snout, sucking, and jaw jerk reflexes were absent.

Conversational speech was characterized by irregular articulatory breakdowns (1,2), reduced rate (1,2), dysprosody (1), occasional excess and equal stress (0,1), reduced pitch (0,1), and nonspecific subtle hoarseness (0,1). Speech AMRs were slow and irregular (1,2). Prolonged "ah" was unsteady (1). Speech intelligibility was normal.

The clinician concluded, "ataxic dysarthria, relatively mild." Both the patient and clinician felt therapy was unnecessary, but she was advised to pursue reassessment and therapy if her speech difficulties progressed.

Neurologic evaluation identified multiple signs of cerebellar involvement, particularly pronounced gait and balance difficulties. Computed tomography (CT) scan and magnetic resonance imaging (MRI) identified marked cerebellar atrophy (Figure 6-4) involving both cerebellar hemispheres and the vermis. Family history established that her brother and father probably had the same condition. It was suspected that the patient had an autosomal dominant cerebellar degenerative disease. Genetic counseling was provided; her three children were felt to have a one-in-two risk of inheriting cerebellar degenerative disease.

Commentary. (1) Ataxic dysarthria is a common and sometimes presenting sign of degenerative cerebellar disease, including inherited conditions. Its accurate diagnosis helps confirm disease localization. (2) Diagnosis of dysarthria and its specific type can be made even when the problem is mild and intelligibility is unaffected.

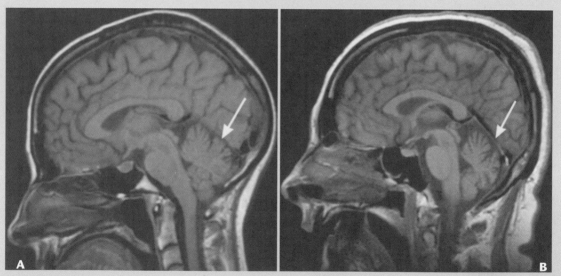

FIGURE 6-4 Midsagittal magnetic resonance imaging demonstrating, **A,** normal adult brain structure and, **B,** mild to moderate cerebellar atrophy in a 54-year-old woman with degenerative cerebellar disease and mild ataxic dysarthria.

Case 6-2

A 27-year-old woman presented with a 10-year history of progressive gait imbalance, incoordination of the hands, and "slurred speech." Her symptoms worsened around her menstrual periods and when she was nervous or fatigued; they had worsened slightly during a pregnancy. Neurologic examination confirmed the presence of ataxic gait, upper limb ataxia, and nystagmus.

During speech examination, she admitted to an approximately 10-year history of "slurred speech," which did not seem to have progressed recently. Conversational speech was characterized by occasional irregular articulatory breakdowns (0,1), which were most apparent during consonant clusters and affricates. Infrequently, rate was mildly slowed and multisyllabic words were produced with excess and equal stress. Prolonged "ah" was unsteady (1). Speech AMRs were slow (1) but not noticeably irregular.

The clinician concluded that the patient had a "mild ataxic dysarthria" that was not pervasively apparent and did not affect intelligibility. Therapy was not recommended.

An electromyelogram revealed a severe disorder of primary sensory neurons and other findings that were consistent with the diagnosis of spinocerebellar degeneration.

She was seen for follow-up 6 years later. There was some worsening of her gait disturbance but no worsening of her other deficits, including speech.

Commentary. (1) Ataxic dysarthria can be among the presenting signs of cerebellar degenerative disease. Its characteristics can be quite subtle, but its recognition can help confirm cerebellar dysfunction. (2) Some degenerative CNS diseases that affect speech may be so slowly progressive that intelligibility is preserved over many years.

Case 6-3

A 56-year-old woman presented for neurologic assessment with a primary complaint of speech difficulty. This had developed gradually, with some progression, over the previous 8 months. It was accompanied by general "awkwardness" when sewing or running and some memory problems. Neurologic examination was normal with the exception of her speech deficit, although questions were raised about depression and possible cognitive decline. Subsequent psychometric assessment was normal. CT and MRI scans were negative. A complete general medical workup was normal. Psychiatric consultation confirmed the presence of depression, probably developed in response to her neurologic or speech difficulties.

Speech examination was notable for the presence of irregular articulatory breakdowns during connected speech (2), irregular speech AMRs (2), and unsteadiness of vowel prolongation (1,2). Intelligibility was mild to moderately reduced. There was no evidence of aphasia.

The clinician concluded "dysarthria, ataxic (cerebellar), moderate-marked."

The neurologist concluded that the patient had a cerebellar dysarthria of undetermined etiology and stated that the underlying disease might "declare itself more clearly with time." She was seen approximately 18 months later for reassessment. Her dysarthria had worsened, and she had a clear-cut gait ataxia. MRI scan was again normal. Repeat psychometric assessment was unchanged, and no other abnormalities were identified during a complete medical workup. Again, the diagnosis was "cerebellar syndrome of unknown origin."

The patient experienced progression of her deficits over the next 18 months, but her only new symptom was a mild and vaguely described swallowing problem. These were reported through correspondence and not observed during formal reassessment. She was not seen for further follow-up.

Commentary. (1) Ataxic dysarthria can be the first and most prominent finding in degenerative neurologic disease. (2) It may precede the development of other signs of disease and may be present in the absence of neuroimaging evidence of cerebellar degeneration or lesions.

Case 6-4

A 63-year-old woman was hospitalized for evaluation and treatment of cardiovascular problems. She had a history of myocardial infarction and had had coronary bypass surgery 6 months previously. Three weeks before admission she developed the sudden onset of speech difficulty and problems with gait. She had no difficulties with language, chewing, or swallowing.

Oral mechanism examination was normal. Speech was characterized by irregular articulatory breakdowns (1,2), irregular speech AMRs (1), and unsteady vowel prolongation (2). Intelligibility was normal.

The clinician concluded that the patient had a "mild ataxic dysarthria." Because intelligibility was essentially normal, and because the patient was compensating well for her deficit and was generally unconcerned about it, therapy was not recommended.

Subsequent CT scan identified a 2-cm area of low attenuation in the right cerebellar hemisphere consistent with a diagnosis of stroke.

Commentary. (1) Ataxic dysarthria can result from cerebellar stroke and may be among the most prominent signs of such an event. (2) Although probably uncommon, ataxic dysarthria sometimes can result from a unilateral lesion affecting the cerebellar hemispheres. (3) Although some studies suggest that ataxic dysarthria resulting from unilateral cerebellar lesions occurs more frequently with lesions of the left cerebellar hemisphere, it can occur with lesions to the right cerebellar hemisphere. (4) The presence of dysarthria does not lead automatically to a recommendation for treatment. Such a recommendation is based on the degree of disability and the patient's judgment about, and compensations for, the problem, among other things.

Case 6-5

A 53-year-old woman presented with a 2- to 3-year history of intermittent "jumping" of her vision. For 9 months she had double vision, imbalance when walking, and mild "slurring" of speech, all of which had gradually worsened.

Neurologic examination revealed nystagmus, mild proximal weakness in all limbs, severe gait ataxia, and moderate limb ataxia. MRI scan revealed several areas of abnormality in the white matter of both hemispheres, suggestive of demyelinating disease. Multiple sclerosis was suspected, but she had a high cerebrospinal fluid white blood cell count. A serum Purkinje cell antibody test was ordered.

The patient felt that her speech was "slightly slurred." It had worsened over the past 5 months and was susceptible to fatigue. She sometimes bit her tongue when eating and occasionally drooled when laughing or crying.

The speech mechanism was normal in size, strength, and symmetry. Jaw and lateral tongue movements were dysmetric. Voluntary cough and glottal coup seemed poorly coordinated. Conversational speech was characterized by irregular articulatory breakdowns (3), dysprosody (3), excess and equal stress (scanning) (2,3), and inappropriate loudness variability (1). Overall speech rate was slow (−2). Speech AMRs were irregular (3) and slow (−2). Vowel prolongation was breathy and unsteady (1,2).

The speech clinician concluded, "Unambiguous, moderately severe ataxic dysarthria suggestive of cerebellar dysfunction. Unless she is emotionally upset while talking, speech intelligibility is good. In fact, the scanning quality to her speech works to her advantage in terms of intelligibility." Speech therapy was not recommended.

Subsequently, her serum Purkinje cell antibody test was positive, strongly suggestive of paraneoplastic cerebellar degeneration associated with underlying malignancy. She was unable to remain at the clinic for a full workup for malignancy, but this was pursued at home. Initial workups there were negative, but an ovarian tumor was discovered approximately 5 months later.

Commentary. (1) Ataxic dysarthria is not uncommon in cerebellar disease and frequently occurs in paraneoplastic syndromes that affect the cerebellum. In such cases, the dysarthria and other neurologic signs may be apparent before detection of the primary malignancy. (2) The presence of ataxic dysarthria (and other dysarthrias) does not dictate that therapy should be undertaken. The patient's intelligibility was normal, and there was nothing obvious about her speech that suggested therapy would alter speech in a direction of greater normalcy. She was advised to pursue therapy if her dysarthria worsened, however.

Case 6-6

A 49-year-old woman presented to neurology with a 1-year history of speech or balance difficulties and cognitive decline. She had also had three episodes of loss of consciousness. Hashimoto's thyroiditis was diagnosed approximately 6 months after the onset of her symptoms, and she subsequently underwent total thyroidectomy. Postoperatively, she was given a small dose of Synthroid.

Neurologic examination noted balance difficulty, speech difficulty, mental status problems, and apparent indifference to her symptoms. It was not certain if her problems were organic or nonorganic in nature.

During speech evaluation, she reported a 2-year history of episodic "garbled" speech with gradual progression to more constant difficulties. She also complained of occasional word retrieval difficulties and problems with spelling and recall. Oral mechanism examination was normal. Her speech pattern was somewhat unusual and included a moderate degree of hoarse-rough voice quality with occasional pitch breaks and unusual variability in pitch and duration. Irregular articulatory breakdowns were also evident. Rate was mildly slowed. Vowel prolongation was unsteady (+2). Speech AMRs were moderately irregular. There was no evidence of aphasic language impairment, but she occasionally forgot stimuli and had to be reinstructed about the nature of tasks. The clinician concluded that the patient's speech problem was organic and that it represented an obvious ataxic dysarthria plus a mild dysphonia; it was noted that the dysarthria and dysphonia could be compatible with hypothyroidism. A recommendation regarding therapy was deferred until the completion of her medical workup.

The patient's electroencephalogram and MRI scan were normal. Assessment of thyroid function confirmed hypothyroidism, and thyroid hormone replacement medications were increased. She noted some improvement in all of her symptoms within several days, although she was advised that full benefit from the thyroid replacement treatment would take some time.

Commentary. (1) Ataxic dysarthria can be associated with hypothyroidism. (2) Dysarthria can be the first sign of neurologic disease, including neurologic signs and symptoms stemming from hypothyroidism. (3) Identification of dysarthria and its type can help establish if speech disturbances are compatible with certain neurologic conditions. Ataxic dysarthria and dysphonia are known possible sequences of hypothyroidism, whereas other MSDs typically are not.

SUMMARY

1. Ataxic dysarthria results from damage to the cerebellar control circuit, most frequently damage to the lateral hemispheres or vermis of the cerebellum. It occurs at a frequency comparable to that for other major single dysarthria types. Although it may reflect deficits at all levels of speech production, it is most perceptible in articulation and prosody. Incoordination and reduced muscle tone appear responsible for the slowness of movement and inaccuracy in the force, range, timing, and direction of speech movements.

2. Degenerative disease probably accounts for the largest proportion of cases of ataxic dysarthria; demyelinating, vascular, and undetermined etiologies are also common. Most patients have clinical evidence of cerebellar involvement other than ataxic dysarthria. When positive, neuroimaging studies frequently identify cerebellar lesions or abnormalities in the brainstem or posterior fossa.

3. People with ataxic dysarthria frequently complain of slurred speech and a "drunken" quality to their speech. Complaints of dysphagia and difficulty with drooling are infrequent.

4. The major clusters of deviant speech characteristics in ataxic dysarthria include articulatory inaccuracy, prosodic excess, and phonatory-prosodic insufficiency. Although many abnormal speech characteristics can be detected in ataxic dysarthria, irregular articulatory breakdowns, irregular speech AMRs, excess and equal stress, distorted vowels, and excess loudness variations are the most distinctive clues to the presence of ataxic dysarthria.

5. In general, acoustic and physiologic studies of ataxic dysarthria have provided quantitative supportive evidence for the clinical perceptual characteristics of the disorder. They have helped to specify more completely the loci and dynamics of abnormal movements underlying the perceived speech disturbance. They support conclusions that slowness of movement and problems with timing are predominant deficits.

6. Ataxic dysarthria can be the only, the first, or among the first or most prominent manifestations of neurologic disease. Its recognition and

correlation with cerebellar dysfunction can aid the localization and diagnosis of neurologic disease and may influence medical and behavioral management.

References

1. Abbs JH, Hunker CJ, Barlow SM: Differential speech motor subsystem impairments with suprabulbar lesions: neurophysiological framework and supporting data. In Berry WR, editor: Clinical dysarthria, San Diego, 1983, College-Hill.
2. Ackermann H, Hertrich I: Speech rate and rhythm in cerebellar dysarthria: an acoustic analysis of syllable timing, Folia Phoniatr Logop 46:70, 1994.
3. Ackermann H, Hertrich I: Voice onset time in ataxic dysarthria, Brain Lang 56:321, 1997.
4. Ackermann H, Hertrich I, Hehr T: Oral diadokokinesis in neurological dysarthrias, Folia Phoniatr Logop 47:15, 1995.
5. Ackermann H, Hertrich I, Scharf G: Kinematic analysis of lower lip movements in ataxic dysarthria, J Speech Hear Res 38:1252, 1995.
6. Ackermann H, Ziegler W: Cerebellar voice tremor: an acoustic analysis, J Neurol Neurosurg Psychiatry 54:74, 1991.
7. Ackermann H, Ziegler W: Acoustic analysis of vocal instability in cerebellar dysfunctions, Ann Otol Rhinol Laryngol 103:98, 1994.
8. Ackermann H et al: Speech deficits in ischaemic cerebellar lesions, J Neurol 239:223, 1992.
9. Ackermann H et al: Kinematic analysis of articulatory movements in central motor disorders, Mov Disord 12:1019, 1997.
10. Ackermann H et al: Phonemic vowel length contrasts in cerebellar disorders, Brain Lang 67:95, 1999.
11. Adams RD, Victor M: Principles of neurology, New York, 1991, McGraw-Hill.
12. Amarenco P et al: Paravermal infarct and isolated cerebellar dysarthria, Ann Neurol 30:211, 1991.
13. Amici R, Avanzini G, Pacini L: Cerebellar tumors: clinical analysis and psysiopathologic correlations, New York, Monographs in neural sciences, vol 4, Basel, Switzerland, 1976, Karger.
14. Anderson NE, Rosenblum MK, Posner JB: Paraneoplastic cerebellar degeneration: clinical-immunological correlations, Ann Neurol 24:559, 1988.
15. Aronson AE: Clinical voice disorders, New York, 1990, Thieme.
16. Baker KG et al: Neuronal loss in functional zones of the cerebellum of chronic alcoholics with and without Wernicke's encephalopathy, Neuroscience 91:429, 1999.
17. Barkovich AJ: Pediatric neuroimaging, ed 2, New York, 1995, Raven Press.
18. Barth A, Bogousslavsky J, Regli F: The clinical and topographic spectrum of cerebellar infarcts: a clinical-magnetic resonance imaging correlation study, Ann Neurol 33:451, 1993.
19. Boutsen FR, Bakker K, Duffy JR: Subgroups in ataxic dysarthria, J Med Speech-Lang Pathol 5:27, 1997.
20. Boutsen FR, Duffy JR: An analysis of tremor in ataxic dysarthria, Presented at the Conference on Motor Speech, Tucson, AZ, January 1998.
21. Brown JR: Localizing cerebellar syndromes, JAMA 141:518, 1949.
22. Brown JR, Darley FL, Aronson AE: Deviant dimensions of motor speech in cerebellar ataxia, Trans Am Neurol Assoc 93:193, 1968.
23. Brown JR, Darley FL, Aronson AE: Ataxic dysarthria, Int J Neurol 7:302, 1970.
24. Chester CS, Reznick BR: Ataxia after severe head injury, Ann Neurol 22:77, 1987.
25. Chiu MJ, Chen RC, Tseng CY: Clinical correlates of quantitative acoustic analysis in dysarthria, Eur Neurol 36:310, 1996.
26. Dalmau JO, Posner JB: Paraneoplastic syndromes, Arch Neurol 56:405, 1999.
27. Darley FL, Aronson AE, Brown JR: Clusters of deviant speech dimensions in the dysarthrias, J Speech Hear Res 12:462, 1969a.
28. Darley FL, Aronson AE, Brown JR: Differential diagnostic patterns of dysarthria, J Speech Hear Res 12:246, 1969b.
29. Darley FL, Aronson AE, Brown JR: Motor speech disorders, Philadelphia, 1975, WB Saunders.
30. Daube JR et al: Medical neurosciences, Boston, 1986, Little, Brown.
31. Diener HC, Dichgans J: Pathophysiology of cerebellar ataxia, Mov Disord 7:95, 1992.
32. Dworkin JP, Aronson AE: Tongue strength and alternate motion rates in normal and dysarthric subjects, J Commun Disord 19:115, 1986.
33. Dworkin LA et al: Cerebellar toxicity following high-dose cytosine arabinoside, J Clin Oncol 3:613, 1985.
34. Erdemoglu AK, Duman T: Superior cerebellar artery territory stroke, Acta Neurol Scand 98:283, 1998.
35. Espir MLE, Walker ME: Carbamazepine in multiple sclerosis, Lancet 1:280, 1969.
36. Evidente VG et al: Hereditary ataxias, Mayo Clin Proc 75:475, 2000.
37. Fadic R et al: Sensory ataxic neuropathy as the presenting feature of a novel mitochondrial disease, Neurology 49:239, 1997.
38. Fiez JA et al: Impaired non-motor learning and error detection associated with cerebellar damage, Brain 115:155, 1992.
39. Gentil M: Acoustic characteristics of speech in Friedreich disease, Folia Phoniatr Logop 42:125, 1990a.
40. Gentil M: Dysarthria in Friedreich's disease, Brain Lang 38:438, 1990b.
41. Gilchrist E, Wilkinson M: Some factors determining prognosis in young people with severe head injuries, Arch Neurol 36:355, 1979.
42. Gilman S, Bloedel JR, Lechtenberg R: Disorders of the cerebellum, Philadelphia, 1981, FA Davis.
43. Gilman S, Kluin D: Perceptual analysis of speech disorders in Friedreich disease and olivopontocerebellar atrophy. In Bloedel JR et al, editors: Cerebellar functions, Berlin, 1984, Springer-Verlag.
44. Gironell A, Arboix A, Marti-Vilalta JL: Isolated dysarthria caused by a right paravermal infarction, J Neurol Neurosurg Psychiatry 61:205, 1996.
45. Grewel F: Classification of dysarthrias, Acta Psychiatr Scand 32:325, 1957.
46. Haggard MP: Speech waveform measurements in multiple sclerosis, Folia Phoniatr Logop 21:307, 1969.

47. Harding AE: Commentary: olivopontocerebellar atrophy is not a useful concept. In Marsden CN, Fahn S, editors: Movement disorders 2, New York, 1987, Butterworth.

48. Hartelius L et al: Temporal speech characteristics of individuals with multiple sclerosis and ataxic dysarthria: "scanning speech" revisited, Folia Phoniatr Logop 52:228, 2000.

49. Hertrich I, Ackermann H: Temporal and spectral aspects of coarticulation in ataxic dysarthria: an acoustic analysis, J Speech Lang Hear Res 42:367, 1999.

50. Hirose H et al: Analysis of abnormal articulatory dynamics in two dysarthric patients, J Speech Hear Disord 4:96, 1978.

51. Holmes G: Clinical symptoms of cerebellar disease, Lancet 2:59, 1922.

52. Jaeckle KA, Cohen ME, Duffner PK: Primary and secondary tumors of the central nervous system: clinical presentation and therapy of nervous system tumors. In Bradley WG et al, editors: Neurology in clinical practice: principles of diagnosis and management, vol 2, ed 3, Boston, 2000, Butterworth-Heinemann.

53. Janvrin F, Worster-Drought C: Diagnosis of disseminated sclerosis by graphic registration and film tracks, Lancet 2:1348, 1932.

54. Joanette Y, Dudley JG: Dysarthric symptomatology of Friedreich's ataxia, Brain Lang 10:39, 1980.

55. Jordan JE: Thyroid disorder, Semin Neurol 5:304, 1985.

56. Judd LL: The therapeutic use of psychotropic medications. In Wilson et al, editors: Harrison's principles of internal medicine, New York, 1991, McGraw-Hill.

57. Kent R: Isovowel lines for the evaluation of vowel formant structure in speech disorders, J Speech Hear Disord 44:513, 1979.

58. Kent R, Netsell R: A case study of an ataxic dysarthric: cineradiographic and spectrographic, J Speech Hear Disord 40:115, 1975.

59. Kent RD, Netsell R, Abbs JH: Acoustic characteristics of dysarthria associated with cerebellar disease, J Speech Hear Disord 22:627, 1979.

60. Kent RD, Rosenbek JC: Prosodic disturbance and neurologic lesion, Brain Lang 15:259, 1982.

61. Kent RD et al: A speaking task analysis of the dysarthria in cerebellar disease, Folia Phoniatr Logop 49:63, 1997.

62. Kent RD et al: The dysarthrias: speech-voice profiles, related dysfunctions, and neuropathology, J Med Speech-Lang Pathol 6:165, 1998.

63. Kent RD et al: Ataxic dysarthria, J Speech Lang Hear Res 43:1275, 2000.

64. Kent RD et al: Clinicoanatomic studies in dysarthria: review, critique, and directions for research, J Speech Lang Hear Res 44:535, 2001.

65. Kent RD et al: Voice dysfunction in dysarthria: application of the Multi-Dimensional Voice Program, J Commun Disord 36:281, 2003.

66. Klein ES, Willbrand ML, Alvord LS: Cerebellar ataxia secondary to high-dose cytosine arabinoside (ARA-C) toxicity in treatment of acute leukemia: a case study, J Med Speech-Lang Pathol 7:243, 1999.

67. Kores B, Lader MH: Irreversible lithium toxicity: an overview, Clin Neuropharmacol 20:283, 1997.

68. Laforce R, Doyon J: Distinct contribution of the striatum and cerebellum to motor learning, Brain Cogn 45:189, 2001.

69. Lechtenberg R, Gilman S: Speech disorders in cerebellar disease, Ann Neurol 3:285, 1978.

70. Lehiste I: Some acoustic characteristics of dysarthric speech, Bibliotheca phonetica, fasc 2, Basel, Switzerland, 1965, Karger.

71. Liepert J et al: Reduced intracortical facilitation in patients with cerebellar degeneration, Acta Neurol Scand 98:318, 1998.

72. Linebaugh CW, Wolfe VE: Relationships between articulation rate, intelligibility, and naturalness in spastic and ataxic speakers. In McNeil MR, Rosenbek JC, Aronson AE, editors: The dysarthrias: physiology, acoustics, perception, management, San Diego, 1984, College-Hill Press.

73. Liss JM et al: Lexical boundary errors in hypokinetic and ataxic dysarthria, J Acoust Soc Am 107:3415, 2000.

74. Liss JM et al: The effects of familiarization on intelligibility and lexical segmentation in hypokinetic and ataxic dysarthria, J Acoust Soc Am 112:3022, 2002.

75. Logeman J: Evaluation and treatment of swallowing disorders, San Diego, 1983, College-Hill Press.

76. Manto M: Isolated cerebellar dysarthria associated with heat stroke, Clin Neurol Neurosurg 98:55, 1996.

77. Marien P, Engelborghs S, DeDeyn P: Cerebellar neurocognition: a new avenue, Acta Neurol Belg 101:96, 2001.

78. Mayo Clinic Department of Neurology: Mayo Clinic examinations in neurology, ed 7, St Louis, 1998, Mosby.

79. McClean MD, Beukelman DR, Yorkston KM: Speech-muscle visuomotor tracking in dysarthric and nonimpaired speakers, J Speech Hear Res 30:276, 1987.

80. McNeil MR et al: Oral structure nonspeech motor control in normal, dysarthric, aphasic, and apraxic speakers: isometric force and static position, J Speech Hear Res 33:255, 1990.

81. Middleton FA, Strick PL: Basal ganglia and cerebellar loops: motor and cognitive circuits, Brain Res Rev 31:236, 2000.

82. Miller RM, Groher ME: Medical speech pathology, Rockville, Md, 1990, Aspen Publishers.

83. Murdoch BE et al: Respiratory kinematics in speakers with cerebellar disease, J Speech Hear Res 34:768, 1991.

84. Murry T: The production of stress in three types of dysarthric speech. In Berry W, editor: Clinical dysarthria, Boston, 1983, College-Hill Press.

85. Netsell R, Kent R: Paroxysmal ataxic dysarthria, J Speech Hear Disord 41:93, 1976.

86. Ozawa Y et al: Symptomatic differences in decreased alternating motion rates between individuals with spastic and with ataxic dysarthria: an acoustic analysis, Folia Phoniatr Logop 53:67, 2001.

87. Paslawski TM, Duffy JR, Vernino SA: Paraneoplastic cerebellar degeneration: a speech retrospective, Presented at the annual convention of the American Speech-Language-Hearing Association, November 2002.

88. Portnoy RA, Aronson AE: Diadochokinetic syllable rate and regularity in normal and in spastic ataxic dysarthria subjects, J Speech Hear Disord 47:324, 1982.

89. Putnam AHB: Review of research in dysarthria. In Winitz H, editor: Human communication and its disorders, a review 1988, Norwood, NJ, 1988, Ablex Publishing Corp.

90. Quinn N: Multiple system atrophy—the nature of the beast, J Neurol Neurosurg Psychiatry Special Supplement:78, 1989.

91. Ropper AH: The Guillain-Barré syndrome, N Engl J Med 326:1130, 1992.

92. Rossor MN: Dementia as part of other degenerative diseases. In Bradley WG et al, editors: Neurology in clinical practice: principles of diagnosis and management, vol 2, ed 3, Boston, 2000, Butterworth-Heinemann.

93. Rust RS: Neurocutaneous disorders. In Noseworthy JH, editor: Neurological therapeutics: principles and practice, vol 2, New York, 2003, Martin Dunitz.

94. Scripture EW: Records of speech in disseminated sclerosis, Brain 39:455, 1916.

95. Simmons N: Acoustic analysis of ataxic dysarthria: an approach to monitoring treatment. In Berry W, editor: Clinical dysarthria, Boston, 1983, College-Hill Press.

96. Tatsumi IF et al: Acoustic properties of ataxic and parkinsonian speech, in syllable repetition tasks, Annu Bull Res Inst Logop Phoniatr 13:99, 1979.

97. Trouillas P et al: International cooperative ataxia rating scale for pharmacological assessment of the cerebellar syndrome, J Neurol Sci 145:858, 1997.

98. von Cramon D: Bilateral cerebellar dysfunctions in a unilateral mesodiencephalic lesion. J Neurol Neurosurg Psychiatry 44:361, 1981.

99. Walshe F: Diseases of the nervous system, ed 11, New York, 1973, Longman.

100. Wood NW, Harding AE: Cerebellar and spinocerebellar disorders. In Bradley WG et al, editors: Neurology in clinical practice: principles of diagnosis and management, vol 2, ed 3, Boston, 2000, Butterworth-Heinemann.

101. Yorkston KM, Beukelman DR: Ataxic dysarthria: treatment sequences based on intelligibility and prosodic considerations, J Speech Hear Disord 46:398, 1981.

102. Yorkston KM et al: Assessment of stress patterning. In McNeil M, Rosenbek J, Aronson A, editors: The dysarthrias: physiology, acoustics, perception, management, Austin, Tex, 1984, Pro-Ed.

103. Yorkston KM et al: Management of motor speech disorders in children and adults, Austin, Tex, 1999, Pro-Ed.

104. Ziegler W: Task-related factors in oral motor control, Brain Lang 80:556, 2002.

105. Ziegler W, Wessel K: Speech timing in ataxic disorders, Neurology 47:208, 1996.

Hypokinetic Dysarthria

"I became conscious that my voice tended to sound flat and lacking in expression . . . . My voice had become softer, and I was unable to enunciate certain words clearly . . . if I went on talking, my voice would fail, and I could do no more than whisper . . . ."[119]

A.W.S. Thompson

CHAPTER OUTLINE

   I. **Anatomy and basic functions of the basal ganglia control circuit**
  II. **Clinical characteristics of basal ganglia control circuit disorders associated with hypokinetic dysarthria**
 III. **Etiologies**
      A. Degenerative diseases
      B. Vascular conditions
      C. Toxic-metabolic conditions
      D. Trauma
      E. Infectious conditions
      F. Other
  IV. **Speech pathology**
      A. Distribution of etiologies, lesions, and severity in clinical practice
      B. Patient perceptions and complaints
      C. Clinical findings
      D. Acoustic and physiologic findings
   V. **Cases**
  VI. **Summary**

Hypokinetic dysarthria is a perceptually distinctive motor speech disorder (MSD) associated with basal ganglia control circuit pathology. It may be manifest in any or all of the respiratory, phonatory, resonatory, and articulatory levels of speech, but its characteristics are most evident in *voice, articulation,* and *prosody.* The disorder reflects the effects of rigidity, reduced force and range of movement, and slow individual but sometimes fast repetitive movements on speech. Decreased range of movement is a significant contributor to the disorder, hence its designation as *hypokinetic* dysarthria.

Hypokinetic dysarthria is encountered as the primary speech pathology in a large medical practice at a rate comparable to that for most other major single dysarthria types. Based on data for primary communication disorder diagnoses within the Mayo Clinic Speech Pathology practice, it accounts for 8.2% of all dysarthrias and 7.6% of all MSDs (see Figure 1-3).

The identification of hypokinetic dysarthria can aid neurologic diagnosis and localization. Its presence is strongly associated with basal ganglia pathology and is often tied to a depletion or relative insufficiency of the neurotransmitter *dopamine. Parkinson's disease (PD)* is the prototypic, but not the only, disease associated with hypokinetic dysarthria.

The clinical features of hypokinetic dysarthria reflect the effects on speech of aberrations in the maintenance of proper background tone and supportive neuromuscular activity on which the quick, discrete, phasic movements of speech are superimposed. The disorder permits inferences about the role of the basal ganglia control circuit in providing an adequate neuromuscular environment for voluntary motor activity. Hypokinetic speech often gives the impression that its underlying movements are "all there" but have been attenuated in range or amplitude and restricted in their flexibility and speed.

ANATOMY AND BASIC FUNCTIONS OF THE BASAL GANGLIA CONTROL CIRCUIT

The basal ganglia control circuit consists of the basal ganglia and their connections. Its components were described in some detail in Chapter 2. Here briefly summarized are its structures, pathways, and functions that are most relevant to speech.

The basal ganglia are located deep within the cerebral hemispheres. They include the *striatum,* composed of the *caudate nucleus* and *putamen,* and the *lentiform nucleus,* composed of the *putamen* and *globus pallidus.* The *substantia nigra* and *subthalamic nuclei* are anatomically and functionally closely related to the basal ganglia. Basal ganglia activities are strongly associated with the actions of the indirect activation pathway or extrapyramidal system.

The interconnections that make up the basal ganglia control circuit are complex. The basic components include: (1) cortical, thalamic, and substantia nigra input to the striatum, with crucial cortical input coming from the frontal lobe premotor cortex; (2) striatum input to the substantia nigra and globus pallidus; (3) globus pallidus input to the thalamus, subthalamic nucleus, red nucleus, and reticular formation in the brainstem. These connections form loops in which information is returned to its origin. For example, basal ganglia input to the thalamus is relayed to the cortex and returned to its origin in the basal ganglia; striatum input to the substantia nigra returns to the striatum; globus pallidus input to the subthalamic nucleus is returned to the globus pallidus. The major efferent pathways of the basal ganglia originate in the globus pallidus.

The functions of the circuit are to *regulate muscle tone; regulate movements that support goal-directed activities* (e.g., the arm swing during walking); *control postural adjustments during skilled movements* (e.g., stabilize the shoulder during writing); *adjust movements to the environment* (e.g., speaking with restricted jaw movement); and *assist in the learning, selection, and initiation of movements.* Damage to the circuit either reduces movement or results in a failure to inhibit involuntary movement. In hypokinetic dysarthria, speech deficits are mostly associated with reductions of movement.

The primary influence of the basal ganglia control circuit on speech is through its connections with motor areas of the cerebral cortex.* Its influence on the cortex appears inhibitory; that is, it damps or modulates cortical output that would otherwise be in excess of that required to accomplish movement goals. The circuit helps to maintain a stable musculoskeletal environment in which discrete movements can occur. Excessive or insufficient damping of cortical output results in movement disorders.

Imbalances among neurotransmitters are responsible for many motor problems associated with basal ganglia control circuit malfunction. The actions of

dopamine are of particular importance to understanding PD and its associated hypokinetic dysarthria. When substantia nigra neurons are destroyed, the dopamine supply to the striatum is reduced and its role in the circuit is diminished. The functional results of this are discussed in the next section.

■ CLINICAL CHARACTERISTICS OF BASAL GANGLIA CONTROL CIRCUIT DISORDERS ASSOCIATED WITH HYPOKINETIC DYSARTHRIA

Parkinsonism serves as a model for discussing the clinical characteristics of basal ganglia control circuit disorders that result in hypokinesia. PD and parkinsonism are by far the most common causes of hypokinetic dysarthria (Box 7-1). The pathophysiology of PD and parkinsonism are discussed in the next section. At this point, only nonoromotor characteristics of parkinsonism are addressed.

The nonspeech motor characteristics of parkinsonism are summarized in Table 7-1. The classic signs are *tremor at rest, rigidity, bradykinesia,* and *a loss of postural reflexes.*

The *tremor* in parkinsonism is a *static* or *resting tremor* that occurs at a rate of approximately 3 to 8 Hz.[7] It is most apparent when the body part is relaxed, and it tends to decrease during voluntary movement. It is often apparent in the limbs and head but may also be evident in the jaw, lips, and tongue. A *pill-rolling* movement between the thumb and forefinger may be present.

Slowness of movement and a feeling of stiffness or tightness characterize *rigidity.* It is apparent during passive stretch on muscles and probably contributes to paucity of movement. It may be the result of excessive central nervous system (CNS) influence on alpha motor neurons, which occurs because excessive cortical motor output is not properly inhibited by the basal ganglia.[4] Unlike spasticity, in which resistance to movement is usually greatest at the beginning of stretch and is biased in direction, rigidity is associated with resistance in all directions and through the full range of movement. *Cogwheel rigidity,* in which resistance of the limbs to passive stretch has a jerky character, is common.

Posture tends to be characterized by involuntary flexion of the head, trunk, and arms. Because postural reflexes are impaired, the patient may be unable to make adjustments to tilting or falling and have difficulty turning in bed or moving from a sitting to standing position.

Bradykinesia is a problem in the speed with which muscles can be activated. It is characterized by delays or false starts at the beginning of movement and slowness of movement once begun. Movement may also be difficult to stop, and repetitive

---

*Sensory motor integration is a component of the operations of the basal ganglia control circuit. Preliminary evidence indicates that these operations include modulation of auditory feedback for the control of vocalization.[71] This may be relevant to clinical observations that speakers with hypokinetic dysarthria and reduced loudness are poorly calibrated in their judgments of the adequacy of their vocal loudness (i.e., they overestimate it).

<table>
<tr><td rowspan="2">box</td><td rowspan="2">7-1</td><td>Etiologies for 167 quasirandomly selected cases with a primary speech pathology diagnosis of hypokinetic dysarthria at the Mayo Clinic from 1969-1990 and from 1999-2001. Percentage of cases for each etiology is given in parentheses. Specific etiologies under each heading are ordered from most to least frequent.</td></tr>
</table>

Degenerative (78%)

Parkinson's disease (36%)
Parkinsonism (22%)
PSP (7%)
Unspecified degenerative CNS disease (5%)
Shy-Drager syndrome (2%)
Multiple systems atrophy (4%)
Lewy body disease (1%)
Parkinsonism + amyotrophic lateral sclerosis (1%)

Vascular (9%)

Nonhemorrhagic stroke (5%)
Nonparenchymal bleeds (subarachnoid hemorrhage, subdural hematoma) (1%)
Ruptured aneurysm (1%)
Small vessel disease (1%)
Anoxia (cardiac arrest) (1%)

Undetermined (4%)

Extrapyramidal disorder (1%)
PD vs. PSP (2%)
PSP vs. stroke (1%)
Multiple (4%)
Parkinsonism + multiple sclerosis or stroke; Alzheimer's disease or dementia + stroke; PD + subdural hematoma or stroke

Toxic or Metabolic (2%)

Drug related (phenothiazines, unspecified) (1%)
Carbon monoxide (1%)

Traumatic (1%)

Closed head injury

Infectious (1%)

Postencephalitic parkinsonism; encephalitis

Other (1%)

Radiation necrosis; basal ganglia calcification

CNS, Central nervous system; *PD*, Parkinson's disease; *PSP*, progressive supranuclear palsy.

table 7-1	Common nonspeech clinical signs of parkinsonism
Primary Deficits	**Examples**
Resting Tremor	Head
	Limb
	Pill-rolling
	Jaw, lip, tongue
Rigidity	Resistance to passive stretch in all directions through full range of movement
	Paucity of movement
Bradykinesia or Hypokinesia	Slow initiation & speed of movements
	"Freezing"
Akinesia	Festinating gait
	Reduced:
	Arm swing during walking
	Limb gestures during speech
	Eye blinking
	Head movement accompanying vertical & horizontal eye movement
	Frequency of swallowing
	Micrographia
	Masked facies
Postural Abnormalities	Stooped posture (flexed head & trunk)
	Poor adjustment to tilting or falling
	Difficulty turning in bed
	Difficulty going from sitting to standing

movements may be decreased in amplitude and speed. In spite of a desire to move, there may be intermittent *"freezing"* or immobility (akinesia). Bradykinesia or akinesia frequently are "the key feature of parkinsonian off-states, periods when brain levels of dopamine are inadequate."[31]

The terms *hypokinesia* (reduced movement) and *akinesia* (absence of movement) are often used interchangeably with bradykinesia. In addition to slowness, however, they also refer to underactivity or reduced range of movement, reduced use of an affected body part, and a reduction of the automatic, habitual movements that accompany natural movement. This probably cannot be attributed solely to weakness because *strength is thought to be relatively unimpaired in parkinsonism.* However, Corcos et al.[24] have shown that withdrawal of antiparkinsonian medications does produce muscle weakness that is attributable to reduced agonist muscle activation and, in some patients, increased antagonist muscle activation. The authors suggested that patients with PD might benefit from exercise programs designed to improve strength and power, a notion embraced by some behavioral programs for treating hypokinetic dysarthria (see Chapter 17).

The underactivity of hypokinesia is reflected in a masked or expressionless and unblinking facial expression *(masked facies),** a classic feature of

---

*Studies have documented that the intensity of spontaneous emotional expression is reduced in PD, but that posed facial expression and emotional feelings generally are not.[15,109]

parkinsonism (Figure 7-1). Similarly, the normal arm swing during walking and the limb gestures that automatically accompany speech may be reduced. Writing may be *micrographic* (small). Walking may be initiated slowly and then characterized by short, rapid shuffling steps, a phenomenon known as *festination*.

It is possible that a number of problems associated with hypokinesia are influenced by deficits in sensory function. Kent et al.[67] reviewed the growing evidence of impaired sensory function in PD, such as difficulties estimating movement displacements on the basis of kinesthetic information, and poor temporal discrimination of auditory, tactile, and visual stimuli. Summarizing the conclusions of Demirci et al.,[29] they stated: "the reduced kinesthesia, combined with reduced motor output and the likelihood of reduced corollary discharges, could mean that the sensorimotor apparatus is 'set' smaller in PD." The possible role of sensory disturbances in hypokinetic dysarthria is addressed in some speech therapy programs for the disorder (see Chapter 17).

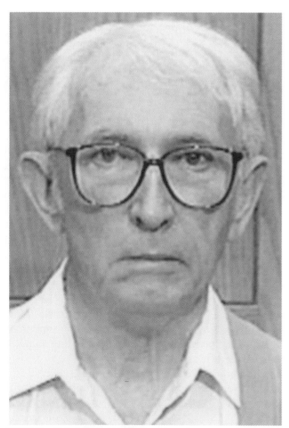

FIGURE 7-1 Masked facial expression associated with Parkinson's disease and hypokinetic dysarthria.

■ ETIOLOGIES

Any process that can damage the basal ganglia control circuit can cause hypokinetic dysarthria. These include degenerative, vascular, traumatic, inflammatory, neoplastic, toxic, and metabolic diseases. The exact distribution of causes of hypokinetic dysarthria is unknown, but degenerative diseases are undoubtedly the most frequent known causes (see Figure 7-1 and Box 7-1).

PD is almost certainly the most frequent cause of hypokinetic dysarthria. Also, in the absence of other influences (e.g., medication effects), hypokinetic dysarthria is *the* dysarthria of PD. This sometimes leads to the use of such terms as "the dysarthria of PD" or "parkinsonian dysarthria." The term *hypokinetic* dysarthria is preferable, however, because conditions other than PD can be associated with it. In addition, patients with PD may have more than hypokinetic dysarthria. For example, medication used to treat PD sometimes causes involuntary movements that result in hyperkinetic dysarthria. Also, some patients with an initial diagnosis of PD ultimately receive a different diagnosis, one indicating the presence of more than basal ganglia dysfunction (e.g., progressive supranuclear palsy [PSP]).

Some of the common neurologic conditions associated with hypokinetic dysarthria with noticeably greater frequency than other dysarthria types are discussed later. Other diseases that can produce it but are more frequently associated with other dysarthria types, especially mixed dysarthrias, are discussed in the chapters that address those specific dysarthria categories.

Degenerative Diseases

PD is a common, slowly progressive idiopathic neurologic disease that affects approximately 50 people per 100,000 older than the age of 50. It usually begins in mid-to-later life; survival from symptom onset is approximately 9 years. Its occurrence can be sporadic, but nearly one third of people with two or more affected first-degree relatives are likely to acquire the disease; unidentified environmental toxins such as herbicides and pesticides are other possible causes.[88] Although dysarthria usually does not emerge for several years after the onset of other signs of PD, Müller et al.[95] found that it did become evident in approximately 90% of autopsy-confirmed cases during the course of the disease, nearly always preceding the onset of dysphagia, which occurred in approximately 40% of cases.

PD may affect more than motor function. Ten to thirty percent of affected people eventually develop significant dementia, and depression occurs in 40%

to 60%.[31] Sometimes akinesia and bradykinesia are mistaken for depression, and the diagnosis of PD is missed.

The pathologic changes of PD most often involve nerve cell loss in the substantia nigra and locus ceruleus, as well as decreased dopamine content in the striatum. The imbalance between dopamine and acetylcholine caused by the depletion of dopamine in the striatum is thought to be responsible for clinical signs of the disease. PD tends to be responsive to *dopaminergic drugs* (known as *dopamine agonists*), but such drugs are not curative. *Carbidopa-levodopa (Sinemet)* is the cornerstone of treatment of PD. It works by increasing dopamine levels in the striatum; the carbidopa component prevents destruction of levodopa in the bloodstream and minimizes side effects. Direct-acting dopamine agonists, including *bromocriptine (Parlodel), pergolide (Permax), pramipexole (Mirapex),* and *ropinirole (Requip)* are sometimes used in place of Sinemet. Some newly diagnosed, mildly impaired PD patients are treated with *amantadine (Symmetrel), selegiline (Eldepryl), trihexyphenidyl (Artane),* or *benztropine (Cogentin),* but those drugs are less potent than Sinemet or direct-acting dopamine agonists.[7] *Anticholinergic drugs* may be used for resting tremor.

Unfortunately, the medications used to treat PD have side effects that include dystonia and dyskinesias, confusion, and *on-off effects.* On-off effects are symptom fluctuations that occur during a dosage cycle; they may include shifts from worsening of parkinsonian symptoms to the development of dystonia or dyskinesias at the beginning, peak, or end of a dosage cycle. Worsening of hypokinetic dysarthria or the emergence of hyperkinetic dysarthria may occur as reflections of on-off effects. Thus the dysarthria encountered in people with PD can represent the effects of the disease itself, as well as the effects of medications used to treat it. The design of clinical and laboratory investigations of hypokinetic dysarthria in PD must take into account medication effects, and they need to control for the time at which observations are made during the dosage cycle, especially in longitudinal investigations.

The term PD is usually reserved for parkinsonism of unknown cause that is responsive to levodopa treatment. In contrast, *parkinsonism* is a more generic term that refers to the clinical signs of the disease regardless of etiology. Parkinsonism is often used to refer to conditions with etiologies and pathophysiology that are different from PD (e.g., vascular, Alzheimer's disease [AD], drug induced), or when symptoms are not responsive to medications that are effective in managing PD.

Degenerative neurologic diseases that include but go beyond signs and symptoms of parkinsonism are often called *parkinsonism-plus syndromes* or *atypical parkinsonian disorders.* They include *multiple system atrophy* (with subtypes of *Shy-Drager syndrome, olivopontocerebellar atrophy,* and *nigrostriatal degeneration), PSP,* and *corticobasal degeneration.* Although hypokinetic dysarthria can be the only MSD encountered in each of these disorders, it is generally more common for a mixed dysarthria to be associated with them. Because of this, further discussion of the parkinsonism-plus conditions is deferred until Chapter 10, which addresses mixed dysarthrias.

Some primary dementing illnesses can be associated with parkinsonian signs. Although AD is marked clinically by its progressive effects on memory, thought, language, and personality, parkinsonian signs have been noted in 35% to 50% of patients with AD.[80,89] *Diffuse Lewy body disease,* characterized early in its course by relatively mild parkinsonian and more severe cognitive symptoms (e.g., dementia, visual hallucinations, paranoid delusions), straddles the boundary between AD and PD. In it, Lewy bodies, a pathologic hallmark of PD, are found not only in the substantia nigra, as in PD, but also in the cerebral cortex.[22] Finally, *Pick's disease,* a dementing illness with primary effects on the frontal and temporal lobes, although not usually associated with motor or sensory deficits, can be associated with signs of parkinsonism late in its course.[96] Thus the development of hypokinetic dysarthria is possible in some degenerative diseases whose primary manifestations are in the cognitive domain.

Vascular Conditions

Although strokes usually do not cause parkinsonism or hypokinetic dysarthria, diffuse frontal lobe white matter lesions and basal ganglia lesions* occasionally are associated with parkinsonian signs; gait difficulty and postural instability, dementia, corticospinal signs, and pseudobulbar affect are more prevalent than in PD.[121,125,126] This entity is frequently called *vascular parkinsonism.* It is not generally responsive to levodopa therapy.[125]

Cerebral hypoxia, including that induced by carbon monoxide poisoning, can also produce parkinsonian syndromes.

Toxic-Metabolic Conditions

Antipsychotic (neuroleptic) and *antiemetic*[†] *medications,* known as *dopamine antagonist drugs,* can

---

*Dysarthria with hypokinetic features has even been reported in bilateral thalamic strokes.[3]

---

†Drugs to relieve nausea or prevent or arrest vomiting.

have prominent blocking effects on dopamine receptors*; such drugs lead to parkinsonism in an estimated 10% to 20% of patients treated with them.[92] Parkinsonism can also be caused by drugs that interfere with the brain's ability to store dopamine *(dopamine depletors); reserpine* and *tetrabenazine*, used to treat tardive dyskinesia and Tourette's syndromes, are such drugs.[†] *Bupropion (Wellbutrin),* an antidepressant, has infrequently been associated with bradykinesia, pseudoparkinsonism, and dysarthria[108]; the dysarthria has not been described, but it is probably hypokinetic. Parkinsonism induced by dopamine antagonist drugs usually develops within the first 2 months of treatment[8] and tends to resolve within weeks to months after withdrawal.[4,92]

Chronic or toxic exposure to heavy metals (e.g., manganese) or to chemicals such as carbon disulfide, cyanide, and methanol can create a parkinsonian syndrome through their effects on the basal ganglia. Temporary parkinsonism can occur during alcohol withdrawal.[92]

Acquired metabolic disorders, including those associated with *liver failure, hypoparathyroidism,* and *central pontine myelinolysis* (discussed in Chapter 10) can damage the basal ganglia and cause parkinsonism.[92]

Wilson's disease, which can lead to abnormal copper depositions in the liver and brain, can produce parkinsonian signs, including hypokinetic dysarthria. Because it may also affect structures outside the basal ganglia, Wilson's disease is frequently associated with mixed dysarthria; it is discussed further in Chapter 10.

Trauma

Bradykinesia, rigidity, and tremor are among the many neuromotor deficits that may be caused by a single-event traumatic brain injury (TBI) that causes loss of consciousness. Repeated head trauma, as can occur in boxers *(dementia pugilistica),* can damage the substantia nigra. Over time, this can lead to parkinsonian-like motor abnormalities (including hypokinetic dysarthria), as well as dementia and ataxia.

Neurosurgery, including stereotactically guided lesioning and deep brain stimulation of the thalamus and globus pallidus, have been effective in relieving limb tremor and dyskinesias associated with PD.

---

*These drugs include phenothiazines (e.g., chlorpromazine), butyrophenones (e.g., haloperidol), thioxanthenes (e.g., thioxene), dibenzazepines (e.g., loxapine), and substituted benzamides (e.g., metoclopramide).[92]

[†]See Molho and Factor[92] for a list of other medications that may cause or worsen parkinsonism.

However, such treatments, especially when bilateral, carry risks for temporary or persisting speech deficits, including the development of dysarthria or worsening of a preexisting dysarthria.[46,107,115]

Infectious Conditions

Many cases of parkinsonism emerged in the aftermath of a viral encephalitis epidemic during and after World War I; this no-longer-occurring condition is known as *postencephalitic parkinsonism.* Today, other viral encephalitides are sometimes associated with parkinsonism.[42] *Acquired immunodeficiency syndrome (AIDS)* is thought to be the most common infectious cause of parkinsonism. Uncommon infectious causes include *Creutzfeldt-Jacob disease, syphilis, tuberculosis, Whipple's disease*, and *mycoplasma pneumoniae.*[92]

Other

Normal pressure hydrocephalus (NPH) (defined in Chapter 6) and *obstructive hydrocephalus* can be associated with parkinsonism, including hypokinetic dysarthria. Ataxic features (including ataxic dysarthria), dementia, and incontinence are also often present.

Parkinsonism can be a significant or minor component of many inherited diseases. Some examples include Wilson's disease, Huntington's disease, familial basal ganglia calcification, some dominantly inherited spinocerebellar ataxias, and some rare inborn errors of metabolism.[92] Some of these conditions are addressed in Chapters 6, 8, and 10.

■ SPEECH PATHOLOGY

Distribution of Etiologies, Lesions, and Severity in Clinical Practice

Box 7-1 and Figure 7-2 summarize the etiologies for 167 quasirandomly selected cases seen at the Mayo Clinic with a speech pathology diagnosis of hypokinetic dysarthria. The cautions expressed in Chapter 4 about generalizing these data to the general population or to all speech pathology practices also apply here.

The data establish that hypokinetic dysarthria can have numerous etiologies, the distribution of which are different from that associated with several other dysarthria types. Degenerative diseases accounted for 78% of the cases, of which three quarters had diagnoses of PD or parkinsonism. Unspecified "CNS degenerative disease" was the diagnosis for several cases; parkinsonism was suspected in some of these, but others had signs of more than basal ganglia degeneration (e.g., dementia or cerebellar findings).

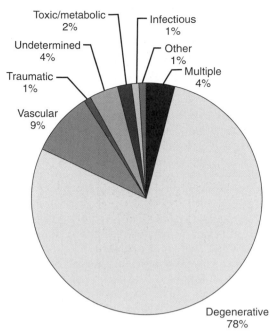

FIGURE 7-2 Distribution of etiologies for 167 quasirandomly selected cases with a primary speech pathology diagnosis of hypokinetic dysarthria at the Mayo Clinic from 1969-1990 and from 1999-2001 (see Box 7-1 for details).

The remaining degenerative diseases included conditions associated with multiple system atrophy or one of its subtypes, Lewy body disease, and parkinsonism plus amyotrophic lateral sclerosis.

Nonhemorrhagic stroke accounted for the largest proportion of the relatively small number of vascular etiologies. This small number is consistent with clinical impressions that hypokinetic dysarthria is an uncommon result of stroke. The remaining vascular etiologies included hemorrhagic events, small vessel disease, and anoxia resulting from cardiac arrest.

The 4% of cases with undetermined etiology had diagnostic possibilities that included PD, PSP, and stroke. In several of these cases, signs and symptoms were of recent onset or were subtle. It is likely that a more definitive diagnosis emerged over time.

The small percentage of cases (2%) with toxic or metabolic etiology is generally consistent with predictions from the literature (e.g., phenothiazine use, carbon monoxide poisoning).

Two cases had closed head injuries, illustrating that the frequent significant effect of head injuries on subcortical structures can produce hypokinetic dysarthria. A few cases had more than one disease, any of which might have caused the dysarthria (i.e., parkinsonism, stroke, and multiple sclerosis). The remaining causes included postencephalitic parkinsonism, encephalitis, basal ganglia calcification, and an unusual case with parkinsonian signs following radiation therapy.

These cases support the status of PD and parkinsonism as prototypes of diseases associated with hypokinetic dysarthria, and they establish that vascular, toxic-metabolic, traumatic, and infectious conditions can also produce the disorder. As might be expected, nearly all patients had nonspeech deficits that were clinically localized to the basal ganglia control circuit, although not necessarily limited to it. Neuroimaging (e.g., computed tomography [CT] scan, magnetic resonance imaging [MRI]) in most cases, however, was either negative or revealed only mild cerebral atrophy or enlarged ventricles. This is common in idiopathic PD and related degenerative diseases that include the basal ganglia. Most vascular and traumatic cases had neuroimaging evidence of lesions in or near the basal ganglia but not always bilaterally; however, patients with only unilateral lesions on neuroimaging nonetheless usually had bilateral clinical signs, indicating the presence of bilateral pathology.

This retrospective review did not permit a precise description of dysarthria severity. However, in those patients for whom a judgment about intelligibility was stated (75% of the sample), *77% had reduced intelligibility*. The degree to which this figure accurately estimates the frequency of intelligibility impairments in the population with hypokinetic dysarthria is unclear. It is likely that many patients for whom an observation of intelligibility was not made had normal intelligibility, but the sample probably contains a larger number of mildly impaired patients than is encountered in many rehabilitation settings. In general, however, it is reasonable to conclude that intelligibility is frequently reduced by hypokinetic dysarthria.

Finally, cognitive impairment was common in this sample. For patients whose cognitive abilities were explicitly commented on or formally assessed (84% of the sample), *72% had some degree of cognitive impairment.**

Patient Perceptions and Complaints

Affected people may describe their speech in ways that provide clues to diagnosis and its localization. Although they frequently report that others tell them their voice is *quieter* or *weak,* they often *deny or minimize such changes* themselves. Complaints that rate is *too fast* or that words are *indistinct* are common. Some report that it is *"hard to get speech started."* Some use the word *stutter* to describe sound, syllable, and word repetitions or difficulty

---

*Bayles et al.[10] found no evidence of language difficulty in a group of 75 people with PD who were not demented. Mildly demented PD patients did have difficulty on several measures of language performance.

initiating speech. It is rare that a patient associates such dysfluencies with anxiety, anticipation of difficulty, or specific word or sound fears.

Complaints about negative effects of *fatigue* on speech are not uncommon. Those with drug-responsive parkinsonism sometimes note *variations in speech during their medication cycle,* frequently characterized by deterioration just before their next dose. *Drooling* and *swallowing complaints* are not uncommon. Some report that their upper lip feels stiff, perhaps reflecting a perception of reduced movement flexibility.

Clinical Findings

Hypokinetic dysarthria usually occurs with other signs of basal ganglia disease, and it occurs frequently enough in parkinsonism for its recognition to serve as confirmatory evidence for the neurologic diagnosis. Even more important, it sometimes is the presenting complaint and only sign of parkinsonism. In such cases, recognition of the dysarthria as hypokinetic can be essential to localization and diagnosis.

Nonspeech Oral Mechanism

The oral mechanism examination can be revealing and often confirmatory of a diagnosis of hypokinetic dysarthria. The eyes may have a *reduced blink frequency.* The face may be *unsmiling, masked,* or *expressionless* at rest (see Figure 7-1) and *lack animation* during social interaction. Movements of the eyes and face, hands, arms, and trunk that normally accompany speech and complement the emotions and indirect meanings conveyed through prosody may be attenuated. Chest and abdominal movements during quiet breathing may be reduced, and excursion may remain reduced even when the patient attempts to breathe deeply.

As the eyes may blink infrequently, so may the patient *swallow infrequently,* perhaps another reflection of rigidity or reduced automatic movements. This may lead to excessive saliva accumulation and *drooling.* When moving the eyes to look to the side or up or down, the normal tendency for head turning to accompany the gaze may be reduced.

A tremor or *tremulousness* of the jaw and lips may be apparent at rest or during sustained mouth opening or lip retraction. Similarly, the tongue is often strikingly tremulous on protrusion or at rest within the mouth. The lips (particularly upper) can appear tight or immobile at rest and during movement, including speech. Jaw, face, and tongue strength may be grossly normal, often surprisingly so given their limited movement during speech. Nonspeech alternating motion rates (AMRs) of the jaw, lips, and tongue may be slowly initiated and completed or rapid and markedly restricted in range. In contrast, range of motion for single movements (e.g., lip retraction) may be normal or distinctly greater than that observed during speech or expected emotional responses.

The occurrence of swallowing problems in PD ranges from approximately 40% to 80%[66]; they are usually preceded by dysarthria. The median latency between disease onset to development of dysphagia is generally longer in PD (130 months) than other degenerative diseases associated with parkinsonism, and latency from disease onset to onset of dysphagia is strongly correlated with overall survival.[95]

The overall impression derived during casual observation and formal oral mechanism examination is one of a lack of vigor or animation in the absence of a degree of weakness that might explain it. At rest, as well as during social interaction and speech, the patient's facial affect appears restricted, unemotional, and sometimes depressed. These appearances may not accurately reflect the inner emotional state. Unfortunately, speech usually mirrors these nonverbal characteristics.

Speech

Conversational speech or reading, speech AMRs, and vowel prolongation all provide useful information about salient and distinguishing speech characteristics. Conversational speech and reading are essential for identifying the prosodic abnormalities that can be so prominent in the disorder. Speech AMRs are particularly useful for observing reductions in range of movement and rate abnormalities; although not always present, *rapid, accelerated, and sometimes "blurred" speech AMRs are distinguishing perceptual characteristics of hypokinetic dysarthria* (Figure 7-3). Vowel prolongation is useful for isolating some of the disorder's phonatory characteristics, especially those associated with loudness and quality.

Hypokinetic dysarthria usually reflects neuromuscular abnormalities at all levels of the speech system, usually related to restriction in the range or speed of movements. The effects of these abnormalities give hypokinetic dysarthria its distinctive characteristics, most of which are associated with phonatory and articulatory activities and the effects of those abnormalities on prosody.

Table 7-2 summarizes the neuromuscular deficits presumed by Darley, Aronson, and Brown (DAB)[27,28] to underlie hypokinetic dysarthria. Speech movements and their timing are generally accurate. Individual movements are slowed, but repetitive movements may be fast, especially when range of movement is limited. The range and force of individual and repetitive movements are reduced.

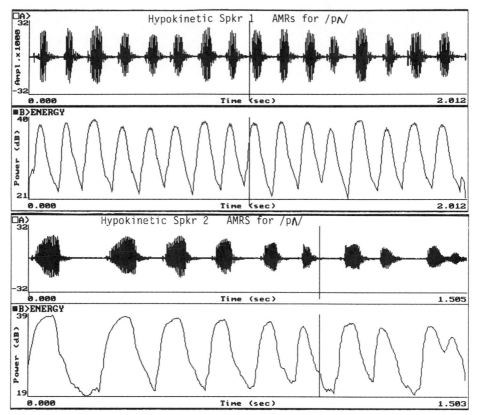

FIGURE 7-3 Raw waveform and energy tracings of speech alternate motion rates (AMRs) for /pʌ/ by two speakers with hypokinetic dysarthria. Speaker 1's AMRs (2 seconds) are regular but rapid (≈8 Hz). Speaker 2's productions (1.5 seconds) are normal in rate (≈6 Hz in the first second) but show a trend toward increased overall rate and reduced amplitude and duration of each pulse, the acoustic correlate of perceived accelerated rate.

table	7-2	Neuromuscular deficits associated with hypokinetic dysarthria					
Direction	**Rhythm**	**Rate**		**Range**		**Force**	**Tone**
Individual Movements	Repetitive Movements	Individual Movements	Repetitive Movements	Individual Movements	Repetitive Movements	Individual Movements	Muscle Tone
Normal	Regular	Slow	Fast	Reduced	Very reduced	Reduced (paretic)	Excessive (balanced)

Modified from Darley FL, Aronson, AE, Brown JR: Clusters of deviant speech dimensions in the dysarthrias, *J Speech Hear Res* 12:462, 1969b.

Muscle tone is often excessive (i.e., rigid) with resistance to movement in all directions, a condition that contributes to decreased range of movement. *Reduced range of movement may be the most significant underlying neuromuscular deficit in hypokinesia as it affects speech.* The relationships among these characteristics and the specific deviant characteristics associated with hypokinetic dysarthria are discussed in the next section. Experimental support for the presumed

underlying neuromuscular deficits are reviewed in the section on acoustic and physiologic findings.

Prominent Deviant Speech Characteristics and Clusters of Deviant Dimensions

A general profile of hypokinetic dysarthria was established by Logeman et al.,[82] who determined the frequency of deviant speech characteristics in a

	Deviant cluster of abnormal speech characteristics found in hypokinetic dysarthria
table 7-3	

Cluster	Speech Characteristics
Prosodic insufficiency	Monopitch
	Monoloudness
	Reduced stress
	Short phrases
	Variable rate*
	Short rushes of speech*
	Imprecise consonants*

Modified from Darley FL, Aronson, AE, Brown JR: Clusters of deviant speech dimensions in the dysarthrias, *J Speech Hear Res* 12:462, 1969b.
*Considered a component of prosodic insufficiency in hypokinetic dysarthria but not in other dysarthria types with prosodic insufficiency.

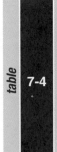

	The most deviant speech dimensions encountered in hypokinetic dysarthria by Darley, Aronson, and Brown,[27] listed in order from most to least severe. Also listed is the component of the speech system associated with each speech characteristic. The component "prosodic" is listed when several components of the speech system may contribute to the dimension.
table 7-4	

Dimension	Speech Component
Monopitch*	Phonatory-prosodic
Reduced stress*	Prosodic
Monoloudness*	Phonatory-respiratory-prosodic
Imprecise consonants	Articulatory
Inappropriate silences*	Prosodic
Short rushes of speech*	Articulatory-prosodic
Harsh voice quality	Phonatory
Breathy voice (continuous)	Phonatory
Low pitch	Phonatory
Variable rate*	Articulatory-prosodic
Other	
Increased rate in segments*	Prosodic
Increase of rate overall*	Prosodic
Repeated phonemes*	Articulatory

*Tend to be distinctive or more severely impaired than in any other single dysarthria type.

group of 200 people with PD. Approximately 90% had a speech deficit, attesting to the high prevalence of dysarthria in the disease. Eighty-nine percent had voice disorders characterized by *hoarseness, roughness, tremulousness,* and *breathiness*, and 45% had articulation problems. Twenty percent had rate abnormalities characterized by *syllable repetitions, shortened syllables, lengthened syllables,* and *excessive pauses*. Ten percent were *hypernasal*. Of interest, 45% had voice abnormalities only, and all patients with articulation problems had voice problems. The authors noted that this might reflect the existence of subgroups of dysarthrias in PD or the tendency for dysarthria to begin with laryngeal manifestations and eventually include articulation and other abnormalities. Zwirner and Barnes[129] also noted the higher frequency of laryngeal than articulatory impairment in PD.

DAB[28] found only one cluster of deviant speech dimensions in their group of parkinsonian patients. They labeled it *prosodic insufficiency* to represent the attenuated patterns of vocal emphasis that result from the combined effects of speech characteristics that make up the cluster. The characteristics include *monopitch, monoloudness, reduced stress, short phrases, variable rate, short rushes of speech,* and *imprecise consonants* (summarized in Table 7-3). Together, these features give hypokinetic dysarthria its distinctive gestalt of a flat, attenuated, and sometimes accelerated quality. The neuromuscular basis for the cluster was attributed by DAB to reduced range of movement and to the fast repetitive movements that are unique to parkinsonism.

Table 7-4 summarizes the most deviant speech characteristics encountered in hypokinetic dysarthria,[27] as well as the component of the speech system most prominently associated with each characteristic. The rankings in the table represent severity ratings of the speech characteristics and not necessarily the features that best distinguish hypokinetic dysarthria from other dysarthria types.

A few additional observations help to complete the picture of the disorder:

1. Logeman and Fisher[81] described the specific features of imprecise consonants. They found a predominance of manner errors, which occurred most frequently for stops, fricatives, and affricates. Stops, especially velars, were most frequently in error and were perceived as fricatives, presumably because of incomplete articulatory contact and continual emission of air during what should have been a stop period; this was also perceived for the stop portion of affricates. Fricatives were perceived as reduced in sharpness, presumably due to a reduced degree of articulatory constriction. These features are related to the acoustic feature of *spirantization* and may be the result of *articulatory undershooting* resulting from accelerated rate or reduced range of movement, or both.

2. Some prominent features of hypokinetic dysarthria are not captured in the cluster of prosodic insufficiency (compare the speech characteristics in Tables 7-3 and 7-4). For

example, frequently occurring *inappropriate silences* are not logically related to the neuromuscular deficits presumed to underlie prosodic insufficiency; they more likely reflect difficulty in initiating movements.

3. Harshness, breathiness, and reduced loudness are sometimes the first sign of hypokinetic dysarthria and parkinsonism. When marked, this dysphonia can have a *mildly strained, tight, aphonic,* or *whispered quality.* Even when not pervasively present, a strained-whispered aphonia will sometimes emerge from a breathy-harsh quality and persist for several seconds toward the end of a maximum vowel prolongation task; in the author's experience, this rarely occurs in other dysarthria types. In general, *dysphonia can be the presenting and most prominent and debilitating speech feature in people with hypokinetic dysarthria.*

4. Rate abnormalities can be a striking and highly distinctive feature of hypokinetic dysarthria. These often are apparent during AMRs, in which rate may be *rapid or accelerated;* combined with reduced range of articulatory excursions, they may have a "blurred" quality, as if all syllables are run together. In conversation or reading, patients may demonstrate *short rushes of speech* in which several words are uttered together, sometimes rapidly, and are separated from the remainder of the utterance by pauses that may occur at inappropriate intervals. Some patients demonstrate an apparent *increased speech rate within segments,* a characteristic that appears analogous to the festinating gait so often present in parkinsonism. Finally, some patients' *overall speech rate is rapid.* Although not always present, features that lead to a perception of rapid rate in hypokinetic dysarthria are unique among the dysarthrias.*

5. Dysfluencies in the form of *repeated phonemes* are not uncommon,[†] and some-

times they are prominent enough to be designated as stuttering.[72] They tend to occur at the beginning of utterances or following pauses. They are usually rapid and sometimes blurred and restricted in range of movement. When vowels and some consonants are "repeated," they may sound more like a prolonged vowel with a tremulous character. These features may be analogous to parkinsonian patients' difficulty in initiating walking ("freezing"), and the rapid, short shuffling steps that may occur as walking begins. Although dysfluencies or stuttering-like behavior can occur in several neurologic conditions (see Chapter 13), the specific character of repeated phonemes in hypokinetic dysarthria tend to be distinctive.

6. A disorder that can be associated with hypokinetic dysarthria and may be strongly related to phoneme repetitions is *palilalia,* a problem characterized by "compulsive reiteration of utterances in a context of increasing rate and decreasing loudness."[74] The repetitions usually involve words and phrases; phoneme repetitions are generally not subsumed in the disorder's definition. Palilalia is usually associated with bilateral subcortical pathology, especially involving the basal ganglia, but has also been noted in bilateral frontal lobe pathology.[14] It is discussed further in Chapter 13.

7. True voice tremor is uncommon in hypokinetic dysarthria. However, the voice may be unsteady and tremorlike in character secondary to the prominent head and upper limb tremor present in some patients. In addition, the voice during vowel prolongation is sometimes characterized by a rapid, low amplitude *tremulousness,* sometimes known as *flutter.* Logeman et al.[82] found vocal tremulousness in 14% of their 200 parkinsonian patients.

8. Abnormal resonance is not usually prominent, but mild hypernasality is probably present in 10% to 25% of patients with hypokinetic dysarthria.[27,28,82] Thus hypernasality and mild "weakening" of pressure consonants because of nasal airflow are acceptable abnormalities in the disorder; that is, they need not raise strong suspicions about another dysarthria type (particularly flaccid or spastic dysarthria) in people whose other deviant speech characteristics are consistent with hypokinetic dysarthria.

What features of hypokinetic dysarthria help distinguish it from other MSDs? Among all of the abnormal characteristics that may be detected,

---

*Note, however, that rapid speech rate can be idiosyncratic or associated with some nondysarthric neurologic and psychiatric conditions.

[†]Dysfluencies, including repetitions of sounds, syllables, and words, sound prolongations, and inappropriate silences and excessive pauses, have been observed in several group studies of hypokinetic speakers with PD.[11,27,82] Some suggest that dysfluencies are exacerbated by levodopa,[83] others suggest that increased dysfluency is associated with increased or decreased dopamine levels,[41] and still others report that dysfluencies are more frequent in PD patients with advanced disease regardless of whether they are in an on or off levodopa state.[11]

monopitch, monoloudness, reduced loudness, reduced stress, variable rate, short rushes of speech, overall increases in rate, increased rate within segments, rapid speech AMRs, repeated phonemes, and *inappropriate silences* are the most common distinctive clues to the presence of the disorder.

Table 7-5 summarizes the primary distinguishing, distinctive speech characteristics and common oral mechanism findings and patient complaints encountered in hypokinetic dysarthria.

Acoustic and Physiologic Findings

Although hypokinetic dysarthria is often clearly distinguishable from other dysarthria types, there is perceptual heterogeneity among patients with the disorder. This variability is also apparent, and perhaps even greater, within and among many acoustic and physiologic measures. Acoustic and physiologic abnormalities often exist in only some dysarthric patients under study, and a number of the abnormalities may also be found in other dysarthria types. In fact, some "abnormalities" may be normal if they are compared to appropriate age and gender-matched normative data. This may be the case for

hypokinetic dysarthria more than for any other dysarthria type, because several of its salient perceptual features (e.g., reduced loudness, hoarseness, breathiness) and acoustic correlates are common in elderly people without neurologic disease. With these caveats in mind, acoustic and physiologic measures have contributed to a richer description and better understanding of the disorder.

Respiration

Respiratory abnormalities occur frequently and are a common cause of death in parkinsonism.[30] Although respiration has received comparatively little attention in acoustic and physiologic studies of speech, it could logically contribute to some of the prominent features of the disorder, particularly those related to loudness and prosody. Reduced vital capacity, reduced amplitude of chest wall movements during breathing, reduced respiratory muscle strength and endurance, irregularities in breathing patterns, and increased respiratory rates have been documented.[55,69,76,111,122] Many abnormalities have been attributed to alterations in the normal agonist-antagonist relationships among respiratory muscles during breathing.

Of direct relevance to speech are data from speech and maximum performance vocal tasks. Reduced maximum vowel duration, reduced airflow volume during vowel prolongation, fewer syllables per breath group, use of greater than average percentage of vital capacity per syllable, and increased breath groups during reading have been documented in some patients with parkinsonism and presumed hypokinetic dysarthria.[12,20,55,69,94] It should be noted, however, that such characteristics could also reflect abnormalities at the laryngeal level. That respiratory abnormalities contribute to these characteristics in at least some patients is suggested by findings of abnormally small rib cage volumes and abnormally large abdominal volumes at the initiation of speech breath groups in PD speakers who produced fewer words per breath group and spoke for less time per breath group than normal speakers.[111] In addition, Murdoch et al.[97] found abrupt movements of chest wall parts and paradoxical movements of the rib cage and abdomen during vowel prolongation and syllable repetition tasks in approximately half of their 19 subjects with hypokinetic dysarthria; there was no unambiguous explanation for the abnormalities, but the authors speculated that rigidity of respiratory muscles might have been responsible. Finally, the presence of impaired respiratory control in some speakers is suggested by documentation of longer latencies before beginning exhalation following forceful inhalation, delayed initiation of phonation once exhalation begins, difficulty altering automatic

table 7-5	Primary distinguishing speech and speech-related findings in hypokinetic dysarthria
Perceptual	
Phonatory-respiratory	Reduced loudness
Articulatory	Repeated phonemes, palilalia, rapid or "blurred" AMRs
Prosodic	Reduced stress, monopitch, monoloudness, inappropriate silences
	Short rushes of speech, variable rate, increased rate in segments, increased overall rate
Physical	Masked facial expression
	Tremulous jaw, lip, tongue
	Reduced range of motion on AMR tasks
	Head tremor
Patient Complaints	Reduced loudness, rapid rate, "mumbling," "stuttering," difficulty initiating speech (often reported as what listeners tell them as opposed to their own perception)
	Stiff lips

AMR, Alternate motion rate.

respiratory rhythms for speech, and difficulty tracking a sinusoidal target with respiratory movements.[35,69,90]

Reduced respiratory excursions, reduced vital capacity, paradoxical respiratory movements, rapid breathing cycles, and difficulty altering vegetative breathing patterns for voluntary activities seem consistent with patterns of rigidity, hypokinesia, and difficulty initiating movements that occur in other muscle groups in parkinsonism. Such difficulties could contribute importantly to reduced physiologic support for speech and some of the disorder's phonatory and prosodic abnormalities, especially reduced loudness, short phrases, short rushes of speech, and inappropriate pauses.

Phonation

A number of acoustic and physiologic studies have examined laryngeal function in hypokinetic dysarthria. In general, they confirm hypotheses generated by perceptual analyses and provide additional insights into mechanisms underlying abnormal voice and speech characteristics.

1. *Fundamental frequency (f_o) and intensity.* Abnormal pitch is usually not a prominent perceptual feature of hypokinetic dysarthria, but several studies have reported elevated f_o.[19-21,53,58,61,68,84,85,106] However, the increase in f_o is not always statistically significant relative to age-matched norms,[68] and in females f_o is sometimes reduced.[53] For example, the median f_o for Canter's[19] male parkinsonian subjects was 129 Hz, compared to 106 Hz for age-matched male controls; Metter and Hanson[91] found that f_o fell mostly within the normal range in their PD patients, although with a tendency for it to increase with increased disease severity. These findings stand in contrast to the perceptual observation of DAB[27] that pitch tended to be perceived as low. The reasons for these discrepancies are not clear. It may be that there is considerable intersubject variability in f_o/pitch, that there are gender differences, or that factors other than f_o lead to a perception of low pitch (i.e., monopitch, monoloudness, and reduced loudness could lead to perceptions of lower pitch). The fact that pitch and f_o are neither generally nor extremely abnormal, however, suggests that they are not reliably sensitive distinguishing features of hypokinetic dysarthria.

    Measures of intensity have been less ambiguous. They generally document reduced vocal intensity during various speech, vowel prolongation, and AMR tasks.[33,39,51,53,58,68,106a] Ho, Iansek, and Bradshaw[51] found that speakers with PD had reduced conversational loudness at various distances from their listeners but did increase loudness as listener distance increased. These results were interpreted as a reflection of normal loudness regulation but within a context of a dampened "motor set" for loudness, analogous to the reduced range of limb movement associated with PD. It is also of interest that the PD patients' perceptual judgments overestimated speaker loudness as distance increased, raising the possibility that perceptual deficits played a role in their ability to set loudness for themselves. Finally, loudness problems (e.g., overall loudness, loudness decay) may be exacerbated under conditions of divided attention, such as speaking while performing a visual-manual tracking task.[52]

2. *f_o and intensity variability and the voice spectrum.* Measures of f_o and intensity variability are much more revealing. They have been examined in a wide variety of tasks, including vowel prolongation, spontaneous speech, reading, word and sentence imitation, emotional expression, pitch glide tasks, and tasks requiring a range of high or low pitch productions. Specific abnormalities are somewhat task dependent, with increased variability found on some measures and decreased variability on others. In general, acoustic findings provide strong support for perceptual ratings of monopitch and monoloudness (Figure 7-4).

    Many long-term measures (e.g., syllables, sentences) consistently document reduced f_o and loudness variability or range.*† The relevance of these findings to clinical practice is illustrated by Bunton et al.,[16] who documented reduced f_o range during sentence production in several speakers with PD. They then used a linear predictive coding (LPC) technique to artificially flatten f_o range during production of sentences in normal speakers and PD speakers. This resulted in reduced intelligibility in all subject groups, with the effect exaggerated in the dysarthric speakers. These findings support the perception of monopitch in hypokinetic dysarthria and

---

*Reduced loudness can interfere with other acoustic measures, as illustrated by Canter's[21] observation that he was unable to measure speech AMR rate in some of his patients because of "flattened intensity peaks."

†References 16, 17, 19, 20, 26, 53, 61, 84, 85, 91, 105.

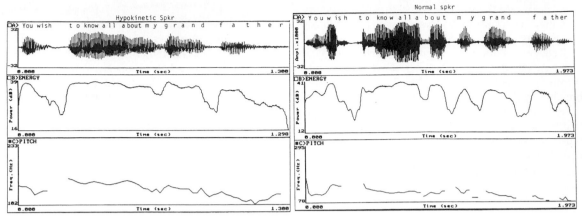

FIGURE 7-4 Raw waveform and energy and pitch (f$_o$) tracings for the sentence "You wish to know all about my grandfather" by a normal male speaker and a male with hypokinetic dysarthria. The normal speaker completes the sentence in approximately 2 seconds, the hypokinetic speaker in 1.3 seconds (66% of the normal speaker's rate, consistent with a perception of rapid rate). The energy tracing for the normal speaker has clearly defined syllables of varying duration; the hypokinetic speaker has few well-defined syllables, possibly reflecting the effects of rapid rate, continuous voicing, spirantization, and monoloudness. The speakers' pitch tracings are similar in contour, but the normal speaker has brief breaks in phonation during stop closure and voiceless consonants. The absence of breaks in phonation after the word "to" for the hypokinetic speaker probably reflects continuous voicing and spirantization.

attest to the perceptual contribution of f$_o$ variation to sentence-level intelligibility.*

In contrast to decreased variability of f$_o$ and intensity during sentence and maximum range tasks, long-term variability within vowel prolongation tasks is generally increased. For example, during vowel prolongation tasks PD speakers tend to have abnormally large standard deviations of f$_o$, and that variability is correlated with perceptual judgments of dysphonia.[32,129,130] In some studies, many hypokinetic speakers have abnormally high percentage variation in f$_o$ and variation in peak amplitude during sustained phonation.[64,68] Larson, Ramig, and Scherer,[75] who found abnormally high long-term amplitude perturbation in two speakers with PD, felt the abnormality might reflect relatively slow innervation fluctuations to laryngeal abductory or adductory muscles, supraglottic structures, or a combination of these.

A promising acoustic measure for capturing some of the abnormalities perceived in hypokinetic dysarthria, especially in connected speech, may lie in long-term average spectrum (LTAS) measures, which capture the shape of the distribution of energy in the

acoustic spectrum. Dromey[33] compared dysarthric speakers with PD to age-matched controls and found that LTAS measures distinguished the two groups on vowel prolongation, reading, and monologue tasks when other acoustic measures, such as sound pressure level and f$_o$ variability, did not. This suggests that some of the prominent qualitative deficits perceived in the hypokinetic voice may be more readily detectable in the spectrum of the voice than in "simpler" measures of frequency and intensity variability.

3. *Voice tremor.* Voice tremor is not a prominent perceptual feature of hypokinetic dysarthria, and the tremor that can be detected seems not to differ substantially from the tremor in normal individuals.[102] Nonetheless, visual and acoustic evidence of voice tremor is not uncommon. Schulz et al.[106] found evidence of laryngeal or arytenoid tremor on videostroboscopy in six people with PD, and Gallena et al.[40] documented laryngeal tremor in three of their six PD speakers. Perez et al.[101] observed that more than 50% of their 29 patients with PD or parkinson's plus syndromes had vertical laryngeal tremor or tremor of the arytenoid cartilages during endoscopic and stroboscopic examination.

Although voice tremor in the range of 4 to 7 Hz has been reported in some speakers with PD,[59] it is not pervasively present perceptu-

---

*Laures and Weismer[77] also demonstrated reduced sentence intelligibility by synthetically flattening f$_o$ in two normal speakers.

ally or acoustically and therefore not essential for a diagnosis of hypokinetic dysarthria. For example, Holmes et al.[53] found tremor in their patients with later-stage but not early-stage PD. Some investigators have found both amplitude and frequency fluctuations in the tremor, but others suggest that tremor is more likely in the frequency than the amplitude domain.[87,102,104,116]

Boutsen, Duffy, and Aronson[13] obtained acoustic confirmation of a perceived high-frequency tremor or flutter (one component in the 5 to 6 Hz range and another in the 9 to 11 Hz range) in a woman with PD, in which the tremor was more evident in amplitude than frequency modulation. The association of flutter with hypokinetic dysarthria is important to differential diagnosis, because flaccid dysarthria is the only other dysarthria type in which it has been observed.

4. *Maximum phonation time (MPT).* Adams[6] suggests that MPT for vowel prolongation may not be different from normal, perhaps because of test methods and inherent variability within and across individuals. However, King et al.[70] studied a group of PD subjects and documented significant longitudinal declines (3 to 36 months) in maximum and average duration of sustained vowel prolongation. Thus reliably obtained MPT may be sensitive to changes within individuals with hypokinetic dysarthria over time but not necessarily sensitive to detection of the disorder itself.

5. *Jitter, shimmer, and other indices of quality.* Speakers with PD may have abnormally high jitter and shimmer or related measures of the regularity of vocal fold vibration, possibly reflecting reduced short-term neuromuscular control of the laryngeal abductory or adductory mechanism.[6,53,75,85] Abnormal shimmer values have been correlated with perceptual measures of breathiness, a relationship that could be related to vocal fold bowing, with subsequent increased airflow turbulence and intensity variations.[85]

Abnormal jitter and shimmer values are not always found in hypokinetic speakers. For example, although Kent et al.[65] found females with PD to differ from female controls in shimmer, measures of jitter and shimmer failed to discriminate PD males from healthy males. They concluded that "there is reason to question the sensitivity of acoustic perturbation measures *[such as shimmer and jitter]* to voice function in

dysarthria, at least for the general purposes of identifying abnormality and classifying clinical groups."

Although abnormal signal-to-noise (S/N) ratios measured in vowels have been reported in some speakers with hypokinetic dysarthria, Adams[6] indicates that such abnormalities are not always present. For example, Kent et al.[65] found that S/N ratio failed to discriminate males with PD from healthy males.

6. *Motor control.* Several acoustic studies suggest that laryngeal control is reduced. There is evidence that some patients are slow to initiate phonation and that such events correlate with perceived inappropriate silences.[85] Relatedly, Lehiste[79] found evidence of voiceless transitions from vowels to following consonants within syllables, possibly attributable to incoordination of articulation and voicing. Canter[21] noted that perceived omission of final consonants in parkinsonian patients could be due to poor phonatory control. Other studies have found evidence of continuous voicing (see Figure 7-4) within sentences or on AMR tasks containing voiceless consonants.[63,85,105] These findings suggest difficulty with the rapid termination of voicing within utterances containing voiceless phonemes. Finally, McClean, Beukelman, and Yorkston's[90] PD patients had difficulty varying vocal pitch to control a cursor in order to track a visually displayed sinusoidal target.

7. *Laryngeal structure, movement, and airflow.* Laryngeal structure and functions for speech have received considerable attention. A comprehensive telescopic cinelaryngoscopy study of 32 unselected patients with PD by Hanson, Gerratt, and Ward[45] documented a number of visible abnormalities. Among the most striking was that only two patients were free of "abnormal phonatory posturing," and they had normal voices and no voice complaints. *Vocal fold bowing* during phonation, represented by a significant glottic gap but with tightly approximated vocal processes, was observed in 30 patients; the increased glottal gap was correlated with perceived breathiness and reduced intensity. Tremulousness of the arytenoid cartilages was apparent during quiet breathing in some subjects, but the perception of voice tremor seemed more strongly related to the secondary effects of head tremor. Laryngeal structure asymmetries were apparent in many patients, with asymmetries occurring in vocal

fold length, degree of bowing, and ventricular fold movements. Some patients exhibited approximation of the ventricular folds during phonation. Voice was often better for patients with supraglottic contraction, which may have assisted adduction and reduced breathiness. The authors noted that the vocal folds appeared solid, in spite of bowing, in contrast to the hypotonicity that may be present with lower motor neuron (LMN) paralyses. The evidence of increased adductor contraction, asymmetric contraction, and vocal fold bowing inconsistent with LMN lesions led to the conclusion that abnormalities in phonatory postures were related to laryngeal muscle rigidity.

The observations of Hanson, Gerratt, and Ward have been largely replicated and refined in subsequent studies. For example, findings of bowing and a glottal gap or incomplete vocal fold adduction during phonation have been replicated.[40,106,110] Perez et al.[101] observed a predominantly open phase configuration of the vocal folds during phonation (consistent with breathiness and reduced loudness); phase asymmetry (consistent with hoarseness) frequently was also evident endoscopically.

Electromyography (EMG) and aerodynamic studies provide further insight about restricted vocal fold movements and, in general, suggest that the voice characteristics of hypokinetic dysarthria may be due to problems other than weakness. Hirose,[47] in a study of EMG patterns in the thyroarytenoid (TA) muscle of a patient with PD and laryngoscopically confirmed limited vocal fold movement, observed that although neuromuscular discharges during phonation were not reduced and there were no pathologic discharge patterns, there was a loss of reciprocal suppression of the TA muscle during inspiration. This suggested that limited vocal fold motion might reflect a loss of appropriate reciprocal activity between agonist and antagonist muscles, rather than weakness. In support of this, observations of vocal fold bowing and impairment of voice onset and offset control by Gallena et al.[40] were associated with increased TA and cricothyroid (CT) activity that could increase vocal fold tension and stiffness and reduce the ability of a speaker to rapidly move the folds for voice onset and offset during speech. The authors concluded that vocal fold bowing was a manifestation of "rigidity due to excessive muscle activity," although they acknowledged that a slight reduction in the abduction action of the posterior cricoarytenoid to oppose the increased action of TA and CT also might contribute to the bowed appearance of the folds.

Aerodynamic studies also suggest that subglottic pressure and laryngeal resistance are abnormally increased during speech in some hypokinetic speakers.[43,60] These findings suggest the presence of increased glottal or supraglottal muscle tension during phonation, caused by phonation with a smaller glottal aperture or by greater resistance to deformation of the folds with decreased pulsing of airflow. Jiang et al.[60] suggested that higher pressures and, presumably, respiratory effort confirm some patients' impressions that they are working harder to produce intensity even when the voice is not as loud as they would like.

In summary, acoustic and physiologic studies of phonatory attributes of hypokinetic dysarthria provide evidence of reduced laryngeal efficiency, flexibility, and control that are, for the most part, consistent with many perceived deviations in voice quality and prosody. Many of these abnormalities can be related to the underlying neuromuscular deficits of rigidity, reduced range of movement, and slowness of movement in the laryngeal muscles.

Resonance

There has been little acoustic or physiologic study of velopharyngeal function in hypokinetic dysarthria, possibly because resonance abnormalities usually are not perceptually prominent. However, a few studies have demonstrated that nasal airflow can be increased in the disorder,[54,118] that nasalization may spread across several consecutive syllables,[63,105] and that the degree and velocity of velar movements during speech tasks can be reduced.[49,50,99] Hirose[47] noted that velar displacement (as measured by x-ray microbeam) became limited and irregular at faster rates and that the velum tended to stay in an elevated posture. He suggested that this might be due to a loss of reciprocal suppression between functionally antagonistic muscle pairs (e.g., velar lowering resisted by action of velar elevators).

Hoodin and Gilbert[54] speculated that the perception of resonance abnormalities might be masked by phonatory problems because their nasal airflow measures did not correlate strongly with perceptual ratings of hypernasality. This seems quite possible, but it is also important to note that hypernasality is perceptually evident in some hypokinetic speakers. For example, 31% of the 23 speakers studied by Theodoros, Murdoch, and Thompson[118] were perceived as mild or moderately hypernasal. However, the fact that 71% of the speakers were more than one standard deviation above control subjects' mean nasal accelerometry scores suggests that instrumental measures may be more sensitive than perceptual measures to velopharyngeal abnormalities.

To summarize, there is acoustic and physiologic evidence of velopharyngeal dysfunction in at least some people with hypokinetic dysarthria. This seems to reflect the effects of slow movement, rigidity, or reduced range of movement. These can lead to the perception of hypernasality and weak intraoral pressure during pressure consonant productions.

Articulation

A number of acoustic and physiologic studies of articulatory dynamics provide considerable support (with some qualifications) for the perception of imprecise articulation and rate abnormalities and reduction in range of articulatory movement. These attributes include, but are not limited to, spirantization, reduced displacements of movements, abnormal movement velocities, increased activation in muscles antagonistic to targeted movement, weakness or fatigue, and tremor or unsteadiness. In general, they support a conclusion that articulatory muscles exhibit rigidity and reduced range of motion.[66]

1. *Precision.* It appears that articulatory "undershoot," or failure to completely reach articulatory targets or sustain contacts for sufficient durations, plays a significant role in imprecision in hypokinetic dysarthria. Numerous acoustic studies have detected evidence of *spirantization* during stop and affricate productions.[2,21,63,123,128] Spirantization, usually taken as evidence of articulatory undershooting, is characterized acoustically by the replacement of a stop gap with low-intensity frication. It is attributed to a failure of complete articulatory closure for stop productions or the stop portion of affricates (see Figure 7-4) and is perceived as aperiodic, fricative-like noise.[123] Its effect is to reduce acoustic contrast and detail, a natural product of undershooting articulators and a reasonable explanation for at least some aspects of perceived imprecise articulation.*

2. *Range of movement.* Several studies provide evidence for reduced range of movement (which could explain articulatory undershooting), rigidity, and abnormal speed of articulator movements. Findings include kinematic evidence of lip muscle stiffness or rigidity, reduced amplitude (range) and velocity of lip and jaw movements, and electromyographic evidence of reduced duration and amplitude of lip muscle action potentials.[18,36,37,43,48-50,56,57,99] EMG studies have also

documented poor reciprocal patterns of activity between jaw opening (e.g., anterior digastric) and jaw closing (e.g., mentalis) muscles during speech tasks[47,93]; simultaneously active jaw opening and closing muscles would tend to slow or restrict range of movement or do both. It has been suggested that such persistent abnormal muscle contractions—reflecting difficulties with reciprocal adjustments of antagonistic muscles or a loss of reciprocal suppression between functionally antagonist muscle pairs—may represent the physiologic basis of hypokinesia and rigidity.[47,78]

Evidence from acoustic studies also supports conclusions that range of articulator movement is reduced. For example, Forrest, Weismer, and Turner[37] found that some parkinsonian speakers have reduced formant transitions. Weismer et al.[124] found that speakers with PD had restricted acoustic vowel space (i.e., the acoustic space covered by the first and second formant values for the corner vowels [/a/, /i/, /æ/, /u/]), suggestive of a smaller "working space" for vowels (i.e., reduced range of movement).

3. *Rate.* Numerous physiologic and acoustic studies have examined speech rate, a phenomenon of considerable interest because increased rate is often perceived in hypokinetic dysarthria. Results have been inconsistent but illuminating because they suggest that listener perceptions may not always reflect underlying movement dynamics.

Some studies demonstrate variability in rate across subjects, ranging from abnormally slow to abnormally fast.[19,21,91] Several studies, however, have failed to find abnormalities in speech rate on various tasks.*

Some studies have found evidence of reduced rate. Dworkin and Aronson[34] and Ludlow, Connor, and Bassich[86] found slow AMRs or slow syllable repetition rates in some subjects. Kruel[73] documented slow reading rate, and Ludlow, Connor, and Bassich[86] found reduced first and second formant transition rates, suggestive of decreased articulatory speed.

As might be expected from perceptual descriptions, numerous studies report acoustic or physiologic evidence for increased or accelerated rate on speech AMR or meaningful connected speech tasks, sometimes with concurrent evidence of reduced

---

*The lack of firm articulatory contact signified by spirantization can make the measurement of voice onset time (VOT) during the production of stop consonants difficult due to lack of a burst signifying the release of the stop.[100]

*References 2, 19, 21, 23, 86, 117, 123, 124, 127, 128.

amplitude of articulator movements, in at least some speakers.[2,5,44,48-50,99] AMRs can be fast (see Figure 7-3), up to 13 per second, with associated decreased range of movement; this extremely fast rate suggests a mode of speech over which there can be no voluntary control.[99] Hirose[47] likened abnormally fast speech rate to festinating gait and speculated that this may reflect a disturbance of CNS inhibitory function, such as an abnormal release of an intrinsic oscillation mechanism.

Finally, at least some speakers with PD have difficulty altering rate when requested.[85,86] For example, speakers studied by Ludlow, Connor, and Bassich[86] had trouble altering sentence and phrase durations when they were asked to speak at faster than conversational rates; that is, there was less of a difference between their conversational and fast rates in comparison to control speakers. The authors speculated that a major problem for these speakers is in controlling alterations in rate, even though the overall temporal organization of speech may be unaffected.

The results of these studies indicate that speech rate is heterogeneous within the population of speakers with hypokinetic dysarthria. Because such variability is probably not simply a function of severity, this raises the possibility of subtypes of the disorder, something that deserves investigation. At this time, however, it is important to recognize that hypokinetic dysarthria is the only dysarthria type in which rate is perceived as, or actually is, rapid or accelerated. The caveat, as Weismer[123] and Kent and Rosenbek[63] have suggested, is that the perception of fast rate could be an artifact of features such as articulatory imprecision and continuous voicing that reduce discrete acoustic contrasts; this "blurring" of acoustic contrasts may lead to a perception of increased rate. Some experimental support for this derives from a study by Torp and Hammen[120] that determined that speaking rate was perceived as faster in PD than control speakers even when actual speaking rates were equivalent. This supports the notion that things within the speech signal can lead to a perception of rapid rate when rate may not actually be rapid. These insights suggest that clinicians may need to tune more finely their perceptual judgments when assessing speech rate in hypokinetic dysarthria.

4. *Strength and endurance.* It appears that weakness (CNS, not peripheral nervous system [PNS]), in addition to rigidity, may contribute to reduced range of movement in hypokinetic dysarthria. Structures in which weakness (and sometimes reduced endurance) have been found include the upper lip and (probably) velum,[99] as well as the tongue.[112-114] Solomon et al.[114] found that a group of patients with mild to moderate PD had reduced tongue strength but not abnormal fatigue when asked to exert maximum lingual pressure on an air-filled bulb (the Iowa Oral Performance Instrument, as defined in Chapter 3). Others have also found evidence of fatigue or reduced tongue endurance.[112,113]

The presence of weakness and fatigue are not necessarily linearly related to abnormal perceptual speech characteristics. For example, Solomon, Robin, and Luschei[112] found no significant relationship between tongue strength and endurance and articulatory precision and overall speech defectiveness, suggesting that modest degrees of tongue weakness and fatigue may not be associated with perceptible (or otherwise measurable) speech deficits. The authors noted that the operating range for speech muscles is approximately 10% to 25% of their maximum strength, so the threshold for weakness to result in functional impairment may not be a straightforward value; tongue strength may need to be impaired beyond a critical level before deficits in speech become evident.

5. *Tremor, control, and steadiness.* Hunker and Abbs[56] found evidence of pathologic tremor in the jaw and lip at rest, during sustained postures, and during active and passive movement. They speculated that prolonged reaction times (i.e., delayed initiation of movement) in PD may be due to an inability to initiate muscle contraction until it coincides with the involuntary burst of a tremor oscillation, and that tremor rate may set limits on maximum rates of syllable production that can be attained without acceleration. Abbs, Hunker, and Barlow[1] also observed lip and jaw tremor during nonspeech tasks involving muscle force. The lips and jaw were otherwise adequate in producing stable forces, although patients had difficulty producing stable tongue elevation forces. Putnam,[103] summarizing the relevant literature, noted that tremor may be involved in acceleration

phenomena in hypokinetic dysarthria, and that patients may have to contend with the effect of tremor on phasic movements during speech.

There is evidence that at least some speakers with hypokinetic dysarthria have reduced oromotor control and reduced steadiness in orofacial structures during speech and nonspeech tasks. For example, McClean, Beukelman, and Yorkston[90] found evidence of poor visuomotor tracking of a sinusoidal signal with both jaw and lip movements. Zwirner and Barnes[129] found acoustic evidence of decreased jaw stability (as reflected in first formant steadiness) during vowel prolongation. Adams,[6] summarizing the results of relevant studies, noted that PD patients have increased instability on isometric oromotor force tasks, and that such instability may vary across orofacial structures (tongue, lip, jaw), perhaps as a function of the degree of tremor in each structure.

Stress, Pause, and Other Durational Characteristics

Findings of rate abnormalities and reduced frequency and intensity variability help explain some of the acoustic factors underlying the perception of prosodic insufficiency in hypokinetic dysarthria. Some additional factors, mostly related to stress, pause, and between-syllable durational differences, help to round out the disorder's prosodic features.

Although Canter[19] found no differences between parkinsonian and control subjects in number of pauses or mean pause duration during reading, several studies have found such abnormalities. Parkinsonian subjects' pauses during speech have been shown to represent a higher percentage of the total time within speech samples.[44,91] Pauses may also occur slightly more frequently.[44]

Illes et al.[58] found an increased frequency and duration of pauses that exceeded 200 ms. These hesitations or pauses tended to be longer and occur more frequently at the beginning of sentences. There was also an increase in number of words between silent intervals, a finding that may be related to the perception of short rushes of speech. Finally, Ludlow and Bassich[85] found reduced differences in word boundary durations between separate nouns and compound nouns (e.g., the boundary between the syllables "sail" and "boats" in the sentences "They were sailboats" vs. "They will sail boats"). This was correlated with the perception of reduced stress.

Murry[98] examined the ability to vary stress in the word initial and final position when answering questions with a standard sentence that established the point of emphasis (e.g., responding "Bob bit Todd" in response to the question, "Who bit Bob?").

Normal subjects tend to increase frequency, intensity, and articulatory effort (e.g., as measured by peak intraoral pressure) to signal stress in the word initial or final position. Murry's hypokinetic speaker demonstrated only minimal increases in frequency and intensity to signal stress, and this occurred at the expense of articulatory effort. Illes et al.[58] found that hypokinetic speakers exhibited fewer interjections and "modalizations" (comments that bear on verbal behavior, such as "you know") during narrative speech. Combined with other findings, this suggests that hypokinetic speakers display silent pauses instead of fillers, and that this loss of verbal "asides" may be analogous to a reduction of the automatic movements that accompany purposeful movements in PD (e.g., masked facial expression, reduced arm swing during walking).

Kent and Rosenbek[63] have provided a useful summary of the acoustic "signature" of hypokinetic dysarthria. They label the pattern, in which the contour across syllables within utterances is flattened or indistinct, as *fused*. This fused or flattened profile is characterized by (1) small and gradual f_o and intensity variations within and between syllables, (2) continuous voicing, (3) reduced variations in syllable durations, (4) syllable reduction, (5) indistinct boundaries between syllables because of faulty consonant articulation, and (6) a spread of nasalization across consecutive syllables. In general, these features represent a reduced ability to use the full range of pitch, intensity, articulatory, and durational options that are used by normal speakers (see Figure 7-4).

Sensory and Perceptual Deficits

People with PD and hypokinetic dysarthria may have sensory or perceptual difficulties that impact on speech production. For example, there is evidence that some individuals with PD have poor temporal discrimination for tactile, auditory, and visual stimuli.[9] Dagenais, Southwood, and Mallonee,[25] examining responses to delayed auditory feedback (DAF) in PD speakers, concluded that "they may have reduced resources to monitor and produce speech concurrently." Forrest et al.[38] found that PD speakers had below normal word identification scores when words were spoken at a slower than normal rate. They suggested that perceptual deficits might be additional factors that contribute to rate variations in PD speech. These findings have implications for the management of hypokinetic dysarthria and are discussed further in Chapter 17.

The general observations derived from the acoustic and physiologic studies reviewed in this section are summarized in Table 7-6.

7-6   Summary of acoustic and physiologic findings in studies of hypokinetic dysarthria*

Speech Component	Acoustic or Physiologic Observation

Respiratory (or respiratory or laryngeal)	Reduced:
	  Vital capacity
	  Amplitude of chest wall movements
	  Strength & endurance
	  Airflow volume during vowel prolongation
	  Intraoral pressure during AMRs
	  Syllables per breath group
	  Maximum vowel duration
	Increased:
	  Respiratory rate
	  Latency to begin exhalation
	  Latency to initiate phonation after exhalation initiated
	  Breath groups during reading
	  Percentage of vital capacity per syllable
	Irregular breathing patterns
	Paradoxical rib cage & abdominal movements
	Difficulty altering automatic breathing patterns for speech
	Poor respiratory control for visuomotor tracking

Laryngeal	Bowed vocal folds in spite of solid, nonflaccid appearance
	Tremulousness of arytenoid cartilages
	Asymmetry of laryngeal structures & movements during phonation, especially in hemiparkinsonism
	Ventricular fold movement during phonation
	Decreased:
	  Intensity
	  Pitch & loudness variability
	  Speed to initiate phonation
	  Intensity peaks across syllables
	  Maximum phonation time over disease course
	Increased:
	  f_o & long-term variability of f_o
	  Glottal resistance & subglottic pressure
	  TA & CT activity (cocontraction)
	Laryngealization
	Shimmer & jitter
	Voice tremor & flutter
	Continuous voicing in segments with voiceless consonants
	Voiceless transitions from vowels to following consonants
	Poor pitch control for visuomotor tracking
	Abnormal long-term average spectrum shape

Velopharyngeal	Increased nasal airflow during nonnasal target productions Reduced velocity & degree of velar movement during speech Abnormal spread of nasalization across syllables

Articulation or Rate or Prosody	Reduced:
	  Amplitude & velocity of lip movement
	  Amplitude & duration of lip muscle action potentials
	  Jaw stability during vowel prolongation
	  Tongue endurance & strength
	  Spectrographic acoustic contrast & detail
	  Speech rate
	  Ability to increase rate on request
	  F1 & F2 formant transition rates
	  Syllable boundary durational differences between separate & compound nouns
	  F_o, intensity, & articulatory effort increases to signal stress
	  Variation in syllable duration

table 7-6	Summary of acoustic and physiologic findings in studies of hypokinetic dysarthria*—cont'd

Speech Component	Acoustic or Physiologic Observation

	Increased or accelerated:
	  Connected speech & AMR rates
	  Rate variability
	  Frequency & duration of pauses during connected speech
	Articulatory undershoot in lip & velum
	Lip rigidity or stiffness
	Poor maintenance of temporal reciprocity between jaw depressors & elevators
	Poor visuomotor tracking with jaw & lip movements
	Abnormal jaw & lip tremor at rest, during sustained postures, & active & passive movement
	Spirantization of stops & affricates
	Continuous voicing
	Indistinct boundaries between syllables
	Spread of nasalization across syllables
	Spread of nasalization across syllables
	Small & gradual f_o & intensity variations within & between syllables

AMR, Alternate motion rates; *CT*, computed tomography; f_o, fundamental frequency; *TA*, thyroarytenoid.
*Many of these observations are based on studies of only one or a few speakers, and not all speakers with hypokinetic dysarthria exhibit these features. These characteristics may not be unique to hypokinetic dysarthria; some may also be found in other motor speech disorders or nonneurologic conditions.

Cases

Case 7-1

A 69-year-old man presented with a 4-year history of progressive difficulty getting in and out of chairs and a 2- to 3-year history of speech difficulty. These had progressed to include slowness in walking and poor handwriting.

Neurologic examination disclosed generalized bradykinesia, some rigidity of the trunk and limbs, and abnormal pursuit and saccadic eye movements. He could barely walk and did so in slow shuffling steps. "Severe speech hesitancy" was also apparent.

During speech examination, the patient described himself as "stuttering" as a child, beginning at 3 years of age and resolving by his ninth year. This problem was mild, and he had never had treatment for it. However, he noted that throughout his life he would "stutter" when excited, although his family had never noticed this. The patient had a brother who also reportedly stuttered as a child, with occasional dysfluencies in adulthood.

The tongue was tremulous on protrusion and during lateral movements. No other abnormalities were noted. Conversational speech, reading, and repetition were characterized by a remarkable degree of dysfluency, characterized by rapid repetition of initial sounds, syllables, and occasionally words and phrases. Sound and syl-

lable repetitions occurred up to 30 to 40 repetitions per dysfluent moment. There was no evidence of associated struggle behavior during dysfluencies, although he did express frustration over them. In addition to the dysfluencies, articulation was moderately imprecise, pitch and loudness variability was reduced, and overall loudness was mildly reduced. Speech AMRs were rapid or accelerated. Prolonged "ah" was hoarse (2).

The clinician concluded: "(1) Hypokinetic dysarthria. (2) Marked to severe stuttering-like behavior associated with CNS disease, including some dysfluencies suggestive of palilalia. I strongly suspect the dysfluencies reflect a component of his hypokinetic dysarthria. In my opinion, this is a variant of hypokinetic dysarthria with associated dysfluencies and does not reflect the reemergence of his reported childhood stuttering."

During the patient's few days at the clinic, speech therapy was undertaken, primarily to modify his dysfluencies. Hand tapping and use of a pacing board were unsuccessful because his limb movements were as accelerated or rapid as his speech. He did, however, respond positively to DAF, with a significant reduction in speech rate and marked reduction of dysfluency. This greatly enhanced efficiency and intelligibility during

Case 7-1—cont'd

conversation. The patient left the clinic with a recommendation to pursue therapy, with consideration given to acquiring a DAF device for use in conversation.

The neurologist concluded that the patient had idiopathic PD.

Commentary. (1) Hypokinetic dysarthria may be among the prominent presenting signs of PD. (2) Dysfluencies occur commonly in hypokinetic dysarthria, and palilalia may also occur. For some patients, their dysfluencies may be the most debilitating component of their hypokinetic dysarthria. (3) The history of early childhood stuttering was of unknown significance in this case. However, recognizing that the patient had a hypokinetic dysarthria with associated dysfluencies helped establish that his speech deficit could probably not be attributed to a reemergence or persistence of childhood stuttering. Rather, it was related to the patient's neurologic disease. (4) Marked dysfluencies associated with hypokinetic dysarthria can be responsive to speech therapy. These approaches are discussed in Chapter 17.

Case 7-2

A 69-year-old man presented with a 5-year history of difficulty getting in and out of chairs, stiffness during walking, and difficulty turning in bed. He also had voice and handwriting difficulty. There was no history of encephalitis, toxic exposure, or drug use that might be related to his symptoms, nor was there any family history of neurodegenerative disorder.

On neurologic examination, the arm swing was diminished and the neck and extremities were rigid. He had a mild static tremor of the left hand, and upper limb movements were bradykinetic. Facial expression was masked, and postural reflexes were mildly impaired. An MRI scan was normal. He was referred for a speech assessment "to see if there are any clues in his voice as to the type of problem that he has."

During speech examination, the patient described a 1-year history of uncertainty if "words would come out." He believed his speech had become quieter and perhaps slower, more so in the evening or after extended speaking. He reported occasional difficulty "getting going" with his speech, even though he knew what he wanted to say.

The jaw, lips, and tongue were mildly tremulous during sustained postures. Breathy-hoarse voice quality (2), reduced loudness (1), and a tendency toward accelerated rate (0,1) characterized speech. Very infrequently, there were rapid repetitions or prolongations of initial phonemes. There was some nasal emission during production of pressure sound–filled sentences, but he was not obviously hypernasal. Speech AMRs were normal. Prolonged "ah" was breathy-hoarse (1,2). Speech did not deteriorate during stress testing.

The speech clinician concluded "hypokinetic dysarthria, mild."

The neurologist concluded that the patient had parkinsonism. However, his symptoms were unresponsive to Sinemet. Because of this, the neurologist believed he might have striatonigral degeneration, "which can appear much like PD at onset but is not Sinemet responsive."

Commentary. (1) Speech change is often associated with parkinsonism and may be among the signs encountered during initial neurologic evaluation. (2) Changes in voice quality and loudness are often among the initial complaints of patients with hypokinetic dysarthria. (3) Identification of hypokinetic dysarthria can provide confirmatory evidence for a diagnosis of parkinsonism.

[handwritten annotations: "excessive pendulum or ROM", "bradykinetic - false starts", "hallolaylia - prolonged initial consonant"]

Case 7-3

A 74-year-old woman presented with a 4-year history of progressive "wobbling" when walking and a tendency to fall backward. Neurologic examination initially suggested prominent proximal muscle weakness. Polymyositis, myasthenia gravis, and myopathy were suspected. Because she complained of "slurred" speech and "hesitation" when speaking, she was referred for speech assessment.

During speech examination she stated, "When I speak, I don't know how it will come out. Sometimes words do not come out at all." Conversational speech was characterized by prolonged silent intervals, occasional whole word repetitions, and repeated syllables (e.g., "I took dic-ta-ta-ta-ta-tion from him"). Rate was mildly accelerated, and articulation was often mildly imprecise, with slighting of consonants when she spoke rapidly. Resonance was normal, but voice quality was harsh. There was no evidence of speech deterioration during 4 minutes of continuous talking.

The clinician concluded, "Speech features are most suggestive of hypokinetic dysarthria. At times, the pattern is almost that of palilalia, also seen in parkinsonian patients. This is not a speech pattern of flaccid dysarthria; no suggestion of myasthenia gravis."

The speech diagnosis prompted additional neurologic investigation. CT scan was normal with the exception of mild generalized cerebral atrophy. Consultation with other neurologists ruled out PNS disease and myopathy and detected postural instability, slight rigidity, and brisk reflexes. Neurologic diagnosis was uncertain, but it was concluded that she had several parkinsonian symptoms but without classic idiopathic PD. A diagnosis of PSP was entertained, but evidence for its diagnosis was considered equivocal.

Commentary. (1) Hypokinetic dysarthria is common in parkinsonism. (2) Diagnosis of hypokinetic dysarthria can be helpful to neurologic diagnosis. In this case, it raised suspicions about CNS degenerative disease, specifically parkinsonism. It helped focus attention on the CNS as opposed to the PNS. (3) Dysfluencies and palilalia can be associated with hypokinetic dysarthria.

Case 7-4

A 29-year-old woman presented to a rehabilitation unit 14 months after cerebral anoxia that developed secondary to cardiac arrest during a tubal ligation. Neurologic examination revealed neck and left upper extremity rigidity, upper extremity dystonia, diffuse hyperactive reflexes, and weakness in all extremities. Gait was slow with short steps. She had difficulty with chewing and swallowing and frequently choked on solid foods.

Speech examination revealed reduced loudness (3), imprecise articulation (3), accelerated speech rate (3), little variation in pitch, loudness, and syllable duration, and reduced range of articulatory movement (3,4). Speech AMRs were "super fast and blurred."

The clinician concluded "hypokinetic dysarthria, severe." There was no evidence of aphasia, but neuropsychological assessment revealed deficits in attention, concentration, new learning, and short-term recall. She received speech therapy while at the rehabilitation unit, with subsequent improved speech intelligibility as long as she was cued to increase loudness and slow rate.

Commentary. (1) Hypokinetic dysarthria can occur in conditions other than parkinsonism and can be encountered in anoxic encephalopathy. In such cases the dysarthria may not be distinguishable from hypokinetic dysarthria associated with idiopathic PD. (2) Cognitive deficits can be present in individuals with hypokinetic dysarthria.

Case 7-5

A 75-year-old man presented with a 3- to 4-year history of shuffling gait, stooped posture, loss of facial expression, tremor, and voice change. Neurologic examination confirmed the presence of these symptoms. The patient also admitted to occasional confusion and reduced memory. Neuropsychological assessment revealed mild to moderate generalized, organic cognitive decline consistent with mild dementia.

During speech examination, the patient complained of "hoarseness" and noted that his voice occasionally "gets to a whisper." Voice quality was characterized by reduced loudness (1,2), continuous breathiness (1,2), and monopitch and monoloudness (1,2). Articulation was equivocally fast during conversation. Speech AMRs were normal.

The clinician concluded, "Mild hypokinetic dysarthria, primarily characterized by reduced pitch and loudness variability, reduced volume, and breathiness."

Because the patient cleared his throat frequently and had prominent dysphonia, he was referred for laryngeal examination; bowing of the vocal folds was observed.

The neurologist concluded that the patient had a degenerative CNS disease that did not fit well with classic idiopathic PD. Sinemet was prescribed. Two years later, although improved on Sinemet, the neurologic examination was unchanged and there was no other evidence of deterioration. Speech was also unchanged, with the exception that tongue tremulousness was apparent on protrusion.

Commentary. (1) Hypokinetic dysarthria frequently manifests as dysphonia and prosodic insufficiency. Such difficulties can remain the only speech symptoms for extended periods. (2) The dysphonia of hypokinetic dysarthria is frequently associated with bowing of the vocal folds. (3) People with hypokinetic dysarthria can also have cognitive impairments.

bowed VF = breathiness

Case 7-6

A 51-year-old man presented for another opinion about his neurologic deficit. His difficulties began 3 years previously, over approximately 10 days, when he had several suspected myocardial infarctions. His symptoms at that time included speech difficulty and problems with gait.

Neurologic examination showed a loss of facial expression, generalized loss of associated movements, generalized bradykinesia, and generalized rigidity, greater on the left than right side.

During speech examination, the patient stated, "I can't talk in long sentences; I repeat myself; bad volume; out of breath fast." He had had three periods of speech therapy, benefiting only temporarily from each.

Examination revealed facial masking, reduced range of movement of the jaw, lips, and tongue, and, perhaps, mild left tongue weakness. Connected speech was characterized by imprecise articulation (3), accelerated rate within utterances (2,3), monopitch and monoloudness (3,4), and breathy-harsh-strained voice quality (2,3). In addition, during conversation he exhibited numerous phoneme and syllable repetitions and fairly frequent word and phrase repetitions, usually with associated accelerated rate, consistent with the characteristics of palilalia. At times, however, these repetitions appeared voluntary, based on his perception that he had not been understood, while at other times they appeared involuntary. Speech AMRs were markedly imprecise and

blurred. Intelligibility was significantly reduced but improved with slowing of rate, which was facilitated by hand tapping.

The clinician concluded, "Marked hypokinetic dysarthria and palilalia."

It was recommended that he resume speech therapy. It was felt that he might benefit from efforts to more consistently slow his rate and prepare himself respiratorily for each utterance. Development of a backup augmentative system was also recommended. The patient had been under the impression that speech therapy was intended to completely remediate his speech difficulty. During a lengthy discussion, it was stressed that speech therapy would not likely restore normal speech but could focus on maximizing intelligibility. The patient accepted this explanation, with disappointment, and did pursue additional speech therapy at a facility near his home.

Additional neurologic workup included an MRI scan that identified small lacunar infarcts in the right putamen and external capsule. The neurologist concluded that the patient had extrapyramidal disease as a result of a previous cerebrovascular event and, perhaps, diffuse cerebral ischemia that was secondary to an episode of hypotension of undetermined etiology. Although clinical findings were somewhat asymmetric and only a unilateral lesion was present on neuroimaging, the clinical picture appeared to reflect bilateral involvement of the basal ganglia.

Case 7-6—cont'd

Commentary. (1) Hypokinetic dysarthria and palilalia can result from cerebral ischemia and infarction. (2) Hypokinetic dysarthria can be among the most debilitating deficits stemming from basal ganglia disease. (3) Although neuroimaging evidence suggested only a unilateral lesion, the dysarthria and associated neurologic findings were strongly suggestive of bilateral involvement. (4) Dysarthric patients sometimes have unrealistic expectations about speech therapy. It is crucial that patients understand the goals of therapy when therapy is recommended. Counseling in this regard is helpful to managing patients' acceptance and understanding of their deficits, as well as to develop an understanding of what may and may not be achieved with treatment.

SUMMARY

1. Hypokinetic dysarthria results from damage to the basal ganglia control circuit. It probably occurs at a rate comparable to that of other single dysarthria types. Its characteristics are most evident in voice, articulation, and prosody. The effects of rigidity, reduced force and range of movement, and slow individual and sometimes fast repetitive movements seem to account for many of its deviant speech characteristics.

2. Parkinsonism, the prototypic condition associated with hypokinetic dysarthria, is most often due to PD, a degenerative condition associated with a depletion of dopamine in the striatum of the basal ganglia. Several symptoms of the disease are often managed by medications that restore the balance between dopamine and acetylcholine within the basal ganglia. Several other neurodegenerative diseases may also cause parkinsonian symptoms and hypokinetic dysarthria.

3. Hypokinetic dysarthria may also result from nondegenerative conditions, most often including vascular disease, neuroleptic and illicit drugs, certain metabolic diseases, chronic exposure to heavy metals, trauma, and infection.

4. Patients or, more often, their significant others frequently complain that their voice is weak or quiet, and sometimes that their rate is too rapid. They may also note dysfluencies and difficulty initiating speech. They often are aware of deterioration with fatigue or toward the end of an antiparkinsonian medication cycle. Drooling and swallowing complaints are common. Facial masking and a general reduction in the visible range of articulator movement during speech are common.

5. Several deviant speech characteristics combine to give many patients a distinctive flat, attenuated, and sometimes accelerated speech pattern. This has been called prosodic insufficiency and is characterized by monopitch, monoloudness, reduced stress, short phrases, variable rate, short rushes of speech, and imprecise articulation. Additional distinctive characteristics that may be present include inappropriate silences, breathy dysphonia, reduced loudness, and increased speech rate. Dysfluencies and palilalia may also be present.

6. In general, acoustic and physiologic studies have provided support for the auditory-perceptual characteristics of the disorder; have specified more precisely the disorder's acoustic and physiologic characteristics; and have documented the role of rigidity, reduced range of movement, slowness of movement, and acceleration phenomena during speech. Data suggest that the perception of accelerated rate may sometimes be an artifact of listener expectations and reduced acoustic contrast.

7. Hypokinetic dysarthria can be the only, the first, or among the first and most prominent manifestations of neurologic disease. Its recognition can aid neurologic localization and diagnosis and may contribute to the medical and behavioral management of the individual's disease and speech disorder.

References

1. Abbs JH, Hunker CJ, Barlow SM: *Differential speech motor subsystem impairments with suprabulbar lesions: neurophysiologic framework and supporting data.* In Berry WR, editor: *Clinical dysarthria,* San Diego, 1984, College-Hill Press.

2. Ackermann H, Hertrich I, Hehr T: *Oral diadokokinesis in neurological dysarthrias,* Folia Phoniatr Logop 47:15, 1995.

3. Ackermann H, Ziegler W, Petersen D: *Dysarthria in bilateral thalamic infarction,* J Neurol 240:357, 1993.

4. Adams RD, Victor H: *Principles of neurology,* New York, 1991, McGraw-Hill.

5. Adams SG: *Accelerating speech in a case of hypokinetic dysarthria: descriptions and treatment.* In Till JA, Yorkston KM, Beukelman DR, editors: *Motor speech disorders: advances in assessment and treatment,* Baltimore, 1994, Brookes Publishing.

6. Adams SG: Hypokinetic dysarthria in Parkinson's disease. In MR McNeil, editor: Clinical management of sensorimotor speech disorders, New York, 1997, Thieme.

7. Ahlskog JE: Approach to the patient with a movement disorder: basic principles of neurologic diagnosis. In Adler CH, Ahlskog JE, editors: Parkinson's disease and movement disorders: diagnosis and treatment guidelines for the practicing physician, Totowa, NJ, 2000, Humana Press.

8. Arana GW, Hyman SE: Handbook of psychiatric drug therapy, ed 2, Boston, 1991, Little, Brown.

9. Artieda J et al: Temporal discrimination is abnormal in Parkinson's disease, Brain 115:199, 1992.

10. Bayles KA et al: The effect of Parkinson's disease on language, J Med Speech-Lang Pathol 5:157, 1997.

11. Benke TH et al: Repetitive speech phenomena in Parkinson's disease, J Neurol Neurosurg Psychiatry 69:319, 2000.

12. Boshes B: Voice changes in parkinsonism, J Neurosurg 24:286, 1966.

13. Boutsen FR, Duffy JR, Aronson AE: Flutter or tremor in hypokinetic dysarthria: a case study. In Cannito MP, Yorkston KM, Beukelman DR, editors: Neuromotor speech disorder, nature, assessment, and management, Baltimore, 1998, Brookes Publishing.

14. Brown JW: Aphasia, apraxia, and agnosia, Springfield, Ill, 1972, Charles C Thomas.

15. Buck R, Duffy RJ: Nonverbal communication of affect in brain-damaged patients, Cortex 16:351, 1980.

16. Bunton K et al: The effects of flattening fundamental frequency contours on sentence intelligibility in speakers with dysarthria, Clin Ling Phonet 15:181, 2001.

17. Caekebeke JFV et al: The interpretation of dysprosody in patients with Parkinson's disease, J Neurol Neurosurg Psychiatry 54:145, 1991.

18. Caligiuri MP: The influence of speaking rate on articulatory hypokinesia in parkinsonian dysarthria, Brain Lang 36:493, 1989.

19. Canter GJ: Speech characteristics of patients with Parkinson's disease: I. Intensity, pitch, and duration, J Speech Hear Disord 28:221, 1963.

20. Canter GJ: Speech characteristics of patients with Parkinson's disease: II. Physiological support for speech, J Speech Hear Disord 30:44, 1965a.

21. Canter GJ: Speech characteristics of patients with Parkinson's disease: III. Articulation, diadochokinesis, and overall speech adequacy, J Speech Hear Disord 30:217, 1965b.

22. Caselli RJ: Parkinsonism in primary degenerative dementia. In Adler CH, Ahlskog JE, editors: Parkinson's disease and movement disorders: diagnosis and treatment guidelines for the practicing physician, Totowa, NJ, 2000, Humana Press.

23. Connor NP, Ludlow CL, Schulz GM: Stop consonant production in isolated and repeated syllables in Parkinson's disease, Neuropsychologia 27:829, 1989.

24. Corcos DM et al: Strength in Parkinson's disease: relationship to rate of force generation and clinical status, Ann Neurol 39:79, 1996.

25. Dagenais PA, Southwood MH, Mallonee KO: Assessing processing skills in speakers with Parkinson's disease using delayed auditory feedback, J Med Speech-Lang Pathol 7:297, 1999.

26. Darkins AW, Fromkin VA, Benson DF: A characterization of the prosodic loss in Parkinson's disease, Brain Lang 34:315, 1988.

27. Darley FL, Aronson AE, Brown JR: Differential diagnostic patterns of dysarthria, J Speech Hear Res 12:246, 1969a.

28. Darley FL, Aronson, AE, Brown JR: Clusters of deviant speech dimensions in the dysarthrias, J Speech Hear Res 12:462, 1969b.

29. Demirci M, Grill S, McShane L, Hallett M: A mismatch between kinesthetic and visual perception in Parkinson's disease, Ann Neurol 41:781, 1997.

30. De Pandis MF et al: Modification of respiratory function parameters in patients with severe Parkinson's disease, Neurolog Sci 23:S69, 2002.

31. Dewey RB: Clinical features of Parkinson's disease. In Adler CH, Ahlskog JE, editors: Parkinson's disease and movement disorders: diagnosis and treatment guidelines for the practicing physician, Totowa, NJ, 2000, Humana Press.

32. Doyle PC et al: Fundamental frequency and acoustic variability associated with production of sustained vowels by speakers with hypokinetic dysarthria, J Med Speech-Lang Pathol 3:41, 1995.

33. Dromey C: Spectral measures and perceptual ratings of hypokinetic dysarthria, J Med Speech-Lang Pathol 11:85, 2003.

34. Dworkin JP, Aronson AE: Tongue strength and alternate motion rates in normal and dysarthric subjects, J Commun Disord 19:115, 1986.

35. Ewanowski SJ: Selected Motor-Speech Behavior of Patients with Parkinsonism [PhD dissertation]. Madison, Wis; University of Wisconsin; 1964.

36. Forrest K, Weismer G: Dynamic aspects of lower lip movement in parkinsonian and neurologically normal geriatric speakers' production of stress, J Speech Hear Res 38:260, 1995.

37. Forrest K, Weismer G, Turner GS: Kinematic, acoustic, and perceptual analyses of connected speech produced by parkinsonian and normal geriatric adults, J Acoust Soc Am 85:2608, 1989.

38. Forrest K et al: Effects of speaking rate on word recognition in Parkinson's disease and normal aging, J Med Speech-Lang Pathol 6:1, 1998.

39. Fox CM, Ramig LO: Vocal sound pressure level and self-perception of speech and voice in men and women with idiopathic Parkinson disease, Am J Speech-Lang Pathol 6:85, 1997.

40. Gallena S et al: Effects of levodopa on laryngeal muscle activity for voice onset and offset in Parkinson disease, J Speech Lang Hear Res 44:1284, 2001.

41. Goberman AM, Blomgren M: Parkinsonian speech dysfluencies: effects of L-dopa-related fluctuations, J Fluency Dis 28:55, 2003.

42. Goetz CG et al: Parkinson's disease, Continuum 1:4, 1995.

43. Gracco LC et al: Aerodynamic evaluation of parkinsonian dysarthria: laryngeal and supralaryngeal manifestations. In Till JA, Yorkston KM, Beukelman DR, editors: Motor speech disorders: advances in assessment and treatment, Baltimore, 1994, Paul H Brookes.

44. Hammen VL, Yorkston KM, Beukelman DR: Pausal and speech duration characteristics as a function of speaking rate in normal and dysarthric individuals. In Yorkston KM, Beukelman DR, editors: Recent advances in clinical dysarthria, Austin, Tex, 1989, Pro-Ed.

45. Hanson DG, Gerratt BR, Ward PH: Cinegraphic observations of laryngeal function in Parkinson's disease, Laryngoscope 94:348, 1984.

46. Higuchi Y, Iacono RP: Surgical complications in patients with Parkinson's disease after posteroventral pallidotomy, Neurosurgery 52:558, 2003.

47. Hirose H: Pathophysiology of motor speech disorders (dysarthria), Folia Phoniatr Logop 38:61, 1986.

48. Hirose H, Kiritani S, Sawashima M: Patterns of dysarthric movement in patients with amyotrophic lateral sclerosis and pseudobulbar palsy, Folia Phoniatr Logop 34:106, 1982a.

49. Hirose H, Kiritani S, Sawashima M: Velocity of articulatory movements in normal and dysarthric subjects, Folia Phoniatr Logop 34:210, 1982b.

50. Hirose H et al: Patterns of dysarthric movement in patients with parkinsonism, Folia Phoniatr Logop 33:204, 1981.

51. Ho AK, Iansek R, Bradshaw JL: Regulation of parkinsonian speech volume: the effect of interlocuter distance, J Neurol Neurosurg Psychiatry 67:199, 1999.

52. Ho A, Iansek R, Bradshaw JL: The effect of a concurrent task on parkinsonian speech, J Clin Exp Neuropsychol 24:36, 2002.

53. Holmes RJ et al: Voice characteristics in the progression of Parkinson's disease, Int J Lang Commun Disord 35:407, 2000.

54. Hoodin RB, Gilbert HR: Parkinsonian dysarthria: an aerodynamic and perceptual description of velopharyngeal closure for speech, Folia Phoniatr Logop 41:249, 1989.

55. Huber JE et al: Respiratory function and variability in individuals with Parkinson disease: pre- and post-Lee Silverman Voice Treatment, J Med Speech-Lang Pathol 11:185, 2003.

56. Hunker CJ, Abbs JH: Physiological analyses of parkinsonian tremors in the orofacial system. In McNeil MR, Rosenbek JC, Aronson AE, editors: The dysarthrias, Austin, Tex, 1984, Pro-Ed.

57. Hunker C, Abbs J, Barlow S: The relationship between parkinsonian rigidity and hypokinesia in the orofacial system: a quantitative analysis, Neurology 32:749, 1982.

58. Illes J et al: Language production in Parkinson's disease: acoustic and linguistic considerations, Brain Lang 33:146, 1988.

59. Jiang J, Lin E, Hanson DG: Acoustic and airflow spectral analysis of voice tremor, J Speech Lang Hear Res 43:191, 2000.

60. Jiang J et al: Aerodynamic measurements of patients with Parkinson's disease, J Voice 13:583, 1999.

61. Kammermeier MA: A Comparison of Phonatory Phenomena Among Groups of Neurologically Impaired Speakers [PhD dissertation]. Minneapolis/St Paul; University of Minnesota; 1969.

62. Kent RD, Kent JF: Task-based profiles of the dysarthrias, Folia Phoniatr Logop 52:48, 2000.

63. Kent RD, Rosenbek JC: Prosodic disturbance and neurologic lesion, Brain Lang 15:259, 1982.

64. Kent RD, Vorperian HK, Duffy JR: Reliability of the Multi-Dimensional Voice Program for the analysis of voice samples of subjects with dysarthria, Am J Speech-Lang Pathol 8:129, 1999.

65. Kent RD et al: Laryngeal dysfunction in neurological disease: amyotrophic lateral sclerosis, Parkinson's disease, and stroke, J Med Speech-Lang Pathol 2:157, 1994.

66. Kent RD et al: The dysarthrias: speech-voice profiles, related dysfunctions, and neuropathology, J Med Speech Lang Pathol 6:165, 1998.

67. Kent RD et al: What dysarthrias can tell us about the neural control of speech, J Phonet 28:273, 2000.

68. Kent RD et al: Voice dysfunction in dysarthria: application of the Multi-Dimensional Voice Program, J Commun Disord 36:281, 2003.

69. Kim R: The chronic residual respiratory disorder in post-encephalitic parkinsonism, J Neurol Neurosurg Psychiatry 31:393, 1968.

70. King JB et al: Parkinson's disease: longitudinal changes in acoustic parameters of phonation, J Med Speech-Lang Pathol 2:29, 1994.

71. Kiran S, Larson CR: Effect of duration of pitch-shifted feedback on vocal responses in patients with Parkinson's disease, J Speech Lang Hear Res 44:975, 2001.

72. Koller WC: Dysfluency (stuttering) in extrapyramidal disease, Arch Neurol 40:175, 1983.

73. Kruel EJ: Neuromuscular control examination (NMC) for parkinsonism: vowel prolongations and diadokokinetic and reading rates, J Speech Hear Res 15:72, 1972.

74. LaPointe LL, Horner J: Palilalia: a descriptive study of pathological reiterative utterances, J Speech Hear Res 46:34, 1981.

75. Larson KK, Ramig LO, Scherer RC: Acoustic and glottographic voice analysis during drug-related fluctuations in Parkinson disease, J Med Speech-Lang Pathol 2:227, 1994.

76. Laszewski A: Role of the department of rehabilitation in preoperative evaluation of parkinsonian patients, J Am Geriatr Soc 4:1280, 1956.

77. Laures JS, Weismer G: The effects of a flattened fundamental frequency on intelligibility at the sentence level, J Speech Lang Hear Res 42:1148, 1999.

78. Leanderson R, Meyerson BA, Persson A: Lip muscle function in parkinsonian dysarthria, Acta Otolaryngol 74:271, 1972.

79. Lehiste I: Some acoustic characteristics of dysarthric speech, bibl phonetica, fasc 2, Basel, Switzerland, 1965, S Karger.

80. Leverenz J, Sumi SM: Prevalence of Parkinson's disease in patients with Alzheimer's disease, Neurology 34(suppl 1):101, 1984.

81. Logemann JA, Fisher HB: Vocal tract control in Parkinson's disease: phonetic feature analysis of misarticulations, J Speech Hear Disord 46:348, 1981.

82. Logemann JA et al: Frequency and occurrence of vocal tract dysfunctions in the speech of a large sample of Parkinson patients, J Speech Hear Disord 43:47, 1978.

83. Louis ED et al: Speech dysfluency exacerbated by levodopa in Parkinson's disease, Mov Disord 16:562, 2001.

84. Ludlow CL, Bassich CJ: The results of acoustic and perceptual assessment of two types of dysarthria. In Berry W, editor: Clinical dysarthria, Boston, 1983, College-Hill Press.

85. Ludlow C, Bassich C: Relationship between perceptual ratings and acoustic measures of hypokinetic speech. In McNeil J, Aronson A, editors: The dysarthrias: physiologic, acoustics, perception, management, Austin, Tex, 1984, Pro-Ed.

86. Ludlow CL, Connor NP, Bassich CJ: Speech timing in Parkinson's and Huntington's disease, Brain Lang 32:195, 1987.

87. Ludlow CL et al: Phonatory characteristics of vocal fold tremor, J Phonet 14:509, 1986.

88. Maraganore DM: Epidemiology and genetics of Parkinson's disease. In Adler CH, Ahlskog JE, editors: Parkinson's disease and movement disorders: diagnosis and treatment guidelines for the practicing physician, Totowa, NJ, 2000, Humana Press.

89. Mayeux R, Stern Y, Stanton S: Heterogeneity in dementia of the Alzheimer type: evidence of subgroups, Neurology 35:453, 1985.

90. McClean MD, Beukelman DR, Yorkston KM: Speech-muscle visuomotor tracking in dysarthric and nonimpaired speakers, J Speech Hear Res 30:276, 1987.

91. Metter EJ, Hanson WF: Clinical and acoustical variability in hypokinetic dysarthria, J Commun Disord 19:347, 1986.

92. Mohlo ES, Factor SA: Secondary causes of parkinsonism. In Adler CH, Ahlskog JE, editors: Parkinson's disease and movement disorders: diagnosis and treatment guidelines for the practicing physician, Totowa, NJ, 2000, Humana Press.

93. Moore CA, Scudder RR: Coordination of jaw muscle activity in parkinsonian movement: description and response to traditional treatment. In Yorkston KM, Beukelman DR, editors: Recent advances in clinical dysarthria, Austin, Tex, 1989, Pro-Ed.

94. Mueller PB: Parkinson's disease: motor-speech behavior in a selected group of patients, Folia Phoniatr Logop 23:333, 1971.

95. Müller J et al: Progression of dysarthria and dysphagia in postmortem-confirmed parkinsonian disorders, Arch Neurol 58:259, 2001.

96. Murdoch BE: Acquired speech and language disorders, New York, 1990, Chapman & Hall.

97. Murdoch BE et al: Respiratory function in Parkinson's subjects exhibiting a perceptible speech deficit: a kinematic and spirometric analysis, J Speech Hear Disord 54:610, 1989.

98. Murry T: The production of stress in three types of dysarthric speech. In Berry W, editor: Clinical dysarthria, Boston, 1983, College-Hill.

99. Netsell R, Daniel B, Celesia GG: Acceleration and weakness in parkinsonian dysarthria, J Speech Hear Disord 40:170, 1975.

100. Ozsancak C et al: Measurement of voice onset time in dysarthric patients: methodological considerations, Folia Phoniatr Logop 53:48, 2001.

101. Perez KS et al: The parkinson larynx: tremor and videostroboscopic findings, J Voice 10:354, 1996.

102. Phillipbar SA, Robin DA, Luschei ES: Limb, jaw, and vocal tremor in Parkinson's patients. In Yorkston KM, Beukelman DR, editors: Recent advances in clinical dysarthria, Boston, 1989, College-Hill Press.

103. Putnam AHB: Review of research in dysarthria. In Winitz H, editor: Human communication and its disorders, a review 1988, Norwood, NJ, 1988, Ablex Publishing.

104. Ramig LO et al: Acoustic analysis of voices of patients with neurologic disease, Ann Otol Rhinol Laryngol 97:164, 1988.

105. Robin DA, Jordan LS, Rodnitzky RL: Prosodic impairment in Parkinson's disease, Presented at the Clinical Dysarthria Conference, Tucson, 1986.

106. Schulz GM et al: Voice and speech characteristics of persons with Parkinson's disease pre- and post-pallidotomy surgery: preliminary findings, J Speech Lang Hear Res 42:1176, 1999.

106a. Schulz GM, Greer M, Freidman W: Changes in vocal intensity in Parkinson's disease following pallidotomy, J Voice, 14:589, 2000.

107. Scott R et al: Neuropsychological, neurological and functional outcome following pallidotomy for Parkinson's disease: a consecutive series of eight simultaneous bilateral and twelve unilateral procedures, Brain 121:659, 1998.

108. Smith E, Faber R: Effects of psychotropic medications on speech and language. Special interest div, ASHA, Neurophysiol Neurogen Speech Lang Disord 2:4, 1992.

109. Smith MC, Smith MK, Ellring H: Spontaneous and posed facial expression in Parkinson's disease, J Int Neuropsych Soc 2:383, 1996.

110. Smith ME et al: Intensive voice treatment in Parkinson disease: laryngostroboscopic findings, J Voice 9:453, 1995.

111. Solomon NP, Hixon TJ: Speech breathing in Parkinson's disease, J Speech Hear Res 36:294, 1993.

112. Solomon NP, Robin DA, Luschei ES: Strength, endurance, and stability of the tongue and hand in Parkinson disease, J Speech Lang Hear Res 43:256, 2000.

113. Solomon NP et al: Tongue function testing in Parkinson's disease: indications of fatigue. In Till JA, Yorkston KM, Beukelman DR, editors: Motor speech disorders: advances in assessment and treatment, Baltimore, 1994, Brookes Publishing.

114. Solomon NP et al: Tongue strength and endurance in mild to moderate Parkinson's disease, J Med Speech-Lang Pathol 3:15, 1995.

115. Solomon NP et al: Effects of pallidal stimulation on speech in three men with severe Parkinson's disease, Am J Speech-Lang Pathol 9:241, 2000.

116. Stewart et al: Speech dysfunction in early Parkinson's disease, Mov Disord 10:562, 1995.

117. Tatsumi IF et al: Acoustic properties of ataxic and parkinsonian speech, in syllable repetition tasks, Annu Bull Res Instit Logop Phoniatr 13:99, 1979.

118. Theodoros DG, Murdoch BE, Thompson EC: Hypernasality in Parkinson's disease: a perceptual and physiological analysis, J Med Speech-Lang Pathol 3:73, 1995.

119. Thompson AWS: On being a parkinsonian. In Kapur N, editor: Injured brains of medical minds: views from within, New York, 1997, Oxford University Press.

120. Torp JN, Hammen VL: Perception of Parkinson speech rate, J Med Speech-Lang Pathol 8:323, 2000.

121. van Zagten M, Lodder J, Kessels F: Gait disorder and parkinsonian signs in patients with stroke related to small deep infarcts and white matter lesions, Mov Disord 13:89, 1998.

122. Weiner P et al: Respiratory muscle performance and the perception of dyspnea in Parkinson's disease, Can J Neurol Sci 29:68, 2002.

123. Weismer G: Articulatory characteristics of parkinsonian dysarthria: segmental and phrase-level timing, spirantization, and glottal-supraglottal coordination. In McNeil MR, Rosenbek JC, Aronson AE, editors: The dysarthrias, Austin, Tex, 1984, Pro-Ed.

124. Weismer G et al: Acoustic and intelligibility characteristics of sentence production in neurogenic speech disorders, Folia Phoniatr Logop 53:1, 2001.

125. Winikates J, Jankovic J: Clinical correlates of vascular parkinsonism, Arch Neurol 56:98, 1999.

126. Yamanouchi H, Nagura H: Neurological signs and frontal white matter lesions in vascular parkinsonism. A clinicopathologic study, Stroke 28:965, 1997.

127. Ziegler W: Task-related factors in oral motor control, Brain Lang 80:556, 2002.

128. Ziegler W et al: Accelerated speech in dysarthria after acquired brain injury: acoustic correlates, Br J Disord Commun 23:215, 1988.

129. Zwirner P, Barnes GJ: Vocal tract steadiness: a measure of phonatory and upper airway motor control during phonation in dysarthria, J Speech Hear Res 35:761, 1992.

130. Zwirner P, Murry T, Woodson GE: Phonatory function of neurologically impaired patients, J Comm Disord 24:287, 1991.

"The flow of speech is often jerky, generated in fits and starts. As they proceed, patients are seemingly on guard against anticipated speech breakdowns, making compensation from time to time as they feel the imminence of glottic closure, respiratory arrest, or articulatory hindrance."

(Description of effects of chorea on speech—Darley, Aronson, and Brown [DAB][36])

CHAPTER OUTLINE

I. Anatomy and basic functions of the basal ganglia control circuit

II. Clinical characteristics of basal ganglia control circuit disorders associated with hyperkinetic dysarthrias
   A. Dyskinesias
   B. Myoclonus
   C. Tics
   D. Chorea
   E. Ballismus
   F. Athetosis
   G. Dystonia
   H. Spasm
   I. Tremor

III. Etiologies
   A. Toxic-metabolic conditions
   B. Degenerative diseases
   C. Infectious processes
   D. Vascular disorders
   E. Neoplasm
   F. Other

IV. Speech pathology
   A. Distribution of etiologies, lesions, and severity in clinical practice
   B. Patient perceptions and complaints
   C. Chorea
   D. Dystonia
   E. Athetosis
   F. Spasmodic torticollis (cervical dystonia)
   G. Palatopharyngolaryngeal myoclonus
   H. Action myoclonus
   I. Tics—Tourette's syndrome
   J. Organic (essential) voice tremor
   K. Spasmodic dysphonia

VI. Cases

VII. Summary

Hyperkinetic dysarthrias are a perceptually distinguishable group of motor speech disorders (MSDs) that are most often associated with diseases of the basal ganglia control circuit. They may be manifest in any or all of the respiratory, phonatory, resonatory, and articulatory levels of speech, and they often have prominent effects on prosody. Unlike most central nervous system (CNS)–based dysarthrias, they can result from abnormalities of movement at only one level of speech production, sometimes only a few muscles at that level. Their deviant speech characteristics are the product of abnormal, rhythmic or irregular and unpredictable, rapid or slow involuntary movements.

The designation of this dysarthria type as a plural disorder, the *hyperkinetic dysarthrias,* is justified by the existence of different kinds of involuntary movements that can cause them. Thus the singular term, hyperkinetic dysarthria, serves to identify a type of MSD that reflects the effects of involuntary movements on speech. Its subtypes designate the specific kind of involuntary movement. As with any classification scheme, there is overlap among subtypes, and clinical distinctions are sometimes difficult to make. Nonetheless, recognizing subtypes is useful for various reasons. This chapter's organization uses the notion of subtypes as a vehicle for discussing the shared features, as well as the remarkable variability among speech problems caused by different involuntary movement disorders.

Hyperkinetic dysarthrias are encountered in a large medical practice at a higher frequency than other major single dysarthria types. Based on data for primary communication disorder diagnoses in the Mayo Clinic Speech Pathology practice, they account for 21.6% of all dysarthrias and 19.9% of all MSDs (see Figure 1-3). However, neurogenic spasmodic dysphonia and organic voice tremor accounted for approximately 75% of the hyperkinetic cases in the database. Thus if those two disorders are excluded, hyperkinetic dysarthrias are encountered somewhat less frequently than the other major single dysarthria types.

Hyperkinetic dysarthrias are perceptually distinguishable from other types of dysarthria, and observing the visible abnormal orofacial, head, and respiratory movements that underlie them often facilitates their diagnosis. The bizarreness of these involuntary movements and resultant speech abnormalities frequently raises suspicions about psychogenic etiology, so proper recognition of these dysarthrias can be essential for accurate medical diagnosis. Their diagnosis implies pathology in the basal ganglia or related portions of the extrapyramidal system or sometimes the cerebellar control circuit. The diversity of lesion loci associated with them (and movement disorders in general) reflects the diversity of abnormal movements that may occur in CNS disease and our limited understanding of their anatomy and pathophysiology.

The clinical features of hyperkinetic dysarthrias illustrate the devastating effects that involuntary movements and variations in muscle tone can have on voluntary movement. Hyperkinetic speech often gives the impression that normal speech is being executed but then is interfered with by regular or unpredictable involuntary movements that distort, slow, or interrupt it.

■ ANATOMY AND BASIC FUNCTIONS OF THE BASAL GANGLIA CONTROL CIRCUIT

The anatomy and functions of the basal ganglia control circuit and other portions of the CNS that may be implicated in this dysarthria type were discussed in Chapter 2 and reviewed in Chapter 7. The anatomy and functions of the circuit are the same as those discussed for hypokinetic dysarthria. They are reviewed briefly here, with specific focus on the possible anatomic and pathophysiologic bases of hyperkinetic dysarthrias.

The ventrolateral nucleus of the thalamus has a primarily excitatory effect on the cortex. The nuclei of the basal ganglia have complex interconnections whose output is channeled to the cortex through the ventrolateral nucleus. The aggregate impulses from the basal ganglia have an inhibitory effect on the thalamus. As a result, they tend to inhibit cortical neuronal firing as well. Many hyperkinesias seem to result from a failure of these pathways to properly inhibit cortical motor discharges. This may happen in a number of ways. For example, the subthalamic nucleus normally exerts an inhibitory effect on the thalamus via its regulation of the globus pallidus. Destruction of the subthalamic nucleus causes reduced inhibitory output from the basal ganglia, with resultant increased thalamic and, subsequently, cortical firing. Consequently, uninhibited abnormal movement commands are "released" through the motor cortex to the corticospinal or corticobulbar pathways. Other movement disorders may have similar explanations. For example, a loss of neurons in the striatum, which normally modulates the globus pallidus, can result in abnormal involuntary movements.

Hyperkinesias can also result from a disruption of the normal equilibrium between excitatory and inhibitory neurotransmitters. For example, a relative increase in dopaminergic activity or a relative decrease in cholinergic activity within the circuit may result in hyperkinesia. Finally, the basal ganglia control circuit's role in movement disorders is demonstrated by the outcome of neurosurgical lesions or stimulators placed in the globus pallidus or ventrolateral nucleus of the thalamus. Such lesions can abolish tremor, rigidity, and involuntary limb movements by interrupting the loop through which the abnormal movements are generated.

Portions of the cerebellar control circuit can be similarly implicated in movement disorders. For example, lesions in cerebellar structures such as the dentate nucleus, or in brainstem structures such as the inferior olive or red nucleus, can alter the circuit's discharge patterns to thalamocortical pathways. The resultant input to the cortex can ultimately lead to abnormal motor cortex discharges through the corticospinal and corticobulbar pathways, with subsequent abnormal, involuntary patterns of movement.

■ CLINICAL CHARACTERISTICS OF BASAL GANGLIA CONTROL CIRCUIT DISORDERS ASSOCIATED WITH HYPERKINETIC DYSARTHRIAS

Some involuntary movements are normal. Startle reactions to loud noises, fear-induced tremor of the hands, shivering in response to cold, and jerking of body parts when falling asleep are all normal involuntary responses to certain intrinsic conditions or external stimuli. *Abnormal involuntary movements* are those that occur in conditions where motor steadiness is expected. They can occur at rest, during static postures, or during voluntary movement. They are usually abolished by sleep and exacerbated by anxiety and heightened emotions. In some cases only specific movements trigger them, and sometimes adopting specific postures can inhibit them. The term *hyperkinesia* refers to these abnormal or excessive involuntary movements. The prefix "hyper" does not necessarily reflect excessive speed of voluntary movement; it indicates the presence of "extra" or involuntary movements that can range in rate from slow to fast. In fact, voluntary movements are generally slowed in body parts affected by hyperkinesias.

The precise location and underlying pathophysiology of many movement disorders are poorly understood. As a result, classifications are descriptive, often based on the speed of the involuntary movements (i.e., quick or slow hyperkinesias). Such divisions are often inadequate, because quick and slow involuntary movements occur on a continuum and often reflect a mixture of slow and quick components. However, some descriptive terms are useful, because they convey something about the predominant character of the abnormal movement. In general, it is important to recognize that some hyperkinesias are rapid, unsustained, and unpatterned, whereas others are slower to develop, may be sustained for seconds (or longer), or may be prolonged to a degree that distorts posture in a constant or waxing and waning manner. Combinations of these characteristics are often apparent.

The varieties of movement disorders that are most relevant to understanding hyperkinetic dysarthrias are discussed as follows. Their basic characteristics are summarized in Table 8-1. Additional concepts that describe some associated nonspeech motor behaviors are also addressed.

Dyskinesias

Dyskinesia is a general term used to refer to abnormal, involuntary movements, regardless of etiology. *Orofacial dyskinesias* are involuntary orofacial movements that can occur without hyperkinesias elsewhere in the body. Most hereditary and acquired diseases that cause orofacial dyskinesias are associated with basal ganglia pathology.

table 8-1	Categories of abnormal movement and their predominant rate and rhythm characteristics and presumed anatomic substrates. All but the movements under "Other" may be associated with hyperkinetic dysarthria.

Designation	Speed	Rhythmicity	Anatomic Substrate
Dyskinesia	Fast or slow	Irregular or rhythmic	Basal ganglia control circuit
Myoclonus	Fast or slow	Irregular or rhythmic	Cortex to spinal cord
Palatopharyngo-laryngeal	Slow	Regular	Brainstem (Guillain-Mollaret triangle)
Action	Fast	Irregular	Basal ganglia or cerebellar control circuit
Tics	Fast	Irregular but patterned	Basal ganglia control circuit
Chorea	Fast	Irregular	Basal ganglia control circuit
Ballism	Fast	Irregular	Area of subthalamic nucleus
Athetosis	Slow	Irregular	Basal ganglia control circuit
Dystonia	Slow	Irregular or strained	Basal ganglia control circuit
Spasmodic dysphonia	Slow	Irregular or sustained	?
Spasmodic torticollis	Slow	Irregular or sustained	? Basal ganglia control circuit
Blepharospasm	Slow	Irregular	? Midbrain, cerebellum, facial nucleus
Spasm	Slow or fast	Irregular	? Basal ganglia control circuit
Hemifacial spasm	Fast	Irregular	Facial nucleus cerebellopontine angle, facial canal
Essential tremor	Slow or fast	Rhythmic	? Striatum
Organic voice	Slow	Rhythmic	Cerebellar control circuit
Spasmodic dysphonia	Slow	Rhythmic	?
Other*			
Fasciculations	Fast	Irregular	LMN
Synkinesis	Fast or slow	Irregular	LMN
Facial myokymia	Intermediate	Rhythmic	LMN

CNS, Central nervous system; *LMN,* lower motor neuron.
*These abnormal movements may be visibly apparent in the speech muscles, but they are not considered hyperkinesias because they do not, by themselves, interfere with voluntary movement. Fasciculations, synkinesis, and facial myokymia may be associated with flaccid, not hyperkinetic, dysarthrias and are signs of LMN, not CNS pathology.

Orofacial dyskinesias are a common side effect of prolonged use of antipsychotic drugs, a condition known as *tardive dyskinesia (TD)*. The most common manifestation of TD is an *oro-buccal-lingual dyskinesia* that can be characterized by involuntary *stereotyped and repetitive lip smacking; pursing; puffing and retraction; tongue protrusion; or opening, closing, or lateral jaw movements*. TD can also affect respiratory function, with subsequent effects on speech.[26,41,99] The emergence of hyperkinetic dysarthria caused by dyskinesias can represent TD, and its early recognition may help prevent a permanent TD if drug withdrawal or dosage modifications are possible.

Akathisia is a condition characterized by an inner sense of motor restlessness, which can be manifest by overt motor restlessness (e.g., weight shifting, pacing) to relieve the sensation. It can occur in parkinsonism and Parkinson's disease (PD) and sometimes in response to dopamine antagonist drugs (e.g., neuroleptic or antiemetic agents). It occurs in approximately 25% of patients with tardive dyskinesia.[19,76]

Myoclonus

Myoclonus is characterized by involuntary single or repetitive brief, lightninglike jerks of a body part; if repetitive, jerks can be rhythmic or nonrhythmic. It cannot be inhibited willfully. Myoclonic movements can be confined to a single muscle or can be multifocal. They may occur spontaneously or be induced by visual, tactile, or auditory stimuli, or, sometimes, by voluntary movements. When brought on by movement, the condition is known as *action myoclonus (AM)*.

Myoclonus can be associated with lesions anywhere from the cortex to the spinal cord. It can occur in epilepsy *(myoclonic epilepsy),* where it is considered a component of a seizure. A common form of acquired myoclonus is *postanoxic myoclonus,* which can occur in the aftermath of cardiorespiratory arrest.[99a]

Hiccups (singultus) are a form of complex myoclonus produced by a brief spasm of the diaphragm with subsequent adduction of the vocal folds. They commonly result from irritation of the peripheral sensory nerves in the stomach, esophagus, diaphragm, or mediastinum and may be associated with some toxic-metabolic conditions, such as uremia. Hiccupping may be a sign of medullary involvement in the region of the tractus solitarius, which has important respiratory control functions.[58]

Palatal or *palatopharyngolaryngeal myoclonus (PM)* (also referred to as *palatal tremor*) is a unique, complex form of myoclonus associated with lesions

in the area of the brainstem known as the *Guillain-Mollaret triangle*. It can be associated with specific speech characteristics and is discussed later in a section on speech pathology.

Tics

Tics are rapid, stereotyped, coordinated, or patterned movements that are under partial voluntary control. They tend to be associated with an irresistible urge to perform them and often can be temporarily voluntarily suppressed. Simple tics are difficult to distinguish from dystonia or myoclonus. Complex tics, however, are coordinated and sometimes include jumping, noises, coprolalia, lip smacking, and touching. The prototypical tic condition is *Gilles de la Tourette's syndrome (TS),* which is discussed later in a section under speech pathology.

Chorea

Chorea is characterized by involuntary rapid, nonstereotypic, random, purposeless movements of a body part. It may be present at rest and during sustained postures and voluntary movement. Choreiform movements can be subtle or can grossly displace body parts. They are sometimes modified by the patient to make them appear intentional in order to mask them and avoid embarrassment. Chorea can be degenerative (e.g., Huntington's chorea) or inflammatory or infectious in origin (e.g., Sydenham's chorea, encephalitis). It can occur in response to drugs, during pregnancy *(chorea gravidarum),* in association with some metabolic abnormalities, sometimes from neoplasm, and occasionally from vascular lesions of the subthalamic nucleus, striatum, or thalamus. Etiology can be undetermined. Rarely, the condition is benign and familial.[27]

Ballismus

Ballismus involves gross, abrupt contractions of axial and proximal muscles of the extremities that can produce wild flailing movements; when unilateral, the condition is called *hemiballismus*. Lesions of the subthalamic nucleus are often responsible, and stroke is the most common cause.[27]

Athetosis

Athetosis is characterized by slow, writhing, purposeless movements that tend to flow into one another. It is often considered a major category of cerebral palsy; when acquired, it may be caused by various conditions. Athetotic movements, especially when acquired, are often considered a combination of chorea and dystonia; when chorea is predominant, the term *choreoathetosis* is sometimes used to describe them.[6]

Dystonia

Dystonia is a relatively slow hyperkinesia characterized by involuntary abnormal postures resulting from excessive cocontraction of antagonistic muscles. The primary abnormal movements tend to be slow and sustained, but there may be superimposed quick movements. The abnormal posture may involve torsion of a body part. Dystonias probably reflect a combination of dopaminergic and cholinergic overactivity in the basal ganglia.[89]

Dystonia may involve only one segment of the body or contiguous regions (segmental). When only orofacial muscles are affected, the condition is often called *focal mouth dystonia* or *orofacial dystonia* or *dyskinesia*. Many occupational cramp syndromes, such as writers' cramp, are probably forms of dystonia. Dystonia can also be generalized and, when not associated with other neurologic deficits, is known as *primary generalized dystonia*.

Torticollis (cervical dystonia) is a segmental dystonia characterized by tonic or clonic spasms of the neck muscles, especially the sternocleidomastoid and trapezius. This causes deviation of the head to the right or left or, less frequently, backward *(retrocollis)* or forward *(antecollis)*. Torticollis is generally considered a basal ganglia disease, and it is most often idiopathic. Cervical spine abnormalities and focal lesions in the putamen, caudate, thalamus, and globus pallidus, or their connecting pathways, have been associated with the condition.[17,90]

Blepharospasm is characterized by a forceful, spasmodic, relatively sustained closure of the eyes. It can occur alone or with other dystonic disorders, particularly those involving orofacial muscles. Its biochemical and neuroanatomic mechanisms are poorly understood, but bilateral lid closure and blinking can be caused by stimulation of the midbrain and cerebellum. It is usually taken as a sign of extrapyramidal disease; it has also been associated with disturbances in the thalamus, putamen, and lower pontine tegmentum.[17]

Spasm

Spasm is a general descriptive term that designates various muscular contractions. Tonic spasms are prolonged or continuous. Clonic spasms are repetitive, rapid in onset, and brief in duration.

Spasms are usually involuntary, even when they result from fear, anxiety, and conversion disorders. They often result in movement, but sometimes they limit motion (e.g., when attempting to avoid back pain that may arise from movement). The term *spasm* is sometimes used to describe the abnormal postures seen in dystonia.

Hemifacial spasm is characterized by paroxysms of rapid, irregular clonic twitching of half of the face. The causative lesion affects the facial nerve in the cerebellopontine angle or facial canal and is often thought to result from a pulsating blood vessel (see Chapter 4). This interesting phenomenon illustrates that not all movement disorders result from primary lesions of the CNS control circuits or extrapyramidal system.

Tremor

Tremor is the most common involuntary movement. It involves the rhythmic (periodic) movement of a body part. It may be characterized as resting, postural, action, or terminal. *Resting tremor* occurs when the body part is in repose, *postural tremor* when the body part is maintained against gravity, *action tremor* during movement, and *terminal tremor* as the body part nears a target. Some clinically observable tremors are *physiologic,* meaning they are exaggerations of the normal tremor that exists in muscle, becoming of sufficient amplitude to be visible under conditions of extreme fatigue or emotion. Physiologic tremor is in the 10- to 12-Hz range until the fifth decade, after which it progressively decreases with age.[66] Toxic tremors can be induced by endogenous toxic states, such as thyrotoxicosis and uremia, or by medications, toxins, or during withdrawal from drugs or alcohol.

Essential (familial) tremor occurs with sustained posture and action and commonly affects the upper limbs, head, or voice. It tends to be reduced by alcohol.

Cerebellar tremor was discussed in Chapter 6. It occurs during sustained postures and action and terminally, and it is primarily due to involvement of the dentatorubrothalamic pathway; lesions of the superior cerebellar peduncle can cause severe tremor.[6] *Wing-beating tremor* (frequently present in Wilson's disease) is a severe proximal postural tremor and is considered a special type of cerebellar tremor. It has a wing-beating appearance when the arms are held in an outstretched or abducted position.[17]

▣ ETIOLOGIES

Hyperkinetic dysarthrias can be caused by any process that damages the basal ganglia control circuit or portions of the cerebellar control circuit or indirect activation pathways that can lead to hyperkinesias. Known causes include degenerative, vascular, traumatic, inflammatory, toxic, and metabolic

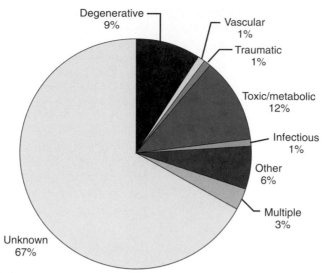

FIGURE 8-1 Distribution of etiologies for 141 quasirandomly selected cases with a primary speech pathology diagnosis of hypokinetic dysarthria at the Mayo Clinic from 1969-1990 and 1999-2001 (see Box 8-1 for details).

diseases. These broad etiologic categories are associated with hyperkinetic dysarthrias with varying frequency, but the exact distribution of etiologies is unknown. Idiopathic, toxic-metabolic, and degenerative causes are probably the most frequent etiologies, however (Figure 8-1 and Box 8-1).

Some of the common neurologic conditions associated with hyperkinetic dysarthrias with noticeably greater frequency than other dysarthria types are discussed as follows; much of the specific information provided is based on known causes of hyperkinesias in general, with an assumption that dysarthria can be caused by them as well. Conditions associated with hyperkinetic dysarthrias but that are more frequently associated with other dysarthria types (e.g., PD) are discussed in chapters dealing with those dysarthrias.

Toxic-Metabolic Conditions

Drugs that affect the balance of neurotransmitters in the basal ganglia are a common cause of acute or delayed-onset involuntary movements. *Neuroleptic* (meaning that which takes on the neuron) or *antipsychotic drugs,* whose actions block (antagonize) dopamine receptors, are the most frequent culprits. In some populations, drug-induced movement disorders are quite common. For example, the overall prevalence of tardive dyskinesia (TD) in schizophrenic patients on long-term treatment is 24%,[93] and the elderly who take antipsychotic drugs are at considerably higher risk for TD than younger people.[61]

TD can be associated with all classes of dopamine-blocking agents, including phenothiazines (e.g., chlorpromazine [Thorazine], thioridazine [Mellaril]) and butyrophenones (e.g., haloperidol [Haldol]).* Dopamine-blocking drugs used to control gastrointestinal disorders (e.g., metoclopramide [Reglan], prochlorperazine [Compazine]) can also cause TD.[94] Although the first step in treating TD is drug withdrawal, the dyskinesia often worsens in the first weeks after withdrawal and sometimes does not emerge until drug use is stopped. Drug withdrawal may be associated with remission of the dyskinesias, perhaps in 60% of patients, but it may take 3 to 5 years.[75] Acute dystonic reactions can also be triggered by dopamine receptor blocking agents.[94] Other drugs that can cause dyskinesias include levodopa, amphetamines, cocaine, tricyclic antidepressants, and phenytoin.[93]

Chorea and dystonia can be caused by antiparkinsonian drugs and usually occur at the time of peak levodopa effect.[7] These dyskinesias are frequently evident in limb and orofacial muscles, and sometimes they alter respiration.[87] L-Dopa–induced dyskinesias seem to reflect effects of excessive dopaminergic stimulation of certain striatal neurons, with subsequent thalamic disinhibition and excessive positive feedback to precentral motor areas, resulting in excessive, involuntary (hyperkinetic) movements.[81]

*A newer generation of "atypical" antipsychotic drugs (e.g., clozapine, risperidone, olanzapine, amisulpride) seem to carry less risk for TD than conventional neuroleptics, even in the elderly.[40,71,101]

box 8-1	Etiologies for 141 quasirandomly selected cases with a primary speech pathology diagnosis of hyperkinetic dysarthria at the Mayo Clinic from 1969-1990 and 1999-2001. Percentage of cases under each heading is given in parentheses. Specific etiologies under each heading are ordered from most to least frequent. Cases with isolated essential voice tremor or isolated neurogenic spasmodic dysphonia are not included, because etiology is nearly always idiopathic in those disorders; if they were included in these data, the percentage of unknown etiologies would be substantially higher.

Unknown (67%)

Orofacial dyskinesia, dystonia, or tremor (21%)
(other descriptors include oromandibular dystonia, lingual-mandibular dystonia, focal dystonia, orallaryngeal dystonia, lingual-pharyngeal dystonia, palatal-pharyngeal-lingual-facial dystonia, oral dyskinesia, buccolingual dyskinesia, extrapyramidal facial movement disorder)
Essential tremor (11%)
Segmental dystonia or tremor (7%)
Spasmodic torticollis or retrocollis or antecollis (6%)
Face or neck or axial dyskinesia (4%)
Chorea (2%)
Meige's syndrome (2%)
Dystonia, not otherwise specified (2%)
Other (12%)
Movement disorder; dyskinesia; extrapyramidal syndrome; acquired basal ganglia disorder; myoclonus; indeterminate brainstem lesion; isolated hyperkinetic dysarthria; torticollis and facial dystonia; respiratory-laryngeal dystonia; abdominal myoclonus; action dystonia; focal seizure disorder; generalized dystonia

Toxic or Metabolic (12%)

Tardive dyskinesia (7%)
Drug-induced dyskinesia (2%)
Other (3%)
Dialysis encephalopathy; hepatic encephalopathy; hypoparathyroidism

Degenerative (9%)

Huntington's chorea (3%)
Other (6%)
Unspecified degenerative CNS disease; dystonia musculorum deformans; amyotrophic lateral sclerosis; multiple sclerosis; Parkinson's disease

Multiple (3%)

Multiple sclerosis + drug-induced parkinsonism; familial ataxia + alcoholism; senile chorea + stroke; tardive dyskinesia + stroke + anxiety

Infectious (1%)

Sydenham's chorea

Trauma (1%)

After cerebellar tumor removal (ataxia and palatal myoclonus)

Vascular (1%)

Brainstem stroke

Other (6%)

Tourette's syndrome; myoclonic epilepsy; focal seizure disorder; familial tremor-dystonia syndrome; seizure-related generalized polymyoclonus; focal myoclonus; paraneoplastic encephalopathy; no neurologic diagnosis

CNS, Central nervous system.

Chorea, including choreiform facial movements, can be associated with oral contraceptive use, alcohol withdrawal, and certain metabolic conditions including hyperthyroidism, anoxic or hepatic encephalopathy, hypernatremia, hypoglycemia, choreoacanthocytosis, and hypoparathyroidism.[3,27,60]

Action or postural tremor can be associated with valproic acid, lithium, and theophylline derivatives and may occur during alcohol or other drug withdrawal states. Tremor (and dystonia) may also occur in Wilson's disease.[77]

A number of toxins can cause myoclonus (e.g., mercury, lead, strychnine, marijuana), as well as a number of drugs (e.g., psychiatric medications, antiinfective agents, narcotics, anticonvulsants, anesthetics, cardiac medications, and antihistamines).[28]

Degenerative Diseases

Huntington's disease is an inherited autosomal dominant degenerative CNS disorder. Because it has complete penetrance, half of the offspring of individuals with the gene are affected. It usually begins insidiously by the fourth or fifth decade, with progression to death within 10 to 20 years.[27] Cellularly, there is severe loss of neurons in the caudate nucleus and putamen and diffuse neuronal loss in the cortex. Functionally, positron emission tomography (PET) has shown impaired activity of the striatum and its frontal projection areas.[14,98] The disease's most characteristic clinical feature is chorea, which can be generalized, but it is sometimes initially manifest only in the face or hands. Dementia, depression, personality changes, and attention deficits are also characteristic, and dysarthria and dysphagia are common.

Primary generalized dystonia (also called *idiopathic torsion dystonia* or *dystonia musculorum deformans*) usually results from autosomal dominant inheritance, with marked variation in clinical expression. It is often associated with gait abnormalities and postural deformities in the neck, trunk, and extremities. Usually beginning in childhood as a focal dystonia, it eventually spreads over months or years to affect other body parts.[88,94]

Involuntary movements may also occur in degenerative diseases that primarily affect cognitive abilities. For example, orofacial dyskinesia in the elderly tends to be associated with dementia.[33] Dyskinesia, especially orofacial dyskinesia, has been reported in 17% of individuals with a diagnosis of Alzheimer's disease.[80]

Infectious Processes

Sydenham's chorea is associated with streptococcal infection or rheumatic fever; it occurs in 26% of patients with rheumatic fever. It affects mostly the young and usually resolves in a relatively short time, but it is sometimes persistent.[25] Single photon emission computed tomography (SPECT) has documented hyperperfusion of the basal ganglia in people with recent onset of symptoms.[13]

Other infectious causes of chorea include diphtheria, rubella, systemic lupus erythematosus, and acquired immune deficiency syndrome (AIDS).[85,89]

Vascular Disorders

Although stroke is the usual cause of hemichorea and hemiballismus, vascular lesions are not a common cause of hyperkinesias.[52] Nonetheless, stroke or other vascular disturbances in the basal ganglia control circuit, and sometimes the cerebellar control circuit, can lead to movement disorders and hyperkinetic dysarthria. For example, dystonia can result from putaminal stroke[49,89]; chorea, dystonia, athetosis, or action tremor can result from lateral-posterior thalamic stroke[65]; and blepharospasm, *Meige's syndrome* (see later discussion), and palatal myoclonus have been reported in brainstem stroke or hypoxic encephalopathy.[37,60a]

Neoplasm

Tumors of the basal ganglia and thalamus have been associated with chorea and dystonia.[89,90]

Other

Movement disorders, particularly dystonias, are often considered *primary* or *unassociated with a known cause or other neurologic abnormalities.* A genetic basis for some primary dystonias has been established and is suspected for others. Primary dystonia can be generalized or focal.[94] Meige's syndrome is a primary focal cranial dystonia characterized by a combination of blepharospasm and oromandibular dystonia. Many spasmodic dysphonias are considered primary focal dystonias.

Although uncommon, some hyperkinetic movement disorders are paroxysmal or evident only during brief (minutes to hours) recurring episodes.* Examples of these disorders include *paroxysmal kinesigenic choreoathetosis,* which is precipitated by sudden movement; *paroxysmal exercise-induced dystonia,* which is induced by prolonged exercise; and *paroxysmal (nonkinesigenic) dystonic choreoathetosis,* which can be triggered by various factors, such as alcohol, coffee, tea, fatigue, stress, and anxiety. Many of these disorders are thought to represent *"channelopathies,"* or dysfunction of ion channels involved in neurotransmission. Cases are frequently idiopathic and sporadic, but a family history with autosomal dominant inheritance is common. Occasionally, paroxysmal dyskinesias are symptomatic of other conditions (e.g., multiple sclerosis, progressive supranuclear palsy [PSP], perinatal hypoxic encephalopathy, endocrine disorders, diabetes mellitus, vascular lesions, traumatic brain injury). In at least some of these disorders, speech can be affected during episodes.[15]

TS is characterized by motor and vocal tics. The disorder has a significant genetic component, and its signs are always apparent before adulthood. Its vocal and speech characteristics are discussed in a section under speech pathology.

Abnormalities of the dental arch in edentulous elderly people have been associated with involuntary chewing movements. Disruption of dental proprioception has been suggested as a general explanatory mechanism.[60]

Facial dyskinesias may be observed in schizophrenic individuals, and they can occur before the introduction of antipsychotic drugs.[60]

Chorea gravidarum is a rare, benign choreiform disorder that occurs during pregnancy, most frequently in women with chronic rheumatic heart disease.[44]

■ SPEECH PATHOLOGY

Distribution of Etiologies, Lesions, and Severity in Clinical Practice

Box 8-1 and Figure 8-1 summarize the etiologies for 141 quasirandomly selected cases seen at the Mayo

---

*Episodic ataxias are discussed in Chapter 6.

Clinic with a primary speech pathology diagnosis of hyperkinetic dysarthria. Cases with organic voice tremor and neurogenic spasmodic dysphonia were not included in the review, because their etiology is nearly always unknown. The cautions expressed in Chapter 4 about generalizing these data to the general population of patients with hyperkinetic dysarthrias or to all speech pathology practices also apply here.

The data establish that hyperkinetic dysarthrias can result from several medical conditions and that distribution of the etiologies is quite different from that for most other dysarthria types. Sixty-seven percent of the cases were of undetermined etiology, with toxic or metabolic causes accounting for an additional 12% of the cases. These percentages illustrate the elusive nature of the neuroanatomic bases of movement disorders, and they suggest that their causes often lie in neurochemical abnormalities rather than structural lesions.

The nature and muscular locus of involuntary movements of unknown etiology illustrate the heterogeneity that exists in this group of speech disorders. The abnormal movements were given numerous descriptive labels, including dyskinesia, dystonia, torticollis, retrocollis, antecollis, chorea, tremor, myoclonus, AM, and action dystonia. In some cases the neurologic diagnosis was limited to general labels such as "movement disorder," "extrapyramidal syndrome," and "acquired basal ganglia disorder."

The largest single diagnosis for the 141 cases was orofacial dyskinesia of unknown etiology (21%). This means that the patients' movement disorders were confined to the face, jaw, tongue, pharynx, or larynx. This highlights the predilection of many movement disorders for the orofacial muscles, the likelihood that many generalized movement disorders may be manifest first in the orofacial area, and the importance of recognizing the meaning of abnormal orofacial movements and associated dysarthria as signs of neurologic disease. The prevalence of movement disorders that are limited to the head and neck muscles in people with dysarthria is further illustrated by the frequency of cases with spasmodic torticollis, retrocollis, or antecollis (6%), face or neck or axial dyskinesia (4%), and tardive dyskinesia (7%). Thus approximately 85% of the group had a dysarthria in which the underlying movement disorder was not evident in the limbs. This percentage would be even higher if organic voice tremor and neurogenic spasmodic dysphonias were included in the sample.

Most cases with toxic or metabolic etiology were drug related, most often involving neuroleptic or anticonvulsive medications. Although most were delayed in onset (tardive), some occurred soon after medication was started. In contrast to the distribution of etiologies for other dysarthria types, drugs were the most frequent known cause of hyperkinetic dysarthrias in this sample.

Huntington's chorea was the most frequent degenerative disease (3% of the entire sample). The remaining etiologic categories (infectious, trauma, vascular) were not frequently represented but did contain conditions with established and prominent associations with hyperkinesias (e.g., TS, myoclonic epilepsy, Sydenham's chorea).

To what extent was dysarthria the only manifestation of an involuntary movement disorder? A substantial minority of the sample had involuntary movements that were confined to the orofacial muscles but present at rest or during nonspeech movements. Several cases had a dysarthria in which the hyperkinesia was triggered by speech and not present during orofacial movements other than speech (this percentage would be considerably higher if cases with organic voice tremor and neurogenic spasmodic dysphonia were included). Thus *movement disorders may become clinically evident only during speech.* Unfortunately, when this is the case, the problem is often diagnosed as psychogenic, and affected people may have a painfully long history of repeated psychiatric assessments and treatment, without any connection emerging between psychopathology and the speech disorder and without benefit from psychotherapy, behavioral interventions, or psychotropic medications. Such cases illustrate a lack of understanding about the possible connection between speech disorders and neurologic disease, especially when speech is the presenting and only obvious physical problem.

What speech structures were involved in these cases, and how often was only a single structure involved? Table 8-2 summarizes the percentage of

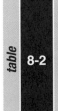

table 8-2	Percentage of patients with involvement of the jaw, face, tongue, palate, larynx, and respiratory muscles—singly and in combination—for 86 cases with hyperkinetic dysarthrias (excluding organic voice tremor and spasmodic dysphonia)

Structure Involved	% in Combination with Other Structures	% Isolated
Jaw	52	3
Face	67	1
Tongue	56	3
Palate	13	0
Larynx	44	1
Respiratory	7	1

cases (among the first 86 cases in the group of 141 reviewed in Box 8-1) in which a clear indication was given about involvement of the jaw, face, tongue, palate, larynx, and respiratory muscles, and the percentage of cases in which only one of those structures was affected. It is clear that more than one speech structure is involved in most cases and that face, tongue, and jaw involvement are most frequently recognized (note again that organic voice tremor and spasmodic dysphonia were not included in the sample, so laryngeal involvement is underrepresented). Combined jaw, face, and tongue hyperkinesia was the most frequently recognized combination of involved structures. It is also apparent that only a single speech structure may be involved in hyperkinetic dysarthria. Nine cases (10%) had only one structure affected; the palate was the only structure not affected in isolation. In a few cases, involuntary movements in the singly involved structure were induced only by speech; for example, two cases with jaw dystonia had abnormal jaw movements only during speech. Thus these data suggest that involuntary movements underlying dysarthria usually involve more than a single speech structure, but they sometimes affect only a single speech structure and sometimes occur only during speech.

Precise anatomic localization of lesions for the patients in this sample, as predicted by the high frequency of undetermined etiologies, was sparse. A majority of those who had computed tomography (CT) or magnetic resonance imaging (MRI) had no identifiable pathology, and detected abnormalities were often nonfocal or not necessarily related to the movement disorder. For example, several cases had evidence of general cerebral or cerebellar atrophy, or both; bilateral white matter changes; or ventricular dilatation. A few had evidence of cortical lesions, but there was no common site among them. Some did have evidence of basal ganglia pathology, and a few had evidence of cerebellar pathology or a thalamic lesion. Even in cases with identifiable lesions in the basal ganglia, cerebellum, and thalamus, it was sometimes concluded that they were not directly responsible for the movement disorder (e.g., one patient's movement disorder was most likely due to tardive dyskinesia). Thus although CT and MRI sometimes reveal abnormalities, the connection between the identified lesion and the movement disorder is not always clear.

This retrospective review did not permit a clear delineation of dysarthria severity. However, in those patients for whom a judgment of intelligibility was explicitly stated (60% of the sample), *49% had reduced intelligibility.* The degree to which this figure accurately estimates the frequency of intelligibility impairments in the population with hyperkinetic dysarthrias is unclear. It is likely that many patients for whom an observation of intelligibility was not made had normal intelligibility, but the sample probably contains a larger number of mildly impaired patients than is encountered in the typical rehabilitation setting. In addition, reduced intelligibility is only one measure of deficit and may not accurately represent degree of handicap or disability. For example, many hyperkinetic dysarthrias significantly reduce efficiency (speed) of communication without affecting intelligibility, and the visible, bizarre involuntary movements that are responsible for many aspects of the dysarthria can have devastating social and emotional consequences. The relatively low frequency of intelligibility impairments in this dysarthria is fortunate, but to conclude that the disorder often does not have a significant impact on verbal and nonverbal communication, and its emotional and social consequences, probably grossly underestimates its impact on affected individuals.

Finally, movement disorders and hyperkinetic dysarthria can occur in conditions that also affect cognitive functions (e.g., Huntington's disease). Of the patients in the sample whose cognitive abilities were explicitly commented on or formally assessed (80% of the sample), *20% had some impairment of cognitive ability.*

Patient Perceptions and Complaints

Patient complaints often depend on the type of movement disorder and the level of the speech system it affects. Those with nonrhythmic hyperkinesias (e.g., chorea, dystonia) affecting the jaw, face, tongue, and larynx tend to describe their speech as slurred, slow, halting, or "hard to get out." Somewhat surprisingly, those with hyperkinesia at several levels of the speech system may not be aware of the abnormal movements, even when they are visibly apparent to the examiner. They may, however, recognize their inability to maintain a steady jaw, face, or tongue posture when requested by the examiner. Failure to spontaneously complain about orofacial hyperkinesias is more frequent in patients whose hyperkinesia is apparent only during speech, chewing, or swallowing (i.e., they complain of difficulty with speech but not the underlying abnormal movement). Chewing and swallowing complaints are common in chorea and dystonia.

Patients whose hyperkinesia is limited to a single or a few structures may complain of abnormal movements, both at rest and during speech. Complaints about abnormal movements at rest may predominate in patients whose hyperkinesias are mild or can be suppressed temporarily during speech. These complaints include feelings of tightness in affected structures, an inability to move a structure, an inability to control or inhibit abnormal movements, or a sense that the structure simply "doesn't work right." Some patients report being able to suppress the abnormal movements for a time but find that they return with a vengeance when their efforts cease.

Patients with prominent laryngeal hyperkinesias (usually associated with tremor or dystonia) often complain that their voice is shaky, tight, closes off, or does not want to come out. Because of increased resistance to airflow with laryngeal spasm during speech, they may complain of shortness of breath or physical exhaustion during speech and associate it with respiratory difficulty. When the problem is isolated to the larynx, however, the patient usually does not note similar fatigue during strenuous nonspeech physical activities. Patients with respiratory hyperkinesias that are triggered only by speaking may be unaware of the locus of the problem, even when they are acutely aware of their abnormal speech.

Some patients learn that the severity of orofacial dystonic posturing or movements can be reduced or eliminated by certain tactile or proprioceptive *sensory tricks*. For example, a patient with torticollis may learn that bringing the hand to the chin or the back of the head allows them to posture the head more normally; a patient with involuntary jaw opening may learn that lightly touching the hand to the jaw may prevent the movement. With increasing severity or duration of the disorder, however, the facilitory effect of these stimuli diminishes. The term "sensory tricks" is descriptive, and the real mechanism for their effect is unknown.[43] Nonetheless,

patient reports of previously successful sensory tricks, or observation of them during examination, are useful diagnostically, because they are rarely developed in other dysarthria types or in psychogenic speech disorders characterized by abnormal movements.

The following sections review the primary oral mechanism and speech characteristics associated with each of a number of movement disorders known to underlie the hyperkinetic dysarthrias. Related acoustic and physiologic findings are summarized when appropriate.

Chorea

Nonspeech Oral Mechanism

The jaw, face, tongue, and palate are usually normal in size, strength, and symmetry. The gag reflex is usually normal, and pathologic oral reflexes are usually absent. Drooling is occasionally observed, and chewing and swallowing difficulties are not uncommon. The most striking abnormality is motor unsteadiness and, often, easily observed choreiform movements. At rest or during attempts to maintain steady orofacial postures, *quick, unpredictable, involuntary movements* may occur. They can range from subtle exaggerations of facial expression to movements that are so pervasive and prominent that affected structures seem never to be at rest (Figure 8-2). Difficulty recognizing these movements as hyperkinesias occur when (1) movements are subtle

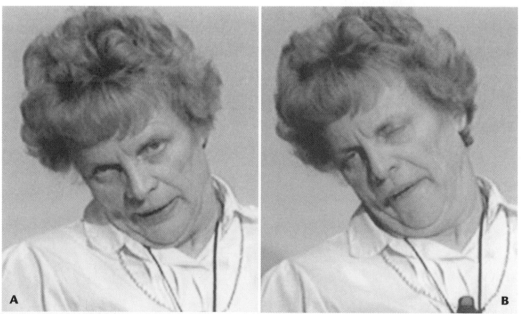

FIGURE 8-2 Quick, involuntary head, jaw, face, lip, and eye movements in a woman with generalized chorea. The depicted movements in panels **A** and **B** were brief and separated from each other by less than 1 second.

and infrequent, because they may be difficult to distinguish from normal unsteadiness, and (2) patients display motor impersistence or cognitive impairments that raise doubts about their ability to sustain adequate effort on the task.

Speech

Conversation, reading, and speech alternate motion rates (AMRs) are useful for eliciting the unpredictable breakdowns of articulation and the abnormalities of rate and prosody that may predominate. Vowel prolongation is indispensable, because it is an opportunity to observe fluctuations in the steady state of the vowel induced by choreiform movements. The open vowel "ah" is particularly useful, because adventitious movements of the jaw, face, tongue, and palate can be easily observed and heard during the sound.

Careful visual observation of the patient during speech is important. It provides confirmatory evidence of abnormal movements as the source of the speech deficit and permits the identification of at least some of the structures involved in the movement disorder.

Table 8-3 summarizes the neuromuscular deficits presumed by DAB[34-36] to underlie the dysarthria of chorea. Nearly all aspects of movement may be disturbed. Involuntary movements may alter the direction and rhythm of movement, and they generally slow rate. Force and range of individual and repetitive movements may vary from reduced to normal to excessive depending on the presence or absence of choreic movements at the moment and the relationship of their direction to that of the intended voluntary speech gesture. Muscle tone may be excessive and, when it is, it tends to be biased. The relationship of these characteristics to specific deviant speech characteristics is discussed in the following section, as are findings from relevant acoustic and physiologic studies.

Clusters of Deviant Dimensions and Prominent Deviant Speech Characteristics

DAB[35] identified several clusters of deviant speech dimensions in their patients with chorea, but a complete review of each is unnecessary to appreciate the major features of the disorder. Only those clusters that are most prominent and distinctive of the hyperkinetic dysarthria of chorea are addressed. Here the focus primarily is on the distinct clusters and most deviant or unique speech characteristics, as well as their relationship to movement abnormalities at each level of the speech system. These characteristics are useful to understanding the disorder's underlying neuromuscular deficits, the components of the speech system that tend to be most prominently involved, and the features that help to distinguish the hyperkinetic dysarthria of chorea from other dysarthria types. The most deviant speech characteristics encountered in the dysarthria of chorea are summarized in Table 8-4.

Respiration. Choreiform movements that affect respiration during speech can be reflected in *sudden, forced, involuntary inspiration or expiration.* Although not pervasive, and not necessarily severe, this feature was not encountered in any other dysarthria type by DAB.[36]

Phonation. Patients may exhibit *harsh voice quality, excess loudness variations*, and *a strained-strangled voice quality.* These features correlated

---

table 8-3	Neuromuscular deficits found in hyperkinetic dysarthria associated with dystonia and chorea

Direction	Rhythm		Rate		Range		Force	Tone
	Individual Movements	Repetitive Movements	Individual Movements	Repetitive Movements	Individual Movements	Repetitive Movements	Individual Movements	Muscle Tone
Dystonia	Inaccurate due to slow involuntary movements	Irregular	Slow	Slow	Reduced to normal	Reduced to normal	Normal	Excessive (biased)
Chorea	Inaccurate due to quick > slow involuntary movements	Irregular	Slow	Slow	Reduced to excessive	Reduced to excessive	Reduced to excessive	Often excessive (biased)

Modified from Darley FL, Aronson AE, Brown JR: Clusters of deviant speech dimensions in the dysarthrias, *J Speech Hear Res* 12:462, 1969.

table 8-4	The most deviant speech dimensions encountered in the hyperkinetic dysarthria of chorea by Darley, Aronson, and Brown,[34] listed in order from most to least severe. Also listed is the component of the speech system associated with each characteristic. The component "prosodic" is listed when several components of the speech system may contribute to the dimension. Characteristics listed under "Other" include speech features not among the most deviant but that may occur and are not typical of most other dysarthria types.

Dimension	Speech Component
Imprecise consonants	Articulatory
Prolonged intervals*	Prosodic
Variable rate*	Prosodic
Monopitch	Phonatory-prosodic
Harsh voice quality	Phonatory
Inappropriate silences*	Prosodic
Distorted vowels	Articulatory-prosodic
Excess loudness variations*	Respiratory-phonatory-prosodic
Prolonged phonemes*	Prosodic
Monoloudness	Phonatory-prosodic
Short phrases	Prosodic
Irregular articulatory breakdowns	Articulatory
Excess and equal stress	Prosodic
Hypernasality	Resonatory
Reduced stress	Prosodic
Strained-strangled quality	Phonatory
Other	
Sudden forced inspiration or expiration*	Respiratory-prosodic
Voice stoppages*	Phonatory-prosodic
Transient breathiness*	Phonatory

*Tend to be distinctive or more severely impaired than in any other single dysarthria type.

with one another in DAB's subjects to form the cluster of *phonatory stenosis,* presumably resulting from relatively brief, random hyperadduction of the vocal folds (excess loudness variations could also result from choreic respiratory movements). Phonatory stenosis may be sufficient to cause *voice stoppages* in some patients. Acoustic analyses of patients with Huntington's disease have documented abnormal fundamental frequency (f_o) variability (often with abrupt changes), abnormally variable voice onset time (VOT), voice arrests, and reduced maximum vowel duration.[56,86,104] These perceptual and acoustic findings mostly reflect instability of laryngeal movements during speech.

Although infrequent, some patients may exhibit *transient breathiness.* This may occur as a result of brief, involuntary vocal fold abduction, poor timing between expiration and phonation, or possibly in response to, or in compensation for, the physically exhausting effects of phonatory stenosis.

Resonance. Chorea may lead to *hypernasality* in some patients, although it is rarely pronounced. Hypernasality was correlated with imprecise consonants and short phrases in DAB's subjects, forming the cluster of *resonatory incompetence.* This suggests that air wastage through the velopharyngeal port may at least partially explain the occurrence of imprecise consonants and short phrases in some speakers.

Articulation. *Imprecise articulation* is the most prominent but not the most distinguishing feature of the dysarthria of chorea. It tends to occur simultaneously with *distorted vowels* and *hypernasality;* in DAB's patients these features formed the cluster of *articulatory-resonatory incompetence. Irregular articulatory breakdowns* also occur frequently. All of these features are presumably the result of various combinations of choreiform movements of the jaw, face, tongue, and palate. Acoustic analyses of people with Huntington's disease have supported this conclusion by documenting disproportionate lengthening of short vowels, slowed* and markedly variable speech AMRs or sentence duration, and abnormal first formant variability (suggestive of abnormal jaw movements) and second formant variability (suggestive of abnormal tongue position and shape) during steady state vowels.[1,56,104] Many of these features have a significant impact on prosody.

Prosody. *Prosodic disturbances are prominent.* They can reflect the primary effects of chorea on speech, as well as the individual's response to the unpredictable movements. As DAB stated, "The flow of speech is often jerky, generated in fits and starts. As they proceed, patients are seemingly on guard against anticipated speech breakdowns, making compensation from time to time as they feel the imminence of glottic closure, respiratory arrest, or articulatory hindrance."[36]

The most prominent cluster of speech characteristics in DAB's study was *prosodic excess,* composed of *prolonged intervals, inappropriate silences, prolonged phonemes,* and *excess and equal stress.* Patients also exhibited *prosodic insufficiency,* characterized by *monopitch, monoloudness, reduced stress,* and *short phrases.* Many patients also had

---

*Reduced syllable repetition rates have been detected before the emergence of other signs of disease in patients with Huntington's disease.[30]

variable rate, possibly reflecting their efforts to complete phrases quickly before the next involuntary movement. The cooccurrence of the seemingly mutually exclusive clusters of prosodic excess and prosodic insufficiency attests to the moment-to-moment variability that occurs in this form of dysarthria, as well as the unpredictability of the effects of relatively quick and variable involuntary movements on speech. They probably also reflect the combined effects of the primary motor disturbance and compensatory or cautious responses to it.

What features of the dysarthria of chorea help identify and distinguish it from other MSDs? Most apparent is the *transient and unpredictable nature of the deviant speech characteristics,* the most obvious of which are *hypernasality, strained-harshness, transient breathiness, articulatory distortions and irregular articulatory breakdowns, loudness variations,* and *sudden forced inspiration or expiration.* These features, often in combination with the speaker's attempt to avoid or compensate for them, lead to *prolonged intervals and phonemes, variable rate, inappropriate silences, voice stoppages,* and *excessive or insufficient stress patterns.* The primary and distinguishing speech and speech-related findings in this form of hyperkinetic dysarthria are summarized in Table 8-5.

Dystonia*

Nonspeech Oral Mechanism

As in chorea, the oral mechanism is often normal in size, strength, and symmetry. Reflexes may be normal. Drooling may occur, and chewing and swallowing complaints are common. Patients frequently complain that food gets stuck in the throat or that chewing is difficult because of involuntary jaw or tongue movements.[53] The striking features of the nonspeech oral mechanism examination are most evident at rest or during attempts to maintain steady facial postures. Dystonic movements are slower than those of chorea, and they have a *waxing and waning* character. Blepharospasm and facial grimacing may be present, as may intermittent, relatively sustained spasms that lead to mouth opening and closing, lip pursing or retraction, and protrusion or rotary movements of the tongue (Figure 8-3). Affected neck muscles may cause elevation of the larynx; torsion of the neck may be marked in patients with torticollis. Recognition of dystonia is most difficult when

---

*This section addresses the general effects of dystonia on speech. Spasmodic dysphonia—because it is encountered fairly frequently in speech pathology practices, and because it often occurs as an isolated problem—is addressed separately in a subsequent section.

table 8-5	Primary distinguishing speech and speech-related findings in the hyperkinetic dysarthria of chorea
Perceptual	
Phonation-respiration	Sudden forced inspiration-expiration, voice stoppages, transient breathiness, strained-harsh voice quality, excess loudness variations
Resonance	Hypernasality (intermittent)
Articulation	Distortions & irregular breakdowns, slow & irregular AMRs
Prosody	Prolonged intervals & phonemes, variable rate, inappropriate silences, excessive-inefficient-variable patterns of stress
Physical	Quick, unpatterned involuntary head or neck, jaw, face, tongue, palate, pharyngeal, laryngeal, thoracic-abdominal movements at rest, during sustained postures & movement
	Dysphagia
Patient Complaints	Effortful speech, involuntary orofacial movements
	Chewing & swallowing problems

AMRs, Alternate motion rates.

movements are subtle or when cognitive or other motor deficits make valid observations difficult.

Patients may use sensory tricks to inhibit dystonic movements, and it is important to ask if they are aware of such tricks when they do not use them spontaneously. These often involve pressure or light touch to the jaw, cheek, or back of the neck; some patients will hold a pipe in the mouth, because it inhibits jaw, lip, or tongue dystonias.

In some cases the nonspeech oral mechanism examination can be entirely normal, with dystonic movements being triggered only by speech. There is a tendency for such patients to have focal dystonic movements that may involve only the jaw, tongue, pharynx, larynx, or respiratory muscles.

Speech

Conversational speech or reading, speech AMRs, and vowel prolongation are useful when assessing the dysarthria of dystonia. Careful visual observation of the patient during speaking is similarly important.

Table 8-3 summarizes the neuromuscular deficits presumed by DAB[34,35] to underlie the dysarthria of

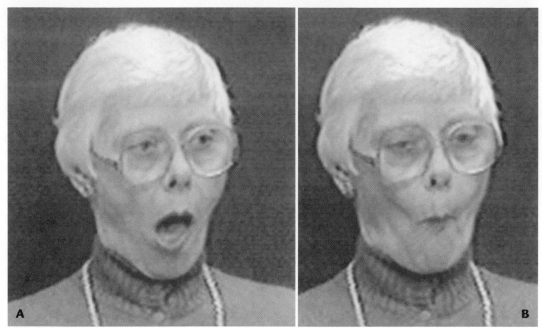

FIGURE 8-3 Woman with oromandibular-lingual dystonia attempting to sit in a relaxed posture with, **A,** relatively slow involuntary jaw opening and tongue lateralization and protrusion and, **B,** involuntary lip pursing.

dystonia. Nearly all aspects of movement may be disturbed. Dystonic movements may alter direction and rhythm of movement, and rate is generally slow. Range of individual and repetitive movements may be normal but can be reduced by excessive and biased muscle tone. The relationship of these characteristics to specific deviant speech characteristics is discussed as follows, as are findings from relevant acoustic and physiologic studies.

Clusters of Deviant Dimensions and Prominent Deviant Speech Characteristics

DAB[35] found several clusters of deviant speech dimensions in their patients with dystonia. Only those that are most prominent and distinctive are addressed here; the focus is on the most deviant or distinctive speech characteristics and their relationship to movement abnormalities at each level of the speech system.* The most deviant speech characteristics encountered in the dysarthria of dystonia are summarized in Table 8-6.

Respiration. The dystonic speakers in DAB's study did not exhibit speech characteristics that

*Golper et al.[53] found a pattern of speech deficits similar to DAB's dystonic patients in a group of 10 patients with focal cranial dystonia (Meige's syndrome).

clearly reflected respiratory dystonia. However, some had *excess loudness variations,* and a small number had mild *alternating loudness.* These features could reflect abnormal respiratory movements or respiratory movements made in an effort to overcome phonatory stenosis.

Phonation. Several phonatory deviations may be present, including *harshness, strained-strangled voice quality, excess loudness variations,* and *voice stoppages.* Combined with *short phrases,* these characteristics combined in DAB's dystonic speakers to form the cluster of *phonatory stenosis,* a cluster also found in speakers with chorea. All of these characteristics can be related to dystonic hyperadduction of the vocal folds during phonation.

Some patients exhibit *audible inspiration,* probably secondary to involuntary vocal fold adduction during inhalation. With the exception of abductor vocal fold weakness, this feature is rarely encountered in other dysarthria types.

Although not prominent in frequency of occurrence or severity, *voice tremor* may be present. In fact, voice tremor was more evident in speakers with dystonic speech than in any other dysarthric group studied by DAB.

Resonance. Although dystonic movements can affect velopharyngeal function during speech, hyper-

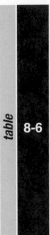

table 8-6	The most deviant speech dimensions encountered in the hyperkinetic dysarthria of dystonia by Darley, Aronson, and Brown,[34] listed in order from most to least severe. Also listed is the component of the speech system associated with each characteristic. The component "prosodic" is listed when several components of the speech system may contribute to the dimension. Characteristics listed under "Other" include speech features not among the most deviant but that may occur and are not typical of most other dysarthria types.

Dimension	Speech Component
Imprecise consonants	Articulatory
Distorted vowels*	Articulatory-prosodic
Harsh voice quality*	Phonatory
Irregular articulatory breakdowns*	Articulatory
Strained-strangled quality*	Phonatory
Monopitch	Phonatory-prosodic
Monoloudness	Phonatory-prosodic
Inappropriate silences*	Prosodic
Short phrases	Prosodic
Prolonged intervals	Prosodic
Prolonged phonemes	Prosodic
Excess loudness variations*	Respiratory-phonatory-prosodic
Reduced stress	Prosodic
Voice stoppages*	Phonatory-prosodic
Slow rate	Articulatory-prosodic
Other	
Audible inspiration*	Phonatory-respiratory
Voice tremor*	Phonatory
Alternating loudness*	Respiratory-phonatory-prosodic

*Tend to be distinctive or more severely impaired than in any other single dysarthria type.

nasality is not a pervasive characteristic and is usually rated as mild when present.[34]

Articulation. *Imprecise consonants, distorted vowels,* and *irregular articulatory breakdowns* may be prominent when dystonia affects articulators. These features formed the cluster *articulatory inaccuracy* in DAB's dystonic speakers. They logically reflect the effects on articulation of adventitious involuntary jaw, face, lip, or tongue movements (Figures 8-4 and 8-5). This conclusion receives support from acoustic analyses that have identified excessive second formant fluctuations during

steady state vowels in patients with tardive dyskinesia.[51] This acoustic variability reflects vocal tract instability induced by orofacial dyskinesia (Figure 8-6).

Prosody. Prosodic disturbances are prominent and are similar to those encountered in chorea. *Monopitch, monoloudness, short phrases,* and *reduced stress* may be present, and in DAB's speakers they combined to form the cluster of *prosodic insufficiency.* Also commonly heard are *prolonged intervals, prolonged phonemes,* and *slow rate,* features that combined to form the cluster of *prosodic excess. Inappropriate silences* and *excess and equal stress* may also be detected, and they contribute to the general perception of exaggerated stress patterns. All of these features may reflect the effect of slowness of movement or interruptions in the flow of normal speech movements.

Similar to chorea, the cooccurrence of clusters of prosodic excess and prosodic insufficiency may reflect the variable nature of dystonia with its underlying cooccurring slowness and reduced range of movement, and the speaker's compensatory or cautious response to the primary disorder.

What features of the dysarthria of dystonia help identify and distinguish it from other motor speech disorders? Most apparent is the variable nature of the deviant speech characteristics, the most prevalent of which are *imprecision and irregular breakdowns of articulation, inappropriate variability of loudness and rate, strained harshness, transient breathiness,* and *audible inspiration.* These features, often in combination with the speaker's attempt to avoid or compensate for dystonic movements, may lead to *slow rate, prolonged intervals and phonemes, inappropriate silences,* and prosodic features that lead to both *excessive and insufficient stress patterns.* The primary and distinguishing speech and speech-related findings in this form of dysarthria are summarized in Table 8-7.

Athetosis

Although athetosis is a major subcategory of cerebral palsy, the term "athetosis" is rarely used to describe acquired movement disorders (possibly because many neurologists consider athetosis to be synonymous with dystonia). As a result, the literature on the dysarthria of athetosis is based exclusively on studies of children or adults with cerebral palsy. The results of such studies suggest that the speech characteristics of athetosis are probably captured within the descriptions of dysarthria associated with dystonia and, perhaps, chorea. Because of this apparent overlap, and because the focus of this book is on acquired MSDs, the literature on the speech of

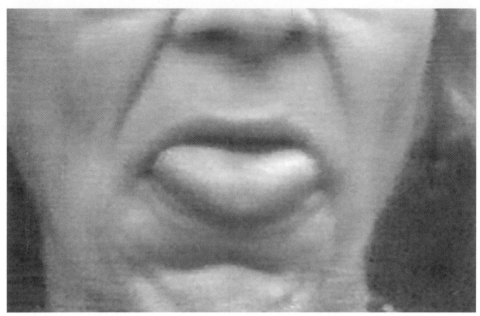

FIGURE 8-4 Woman with predominantly lingual dyskinesia during normally rapid production of alternate motion rates for /pʌ/; involuntary tongue protrusion prevents bilabial closure.

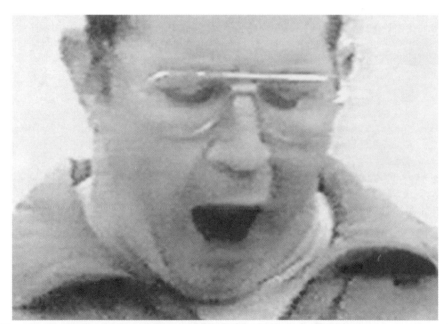

FIGURE 8-5 Man with jaw opening dystonia during production of the /æ/ in "grand." Excessive jaw opening and lingual retraction occurred only during speech and were associated almost exclusively with production of open vowels or velar consonants (see Case 8-2 for complete description).

individuals with athetotic cerebral palsy is not discussed here.*

*The interested reader is referred to reviews or comprehensive descriptive studies by DAB[36]; Hardy[54]; Kent and Netsell[62]; Nielson and O'Dwyer[81a]; Platt, Andrews, and Howie[82]; Platt et al.[83]; and Putnam.[84]

Spasmodic Torticollis (Cervical Dystonia)

Spasmodic torticollis (ST) affects the cervical neck muscles and not the cranial nerve–innervated speech muscles. Unless accompanied by dystonia that directly affects the speech muscles, any ST-related speech abnormalities are presumably secondary to the effects of neck postural deviations

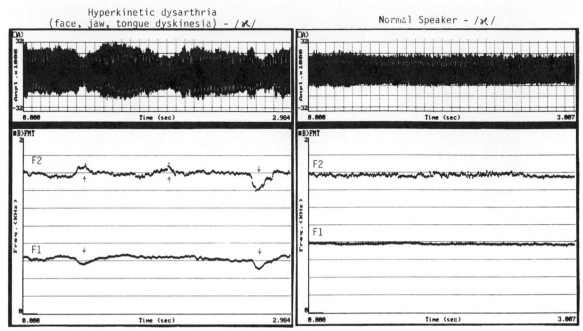

FIGURE 8-6 Raw acoustic waveform and first *(F1)* and second *(F2)* formant tracings for a 3-second prolongation of the vowel /ɚ/ by a man with face, jaw, and tongue dyskinesia *(left side)* and a normal male speaker *(right side)*. Maintenance of steady vocal tract posture is reflected in all tracings for the normal speaker. In contrast, the hyperkinetic speaker's abnormal movements are reflected in the raw waveform and in the relatively sustained (≈230 to 280 ms) fluctuations in F1 and F2 (see *arrows*). The fluctuations are sometimes apparent in F1 and F2 simultaneously, but not always, and there is variability in their amplitude and direction. The fluctuations reflect auditorily perceptible abnormal movements of the tongue, lips, or jaw.

---

table 8-7   Primary distinguishing speech and speech-related findings in the hyperkinetic dysarthria of dystonia

Perceptual

Phonation-respiration	Strained-harsh voice quality, voice stoppages, audible inspiration, excess loudness variations, alternating loudness, voice tremor
Resonance	Hypernasality
Articulation	Distorted vowels, irregular articulatory breakdowns, slow irregular AMRs
Prosody	Inappropriate silences, excess loudness variations, excessive-inefficient-variable patterns of stress
Physical	Relatively slow, waxing & waning head-neck, jaw, face, tongue, palate, pharyngeal, laryngeal, thoracic-abdominal movements
	Present at rest, during sustained postures & movement, but sometimes only during speech
	Improvement with "sensory tricks"
	Dysphagia
Patient Complaints	Effortful speech, involuntary orofacial movements
	"Tricks" that improve speech temporarily
	Chewing & swallowing problems (e.g., food "sticks" in throat)

AMRs, Alternate motion rates.

---

on primary speech muscle activity, or to alterations in the shape of the subglottic, glottic, or supraglottic vocal tract induced by abnormal neck postures (Figure 8-7). Given the severe distortions of neck posture that may occur in ST, it is surprising

that speech is not affected more frequently and dramatically.

The most detailed study of speech in people with ST is that by LaPointe, Case, and Duane.[70] In comparison to age-matched controls, their group

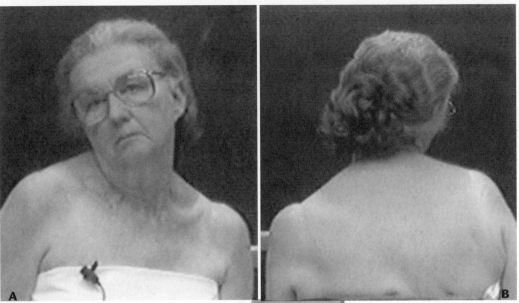

FIGURE 8-7 A, Front and **B,** back views of a woman with spasmodic torticollis attempting to sit in a normal resting posture. The neck rotation and head turning are sustained and involuntary.

of 70 people with ST exhibited reduced reading rate; reduced speech AMRs and sequential motion rates (SMRs); reduced maximum duration of /s/, /z/, and vowel prolongation; reduced phonation reaction time; and, in women, reduced habitual pitch, highest pitch, and pitch range. Intelligibility was also reduced, although the authors stated the overall impression "was that it was functional and intelligible, even if subtly different along some parameters." Increased vocal jitter and shimmer and decreased harmonic-to-noise ratio during vowel prolongation has also been reported.[103] In general, these studies suggest that the speech of some speakers with ST may be perceived as *slowly initiated, reduced in maximum duration of utterances, reduced in pitch and pitch variability, dysphonic,* and *reduced in rate.* These deficits, when present, are usually mild, and intelligibility is usually maintained.

The exact manner in which ST affects speech movements or vocal tract configurations is unclear. The speech characteristics of the disorder deserve further study, however, as much to establish how speakers adapt so well to abnormal head or neck postures as to understand the physiologic bases of the relatively mild speech abnormalities that may occur. The primary speech and speech-related findings associated with ST are summarized in Table 8-8.

Palatopharyngolaryngeal Myoclonus

PM is a rare disorder characterized by relatively abrupt rhythmic or semirhythmic unilateral or bilat-

table 8-8	Primary distinguishing speech and speech-related findings in the hyperkinetic dysarthria of spasmodic torticollis
Perceptual	
Phonation-respiration	Reduced pitch & pitch variability
	Dysphonia
Articulation-prosody	Reduced rate, delayed speech initiation, slow AMRs
Physical	Relatively sustained deviation of head to right or left, forward or back
	Sensory tricks reduce abnormal posturing
Patient Complaints	Speech often reported as normal
	Complaints related to neck movement & pain
	Occasional dysphagia
	Aware of sensory tricks that reduce spasm temporarily

AMRs, Alternate motion rates.

eral movements of the soft palate, pharyngeal walls, and laryngeal muscles.* The lesion causing it has

---

*Because PM is rhythmic and not lightninglike, neurologists have argued that the preferred term for this disorder should be "palatal tremor."[38]

been localized to an area of the brainstem and cerebellum known as the Guillain-Mollaret triangle, encompassing the loop among the dentate nucleus, red nucleus, and inferior olive (the dentato-rubro-olivary tracts). PM is sometimes regarded as the prototypic movement disorder that depends on a central pacemaker that generates myoclonic jerks time-locked in different muscles. The inferior olive is thought to be the pacemaker, and hypertrophic degeneration of it is a common autopsy finding in people with the condition.[38] The MRI image in Figure 8-8 illustrates hypertrophy of the inferior olives that can be associated with PM.

PM is usually caused by a brainstem or cerebellar vascular event, but neoplasm, multiple sclerosis, encephalitis, and other degenerative diseases affecting the same general areas have been reported as causes.[17] When caused by an acute lesion, there may be a delay of several months to years before the PM emerges.[78]

PM can also be idiopathic. Deuschl et al.[38] found 27% of 287 cases with PM to have unknown etiologies. They referred to this condition as "essential rhythmic palatal myoclonus," similar to other benign extrapyramidal conditions of undetermined origin, such as essential tremor (which includes essential

or organic voice tremor). Patients with this idiopathic condition had a much higher frequency of "earclicks" (explained later) and a slower rate of myoclonus (<120/min) than patients with symptomatic PM (i.e., PM with established etiology). They were generally younger than 40 years of age at onset and frequently also had myoclonus of the chin or perioral area.

Nonspeech Oral Mechanism

PM is present at rest, during sustained postures and movement, and during sleep. In some cases the eyeballs, diaphragm, tongue, lips, and jaw are also involved. The most common finding in PM is *abrupt, rhythmic, beatinglike elevation of the soft palate at a rate of 60 to 240 per minute.* Pharyngeal contractions also may be apparent and, because of activity of the tensor veli palatini, may produce opening and closing of the eustachian tube with an associated clicking sound that sometimes can be heard by others. These *"earclicks"* are a frequent complaint when PM is idiopathic but uncommon when PM is symptomatic.[38]

Myoclonic movements of the larynx can sometimes be seen on the external surface of the neck, and patients may complain of a clicking sensation in the larynx or a sensation of laryngeal spasm. It is important to distinguish myoclonic movements in the external neck from carotid pulses, which are usually slower and do not visibly displace the laryngeal cartilages. Myoclonic movements of the lips and even the nares are sometimes present. Apparent lingual myoclonus may be seen, but lingual jerks may be secondary to laryngeal myoclonus.

Speech

The effects of PM on speech, even when it affects the jaw, lips, tongue, palate, pharynx, and larynx, are not apparent under most circumstances and may not be detectable at all during conversational speech, because they are so brief and relatively low in amplitude. If apparent during connected speech, it is perceived as a slow voice tremor and, less frequently, as intermittent hypernasality.[36] However, the effects of PM can usually be heard during vowel prolongation as *momentary rhythmic arrests or tremorlike variations* at a rate that matches the rate of palatal myoclonus. Myoclonic variations can be distinguished from those of essential voice tremor by their slower frequency and the relatively abrupt character of each cycle (voice tremor has a slower, more sinusoidal, waxing and waning character). Rarely, a clicking noise is audible at rest, reflecting eustachian tube opening. There may be occasional prolonged

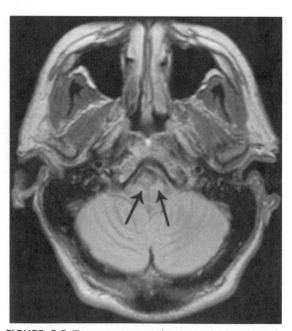

FIGURE 8-8 Transverse magnetic resonance image at the level of the medulla and cerebellum illustrating bilateral hypertrophy of the inferior olives *(arrows)* in a 45 year-old man with palatopharyngolaryngeal myoclonus (and ataxic dysarthria). See Case 8-7 for an illustrative case.

silent intervals or inappropriate silences during speech if myoclonic vocal fold adduction occurs before inhalation at phrase boundaries is completed.[9] If the diaphragm is involved, there may be momentary interruptions in phonation due to interrupted airflow.

The dysarthria of PM is probably rare as an isolated speech disturbance. Except when idiopathic, PM is usually accompanied by other signs of posterior fossa damage. As a result, PM probably most often occurs as one part of a speech disturbance that may include spastic, ataxic, flaccid, or unilateral upper motor neuron (UMN) dysarthria. Table 8-9 summarizes the primary speech and speech-related findings associated with PM.

Action Myoclonus

The effect of AM on speech has received little attention, but dysarthria can result from it.[12] The character of AM is quite different from that of PM, and its effects can have a greater functional impact on speech than PM.

Dysarthria is apparently common in patients with AM in nonspeech muscles. Fahn, Davis, and Rolland[42] noted that at least 40% of their 59 cases with AM had dysarthria; it is unclear, however, whether the dysarthria was due to the AM or other cooccurring neuromuscular deficits.

AM is distinguished from other myoclonic conditions because it is induced by volitional muscle activity and is less generalized and rhythmic than other forms. In their classic description of four cases, Lance and Adams[69] noted that "the essential clinical picture was that of an arrhythmic fine or coarse jerking of a muscle or group of muscles in disorderly fashion, excited mainly by muscular activity when a conscious attempt at precision was required, worsened by emotional arousal, suppressed by barbiturates, and superimposed on a mild cerebellar ataxia." The jerks were typically less than 200 ms in duration and occurred singly or in series. Each patient had slow and "slightly slurred" speech.

AM is often associated with cerebellar, basal ganglia, or pyramidal system involvement. Lance and Adams[69] suggested that it might be a product of unrestrained synchronous or repetitive firing of thalamocortical neurons in the ventrolateral thalamus, the main relay nucleus from the cerebellum to the cortex. These abnormal discharges are then relayed from the cortex to the corticospinal and corticobulbar tracts, where they result in AM. Abnormal thalamocortical activity may be explained by inadequate control from the pontine reticular formation or by abnormal synchronous impulses through dentatothalamic pathways.

table 8-9	Primary distinguishing speech and speech-related findings in the hyperkinetic dysarthria of palatopharyngolaryngeal myoclonus
Perceptual	
Phonation-respiration	Often no apparent abnormality
	Momentary voice arrests during contextual speech when severe
	Voice arrests or myoclonic beats at 60-240 Hz during vowel prolongation
Resonance	Usually normal, but occasional intermittent hypernasality
Articulation-prosody	Usually normal, but brief silent intervals if myoclonus interrupts inhalation or initiation of exhalation, phonation, or articulation
Physical	Myoclonic movements of palate, pharynx & larynx, & sometimes lips, nares, tongue, & respiratory muscles
	Laryngeal or pharyngeal myoclonus sometimes observable beneath neck surface
Patient Complaints	Earclicks
	Patient often unaware of myoclonic movements & usually does not complain of speech difficulty

The most common etiology of AM is anoxic encephalopathy (e.g., due to cardiorespiratory arrest), in which the principal findings have been degeneration of cells and fibers in the globus pallidus, hippocampus, deep folia in the cerebellum, and the deep layers of the cerebral cortex, especially the parietal and occipital lobes.[69] Multiple other causes also have been documented, including myoclonic epilepsy, toxic-metabolic disturbances (e.g., lithium exposure, immunosuppressive drugs in transplant patients), infectious processes (e.g., encephalitis), paraneoplastic cerebellar degeneration, stroke, and multiple sclerosis.[29,68,100]

Nonspeech Oral Mechanism and Speech

By definition, AM is not present at rest, and nonspeech oral mechanism examination may be entirely normal unless deficits in addition to the AM are present.

Aronson, O'Neill, and Kelly[12] have presented the only specific description of the dysarthria of AM. The disorder appears to have its primary perceptual effects on articulation (labial) and phonation. Their four cases were described as having stable orofacial muscles at rest but quick, gross, or fine jerky movements during attempts to speak. *"Repetitive fluctuation of phonation"* and *adductor voice arrests,* which were synchronous with myoclonic spasms of the lips, were characteristic. Slow speech rate was apparent in each case, and the myoclonic movements worsened with increased speech rate. Slow rate could be compensatory, although the authors noted that, consistent with the general physiology of myoclonus, it could also reflect brief periods of inability to contract muscles following myoclonic jerks. These observations suggest that patients suspected of having the disorder should be asked to speak at slow, average, and rapid rates. Noticeable deterioration of voice quality or articulatory adequacy with increased rate or the emergence of myoclonic facial movements with increased rate can help confirm the diagnosis, because other dysarthrias are generally not triggered by increases in rate; intelligibility may improve at slowed rates, but the underlying disordered movements are generally not altered. Speech AMRs may be particularly useful for making such observations. Table 8-10 summarizes the primary speech and speech-related findings associated with the dysarthria of AM.

Tics—Tourette's Syndrome

Tics may occur as an isolated, nonspecific disorder, but TS is the prototypic tic disorder. It is defined operationally in the *Diagnostic and Statistical Manual of Mental Disorders*[39] as including: (1) multiple motor and one or more vocal tics, (2) tic-free periods not exceeding 3 months, (3) marked distress or impairment in daily functioning, (4) onset before 18 years of age, and (5) not due to physiologic effects of a substance (e.g., stimulants) or other medical condition (e.g., Huntington's disease, postviral encephalitis). It is generally felt that most cases are genetically determined and suspected that pathophysiology involves striatal dopamine receptor supersensitivity. Although traditionally viewed as severe and disabling, TS is now recognized as a clinically heterogeneous disorder with motor and behavioral features that vary along a severity continuum.[67]

TS, which affects mostly males ($\approx$3:1 ratio), frequently cooccurs with obsessive-compulsive disorder or attention deficit hyperactivity disorder.[67] Stuttering, dyslexia, conduct disorder, panic attacks,

table 8-10	Primary distinguishing speech and speech-related findings in the hyperkinetic dysarthria of action myoclonus
Perceptual	
Phonation-respiration	Occasional adductor voice arrests
Articulation-prosody	Slow rate, decreased precision with increased rate
	Marked deterioration of AMR regularity with increased rate
Physical	Normal at rest unless other neuromuscular deficits present
	Quick, gross, or fine jerky movements of orofacial muscles during speech—especially lips—worsening with increased rate
Patient Complaints	Awareness of imprecise speech & inability or reluctance to speak at normal or rapid rates

AMR, Alternate motion rate.

multiple phobias, depression, and mania reportedly are more common than in control subjects.[31]

Tics are brief involuntary movements or sounds that occur over normal background motor activity. They can be brief and isolated (e.g., eye blink, head twitch, facial grimace) or can consist of coordinated and seemingly purposeful movements (e.g., touching, jumping, obscene gestures). Some patients experience "sensory tics," which are somatic sensations, such as pressure, tickling, and temperature changes, that may lead to movements intended to relieve the sensation, such as tightening or stretching of muscles.[67] Tics are often bizarre appearing and frequently misinterpreted as signs of psychiatric disease.

In addition to motor tics and behavioral disorders, TS is characterized by *vocal tics* that can be isolated or embedded within voluntary verbal utterances. Vocal tics are unique, because they represent *the only dysarthria in which specific sounds or spoken words represent the disorder.*

Simple vocal tics include noises and sounds that are made repetitively and sometimes can be suppressed temporarily. The most common of these are throat clearing and *grunting,* but *yelling-screaming, sniffing, barking, snorting, coughing, spitting, squeaking,* and *humming* can also occur.[32] These sounds are usually executed rapidly, and some of them may reflect a response to a sensation in the larynx or throat.[67] More complex vocal tics may include *echolalia* (repetition of other's utterances), *palilalia* (discussed in Chapter 7), and *coprolalia*.

Coprolalia (copro = feces; lalia = lips), or involuntary, compulsive, repetitive, almost ritualistic swearing, is one of the most dramatic, although not universally present, features of TS (the words "fuck," "shit," and "piss" are the most common scatological utterances, according to Comings[32]). The words are often said softly or incompletely and are sometimes accompanied by throat clearing or other noises, possibly reflecting an attempt to suppress or mask the coprolalia. They may emerge independent of any volitional verbal expression or at the start of or within volitional utterances. They sometimes may appear socially acceptable or even humorous, but the social and psychologic consequences for the patient are often tragic.

The primary speech and speech-related characteristics of TS are summarized in Table 8-11.

Organic (Essential) Voice Tremor

Organic or essential (idiopathic) voice tremor is often simply viewed as a voice disorder and not a neurologic disorder or a dysarthria. However, it occurs in approximately 20% of patients with essential tremor elsewhere.[60] and clearly can be classified as a hyperkinetic dysarthria of tremor.*

Essential tremor is the most common movement disorder, and a family history of tremor is present in 17% to 96% of affected people.[59] It can begin at any age, often before 50 years, and incidence increases with age. It occurs most frequently in the hands but, on average, is present in the voice in approximately 14% of affected people.[59] Although generally benign, it usually slowly progresses in severity (tremor amplitude). A focal presentation of the disorder (e.g., voice tremor) sometimes spreads to include other body parts, and it is sometimes a precursor to, or associated with, other movement disorders such as focal dystonias, dystonia musculorum deformans, and ST.[45,66]

The localization of essential tremor is unknown, but it is probably related to a CNS oscillatory abnormality. The red nucleus, cerebellum, and inferior olivary and ventrolateral thalamic nuclei are possible sites on the basis of their inherent rhythmic physiology, the results of PET studies in people with the

table 8-11	Primary distinguishing speech and speech-related findings in the hyperkinetic dysarthria of *Tourette's* syndrome
Perceptual	
Phonation-respiration	Coughing, grunting, throat clearing, screaming, moaning, etc.
Resonance	Sniffing
Articulation-prosody	Humming, whistling, lip smacking, echolalia, palilalia, coprolalia
Physical	Multiple motor tics (e.g., eyeblinks, head twitch, facial grimacing, jumping, touching, obscene gestures)
Patient Complaints	Awareness of vocal and motor tics, compulsion to perform them, & inability to inhibit them for sustained periods
	Behavioral & psychiatric disorders may be present (e.g., obsessive-compulsive, phobias, hyperactivity & attention deficit disorder, learning disability)

disorder, or known sites of surgical or vascular lesions that may abolish or cause it.*[59]

The onset of essential voice tremor is usually gradual. When mild, patients may not be aware of its presence. Those who are aware often note that it worsens with fatigue and psychologic stress and improves with alcohol intake. The voice tremor can be an isolated problem, but more often is accompanied by head or extremity tremor. When isolated, it is sometimes misdiagnosed as a psychogenic disorder.

Nonspeech Oral Mechanism

Lingual tremor may be apparent at rest or on protrusion in patients with organic voice tremor. When present during phonation, it may represent genuine

---

*Essential tremor can affect the tongue, sometimes in isolation, but essential lingual tremor is rare in comparison to essential voice tremor. Patients with lingual tremor are usually unaware of it. It occurs at a rate of 4 to 8 Hz, is generally apparent on protrusion but not at rest, and is often alcohol responsive.[16] Its effects on speech are unclear.

---

*Patients with cerebellar disease sometimes have voice tremor. The tremor frequency is in the range of 3 Hz, similar in frequency to other forms of cerebellar postural tremor.[2] This is slower than that of essential voice tremor and usually occurs with an ataxic dysarthria. Although its frequency is in the general range of palatal-laryngeal myoclonus, it can occur without evidence of myoclonic movements at rest.

lingual tremor or be secondary to vertical oscillations of the larynx. Tremulous movements of the jaw and lips are often apparent at rest, during sustained postures, and during vowel prolongation. Palatal and pharyngeal tremor are often obvious during sustained "ah," synchronous with the perceived voice tremor; this can be evident even when resonance is perceived as normal. Fiberscopic observation of the larynx may reveal rhythmic vertical laryngeal movements and adductor and abductor oscillation of the vocal folds, synchronous with the perceived voice tremor. Vertical oscillations of the larynx also can often be seen on the external neck during vowel prolongation. Tomoda et al.[96] recorded electromyographic evidence of tremor in the cricothyroid muscle and expiratory muscles (rectus abdominis) in three patients with organic voice tremor, synchronous with voice tremor. They suggested that voice tremor may be an action tremor of voluntary expiratory muscles that affects phonatory function. Although respiratory tremor should be considered a possible source of voice tremor, it is probably not a primary factor in most cases of organic voice tremor.

Speech

Aronson[9] describes three effects of essential tremor on voice: (1) a "typical" organic voice tremor when the adductor and abductor vocal fold tremor components are relatively equal, (2) an adductor spasmodic dysphonia when the adductor component is predominant, and (3) an abductor spasmodic dysphonia when the abductor component is predominant. Only the typical voice tremor is addressed here (spasmodic dysphonias associated with tremor are discussed in the next section).

Voice tremor may not be apparent during contextual speech, especially when mild, which may be why some patients are unaware of it. Its rhythmic fluctuations are most easily perceived during vowel prolongation. To rule out a respiratory contribution to the voice tremor, it is often useful to have the patient prolong /s/ and /z/. If the /s/ is steady and the /z/ or vowel contains tremor, a prominent respiratory contribution to the voice tremor is unlikely.

Organic voice tremor most often occurs at a frequency of 4- to 7-Hz, most often in the 5- to 6-Hz range, with a tendency for tremor frequency to be slower with increasing age.[10,18] The tremor has a *sinusoidal, quavering,* or *rhythmic waxing and waning character* during vowel prolongation, presumably due to rhythmic alterations in pitch, loudness, or both (Figure 8-9). When severe, there may be abrupt, staccato voice arrests that, in most cases, are rhythmic. However, the tremor may lose its rhythmic character when arrests are present, pos-

sibly because of the speaker's efforts to avoid or otherwise compensate for them. In such cases, having the patient prolong a vowel at a higher pitch may abort the arrests and allow the tremor to be heard more easily. Additional acoustic attributes associated with essential voice tremor include increased jitter, reduced harmonic or noise ratio, and reduced dynamic range at the natural frequency of phonation.[50]

Patients with marked to severe organic voice tremor may have *reduced speech rate* secondary to phonatory interruptions; speech rate may also be reduced secondary to jaw, lip, and tongue tremor. When voice and oromandibular tremor occur simultaneously and are marked, the effects on speech can be pronounced, and the disorder can become more complex than the smooth modulations of a sinusoidal tremor. Kent et al.[63] reported such a case with severely reduced intelligibility. Acoustic analyses documented variable patterns of phonation, with dysphonic intervals, harmonic doubling, and noise. Single word rates and AMRs were slow and variable, and the jaw tremor interfered with stability of articulation. Of interest, articulatory movements sometimes seemed timed to the 3- to 5-Hz tremor cycle; Kent et al.[64] note that one way an individual with tremor can contend with it "is to coordinate voluntary movements with the tremor, which then acts as an internal pacemaker."

The primary speech and speech-related characteristics associated with organic voice tremor are summarized in Table 8-12.

Spasmodic Dysphonia

Spasmodic dysphonia (SD) designates a group of voice disorders that are characterized by strained or breathy voice qualities resulting from adductor or abductor laryngospasm. Concepts of the disorder have an interesting history. For a number of years SD was thought to be a manifestation of psychopathology, usually stemming from psychologic trauma, stress, or anxiety. Neurologic etiologies were rarely considered. Over the past 2 decades the etiologic pendulum has swung to a point where many investigators and clinicians assume that the disorder is always neurogenic, with only lesion loci and the specific neurophysiologic nature of the disorder in question. Along with this trend has come a shift from use of the term "spastic" to the term "spasmodic" to characterize the dysphonia. This latter trend is useful, because, although the term "spastic" describes the strained character of the adductor form of the disorder, it does not appear that spasticity (in the physiologic sense) is responsible for most cases of SD. The term "spasmodic" retains descriptive power and at the same time suggests that spasm (or

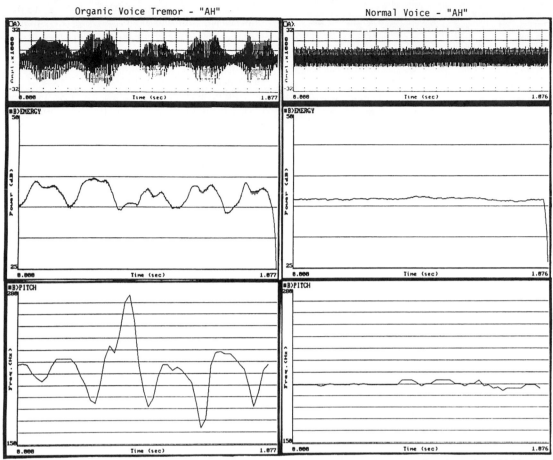

FIGURE 8-9 Raw acoustic waveform, energy, and pitch contours for an approximately 1-second prolongation of /a/ by a female speaker (see Case 8-4 for full clinical description) with an approximately 5-Hz organic voice tremor *(left side)* and a normal female speaker *(right side)*. The fairly regular tremor is apparent in all tracings and stands in marked contrast to the steady maintenance of the same parameters by the normal speaker.

dystonia) is the basis for at least some or many forms of the disorder.

Aronson[9] has argued that any diagnosis of SD should be modified to specify likely etiology. There are three broad etiologic possibilities: *neurogenic, psychogenic,* and *idiopathic*. This recognizes that SD can have at least two etiologies—neurogenic and psychogenic—and that etiology sometimes cannot be specified with any degree of confidence (hence is idiopathic). Importantly, psychogenic and neurogenic SD may not be distinguished on the basis of auditory perceptual characteristics; the distinction is often made on the basis of history and other examination findings. Evidence that SD can have a psychogenic etiology is discussed in Chapter 14. Here are addressed only neurogenic varieties of SD, which justifiably can be considered a subtype of hyperkinetic dysarthria.

It is also important to establish if SD is *adductor, abductor,* or *mixed* in form. Adductor SD, by far the most common variety, is characterized by adductor laryngospasms that give the voice a *strained, tight* character. Abductor SD is characterized by abductor laryngospasms that give it an *intermittent breathy* or *aphonic* character. Some patients have a mixed form, with both intermittent strained and breathy qualities. There is no evidence that these symptomatic types vary in distribution as a function of neurogenic versus psychogenic etiology.

Ignoring possible etiologic differences, SD has an average age of onset of approximately 45 to 50 years, but it can develop anywhere from the third to eighth decades. Male-to-female ratio ranges from 1:1 to 1:4. It may develop suddenly but usually begins insidiously, often taking a year or longer to develop into its full-blown state. Remissions are rare when

table 8-12	Primary distinguishing speech and speech-related findings in the hyperkinetic dysarthria of organic voice tremor

Perceptual

Phonation-respiration	Quavering, rhythmic, waxing & waning tremor, most evident on vowel prolongation, at a rate of ≈4 to 7 Hz
	Voice arrests may occur in severe forms but may disappear if pitch is raised
Articulation	Usually normal, but rate may be slowed
Prosody	Normal pitch & loudness variability may be restricted or altered by tremor
Physical	Rhythmic, vertical laryngeal movements & adductor & abductor oscillations of the vocal folds synchronous with voice tremor.
	Tremor of jaw, lips, tongue, & palate or pharynx may be present, especially during phonation. Lingual & jaw tremor may be secondary to laryngeal tremor.
Patient Complaints	Shaky or jerky voice
	Worse with fatigue or anxiety
	Improves with alcohol
	Frequent family history of tremor

the cause is neurologic. It is not unusual for the disorder to begin during a flulike illness or during a period of acute or chronic psychologic stress; this may be the case even when SD is clearly neurogenic in origin.

In an extensive review of evidence for the neurologic underpinnings of SD, Cannito[21] concluded that SD probably results from an impairment of the volitional motor system, rather than the limbic or lower brainstem centers for vocal control. He based this conclusion on evidence from several studies of (1) a relatively high incidence of extrapyramidal and pyramidal motor signs in patients with SD, (2) neuroimaging evidence for such lesions,*[46] (3) the tendency for the disorder's manifestations to be greater for complex than simple verbal activities, and (4) a strong association between SD voice and speech characteristics and those found in spastic

dysarthria and the dysarthrias of dystonia and chorea. He tied these data to models of hyperkinesias that implicate cortical premotor-striatal-pallidal-thalamic control circuits that are normally involved in the control of complex, voluntary sequential movements.

Numerous factors influence SD, and wide intraindividual fluctuations are common. Emotional stress, anxiety, depression, and physical exertion often make symptoms worse. These influences are superficially suggestive of psychogenic etiology, but it is important to note that many of them also affect severity in people with unambiguous neurogenic movement disorders, and that they are common complaints in many patients with other dysarthria types. In contrast to most other dysarthria types, however, voice in SD may be normal during singing or laughter, and under conditions of surprise or quickly emitted "automatic" utterances. Most often, the movement disorder underlying neurogenic SD is *action induced,* the triggering action being volitional speech.

Tremor and dystonia have a strong causal association with neurogenic SD. This suggests that SD is related to extrapyramidal system dysfunction in the broad sense, more specifically to dysfunction in the basal ganglia or cerebellar control circuit. SD may be an isolated, focal manifestation of tremor or dystonia, or may coexist with more widespread manifestations of them.

That dystonia or tremor can be focal to the larynx receives support from other focal manifestations of tremor and dystonia (e.g., blepharospasm, oromandibular dystonia or tremor, torticollis) and the fact that the basal ganglia have a somatotopic organization. Jankovic[60] notes that the somatotopic organization of the basal ganglia plays an important role in the muscular distribution of hyperkinesias and the preferential involvement of head and orofacial structures in them.

SD of essential voice tremor presumably occurs (1) when the adductor component of the tremor predominates and causes adductor laryngospasms and squeezing of the glottis (adductor SD of essential voice tremor), (2) when the abductor component of the tremor predominates and causes abductor laryngospasm and widening of the glottis (abductor SD of

---

*The interested reader is referred to the work of Finitzo and Freeman[46] and an exchange of letters between Aronson and Lagerlund[11] and Finitzo et al.[47] for a comprehensive and critical overview of approaches to establishing the neurologic locus of SD and the methodological and interpretive challenges and controversies faced by such efforts.

essential voice tremor), or (3) when the tremor amplitude is relatively balanced in adductor and abductor muscles but sufficient to cause both abductor and adductor laryngospasm (mixed adductor and abductor SD of essential voice tremor). Thus there appears to be a continuum along which a diagnosis of essential voice tremor can merge into a diagnosis of SD. The continuum seems to include severity as well as the balance of muscle forces involved in adductor and abductor laryngeal activity. In addition to perceptual evidence, a link between SD and essential tremor comes from evidence of nonlaryngeal tremor in patients with SD. For example, approximately one third of patients with SD have evidence of essential tremor elsewhere[60]; Aronson and Hartman[11] found a similar tremor frequency between patients with essential voice tremor and patients with SD and voice tremor, and their SD patients had a high incidence of tremor elsewhere in the body.

Nonspeech Oral Mechanism

Affected patients often have a normal oral mechanism examination. If associated with generalized or other orofacial tremor or dystonia, Meige's syndrome, or ST, manifestations of those problems will be apparent. Soft neurologic signs such as facial or palatal asymmetry, mild weakness, or pathologic oral reflexes can be present, but not usually, and probably not as a reflection of any causal relationship. *Because SD is an action-induced disorder, evidence for it might be found only during voluntary speech.*

Speech (Adductor Spasmodic Dysphonia)

The primary perceptual feature of adductor SD is a *strained, jerky, grunting, squeezed, groaning,* and *effortful* voice quality. When mild, there may be no more than a mild strained quality. These qualities can be intermittent or relatively continuous. *Silent articulatory movements* or *sound repetitions,* presumably as a result of unanticipated laryngospasms, may be present. Additional dysfluent characteristics, such as tense pauses, dysrhythmic phonation, part and whole word repetitions, and revisions have been documented and contribute to clinical impressions of overall severity.[24]

When tremor underlies adductor SD, there may be a *staccato quality* or *an obvious tremor or rhythmic character* to the laryngospasms. This is heard most easily during vowel prolongation; when voice arrests are prominent, having the patient phonate at a higher pitch may attenuate the arrests and permit perception of the tremor. There may be associated head, jaw, lip, tongue, palatal, pharynx, and thoracic tremor during vowel prolongation.

When dystonia underlies the laryngospasm, the spasmodic voice may be continuous, or arrests may be unpredictable. Speech rate may be slow secondary to laryngospasm, or perhaps, in some cases, because of involvement of supralaryngeal muscles.[20,22] Intermittent or fairly constant *hypernasality* is perceptually evident in some patients. Jerky and dysrhythmic movements of the thorax and abdomen may be apparent during speech, synchronous with strained voice and voice arrests; these are probably a secondary effect of uncontrolled glottic closure.

When adductor SD is severe, there may be *facial grimacing,* associated *neck contractions,* and *movements of the shoulder girdle and upper arms.* The overall picture may be one of *extreme physical effort* during speech. This may be one of the primary complaints of people with the disorder, sometimes exceeding their dissatisfaction with the voice itself.

Patients with adductor SD can have abnormally increased subglottal air pressure, abnormal variability of phonatory airflow, and increased laryngeal resistance during speech.[5,48,57] Electromyogram (EMG) examinations have revealed delays in speech initiation and overactivity of laryngeal muscles.[72] Videofiberoptic laryngoscopy during speech may reveal rhythmic, arrhythmic, or relatively sustained adductor spasms of the true vocal folds and arytenoids, but as severity increases, spasm of the false folds and even the inferior pharyngeal constrictor muscles may be observed. In some cases the entire larynx may move upward, implicating spasmodic activity in the extrinsic laryngeal muscles as well. High-amplitude muscle burst activity in the 6- to 7-Hz range, synchronous with fluctuations in the speech waveform, have been observed in the thyroarytenoid and levator palatini muscles.[46,97] Lundy et al.,[74] using fiberoptic videonasolaryngoscopy, found abnormal soft palate posturing during speech in 84% of 83 patients with laryngeal movement disorders who did not have perceptually abnormal oral or nasal resonance; speech diagnoses included adductor, abductor, and mixed SD and voice tremor. The findings suggest that the abnormal soft palate posturing reflects compensatory behavior or an additional area of primary involvement. Similar explanations may apply to a finding of abnormal kinematic patterns of lip movements during speech in two speakers with adductor SD (and another with abductor SD).[95]

table 8-13	Primary distinguishing speech and speech-related findings in the hyperkinetic dysarthria of spasmodic dysphonia
Perceptual	
Phonation-respiration	*Adductor:* Continuous or intermittent strained, jerky, squeezed, effortful quality, with voice arrests when severe. If tremor based, voice tremor may be apparent, especially during vowel prolongation at higher pitches.
	Abductor: Brief, breathy or aphonic segments, most obvious at beginning of utterances or in voiceless consonant environments
Resonance	*Adductor:* Usually normal but occasionally hypernasal
	Abductor: Usually normal, but occasionally hypernasal
Articulation-prosody	*Adductor:* Inappropriate silences, silent articulatory movements, & sound repetitions, especially when voice arrests are prominent
	Contextual speech and AMRs may be slow secondary to laryngospasms
	Abductor: Short due to air wastage through glottis during abductor spasms
Physical	Nonlaryngeal muscles are usually normal, unless tremor or dystonia present elsewhere (e.g., head or limb tremor, orofacial dyskinesia, torticollis)
	Rhythmic or arrhythmic spasms of true folds & arytenoids, & sometimes false folds & pharyngeal constrictors, usually only during speech
	Jerky & arrhythmic thoracic or abdominal movements, usually secondary to adductor laryngospasm
	Facial grimacing & neck or shoulder movements secondary to severe adductor laryngospasms
Patient Complaints	*Adductor:* Tight, strained voice
	Abductor: Intermittent, weak, breathy, aphonic voice
	Adductor & abductor: Increased physical effort & fatigue associated with speaking
	Occupational, social, & emotional impact may be significant. Voice may improve with alcohol when tremor based.

Acoustic analyses have documented phonatory breaks, aperiodicity, breakdown in formant structure, elevated standard deviation of f_o, abnormal frequency shifts and intensity fluctuations, widely spaced vertical striations at irregular intervals (reflecting reduced f_o and aperiodicity of phonation), increased jitter and shimmer, interruptions in articulation, separation of sounds in syllables, delayed onset of phonation in vowels, and a tendency toward reduced f_o and loudness (e.g., Adams et al.[4]; Cimino-Knight and Sapienza, 2001[29a]; Hertegard, Granqvist, and Lindestad[55]; Ludlow and Connor[73]; Sapienza, Walton, and Murry[91]; Sapienza et al.[92]; Wolfe and Bacon[102]; Zwirner, Murry, and Woodson[105]).* A number of these acoustic measures have served as indices of change in response to treatment with botulinum toxin. These acoustic and physiologic attributes are generally consistent with and further refine perceptual descriptions of the disorder.

*Despite evidence of phonatory instability or unsteadiness in the disorder, the number of phonatory breaks, frequency shifts, and aperiodic segments seems consistent across repeated trials and over time (Cimino-Knight and Sapienza, 2001).[29a] However, the relative predominance of acoustic abnormalities may vary as a function of speech task (e.g., reading versus vowel prolongation).[91]

Speech (Abductor Spasmodic Dysphonia)

In abductor SD, the voice is interrupted by brief, inappropriate breathy or aphonic segments that are most easily triggered by voiceless consonants in the beginning of an utterance or syllable. During these segments airflow increases, speech rate may be slowed.[79] As in adductor SD, dysfluencies and hypernasality are sometimes apparent.

Acoustic analyses have revealed increased aspiration time for initial stops, a loss of energy in the higher formants, intensity fluctuations, prolonged VOT for voiceless consonants, elevated average f_o, and increased sentence articulation times.[23,102] Direct observation of the larynx may show abduction of the vocal folds during phonation, resulting in a wide glottal chink; these coincide with breathy releases. If tremor is present, abductor movements may be rhythmic. EMG has identified increased activity in the thyroarytenoid and posterior cricoarytenoid muscles in speakers with this form of SD.[97] There can be a breakdown of formant structure or superimposed noise on vertical striations in spectrograms of affected speakers.[102]

The primary speech and speech-related findings associated with SD are summarized in Table 8-13.

Cases

Case 8-1

A 73-year-old man presented with a 5-month history of "hesitation" in speech, which had initially worsened for a few months and then plateaued. Neurologic examination was normal with the exception of abnormal orofacial movements. His CT scan and electroencephalogram were normal. Routine laboratory studies and screening for heavy metal poisoning were within normal limits. He had never taken neuroleptic medications.

During speech examination, he complained of halting and slurred speech as well as involuntary mouth movements. Examination revealed tremor of the lips at rest and on lip rounding and semirhythmic movement of the tongue at rest. A regular voice tremor was present during vowel prolongation. Relatively rapid chewing and smacking and rounding movements of the lips interrupted contextual speech. They were noticeably reduced if the patient spoke while biting on a tongue depressor or with some pressure at the angle of the mouth.

The clinician concluded that the patient had a "hyperkinetic dysarthria associated with oro-facial dyskinesia with an accompanying tremor component."

The patient was advised to speak while holding a pipestem in his mouth and biting down, and he was given some practice at doing it. The neurologist recommended a trial of Inderal for the movement disorder. Several weeks later, the patient wrote to indicate that the Inderal had significantly reduced, but not eliminated, his facial grimacing. He also noted that "a pipe held between my teeth is definitely effective and socially acceptable." — dystonia

Commentary. (1) Orofacial dyskinesias or focal mouth dystonias often develop without a clear etiologic explanation. They can be present in the absence of any other neurologic symptoms and in the absence of abnormalities on neuroimaging studies. (2) Orofacial dyskinesias can affect speech. (3) Sensory tricks, such as biting down or exerting some pressure on the cheek, can be effective (temporarily) in relieving abnormal movements and improving speech.

Case 8-2

A 53-year-old man presented with an 18-month history of speech difficulty and a right upper and lower limb movement disorder. The course was one of gradual onset and progression. A question had been raised about manganese intoxication, possibly secondary to exposure when welding or from materials used in refinishing a boat.

Neurologic evaluation revealed the presence of torsion dystonia of the right foot during walking and right upper extremity cogwheel rigidity. A jaw-opening dystonia during speech was also apparent. He was referred for speech evaluation.

The patient was aware of abnormal jaw movements during speech but was unaware of difficulty at other times, including during chewing and swallowing. His speech tended to worsen when he was anxious, excited, or consuming alcohol. Speech was better in the morning, following relaxation exercises, and when writing or drawing while speaking; he felt this latter activity distracted his attention from speech.

Oral mechanism examination at rest and during non-speech sustained postures was normal. During speech he had intermittent marked jaw opening and tongue retraction. Superficially, these movements were random, but careful analysis established that they were strongly associated with the occurrence of open vowels and velar consonants (i.e., sounds requiring jaw opening or back-of-tongue elevation). Speech improved somewhat during whispering and noticeably when he clenched his jaw during speaking. It improved moderately when he wrote while talking. His jaw opening was often sufficient to arrest speech, with continuation possible only after the dystonic interval passed.

MRI and SPECT scans were normal. Additional laboratory and radiologic studies were negative. An EMG revealed normal blink and facial nerve conduction and a normal masseter-inhibiting reflex. There was no evidence of abnormal activity in the lateral pterygoid muscles and digastric muscles at rest or during chewing and drinking, but tonic spasms of 500 to 3000 ms were present in those muscles during speech.

It was concluded that the patient had a progressive extrapyramidal disorder of unclear etiology. It was recommended that he avoid welding, painting, and other heavy metal exposure. Sinemet was prescribed. There was some improvement in the patient's limb symptoms but no change in speech. Subsequent examination of the paint and several metals to which he had been exposed

Case 8-2—cont'd

failed to provide convincing evidence that his disorder was due to heavy metal intoxication.

Commentary. (1) Dystonia affecting speech can be specific to small groups of muscles (jaw and possibly tongue in this case) and, in fact, may be present only during speech. In some cases focal, speech-induced dystonias can be relatively pho-neme specific; in this case they were triggered by open vowels and back of tongue

elevation. (2) Focal speech-induced dystonias sometimes improve with altered postures and distraction and are generally better under conditions of relaxation. The worsening of dystonia or speech difficulty under conditions of anxiety does not establish anxiety as a cause of the speech problem. (3) Perhaps more frequently than any other dysarthria type, the cause of hyperkinetic dysarthria may be indeterminate.

Case 8-3

A 49-year-old woman presented with a 1-year history of ataxia and movement difficulties, including speech. Her problems had begun suddenly with a severe headache and "drunken" speech. Within days she noticed some twitching of the right facial muscles and shaking and twitching in her hands. Medical workup shortly after onset suggested a diagnosis of myoclonic epilepsy of cortical origin.

During speech examination she complained of slurred speech. She noted a feeling of "tightness" in her face and neck intermittently when speaking. Oral mechanism examination was normal at rest. Myoclonic or tremorlike movements of the tongue were present during protrusion and lateral movements. There was no obvious palatal or pharyngeal myoclonus. Jaw and perioral myoclonus was more apparent during sustained phonation than when her mouth was open without phonation. Traces of nasal emission were apparent during pressure sound production. Some dystonic-like perioral movements were also apparent during speech. Her speech was characterized by reduced rate (3), and imprecise articulation (3), with difficulty achieving bilabial closure during connected speech, apparently secondary to dystonic lip contractions. Voice quality was strained-hoarse (2,3) with monopitch and monoloudness (3). Prosody was characterized by excess and equal syllabic stress. Prolonged "ah" was unsteady (2). Speech AMRs were regular when produced

at a rate of one per second but markedly irregular when she attempted to maximize rate. Intelligibility was reduced.

The clinician concluded that the patient had a "hyperkinetic dysarthria of AM. In addition, there appear to be some dystonic perioral movements during speech that make it difficult for her to achieve bilabial closure. Speech clearly worsens during attempts to increase speech rate, and she has consciously reduced her rate because of this." Some suspicion was raised about accompanying ataxic and spastic components to her dysarthria, although it was felt that her scanning prosody and strained voice could well be secondary to efforts to compensate for her hyperkinetic dysarthria.

Neurologic evaluation indicated the presence of ataxia in the limbs, hyperreflexia, and action-induced myoclonus of the trunk, extremities, and face.

A complete workup confirmed a diagnosis of myoclonus epilepsy of cortical origin. Etiology was unclear, but an undiagnosed viral illness was felt to be the most likely cause.

Commentary. (1) Some movement disorders may be speech specific. (2) AM can cause dysarthria, one whose manifestations are noticeably exacerbated by increased speaking rate. In some cases, the myoclonus is associated with dystonic-like movements.

Case 8-4

A 35-year-old woman presented with a 2-year history of gradual mental deterioration, handwriting difficulty, reduced ability to concentrate, and reduced personal hygiene. She complained of speech difficulty, stating, "Nobody can understand me." There was a family history of Huntington's disease, most convincingly present in the patient's father, who died at age 45. Neurologic evaluation identified difficulty with balance and the presence of involuntary movements, generalized motor impersistence, mild cogwheel rigidity, and probable dementia. Neuropsychological assessment confirmed the presence of significant cognitive or memory limitations.

MRI showed an abnormality in the right putamen that could represent the iron deposition sometimes seen in Huntington's disease. Mild generalized atrophy was also present.

During speech examination, rapid, unsustained, choreic-like movements of the lower face, jaw, and tongue were present at rest. Involuntary tongue clicking was noted. She had difficulty maintaining a protruded tongue, open mouth, and lip retraction, as much because of motor impersistence as involuntary movements. Speech was characterized by accelerated rate (1,2), imprecise articulation with irregular articulatory breakdowns (1,2), dysprosody (2), and variable rate (1,2). Choreiform movements tended to delay the initiation of speech or delay continuation of speech at phrase boundaries. Vowel prolongation was characterized by a low amplitude tremor. Speech AMRs were irregular (1,2).

Pitch and loudness variability was reduced, but pitch and loudness occasionally varied inappropriately.

The clinician concluded, "hyperkinetic dysarthria associated with dyskinetic or choreiform movements of the lower face, jaw, and tongue. Her tendency toward accelerated rate and monopitch and monoloudness raise the possibility of an accompanying hypokinetic component, although it is possible that those characteristics are secondary to efforts to race through speech before the next occurrence of orofacial involuntary movements." The clinician also noted that the patient seemed impaired cognitively and often responded impulsively. She was seen for one session of speech therapy, during which she demonstrated an ability to slow her rate and improve articulatory precision. She was unable to do this without constant reminders, however. The family was counseled about the best strategy to use when they were unable to understand the patient; this focused primarily on cueing her to reduce speech rate.

Commentary. (1) Hyperkinetic dysarthria and orofacial choreiform movements may be among the presenting signs of Huntington's disease. (2) Cognitive deficits and personality changes often accompany the dysarthria in Huntington's disease. (3) People with chorea affecting speech sometimes accelerate rate in order to complete a statement before the next involuntary movement. This may give the appearance of an accompanying hypokinetic component to their dysarthria; the distinction between hypokinetic dysarthria and such compensatory efforts can be difficult to make in such cases.

Case 8-5

A 70-year-old woman presented with a 1-year history of voice difficulty. She denied chewing or swallowing difficulty. She had never smoked and did not abuse alcohol. An ear, nose, and throat (ENT) examination was normal. She was referred for speech evaluation.

During speech assessment, she reported the gradual emergence of voice difficulty that she described as "a quiver." This worsened under conditions of stress and fatigue. She denied other speech difficulties or problems with chewing or swallowing. She felt self-conscious about her voice, and it occasionally made her reluctant to speak. She reported that her father had "parkinsonism" and that her 71-year-old brother had some "shaking in his hands."

Oral mechanism examination was normal in size, strength, and symmetry. There was a subtle low-amplitude tremor of her lips at rest, and tremor of her jaw, tongue, palate, and pharynx were quite apparent during vowel prolongation. Articulation and resonance were normal. During conversation, a voice tremor with occasional voice interruptions was apparent. The tremor was particularly apparent during vowel prolongation. There was no evidence of respiratory tremor during prolonged voiceless fricatives or prolonged audible exhalations.

The clinician concluded, "Organic voice tremor with tremor frequency in the 5- to 8-Hz range. No other speech-language abnormalities detected. There are no

Case 8-5—cont'd

other deviant speech characteristics to suggest the presence of hypokinetic dysarthria, which might reflect early Parkinson's disease." This impression was discussed with the patient, who was relieved to have a diagnosis. She expressed concern, however, that her voice difficulty might reflect Parkinson's disease. She was referred for neurologic assessment to rule out PD. Neurologic examination was normal, with the exception of the voice tremor. There was no evidence of parkinsonism. Propranolol was prescribed in an effort to reduce the voice tremor but was ineffective.

Commentary. (1) Voice tremor can be an isolated manifestation of dysarthria. (2) Laryngeal tremor may not be apparent (or may be missed) during laryngeal examination, and correct diagnosis is often made solely on the basis of perception of voice tremor. (3) Organic voice tremor can occur in the absence of other neurologic signs. (4) In addition to voice tremor's effect on communication ability, it often raises concerns in the patient about more serious neurologic disease. In this case the patient could be reassured that her condition was probably benign. The speech pathologist's impression was confirmed during neurologic evaluation. (5) In some cases the most effective management of a speech problem is correct diagnosis. This patient expressed relief about her diagnosis and a relative lack of concern about the minor difficulties her voice problem was causing her in some social situations.

Case 8-6

A 73-year-old woman presented with a 10-year history of voice difficulty that was present upon awakening one day, without obvious explanation. The problem worsened but had been stable for 3 to 4 years. She had had several periods of speech therapy, without benefit. Neurologic evaluation identified the presence of a head tremor, postural upper extremity tremor, and "spastic speech." A cause for these abnormal movements was not identified during a complete neurologic workup.

During speech examination, the patient associated onset of her voice problem with a period of considerable psychologic stress (her adopted son was having difficulty with drugs and was in the process of attempting to locate his biologic parents). She also noted that her voice worsened when she was anxious or spoke in a group. She noted mild improvement in her voice when she had a glass of wine.

Her voice was characterized by a tremor that consistently interrupted her voice and mildly slowed speech rate. Prolonged "ah" contained consistent, somewhat irregular, and strained voice interruptions. At higher pitches, voice interruptions disappeared and a tremor became apparent. Tremor was not apparent during prolongation of voiceless fricatives.

The clinician concluded, "Adductor spasmodic dysphonia of essential voice tremor, moderate to marked in severity."

Botox injection (discussed in Chapter 17) was recommended. Her voice improved significantly after several weeks of a weak-breathy dysphonia and mild swallowing difficulty. She noted a marked reduction in physical effort to speak and was pleased with her voice quality. Voice quality was indeed markedly improved, although evidence of mild voice tremor persisted, but without voice interruptions.

Commentary. (1) Adductor spasmodic dysphonia can develop in association with organic voice tremor. Voice tremor may be accompanied by tremor elsewhere in the body, particularly in the jaw, face, tongue, palate, and pharynx. (2) The onset of spasmodic dysphonia is often associated with psychologic stress, even when examination reveals an organic basis for the problem. The relationship between psychologic stress and neurogenic spasmodic dysphonia is unclear, but the presence of psychologic stress at the time of onset does not rule out the possibility of neurogenic etiology for persistent voice difficulty. (3) Proper diagnosis of adductor spasmodic dysphonia can lead to fairly effective treatment of the disorder. A 68-year-old man presented with complaints of gradually progressive dizziness, visual difficulties, and slurred speech and mild swallowing difficulty. He had had a "mild" stroke and subsequent left carotid endarterectomy 8 years previously, but his speech and visual difficulties did not emerge until 2 years later. Neurologic examination was normal except for abnormal speech. Concern was raised about motor neuron disease. The patient was referred for EMG, MRI, and ENT and speech consultations.

During speech evaluation the patient reported having some mild difficulty with speech following his stroke, with subsequent improvement, but then worsening in recent years, characterized by voice difficulty and occasional problems with pronunciation. He did not complain of swallowing difficulties during meals but felt he was having problems controlling saliva.

Case 8-7

Oral mechanism examination was normal with the exception of some quick myoclonic-like movements of the tongue and 2- to 4-Hz myoclonic movements of the palate at rest and during phonation. Hoarse-rough voice quality (2,3), sporadic voice breaks, and inconsistent, imprecise articulation (1) of lingual fricatives and affricates characterized speech. Speech AMRs and SMRs were normal in rate and rhythm. Vowel prolongation was variable but consistent with the rate of the palatal myoclonus.

The clinician concluded: "The patient has a palatolaryngeal and perhaps lingual myoclonus suggestive of dysfunction in the Guillain-Mollaret triangle (brainstem or cerebellum). I think his myoclonus can explain some of the variability in his voice and some of his inconsistent articulatory imprecision. I do not think it explains very well his rough-hoarse voice quality."

EMG and ENT evaluations were normal. MRI showed old lacunar strokes in the thalami and right caudate nucleus but no lesion in the brainstem or cerebellum. His speech difficulties may have resulted from an undetectable brainstem stroke, but a degenerative neurologic disorder could not be ruled out. Clonazepam was prescribed in the hope that it would help the myoclonus.

The patient returned for neurologic reassessment 1 year later with worsening of symptoms. He had been unable to tolerate the side effects of Clonazepam and had discontinued it. Examination revealed palatal myoclonus and obvious but mild gait unsteadiness. An MRI now showed clear evidence of hypertrophic olivary degeneration (see Figure 8-8 for illustration of hypertrophic olivary degeneration). He was not seen for speech reassessment. It was concluded that he had a neurodegenerative disorder that, at the present time, could not be more clearly defined.

Commentary. (1) Palatal-laryngeal myoclonus is a well-localized disorder. Its presence in this case predicted the MRI abnormality that eventually emerged. (2) Although uncommon, PM can be the result of degenerative neurologic disease. (3) Changes in speech and oral mechanism examination can be among the first signs of neurologic disease.

SUMMARY

1. Hyperkinetic dysarthrias are usually associated with dysfunction of the basal ganglia control circuit, but can also be related to involvement of the cerebellar control circuit or other portions of the extrapyramidal system. They probably occur somewhat less frequently in speech pathology practices than other dysarthria types, but if organic voice tremor and neurogenic spasmodic dysphonias are included in such comparisons, they may be more prevalent than all other single dysarthria types. Their characteristics can be manifest in the respiratory, phonatory, resonatory, and articulatory levels of speech, and prosody is often prominently affected. The deviant speech characteristics of hyperkinetic dysarthrias reflect the effects on speech of abnormal rhythmic or irregular and unpredictable, rapid or slow involuntary movements.

2. Hyperkinetic dysarthrias are heterogenous, both in terms of the various abnormal movements that can lead to it and the particular speech muscles affected by the involuntary movements. The movement disorders underlying them are often categorized by the degree to which they vary in speed and rhythmicity. The most common abnormal movements associated with hyperkinetic dysarthrias include chorea, dystonia, athetosis, ST, myoclonus, tics, and tremor.

3. The cause of hyperkinetic dysarthrias is often unknown. This is particularly true when the movement disorder is limited to the speech or cervical muscles. Toxic and metabolic conditions are frequent known causes, with antipsychotic or neuroleptic medications representing the most frequent toxic cause. Orofacial dyskinesias and dysarthria are often the first or only manifestation of drug toxicity and tardive dyskinesia. Hyperkinetic dysarthrias are not uncommonly associated with degenerative neurologic conditions. Infection, neoplasm, trauma, and stroke are possible but infrequent causes.

4. The jaw, face, and tongue are frequently affected by hyperkinesias, usually in combination, but sometimes only a single speech structure is involved. Organic voice tremor and spasmodic dysphonias frequently have speech abnormalities that are perceptually limited to phonatory functions. Sometimes the involuntary movements are action induced and occur only during speech. In such cases the dysarthria is sometimes misdiagnosed as psychogenic in origin.

5. Patient complaints and specific deviant speech characteristics are quite variable, and they depend on the type of involuntary movement and the specific levels of the speech system affected. Distinctions can generally be made among dysarthrias that are due to chorea, dystonia, athetosis, ST, PM, AM, tics, organic voice tremor, and spasmodic dysphonias. These distinctions are what justify consideration of hyperkinetic dysarthria as a plural disorder, with subtypes based on the nature of the underlying involuntary movement.

6. In general, acoustic and physiologic studies have provided support for the auditory-perceptual characteristics of hyperkinetic dysarthrias, have specified more precisely the disorder's acoustic and physiologic characteristics, and have established approaches to documenting and quantifying relevant parameters of the disorder.

7. Hyperkinetic dysarthria can be the only, the first, or among the first and most prominent manifestations of neurologic disease. Its recognition can aid neurologic localization and diagnosis and may contribute to the medical and behavioral management of the individual's disease and speech disorder.

References

1. Ackermann H, Hertrich I, Hehr T: Oral diadokokinesis in neurological dysarthrias, Folia Phoniatr Logop 47:15, 1995.
2. Ackerman H, Ziegler W: Cerebellar voice tremor: an acoustic analysis, J Neurol Neurosurg Psychiatry 54:74, 1991.
3. Adams RD, Victor M: Principles of neurology, New York, 1991, McGraw-Hill.
4. Adams SG et al: Comparison of botulinum toxin injection procedures in adductor spasmodic dysphonia, J Otolaryngol 24:345, 1995.
5. Adams SG et al: Effects of Botulinum toxin type A injections on aerodynamic measures of spasmodic dysphonia, Laryngoscope 106:296, 1996.
6. Ahlskog JE: Approach to the patient with a movement disorder: basic principles of neurologic diagnosis. In Adler CH, Ahlskog JE, editors: Parkinson's disease and movement disorders: diagnosis and treatment guidelines for the practicing physician, Totowa, NJ, 2000, Humana Press.
7. Ahlskog JE: Initial symptomatic treatment of Parkinson's disease. In Adler CH, Ahlskog JE, editors: Parkinson's disease and movement disorders: diagnosis and treatment guidelines for the practicing physician, Totowa, NJ, 2000, Humana Press.
8. Arana GW, Hyman SE: Handbook of psychiatric drug therapy, ed 2, Boston, 1991, Little, Brown & Company.
9. Aronson AE: Clinical voice disorders, New York, 1990, Thieme.
10. Aronson AE, Hartman DE: Adductor spastic dysphonia as a sign of essential (voice) tremor, J Speech Hear Disord 46:52, 1981.
11. Aronson AE, Lagerlund TC: Neuroimaging studies do not prove the existence of brain abnormalities in spastic (spasmodic) dysphonia, J Speech Hear Res 34:801, 1991.
12. Aronson AE, O'Neill BP, Kelly JJ: The dysarthria of action myoclonus: a new clinical entity, Presented at the Clinical Dysarthria Conference, Tucson, Ariz, February 1984.
13. Barsottini OG et al: Brain SPECT imaging in Sydenham's chorea, Braz J Med Biol Res 35:431, 2002.
14. Bartenstein P et al: Central motor processing in Huntington's disease: a PET study, Brain 120:1553, 1997.
15. Bhatia KP: The paroxysmal dyskinesias, J Neurol 246:149, 1999.
16. Biary N, Koller WC: Essential tongue tremor, Mov Disord 2:25, 1987.
17. Brazis P, Masdeu JC, Biller J: Localization in clinical neurology, ed 4, Philadelphia, 2001, Lippincott Williams & Wilkins.
18. Brown JR, Simonson J: Organic voice tremor: a tremor of phonation, Neurology 13:520, 1963.
19. Burke RE: Tardive dyskinesia: current clinical issues, Neurology 34:1348, 1984.
20. Cannito MP: Vocal tract steadiness in spasmodic dysphonia. In Yorkston KM, Beukelman DR, editors: Recent advances in clinical dysarthria, Boston, 1989, College-Hill Press.
21. Cannito MP: Neurobiological interpretations of spasmodic dysphonia. In Vogel D, Cannito MP, editors: Treating disordered speech motor control, Austin, Tex, 1991, Pro-Ed.
22. Cannito MP, Kondraske GV, Johns DF: Oral-facial sensorimotor function in spasmodic dysphonia. In Moore CA, Yorkston KM, Beukelman DR, editors: Dysarthria and apraxia of speech: perspective on management, Baltimore, 1991, Brooks Publishing Company.
23. Cannito MP, McSwain LS, Dworkin JP: Abductor spasmodic dysphonia: acoustic influence of voicing on connected speech. In Robin DA, Yorkston KM, Beukelman DR, editors: Disorders of motor speech: assessment, treatment, and clinical characterization, Baltimore, 1996, Brookes Publishing Company.
24. Cannito MP et al: Dysfluency in spasmodic dysphonia: a multivariate analysis, J Speech Lang Hear Res 40:627, 1997.
25. Cardoso F et al: Persistent Sydenham's chorea, Mov Disord 14:805, 1999.
26. Casey DE, Robins P: Tardive dyskinesia as a life-threatening illness, Am J Psychiatry 135:486, 1978.
27. Caviness JN: Huntington's disease and other choreas. In Adler CH, Ahlskog JE, editors: Parkinson's disease and movement disorders: diagnosis and treatment guidelines for the practicing physician, Totowa, NJ, 2000, Humana Press.
28. Caviness JN: Myoclonus. In Adler CH, Ahlskog JE, editors: Parkinson's disease and movement disorders: diagnosis and treatment guidelines for the practicing physician, Totowa, NJ, 2000, Humana Press.

29. Caviness JN, Evidente VG: Cortical myoclonus during lithium exposure, Arch Neurol 60:401, 2003.

29a. Cimino-Knight AM, Sapienza CM: Consistency of voice produced by patients with adductor spasmodic dysphonia: a preliminary investigation, J Speech Lang Hear Res, 44:793, 2001.

30. Coleman, R, Anderson D, Lovrien E: Oral motor dysfunction in individuals at risk for Huntington's disease, Am J Med Genet 37:36, 1990.

31. Comings DE: A controlled study of Tourette syndrome. VII. Summary: a common genetic disorder causing disinhibition of the limbic system, Am J Hum Genet 41:839, 1987.

32. Comings DE: Tourette syndrome and human behavior, Duarte, Calif, 1990, Hope Press.

33. D'Alessandro R et al: The prevalence of lingual-facial-buccal dyskinesias in the elderly, Neurology 36:1350, 1986.

34. Darley FL, Aronson AE, Brown JR: Differential diagnostic patterns of dysarthria, J Speech Hear Res 12:246, 1969a.

35. Darley FL, Aronson AE, Brown JR: Clusters of deviant speech dimensions in the dysarthrias, J Speech Hear Res 12:462, 1969b.

36. Darley FL, Aronson AE, Brown JR: Motor speech disorders, Philadelphia, 1975, WB Saunders.

37. Day TJ, Lefroy RB, Mastaglia FL: Meige's syndrome and palatal myoclonus associated with brain stem stroke: a common mechanism? J Neurol Neurosurg Psychiatry 49:1324, 1986.

38. Deuschl G et al: Symptomatic and essential rhythmic palatal myoclonus, Brain 113:1645, 1990.

39. First MB, editor: Diagnostic and statistical manual of mental disorders, ed 4, revised, Washington, DC, 1994, American Psychiatric Association.

40. Dolder CR, Jeste DC: Incidence of tardive dyskinesia with typical versus atypical antipsychotics in very high risk patients, Biol Psychiatry 53:1142, 2003.

41. Faheem DA et al: Respirator dyskinesia and dysarthria from prolonged neuroleptic use: tardive dyskinesia? Am J Psychiatry 139:517, 1982.

42. Fahn S, Davis JM, Rolland LP: Cerebral hypoxia and its consequences. In Fahn S, David JM, Rolland, editors: Advances in neurology, New York, 1979, Raven Press.

43. Fahn S, Marsden C, Calne DB: Classification and investigation of dystonia. In Marsden CD, Fahn S, editors: Movement disorders 2, London, 1987, Butterworth-Heinemann.

44. Fam NP, Chisholm RJ: Chorea in a pregnant woman with rheumatic mitral stenosis, Can J Cardiol 19:719, 2003.

45. Findley LJ, Koller WC: Essential tremor: a review, Neurology 37:1194, 1987.

46. Finitzo T, Freeman F: Spasmodic dysphonia, whether and where: results of seven years of research, J Speech Hear Res 32:541, 1989.

47. Finitzo T et al: Whether and wherefore: a response to Aronson and Lagerlund, J Speech Hear Res 34:806, 1991.

48. Finnegan EM et al: Increased stability of airflow following botulinum toxin injection, Laryngoscope 109: 1300, 1999.

49. Fross RD et al: Lesions of the putamen: their relevance to dystonia, Neurology 37:1125, 1987.

50. Gamboa J et al: Acoustic voice analysis in patients with essential tremor, J Voice 12:444, 1998.

51. Gerratt BR: Formant frequency fluctuation as an index of motor steadiness in the vocal tract, J Speech Hear Res 26:297, 1983.

52. Ghika-Schmid F et al: Hyperkinetic movement disorders during and after acute stroke: the Lausanne stroke registry, J Neurol Sci 146:109, 1997.

53. Golper LA et al: Focal cranial dystonia, J Speech Hear Disord 48:128, 1983.

54. Hardy JC: Cerebral palsy, Englewood Cliffs, NJ, 1983, Prentice-Hall.

55. Hertegrad S, Granqvist S, Lindestad P: Botulinum toxin injections for essential voice tremor, Ann Otol Rhinol Laryngol 109:204, 2000.

56. Hertrich I, Ackermann H: Acoustic analysis of speech timing in Huntington's disease, Brain Lang 47:182, 1994.

57. Higgins MB, Chait DH, Schulte L: Phonatory air flow characteristics of adductor spasmodic dysphonia and muscle tension dysphonia, J Speech Lang Hear Res 42:101, 1999.

58. Howard RS et al: Respiratory involvement in multiple sclerosis, Brain 115:479, 1992.

59. Hubble JP: Essential tremor: diagnosis and treatment. In Adler CH, Ahlskog JE, editors: Parkinson's disease and movement disorders: diagnosis and treatment guidelines for the practicing physician, Totowa, NJ, 2000, Humana Press.

60. Jankovic J: Cranial-cervical dyskinesias. In Appel SH, editor: Current neurology, vol 6, Chicago, 1986, Year Book Publishers.

60a. Jankovic J, Patel SC: Blepharospasm associated with brainstem lesions. Neurology 33:1237, 1983.

61. Jeste DV: Tardive dyskinesia in older patients, J Clin Psychiatry 61(Suppl 4):27, 2000.

62. Kent R, Netsell R: Articulatory abnormalities in athetoid cerebral palsy, J Speech Hear Disord 43:353, 1978.

63. Kent RD et al: Severe essential vocal and oromandibular tremor: a case report, Phonoscope 1:237, 1998.

64. Kent RD et al: What dysarthrias can tell us about the neural control of speech, J Phonet 28:273, 2000.

65. Kim JS: Delayed onset mixed involuntary movements after thalamic stroke: clinical, radiological and pathophysiological findings, Brain 124:299, 2001.

66. Koller WC: Diagnosis and treatment of tremors, Neurol Clin 2:499, 1984.

67. Kurlan R: Tourette's syndrome and tic disorders. In Noseworthy JH, editor: Neurological therapeutics: principles and practice, vol 2, New York, 2003, Martin Dunitz.

68. Lance JW: Action myoclonus, Ramsay Hunt syndrome, and other cerebellar myoclonic syndromes. In Fahn S, editor: Advances in neurology, vol 43, myoclonus, New York, 1986, Raven Press.

69. Lance JW, Adams RD: The syndrome of intention or action myoclonus as a sequel to anoxic encephalopathy, Brain 87:111, 1963.

70. LaPointe LL, Case JL, Duane DD: Perceptual-acoustic speech and voice characteristics of subjects with spasmodic torticollis. In Till JA, Yorkston KM, Beukelman DR, editors: Motor speech disorders: advances in assessment and treatment, Baltimore, 1994, Paul H Brookes.

71. Llorca PM et al: Tardive dyskinesias and antipsychotics: a review, Eur Psychiatry: J Assoc Eur Psychiatrists 17:129, 2002.

72. Ludlow CL: Treatment of speech and voice problems with botulinum toxin, JAMA 264:2671, 1990.

73. Ludlow CL, Connor NP: Dynamic aspects of phonatory control in spasmodic dysphonia, J Speech Hear Res 30:197, 1987.

74. Lundy DS et al: Abnormal soft palate posturing in patients with laryngeal movement disorders, J of Voice 10:348, 1996.

75. Marsden CD: Is tardive dyskinesia a unique disorder? In Casey DE et al, editors: Dyskinesias: research and treatment, New York, 1985, Springer-Verlag.

76. Marsden CD, Fahn S: Problems in the dyskinesias. In Marsden CE, Fahn S, editors: Movement disorders Vol 2, London, 1987, Butterworth-Heinemann.

77. Matsumoto JY: Tremor disorders: overview. In Adler CH, Ahlskog JE, editors: Parkinson's disease and movement disorders: diagnosis and treatment guidelines for the practicing physician, Totowa, NJ, 2000, Humana Press.

78. Matsuo F, Ajax ET: Palatal myoclonus and denervation supersensitivity in the central nervous system, Ann Neurol 5:72, 1978.

79. Merson RM, Ginsberg AP: Spasmodic dysphonia: abductor type; a clinical report of acoustic, aerodynamic and perceptual characteristics, Laryngoscope 89:129, 1979.

80. Mölsä PR, Marttila RJ, Rinne UK: Extrapyramidal signs in Alzheimer's disease, Neurology 34:1114, 1984.

81. Murdoch BE: Subcortical brain mechanisms in speech and language, Folia Phoniatr Logop 53:233, 2001.

81a. Nielson P, O'Dwyer N: Reproducibility and variability of speech muscle activity in athetoid dysarthria of cerebral palsy, J Speech Hear Res 27:502, 1984.

82. Platt LJ, Andrews G, Howie P: Dysarthria of adult cerebral palsy: II. analysis of articulation errors, J Speech Hear Res 23:41, 1980.

83. Platt LJ et al: Dysarthria of adult cerebral palsy: I. intelligibility and articulatory impairment, J Speech Hear Res 23:28, 1980.

84. Putnam AHB: Review of research in dysarthria. In Winitz H, editor: Human communication and its disorders, a review 1988, Norwood, NJ, 1988, Ablex Publishing.

85. Quinn N, Schrag A: Huntington's disease and other choreas, J Neurol 245:709, 1998.

86. Ramig LO: Acoustic analysis of phonation in patients with Huntington's disease, Ann Otol Rhinol Laryngol 95:288, 1986.

87. Rice JE, Antic R, Thompson PD: Disordered respiration as a levodopa-induced dyskinesia in Parkinson's disease, Mov Disord 17:524, 2002.

88. Rosenberg RN, Pettegrew JW: Genetic neurologic disease. In Rosenberg RN, editor: Comprehensive neurology, New York, 1991, Raven Press.

89. Rosenfield DB: Pharmacologic approaches to speech motor disorders. In Vogel D, Cannito MP, editors: Treating disordered speech motor control, Austin, Tex, 1991, Pro-Ed.

90. Rothwell JC, Obeso JA: The anatomical and physiological basis of torsion dystonia. In Marsden CF, Fahn S, editors: Movement disorders Vol 2, London, 1987, Butterworth-Heinemann.

91. Sapienza CM, Walton S, Murry T: Acoustic variations in adductor spasmodic dysphonia as a function of speech task, J Speech Lang Hear Res 42:127, 1999.

92. Sapienza CM et al: Acoustic variations in reading produced by speakers with spasmodic dysphonia pre-Botox injection and within early stages of post-Botox injection, J Speech Lang Hear Res 45:830, 2002.

93. Sethi KD: Tardive dyskinesias. In Adler CH, Ahlskog JE, editors: Parkinson's disease and movement disorders: diagnosis and treatment guidelines for the practicing physician, Totowa, NJ, 2000, Humana Press.

94. Tarsy D: Dystonia. In Adler CH, Ahlskog JE, editors: Parkinson's disease and movement disorders: diagnosis and treatment guidelines for the practicing physician, Totowa, NJ, 2000, Humana Press.

95. Tingley S, Dromey C: Phonatory-articulatory relationships: Do speakers with spasmodic dysphonia show aberrant lip kinematic profiles? J Med Speech-Lang Pathol 8:249, 2000.

96. Tomoda H et al: Voice tremor: dysregulation of voluntary expiratory muscles, Neurology 37:117, 1987.

97. Watson BC et al: Laryngeal electromyographic activity in adductor and abductor spasmodic dysphonia, J Speech Hear Res 34:473, 1991.

98. Weeks RA et al: Corticol control of movement in Huntington's disease. A PET activation study, Brain 120:1569, 1997.

99. Weiner WJ et al: Respiratory dyskinesias: extrapyramidal dysfunction and dyspnea, Ann Intern Med 88:327, 1978.

99a. Werhahn KJ et al: The clinical features and prognosis of chronic posthypoxic myoclonus, Mov Disord 12:216, 1997.

100. Wijdicks EF, Weisner RH, Krom RA: Neurotoxicity in transplant recipients with cyclosporine immunosuppression, Neurology 45:1962, 1995.

101. Wirshing WC: Movement disorders associated with neuroleptic treatment, J Clin Psychiatry 62 (Suppl 21):15, 2001.

102. Wolfe VI, Bacon M: Spectrographic comparison of two types of spastic dysphonia, J Speech Hear Disord 41:325, 1976.

103. Zraik RI et al: Acoustic correlates of voice quality in individuals with spasmodic torticollis, *J Med Speech-Lang Pathol* 1:261, 1993.

104. Zwirner P, Barnes GJ: Vocal tract steadiness: a measure of phonatory and upper airway motor control during phonation in dysarthria, *J Speech Hear Res* 35:761, 1992.

105. Zwirner P, Murry T, Woodson GE: Perceptual-acoustic relationships in spasmodic dysphonia, *J Voice* 7:165, 1993.

Unilateral Upper Motor Neuron Dysarthria

"I didn't even know anything happened except I was talkin' to this gal, and I said, 'somethin's happened to me and I can't talk real good!'"

(82-year-old woman describing the onset of her right internal capsule lacunar stroke)

CHAPTER OUTLINE

  I. **Anatomy and basic functions of the upper motor neuron system**

 II. **Clinical characteristics associated with unilateral upper motor neuron lesions**

III. **Etiologies**

IV. **Speech pathology**

    A. Distribution of etiologies, lesions, and severity in clinical practice

    B. Patient perceptions and complaints

    C. Clinical findings

    D. Acoustic and physiologic findings

 V. **The distinctiveness of unilateral upper motor neuron dysarthria: conclusions and clinical suggestions**

VI. **Cases**

VII. **Summary**

Unilateral upper motor neuron (UUMN) dysarthria is an often distinguishable motor speech disorder associated with damage to the upper motor neuron (UMN) pathways that carry impulses to the cranial and spinal nerves that supply the speech muscles. It may be manifest in any component of speech but is most often apparent in articulation, phonation, and prosody. Its deviant characteristics usually reflect the effects of weakness on speech, but sometimes spasticity and incoordination are implicated. The identification of a UUMN dysarthria can aid the diagnosis of neurologic disease and its localization to central nervous system (CNS) motor pathways.

In contrast to other dysarthria types, the label for this dysarthria is anatomic rather than pathophysiologic. This is because only in recent years have we begun to carefully describe its clinical perceptual characteristics and understand its anatomic and physiologic correlates. We do know that the disorder's clinical features and anatomic and physiologic correlates can vary considerably among affected people. It thus seems best to avoid a single physiologic label until clinical characteristics and their underpinnings are better defined and to use a label that conveys what is most certain about it, hence its designation as *UUMN dysarthria*. The reasons for the variability associated with UUMN dysarthria, as well as some related practical clinical issues, are tied together at the end of this chapter.

Why has UUMN dysarthria received limited attention? One reason is that historically it has been considered a mild and temporary problem (e.g., Darley, Aronson, and Brown [DAB][18]; Metter[48]). Although this is not always the case, disorders that frequently are mild and short-lived in their clinical manifestations are naturally difficult to study. In addition, UUMN dysarthria often occurs simultaneously with aphasia or apraxia of speech when the lesion is in the left hemisphere and with cognitive or nondysarthric speech deficits when the lesion is in the right hemisphere. Such disorders can be devastating in their effects on communication; as a result, a dysarthria may be masked by them or made more difficult to study because of their presence. In general, therefore, UUMN dysarthria has probably received little attention because of its presumed mildness and short duration, and its frequent cooccurrence with deficits that may mask or over-whelm its manifestations, minimizing its functional importance and making it difficult to isolate and study.

It should be recognized, however, that UUMN dysarthria is sometimes a person's only or most obvious communication disorder and sometimes the only or most obvious manifestations of neurologic disease.* Its recognition is especially important when it is a relatively isolated sign, because the offending lesion tends to be small and can escape detection by neuroimaging techniques, especially early after onset. An understanding of UUMN dysarthria's char-acteristics is also important, because it can occur simultaneously and be difficult to distinguish from other speech disorders associated with unilateral CNS disease, such as apraxia of speech (left hemi-sphere lesions) and aprosodia (right hemisphere lesions).

UUMN dysarthria is encountered in a large medical practice at a rate comparable to that of the other major single dysarthria types. Based on data for primary communication disorder diagnoses in the Mayo Clinic speech pathology practice, it accounts for 8.5% of all dysarthrias and 7.8% of all motor speech disorders (MSDs) (see Figure 1-3). This is almost certainly an underestimate of its actual prev-alence in clinical practice, because it occurs fre-quently as a secondary diagnosis for people with aphasia, apraxia of speech, or nonaphasic cognitive-communication deficits.

The clinical features of UUMN dysarthria nearly always reflect, at least in part, the effects of unilat-eral UMN weakness in the face and tongue, and sometimes other levels of the speech system. In some cases, however, deviant speech characteristics also suggest effects of spasticity, incoordination, or both, sometimes making the overall speech pattern difficult to distinguish from spastic or ataxic dysarthria. These perceptual ambiguities can usually be clarified by additional clinical data.

◼ ANATOMY AND BASIC FUNCTIONS OF THE UPPER MOTOR NEURON SYSTEM

The UMN system includes the *direct and indirect activation pathways*. They were described in detail

---

*Urban et al.[74] reported that, in 69 consecutive patients with the sudden onset of dysarthria due to a single stroke, isolated dysarthria or dysarthria with central facial and lingual paresis occurred in 3% and 10%, respectively; dysarthria-clumsy hand syndrome in 12%; and dysarthria with pure motor hemiparesis or ataxic hemiparesis in 28%. Lesions were in the lower part of the primary motor cortex, the centrum semiovale, the internal capsule, the cerebral peduncle, the base of the pons, or the ventral pon-tomedullary junction. All of these locations are along the course of the pyramidal tract.

---

in Chapter 2 and reviewed again in Chapter 5 when the effects on speech of bilateral UMN lesions (spastic dysarthria) were addressed. These pathways are reviewed here only with reference to their impli-cations for understanding UUMN dysarthria and the neurologic deficits that frequently accompany it. Their relevant anatomy and functions can be sum-marized as follows:

1. The UMN system is bilateral, half originat-ing in the right hemisphere and half in the left hemisphere.

2. The *direct activation pathway* of the UMN system passes directly as corticobulbar and corticospinal tracts to the cranial and spinal nerves, respectively, mostly to the side oppo-site their origin. It emerges from the *cerebral cortex* and begins its descent in the *corona radiata*. The corona radiata converges into the *internal capsule* in the vicinity of the basal ganglia and thalamus (corticobulbar fibers are grouped primarily in the *genu,* or midportion, of the internal capsule). From there it descends to the brainstem, where cor-ticobulbar fibers cross to the opposite side just before reaching the cranial nerve nuclei they are to innervate; corticospinal fibers cross in the pyramids of the medulla. The impulses traveling in the direct pathway appear *crucial for finely coordinated skilled movements*.

3. The *indirect activation pathway* of the UMN system has the same predominantly con-tralateral destinations, and it crosses in the brainstem in the same general areas as the direct activation pathway. However, along its route to the cranial and spinal nerves are synaptic connections in several interven-ing structures, lying mostly in the *reticular formation* and *other brainstem nuclei*. This pathway appears *crucial for regul-ating reflexes and controlling posture and tone,* upon which skilled movements are superimposed.

4. In the bulbar speech muscles of most people, *the general principle of contralateral inner-vation holds true only for the lower face and, to a lesser and probably variable degree, the tongue.* The trigeminal nerve, the fibers of the facial nerve going to the upper face, and the glossopharyngeal, vagus, accessory, and, at least in some individuals, hypoglossal nerves receive both contralateral and ipsilateral UMN innervation. This bilateral input to most of the speech cranial nerves provides a degree of redundancy that helps to preserve breathing, feeding, and motor speech func-tions when UMN lesions are confined to one

Primary clinical features of UUMN lesions. All features are present on the side of the body contralateral to the lesion.

Direct Activation Pathway (Pyramidal Tract)

Hemiplegia or hemiparesis
Loss/impairment of fine, skilled movements
Absent abdominal reflex
Babinski's sign
Hyporeflexia
Central facial weakness at rest and during voluntary movement
Lingual weakness

Indirect Activation Pathway (Extrapyramidal Tract)

Increased muscle tone
Spasticity
Clonus
Hyperactive stretch reflexes
Decerebrate or decorticate posturing
Central facial weakness apparent during emotional expression

UUMN, Unilateral upper motor neuron.

side of the brain. However, this redundancy is not always all protective. Evidence suggests that *at least some individuals with UUMN lesions have detectable contralateral weakness of the jaw, palate, vocal folds, and, most frequently and obviously, the tongue;* in some cases, even ipsilateral weakness can be measured. This is important to remember, because it helps explain several of the deviant speech characteristics that can be present in UUMN dysarthria. This is addressed later in the speech pathology section.

CLINICAL CHARACTERISTICS ASSOCIATED WITH UNILATERAL UPPER MOTOR NEURON LESIONS

The distinctive effects of UUMN lesions affecting the direct and indirect activation pathways are summarized in Box 9-1.* Briefly, such lesions are often associated with contralateral hemiplegia or hemiparesis. A *Babinski reflex* is usually present on the affected side.

A combination of weakness and spasticity is usually present in the affected limbs. Weakness, hyporeflexia, and hypotonia in the limbs tend to predominate shortly after the onset of acute lesions,

with spasticity, hyperactive stretch reflexes, and increased muscle tone often emerging over time. Limb motor deficits tend to be worse when muscle flaccidity (as opposed to spasticity) is prolonged following stroke. Evidence suggests that prolonged flaccidity is associated with a higher prevalence of structural involvement of the lentiform nucleus and reduced cerebral blood flow in the lentiform nucleus, thalamus, and contralateral cerebellum.[58] Whether or not structural or physiologic involvement of these basal ganglia and cerebellar control circuits predicts specific deviant features of UUMN dysarthria, or its severity and prognosis, has yet to be determined.

Corticobulbar involvement is often manifest by varying degrees of *contralateral lower facial weakness.* This is usually called *central (or supranuclear) facial weakness* to distinguish it from peripheral cranial nerve VII lesions that usually affect the upper and lower face. Similarly, when contralateral lingual weakness is present, it is often called *central lingual weakness.*

A combination of direct and indirect pathway lesion effects are usually present, at least in the limbs. Depending on the specific site of lesion, however, there may be relative sparing of the upper or lower limb or bulbar muscles. For example, some lesions affect only the bulbar muscles or only the bulbar muscles and hand.

ETIOLOGIES

Any process that can damage UMNs unilaterally can cause UUMN dysarthria. Because degenerative, inflammatory, and toxic-metabolic diseases usually produce diffuse effects, they are rarely associated with focal unilateral signs, including UUMN dysarthria. Tumors confined to one side of the CNS can cause UUMN dysarthria when they invade or produce mass effects on UMN structures and pathways unilaterally. Trauma, particularly surgical trauma, can produce focal deficits, including UUMN dysarthria; the typical multifocal, bilateral, or diffuse deficits associated with closed head injury are usually associated with other dysarthria types.

Stroke is by far the most common cause of UUMN damage, and dysarthria is a frequent consequence of stroke, occurring in 29% of patients with stroke associated with hemiparesis.[46] It is thus appropriate to review some of the vascular conditions that can produce relatively isolated UMN deficits.

Left carotid or middle cerebral artery occlusions are the most common causes of strokes leading to UMN deficits that are also accompanied by aphasia or apraxia of speech. Right carotid or middle cerebral artery occlusions are the most common cause of

---

*These features are discussed in more detail in Chapter 5.

strokes leading to UMN deficits that are also accompanied by neglect and cognitive disturbances characteristic of right hemisphere pathology. Unilateral strokes in the distribution of the posterior cerebral, basilar, and, less frequently, anterior cerebral arteries can also cause UUMN deficits.

Sometimes small infarcts occur in the brainstem or cortical or subcortical areas of the cerebral hemispheres as the result of occlusion of the small penetrating branches of the large cerebral arteries. These small infarcts are often called *lacunes* or *lacunar infarcts* because, in healing, they leave behind a small cavity (lacune).* They most often involve the lenticulostriate branches of the anterior and middle cerebral arteries, the thalamoperforant branches of the posterior cerebral arteries, and the paramedian branches of the basilar artery. The most common sites of lacunar strokes are the putamen, caudate nucleus, thalamus, pons, internal capsule, and white matter below the cerebral cortex.[23] These locations establish the relevance of lacunes as a mechanism for producing UUMN dysarthria (and spastic dysarthria, when lesions are bilateral); that is, most of them are part of the UMN pathways.[†] In addition, because of their location, lacunes often are not associated with aphasia, neglect, visual field deficits, severe memory impairment, or alterations in consciousness; their signs usually are primarily motor or sensorimotor. Lacunar stroke is probably the most frequent cause of UUMN dysarthria when dysarthria is a relatively isolated sign of stroke.[‡]

Fisher[23] has outlined a number of "lacunar syndromes." Dysarthria (presumably UUMN dysarthria) is among the defining characteristics for several of them.[§] The most relevant of these are:

1. *Pure motor hemiparesis.* A pure motor stroke involving the face, arm, and leg on one side in the absence of sensory deficit, homonymous hemianopia, aphasia, agnosia, or apraxia. The lesion may be in the corona radiata, internal capsule, cerebral peduncle,

or pons. The vascular origin is usually a branch of the middle cerebral artery or vertebrobasilar system.

2. *Ataxic hemiparesis.* This involves signs of pure motor hemiparesis plus cerebellar dysmetria in the affected limbs. The lesion is often in the pons, internal capsule, or corona radiata.[22,32,41,44] It has also been reported in people with thalamic lesions, often including the posterior limb of the internal capsule.[47,76]

3. *Dysarthria clumsy hand syndrome.* Facial weakness, dysarthria, and dysphagia are prominent, but there is also slight weakness and clumsiness of the hand. The lesion is usually in the pons; genu or posterior limb of the internal capsule; or the adjacent corona radiata, caudate nucleus, or cerebral peduncle.[27,41,42,44,62,71] This syndrome may account for 6% of lacunar infarcts.[13]

4. *Pure dysarthria.* The sudden onset of dysarthria without other signs (except for face and tongue weakness). This syndrome, which may be a variant of the dysarthria clumsy-hand syndrome,[40] was found in approximately 1% of 670 consecutive cases of stroke.[4] The genu of the internal capsule or the adjacent corona radiata are probably the most frequent lesion sites in cases of pure dysarthria resulting from a unilateral stroke, but lesions in the basal ganglia,* base of the pons, and cortical-subcortical motor area have also been reported.[9,31,34,40,41,44,56,57,73] Urban et al.[73] concluded, "interruption of the cortico-lingual pathways is crucial in the pathogenesis of isolated dysarthria after extracerebellar lacunar stroke"; affected patients had no involvement of corticospinal tracts and no cerebellar diaschisis.

◼ SPEECH PATHOLOGY

It is unfortunate that the neurology literature's often-refined descriptions of lesion loci associated with dysarthria are not matched by clear descriptions of specific speech deficits. Beyond describing speech as dysarthric, description is usually limited to vague terms such as "slow dysarthria," "slurred," "unintelligible," or "thick."

Systematic prospective studies of UUMN dysarthria providing detailed descriptions of speech and oral mechanism findings are few in number, and their data are based on small numbers of subjects. In this section, the results of a relatively large retrospective study of 56 patients with UUMN

---

*Lacunes account for approximately 25% of all strokes in some clinical practices.[13] They range in size from 0.2 to 15 mm³; the smallest lacunes may escape detection by computed tomography (CT) scan.[50]

†Dysarthria has been found in 25% of patients with lacunar infarcts[3] and occurs in approximately 30% of patients with stroke in the internal capsule.[24]

‡For example, Urban et al.[74] reported that in 69 consecutive patients with the sudden onset of dysarthria due to a single stroke, lacunar stroke was the cause in 53%.

§Dysarthria can also be a defining feature of nonlacunar infarcts. For example, Kataoka et al.[35] found that it was the most common clinical sign among 49 patients with acute paramedian pontine infarcts, occurring in 55% of the patients.

---

*Facial weakness is apparently common (50%) in unilateral putaminal lacunar strokes.[26]

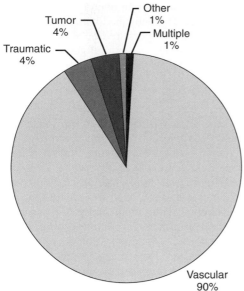

FIGURE 9-1 Distribution of etiologies for 98 Mayo Clinic patients with a primary speech pathology diagnosis of unilateral upper motor neuron dysarthria (see text for description of data sources and Box 9-2 for other details).

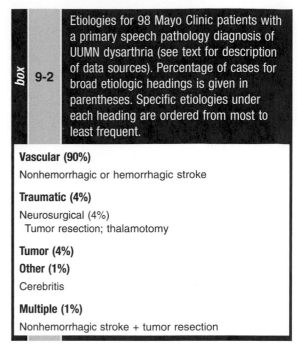

box 9-2

Etiologies for 98 Mayo Clinic patients with a primary speech pathology diagnosis of UUMN dysarthria (see text for description of data sources). Percentage of cases for broad etiologic headings is given in parentheses. Specific etiologies under each heading are ordered from most to least frequent.

Vascular (90%)
Nonhemorrhagic or hemorrhagic stroke

Traumatic (4%)
Neurosurgical (4%)
  Tumor resection; thalamotomy

Tumor (4%)
Other (1%)
Cerebritis

Multiple (1%)
Nonhemorrhagic stroke + tumor resection

UUMN, Unilateral upper motor neuron.

dysarthria*[21] serve as the primary vehicle for describing the disorder. Findings from prospective studies are used to support, supplement, and qualify or modify the observations of Duffy and Folger as appropriate.

Distribution of Etiologies, Lesions, and Severity in Clinical Practice

Etiology

Figure 9-1 and Box 9-2 summarize the etiologies for 98 Mayo Clinic patients with a primary speech pathology diagnosis of UUMN dysarthria. Duffy and Folger[21] described 56 of the cases in their retrospective study. The remaining 42 cases were quasirandomly selected from cases seen from 1999-2001. The cautions expressed in Chapter 4 about generalizing these observations to the general population or all speech pathology practices apply here as well.

*Duffy and Folger's patients were selected on the basis of their speech diagnosis and clinical or neuroimaging evidence of only a single lesion confined to one side of the brain. Patients with parkinsonism and cerebellar lesions were excluded, as were all patients with apraxia of speech. Patients with aphasia that was severe enough to preclude obtaining a sufficient speech sample also were excluded (18% of the sample had aphasia, but it was usually mild).

The data establish that UUMN dysarthria is almost always due to stroke, tumor, or neurosurgery, and stroke is the overwhelmingly predominant cause (90%). Nonhemorrhagic strokes, which account for the highest proportion of neurovascular disturbances in general, accounted for most of the vascular causes. The predominance of stroke as an etiology is consistent with most other studies that have carefully examined the dysarthria associated with UUMN lesions.*[7,28,33,36,66,67,38]

Lesion Loci

The lesion sites for Duffy and Folger's patients are summarized in Box 9-3. Lesions were supratentorial in approximately 95% of the cases. The internal capsule, pericapsular regions, and regions affecting all or portions of cerebral hemisphere lobes were the most common lesion sites. Larger lesions in the cerebral hemispheres nearly always included the frontal lobes. A few patients had lesions in the thalamus, midbrain, or pons. These lesion loci are consistent with the anatomy of the UMN system, its vascular

*The exclusive stroke etiology in some studies may reflect a desire to study patients with small, focal lesions rather than the natural distribution of etiologies of the disorder. Small strokes are ideal for investigating UUMN dysarthria, because their anatomic boundaries are easier to define than those of diseases with more difficult-to-localize effects, such as traumatic brain injury, tumor, or infection.

supply, and the literature on the locus of lacunar strokes that can produce dysarthria. It is also important to recognize that unilateral stroke affecting regions of the basal ganglia, sometimes including portions of the internal capsule, have also been associated with dysarthria and facial weakness.[7,12,33]

Regarding side of lesion, 61% had lesions in the left hemisphere and 34% had lesions in the right hemisphere. This is consistent with some other studies reporting that dysarthria resulting from single small strokes in UMN pathways occur more frequently when the lesions are on the left, thus suggesting a greater influence of left descending motor fibers on speech.[33,63,69] However, the greater percentage of cases with left side lesions, at least in the Hwang et al.[33] and Duffy and Folger studies, could simply reflect referral bias (e.g., many patients may have been referred primarily because of their aphasia) or differences in the distribution of left- and right-sided strokes that come to medical attention. In addition, at least one study has reported that dysarthria occurs more frequently or is more pronounced when the lesion is in the right than in the left hemisphere.[25] Thus although the possibility of left side dominance for UMN pathway control of speech is intriguing, and logical to the extent that the left hemisphere is dominant for language and motor speech programming, current evidence is insufficient to support such a conclusion. What is clear is that *UUMN dysarthria can result from lesions on either side of the brain.*

Severity

The literature does not permit a precise description of dysarthria severity. Dysarthria severity in Duffy and Folger's patients could not always be ascertained from their records, but it was probably mild in many cases. For example, the median severity ratings across the individual deviant speech characteristics that were detected were almost always mild or mild to moderate. These observations are in general agreement with indices of severity reported in other studies.[28,33,36,65,66,68] However, moderate to severe dysarthria was reported for some cases in several of the just-cited studies (and that of Ropper[61]), and a moderate or severe reduction of intelligibility can sometimes occur.[33,67]

It has been suggested that UUMN dysarthria is a transient problem.*[7,18,19,78] Although clinical experi-

---

*Recovery of limb motor function following unilateral capsular stroke is generally good. Limb motor recovery from unilateral stroke is less adequate when multiple motor areas, their descending pathways, or thalamic circuitry are affected.[8,24]

ence indicates that this frequently is the case, clinical experience and published data also indicate that the dysarthria can persist. For example, approximately 45% of Duffy and Folger's patients were evaluated more than 1 month after onset, and all subjects in some studies have been evaluated at least 3 months after onset.[65-68]

These observations suggest that UUMN dysarthria due to stroke is often mild and that significant recovery often takes place, but it sometimes can be markedly severe, chronic, or both. Why some patients can have a markedly severe or persisting UUMN dysarthria following stroke is not entirely clear, but Takahashi et al.,[63] observing that 41% of their patients with small unilateral strokes had asymptomatic strokes on the contralateral side, noted that when such "silent" strokes were present, dysarthria lasted longer and dysphagia occurred more frequently. Those data, plus clinical experience, suggest that *persistent severe dysarthria following a presumed unilateral stroke should raise suspicions about a lesion or lesions on the other side of the brain.* The effects of "silent" strokes (presumably in areas relevant to speech) may be unmasked by the occurrence of a new lesion elsewhere in the brain, making the effects of the new lesion more severe than predicted by the new lesion alone.

How frequently is UUMN dysarthria associated with aphasia, apraxia of speech, aprosodia, or nonaphasic cognitive deficits? Available data are not satisfactory because studies have not been specifically designed to examine those relationships, but some inferences are possible. Duffy and Folger reported that 24% of their patients with left hemisphere lesions had evidence of aphasia, although they had excluded patients whose aphasia, apraxia of speech, or nonaphasic cognitive problems precluded valid assessment of dysarthria. Among 48 patients with a primary diagnosis of UUMN dysarthria seen in the Mayo Clinic speech pathology practice from 1999-2001, 10% had a less severe aphasia, 2% had a less severe apraxia of speech, and 10% had less severe nonaphasic cognitive impairments. It thus appears that *when UUMN dysarthria is the primary communication deficit, aphasia, apraxia of speech, and nonaphasic communication deficits are not frequently present.* The prevalence of UUMN dysarthria when aphasia or nonaphasic cognitive deficits are more prominent than the dysarthria is unknown, but it is likely to be more prevalent than when UUMN dysarthria is the primary diagnosis, at least in patients with accompanying unilateral limb motor deficits. The occurrence of UUMN dysarthria in people with apraxia of speech is addressed in Chapter 11.

Patient Perceptions and Complaints

People with UUMN dysarthria are usually aware of their speech difficulty. They may minimize its effects, however, especially when intelligibility is preserved. When the etiology is stroke, by the time they are seen for formal speech assessment in the acute setting, they are sometimes more impressed with the improvement they have made than the degree of deficit that remains. When the dysarthria is more severe, they may express distress over its effect on intelligibility or efficiency of communication. They often describe their speech as *slurred, thick,* or *slow.* As with most other dysarthria types, patients tend to complain that *speech deteriorates under conditions of fatigue or psychologic stress.*[*]

Patients frequently complain of *drooling* or a *heavy feeling* on the affected side of the face or corner of the mouth and sometimes of heaviness or thickness in the tongue, especially when speaking. *Chewing* and *swallowing difficulty* are not unusual,[29] especially early after onset. Many complain of *drooling* from the affected side of the mouth. Although less frequent than in people with bilateral UMN lesions and spastic dysarthria, some patients complain of and exhibit *pseudobulbar crying* or *laughter.*[5] Patients with clinically apparent aphasia or apraxia of speech often do not complain of their dysarthria because the language or motor programming deficits overwhelm its functional effects.

Clinical Findings

The lesions leading to UUMN dysarthria usually produce a constellation of physical signs and symptoms on the side of the body contralateral to the lesion (see Box 9-1). For example, 79% of Duffy and Folger's patients had hemiplegia or hemiparesis, and 20% had sensory deficits (Box 9-3). Language and other cognitive disturbances may be present and can and often do have a greater impact on spoken communication than the dysarthria. When aphasia results from left subcortical lesions, an accompanying dysarthria is frequently present.[17,55]

---

[*]Brodal,[10] an anatomist, and Aronson,[5] a speech pathologist, made observations following their own right hemisphere strokes that provide sophisticated testimonial support for many common patient complaints. Brodal spoke of feelings of decreased force of innervation and problems with skilled movements, as if they were no longer automatic, requiring increased volitional energy to generate movement. Even 6 months after his stroke, he felt that his speech deteriorated under conditions of fatigue. Aronson spoke of his "emotional incontinence" and its similarities and differences from normal crying and laughter. He also described his sense of a spastic voice, with an accompanying feeling of overpressure in the thorax and abdomen, and its exacerbation by stress and fatigue.

---

box 9-3

Primary oral mechanism, clinical neurologic findings, and confirmed or presumed lesion locus for 56 cases with a primary speech diagnosis of UUMN dysarthria.[21] Percentage of cases is given in parentheses.

Oral Mechanism Findings

Unilateral lower facial weakness (82%)
Unilateral lingual weakness (52%)
Unilateral palatal weakness (5%)

Clinical Neurologic Findings

Hemiplegia/hemiparesis (79%)
Sensory deficits (20%)
Dysarthria and clumsy hand only (13%)
Dysarthria and bulbar weakness only (lower face or tongue) (5%)

Lesion Locus*

Internal capsule (34%)
Internal capsule or pons (4%)
Pericapsular (11%)
Lobar, cortical, and subcortical (nearly always including frontal lobe) (27%)
Lobar, cortical (always including frontal lobe) (7%)
Lobar, subcortical (always including frontal lobe) (7%)
Pericapsular, subcortical, and lobar (7%)
Brainstem (2%)
Thalamus and midbrain (2%)

UUMN, Unilateral upper motor neuron.
*Lobar—region affecting all or portions of a lobe in a cerebral hemisphere, divisible into cortical and subcortical subcategories when possible; pericapsular—region of the internal capsule plus adjacent structures projecting to or from the cerebral cortex, including the corona radiata.

Thirteen percent of Duffy and Folger's patients had dysarthria and a clumsy hand only, and 5% had dysarthria and face and tongue weakness as their only neurologic abnormality (see preceding discussion of related lacunar syndromes).

Nonspeech Oral Mechanism

Box 9-3 summarizes the primary oral mechanism findings in Duffy and Folger's patients. Unilateral central facial weakness was present in 82% of patients, a figure comparable to that reported in other studies.[*] This weakness is often apparent at rest and

---

[*]This is comparable to the 75% and 79% frequency of central facial weakness in large series of patients with unilateral stroke studied by Willoughby and Anderson[77] and Melo et al.,[46] respectively, and the 86% frequency of facial weakness in 14 dysarthric patients with single unilateral stroke prospectively studied by Hwang et al.[33] Melo et al.[46] reported that 93% of their dysarthric

during movement. If components of both the direct and indirect activation pathways are involved, weakness is apparent during voluntary and emotional facial movements. If the indirect pathway is relatively spared, emotional facial expression, such as smiling, may be relatively symmetric, reflecting the ability of the indirect pathway to drive emotional expression even when voluntary control is impaired. The converse can also occur. These disparities between voluntary and emotional facial expression are not unusual in UUMN dysarthria. In general, *unilateral central facial weakness seems to be a fairly good predictor of dysarthria in people with stroke.*

It is rare to find unilateral central lingual weakness in the absence of unilateral central facial weakness, and unilateral lingual weakness appears to be a good predictor of dysarthria and a fairly good predictor of dysphagia in people with acute stroke.* Unilateral lingual weakness was apparent in 52% of Duffy and Folger's patients.† It is most easily detected as deviation of the tongue to the weak side on protrusion. It can also be detected on attempts to lateralize the tongue, or on lateral strength testing. Difficulty turning or pushing the tongue to one side is occasionally detectable when tongue deviation on protrusion is not apparent.

The reason lingual weakness is observed less frequently than facial weakness may reflect individual variability in the degree to which the twelfth cranial nerve receives contralateral versus bilateral UMN innervation. This variability may also explain some of the variability in deviant speech characteristics among people with UUMN dysarthria.‡

---

patients had unilateral facial weakness. The frequency of unilateral facial weakness has been comparably high or higher in other (small N) prospective studies of patients with dysarthria and UUMN lesions that have made clinical observations of facial weakness.[28,36]

---

*For example, Umapathi et al.[70] found a 29% incidence of tongue deviation in 300 patients with acute stroke that did not include the lower brainstem (i.e., the weakness was central). All patients with tongue deviation also had a central facial weakness on the same side. Dysphagia occurred in 43% and dysarthria in 90% of those with tongue deviation.

---

†This is somewhat less than the 64% frequency of lingual weakness in 14 patients prospectively studied by Hwang et al.[33] Unilateral lingual weakness was also present frequently in the six patients studied by Hartman and Abbs.[28]

---

‡The existence of bilateral UMN input to the hypoglossal nerve, but with variability in degree among individuals, receives support from recent studies using motor-evoked potential and magnetic stimulation methods.[14,53] In addition, Umapathi et al.[70] noted that tongue deviation in people with acute unilateral stroke occurred more frequently in those with a history of prior stroke on the contralateral side, suggesting that bilateral involvement may be necessary to produce clinically obvious lingual weakness in some people.

The jaw is usually normal on clinical examination. For example, jaw weakness was not reported for any of the patients studied by Duffy and Folger or Hwang et al.[33] However, contralateral jaw weakness is occasionally apparent clinically,[9,77] usually as reduced ability to clench or deviation to the weak side on opening. It has also been demonstrated electrophysiologically.[15,28]

Velopharyngeal function has usually been assumed to be normal in UUMN lesions, but recent observations indicate this is not always the case. For example, Duffy and Folger observed palatal weakness (usually manifest as asymmetry at rest or during movement) in 5% and Hwang et al.[33] in 29% of their patients with UUMN strokes. Thompson and Murdoch[65] reported mildly impaired soft palate movement in three out of seven patients with a single unilateral stroke, and Kennedy and Murdoch[36] made similar observations in all four of their patients with unilateral subcortical stroke. Thus palatal asymmetry is clinically apparent more often than predicted by the presumed protective redundancy of bilateral UMN neuron supply to the vagus nerve.

Vocal fold weakness has also been assumed to be rare or nonexistent, but an assumption that bilateral UMN supply to the vagus nerve invariably spares laryngeal functions in UUMN lesions is questionable. For example, Bogousslasky and Regli[9] reported hypotonia and decreased movement of the vocal fold contralateral to an internal capsule lesion in one patient. More convincingly, in a study of patients within 48 hours after a first-ever ischemic stroke, 11% of 35 patients with a lacunar stroke in the internal capsule, corona radiata, or paramedian pons, and 16% of 12 patients with cortical or large subcortical stroke had evidence of contralateral vocal fold paresis on flexible endoscopic examination. All patients with dysphonia had vocal fold weakness, and several also had palatal weakness. The weakness resolved in a majority of patients within 1 month. The authors concluded, "the long-held belief of the invariable bilateral innervation of the nucleus ambiguous may be incorrect."[75] It thus appears that *a minority but not insignificant percentage of patients with UUMN lesions can have contralateral vocal fold weakness.* These are important observations because they help to explain at least some of the deviant voice characteristics that can occur in UUMN dysarthria (described in the next section).

It has been well documented that dysphagia, as well as audible or silent aspiration, can occur with UUMN lesions.[9,29,30,45] Similar to the dysarthria, these problems are often mild and recovery is good.

Motor impersistence may be apparent during oral mechanism examination, especially in patients with right hemisphere lesions. Motor impersistence is discussed in Chapter 3.

Deviant speech characteristics observed in 2 or more of 56 cases with a primary speech diagnosis of UUMN dysarthria (modified from Duffy and Folger[21]). Percentage of cases exhibiting each characteristic is given in parentheses. Confirmatory observations from other studies* are referenced, and observations from those studies not noted by Duffy and Folger and usually noted in only one or a few patients are listed under *"Other characteristics."*

Articulation (98%)

Imprecise consonants (95%)[7,28,33,36,61,66-68]
Irregular articulatory breakdowns (14%)[33]
Imprecise consonants and irregular articulatory breakdowns (11%)
Other characteristics: vowel distortions

Speech AMRs (91%)

Slow (72%)[28,33,38,61]
Imprecise (33%)
Irregular (33%)[28,33,38]
Two or more of above (50%)

Phonation (57%)

Harshness (39%)[7,33,54,61,68]
Reduced loudness (9%)[7,33,61,68]
Strained-harshness (5%)[33,54,68]
Wet hoarseness (4%)[33,54,68]
Breathiness (4%)[33,54]

Monopitch (4%)[33,68]
Monoloudness (4%)[33]
"Unsteady" voice (4%)[33]
Two or more of the above (13%)
Other characteristics: high pitch, low pitch, glottal fry, pitch breaks, increased loudness, loudness decay, reduced maximum vowel duration

Rate and Prosody (23%)

Slow rate (18%)[7,28,33,68]
Increased rate in segments (4%)
Excess and equal stress (4%)
Two or more of above (4%)
Other characteristics: variable rate, short phrases, reduced stress, excess loudness variations

Resonance (14%)

Hypernasality, nasal emission, or both (14%)[7,33,36,65]
Other characteristics: hyponasality

AMRs, Alternate motion rates; *UUMN,* unilateral upper motor neuron.
*Benke and Kertesz studied 35 patients with left hemisphere lesions and 35 patients with right hemisphere lesions and speech deficits (their observations of dysarthria are confounded by the presence of apraxia of speech and aphasia, and perhaps "aprosodia," in some patients). Hartman and Abbs[28] studied six patients with UUMN lesions and dysarthria. Hwang et al.[33] described the dysarthria in 14 patients with a single, unilateral stroke. Kennedy and Murdoch[36] described the speech and language disorders in four patients with left hemisphere subcortical stroke. Ropper[61] described 10 patients with severe dysarthria resulting from right hemisphere lesions. Thompson and Murdoch[65] studied disorders of nasality in seven dysarthric patients (among others) with single, unilateral stroke. Thompson, Murdoch, and Stokes[66] studied lip function in eight dysarthric patients (among others) with single, unilateral stroke. Thompson, Murdoch, and Theodoros[68] studied the perceptual and physiologic attributes of four dysarthric patients (among five patients) with single, unilateral stroke.

Speech

The speech characteristics of UUMN dysarthria, as identified by Duffy and Folger, are summarized in Box 9-4. Confirmatory observations from studies that have provided more than vague descriptions of speech are also referenced. Some speech characteristics noted in those studies but not noted by Duffy and Folger are also listed.

The most pervasive deficit, present in 98% of the patients, was *imprecise consonants.* A smaller percentage of patients had *irregular articulatory breakdowns* in contextual speech, and approximately one third had *irregular alternate motion rates (AMRs).* *Imprecise AMRs* were also apparent in one third of patients. When severity of these characteristics was noted, it was usually rated as mild, although some patients had moderate to marked imprecision. Imprecise articulation is often attributed to the unilateral lower facial and tongue weakness that is apparent in many patients.

Irregular articulatory breakdowns and irregular AMRs are usually associated with ataxic dysarthria.* The reasons for their presence in UUMN dysarthria are not entirely clear. They could reflect clumsiness that occurs as a normal byproduct of weakness[43] or because of imbalance of muscle forces in midline structures (jaw, tongue) or structures that move asynchronously (right and left face) when unilateral weakness is present. They could also reflect *ataxic-like incoordination* resulting from damage to cerebellocortical fibers that intermingle with UMN fibers in white matter pathways.† Regardless of the reason

---

*It is interesting in this regard that Ropper's[61] description of dysarthria in patients with right hemisphere lesions noted that "the overall pattern had some resemblance to the speech of an intoxicated individual."

†The internal capsule and white matter pathways between the thalamus and cortex, for example, contain cerebellocortical and proprioceptive pathways that might, when damaged, contribute to

for such irregularities, these clinical observations indicate that *some patients with UUMN lesions and dysarthria can exhibit perceptual speech attributes that are ataxic.*

The second most prominent deviant feature was *slow AMRs,* which were usually mildly slowed. Such slowness was not as striking in contextual speech, where it was noted in only 18% of patients. The reasons for slowness are not entirely clear, but weakness, compensatory efforts to maintain precision and regularity, and spasticity are possible explanations. These clinical observations suggest that *some patients with UUMN lesions and dysarthria can exhibit perceptual speech attributes that are spastic.*

Somewhat surprisingly, 57% of patients had phonatory abnormalities, 39% with a mild to moderate dysphonia that was described as *harsh* or, less frequently, *strained to harsh.* Nine percent of the patients had *reduced loudness,* possibly also reflecting phonatory or respiratory-phonatory dysfunction. In addition, several characteristics noted in other studies (see Box 9-4) are suggestive of phonatory dysfunction. These findings are surprising in light of the common assumption that the vocal folds are spared from deficits because the tenth nerve receives bilateral UMN input.* The observation nonetheless suggests several possible explanations, none of which are mutually exclusive, including (1) unilateral vocal fold weakness; (2) spasticity[†]; (3) age-related dysphonia, because the elderly are the most

frequent victims of stroke and (4) other factors unrelated to the specific effects of UUMN lesions on speech (e.g., the general effects of illness or inactivity). Relative to the first possibility, vocal fold weakness in some patients with UUMN lesions has been documented (see discussion in the previous section). Similar mechanisms could also contribute to spasticity. It is reasonable to assume that the dysphonia in at least some people with UUMN dysarthria is neurologic in origin, and that many of the observed perceptual attributes can be linked to laryngeal hypofunction or hyperfunction. It thus appears that *some or many of the phonatory abnormalities in at least some people with UUMN dysarthria reflect weakness, spasticity, or both.*

Mild *hypernasality* or *nasal emission* was present in 11% of patients and has been observed in several other studies, again somewhat surprising in light of the presumed bilateral UMN supply to cranial nerve X. The reasons for its occurrence are probably similar to those offered in the previous paragraph for the occurrence of dysphonia.

Rate and prosodic abnormalities were present in 23% of patients, and most often were reflected in mildly *slowed rate.* Other prosodic abnormalities were uncommon, but they did encompass features tied to rate, loudness, pitch, and duration. The presence of irregular articulatory breakdowns almost certainly altered prosody in some patients.

Table 9-1 summarizes the primary clinical speech characteristics and common oral mechanism exami-

---

ataxic-like movements. Attig[6] and Mori et al.[51] have suggested that limb ataxia induced by capsular or corona radiata lesions may reflect disruption of cerebellocortical or thalamocortical projections. Brodal[10] stated: "it is extremely likely that the interruption of pathways other than the direct corticobulbar pathways is of importance . . . the cerebrocerebellar pathways are presumably important and involved in achieving smooth movements."

---

*Metter's[48] clinical description of UUMN dysarthria included breathiness, hypophonia, and sometimes reduced loudness. Reduced loudness, breathiness, and hoarseness have also been noted in studies of aphasia resulting from unilateral subcortical lesions (e.g., Alexander and LoVerme[2]; Damasio, Eslinger, and Adams[16]; Damasio et al[17]; Metter et al.[49]). The lesions in these studies usually included the basal ganglia, thalamus, and internal capsule or corona radiata.

Dysphonia may be an important marker of dysphagia for patients with UUMN lesions. For example, Horner and Massey[29] found dysphonia in 91% of their aspirating patients with UUMN lesions. Dysphonia was less frequently present in nonaspirating patients.

[†]The possibility of an undetected lesion or lesions in the contralateral hemisphere in some cases cannot be excluded. It has also been shown that cerebral blood flow can be diminished in the hemisphere contralateral to a unilateral stroke.[20] This evidence of "transhemispheric diaschisis" might explain the presence of a strained to harsh voice quality in some people with UUMN lesions, especially early after onset.

---

table 9-1	Primary clinical speech and speech-related findings in UUMN dysarthria
Perceptual	
Articulation & prosody	Imprecise articulation
	Irregular articulatory breakdowns
	Slow rate
	Slow AMRs
	Imprecise AMRs
	Irregular AMRs
Phonation	Harshness
	Decreased loudness
Resonance	Hypernasality (infrequent)
Physical	Unilateral lower facial weakness
	Unilateral lingual weakness
Patient Complaints	Slurred speech/difficulty with pronunciation
	Drooping lower face/"heavy" lower face
	"Thick" or heavy tongue
	Drooling
	Dysphagia (relatively mild)
	May not complain of dysarthria if aphasia predominates

AMRs, Alternate motion rates; *UUMN,* unilateral upper motor neuron.

nation findings and patient complaints encountered in UUMN dysarthria.

Acoustic and Physiologic Findings

Acoustic and physiologic studies of patients with UUMN dysarthria are limited. In recent years, however, several such studies have been helpful in establishing the nature of speech subsystem impairment and, in combination with perceptual assessment, they have contributed to treatment planning.[68] The results of these studies are summarized in Table 9-2.

table 9-2	Summary of acoustic and physiologic findings in studies of UUMN dysarthria*
Speech Component	**Acoustic or Physiologic Observation**
Respiratory	Reduced respiratory drive/weakness
Laryngeal	Unilateral vocal fold weakness
	Decreased:
	Glottal airflow
	Laryngeal airway resistance
	Rate of adduction/abduction
	f_o variation
	Increased:
	Glottal airflow
	Laryngeal airway resistance
	f_o variation
	Jitter
	Shimmer
Velopharyngeal	Increased nasal airflow
Articulatory/Rate/ Prosody	Reduced:
	Speech rate
	AMR rates
	Force of contralateral jaw movement
	Strength, endurance, & speed of lip & tongue movement
	Increased:
	Syllable & intersyllable gap duration & variability
	Variability of minimum & maximum waveform amplitude envelopes
	Acoustic energy during stop gap of voiceless consonants (spirantization)
	Irregular AMRs

*AMRs, Alternate motion rates; UUMN, unilateral upper motor neuron. *Note that many of these observations are based on studies of only one or a few speakers, and that not all speakers with UUMN dysarthria exhibit all of these features. Note also that these characteristics may not be unique to UUMN dysarthria; several can be observed in other motor speech disorders or nonneurologic conditions.

Respiration

There is little information about respiration during speech. It is usually assumed that respiratory muscles are under bilateral UMN control and thus not significantly influenced by unilateral lesions. However, Przedborski et al.[60] established with electromyogram (EMG) recordings that most of their 25 patients with flaccid hemiplegia within 12 hours of a unilateral hemispheric stroke had abnormal neural respiratory drive of the contralateral parasternal intercostal muscles. It was not clear if their subjects were dysarthric. The data suggest that the parasternal intercostal muscles and diaphragm are predominantly under the control of contralateral corticospinal pathways in many people.

In a spirometric and kinematic study of two dysarthric patients (among others) with a single unilateral stroke, Thompson, Murdoch, and Theodoros[68] found that both patients had general respiratory impairment and one had impaired respiratory function for speech. Thus the limited data suggest that nonspeech respiratory functions can be affected in at least some patients with UUMN lesions and respiratory functions for speech can also be affected. Although clinical observation suggests that respiratory weakness is not usually of major consequence for speech, when unilateral respiratory weakness is present it could possibly contribute to the short phrases, reduced loudness, loudness decay, and reduced maximum vowel duration that are perceived in some patients.

Laryngeal Function

Endoscopic documentation of vocal fold weakness following unilateral stroke in some patients has already been discussed. Several acoustic and other instrumental measures also support a conclusion that laryngeal function can be abnormal. Similar to perceptual judgments, these findings by no means apply to all people with UUMN dysarthria; substantial variability within and among patient samples has been noted.[37]

Acoustic analyses have documented both reduced and increased fundamental frequency (f_o) variation, as well as abnormalities on several amplitude (e.g., shimmer) and frequency (e.g., jitter) perturbation measures.[11,37,39] Such abnormalities suggest laryngeal subsystem impairment. At least some of these abnormalities could reflect functional differences between the two vocal folds. For example, hoarseness, as reflected in the acoustic measure of jitter, could reflect asymmetric laryngeal hypotonia leading to differences between the vocal folds in overall tension or vibrating mass, with subsequent irregular vocal fold oscillation.[1]

Aerodynamic and electroglottographic measures of laryngeal function during speech have documented abnormalities in a small number of patients with unilateral stroke and dysarthria.[68] The dynamics of abnormal laryngeal movement and airflow seem to vary among patients, sometimes suggesting weakness and sometimes suggesting hypertonicity. For example, Murdoch, Thompson, and Stokes[54] found that half of their 10 patients with dysarthria from UUMN stroke had instrumental findings suggestive of laryngeal hyperfunction, including elevated laryngeal airway resistance and subglottal air pressure, reduced laryngeal airflow, and a slower rate of adduction/abduction (the perceptual correlates of such findings would be harshness and strained voice quality). The remaining half had nearly opposite instrumental findings suggestive of laryngeal hypofunction (the perceptual correlates of such findings would be hoarseness, glottal fry, and breathiness). The authors concluded that differences between the hyperfunctional and hypofunctional subgroups could reflect differences in lesion site or compensation. For example, the instrumental evidence for hypofunction in some cases might have been attributable to increased stiffness/hypertonus preventing vocal fold approximation versus compensation for hyperadduction of the vocal folds. Although the explanation for these findings is not entirely clear, it does provide some support for perceptual voice attributes suggestive of weakness in some cases and spasticity in others.

Velopharyngeal Function

Observations that hypernasality is present only in a minority of people with UUMN dysarthria may explain why there has been only a single study of velopharyngeal function. Thompson and Murdoch[65] used nasal accelerometry and perceptual ratings to study velopharyngeal functions for speech in seven patients (among others) who had dysarthria from a single, unilateral stroke. Two of the seven patients were judged perceptually as hypernasal, and two of the seven had abnormally high nasal accelerometric indices, but for only one patient did both the perceptual and accelerometric indices identify velopharyngeal inadequacy/weakness. These findings agree with other perceptual observations of a relatively low frequency of perceived hypernasality in UUMN dysarthria. They also highlight the frequent incongruities between the results of perceptual and instrumental measures of velopharyngeal function for speech.

Articulation, Rate, and Prosody

Acoustic and physiologic measures of articulation and rate have established that at least some patients have weakness of the articulators contralateral to the side of lesion. Other patients have characteristics suggestive of spasticity or ataxia.

EMG and various other measures of strength, force, and endurance in people with UUMN lesions and dysarthria have demonstrated reduced magnitude of EMG signals and force of movement in the contralateral jaw, as well as reduced strength, endurance, and speed of lip and tongue movements.[28,66-68] Although Thompson, Murdoch, and Stokes felt that the apparent lingual weakness in their patients could represent spasticity, they did not find evidence of lingual hypertonicity. They suggested that UMN weakness could account for reduced weakness and speed of lingual movement because reduced strength reduces the maximum shortening velocity of muscle fibers, with a subsequent reduction in speed of movement. Their results also suggest that fatigue contributes to lingual problems, consistent with frequent patient complaints that speech deteriorates with increased speaking time or general fatigue. It should be noted that their findings for lip and tongue strength, endurance, and speed did not correlate with perceptual measures of intelligibility, articulatory precision, or length of phonemes, leading them to suggest that measures of fine force control may be more relevant to perceptual measures. Nonetheless, these findings of reduced force and endurance are generally supportive of clinical observations of lower facial weakness in many patients and the presence of unilateral jaw weakness in some.

Acoustic measures have documented slow reading rate and slow and sometimes irregular AMRs,[28,37,38] although Kent and Kent[37] note that the slow AMRs are generally not as slow as in ataxic dysarthria. Hartman and Abbs[28] found that slow AMRs were matched by perceptual ratings of AMRs, but that irregular AMRs were not perceived in their patients; irregular AMRs were perceived in some of Duffy and Folger's patients, however.

Kent et al.[38] examined AMRs in depth and found that syllable and intersyllable gap durations were lengthened and more variable than normal, that variability tended to increase as syllable duration increased, and that maximum and minimum waveform amplitude envelopes were more variable than normal. There was also evidence of acoustic energy during the stop gap of voiceless stops, a reflection of incomplete articulatory closure or spirantization, a correlate of perceived articulatory imprecision.

■ THE DISTINCTIVENESS OF UNILATERAL UPPER MOTOR NEURON DYSARTHRIA: CONCLUSIONS AND CLINICAL SUGGESTIONS

What features of UUMN dysarthria help distinguish it from other MSDs? If one attends to auditory-perceptual attributes alone, there do not appear to be any clear distinguishing features. Its most common deviant speech characteristics are not unique relative to other dysarthria types, and some are distinguishing features of other types. However, *if the speech characteristics are viewed in the context of their relative severity and other clinical findings, a cluster of distinguishing features emerges.* That is, UUMN dysarthria may best be distinguished from other dysarthria types by its common association with *unilateral central face and tongue weakness;* its predominant *stroke etiology;* its nearly-always-present but rarely-worse-than-moderate *articulatory imprecision;* and sometimes mild *irregular articulatory breakdowns, slow rate, slow and sometimes irregular AMRs, harsh, strained or hoarse-breathy dysphonia,* and *reduced loudness.* The gestalt impression from its auditory perceptual characteristics is therefore variable but most often suggestive of mild or moderate UMN weakness, sometimes spasticity or incoordination (ataxia), or sometimes various combinations of them. Indeed, studies of the dysarthria in people with UUMN lesions, while usually describing the dysarthria as UUMN in type, have sometimes labeled or at least noted its similarity to flaccid, spastic, ataxic, or mixed dysarthria.[28,33,36,38,68]

It thus appears that a confident clinical diagnosis of UUMN dysarthria is probably best made on the basis of its auditory-perceptual features plus "the company it keeps," such as oral mechanism findings, other neurologic deficits, history, and neuroimaging results. To some extent this is how a confident clinical diagnosis of any dysarthria type is often made, but *reliance on confirmatory signs and other clinical clues is probably necessary more frequently for UUMN dysarthria than other dysarthria types.*

That a diagnosis of UUMN dysarthria is not always possible on the basis of speech features alone is not satisfying to the diagnostic purist, but the reasons this is the case *do* have a logical basis in what we know about the functions of commonly damaged structures. The reasons include the following:

1. Many patients with UUMN lesions have speech characteristics suggestive of weakness because damage to the direct activation pathways produces weakness that most often includes the face and tongue; sometimes the larynx; and less frequently the velopharynx, jaw, and respiration.

2. Some patients (perhaps fewer than those with weakness only) with UUMN lesions have speech characteristics suggestive of spasticity for several possible reasons, including (a) significant damage to the indirect activation pathway and its role in tone, reflexes, and posture; (b) individual variability in the degree to which unilateral UMN lesions have bilateral effects on speech cranial nerves* or the degree to which UMNs to speech cranial nerves are crossed and uncrossed; and (c) effects of altered blood flow to the contralateral hemisphere following stroke or the presence of undetected lesions in the contralateral hemisphere. If all of these explanations are valid, they suggest that speech features suggestive of spasticity sometimes result from the effects of a UUMN lesion alone on contralateral side muscles, the effects of the UUMN lesion alone on contralateral and ipsilateral side muscles, or the combined effects of the UUMN lesion plus influences (e.g., from lesions, altered blood flow/metabolism) of abnormalities on the "unaffected" side of the brain.

3. Some patients (perhaps fewer than those with weakness alone) with UUMN lesions have speech characteristics suggestive of ataxia possibly because of (a) damage to afferent cerebellocortical and proprioceptive tracts (e.g., in the internal capsule), or efferent frontopontocerebellar tracts,† resulting in uncoordinated speech movements, much like damage to such pathways can lead to ataxia in the limbs; or (b) clumsiness that occurs as a byproduct of weakness or imbalance of muscle forces in midline structures (jaw, tongue) or structures that move asynchronously

---

*In a transcranial magnetic stimulation (with CT and magnetic resonance imaging [MRI]) study of patients with dysarthria due to stroke in the lower motor cortex, corona radiata, and genu or posterior limb of the internal capsule, Urban et al.[72] concluded that the effect of stimulation was absent or delayed bilaterally in 17 of their 18 patients.

†Ataxia has been described with lesions in the frontal lobes, presumably attributable to interruption of the frontopontocerebellar tracts. Dysarthria has been reported with such lesions, but its characteristics have not been described well.[64] Moulin et al.,[52] in a study of 100 patients with lacunar infarcts and ataxic hemiparesis and dysmetria, found facial weakness in 60% of patients with pontine lesions, 50% with corona radiata lesions, and 40% with thalamic lesions. Dysarthria was also present with lesions in the internal capsule, pons, thalamus, corona radiata, lentiform nucleus, and cerebellum. Unfortunately, the characteristics of the dysarthria were not described, but the association of dysarthria with apparent ataxia and dysmetria in the limbs suggests that ataxic speech features could be associated with such lesions.

(right and left face) when unilateral weakness is present.

How might a clinician discuss a diagnosis of UUMN dysarthria, knowing that its perceptual characteristics may reflect weakness, spasticity, incoordination, or various combinations of them? When confident that the speech features, confirmatory signs, and clinical context are compatible with the diagnosis, the following may help frame diagnostic statements:

1. When the speech characteristics are all consistent with what can be explained by weakness, using the designation *"UUMN dysarthria with speech features consistent with (right or left side) UMN weakness,"* or, more concisely, *"UUMN dysarthria, flaccid variant,"* seems to convey information about general lesion locus and presumed pathophysiology.

2. When speech characteristics are suggestive of spasticity, using the designation *"UUMN dysarthria with predominant speech features suggestive of hypertonicity,"* or, more concisely, *"UUMN dysarthria, spastic variant,"* conveys information about general lesion locus (and implies that the lesion need not be bilateral, as is usually assumed for spastic dysarthria) and presumed pathophysiology.

3. When speech characteristics are suggestive of ataxia, using the designation *"UUMN dysarthria with predominant speech features suggestive of incoordination,"* or, more concisely, *"UUMN dysarthria, ataxic variant,"* conveys information about general

lesion locus (and implies that the lesion need not be in the cerebellum, as is often assumed for ataxic dysarthria) and presumed pathophysiology.

4. When features of two or more characteristics are present, the designations can be combined (e.g., *"UUMN dysarthria with speech features consistent with weakness and incoordination"* or *"UUMN dysarthria, mixed [specify] variant"*).

In the author's experience, the most frequent designations are likely to be the first or fourth.

It is not uncommon that confidence about the diagnosis of UUMN is low. This is most often the case when the dysarthria is relatively severe and contains features suggestive of spasticity, ataxia, or both that are marked in severity, even when confirmatory signs and other clinical evidence suggest only a UUMN lesion. It is best under these circumstances to highlight the ambiguity with statements such as "although the patient's dysarthria could be explained by a UUMN lesion, the degree of spastic speech characteristics in this case is unusual for unilateral lesions and raises the possibility of bilateral damage," or "although speech characteristics suggestive of ataxia can be present with UUMN lesions, the degree of ataxic characteristics in this case is more commonly encountered with cerebellar lesions." These qualified diagnostic conclusions are most important when lesion site is uncertain or when there are few other lateralizing signs. The ability to draw these confident or qualified conclusions probably requires considerable clinical experience.

Cases

Case 9-1

A 55-year-old right-handed man was admitted to the hospital with a 4-day history of progressive right hemiparesis and dysarthria. Neurologic evaluation revealed dysarthria, right hemiparesis, and mild sensory loss in the right face and upper limb. CT scan showed evidence of an infarct in the posterior limb of the left internal capsule.

Speech evaluation $2\frac{1}{2}$ weeks after onset revealed a right central facial weakness. Speech was characterized by imprecise articulation (2,3), harsh voice quality (0,1), and slow speech AMRs (−1,2). Intelligibility was moderately reduced. There was no evidence of aphasia or any other cognitive disturbance.

The clinician concluded the patient had a UUMN dysarthria. The patient was seen for only one session of speech therapy before his discharge from the hospital. He did not return for follow-up.

Commentary. (1) UUMN dysarthria commonly affects articulation and sometimes voice quality and frequently seems predominantly explained by CNS weakness. (2) It can be associated with moderate reductions of speech intelligibility. (3) The internal capsule is a common site for lesions that cause UUMN dysarthria. Isolated internal capsule lesions in the dominant hemisphere are rarely, if ever, associated with aphasic language impairment or other cognitive disturbances.

Case 9-2

A 70-year-old right-handed man was hospitalized because of a sudden onset of inability to express himself, a right facial droop, and weakness in his right upper extremity. History and clinical evaluation were consistent with a middle cerebral artery stroke. CT scan identified an area of decreased attenuation in the left frontal lobe consistent with recent infarction.

Speech and language evaluation 3 days after onset revealed a mild to moderate aphasia with deficits apparent in verbal formulation and comprehension, as well as reading and writing. Verbal communication, however, was functional. Right facial and tongue weakness was apparent. There was no evidence of apraxia of speech. The patient's speech was characterized by imprecise articulation (1), reduced loudness (0,1), and hoarseness (1,2). Speech intelligibility was normal. The patient began speech-language therapy. Within 1 week his dysarthria had resolved, and the only evidence of aphasia was infrequent word-finding difficulties.

Commentary. (1) UUMN dysarthria associated with dominant hemisphere lesions is frequently associated with aphasia. In this case, the dysarthria and aphasia were approximately equal in severity at onset. (2) UUMN dysarthria frequently resolves rapidly and completely (in this case, within 1 week after onset). (3) The frontal lobe is most often implicated when UUMN dysarthria is the result of a cortical lesion.

Case 9-3

A 73-year-old right-handed man was admitted to the hospital with a 1-day history of slurred speech and difficulty using his right hand. Neurologic examination demonstrated only dysarthria and mild right upper extremity weakness and clumsiness. The neurologist felt that the patient's presentation was consistent with a "dysarthria–clumsy hand syndrome." Subsequent CT scan demonstrated a lacunar infarct in the area of the left lateral basal ganglia and centrum semiovale.

Speech examination the following day identified mild right lower central facial weakness and mild deviation of the tongue to the right on protrusion. Speech was characterized by breathy-hoarse voice quality (0,1), reduced loudness (−1,2), irregular articulatory breakdowns (2), monopitch and loudness (1,2), and equivocal acceleration of speech rate. Speech AMRs were normal in rate but imprecise (1,2) and irregular (2). Speech intelligibility was moderately reduced. There was no evidence of aphasia or apraxia of speech.

The clinician concluded that the patient had "a moderately severe UUMN dysarthria." Speech therapy was recommended, and improvement in speech was noted before discharge several days later.

Commentary. (1) UUMN dysarthria can be the only or among only a few signs of unilateral neurologic disease. (2) UUMN dysarthria is often associated with subcortical lesions.

Case 9-4

A 57-year-old man was seen in the clinic for evaluation of residual symptoms stemming from a stroke approximately 3 years earlier. Neurologic examination revealed dysarthria and left hemiparesis. The neurologist concluded that the patient had a "pure motor hemiparesis, almost like a capsular infarct."

Speech evaluation revealed mild left lower face and tongue weakness. Imprecise articulation and imprecise AMRs (1) characterized speech. Articulatory precision improved noticeably with a moderate slowing of speech rate. Phonation and resonance were normal.

The clinician concluded that the patient demonstrated a "mild UUMN dysarthria." Some time was spent demonstrating to the patient the advantages of slowing his speech rate. He appreciated the benefits of this speaking strategy but did not believe speech therapy was necessary. The clinician agreed.

Commentary. (1) UUMN dysarthria can result from lesions on the right or left side of the brain. (2) It can persist long after the spontaneous recovery period. (3) Persistent UUMN dysarthria is often mild, and clinicians and patients frequently feel that therapy is unnecessary.

Case 9-5

An 81-year-old right-handed man was admitted to the hospital with a 2-day history of "garbled speech" and left facial weakness. Neurologic examination revealed left facial weakness and mild left upper extremity weakness. A CT scan 1 week after onset revealed a lesion in the right posterior frontal lobe that was consistent with a recent stroke. A complete neurologic workup led to a right carotid endarterectomy 2 weeks later, without any deterioration in neurologic status.

Speech evaluation 12 days after surgery demonstrated a left central facial weakness (2,3) and deviation of the tongue to the left on protrusion. The patient wore loose-fitting dentures. Speech was characterized by hoarse-rough voice quality (2), imprecise articulation (1), occasional acceleration of speech rate (1,2), and slowed and imprecise AMRs (0,1). Speech intelligibility was, at worst, mildly reduced. The patient believed that his speech was quite adequate and did not want speech therapy. His wife and daughter felt that his speech was almost back to the level before the stroke, and they had only occasional mild difficulty understanding him. Although the clinician felt that therapy might be beneficial, the patient chose not to pursue it.

Commentary. (1) UUMN dysarthria can affect voice quality as well as articulation. (2) The effects of dysarthria on intelligibility can be exacerbated by non-neurologic factors, such as loose-fitting dentures. Problems with dentures frequently become more pronounced after a stroke that affects oromotor function, and they can present additional barriers to adequate articulation. (3) Recommendations for speech therapy must consider patient needs and wishes as well as the clinician's judgment about the possible benefits of therapy.

Case 9-6

A 66-year-old right-handed man with a 20-year history of hypertension was admitted to the hospital after the sudden onset of right hemiplegia, right facial weakness, and inability to speak. A CT scan 3 weeks after onset showed an area of low attenuation in the left centrum semiovale that extended down into the adjacent lentiform nucleus, consistent with stroke.

Language examination 3 weeks after onset was normal. The patient had a right lower facial weakness. Tongue protrusion was midline, but lateral movements were mildly slowed. Voice quality was harsh-breathy (1). Articulation was imprecise (1). In addition, the patient occasionally repeated the first phoneme of a word and was mildly hesitant, but there were no obvious trial-and-error misarticulations or clear-cut substitutions of sounds.

The clinician concluded that the patient had a "flaccid UUMN dysarthria." The possibility of an accompanying apraxia of speech was considered, but evidence for it was considered equivocal. The patient received four sessions of speech therapy that focused on improving articulation through increased self-monitoring and slowing of rate. He improved and asked that therapy be terminated so that he could devote more time to physical therapy.

Commentary. (1) UUMN dysarthria is often associated with subcortical lesions. (2) When the lesion is in the presumed dominant hemisphere, questions about the presence of aphasia and apraxia of speech often arise. There was no evidence of aphasia in this patient, but he did exhibit a few speech characteristics that were suggestive of apraxia of speech. Although it was concluded that apraxia of speech was not present, this case illustrates the difficulty that may be encountered in distinguishing between dysarthria and apraxia of speech. (3) Improvement in speech is usually noted in patients with UUMN dysarthria. It is not unusual for patients to terminate therapy on their own once speech becomes intelligible and sufficiently efficient. Evidence of dysarthria may persist, however.

SUMMARY

1. UUMN dysarthria results from unilateral damage to UMN pathways. It occurs at a frequency comparable to that of other major single dysarthria types. It is most often apparent in articulation, phonation, and prosody. Its deviant characteristics usually reflect the effects of weakness on speech, but sometimes spasticity and incoordination are implicated.

2. The anatomic designation of this dysarthria type is based on the locus of lesions associated with it. The fact that its clinical characteristics and pathophysiologic underpinnings are variable and not well understood precludes a single

pathophysiologic designation for the disorder at this time. It is possible, however, that its deviant characteristics reflect the effects of weakness and sometimes spasticity or incoordination on speech movements.

3. Stroke is by far the most common cause of UUMN dysarthria. Lesions on either side of the brain anywhere along the UMN pathways from the cortex to the brainstem can cause it, but lesions are probably most often in the cerebral hemispheres, usually in the posterior frontal lobe, internal capsule, or related white matter pathways.

4. Lower facial weakness and hemiparesis often accompany UUMN dysarthria. Contralateral lingual weakness is also common, and drooling and dysphagia may be present.

5. UUMN dysarthria is usually only mild to moderate in severity, and recovery from it is often quite good. However, it sometimes is marked in severity and can persist as a significant deficit beyond the period of spontaneous recovery.

6. The most common deviant speech characteristics are imprecise articulation and, less frequently, irregular articulatory breakdowns; slow rate; slow and sometimes irregular AMRs; harsh, strained, or hoarse-breathy dysphonia; and reduced loudness. Hypernasality occurs infrequently.

7. Physiologic studies have documented, with varying frequency, respiratory weakness, vocal fold weakness or hyperfunction, or both, with associated acoustic and aerodynamic abnormalities; velopharyngeal inadequacy; and reduced strength, endurance, or speed of jaw, lip, and tongue movements. Acoustic analyses have documented reduced speech rate and slow and irregular speech AMRs.

8. UUMN dysarthria can be the only or among the first and most prominent signs of neurologic disease. Its recognition and correlation with UUMN dysfunction can aid the localization and diagnosis of neurologic disease. Its specific diagnosis may require reliance on confirmatory clinical signs and clinical context more frequently than other dysarthria types because of the varying degree to which weakness and apparent spasticity or incoordination can be associated with it. Improved understanding of this dysarthria may assist efforts to study other speech and communication deficits that may be associated with unilateral neurologic disease, disorders whose manifestations may be masked or confounded by UUMN dysarthria.

References

1. Ackermann H, Ziegler W: Acoustic analysis of vocal instability in cerebellar dysfunctions, Ann Otol Rhinol Laryngol 103:98, 1994.

2. Alexander M, LoVerme S: Aphasia after left intracerebral hemorrhage, Neurology 30:1193, 1980.

3. Arboix JL, Martí-Vilata, García JH: Clinical study of 227 patients with lacunar infarcts, Stroke 21:842, 1990.

4. Arboix A et al: Isolated dysarthria, Stroke 22:531, 1991.

5. Aronson AE: Dysarthria, crying, and laughing in pseudobulbar palsy from right middle cerebral artery CVA: overview and personal account, J Med Speech-Lang Pathol 6:111, 1998.

6. Attig E: Parieto-cerebellar loop impairment in ataxic hemiparesis: proposed pathophysiology based on an analysis of cerebral blood flow. Can J Neurol Sci 21:15, 1994.

7. Benke T, Kertesz A: Hemispheric mechanisms of motor speech, Aphasiology 3:627, 1989.

8. Binkofsky F et al: Thalamic metabolism and corticospinal tract integrity determine motor recovery in stroke, Ann Neurol 39:460, 1996.

9. Bogousslavsky J, Regli F: Capsular genu syndrome, Neurology 40:1499, 1990.

10. Brodal A: Self-observations and neuro-anatomical considerations after a stroke, Brain 96:675, 1973.

11. Bunton K et al: The effects of flattening fundamental frequency contours on sentence intelligibility in speakers with dysarthria, Clin Linguist Phon 15:181, 2001.

12. Caplan LR et al: Caudate infarcts, Arch Neurol 47:133, 1990.

13. Chamorro A et al: Clinical-computed tomographic correlations of lacunar infarction in the Stroke Data Bank, Stroke 22:175, 1991.

14. Chen CH, Wu T, Chu NS: Bilateral cortical representation of the intrinsic lingual muscles, Neurology 52:411, 1999.

15. Cruccu G, Fornarelli M, Manfredi M: Impairment of masticatory function in hemiplegia, Neurology 38:301, 1988.

16. Damasio H, Eslinger P, Adams HP: Aphasia following basal ganglia lesions: new evidence, Semin Neurol 4:151, 1984.

17. Damasio AR et al: Aphasia with nonhemorrhagic lesions in the basal ganglia and internal capsule, Arch Neurol 39:15, 1982.

18. Darley FL, Aronson AE, Brown JR: Motor speech disorders, Philadelphia, 1975, WB Saunders.

19. DeJong RN: Case taking and the neurologic examination. In Baker AB, Joynt RJ, editors: Clinical neurology, vol 1, Philadelphia, 1986, Harper & Row.

20. Dobkin JA et al: Evidence for transhemispheric diaschisis in unilateral stroke, Arch Neurol 46:1333, 1989.

21. Duffy JR, Folger WN: Dysarthria associated with unilateral central nervous system lesions: a retrospective study, J Med Speech-Lang Pathol 4:57, 1996.

22. Fisher CM: Ataxic hemiparesis, Arch Neurol 35:126, 1978.

23. Fisher CM: Lacunar strokes and infarcts: a review, Neurology 32:871, 1982.

24. Fries W et al: Motor recovery following capsular stroke, Brain 116:369, 1993.

25. Fromm D et al: Various consequences of subcortical stroke: prospective study of 16 consecutive cases, Arch Neurol 42:943, 1985.

26. Giroud M et al: Unilateral lenticular infarcts: radiological and clinical syndromes, aetiology, and prognosis, J Neurol Neurosurg Psychiatry 63:611, 1997.

27. Glass JD, Levy AI, Rothstein JD: The dysarthria-clumsy hand syndrome: a distinct clinical entity related to pontine infarction, Ann Neurol 27:487, 1990.

28. Hartman DE, Abbs JH: Dysarthria associated with focal unilateral upper motor neuron lesion, Eur J Disord Commun 27:187, 1992.

29. Horner J, Massey W: Silent aspiration following stroke, Neurology 38:317, 1988.

30. Horner J et al: Aspiration following stroke: clinical correlates and outcome, Neurology 38:1359, 1988.

31. Huang C, Broe G: Isolated facial palsy: a new lacunar syndrome, J Neurol Neurosurg Psychiatry 47:84, 1984.

32. Huang CY, Lui FS: Ataxic-hemiparesis, localization and clinical features, Stroke 15:363, 1984.

33. Hwang M et al: Dysarthria associated with a single unilateral stroke, Paper presented at the American Speech-Language-Hearing Association convention, Washington, DC, November, 2000.

34. Ichikawa K, Kageyama Y: Clinical anatomic study of pure dysarthria, Stroke 22:809, 1991.

35. Kataoka S et al: Paramedian pontine infarction: neurological/topographical correlation, Stroke 28:809, 1997.

36. Kennedy M, Murdoch BE: Speech and language disorders subsequent to subcortical capsular lesions, Aphasiology 3:221, 1989.

37. Kent RD, Kent JF: Task-based profiles of the dysarthrias, Folia Phoniatr Logop 52:48, 2000.

38. Kent RD et al: Quantification of motor speech abilities in stroke: Time-energy analyses of syllable and word repetition, J Med Speech-Lang Pathol 7:83, 1999.

39. Kent RD et al: Voice dysfunction in dysarthria: application of the Multidimensional Voice Program, J Commun Disord 36:281, 2003.

40. Kim JS: Pure dysarthria, isolated facial paresis, or dysarthria-facial paresis syndrome, Stroke 25:1994, 1994.

41. Kim JS et al: Syndromes of pontine base infarction. A clinico-radiological correlation study, Stroke 26:950, 1995.

42. Koppel BS, Weinberger G: Pontine infarction producing dysarthria–clumsy hand syndrome and ataxic hemiparesis, Eur Neurol 26:211, 1987.

43. Landau WM: Ataxic hemiparesis: special deluxe stroke or standard brand? Neurology 38:1799, 1988.

44. Luijckx GJ et al: Isolated hemiataxia after supratentorial brain infarction, J Neurol Neurosurg Psychiatry 57:742, 1994.

45. Meadows JC: Dysphagia in unilateral cerebral lesions, J Neurol Neurosurg Psychiatry 36:853, 1973.

46. Melo TP et al: Pure motor stroke: a reappraisal, Neurology 42:789, 1992.

47. Melo TP et al: Thalamic ataxia, J Neurol 239:331, 1992.

48. Metter EJ: Speech disorders: clinical evaluation and diagnosis, Jamaica, NY, 1985, Spectrum Publications.

49. Metter EJ et al: Left hemisphere intracerebral hemorrhages studied by (F-18)-fluorodeoxyglucose PET, Neurology 36:1155, 1986.

50. Mohr JP: Lacunes, Stroke 13:3, 1982.

51. Mori E et al: Ataxic hemiparesis from small capsular hemorrhage: computed tomograph and somatosensory evoked potentials, Arch Neurol 41:1050, 1984.

52. Moulin T et al: Vascular ataxic hemiparesis: a re-evaluation, J Neurol Neurosurg Psychiatry 58:422, 1995.

53. Muelbacher W, Artner C, Mamoli B: Motor evoked potentials in unilateral lingual paralysis after monohemispheric ischaemia, J Neurol Neurosurg Psychiatry 65:755, 1998.

54. Murdoch BE, Thompson EC, Stokes PD: Phonatory and laryngeal dysfunction following upper motor neuron vascular lesions, J Med Speech-Lang Pathol 2:177, 1994.

55. Naeser MA et al: Aphasia with predominantly subcortical lesion sites: description of three capsular/putaminal aphasia syndromes, Arch Neurol 39:2, 1982.

56. Ozaki I et al: Pure dysarthria due to anterior internal capsule and/or corona radiata infarction: a report of five cases, J Neurol Neurosurg Psychiatry 49:1435, 1986.

57. Ozaki I et al: Capsular genu syndrome, Neurology 41:1853, 1991.

58. Pantano P et al: Prolonged muscular flaccidity after stroke: morphological and functional brain alterations, Brain 118:1329, 1995.

59. Portnoy RA, Aronson AE: Diadochokinetic syllable rate and regularity in normal and in spastic ataxic dysarthric subjects, J Speech Hear Disord 47:324, 1982.

60. Przedborski S et al: The effect of acute hemiplegia on intercostal muscle activity, Neurology 38:1882, 1988.

61. Ropper AH: Severe dysarthria with right hemisphere stroke, Neurology 37:1061, 1987.

62. Schonewille WJ et al: Diffusion-weighted MRI in acute lacunar syndromes: a clinical-radiological correlation study, Stroke 30:2066, 1999.

63. Takahashi S et al: Dysarthria due to small cerebral infarction—the localization of lesion and clinical characteristics, Rinsho Shinkeigaku 35:352, 1995.

64. Terry JB, Rosenberg RN: Frontal lobe ataxia, Surg Neurol 44:583, 1995.

65. Thompson EC, Murdoch BE: Disorders of nasality in subjects with upper motor neuron type dysarthria following cerebrovascular accident, J Comm Dis 28:261, 1995.

66. Thompson EC, Murdoch BE, Stokes PD: Lip function in subjects with upper motor neuron type dysarthria following cerebrovascular accidents, Euro J Disord Commun 30:451, 1995a.

67. Thompson EC, Murdoch BE, Stokes PD: Tongue function in subjects with upper motor neuron type dysarthria following cerebrovascular accident, J Med Speech-Lang Pathol 3:27, 1995b.

68. Thompson EC, Murdoch BE, Theodoros DG: Variability in upper motor neuron type dysarthria: an examination of five cases with dysarthria following cerebrovascular accident, Euro J Disord Commun 32:397, 1997.

69. Tohgi H et al: The side and somatotopical location of single small infarcts in the corona radiata and pontine base in relation to contralateral limb paresis and dysarthria, Euro Neurol 36:338, 1996.

70. Umapathi T et al: Tongue deviation in acute ischaemic stroke: a study of supranuclear twelfth cranial nerve palsy in 300 stroke patients, Cerebrovasc Dis 10:462, 2000.

71. Urban PP et al: Dysarthria-clumsy hand syndrome due to infarction of the cerebral peduncle, J Neurol Neurosurg Psychiatry 60:231, 1996.

72. Urban PP et al: Impaired cortico-bulbar tract function in dysarthria due to hemispheric stroke. Functional testing using transcranial magnetic stimulation, Brain 120:1077, 1997.

73. Urban PP et al: Isolated dysarthria due to extracerebellar lacunar stroke: a central monoparesis of the tongue, J Neurol Neurosurg Psychiatry 66:495, 1999.

74. Urban PP et al: Dysarthria in acute ischemic stroke: lesion topography, clinicoradiologic correlation, and etiology, Neurology 56:1021, 2001.

75. Venketasubramanian N, Seshardi R, Chee N: Vocal cord paresis in acute ischemic stroke, Cerebrovasc Dis 9:157, 1999.

76. Verma AK, Maheshwari MC: Hypoesthetic-ataxic-hemiparesis in thalamic hemorrhage, Stroke 17:49, 1986.

77. Willoughby EW, Anderson NE: Lower cranial nerve motor function in unilateral vascular lesions of the cerebral hemisphere, BMJ 289:791, 1984.

78. Yorkston KM, Beukelman D, Bell K: Clinical management of dysarthric speakers, San Diego, 1988, College-Hill Press.

10 Mixed Dysarthrias

"It was normal at first. Now it's gotten worse. I don't pronounce my words right. Some words I can't even say, and my voice is even different."

(64-year-old man with a mixed spastic-hypokinetic dysarthria associated with an unspecified neurodegenerative disease)

CHAPTER OUTLINE

I. **Etiologies**
   A. Degenerative diseases
   B. Toxic-metabolic conditions
   C. Vascular disorders
   D. Trauma
   E. Tumor
   F. Infectious and autoimmune diseases

II. **Speech pathology**
   A. Distribution of etiology, types, and severity in clinical practice
   B. Motor neuron disease—amyotrophic lateral sclerosis
   C. Multiple sclerosis
   D. Friedreich's ataxia
   E. Progressive supranuclear palsy
   F. Multiple system atrophy
   G. Corticobasal degeneration
   H. Wilson's disease
   I. Traumatic brain injury

III. **Cases**

IV. **Summary**

Imposing functional and anatomic divisions on the nervous system helps us understand the brain's operations and establish a framework for localizing and categorizing nervous system diseases. Unfortunately, however, there is no rule of nature that obligates neurologic disease to restrict itself to the divisions we impose upon it. As a result, the effects of neurologic disease can be "mixed" or distributed across two or more divisions of the nervous system.

The frequent refusal of neurologic disease to be focal and compartmentalized has implications for motor speech disorders (MSDs). Chapters 4 through 9 focused on "pure" dysarthrias that reflect damage to only one of the divisions of the motor speech system. For practical clinical purposes at least, many people do have only a single type of dysarthria. However, it is often the case that the damage that causes dysarthria is not confined to a single component of the motor system. Thus many people with dysarthria have a *mixed dysarthria,* or combination of two or more of the types that have already been discussed.

Mixed dysarthrias are common. They are encountered as the primary speech disorder in a large medical practice at a considerably higher rate than any single dysarthria type. Based on data for primary communication disorder diagnoses within the Mayo Clinic Speech Pathology practice, it accounts for 29.1% of all dysarthrias and 26.9% of all MSDs (see Figure 1-3).

Does the fact that many dysarthrias are mixed minimize the value of categorizing them into types? No. In fact, because dysarthria type reflects underlying neuropathology, recognizing its mixed forms is also valuable to neurologic localization and diagnosis. For example, a patient with a diagnosis of Parkinson's disease (PD) who has a mixed hypokinetic-ataxic dysarthria may not have PD, or may have more than PD, because PD should not be associated with ataxic dysarthria. Thus the recognition of each component of a mixed dysarthria may help rule out certain neurologic diagnoses or make other diagnoses more likely.

Mixed dysarthrias represent a heterogeneous group of speech disorders and neurologic diseases. Virtually any combination of two or more of the single dysarthria types is possible, and in any particular mix any one of the components may predominate. In spite of its heterogeneity, and the fact that sorting out the various components of mixed dysarthrias can be quite difficult, many mixed dysarthrias are perceptually distinguishable. Also, like pure forms, they may be the first or among the first signs of neurologic disease.

In this chapter, common etiologies of mixed dysarthrias are reviewed, with an emphasis on diseases that are frequently encountered in neurology and medical speech pathology practices. The most common types of mixed dysarthrias and their relation to specific neurologic diseases are also addressed. Finally, the mixed dysarthrias that are encountered in several specific neurologic diseases are discussed because they have been studied sufficiently to permit clinical descriptions of their most salient characteristics. Their description helps establish that they are lawfully derived from diseases that affect more than one component of the brain's motor system.

▧ ETIOLOGIES

Mixed dysarthrias can be caused by many conditions within each of the broad categories of neurologic disease. More than any other dysarthria type, they can result from combined neurologic events (e.g., multiple strokes) or the cooccurrence of two or more neurologic diseases (e.g., stroke plus PD). Also, they occur commonly in a number of degenerative diseases that affect more than one portion of the nervous system.

This section addresses conditions that can cause mixed dysarthrias more frequently than any single dysarthria type. The definition and description of conditions whose speech manifestations have been studied in some detail are emphasized. The specific speech characteristics associated with several of these disorders are addressed later in the section on speech pathology.

Degenerative Diseases

Because a number of degenerative diseases affect more than one portion of the motor system, they are commonly associated with mixed dysarthrias. Some of these diseases primarily affect motor functions. Others are more diffuse in their effects, also producing autonomic, sensory, and cognitive impairments.

Motor Neuron Disease—Amyotrophic Lateral Sclerosis

Motor neuron diseases (MNDs) are disorders characterized by progressive loss of upper motor neurons (UMNs) or lower motor neurons (LMNs), or both.

Spinal muscle atrophies are MNDs that affect LMNs only. Progressive limb wasting and weakness, with or without cranial nerve weakness, characterize them. They can be inherited or occur sporadically and may be congenital or develop in childhood or adulthood.[168] When dysarthria is present, it is flaccid, not mixed, so it is not discussed here further.

Progressive bulbar palsy (PBP) is a syndrome dominated by LMN weakness of cranial nerve muscles. Dysarthria and dysphagia are its predominant signs. UMN signs in the bulbar muscles may or may not be present.[131] When it is confined to the LMNs, PBP is associated with flaccid, not mixed dysarthria. In a sense, PBP can be thought of as amyotrophic lateral sclerosis (ALS) without limb involvement.

Primary lateral sclerosis (PLS), or *progressive pseudobulbar palsy* when bulbar muscles are predominantly affected, is an MND that affects UMNs only. They are characterized by corticospinal or corticobulbar tract signs, or both, but without LMN involvement. They can be difficult to distinguish from ALS. They may be associated with spastic dysarthria (see Chapter 5).

ALS is the most common MND. It is characterized clinically by UMN and LMN signs in the limbs or bulbar muscles, or both, and neuropathologically by loss of motor neurons in the precentral and postcentral cortex, the corticospinal tracts, motor nuclei of cranial nerves, and anterior horns of the spinal cord. Atrophic PNS motor fibers and evidence of denervation are also present.[167] Because it is a mixed UMN and LMN disease that often affects the bulbar muscles, *ALS has a natural and common association with mixed spastic-flaccid dysarthria.*

The incidence of ALS is approximately 1 to 5 per 100,000 population. More men than women are affected. It usually occurs sporadically, but approximately 5% of cases are familial.[131,168] Exact time of onset is often difficult to establish because more than half of the anterior horn cells must be lost before weakness is apparent and patients may adapt well to weakness.[110] Approximately 80% of affected individuals develop symptoms between 40 and 70 years of age, and the peak rate of occurrence is between 60 and 70 years.[84,110] The course of the disease is usually 1 to 5 years, but up to 25% of affected people live beyond 12 years.[21] Death is usually related to respiratory failure.

Although its first signs and symptoms are usually in the limbs, *approximately 25% of patients have their initial problems in the bulbar muscles, most often first represented by dysarthria, and sometimes by dysphagia.*[158,159] Patients with bulbar deficits as the first symptoms tend to have a more rapid course because dysphagia and airway problems represent major threats to life.

The diagnosis of ALS is made on the basis of its clinical profile and electrophysiologic confirmation. General clinical features include fatigue, cramping, fasciculations, weakness, and muscle atrophy, as well as hyperactive deep tendon reflexes with spasticity. Weakness is often focal initially. Electromyogram (EMG) findings of denervation (fibrillations) and reinnervation (large polyphasic motor unit action potentials) from two or more extremities (with the bulbar muscles counted as an extremity) are considered diagnostic of the disease.[131] Eye movements and autonomic and cognitive functions are usually spared, but some patients have cognitive deficits or signs of parkinsonism.[168] Cognitive deficits tend to be greater and more frequently evident in people with bulbar onset of symptoms.[98,144]

Multiple Sclerosis

Multiple sclerosis (MS) is the commonest acquired demyelinating central nervous system (CNS) disease and the commonest serious CNS disorder in young and middle-aged adults, affecting approximately 0.1% to 0.2% of the U.S. population. It affects women more often than men and usually begins between 20 and 40 years of age. Its cause is unknown, but it is believed to be an autoimmune disease triggered by environmental and genetic interactions.[117]

The disease affects scattered and diverse areas of the nervous system, with a predilection for white matter and periventricular areas, the brainstem, spinal cord, and optic nerves. MS plaques are characterized by demyelination (destruction of myelin sheaths with preservation of axons) and death of oligodendrocytes (cells that produce myelin) within the lesion.[130] Some lesions may be acute, with active myelin breakdown, whereas others reflect chronic, inactive demyelinated glial scars. In acute plaques, edema occurs in the area of affected nerve fibers. Resolution of edema may explain some of the recovery from deficits after an exacerbation.

Diagnosis can be difficult, and approximately 10% of MS patients are misdiagnosed,[58] with misdiagnosis sometimes including hysteria.[60,136] Current recommended diagnostic criteria[100] emphasize objective demonstration of disseminated lesions in both time and space, but clinical observations and other objective tests are also important. For example, a diagnosis of MS can be made if there is evidence of two or more attacks and objective evidence of two or more lesions. Various combinations of clinical findings and objective evidence of lesions can also permit the diagnosis, although with varying degrees of confidence. Among objective tests, magnetic resonance imaging (MRI) is emphasized because of its sensitivity to white matter lesions, but cerebrospinal fluid examination and visual evoked potentials are also helpful.

The course of MS is unpredictable. Some people have a benign course, with one or only a few attacks, and complete or nearly complete remission. Others have a relapsing-remitting course, with episodes of deterioration followed by near-complete recovery, a pattern that may persist for years. Still others have a remitting-progressive course with a slow accumulation of deficits. Finally, some have a progressing course, with the insidious onset and slow progression of disease without remission.[117]

MS can produce any sign or symptom of CNS disease. Problems with gait are common, as are visual and other sensory difficulties. Cerebellar dysfunction is often but not invariably present. Cranial nerve abnormalities may occur and can include trigeminal neuralgia, Bell's palsy, and facial myokymia. Psychiatric problems are not unusual and most often reflect affective disorders, which may be a direct consequence of the demyelinating process or a reaction to the disability caused by the disease.[122] Cognitive deficits occur in as many as 25% of people with progressive MS.[139] Aphasia and apraxia of speech are rare but have been reported,[57,92,119,124] as have difficulties with higher-level language functions that are not specifically aphasic in character.[91]

Dysphagia is relatively uncommon in patients who are ambulatory, but it does occur in others.[99] Dysarthria may occur in 50% of people with MS[133]; it is uncommon at the onset of the disease but can be the presenting symptom (see Chapter 6 for a discussion of paroxysmal ataxic dysarthria). When present, *dysarthria may reflect nearly any single type or combination of single types.* A *spastic-ataxic* dysarthria may be the most common mixed dysarthria associated with MS, but it should not be considered *the* dysarthria of MS.

---

*Initial presentation in the bulbar muscles aids neurologic differential diagnosis, because it is unusual in conditions that can mimic ALS, such as multifocal motor neuropathy, motor neuropathy, spinomuscular atrophy, or hyperthyroidism.[157]

Friedreich's Ataxia

Friedreich's ataxia (FA) is an inherited degenerative disease that is predominantly spinocerebellar, but it may also be associated with spasticity, LMN weakness, and extrapyramidal movement disorders. It was discussed in Chapter 6 , but it clearly can be associated with mixed dysarthria, most often *ataxic* and *spastic*.

Progressive Supranuclear Palsy

Progressive supranuclear palsy (PSP) is a multisystem neurodegenerative disease that is often mistaken for PD. Its incidence is approximately 1 to 6.5 per 100,000 population. It affects more men than women and usually begins after age 50; incidence increases with age. Average survival from symptom onset to death is approximately 6 to 7 years. It usually occurs sporadically rather than within families. Etiology is unknown.[20,152]

Neuropathologic characteristics include cell loss in numerous areas of the brain, including structures and pathways of the motor system, such as the globus pallidus, substantia nigra, thalamus, subthalamic nucleus, midbrain, a number of brainstem nuclei, and the cerebellum. The cranial nerves and the cerebral cortex, with the exception of the frontal lobes, are usually spared.[88,152]

Clinically, PSP is characterized by supranuclear ophthalmoparesis (paralysis of vertical gaze, especially downgaze), postural instability, and signs of parkinsonism (e.g., rigidity, bradykinesia). In spite of parkinsonian signs, tremor is usually not prominent, and responsiveness to antiparkinsonism drugs is usually poor or absent. *Dysarthria and dysphagia are common and often early and prominent signs.* Personality and cognitive changes associated with frontal lobe dysfunction (e.g., apathy, irritability, difficulty in planning and sequencing) can be quite evident.[48,94]

The clinical signs and pathology of PSP are indicative of multisystem degeneration. Several dysarthria types are possible. Mixed dysarthria occurs frequently, most often in the form of various combinations of *hypokinetic, spastic,* and *ataxic* types.

Multiple System Atrophy

Multiple system atrophy (MSA) is a sporadic neurodegenerative condition characterized by varying combinations of parkinsonism, ataxia, spasticity, and autonomic dysfunction. Similar to PSP, it is sometimes mistaken for PD, but response to levodopa is suboptimal. Incidence is approximately 3 per 100,000 population. Onset is usually after 50 years of age, and average survival from symptom onset until death is approximately 9 years.[20,38]

Neuropathologic localization varies somewhat across MSA subtypes (discussed later), but the range of involvement includes neuronal loss and gliosis in the basal ganglia, substantia nigra, cerebellum, inferior olives, middle cerebellar peduncles, pontine nuclei, corticospinal tracts, and intermediolateral and anterior horn cells. Cerebral atrophy, especially in the frontal lobes, has also been documented.[38] These loci implicate the basal ganglia and cerebellar control circuits, as well as UMN pathways. As a result, *hypokinetic, hyperkinetic, ataxic,* or *spastic* dysarthria may be encountered in MSA.

MSA recently has become the preferred designation for three previously separated conditions, including *striatonigral degeneration, olivopontocerebellar atrophy (OPCA),* and *Shy-Drager syndrome.* Two MSA subtypes are now identified, *MSA-P when parkinsonian features predominate* and *MSA-C when cerebellar features predominate.* Because the literature contains references to both sets of terminology, the labels of Shy-Drager syndrome, olivopontocerebellar atrophy, and striatonigral degeneration are retained when discussing studies that have used those designations.

In general, MSA-P (and striatonigral degeneration) reflects predominant, although not exclusive, nerve cell loss and gliosis in the basal ganglia and substantia nigra. As a result, parkinsonian features tend to dominate clinical signs and symptoms. When dysarthria is present, the hypokinetic type would most often be expected, either as the only dysarthria type or in combination with spastic or ataxic dysarthria, or both. Similarly, MSA-C and OPCA reflect predominant, although not exclusive, cerebellar involvement. When dysarthria is present, ataxia would most often be expected, either as the only dysarthria type or in combination with spastic or hypokinetic types, or both. In Shy-Drager syndrome, there are usually prominent autonomic nervous system deficits (dysautonomia), such as orthostatic hypotension,[†] incontinence, reduced respiration, and impotence. These problems stem from loss of preganglionic sympathetic neurons in the intermediolateral horns. Because the substantia nigra, striatum, cerebellum, and corticospinal tracts are also affected, various combinations of parkinsonism, ataxia, and spasticity, along with their associated dysarthrias (and, sometimes, laryngeal stridor), may predominate.

---

[*]Based on recommendations of a Consensus Committee of the American Autonomic Society and the American Academy of Neurology.[146]

[†]Orthostatic hypotension is characterized by a decrease in blood pressure upon standing.

Corticobasal Degeneration

Corticobasal degeneration (CBD) is an uncommon neurodegenerative disease of unknown etiology that is characterized by asymmetric cortical and extrapyramidal signs. A striking feature is the asymmetry with which CBD presents, even though its progressive course eventually includes the cortex (frontal and parietal lobes most prominently) and basal ganglia bilaterally. Onset is usually between 50 and 70 years of age, usually with a 5- to 15-year progression to death.[13,17,38]

The most consistent clinical features of CBD are asymmetric limb rigidity and apraxia. Asymmetric dystonic limb posturing, myoclonus, tremor, and cortical sensory loss are also common. Other fairly distinctive signs include *alien limb phenomena* and *mirror movements.** Frontal release signs, ataxia, postural instability, nonaphasic cognitive deficits, aphasia, apraxia of speech, and dysarthria can also occur.[16] The dysarthria is usually mixed, with *spastic* and *hypokinetic* types being most common, but *hyperkinetic* and *ataxic* components are possible.

Toxic-Metabolic Conditions

When toxic and metabolic diseases alter neurologic functions, their effects tend to be diffuse. When they affect the motor system, they commonly affect more than one of its components. When motor speech is affected, the result is often a mixed dysarthria. Some toxic-metabolic conditions that may be associated with mixed dysarthrias are described as follows.

Wilson's Disease

Wilson's disease (WD) is a rare autosomal recessive genetic metabolic disorder associated with inadequate processing of dietary copper. It is also known as *hepatolenticular degeneration* to indicate liver involvement and the consistent postmortem findings of degeneration in the lenticular nuclei of the basal ganglia. The metabolic inadequacy in WD leads to a buildup of copper in the liver, brain, and cornea of the eye, with the appearance of neuromotor signs by late adolescence or early adulthood. WD can be fatal if it goes undiagnosed.

WD may present with a hepatic, neurologic, or mood disturbance.[49] The pathognomonic sign of the disease is a golden brown ring *(Kayser-Fleischer*

rings) around the cornea of the eyes, reflecting copper deposits. Its classic neurologic manifestations are motor in nature and most frequently include a wing-beating tremor when the arms are outstretched; truncal rigidity; slowness of movement; incoordination; dystonia; dysarthria; drooling; and facial masking or a grinning, vacuous smile.[2,49] The basal ganglia are usually the most severely affected structures. If diagnosed before permanent damage occurs, a low copper diet, substances such as zinc to reduce copper absorption, and agents such as penicillamine to promote urinary excretion of copper can control copper balance and reverse many of the neurologic manifestations. Unfortunately, dysarthria is one of the neurologic signs that tend to be resistant to these treatments.[121] Liver transplant is pursued with fulminant liver failure.[49]

Dysarthria is considered a cardinal feature of WD, and it may be its initial sign.[118] The most common types of dysarthria associated with WD are *hypokinetic, spastic,* and *ataxic.*

Hepatocerebral Degeneration

Hepatocerebral degeneration can occur in people who have survived episodes of hepatic coma or in people with chronic liver disease. Common clinical manifestations include limb tremor, chorea or choreoathetosis in the face and limbs, unsteady gait, ataxia, and dysarthria. Corticospinal signs and mental deterioration may also be present. Pathologically, abnormalities are noted in the cerebral cortex, the lenticular nuclei, thalamus, and a number of brainstem nuclei. The lesions are similar to those encountered in WD.[2]

The dysarthrias associated with this condition have not been studied. The presence of *hypokinetic, hyperkinetic, spastic,* or *ataxic* forms seems possible.

Hypoxic Encephalopathy

Hypoxic encephalopathy is a diffuse neurologic condition resulting from a lack of oxygen to the brain because of failure of the heart and circulation or failure of the lungs and respiration. These failures most often involve myocardial infarction or cardiac arrest, carbon monoxide poisoning, suffocation (e.g., drowning, strangulation), diseases that paralyze respiratory muscles (e.g., Guillain-Barré syndrome), or diffuse CNS damage (e.g., traumatic brain injury [TBI]).

In general, when consciousness is lost and oxygen deprivation exceeds several minutes, permanent neurologic damage occurs. If consciousness and responsiveness are regained, several clinical abnormalities may emerge. Among the most common are memory

---

*The alien limb phenomenon is characterized by involuntary extremity movements such as elevation of the arm or grasping of objects, with the limb often described by patients as having a mind of its own. Mirror movements are characterized by inappropriate, involuntary movements of a limb that crudely mirror those of the contralateral limb as it performs volitional activity; they are usually associated with parietal lobe damage.[17]

disturbances, personality changes and disruptive behavioral problems, poor insight, visuospatial problems, spasticity, ataxia, dystonia, parkinsonism, tremor, action myoclonus, and pseudobulbar palsy. *Delayed postanoxic encephalopathy,* characterized by mental status changes and parkinsonism, occurs in some patients, most often days to weeks after carbon monoxide poisoning.[27]

The dysarthrias associated with hypoxic encephalopathy have not been described. The involvement of cortical, extrapyramidal, and cerebellar structures predicts the possible emergence of a number of dysarthria types that could include, at the least, *hypokinetic, hyperkinetic,* and *ataxic* forms, either singly or in combination.

Central Pontine Myelinolysis

Central pontine myelinolysis (CPM) is a serious metabolic condition characterized by destruction of myelin in the base of the pons. It also can affect the thalamus, subthalamus, amygdala, striatum, internal capsule, lateral geniculate bodies, white matter of the cerebellum, and deep layers of the cerebral cortex and adjacent white matter.

CPM is often associated with alcoholism and other conditions associated with malnutrition. It can occur in people with chronic liver or kidney disease or after organ transplant. It is believed that the basis pontis and other affected structures are especially susceptible to some acute metabolic fault, such as rapid correction or overcorrection of a profound electrolytic disturbance, such as hyponatremia.[2,97]

A number of neurologic signs are possible in CPM. Quadriplegia, spasticity, pseudobulbar palsy, and dysarthria or anarthria are common.

The dysarthrias of CPM have not been studied. Clinical experience suggests that *spastic, ataxic*, and *hyperkinetic* forms, at the least, can occur.

Vascular Disorders

Multiple strokes that affect various components of the motor system have a natural association with mixed dysarthrias. They can produce any combination of dysarthria types. Single brainstem strokes can also result in mixed dysarthrias because of the close proximity of pyramidal and extrapyramidal fibers, the cerebellar control circuit, and cranial nerve nuclei in that area of the brain. As a result, various combinations of *spastic, ataxic,* and *flaccid* dysarthria are not uncommon in brainstem stroke and can even occur in hemispheric stroke. *Hyperkinetic* dysarthria (e.g., secondary to palatal myoclonus) can also occur.

Trauma

The diffuse or multifocal lesions associated with traumatic and closed head injuries (CHIs) can produce virtually any combination of dysarthrias. Trauma from neurosurgery, especially if it involves posterior fossa structures, can also result in various mixed dysarthrias.

Tumor

Tumors, especially in the brainstem, can cause mixed dysarthrias because they can invade or produce mass effects on multiple components of the nervous systems. Brainstem tumors can be associated with various combinations of *spastic, ataxic,* and *flaccid* dysarthria.

Infectious and Autoimmune Diseases

The diffuse or multifocal effects of infectious and autoimmune diseases such as meningitis, encephalitis, and acquired immunodeficiency syndrome (AIDS) can be associated with various mixed dysarthrias. Two examples of such conditions, *progressive multifocal leukoencephalopathy** and *systemic lupus erythematosus,* are addressed here.

Progressive multifocal leukoencephalopathy (PML) is a rare, usually viral demyelinating CNS disease. It tends to occur in people with autoimmune disorders (e.g., AIDS, lymphoma, chronic lymphocytic leukemia) or in people receiving immunosuppressive therapy. The predominantly white matter lesions in PML are most prominent in cerebral subcortical areas and the posterior fossa. Clinical features include personality changes; motor deficits; ataxia; visual and other sensory deficits; and speech, language, and cognitive problems.[8,91]

The dysarthrias of PML have not been studied in detail. Lethlean and Murdoch,[91] describing the language deficits of one woman with PML, noted the presence of severe dysarthria; type was not identified, but clinical features suggest it was mixed, possibly with spastic and ataxic components. Dysarthria has been among the initial neurologic manifestations of PML in people undergoing chemotherapy (5-fluorouracil and levamisole) for colon cancer.[62,78] The presence of multiple and scattered hemispheric and brainstem lesions makes it likely that the dysarthrias were mixed. Because patients improved when chemotherapy was discontinued or modified, toxic effects of chemotherapy were the suspected cause.[†]

---

*Leukoencephalopathy is also discussed briefly in Chapter 5.

†Mixed hypokinetic, spastic, and ataxic dysarthria, plus apraxia of speech, have been reported in a patient without PML or any other structural lesions who was receiving the immunosuppressive agent FK-506 following liver transplantation.[18]

It appears that recognition of a developing dysarthria may be an early indication of neurotoxicity in this type of chemotherapy.

Systemic lupus erythematosus (SLE) is an autoimmune disease that can affect any organ, including the nervous system. Its effects on the nervous system can be temporary or permanent, and it can affect multiple, diffuse areas of the nervous system. Mechanisms of damage can be multiple and complex but are usually vascular. Various speech, language, and cognitive-communication disorders can result from SLE,[175] including dysarthria, which, on the basis of clinical experience, can be mixed. Specific speech characteristics and dysarthria types have not been studied carefully, however.

SPEECH PATHOLOGY

Sorting out the individual components of mixed dysarthrias can be difficult. Clinical uncertainty about all or some of the components of a mixed dysarthria probably occurs much more frequently than for the diagnosis of any single dysarthria type. It is not unusual, for example, to identify with confidence one of the components but to be uncertain if a second or third or fourth component is also present. Diagnostic impressions such as "the patient has an unambiguous mixed spastic-ataxic dysarthria, possibly with an accompanying flaccid component," or "ataxic dysarthria versus mixed spastic-ataxic dysarthria" are not unusual in clinical practice. This uncertainty probably reflects combinations of the natural overlap among manifestations of diseases affecting several portions of the motor system, the shortcomings of perceptual methods, and the "true" equivocal presence of certain neurologic signs in some cases. The need to draw equivocal or qualified conclusions can be unsettling to a clinician's desire for certainty and precision, but there is little choice when uncertainty reflects clinical reality. It may be reassuring, or equally as unsettling, to know that clinical neurologic examinations frequently reach similar tenuous interpretations of signs and symptoms.

Table 10-1 summarizes the types of dysarthria that can be encountered in a number of neurologic diseases that can produce mixed dysarthrias. It may be useful for setting a range of expectations for types of dysarthria that may be present when a neurologic diagnosis is relatively unambiguous and for identifying mixed dysarthrias that may be incompatible with particular neurologic diagnoses. Chapter 15, which addresses differential diagnosis, summarizes distinctive features of each of the single dysarthria types in a manner that helps identify each component that makes up a mixed dysarthria (in particular, see Tables 15-3 and 15-4).

table 10-1 Types of dysarthria that may be present in neurologic diseases that can produce mixed dysarthrias. Dysarthria is not inevitably present in all people with these diseases, and the listed diseases are not exhaustive.

	Dysarthria					
Disease	**Flaccid**	**Spastic**	**Ataxic**	**Hypokinetic**	**Hyperkinetic**	**UUMN**
Degenerative						
ALS*	++	++	?	–	–	–
MS	+	+/++	+/++	+	+	+
Friedreich's ataxia	?/+	+	++	–	–	–
PSP	–	++	+	++	–	–
Multiple system atrophy	+/?	+/++	++	++	+/?	–
Corticobasal degeneration*	–	+/++	+	+/++	?	?
Toxic-metabolic						
Wilson's disease	–	+/++	+/++	++	?/+	–
Hepatocerebral degeneration†	–	+	+	+	+	–
Hypoxic encephalopathy†	–	?	+/++	+/++	+/++	–
CPM†	–	+/++	+/++	?	+/++	–
Vascular†	+	+/++	+/++	+	+	+/++
Tumor*†	+	+	+	+/?	+/?	+
Infectious*†	+	+	+	+	+	+
Traumatic*	+	+/++	+/++	+/++	+	+

ALS, Amyotrophic lateral sclerosis; *CPM,* central pontine myelinolysis; *MS,* multiple sclerosis; *PSP,* progressive supranuclear palsy; *UMN,* unilateral upper motor neuron; ++, often present when dysarthria is present—may be quite typical for a particular disease; +, sometimes present, but not necessarily "typical" for a particular disease; ?, uncommon or of uncertain presence; –, not present.
*Apraxia of speech may also be present.
†Dysarthria has not been explicitly studied in the particular disorder.

| box 10-1 | Etiologies for 406 quasirandomly selected cases with a primary speech pathology diagnosis of mixed dysarthria at the Mayo Clinic from 1969-1990 and 1999-2001. Percentage of cases under each broad etiologic heading is given in parentheses. |

Degenerative (66%)

ALS (includes diagnoses of MND and progressive bulbar palsy) (43%)
Nonspecific CNS degenerative disease (8%)
PSP (4%)
PD or parkinsonism (2%)
Olivopontocerebellar degeneration (2%)
Multiple systems atrophy (2%)
Other (Wilson's disease, asymmetric cortical degeneration, Shy-Drager syndrome, cerebellar degeneration, striatonigral degeneration, hepatocerebral degeneration, Creutzfeldt-Jakob disease, PD vs. Shy-Drager disease, PD vs. PSP) (6%)

Vascular (11%)

Multiple strokes (7%)
Single stroke (4%)
Vascular malformation (<1%)

Traumatic (5%)

CHI (3%)
Surgical (<1%)

Multiple Causes (5%)

Various combinations of stroke, encephalopathy, cerebellar degeneration, Shy-Drager syndrome, postthalamotomy or other neurosurgery, PD, parkinsonism, drug toxicity, CHI, primary lateral sclerosis

Demyelinating (4%)

Multiple sclerosis (3%)
Other (1%)

Tumor (4%)

Mass (mostly posterior fossa) (4%)
Paraneoplastic (<1%)

Undetermined (3%)

Toxic/Metabolic (1%)

Hypothyroidism, central pontine myelinolysis, gangliosidosis, neuroleptic toxicity, hypoxic encephalopathy, hepatic or metabolic encephalopathy, undetermined metabolic disease

Inflammatory (1%)

Postviral encephalopathy, progressive encephalopathy, spongioform encephalopathy

ALS, Amyotrophic lateral sclerosis; *CHI*, closed head injury; *CNS*, central nervous system; *MND*, motor neuron disease; *PD*, Parkinson's disease; *PSP*, progressive supranuclear palsy.

In the remainder of this section, common etiologies of mixed dysarthrias and the most common mixed dysarthrias encountered in clinical practice are discussed. The dysarthrias encountered in specific neurologic diseases, the speech characteristics of which have been studied in some detail, are also summarized.

Distribution of Etiology, Types, and Severity in Clinical Practice

Etiologies

Box 10-1 and Figure 10-1 summarize the etiologies for 406 quasirandomly selected cases seen at the Mayo Clinic with a primary speech pathology diagnosis of mixed dysarthria. The cautions expressed in Chapter 4 about generalizing these data to the general population or all speech pathology practices apply here as well.

The data establish that mixed dysarthrias can be caused by a wide variety of neurologic conditions. Approximately two thirds of the cases were accounted for by degenerative diseases, and nearly 80% were accounted for by degenerative and vascular diseases.

By far, ALS was the most frequent degenerative neurologic disease associated with mixed dysarthria (43% of all cases).* Eight percent of cases clearly had degenerative CNS disease, but the diagnosis was otherwise nonspecific. The remaining degenerative cases were spread across many of the neurodegenerative diseases discussed earlier in this chapter.

Multiple strokes accounted for more than half of the vascular cases (11% of all cases). The sites of the strokes were widely distributed within the CNS and included both hemispheres, the brainstem, and cerebellum. Single strokes causing mixed dysarthrias were nearly always in the brainstem.

CHIs accounted for most of the traumatic etiologies (4% of all cases). Lesions, when identifiable, were widely distributed in the brain, most

*Although this figure may approximate that encountered in large tertiary medical care centers, it is almost certainly an overestimate of the percentage of cases seen in speech pathology practices in rehabilitation or primary care settings.

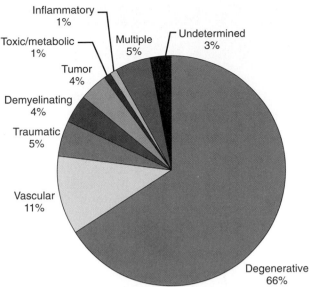

FIGURE 10-1 Distribution of etiologies for 406 quasirandomly selected cases with a primary speech pathology diagnosis of mixed dysarthria at the Mayo Clinic from 1969-1990 and 1999-2001 (see Box 10-1 for details).

often in subcortical areas, the brainstem, or cerebellum. Tumors accounted for 4% of the cases; a majority of the tumors were located in the posterior fossa.

Demyelinating diseases accounted for 4% of the cases. The majority of those cases had MS.

A combination of diseases was present in approximately 5% of the cases. These included various combinations of vascular, inflammatory, degenerative, traumatic, and toxic/metabolic conditions. Toxic/metabolic and inflammatory etiologies, by themselves, were responsible for only a small percentage of cases. Finally, approximately 3% of cases had undetermined neurologic diagnoses. The indeterminate nature of these disorders ranged from unexplained signs and symptoms (e.g., dysarthria, dystonia, blepharospasm) to identifiable lesions of undetermined etiology (e.g., undetermined posterior fossa lesion).

Types of Mixed Dysarthrias

The combination of dysarthria types was examined for the first 300 cases encountered within the sample summarized in Box 10-1. A combination of two dysarthrias represented 84% of the cases. Fourteen percent had three dysarthria types, and 2% had a combination of four types. The dominance of two dysarthria types in mixed dysarthria reflects either the "reality" of localization of neurologic disease in the sample or the limitations on auditory perceptual abilities to detect more than two dysarthria types in

any one person; a combination of these explanations is likely.*

Table 10-2 summarizes the frequency of occurrence of each single dysarthria type within the 300 patients. Because ALS occurred so frequently, the distribution for the entire sample and that portion of the sample minus ALS cases are also given. Spastic dysarthria was the most common type encountered, being present in 91% of the entire sample and 85% of the sample without ALS. Across both samples, ataxic dysarthria was the next most frequently encountered. Flaccid dysarthria was present in a majority of the entire sample but only one quarter of the sample without ALS. Hypokinetic dysarthria was present somewhat less frequently, although present in 35% of the sample without ALS. Hyperkinetic dysarthria was the least frequently encountered but nonetheless was present in far more than a few patients in both samples.

Table 10-3 summarizes the most common types of mixed dysarthria for the sample of 300 patients. The most common neurologic diagnosis for each mixed type is also given. Mixed flaccid-spastic dysarthria was the most frequent mixed dysarthria, accounting for 42% of the entire sample. The vast

*The difficulty that can be encountered in sorting out types in mixed dysarthrias is highlighted by the fact that one component of the mixed dysarthria was considered questionably or equivocally present in approximately 6% of the 300 cases. This uncertainty was associated with flaccid, spastic, ataxic, and hypokinetic types.

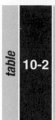

table 10-2	Distribution of individual dysarthria types encountered in a sample of 300 people with a primary speech pathology diagnosis of mixed dysarthria. Percentages are given for the entire sample and the portion of the sample without a diagnosis of ALS.	
Type	**Entire Sample**	**Sample without ALS**
Flaccid	54%	25%
Spastic	91%	85%
Ataxic	43%	66%
Hypokinetic	21%	35%
Hyperkinetic	13%	21%

ALS, Amyotrophic lateral sclerosis.

table 10-3	The most common types of mixed dysarthria and the most frequent neurologic diagnoses in a sample of 300 people with a primary speech pathology diagnosis of mixed dysarthria.	
Type (% of Entire Sample)	**Neurologic Diagnosis (% of Category)**	
Flaccid-Spastic (42%)	ALS (88%)	
	Vascular (5%)	
	Tumor (2%)	
	Other (5%)	
Ataxic-Spastic (23%)	Vascular (17%)	
	Demyelinating (13%)	
	CNS degenerative disease (12%)	
	Inflammatory (9%)	
	Cerebellar degeneration (7%)	
	Spinocerebellar degeneration (6%)	
	Tumor (6%)	
	Trauma (6%)	
	Other (24%)	
Hypokinetic-Spastic (7%)	Degenerative CNS disease (30%)	
	PSP (20%)	
	Vascular (20%)	
	Multiple (15%)	
	Other (15%)	
Ataxic-Flaccid-Spastic (6%)	ALS (59%)*	
	Vascular (18%)	
	Other (23%)	
Hyperkinetic-Hypokinetic (3%)	Parkinson's disease (67%)†	
	Other (33%)	
Other Types (19%)	—	

ALS, Amyotrophic lateral sclerosis; *CNS,* central nervous system;
PSP, progressive supranuclear palsy.
*The ataxic component was equivocal in about half of these cases.
†Often associated with on-off medication effects.

majority (88%) of these cases had ALS. This suggests that *gradual onset and progression of a mixed flaccid-spastic dysarthria should generate a high index of suspicion about ALS.* The association of ALS with mixed flaccid-spastic dysarthria represents the strongest association of any mixed dysarthria with a specific neurologic disease in the sample.

Mixed ataxic-spastic dysarthria accounted for 23% of the mixed dysarthrias. Neurologic diagnoses were quite variable, with a majority of cases associated with vascular, demyelinating (usually MS), degenerative, and inflammatory etiologies.

Hypokinetic-spastic dysarthria accounted for 7% of the cases. Again, neurologic diagnoses were quite variable, although approximately 50% were associated with PSP or undefined degenerative CNS diseases.

Mixed ataxic-flaccid-spastic dysarthria accounted for 6% of the mixed dysarthrias. Of interest, 59% of these cases had a neurologic diagnosis of ALS. This supports the clinical impression that *ataxic-like speech features may be perceived in individuals with ALS, particularly when their dysarthria is mild.* This is discussed further when the specific speech characteristics of ALS are addressed.

Mixed hyperkinetic-hypokinetic dysarthria accounted for 3% of the cases. Approximately two thirds of these cases had a diagnosis of PD. The mixed dysarthrias probably reflected on-off medication effects.

Many other mixed dysarthrias were encountered. In fact, a total of 29 different combinations of single dysarthria types were documented. Other than the mixed types just discussed, however, none of the other mixed types occurred frequently.

Severity and Other Characteristics

This retrospective review did not permit a precise delineation of dysarthria severity. However, intelligibility was specifically commented on in 68% of the first 300 cases encountered within the sample summarized in Box 10-1. In those cases, *76% had reduced intelligibility.* The degree to which this figure accurately estimates intelligibility impairments in mixed dysarthrias is unclear. It is likely that many patients for whom an observation of intelligibility was not made had normal intelligibility. However, the sample probably contains a larger number of mildly impaired patients than is encountered in a typical rehabilitation setting.

Because of its association with damage to more than one portion of the nervous system, it is reasonable to expect that some people with mixed dysarthrias will have cognitive disturbances. For the patients whose cognitive abilities were explicitly judged or formally assessed in the sample summarized in Box 10-1 (83% of the sample), *26% exhibited some impairment of cognitive ability. The proportion of patients with cognitive impairments was much higher among those whose etiology was not ALS.*

Finally, among the first 300 patients summarized in Box 10-1, dysarthria was the initial symptom in 20% and among the initial symptoms of neurologic disease in 25%. Perhaps more important, for 12% of that sample, dysarthria (sometimes with accompanying dysphagia) was the only complaint and neurologic finding at the time the patient presented for neurology and speech pathology diagnosis.

Motor Neuron Disease—Amyotrophic Lateral Sclerosis

Dysarthria may be the first manifestation of ALS, and it usually develops at some point during the disease's course. When dysarthria and dysphagia are the initial symptoms of ALS, they tend to remain the most functionally limiting symptoms as the disease progresses.[173] It has been estimated that approximately half of people with ALS who are receiving hospice care have reduced intelligibility, and only approximately 25% are intelligible just before death.[135] People requiring augmentative communicative devices need them within an average of 3 years following diagnosis and use them for an average of 2 years.[138] Once speech is affected, its decline is inevitable but not necessarily steady.[33] It is important to recognize that dysarthria in ALS may not be perceived as mixed at all points during the disease. It may present as either flaccid or spastic dysarthria; when mixed, either type may predominate.

Oral mechanism abnormalities are typically bilateral and generally consistent with those encountered in people with flaccid or spastic dysarthria of any etiology. Thus if spasticity is present, a jaw jerk, sucking reflex, hyperactive gag reflex, slow orofacial movements, and pseudobulbar affect may be evident. If LMNs are affected, the gag reflex may be reduced, the cough weak, and the face lacking in tone. Lingual fasciculations and atrophy can be prominent and early signs. Fasciculations may also be apparent in the chin and perioral area. Dysphagia may be present on UMN or LMN bases. It is not unusual for ALS patients with flaccid-spastic dysarthria to have an *audible reflexive dry swallow*. Some patients complain of shortness of breath, especially when lying down, and pulmonary function studies may demonstrate reduced vital capacity.

Nonspeech oral mechanism abnormalities are clearly relevant to speech findings. Clinical measures of strength and speed of tongue and lip movements, and other indices of respiratory and oromotor structure and function during nonspeech activities (e.g.,

lingual atrophy, dysphagia, velar movement, vital capacity) correlate strongly with measures of speech function, including intelligibility.[25,169]

Darley, Aronson, and Brown (DAB)[28,29] studied 30 people with ALS and found a combination of the deficits that were present in their groups with flaccid dysarthria alone and spastic dysarthria alone. The primary speech dimensions and clusters of deviant speech dimensions for these ALS patients are summarized in Table 10-4. It is apparent that some features are clearly associated with spastic or flaccid dysarthria and that others can be attributed to either type. The six clusters of deviant dimensions that were identified match with clusters found in spastic

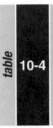

table 10-4	The clusters and most deviant speech dimensions, ranked from most to least severe, associated with the mixed flaccid-spastic dysarthria of ALS, as well as the degree to which the flaccid versus spastic component probably contributes to each feature.

Dimension/Cluster	Component
Dimension	
Imprecise consonants	Either or both
Hypernasality	Flaccid > spastic
Harshness	Spastic > flaccid
Slow rate	Spastic
Monopitch	Either or both
Short phrases	Either or both
Distorted vowels	Spastic
Low pitch	Spastic
Monoloudness	Spastic > flaccid
Excess and equal stress	Spastic
Prolonged intervals*	Combined
Reduced stress	Spastic
Prolonged phonemes*	Combined
Strained-strangled quality	Spastic
Breathiness	Flaccid > spastic
Audible inspiration	Flaccid
Inappropriate silences*	Combined
Nasal emission	Flaccid
Clusters	
Prosodic excess	Spastic
Prosodic insufficiency	Spastic
Articulatory-resonatory incompetence	Spastic
Phonatory stenosis	Spastic
Phonatory incompetence	Flaccid
Resonatory incompetence	Flaccid

Data from Darley FL, Aronson AE, Brown JR: Clusters of deviant speech dimensions in the dysarthrias, *J Speech Hear Res* 12:462, 1969a and Darley FL, Aronson AE, Brown JR: Differential diagnostic patterns of dysarthria, *J Speech Hear Res* 12:246, 1969b.
*Not a prominent dimension in either flaccid or spastic dysarthria. May represent the combined effects of both dysarthria types.

and flaccid dysarthria and provide further support to the types of dysarthria that are prominent in the disorder.

In addition, three features were present that were not found in flaccid or spastic dysarthria alone: *prolonged intervals, prolonged phonemes,* and *inappropriate silences.* These mainly prosodic features may reflect a summation of flaccid and spastic influences on speech. The combined effects of UMN and LMN deficits on speech are also reflected in the finding that distorted vowels, slow rate, short phrases, and imprecise consonants were rated as more severe in the ALS group than in any other group studied by DAB.

Phonatory abnormalities are frequently present but are quite variable across speakers. Perceptual attributes of dysphonia that receive frequent mention include harshness, breathiness, tremor, strained-strangled quality, audible inhalation, and abnormally high or low pitch.[25] Even highly intelligible speakers have a relatively high frequency of voicing contrast errors, suggesting vulnerability of the laryngeal subsystem early in the disease course.[128] The specific phonatory (and other) acoustic attributes may not be uniform across ALS speakers, however,[143] possibly reflecting varying degrees to which spasticity and weakness are present. It also appears that gender may be related to certain patterns of phonetic contrast errors[71,128]; for example, errors related to laryngeal functions are more frequent in men than in women.[71]

The frequent presence of tremor noted by Carrow et al.[25] is curious, because tremor is not a finding in flaccid or spastic dysarthria associated with other diseases. However, Aronson[4] observed the presence of a *rapid tremor or "flutter"* in some people with ALS, a feature detectable during vowel prolongation but usually not during connected speech; perceptually it seems to fall in the 7 to 10 Hz range. Demodulation and spectral analysis of the vowel prolongations of ALS patients with perceived flutter has documented frequency and amplitude modulations ranging from 0 to 25 Hz, with most patients having amplitude or frequency peaks in the 6 to 12 Hz range.[5] The physiologic cause of the vocal flutter associated with ALS is uncertain, but it is generally thought to reflect an LMN deficit rather than a "central" tremor.*

The vocal harshness perceived in mixed flaccid-spastic dysarthria often has a *"wet" or "gurgly"* character. This is presumably due to turbulence during speech from saliva that has accumulated in the pyriform sinuses and on the vocal folds because of reduced frequency of swallowing or inadequate clearing of secretions.

Occasionally, when the dysarthria is mild, a patient may exhibit irregular articulatory breakdowns during contextual speech, leading to a perception of *ataxic* or *ataxic-like dysarthria.* The reasons for this are unclear, but they may be similar to those offered in Chapter 9 for the ataxic-like characteristics that may be perceived in unilateral upper motor neuron dysarthria.

Several studies shed light on the articulatory abnormalities that contribute most to reduced intelligibility in ALS.[72,75,76,80] Among patients with varying degrees of intelligibility impairment, the most disturbed features tended to be related to velopharyngeal function (nasal-oral distinctions), lingual functions for articulatory manner contrasts (stop versus affricate), syllable shape, voicing contrasts, regulation of tongue height for vowels, and production of syllable final consonants. Data suggest that features affecting intelligibility tend to be consistent within speakers over time but may differ among speakers.[80] The findings demonstrate that all speech functions are not affected uniformly and, specifically, that some lingual functions are affected less than others are. For example, front versus back vowel, long versus short vowel, and general place of articulation distinctions seem relatively resistant to intelligibility problems.* Finally, it is noteworthy that perceptual ratings of speech alternate motion rate (AMR) articulatory precision and rhythmic consistency correlate strongly with ratings of sentence intelligibility.[132]

The physiologic and acoustic characteristics of speech in ALS have received some attention. Findings have confirmed or modified perceptual hypotheses and extended our understanding of the disorder. The primary findings of these studies are summarized in Table 10-5.

Kinematic studies have identified increased nasal airflow, difficulty maintaining velar elevation for sequences requiring velopharyngeal closure, slow single and repetitive articulatory movements, reduced velocity of articulator movement, limited range of movement, and reduced maximum strength of voluntary jaw, lip, and tongue movement.[31,32,34,36,61,85] Kinematic findings of slow rate

---

table 10-5	Summary of acoustic and physiologic findings in studies of ALS*

Speech Component	Acoustic or Physiologic Observation
Respiratory	Reduced vital capacity
	Chest wall muscle weakness
Laryngeal	Abnormal f_o (too high or low)
	Abnormal jitter, shimmer, harmonic/noise ratio
	Decreased maximum phonatory frequency range
	Decreased maximum vowel prolongation
Velopharyngeal	Difficulty maintaining velar elevation
	Increased nasal airflow
Articulation, Rate, Prosody	Slow single & repetitive articulatory movements
	Reduced velocity & range of articulatory movements
	Reduced maximum strength of tongue, lip, & jaw movements
	Excessive jaw movement (probably compensatory)
	Lengthened segment and sentence duration
	Increased stop-gap duration
	Blurring of voiced-voiceless VOT distinctions (articulatory-laryngeal)
	Reduced spectral distinctiveness among lingual fricatives
	Increased vowel duration within syllables
	Reduced/shallow/flattened F2 slope within words
	Reduced vowel space
	Exaggerated formant trajectories at vowel onset within syllables
	Frequency or amplitude fluctuations, or both, during vowel prolongation related to perceived vocal flutter

ALS, Amyotrophic lateral sclerosis; f_o, fundamental frequency; F2, second formant; VOT, voice onset time.
*Note that many of these findings are based on only a few speakers and that not all speakers with ALS (or mixed spastic-flaccid dysarthria) exhibit all features. Note also that many of these characteristics are probably not unique to ALS or mixed spastic-flaccid dysarthria; some may be found in other motor speech disorders or other neurologic or nonneurologic conditions.

have been confirmed by acoustic studies that document abnormally slow segment and sentence duration.[153,159,162,163] In general, physiologic findings suggest that *tongue functions are more severely affected than those of the lips and jaw.*[74] Taken together, the movement abnormalities identified in physiologic studies are consistent with the slow rate, imprecise articulation, vowel distortions, hypernasality, and nasal emission commonly perceived in speakers with ALS.

People with ALS may complain of shortness of breath when supine, and they can have reduced vital capacity in the upright position. Studies of respiration have documented chest wall muscle weakness, especially in inspiratory muscles. Low lung volumes can reduce utterance length and loudness, and respiratory weakness can lead to reduced loudness and stress contrasts, short phrases, and reduced power for coughing.[125] Respiratory decline can be expected in all people with ALS, and, unfortunately, severe compromise of bulbar functions is associated with severe compromise in respiratory status, an association that exacerbates dysarthria and dysphagia.[170]

The relationship between weakness and speech disability in ALS is neither simple nor direct, at least partly because of the ability of some muscle groups to compensate for weakness in others. For example, kinematic studies have documented excessive jaw displacements during speech-related lip and tongue movements[61] and exacerbation of speech deficits when the jaw is fixed, suggesting that under normal speaking conditions the jaw is able to compensate for weakness in other articulators, because its strength is relatively preserved.[34] The complex relationship may also be related to the fact that patients with ALS can have significantly reduced muscle force before obvious effects on speech, probably because only approximately 10% of maximum muscle contraction forces are recruited during speech.[85]

Acoustic studies have documented a number of abnormalities, although with substantial variability across patients.[74] Among the common findings are: abnormal fundamental frequency (f_o) (too high or low); abnormal jitter, shimmer, and harmonic/noise ratio; reduced maximum phonatory frequency range; longer stop-gap durations*; longer vowel duration in syllables; decreased maximum vowel duration;

---

*Stop-gap duration is the time from cessation of acoustic energy in a preceding vowel to the onset of acoustic energy from the articulatory burst for a subsequent initial stop-plosive.

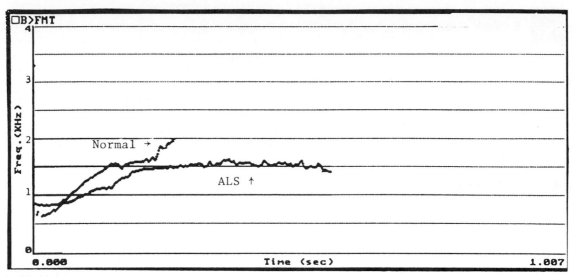

FIGURE 10-2 Second formant (F2) tracings for the vowel /æ/ in the word "wax" for a normal male speaker and a man with mixed spastic-flaccid dysarthria associated with ALS (analysis based on method described by Kent et al.[77]). Relative to the normal speaker, the F2 slope for the dysarthric speaker is only approximately half as steep, covers a smaller frequency range, and takes approximately twice the time to complete. This long and flattened F2 trajectory is an acoustic correlate of slow speaking rate and slowed and restricted range of articulatory movements that can underlie mixed spastic-flaccid dysarthria.

abnormal rate and periodicity of vocal fold diadochokinesis (i.e., rapid repetitions of /hʌ/); slow and short phrase duration; reduced spectral distinctiveness between lingual fricatives; and longer segment and utterance durations.* Some studies document a blurring of the voice onset time (VOT) distinctions between initial voiced and voiceless stops,[137] but others do not,[26] and not all studies find consistent abnormalities in jitter, shimmer, and harmonic/noise ratio.[72,75] This variability in findings probably reflects differences in severity across various speech subsystems and perhaps the degree to which weakness versus spasticity is predominant among the speakers who have been studied. Gender differences have also been noted for some measures.[72] In general, however, these acoustic findings are indicative of slow lingual or laryngeal movements, aperiodicity, or instability of movements and weakness of movements during speech.

The acoustic characteristics of the vocal flutter that is present in some patients have been examined acoustically using fast Fourier transformation (FFT) after the signal from vowel prolongations with perceived flutter was demodulated into frequency and amplitude components.[†5] Results demonstrated mul-

tiple frequency and amplitude modulations, with more prominent modulations in ALS than control subjects. The prominent frequencies spanned the range from 0 to 25 Hz, but most had peaks in the 6 to 12 Hz range. These findings provide support for the perception of flutter in some ALS patients, but they do not clarify the basis for the phenomenon. Aronson et al.[5] speculated that the flutter is probably not central, because tremor is not typically heard in spastic dysarthria alone, the only obvious CNS dysarthria present in ALS. They noted that people with peripheral neuropathy could have tremor in the 8 to 12 Hz range. In addition, the flutter could be a sign of loss of motor units, resulting in an intermittent absence of motor unit firing that, when it affects intrinsic laryngeal muscles, might be perceived as a tremor or flutter.

Studies of the slope of the second formant (F2) in intelligibility test words have revealed reliable and useful findings. For people with ALS, the *F2 slope* seems to be a sensitive index of lingual function, and perhaps speech proficiency in general, because it probably reflects the rate at which lingual movements occur and, by inference, the rate at which motor units can be recruited. F2 slope declines along with intelligibility in subjects followed longitudinally and in groups of men and women with a range of intelligibility impairments[71,75,77,112,162] (see Figure 10-2). Weismer et al.[164] found shallower slopes of formant transitions, exaggerations of formant trajectories at the onset of vocalic nuclei, and greater inter-

---

*References 26,71,72,75,126,127,129,153,154,160,162.

†They also observed tremulous movements of the true folds and supraglottic muscles on fiberscopic examination of ALS patients with vocal flutter.

speaker variability in ALS speakers than in control subjects. Patients who were less than 70% intelligible had more aberrant trajectory characteristics than those with better intelligibility. Poorly intelligible speakers tended to have flat trajectories or shallow slopes. It thus appears that measures of formant transitions, particularly F2, may be a useful index for monitoring the course of ALS and for making predictions about intelligibility impairments. It should be noted, however, that the F2 slope-intelligibility relationship may not be linearly correlated across the full range of intelligibility,[77,112] so measures other than F2 may be required to predict the full range of intelligibility scores in people with ALS.*

Vowel space† appears to be another useful acoustic correlate of impairment. In comparison to normal speakers, vowel space is reduced in some speakers with ALS at habitual, slow, and fast rates, and it is moderately correlated with speech intelligibility.[159,162,163]

Is the typically slow speaking rate of speakers with ALS a primary problem or does it reflect a compensatory response to maintain intelligibility? Although both explanations could be true within or across speakers, it has been shown acoustically and perceptually that although ALS speakers can increase their rate when asked, they nonetheless remain slower than normal. Importantly, vowel space is compressed at habitual and faster rates, and perceptual measures of intelligibility and severity does not show any change between habitual and faster rates. This latter finding suggests that the habitually slow speech rate in speakers with ALS is not a product of compensation.[163]

To summarize the primary speech findings commonly associated with ALS, the dysarthria associated with the disease may be *flaccid, spastic,* or, most often, *mixed flaccid-spastic.* The overall pattern of the mixed form, beyond mild degrees of impairment, is one of *labored, slowly produced speech with short phrases and intervals between words and phrases, grossly defective articulation, hypernasality, strained-strangled and groaning voice quality, and monopitch and monoloudness.* Although all levels of speech production are often affected in ALS, the degree of impairment across levels is not uniform, at least relative to their impact on intelligibility.

*Yorkston et al.[173] present data that suggest that reductions in speaking and AMR rates in people with ALS may be precursors of reduced intelligibility.

†The vowel space is the area of the quadrilateral formed by plotting F1 against F2 for the point vowels [i], [u], [a], and [æ].[73] Reduced vowel space implies reduced acoustic and perceptual distinctiveness among the plotted vowels and reduced distinctiveness among the articulatory movements that generate them.

Multiple Sclerosis

Dysarthria is the most common communication disorder associated with MS, occurring in 40% to 50% of people with the disease.[12,53,107] Severity varies but is generally related to the overall severity of neurologic deficit, including physical and cognitive deficits, and to the number of neurologic systems involved. On average, communication deficits are mild, but a small percentage of affected people have moderate to severe difficulties, with some requiring augmentative or alternative means of communication.[12,30,171] The type of dysarthria is also variable, consistent with the variable presentations of MS in general. *Ataxic and spastic dysarthria, often combined, are probably most common.*

Nonspeech findings in MS that have implications for speech production include the occasional presence of reduced vital capacity and inadequate ventilation.[30,63] Respiratory complications are frequent in the terminal stages of MS and may also occur during disease relapses. Such impairments can include generalized or diaphragmatic respiratory muscle weakness, disordered regulation of automatic and voluntary breathing, and bulbar weakness leading to aspiration and infection. Some patients have obstructive sleep apnea, and some require mechanical respiratory support.[63] Facial paralysis similar to Bell's palsy occurs in approximately 10% of people with MS, and facial myokymia and trigeminal neuralgia may also be present.[139] Although tremor in speech system muscles is not generally present in MS, tremor elsewhere in the body occurs frequently (especially in the upper extremity), and its severity correlates with dysarthria severity.[3] In general, it appears that lingual functions are more severely affected than lip functions, and abnormalities in lingual strength, endurance, and rate of repetitive movements have been demonstrated, even in nondysarthric MS speakers.[52,115]

Table 10-6 summarizes the deviant speech characteristics and some of the related dysfunctions found in Darley, Aronson, and Goldstein's[30] study of 168 people with MS. The presence of impaired loudness and pitch control and sudden articulatory breakdowns are suggestive of ataxic dysarthria, but the dysarthria was spastic in some patients. The presence of spastic dysarthria in MS is also suggested by the findings of Farmakides and Boone,[37] who reported hypernasality, reduced pitch variability, and slow rate in some of their 82 people with MS.

It should be noted that *scanning speech,* as it may occur in some speakers with ataxic dysarthria,* is not

*See Chapter 6 for a discussion of scanning speech. The explanation provided for scanning speech by Hartelius et al.[54] was based on data obtained from speakers with MS.

table 10-6	Speech deviations and related functions in a sample of 168 people with multiple sclerosis	
Deviation		**% of Sample**
Speech		
Impaired loudness control		77
Harshness		72
Defective articulation		46
Impaired emphasis		39
Impaired pitch control		37
Hypernasality		24
Inappropriate pitch level		24
Breathiness		22
Sudden articulatory breakdowns		9
Related Functions		
Decreased vital capacity		35
Nasal escape (on oral manometer) manometer)		2
Inadequate ventilation		2

Based on Darley FL, Aronson AE, Goldstein NP: Dysarthria in multiple sclerosis, *J Speech Hear Res* 15:229, 1972.

a pathognomonic feature of dysarthria in MS. For example, only a small percentage of patients studied by Darley, Aronson, and Goldstein[30] had increased stress on unstressed syllables, the feature that is most relevant to a perception of scanning speech. This should temper descriptions of scanning speech as *the* speech of MS.

Instrumental measures of dysarthria in MS are quite limited, but they do support the ability of acoustic and kinematic measures to identify abnormalities at the phonatory and articulatory levels. For example, it has been established that measures of long-term phonatory instability during vowel prolongations can distinguish MS speakers with perceptible dysphonia from matched control speakers,[51] and that temporal measures of speech AMRs and sequential motion rates (SMRs) are sensitive to distinctions between MS speakers and normal speakers and speakers with PD.[155] Electropalatography has also detected temporal abnormalities (articulatory "overshooting") in tongue movements during speech in one speaker with MS.[113]

It seems reasonable to conclude that *ataxic* and *spastic dysarthria* and *mixed ataxic-spastic dysarthria* are among the most frequent dysarthria types encountered in MS. Perhaps more than in any other of the degenerative diseases discussed here, however, the dysarthrias of MS are unpredictable. It is prudent to consider virtually any dysarthria type or combination of types as possible in people with the disease.

Friedreich's Ataxia

The few studies of speech in FA establish that, despite the disease's label, its associated dysarthria is not always ataxic and that the dysarthria can be mixed. This is a logical consequence of the disease's capacity to affect more than cerebellar structures.

The prominent deviant speech dimensions that have been noted in perceptual studies of FA include abnormal respiratory synchrony, harshness, breathiness, strained-strangled voice quality, audible inspiration, monopitch, pitch breaks, fluctuating pitch, inappropriate pitch level, monoloudness, excess loudness variation, hypernasality, imprecise consonants, distorted vowels, irregular articulatory breakdowns, prolonged phonemes, abnormal rate, excess and equal stress, inappropriate silences, prolonged intervals, slow rate, and slow AMRs.[43,70] Acoustic analysis has quantified abnormal f_o and intensity variability in vowel prolongation, abnormal variability in AMRs, slow speaking rate, and longer word durations and slower AMRs.[1,42,87] Taken together, these observations suggest that more than a single dysarthria type can be present in FA. For example, the statistical analysis by Joanette and Dudley[70] of 22 patients with FA identified a cluster of features suggestive of underlying ataxia with predominant effects on articulation, as well as phonatory stenosis, which could reflect a spastic component (although the authors did not explicitly conclude that the phonatory abnormalities reflected spasticity). The presence of breathiness and audible inspiration raises the possibility of a flaccid component as well. These data plus clinical experience suggest that ataxic dysarthria is not *the* dysarthria of FA.

To summarize, the results of a few perceptual and acoustic studies, combined with the known sites of nervous system degeneration in people with FA, suggest that *ataxic dysarthria* may be the most frequently encountered dysarthria in FA, but that other types can also be present, particularly *spastic dysarthria*. Thus mixed dysarthria can be present in FA, and it seems that the most common mix is an *ataxic-spastic dysarthria*.

Progressive Supranuclear Palsy

Dysarthria is probably the least well described clinical sign of PSP, in spite of it being a frequent, early (often within 2 years), and prominent manifestation of the disease.[88,95,96,108,111,123,140] It is more frequently among the initial manifestations of disease in PSP than PD and more prevalent overall in PSP than PD[69]; dysarthria is present in 70% to 100% of unselected patients with PSP in several reports. Given the predilection of PSP to produce parkinsonian, pseudobulbar, and sometimes ataxic features, it is reasonable to predict several types of dysarthria in PSP.

Oral mechanism examination can reveal various confirmatory signs encountered in people with hypokinetic, spastic, and ataxic dysarthria. Although orofacial manifestations of parkinsonism (e.g., facial masking) are most frequent, evidence of pseudobulbar palsy (e.g., pseudobulbar affect, hyperactive jaw jerk) are common. In addition, in contrast to the flexed neck posture often seen in PD, people with PSP may exhibit neck extension, with the head pointed upward.[88] Dysphagia is common,* with some studies suggesting it is more common than dysarthria,[95] and others suggesting it is less common.[83] Latency from disease onset to complaints of dysphagia is strongly correlated to total survival time.[111]

The dysarthrias of PSP have been delineated in several group studies.[82,83,96,108,140] Hypokinetic, spastic, and ataxic types (generally in that order of frequency) are consistently identified, sometimes singly, but more often in various combinations. A combination of all three types is common in some reports. The severity of the hypokinetic component is related to the degree of neuronal loss in the substantia nigra.[82] In general, the combination of spastic, hypokinetic, and ataxic components coincides with the loci of neuropathologic changes found in PSP, and their recognition is considered important to clinical diagnosis.[83]

Because PSP is often misdiagnosed as PD,[68] some attention to speech findings that seem to distinguish PSP from PD is warranted. Retrospective data suggest that characteristics found more frequently in PSP than PD include monopitch, hoarseness, nasal emission, excess and equal stress, hypernasality, imprecise articulation, and slow rate. Characteristics found more frequently in PD than PSP include vocal flutter, reduced loudness, reduced stress, tremor, breathiness, and rapid rate (Lu, Duffy, and Maraganore, 1992). These differences are logically related to the relative exclusivity of features of hypokinetic dysarthria in PD and the frequent added presence of features of other dysarthria types in PSP, particularly spastic dysarthria. These distinctions suggest that *the presence of a dysarthria type other than hypokinetic in people with a neurologic diagnosis of PD should raise questions about the accuracy of the PD diagnosis;* PSP would be an alternative diagnosis.

Speech difficulties that extend beyond those that can be explained by dysarthria can be present. *Palilalia* is frequently noted,* and *"stuttering" dysfluencies* and *echolalia* are mentioned in some reports (Testa et al., 2001)[83,86,88,108]; recall, however, that palilalia and certain dysfluencies have a strong association with hypokinetic dysarthria (see Chapter 7). Some patients produce *involuntary vocalizations* such as groaning or humming sounds,[152] and some patients have language and cognitive deficits commonly associated with frontal lobe pathology.[38,123] A single atypical case with apraxia of speech has been reported.[16]

To summarize, perceptual observations establish that dysarthria, often mixed dysarthria, is common and tends to appear early in PSP. *Hypokinetic, spastic,* and *ataxic* dysarthria are most commonly present, most often in varying combinations. Recognition of a mixed dysarthria in people with suspected PSP versus PD may be particularly helpful to differential diagnosis. Early in the course of neurologic disease, the presence of hypokinetic dysarthria or, especially, a mixed dysarthria with hypokinetic, spastic, or ataxic components, may be more strongly associated with PSP than with other degenerative neurologic diseases, particularly PD.

Multiple System Atrophy

The dysarthrias associated with MSA and its subtypes—MSA-P and MSA-C—have been sufficiently described to develop a picture of their prevalence, severity, and salient features. This can be supplemented by descriptions of the dysarthrias associated with striatonigral degeneration, OPCA, and Shy-Drager syndrome, conditions now encompassed by the MSA designation.

Dysarthria is common in MSA,† present in 100% of unselected patients in some series.[81] It tends to emerge earlier in the disease course than it does in PD, within the first 2 years in approximately half of affected people. On average, dysarthria seems to be more severe than in PD.[38,81,111,165]

Dysarthria type is usually correlated with other motor signs of MSA and is therefore, often mixed.

---

*Kluin et al.[83] reported that 73% of their patients with PSP had dysphagia. Litvan, Sastry, and Sonies[95] reported that 96% of their PSP patients had abnormal swallowing studies, although only 19% aspirated. A majority of their patients had delayed initiation of the swallow reflex, impaired tongue mobility, premature dripping into the pharynx, and pooling in the valleculae.

---

*Palilalia has been reported as an early-appearing clinical feature that helps distinguish patients with PSP from those with MSA.[145]

†In spite of involvement of multiple systems, apraxia of speech and aphasia are rarely, if ever, encountered in MSA.[38]

Hypokinetic, ataxic, and spastic types (generally in that order of frequency of occurrence) are most often noted. All three types were present in a majority of 46 unselected patients reported by Kluin et al.[81] Recognizing dysarthria types other than hypokinetic can help distinguish MSA from PD.

Before it was absorbed under the heading of MSA, the dysarthrias associated with striatonigral degeneration (MSA-P) were not well described. Hypokinetic dysarthria is the most common expected type, but hyperkinetic and perhaps spastic dysarthria are possible based on the common loci of pathology.

The dysarthrias associated with OPCA have been well described in only a few patients.[43,55] The reported deviant speech features are suggestive of mixed ataxic-spastic dysarthria, perhaps with a flaccid component based on observations in some patients of audible inspiration and vocal flutter.* Because OPCA (MSA-C) may also be associated with parkinsonian features, a hypokinetic dysarthria is also possible. Thus *ataxic, spastic, hypokinetic,* and, less frequently, *flaccid dysarthria,* singly or in combination, are the common expected dysarthria types. Additional but less consistently present deficits that can affect speech and communication include palatal myoclonus and dementia.[35]

The dysarthrias associated with Shy-Drager syndrome are most adequately described in Line-baugh's[93] study of 80 people with the disorder. Forty-four percent had dysarthria. Among those with dysarthria, 43% had ataxic dysarthria, 31% had hypokinetic dysarthria, and 26% had various combinations of mixed dysarthrias. Three forms of mixed dysarthria were present, including *hypokinetic-ataxic, ataxic-spastic,* and *spastic-ataxic-hypokinetic.* These mixes are consistent with the involvement of direct and indirect motor systems and the basal ganglia and cerebellar control circuits that occurs in the disease.

An association of laryngeal stridor with Shy-Drager syndrome has long been recognized, and as many as one third of people with MSA may have stridor.[19] Recognizing stridor within various combinations of spastic, ataxic, and hypokinetic dysarthria is diagnostically valuable because that combination of signs is probably uncommon in degenerative diseases other than MSA. Excessive snoring and sleep apnea are commonly associated with inhalatory stridor, but stridor can sometimes be heard just before speech is initiated or at phrase boundaries during ongoing speech; when more serious, it can be evident during quiet awake breathing. When severe upper airway obstruction occurs, continuous positive airway pressure or tracheostomy may be recommended. The cause of inhalatory stridor is traditionally thought to reflect abductor (posterior cricoarytenoid) laryngeal weakness secondary to involvement of the nucleus ambiguus,[6] hence its frequent recognition as a sign of flaccid dysarthria.* However, recent evidence suggests that laryngeal dystonia may at least sometimes be the cause of stridor, at least as it occurs in MSA.[†7,65]

Corticobasal Degeneration

Communication deficits are common in CBD, and dysarthria is among the most frequent communication problems. For example, among 60 papers that have described speech and language characteristics in a total of 457 people with CBD, dysarthria was reported as present in 42%.[90] Dysarthria and other communication disorders can be early and prominent manifestations of CBD, and the prevalence of dysarthria increases with disease progression.[9,39,90,166] Severity of dysarthria is related to overall disease severity[120] but is not necessarily correlated with disease duration.[39]

Dysarthria type varies, but more often than not it is mixed. *Hypokinetic and spastic types are most common,* but ataxic dysarthria has also been reported, most often in combination with hypokinetic or spastic types, or both.[39,90,120] *Apraxia of speech* may also be present, either as the sole MSD or in combination with dysarthria. Nonverbal oral apraxia is frequently reported, and echolalia and palilalia have been noted.[39,90]

It is important to note that aphasia occurs frequently in CBD, in more than half of patients in some reports, and that aphasia type is most often described as nonfluent or anomic. Aphasia can be the first manifestation of the disease; when this is the case, it is frequently called *primary progressive aphasia.*[41,64,90,106,109]

Patients with CBD may exhibit a behavior that has been called *yes-no reversals,* in which they spontaneously complain that they say or gesture "yes" when they mean "no," and vice versa, when responding to questions during social discourse; the behavior is often confirmed during examination.[40] This can occur in the absence of obvious aphasia, but it does occur more frequently in patients with predominant

---

*Hartman and O'Neill[55] described a man with OPCA whose speech characteristics suggested a mixed flaccid-spastic dysarthria plus stuttering-like dysfluencies, which may or may not have reflected a reemergence of developmental stuttering.

---

*Loss of myelinated nerve fibers in the laryngeal branch of the recurrent laryngeal nerve has been documented in patients with MSA.[56]

†It is known that dystonia can be present in cervical and limb muscles in people with MSA.[15]

left hemisphere involvement. It is correlated with frontal lobe functions related to mental flexibility, inhibitory control, and motor programming. Yes-no reversals in the absence of significant aphasia can be a useful differential diagnostic sign, because among people with degenerative neurologic diseases, they most often occur in CBD and PSP.[40]

To summarize, mixed or isolated dysarthria types are common in CBD, with hypokinetic, spastic, and ataxic types being the most common. When the common asymmetry of the disease involves the left hemisphere, communication deficits are frequently mixed beyond dysarthrias, with frequent occurrence of aphasia and apraxia of speech. Communication can also be affected by additional problems that probably reflect frontal lobe dysfunction (e.g., yes/no reversals, reduced mental flexibility, impaired motor programming). This constellation of deficits can make the communication difficulties encountered in CBD more complex than in many other degenerative neurologic diseases.

Wilson's Disease

Wilson's disease (WD) often affects the bulbar muscles. Dysarthria is one of the most frequent and sometimes the only manifestation of the disorder.[141,156] Oral mechanism findings in people with WD can be similar to those encountered in people with hypokinetic, ataxic, or spastic dysarthria. Dystonia also may be present and is considered responsible for the inappropriate and fixed vacuous or "pseudo smile" exhibited by some patients.[141] Dysphagia and drooling are not unusual.

Berry et al.[10] studied 20 patients with WD who had various combinations of ataxia, rigidity, and spasticity. The most prominent deviant speech characteristics and clusters of speech characteristics (based on factor analysis) derived from the study are summarized in Table 10-7. It was concluded that the dysarthria of WD can be mixed, containing various combinations of *hypokinetic, ataxic,* and *spastic,* but that each single type can occur alone in some people with the disease.

Monitoring the speech of patients undergoing penicillamine and low copper diet management of their WD has established a correlation between improvement in deviant speech characteristics and general neurologic improvement.[11] This suggests that careful monitoring of speech during medical treatment of WD can serve as an index of the effectiveness of treatment for the disease.

Traumatic Brain Injury

Communication deficits are common in TBI. They can include nonaphasic cognitive-communication

table 10-7	Prominent deviant characteristics and clusters of speech characteristics associated with Wilson's disease		
Features	**Hypokinetic**	**Ataxic**	**Spastic**
Characteristics			
Reduced stress	X		X
Slow rate		X	X
Excess and equal stress		X	X
Low pitch	X		X
Irregular articulatory breakdowns		X	
Hypernasality			X
Inappropriate silences	X		
Prolonged phonemes		X	
Prolonged intervals		X	
Strained voice			X
Short phrases			X
Clusters (Based on Factor Analysis)			
Prosodic insufficiency	X		X
Phonatory stenosis			X
Prosodic excess		X	
Articulatory-resonatory incompetence	X		X

Based on Berry WR et al: Dysarthria in Wilson's disease, *J Speech Hear Res* 17:169, 1974a. Only those characteristics that are *not* common to all three dysarthria types are listed (see the original study for a listing of all deviant characteristics).

disorders, aphasia, and MSDs. Our focus here is on the dysarthrias, which occur in approximately one third of the TBI population overall,[134] with approximately 60% having dysarthria early after onset and approximately 10% chronically.[174] Yorkston et al.[172] point out that the dysarthria varies significantly in severity and persistence, may or may not be accompanied by language and other cognitive disorders, and has a more positive outcome in people younger than the age of 20. They also note that although a major portion of recovery tends to occur within the first several months, significant changes in speech can occur over many months or years.

Virtually any type of dysarthria can result from TBI, and mixed dysarthria is probably more common than any isolated dysarthria type. This is a logical consequence of the diffuse or multifocal injuries that are so often associated with the condition, and it is congruent with motor deficits that occur elsewhere in the body, including weakness, spasticity, ataxia, bradykinesia, rigidity, tremor, and dystonia. The locus of CNS lesions is diverse, but it appears that a majority of lesions in people with dysarthria from TBI are subcortical and that the dysarthria is less severe when lesions are predominantly cortical.[89] It

Speech Component	Acoustic or Physiologic Observation
Respiratory	Reduced vital capacity & forced expiratory volumes
	Difficulty coordinating rib cage & abdominal movements
Laryngeal	Increased f_o
	Abnormal vocal fold closing time & phonatory flow rate
	Decreased rate of adduction/abduction
	Increased or decreased subglottal pressure or laryngeal airway resistance
	Increased jitter, shimmer, amplitude perturbation, voice turbulence, & noise/harmonic ratio
	Continuous voicing during connected speech
Velopharyngeal	Increased nasal airflow & nasalance
Articulation, Rate, Prosody	Decreased strength, endurance, speed, & control of tongue & lip movements
	Increased articulatory effort during lip movements
	Syllable lengthening
	Reduced syllable & overall speech rate
	Slow AMR rates, with lengthened syllables & intersyllabic gaps
	Temporal & energy irregularities during AMRs
	Abnormal variability in VOT
	Multiple or missing stop bursts
	Spirantization

AMR, Alternate motion rate; *f_o*, fundamental frequency; *TBI*, traumatic brain injury; *VOT*, voice onset time.
*Note that many of these findings are based on only a few speakers and that not all speakers with TBI exhibit these features. Note also that most, if not all, of these characteristics are not unique to dysarthria in TBI; many may be found in other motor speech disorders or other neurologic or nonneurologic conditions.

is noteworthy that injury is not always confined to the CNS; approximately one third of people with severe TBI can have cranial nerve deficits,[69] sometimes with associated flaccid dysarthria. As with many dysarthria types, all levels of the speech system can be affected but not necessarily to the same degree. Sometimes impairment is evident at only a single level.

Many reports of dysarthria associated with TBI in both children and adults* fail to describe a dysarthria type, but those that do most often document flaccid, spastic, ataxic, hypokinetic, and hyperkinetic types.[22,23,161,172] The reported mixed dysarthrias include spastic-ataxic, flaccid-spastic, flaccid-ataxic, spastic-hypokinetic, hypokinetic-ataxic, ataxic-hyperkinetic (palatal-laryngeal myoclonus), and spastic-hyperkinetic (dystonia and palatal-laryngeal myoclonus). More than two components are sometimes present. Also, because of the complexity of the motor impairments that can occur with TBI, it is not

unusual for a dysarthria type to be described as "undetermined."

A number of physiologic and acoustic studies have confirmed, refined, or modified perceptual findings and inferences about underlying deficits. The findings of these studies are quite variable across speakers within and among studies, at least partly secondary to differences in dysarthria type and subsystem impairments. Most studies have focused on adults, but similar abnormalities have also been demonstrated in children.[150] These findings are summarized in Table 10-8.

At the respiratory level, lower vital capacity, lower forced respiratory volumes, and problems coordinating rib cage and abdominal movements during speech have been documented.[116,149] Such deficits may be related to a tendency to breathe at ungrammatical locations in some dysarthric speakers.[50]

Phonatory dysfunctions are common in TBI[101,147] but not homogeneous. Among patients with various perceived phonatory abnormalities, electrolaryngographic and aerodynamic assessments have demonstrated increased f_o, abnormalities in vocal fold closing time and phonatory flow rate, decreased adduction/abduction rate, and increased or decreased subglottal pressure or laryngeal airway resistance.[104,147-149] Acoustic abnormalities indicative of phonatory problems most often include abnormal values for jitter and shimmer, increased amplitude

*Cahill, Murdoch, and Theodoros (2003) studied 24 children between 5 and 18 years of age with TBI. Sixteen were dysarthric. Various dysarthria types were evident, and severity ranged from mild to severe. The authors concluded that the profile of speech deficits in children with TBI mirrors that of their adult counterparts. Thirty percent of the children with TBI reported by Stierwalt et al.[142] were dysarthric, similar to the incidence reported for adults.

perturbation, voice turbulence, and noise-to-harmonics ratio.[66,101] Several of these physiologic and acoustic abnormalities are suggestive of laryngeal hyperfunction (e.g., strained voice quality) and are consistent with spasticity, but others suggest laryngeal hypofunction (e.g., breathiness) and, possibly, weakness.* Theodoros and Murdoch[148] noted that some intersubject differences on their instrumental measures could reflect compensatory adjustments for laryngeal spasticity or strategies to compensate for problems elsewhere in the system. These appropriate cautions about data interpretation highlight the importance of recognizing that abnormalities heard in dysarthric speakers, as well as abnormalities detected aerodynamically and kinematically, can reflect underlying pathophysiology, as well as, possibly, compensatory responses to the pathophysiology.

Problems at the velopharyngeal level have been documented with aerodynamic measures of nasal airflow, and, in general, they correlate with the perception of hypernasality.[102,103,149,151] For clinicians who rely heavily on perceptual ratings, it is important to note that a perception of hypernasality sometimes can be an artifact of slow speech rate; that is, when hypernasality is perceived in the absence of instrumental findings of increased nasalance, rate of speech tends to be slow.[103]

A number of instrumental studies document abnormalities at the articulatory level. Results vary among affected speakers, but a variety of kinematic and acoustic measures have identified decreased strength, endurance, speed or control of tongue or lip movements, increased effort to achieve normal articulatory (lip) pressures, and syllable lengthening and reduced syllable and overall speech rates.[24,44,45,47,67,114,142,149] In general, tongue movements appear more severely affected than lip or jaw movements.[67] Findings generally suggest that dysarthria in TBI is often associated with reduced speed, force, and endurance of movements, and these abnormalities generally correlate with the perception of slow rate and increased sound, syllable, and word durations. However, physiologic data do not always correlate with all perceptual ratings. Although Stierwalt et al.[142] found that measures of tongue strength and endurance were significantly correlated with perceptual judgments of articulatory imprecision and overall speech defectiveness, other studies have failed to find a strong relationship between perceptual and kinematic measures.[46,105] Goozée, Murdoch, and Theodoros[46] suggested that their dysarthric speakers might have been compensating in different ways for their physiologic impairments, thus weakening the ability of physiologic and perceived articulatory abnormalities to predict each other.

Speech AMRs, analyzed acoustically, can distinguish TBI speakers with dysarthria from normal control speakers.[14] Wang et al.[161] found that TBI speakers had slowed syllable AMR rates that were due to lengthened syllables and, to a lesser extent, lengthened intersyllable gaps. AMR syllable rates were correlated with conversational speech rates, overall dysarthria severity, intelligibility, and prosody. There were also irregularities in temporal and energy parameters within repetition sequences and abnormal variability in VOT. Qualitative analyses revealed evidence of explosive speech quality, breathiness, phonatory instability, multiple or missing stop bursts, continuous voicing, and spirantization. The detection of a large number of motor abnormalities on the basis of AMR data alone may be particularly valuable, because AMRs are probably less susceptible than many other speech tasks to the contaminating influences of the often-present and significant cognitive and linguistic deficits in the TBI population.

---

*It appears that laryngeal abnormalities are less pronounced or occur less frequently in children than adults with TBI. Cahill et al.[23] studied 16 speakers with TBI who were younger than 16 years old at the time of injury. They had normal or only minimally impaired laryngeal function compared to that reported for adults after TBI. The authors noted that the reasons for this are uncertain but could include different dynamics of TBI in children versus adults, better potential for recovery in children, or better ability in children to compensate for impairments because the pediatric larynx is still developing.

Case 10-1

A 68-year-old man presented stating: "I don't know what's the matter with me. If you have a cure, I'd be delighted." During the previous 4 years he had developed impotence, occasional stumbling and falling, dysphagia with aspiration of liquids, and occasional laryngeal stridor. He had recently developed urinary urgency and clumsiness in his hand.

Neurologic examination revealed axial rigidity, poor station, orthostatic hypotension, reduced upward gaze, and dysarthria. EMG revealed a mild, predominantly motor peripheral neuropathy. Autonomic reflex testing identified a generalized autonomic neuropathy. Laryngeal examination revealed left vocal fold paresis.

During speech examination, he noted a 1-year history of a "higher and weaker" voice and a sense that his speech was "clumsy." He reported choking on liquids and having occasional "laryngospasms" during sleep. He was no longer able to play the trumpet or flute because of respiratory fatigue; he stated, "I get out of breath for no good reason." Finally, he complained that his lips were "tight and being stretched across my mouth."

Examination revealed a slight left lower facial droop, equivocal bilateral reduction in tongue strength, a weak cough and glottal coup, and inhalatory laryngeal stridor at phrase boundaries during speech and when inhaling rapidly. His speech was characterized by accelerated rate (1), monopitch and monoloudness (3), imprecise articulation (1), and reduced loudness (1). Pitch was mildly elevated. Vowel prolongation was strained-harsh (1) and unsteady (1,2). Vocal flutter was sometimes evident.

Speech AMRs were irregular (1,2) and occasionally accelerated and "blurred."

The clinician concluded: "mixed dysarthria in which a hypokinetic component is most prominent. His mildly irregular AMRs and vocal unsteadiness suggest an ataxic component. The subtle strained component to his voice could represent a mild spastic component, although there are no other features of spasticity. His laryngeal stridor suggests posterior cricoarytenoid weakness, and his vocal flutter may reflect weakness of laryngeal adductors."

Pulmonary function tests were abnormal but nonspecific. MRI of the head showed moderate cerebellar atrophy and periventricular atrophy.

The neurologist concluded that the patient had MSA that most closely corresponded to Shy-Drager syndrome. Several drugs whose action would stimulate dopamine receptors were recommended. The patient declined speech therapy. He was told that therapy might help maintain intelligibility or could help develop augmentative means of communication if it became necessary.

Commentary. (1) Mixed dysarthria occurs commonly in degenerative neurologic disease. (2) A number of dysarthria types may be perceptually evident in mixed dysarthria. This patient had unequivocal hypokinetic and flaccid dysarthria, probable ataxic dysarthria, and possible spastic dysarthria. All of these types were compatible with the diagnosis of MSA or Shy-Drager syndrome. (3) Many people with obvious dysarthria decline speech therapy when intelligibility and speech efficiency are relatively well maintained.

Case 10-2

A 35-year-old woman with a 10-year history of chronic progressive MS presented for consideration of thalamotomy to control a severe bilateral upper limb tremor. Neurologic examination revealed hyperreflexia; pathologic reflexes; bilateral weakness; spasticity; impaired coordination; nystagmus and optic neuritis; and severe resting, postural, and movement tremor of the upper and lower extremities. Neuropsychological assessment demonstrated severe impairment of new learning and memory and a generalized loss of intellectual abilities.

During speech evaluation, the patient noted a 1-year history of progressive speech difficulty. She had reduced facial and lingual strength. Speech was characterized by slow rate (3), irregular articulatory breakdowns (2), breathy-hoarse voice quality (2), and hypernasality with nasal emission (2). Speech intelligibility was significantly reduced.

The clinician concluded that the patient had a "mixed spastic-ataxic dysarthria of moderate severity."

Unfortunately, the presence of abnormal somatosensory evoked potentials precluded adequate localization within the thalamus for lesion placement to abolish her tremor. Surgery was not recommended. She was not motivated to pursue speech therapy.

Commentary. (1) Mixed dysarthria is not uncommon in people with MS who are dysarthric. Mixed spastic-ataxic dysarthria may be the most common mixed dysarthria encountered in MS. (2) Cognitive deficits may be present in MS, and they can compound difficulties with communication. (3) In spite of reduced intelligibility, not all patients are motivated or interested in speech therapy.

Case 10-3

A 49-year-old woman was referred by her internist because of a 2-month history of speech difficulty that her family interpreted as a response to psychologic stress. During speech evaluation, she admitted to considerable family stress but felt she was handling it well. Her difficulty began with a cold. She described its initial character as "nasal." She had also developed swallowing difficulty characterized by food sticking in her throat after a swallow had been initiated and the need to swallow several more times to get it down. She had recently begun to choke on liquids. She admitted that food occasionally squirreled in her cheeks and that sometimes she needed to use a finger to remove it. She had begun to gag when brushing her teeth or swallowing saliva and reported "crying a lot" even when she did not feel sad. She admitted to some "twitching" around her eyes and left upper lip.

Oral mechanism examination revealed bilateral lower face and tongue weakness and reduced lateral tongue AMRs. Nasal emission was evident during pressure consonant production. Her gag reflex was hyperactive, but her cough and glottal coup were weak. A sucking reflex was present.

Contextual speech was characterized by groaning and strained voice quality (1), reduced loudness (−2), hypernasality (2), imprecise and weak pressure consonants (2,3), reduced rate (2), and short phrases and monopitch and monoloudness (2,3). Speech AMRs were slow but regular (2,3). Vowel prolongation was mildly strained and breathy.

The clinician concluded that the patient had a "mixed flaccid-spastic dysarthria of moderate severity." She was referred for neurologic evaluation. She declined a recommendation for speech therapy because her primary concern at the time was diagnosis.

Neurologic examination showed evidence of hyperreflexia and pathologic reflexes in all limbs and weakness in her face. EMG examination failed to provide evidence for LMN disease in the limbs. A computed tomography (CT) scan of the head was normal.

Her speech continued to worsen. Two months later she was writing to communicate much of the time. She had moderate bilateral lower facial weakness, equivocal jaw weakness, markedly reduced tongue strength, and possible lingual atrophy. The gag reflex was hyperactive, and cough and glottal coup were markedly weak. She had an audible reflexive swallow and inhalatory stridor. Connected speech was characterized by strained-hoarseness (2), reduced loudness (2), hypernasality (2), and imprecise articulation (3). Rate was slow (2,3), and phrases were short, with monopitch and monoloudness (3). Stridor was present at phrase boundaries. Vowel prolongation was strained-harsh-wet. Speech AMRs were slow (3). She had pseudobulbar crying.

Speech therapy was recommended. Speech intelligibility improved for approximately 1 month but then deteriorated. EMG 1 month later demonstrated abnormalities in all limbs, consistent with ALS. The patient communicated fairly efficiently by writing until her death from respiratory and cardiac arrests approximately 6 months later.

Commentary. (1) Dysarthria can be the initial manifestation of neurologic disease and fairly frequently is the presenting sign of ALS. It can progress for some time before diagnosis is confirmed. (2) Initial signs of neurologic disease are sometimes misinterpreted as responses to psychologic stress. When the symptom is speech difficulty, careful examination can help distinguish a motor speech disorder from a psychogenic speech disturbance. (3) Mixed spastic-flaccid dysarthria is the "prototypic" mixed dysarthria of ALS. Its effects on intelligibility can be dramatic and often lead to a need for augmentative/alternative forms of communication. (4) Rate of decline can be quite rapid in some people with ALS.

Case 10-4

A 77-year-old woman developed difficulty with speech, swallowing, and right leg and left arm weakness. She was subsequently hospitalized for an apparent exacerbation of longstanding myasthenia gravis. Her prior symptoms of myasthenia gravis were predominantly ophthalmic, and the disease had been well controlled with Mestinon. Steroids and an increase in Mestinon dose did not help. Her lack of response to these treatments raised the possibility that myasthenia gravis might not be the only cause of her new difficulties.

During speech evaluation, the patient reported a 3-month history of speech and swallowing problems. She was frequently choking, with occasional nasal regurgitation. She also complained of increased ease of crying, even when she did not feel sad. She did not complain of dramatic worsening of her speech with extended talking.

Examination revealed mild jaw and lower facial weakness. The tongue was weak bilaterally, but fasciculations and atrophy were not evident. Palatal movement during vowel prolongation was minimal. A gag reflex could not be elicited. A sucking reflex was present. She had a prominent audible reflexive swallow. Her speech was characterized by slow rate (3), reduced phrase length, strained-harsh voice quality (3), hypernasality (3) with audible nasal emission on pressure sounds, and monopitch and monoloudness (3). Speech AMRs were slow (3), slower than expected for her degree of weakness. Vowel prolongation was strained-hoarse and occasionally characterized by flutter.

The clinician concluded that the patient had: "mixed spastic-flaccid dysarthria. I believe the spastic compo-nent predominates and that respiratory weakness reflects the most significant flaccid component. The spastic component and her pseudobulbar affect are suggestive of UMN involvement and cannot be explained on the basis of weakness secondary to myasthenia gravis. On the basis of this examination, it is not possible to determine if the LMN component of her dysarthria is secondary to neuromuscular junction disease or some other disturbance in LMN function. However, there is no significant deterioration of her speech with stress testing."

Based on the speech evaluation, EMG studies were conducted. They failed to show evidence of ALS. A CT scan of the head showed moderate diffuse cerebral and cerebellar atrophy and a small lacunar infarct in the left basal ganglia. The neurologist concluded that the patient's difficulties were probably due to a combination of her myasthenia gravis and pseudobulbar palsy of undetermined origin. However, multiple small infarctions were suspected as the cause of her pseudobulbar palsy.

Commentary. (1) By definition, mixed spastic-flaccid dysarthria identifies the presence of upper and lower motor neuron dysfunction. In this case, the speech diagnosis helped establish that myasthenia gravis could not be the sole explanation for the patient's difficulties. (2) Mixed dysarthrias can result from the cooccurrence of two or more diseases. In this case, the patient had a confirmed diagnosis of myasthenia gravis and, possibly, vascular disease leading to multiple CNS strokes.

Case 10-5

A 55-year-old woman presented with a 9-month history of cervical pain and hoarseness following a motor vehicle accident. Laryngeal examination was normal. She was referred to speech pathology for evaluation of her hoarseness.

During speech evaluation, the patient noted that her dysphonia developed immediately after her motor vehicle accident and that vocal fold polyps were identified and removed by laser 4 months later. Her voice gradually returned to normal over the next few months, but hoarseness then returned, with an occasional "slurry" quality to her speech. She denied swallowing difficulty or problems with emotional expressiveness.

Examination revealed equivocal lingual weakness but bilateral lingual fasciculations. There was significant nasal emission during production of pressure-filled sentences, although the palate was symmetric and mobile. Speech was characterized by hypernasality (1), imprecise articulation (0,1), and hoarse-rough voice quality (1,2) with occasional diplophonia. Vowel prolongation was breathy-hoarse-rough-strained (1). Speech AMRs were normal, except for equivocal slowing on "tuh." There was a subtle vocal "flutter" during vowel prolongation.

The clinician concluded: "I believe the patient has a flaccid dysarthria that includes the cranial nerve X and cranial nerve XII. A component of her dysphonia may

Case 10-5—cont'd

indeed be due to excessive musculoskeletal tension in the laryngeal area, perhaps due to efforts to compensate for laryngeal trauma or weakness. However, findings are very suspicious for cranial nerve X and XII weakness. Neurologic examination is strongly recommended."

On neurologic examination, in addition to her speech and cranial nerve findings, phrenic nerve weakness was suspected, because she complained of shortness of breath when lying supine. On EMG, the phrenic nerve was normal, but mild neurogenic changes in the tongue bilaterally, of indeterminate duration and origin, were noted.

Eight months later the patient returned for follow-up assessment. She had had increased episodes of choking, and it had become "more difficult to form words and letters" when speaking. She complained that her swallow was often audible and that she swallowed more slowly, and that "when I cry my mouth wants to start laughing." Examination revealed bilateral chin fasciculations, lower facial weakness, lingual weakness, fasciculations and atrophy, nasal escape during pressure sound production, and a weak cough and glottal coup. A sucking reflex and subtle "on the verge of crying" facial expression were present. Speech was characterized by slow rate (1,2), excess and equal stress (1,2), hypernasality with nasal emission (1), vocal "flutter"; strained-harsh voice quality (1), and reduced pitch (2). Vowel prolongation was characterized by flutter and a rough, strained voice quality. Speech AMRs were slow (1). Speech intelligibility was normal.

The clinician concluded: "mixed flaccid-spastic dysarthria, with clear worsening of speech difficulty and the emergence of a spastic component since she was last seen. Strongly suspect mixed bilateral upper and lower motor neuron dysfunction." The patient denied a need for speech therapy, and the clinician concurred. She was advised to seek reevaluation if her speech problems worsened.

Subsequent neurologic evaluation identified the presence of diffuse hyperreflexia and pathologic reflexes and weakness in her upper and lower extremities. EMG showed widespread denervation in three extremities, as well as the tongue, consistent with ALS.

Commentary. (1) Dysphonia may be the first sign of neurologic disease. It can occur simultaneously with or be mistaken for vocal abuse or musculoskeletal tension-related dysphonias. (2) Dysarthria associated with ALS does not always present initially as a mixed dysarthria. (3) When dysarthria is present in ALS, it is usually mixed flaccid-spastic in character eventually.

Case 10-6

A 51-year-old woman presented with a 13-year history of PD with marked fluctuations in her neurologic signs and symptoms during her parkinsonian medication cycle. Neurologic examination revealed dysarthria, right arm dystonia and rigidity, bradykinesia, and left arm and leg tremor.

The patient was seen for speech evaluation 1.5 hours after her last Sinemet dose. Severe limb, torso, and head dyskinesias were present. The oral mechanism was normal in size, strength, and symmetry. Dyskinetic movements of her jaw, face, and tongue were apparent but not prominent during speech. Her speech was characterized by accelerated rate (2,3), reduced loudness (1,2), imprecise articulation (1,2), monopitch and monoloudness (1,2), variable rate (1,2), and occasional inappropriate silences (1). Vowel prolongation was unsteady and intermittently mildly strained. Speech AMRs were irregular (1). Speech intelligibility was mildly reduced.

The clinician concluded that the patient had a "moderately severe mixed hypokinetic-hyperkinetic dysarthria, with the hypokinetic component predominating." It was recognized that her speech probably fluctuated with Sinemet effects, and the patient was quite certain that it was more difficult to talk when her medication wore off. Speech therapy was undertaken, and the patient was quite successful in slowing her speech rate, with subsequent improvement in intelligibility and quality. With some adjustments in medication dosage and timing, there were fewer fluctuations in her speech and other neurologic signs.

Commentary. (1) A mixed hypokinetic-hyperkinetic dysarthria can occur in PD, reflecting the direct effects of the disease on speech and its interaction with medication effects. (2) Fluctuations in the severity and nature of dysarthria in people with PD can occur, sometimes dramatically, as a result of "on and off" effects associated with fluctuating medication effects. (3) Careful monitoring of speech can be a useful way to monitor medication effects in certain neurologic diseases.

Case 10-7

A 61-year-old woman presented with a 6-year history of progressive coordination difficulty and 18-month history of dysarthria. Clinical neurologic examination confirmed the presence of gait ataxia, upper limb incoordination, slowed and ataxic eye movements, and dysarthria.

During speech evaluation the patient described speaking as a "real effort." She felt she had to speak more slowly to be understood but admitted that she was unable to talk more rapidly. She had no chewing or swallowing complaints and denied drooling or difficulty with emotional control. Oral mechanism examination was normal, except that her cough and glottal coup were poorly coordinated. Speech was characterized by slow rate (2); irregular articulatory breakdowns (2); excess and equal stress (2); abnormal alterations in pitch, loudness, and duration of words and syllables (3); and strained voice quality (1). Vowel prolongation was hoarse and unsteady. Speech AMRs were slow and irregular (2).

The clinician concluded that the patient had a "mixed dysarthria, predominantly ataxic, but with a mild spastic component." Intelligibility was minimally compromised, and the patient denied a need or desire for speech therapy. She was advised to pursue reassessment if her speech difficulty worsened.

Head CT scan demonstrated cerebellar and pontine atrophy. The neurologist concluded that the patient had OPCA. The patient's mother probably had a similar disease.

Commentary. (1) OPCA (MSA-C) is often associated with a mixed dysarthria, in this case a mixed ataxic-spastic dysarthria with the ataxic component predominating. This mix logically reflects the sites of prominent degeneration in MSA-C, and in this case it served as a confirmatory sign for the neurologic diagnosis. (2) Mixed ataxic-spastic dysarthria is not diagnostic of any particular neurologic disease. As in most cases, the speech diagnosis can contribute to localization and provide support for neurologic diagnosis.

Case 10-8

A 64-year-old woman with von Hippel-Lindau syndrome (defined in Chapter 6) was referred by a geneticist for speech assessment and recommendations. Her speech difficulty began following neurosurgery for removal of multiple cerebellar hemangioblastomas 2 years previously. She had a vocal fold paralysis as a complication of her neurosurgery.

She described her speech as sounding "drunk." She denied difficulty with chewing, swallowing, or saliva control. Examination revealed subtle myoclonic twitches in the right chin and tongue. The tongue was normal in strength and range of motion, and there was no atrophy or fasciculations. Palatal myoclonus was evident at rest and during phonation. Myoclonic movements in the external neck were also apparent. There were no pathologic oral reflexes. Her speech was characterized by: reduced rate (−1,2); brief voice interruptions or near-interruptions on a periodic basis, at a rate of approximately 2 to 4 Hz, consistent with myoclonus; infrequent subtle hypernasality and hyponasality; irregular articulatory breakdowns (1); and inhalatory stridor (2). Vowel prolongation was characterized by myoclonic variability at 2.5 to 3 Hz (measured acoustically). Speech AMRs were mildly irregular. Intelligibility was normal in the quiet one-to-one setting.

The clinician concluded: "mixed ataxic-hyperkinetic dysarthria. The hyperkinetic component is represented by a palatal laryngeal myoclonus. This latter problem is, in all likelihood, what is most bothersome to the patient.

She also has some inhalatory stridor, about which she does not complain, which could reflect the laryngeal myoclonus and/or a residual of her vocal fold paralysis."

The nature of the patient's speech difficulty was reviewed in detail with her, with particular attention paid to having her understand her palatal-laryngeal myoclonus. She was counseled that the myoclonus was not subject to behavioral management. Although Botox injection might have helped to manage palatal-laryngeal myoclonus in isolation, it was not recommended in her case because of the other components of her dysarthria, which were felt to put her at greater than average risk for significant dysphagia. A number of suggestions were made regarding strategies to maximize comprehensibility of speech. Formal therapy was not recommended because she was otherwise compensating well for her dysarthria.

Commentary. (1) Mixed dysarthria sometimes has more than a single cause. In this case, the dysarthria probably reflected the effects of the underlying disease as well as complications arising from the neurosurgery that was done to treat it. (2) Some speech abnormalities can have more than a single cause. The patient's stridor may have been a product of vocal fold weakness, laryngeal myoclonus, or a combination of the two. (3) Patient education is an important component of management, as much to promote understanding of why certain things cannot or should not be done as to promote understanding of what can be done.

Case 10-9

A 45-year-old man presented to his family physician complaining of a several-month history of speech difficulty. A general medical examination was normal, and it was thought that the patient's symptoms reflected anxiety. Two weeks later, he called to report that his speech was getting worse. He was referred for neurologic assessment, which was judged normal, including speech. However, because of his complaint, a speech pathology consultation was requested. Testing for myasthenia gravis was also ordered; the results were negative.

The patient was seen 2 weeks later for speech evaluation. He reported an approximately 5-month history of difficulty articulating words normally. He felt the problem had worsened. Only within the past several weeks had his wife agreed that there was some "thickness" in his speech.

An oral mechanism examination was normal. His speech was characterized by nonspecific hoarseness with occasional pitch breaks, equivocal hypernasality, and occasional lingual articulatory imprecision, especially for lingual affricates. Speech AMRs were equivocally slow but regular. Vowel prolongation was rough-hoarse with some vocal flutter. There was a trace of nasal airflow on a mirror held at the nares during repetition of sentences with pressure consonant sounds. During 4.5 minutes of continuous reading, there was no dramatic deterioration of voice or speech.

The clinician concluded that the patient had a subtle dysarthria of undetermined type, although with features suggestive of weakness and possible spasticity. Because the patient felt that his dysarthria was often at its worst later in the day, he was asked to call the clinician at home in the evening if he felt that his speech problem was more apparent.

The patient called the clinician several days later in the evening. His speech characteristics were similar to those noted during formal evaluation but worse and strongly suggestive of mixed spastic-flaccid dysarthria. When that observation was communicated to the referring neurologist, additional tests were ordered. Unfortunately, EMG revealed fasciculations and fibrillations in the left upper extremity, left tongue, and bilateral thoracic paraspinal musculature. An MRI was normal. A tentative diagnosis of ALS was made. Subsequent evaluation failed to identify other possible causes for his speech difficulty, and a definite diagnosis of ALS was eventually made. A session of speech therapy established that he would benefit from use of an amplifier in his work as a teacher, primarily to minimize fatigue. Arrangements were made to follow him on an as-needed basis to help manage his communication difficulties.

Commentary. (1) Changes in speech may herald neurologic disease. (2) Subtle changes in speech, in the absence of other symptoms, are fairly frequently misidentified as a reflection of stress or anxiety. (3) Speech changes can be subtle enough to defy a confident, specific speech diagnosis by an experienced clinician, but they may nonetheless be sufficient to warrant a diagnosis of dysarthria and neurologic disease. (4) Accurate recognition of dysarthria type can contribute significantly to a neurologist's decisions about the specifics of a neurologic workup. (5) Early identification of speech deficits in degenerative neurologic disease can establish strategies to maintain intelligible, efficient verbal communication, as well as anticipate and prepare for future communication needs.

SUMMARY

1. Mixed dysarthrias reflect various combinations of individual dysarthria types. They occur more frequently than single dysarthria types, highlighting the fact that dysarthria often reflects damage to more than one component of the speech motor system.
2. Mixed dysarthrias can be caused by many conditions that damage more than one portion of the nervous system, but degenerative diseases are probably their most frequent cause. Single strokes and neoplasms leading to mixed dysarthrias tend to occur in the posterior fossa. Mixed dysarthrias resulting from toxic-metabolic conditions, infection, multiple strokes, and trauma may be the product of diffuse or multifocal damage in many portions of the nervous system.
3. Because a number of diseases are associated with damage to specific parts of the nervous system, the types of mixed dysarthrias encountered in them are somewhat predictable. This is best exemplified by the mixed spastic-flaccid dysarthria that is classically associated with ALS. It should be noted, however, that although most mixed dysarthrias help identify the locus of their causative underlying lesions, they do not, by themselves, usually indicate their specific etiology.

4. Spastic dysarthria is probably the most frequently occurring type of dysarthria encountered within mixed dysarthrias. Flaccid and ataxic dysarthrias also occur frequently. Hypokinetic, hyperkinetic, and unilateral UMN dysarthrias are also encountered in mixed dysarthrias but less frequently than the other dysarthria types.

5. Intelligibility is often affected in mixed dysarthrias. Patients with mixed dysarthrias, excluding those with ALS, frequently also have associated cognitive deficits.

6. Even though mixed dysarthrias reflect damage to more than one component of the motor system, they are fairly frequently the presenting complaints or among the earliest manifestations of neurologic disease. Thus accurate recognition of the components of mixed dysarthrias can aid the localization and diagnosis of neurologic disease and may contribute to the medical and behavioral management of affected individuals.

References

1. Ackermann H, Hertrich I, Hehr T: Oral diadokokinesis in neurological dysarthrias, Folia Phoniatr Logop 47:15, 1995.
2. Adams RD, Victor M: Principles of neurology, New York, 1991, McGraw-Hill.
3. Alusi SH et al: A study of tremor in multiple sclerosis, Brain 124:720, 2001.
4. Aronson AE: Clinical voice disorders, New York, 1990, Thieme.
5. Aronson AE et al: Rapid voice tremor, or "flutter," in amyotrophic lateral sclerosis, Ann Otol Rhinol Laryngol 101:511, 1992.
6. Bannister R et al: Laryngeal abductor paralysis in multiple system atrophy. A report on three necropsied cases, with observations on the laryngeal muscles and the nuclei ambigui, Brain 104:351, 1981.
7. Benarroch EE, Schmeichel AM, Parisi JE: Preservation of branchimotor neurons of the nucleus ambiguus in multiple system atrophy, Neurology 60:115, 2003.
8. Berger JR: Immunodeficiency diseases. In Noseworthy JH, editor: Neurological therapeutics: principles and practice, vol 1, New York, 2003, Martin Dunitz.
9. Bergeron C et al: Unusual clinical presentations of cortical basal ganglionic degeneration, Ann Neurol 40:893, 1996.
10. Berry WR et al: Dysarthria in Wilson's disease, J Speech Hear Res 17:169, 1974a.
11. Berry WR et al: Effects of penicillamine therapy and low-copper diet on dysarthria in Wilson's disease (hepatolenticular degeneration), Mayo Clin Proc 49:405, 1974b.
12. Beukelman DR, Kraft GH, Freal J: Expressive communication disorders in persons with multiple sclerosis: a survey, Arch Phys Med Rehabil 66:675, 1985.
13. Blake ML et al: Speech and language disorders associated with corticobasal degeneration, J Med Speech-Lang Pathol 11:131, 2003.
14. Blumberger J, Sullivan SJ, Clement N: Diadokokinetic rate in persons with traumatic brain injury, Brain Inj 9:797, 1995.
15. Boesch SM et al: Dystonia in multiple system atrophy, J Neurol Neurosurg Psychiatry 72:300, 2002.
16. Boeve B et al: Progressive nonfluent aphasia and subsequent aphasic dementia associated with atypical progressive supranuclear palsy pathology, Eur Neurol 49:72, 2003.
17. Boeve BF: Corticobasal degeneration. In Adler CH, Ahlskog JE, editors: Parkinson's disease and movement disorders: diagnosis and treatment guidelines for the practicing physician, Totowa, NJ, 2000, Humana Press.
18. Boeve BF et al: Dysarthria and apraxia of speech associated with FK-506 (tacrolimus), Mayo Clin Proc 71:969, 1996.
19. Bower JH: Multiple system atrophy. In Adler CH, Ahlskog JE, editors: Parkinson's disease and movement disorders: diagnosis and treatment guidelines for the practicing physician, Totowa, NJ, 2000, Humana Press.
20. Bower JH et al: Incidence of progressive supranuclear palsy and multiple system atrophy in Olmsted County, Minnesota, 1976 to 1990, Neurology 49:1284, 1997.
21. Bromberg M: Accelerating the diagnosis of amyotrophic lateral sclerosis, Neurologist 5:63, 1999.
22. Cahill LM, Murdoch BE, Theodoros DG: Perceptual and instrumental analysis of laryngeal function after traumatic brain injury in childhood, J Head Trauma Rehabil 18:268, 2003.
23. Cahill LM et al: Perceptual analysis of speech following traumatic brain injury in childhood, Brain Inj, 16:415, 2002.
24. Campbell TF, Dollaghan CA: Speaking rate, articulatory speed, and linguistic processing in children and adolescents with severe traumatic brain injury, J Speech Hear Res 38:864, 1995.
25. Carrow E et al: Deviant speech characteristics in motor neuron disease, Arch Otolaryngol 100:212, 1974.
26. Caruso AJ, Burton EK: Temporal acoustic measures of dysarthria associated with amyotrophic lateral sclerosis, J Speech Hear Res 30:80, 1987.
27. Commichau C: Hypoxic-ischemic encephalopathy. In Noseworthy JH, editor: Neurological therapeutics: principles and practice, vol 1, New York, 2003, Martin Dunitz.
28. Darley FL, Aronson AE, Brown JR: Clusters of deviant speech dimensions in the dysarthrias, J Speech Hear Res 12:462, 1969a.
29. Darley FL, Aronson AE, Brown JR: Differential diagnostic patterns of dysarthria, J Speech Hear Res 12:246, 1969b.
30. Darley FL, Aronson AE, Goldstein NP: Dysarthria in multiple sclerosis, J Speech Hear Res 15:229-245, 1972.
31. Delorey R, Leeper HA, Hudson AJ: Measures of velopharyngeal functioning in subgroups of individuals with amyotrophic lateral sclerosis, J Med Speech-Lang Pathol 7:19, 1999.

32. DePaul R, Brooks R: Multiple orofacial indices in amy-
    otrophic lateral sclerosis, J Speech Hear Res 36:1158,
    1993.

33. DePaul R et al: A nine-year progression of speech and
    swallowing dysfunction in a case of ALS, J Med Speech
    Lang Pathol 7:161, 1999.

34. DePaul R et al: Hypoglossal, trigeminal, and facial
    motoneuron involvement in amyotrophic lateral sclero-
    sis, Neurology 38:281, 1988.

35. Duvoisin RC: The olivopontocerebellar atrophies. In
    Marsden CD, Fahn S, editors: Movement disorders, vol
    2, Boston, 1987, Butterworth-Heinemann.

36. Dworkin JP, Aronson AE, and Mulder DW: Tongue force
    in normals and dysarthric patients with amyotrophic
    lateral sclerosis, J Speech Hear Res 23:828, 1980.

37. Farmakides MN, Boone DR: Speech problems of
    patients with multiple sclerosis, J Speech Hear Disord
    25:385, 1960.

38. Frattali C, Duffy JR: Characterizing and assessing
    speech and language disturbances. To appear in Litvan
    I, editor: Atypical parkinsonian disorders: clinical and
    research aspects, Totowa, NJ, (in press), Humana Press.

39. Frattali CM, Sonies BC: Speech and swallowing distur-
    bances in corticobasal degeneration. In Litvan I, Goetz
    CG, Lang AE, editors: Advances in neurology, corti-
    cobasal degeneration and related disorders, vol 82,
    Philadelphia, 2000, Lippincott Williams & Wilkins.

40. Frattali CM et al: Yes/no reversals as neurobehavioral
    sequela: a disorder of language, praxis or inhibitory
    control? Eur J Neurol 2003;103, 2003.

41. Frattali CM et al: Language disturbances in corti-
    cobasal degeneration, Neurology 54:990, 2000.

42. Gentil M: Dysarthria in Friedreich disease, Brain Lang
    38:438, 1990.

43. Gilman S, Kluin D: Perceptual analysis of speech dis-
    orders in Friedreich disease and olivopontocerebellar
    atrophy. In Bloedel JR et al, editors: Cerebellar func-
    tions, New York, 1984, Springer-Verlag.

44. Goozée JV, Murdoch BE, Theodoros DG: Elec-
    tropalatographic assessment of tongue-to-palate con-
    tacts exhibited in dysarthria following traumatic brain
    injury: spatial characteristics, J Med Speech Lang
    Pathol 11:115, 2003.

45. Goozée JV, Murdoch BE, Theodoros DG: Interlabial
    contact pressures exhibited in dysarthria following trau-
    matic brain injury during speech and nonspeech tasks,
    Folia Phoniatr Logop 54:177, 2002.

46. Goozée JV, Murdoch BE, Theodoros DG: Physiological
    assessment of tongue function in dysarthria following
    traumatic brain injury, Logoped Phoniatr Vocol 26:51,
    2001.

47. Goozée JV et al: Kinematic analysis of tongue move-
    ments in dysarthria following traumatic brain injury
    using electromagnetic articulography, Brain Inj 14:153,
    2000.

48. Grafman J et al: Frontal lobe function in progressive
    supranuclear palsy, Arch Neurol 47:553, 1990.

49. Gwinn-Hardy K: Wilson's disease. In Adler CH, Ahlskog
    JE, editors: Parkinson's disease and movement
    disorders: diagnosis and treatment guidelines for the
    practicing physician, Totowa, NJ, 2000, Humana
    Press.

50. Hammen VL, Yorkston KM: Respiratory patterning and
    variability in dysarthric speech, J Med Speech-Lang
    Pathol 2:253, 1994.

51. Hartelius L, Buder EH, Strand EA: Long-term phona-
    tory instability in individuals with multiple sclerosis, J
    Speech Lang Hear Res 40:1056, 1997.

52. Hartelius L, Lillvik M: Lip and tongue function differ-
    ently affected in individuals with multiple sclerosis,
    Folia Phoniatr Logop 55:1, 2003.

53. Hartelius L, Runmarker B, Andersen O: Prevalence and
    characteristics of dysarthria in a multiple-sclerosis inci-
    dence cohort: relation to neurological data, Folia Pho-
    niatr Logop 52:160, 2000.

54. Hartelius L et al: Temporal speech characteristics of
    individuals with multiple sclerosis and ataxic
    dysarthria: 'scanning speech' revisited, Folia Phoniatr
    Logop 52:228, 2000.

55. Hartman DE, O'Neill BP: Progressive dysfluency, dys-
    phagia, dysarthria: a case of olivopontocerebellar
    atrophy. In Yorkston KM, Beukelman DR, editors:
    Recent advances in dysarthria, Boston, 1989, College-
    Hill.

56. Hayashi M et al: Loss of large myelinated nerve fibers
    of the recurrent laryngeal nerve in patients with multi-
    ple system atrophy and vocal cord palsy, J Neurol Neu-
    rosurg Psychiatry 62:234, 1997.

57. Henderscheê D, Stam J, Derix MMA: Aphemia as a first
    symptom of multiple sclerosis, J Neurol Neurosurg Psy-
    chiatry 50:499, 1987.

58. Herndon RM: Multiple sclerosis. In Johnson RT, editor:
    Current therapy in neurologic disease, Philadelphia,
    1990, BC Decker.

59. Herndon RM: Pathology and pathophysiology of multi-
    ple sclerosis, Semin Neurol 5:99, 1985.

60. Herndon RM, Brooks B: Misdiagnosis of multiple scle-
    rosis, Semin Neurol 5:94, 1985.

61. Hirose H, Kiritani S, Sawashima M: Patterns of
    dysarthric movement in patients with amyotrophic
    lateral sclerosis and pseudobulbar palsy, Folia Phoni-
    atr 34:106, 1982.

62. Hook CC et al: Multifocal inflammatory leukoen-
    cephalopathy with 5-fluorouracil and levamisole, Ann
    Neurol 31:262, 1992.

63. Howard RS et al: Respiratory involvement in multiple
    sclerosis, Brain 115:479, 1992.

64. Ikeda K et al: Corticobasal degeneration with primary
    progressive aphasia and accentuated cortical lesion in
    superior temporal gyrus: case report and review, Acta
    Neuropathol 92:534, 1996.

65. Isono S et al: Pathogenesis of laryngeal narrowing in
    patients with multiple system atrophy, J Physiol
    536:237, 2001.

66. Jaeger M et al: Dysphonia subsequent to severe trau-
    matic brain injury: comparative perceptual, acoustic
    and electroglottographic analysis, Folia Phoniatr
    Logop 53:326, 2001.

67. Jaeger M et al: Speech disorders following severe trau-
    matic brain injury: kinematic analysis of syllable repe-
    titions using electromagnetic articulography, Folia
    Phoniatr Logop 52:187, 2000.

68. Jankovic J: Progressive supranuclear palsy, clinical and
    pharmacological update, Neurol Clin 2:473, 1984.

69. Jennett B, Teasdale G: Management of head injuries, Philadelphia, 1981, FA Davis.

70. Joanette J, Dudley JG: Dysarthric symptomatology of Friedreich's ataxia, Brain Lang 10:39, 1980.

71. Kent JF et al: Quantitative description of the dysarthria in women with amyotrophic lateral sclerosis, J Speech Hear Res 35:723, 1992.

72. Kent RD: Laryngeal dysfunction in neurological disease: amyotrophic lateral sclerosis, Parkinson's disease, and stroke, J Med Speech-Lang Pathol 2:157, 1994.

73. Kent RD, Reed C: The acoustic analysis of speech, San Diego, 1992, Singular.

74. Kent RD et al: The dysarthrias: speech-voice profiles, related dysfunctions, and neuropathology, J Med Speech-Lang Pathol 6:165, 1998.

75. Kent RD et al: Speech deterioration in amyotrophic lateral sclerosis: a case study, J Speech Hear Res 34:1269, 1991.

76. Kent RD et al: Impairment of speech intelligibility in men with amyotrophic lateral sclerosis, J Speech Hear Disord 55:721, 1990.

77. Kent RD et al: Relationship between speech intelligibility and the slope of second-formant transitions in dysarthric subjects, Clin Linguist Phon 3:347, 1989.

78. Kimmel DW, Schutt AJ: Multifocal leukoencephalopathy: occurrence during 5-fluorouracil and levamisole therapy and resolution after discontinuation of chemotherapy, Mayo Clin Proc 68:363, 1993.

79. Klasner ER, Yorkston KM: Dysarthria in ALS: a method for obtaining the everyday listener's perception, J Med Speech-Lang Pathol 8:261, 2000.

80. Klasner ER, Yorkston KM, Strand EA: Patterns of perceptual features in speakers with ALS: a preliminary study of prominence and intelligibility consideration, J Med Speech-Lang Pathol 7:117, 1999.

81. Kluin K et al: Characteristics of the dysarthria of multiple system atrophy, Arch Neurol 53:545, 1996.

82. Kluin KJ et al: Neuropathological correlates of dysarthria in progressive supranuclear palsy, Arch Neurol 58:265, 2001.

83. Kluin KJ et al: Perceptual analysis of speech disorders in progressive supranuclear palsy, Neurology 43:563, 1993.

84. Kurtzke JF: Risk factors in amyotrophic lateral sclerosis. In Rowland LP, editor: Advances in neurology, vol 56, New York, 1991, Raven Press.

85. Langmore SE, Lehman ME: Physiologic deficits in the orofacial system underlying dysarthria in amyotrophic lateral sclerosis, J Speech Hear Res 37:28, 1994.

86. Lebrun Y, Devreux F, Rousseau J: Language and speech in a patient with a clinical diagnosis of progressive supranuclear palsy, Brain Lang 27:247, 1986.

87. Le Dorze et al: A comparison of the prosodic characteristics of the speech of people with Parkinson's disease and Friedreich's ataxia with neurologically normal speakers, Folia Phoniatr Logop 50:1, 1998.

88. Lees AJ: The Steele-Richardson-Olszewski syndrome (progressive supranuclear palsy). In Marsden CD, Fahn S, editors: Movement disorders, vol 2, Boston, 1987, Butterworth-Heinemann.

89. Lefkowitz D, Netsell R: Correlation of clinical deficits with anatomical lesions: postraumatic speech disorders and MRI, J Med Speech-Lang Pathol 2:1, 1994.

90. Lehman Blake M et al: Speech and language disorders associated with corticobasal degeneration, J Med Speech-Lang Pathol 11:131, 2003.

91. Lethlean BJ, Murdoch BE: Language dysfunction in progressive multifocal leukoencephalopathy: a case study, J Med Speech-Lang Pathol 1:27, 1993.

92. Lethlean JB, Murdoch BE: Language problems in multiple sclerosis, J Med Speech-Lang Pathol 1:47, 1993.

93. Linebaugh C: The dysarthrias of Shy-Drager syndrome, J Speech Hear Disord 44:55, 1979.

94. Litvan I: Progressive supranuclear palsy: staring into the past, moving into the future, Neurologist 4:13, 1998.

95. Litvan I, Sastry N, Sonies BC: Characterizing swallowing abnormalities in progressive supranuclear palsy, Neurology 48:1654, 1997.

96. Lu FL, Duffy JR, Maraganore D: Neuroclinical and speech characteristics in progressive supranuclear palsy and Parkinson's disease: a retrospective study. Paper presented at the Conference on Motor Speech, Boulder, Colo, 1992.

97. Mancall EL: Central pontine myelinolysis. In LP Rowland, editor: Merritt's textbook of neurology, Philadelphia, 1989, Lea & Febiger.

98. Massman PJ et al: Prevalence and correlates of neuropsychological deficits in amyotrophic lateral sclerosis, J Neurol Neurosurg Psychiatry 61:450, 1996.

99. Matthews WB et al: McAlpine's multiple sclerosis, New York, 1985, Churchill Livingstone.

100. McDonald WI et al: Recommended diagnostic criteria for multiple sclerosis: guidelines from the international panel on the diagnosis of multiple sclerosis, Ann Neurol 50:121, 2001.

101. McHenry M: Acoustic characteristics of voice after severe traumatic brain injury, Laryngoscope 110:1157, 2000.

102. McHenry M: Velopharyngeal airway resistance disorders after traumatic brain injury, Arch Phys Med Rehabil 79:545, 1998.

103. McHenry MA: Aerodynamic, acoustic, and perceptual measures of nasality following traumatic brain injury, Brain Inj 13:281, 1999.

104. McHenry MA: Laryngeal airway resistance following traumatic brain injury. In Robin DA, Yorkston KM, Beukelman DR, editors: Disorders of motor speech: assessment, treatment, and clinical characterization, Baltimore, 1996, Paul H Brookes.

105. McHenry MA et al: Intelligibility and nonspeech orofacial strength and force control following traumatic brain injury, J Speech Hear Res 37:1271, 1994.

106. McNeil MR, Duffy JR: Primary progressive aphasia. In Chapey R, editor: Language intervention strategies in aphasia and related disorders, ed 4, Philadelphia, 2001, Lippincott Williams & Wilkins.

107. Merson RM, Rolnick MI: Speech-language pathology and dysphagia in multiple sclerosis, Phys Med Rehabil Clin N Am 9:631, 1998.

108. Metter EJ, Hanson WR: Dysarthria in progressive supranuclear palsy. In Moore CA, Yorkston KM, Beukelman DR, editors: Dysarthria and apraxia of speech:

perspectives on management, Baltimore, 1991, Paul H Brookes.

109. Mimura M et al: Corticobasal degeneration presenting with nonfluent primary progressive aphasia: a clinico-pathological study, J Neurol Sci 183:19, 2001.

110. Mulder DW: Clinical limits of amyotrophic lateral sclerosis. In Rowland LP, editor: Advances in neurology, vol 36, human motor neuron diseases, New York, 1982, Raven Press.

111. Müller J et al: Progression of dysarthria and dysphagia in postmortem-confirmed parkinsonian disorders, Arch Neurol 58:259, 2001.

112. Mulligan et al: Intelligibility and the acoustic characteristics of speech in amyotrophic lateral sclerosis (ALS), J Speech Hear Res 37:496, 1994.

113. Murdoch BE, Gardiner F, Theodoros DG: Electropalatographic assessment of articulatory dysfunction in multiple sclerosis: a case study, J Med Speech-Lang Pathol 8:359, 2000.

114. Murdoch BE, Goozée JV: EMA analysis of tongue function in children with dysarthria following traumatic brain injury, Brain Inj 17:79, 2003.

115. Murdoch BE et al: Lip and tongue function in multiple sclerosis: a physiological analysis, Motor Control 2:148, 1998.

116. Murdoch BE et al: Abnormal patterns of speech breathing in dysarthric speakers following severe closed head injury, Brain Inj 7:295, 1993.

117. Noseworthy JH, Hartung HP: Multiple sclerosis and related conditions. In Noseworthy JH, editor: Neurological therapeutics: principles and practice, vol 1, New York, 2003, Martin Dunitz.

118. Oder W et al: Neurologic and neuropsychiatric spectrum of Wilson's disease: a prospective study of 45 cases, J Neurol 238:281, 1991.

119. Olmos-Lau N, Ginsberg MD, Geller JB: Aphasia in multiple sclerosis, Neurology 27:623, 1977.

120. Ozsancak C, Auzou P, Hannequin D: Dysarthria and orofacial apraxia in corticobasal degeneration, Mov Disord 15:905, 2000.

121. Pellecchia MT et al: Clinical presentation and treatment of Wilson's disease: a single centre experience, Eur Neurol 50:48, 2003.

122. Petersen RC, Kokmen E: Cognitive and psychiatric abnormalities in multiple sclerosis, Mayo Clin Proc 64:657, 1989.

123. Podoll K, Schwarz M, Noth J: Language functions in progressive supranuclear palsy, Brain 114:1457, 1991.

124. Poser S: Multiple sclerosis, New York, 1978, Springer-Verlag.

125. Putnam AHB, Hixon TJ: Respiratory kinematics in speakers with motor neuron disease. In McNeil MR, Rosenbek JC, Aronson AE, editors: The dysarthrias: physiology, acoustics, perception, management, San Diego, 1984, College-Hill Press.

126. Ramig LO et al: Acoustic analysis of voice in amyotrophic lateral sclerosis: a longitudinal case study, J Speech Hear Res 55:2, 1990.

127. Renout KA et al: Vocal fold diadochokinetic function of individuals with amyotrophic lateral sclerosis, Am J Speech-Lang Pathol 4:73, 1995.

128. Riddel J et al: Intelligibility and phonetic contrast errors in highly intelligible speakers with amyotrophic lateral sclerosis, J Speech Hear Res 38:304, 1995.

129. Robert D et al: Quantitative voice analysis in the assessment of bulbar involvement in amyotrophic lateral sclerosis, Acta Otolaryngol 119:724, 1999.

130. Rodriguez M: Multiple sclerosis: basic concepts and hypothesis, Mayo Clin Proc 64:570, 1989.

131. Rowland LP: Ten central themes in a decade of ALS research. In Rowland LP, editor: Advances in neurology, vol 56, New York, 1991, Raven Press.

132. Samlan RA, Weismer G: The relationship of selected perceptual measures of diadochokinesis to speech intelligibility in dysarthric speakers with amyotrophic lateral sclerosis, Am J Speech-Lang Pathol 4:9, 1995.

133. Sandyk R: Resolution of dysarthria in multiple sclerosis by treatment with weak electromagnetic fields, Int J Neurosci 83:81, 1995.

134. Sarno, MT, Buonaguro A, Levita, E: Characteristics of verbal impairment in closed head injured patients, Arch Phys Med Rehabil 67:400, 1986.

135. Saunders C, Walsh T, Smith M: Hospice care in the motor neuron diseases. In Saunders C, Teller JC, editors: Hospice: the living idea, Dunton Green, Sevenoaks, Kent, UK, 1981, Edward Arnold Publishers.

136. Schiffer RB, Slater RJ: Neuropsychiatric features of multiple sclerosis, Semin Neurol 5:127, 1985.

137. Seikel JA, Wilcox KA, Davis J: Dysarthria of motor neuron disease: longitudinal measures of segmental durations, J Commun Disord 24:393, 1991.

138. Sitver MS, Kratt A: Augmentative communication for the person with amyotrophic lateral sclerosis (ALS), ASHA 24:783, 1982.

139. Smith CR, Scheinberg LC: Clinical features of multiple sclerosis, Semin Neurol 5:85, 1985.

140. Sonies BS: Swallowing and speech disturbances. In Litvan I, Agid Y, editors: Progressive supranuclear palsy: clinical and research approaches, New York, 1992, Oxford University Press.

141. Sternlieb I, Giblin DR, Scheinberg H: Wilson's disease. In Marsden CD, Fahn S, editors: Movement disorders, vol 2, Boston, 1987, Butterworth-Heinemann.

142. Stierwalt JAG et al: Tongue strength and endurance: relation to the speaking ability of children and adolescents following traumatic brain injury. In Robin DA, Yorkston KM, Beukelman DR, editors: Disorders of motor speech: assessment, treatment, and clinical characterization, Baltimore, 1996, Paul H Brookes.

143. Strand EA et al: Differential phonatory characteristics of four women with amyotrophic lateral sclerosis, J Voice 8:327, 1994.

144. Strong MJ et al: A prospective study of cognitive impairment in ALS, Neurology 53:1665, 1999.

145. Testa D et al: Comparison of natural histories of progressive supranuclear palsy and multiple system atrophy, Neurol Sci 22:247, 2001.

147. The Consensus Committee of the American Autonomic Society and the American Academy of Neurology: Consensus statement on the definition of orthostatic hypotension, pure autonomic failure, and multiple system atrophy, Neurology 46:1470, 1996.

148. Theodoros DG, Murdoch BE: Differential patterns of hyperfunctional laryngeal impairment in dysarthric speakers following severe closed head injury. In Robin DA, Yorkston KM, Beukelman DR, editors: Disorders of motor speech: assessment, treatment, and clinical characterization, Baltimore, 1996, Paul H Brookes.

149. Theodoros DG, Murdoch BE: Laryngeal dysfunction in dysarthric speakers following severe closed-head injury, Brain Inj 8:667, 1994.

150. Theodoros DG et al: Hypernasality in dysarthric speakers following severe closed head injury: a perceptual and instrumental analysis, Brain Inj 7:59, 1993.

151. Theodoros DG, Murdoch BE, Stokes PD: Variability in the perceptual and physiologic features of dysarthria following severe closed head injury: an examination of five cases, Brain Inj 9:671, 1995.

152. Theodoros DG, Shrapnel N, Murdoch BE: Motor speech impairment following traumatic brain injury in childhood: a physiological and perceptual analysis of one case, Pediatr Rehabil 2:107, 1998.

153. Thomas M, Jankovic J: Parkinsonism plus disorders. In Noseworthy JH, editor: Neurological therapeutics: principles and practice, vol 1, New York, 2003, Martin Dunitz.

154. Tjaden K, Turner G: Segmental timing in amyotrophic lateral sclerosis, J Speech Lang Hear Res 43:683, 2000.

155. Tjaden K, Turner GS: Spectral properties of fricatives in amyotrophic lateral sclerosis, J Speech Lang Hear Res 40:1358, 1997.

156. Tjaden K, Watling E: Characteristics of diadochokinesis in multiple sclerosis and Parkinson's disease, Folia Phoniatr Logop 55:241, 2003.

157. Topaloglu H et al: Tremor of tongue and dysarthria as the sole manifestation of Wilson's disease, Clin Neurol Neurosurg 92:295, 1990.

158. Traynor BJ et al: Amyotrophic lateral sclerosis mimic syndromes: a population-based study, Arch Neurol 57:109, 2000a.

159. Traynor BJ et al: Clinical features of amyotrophic lateral sclerosis according to the El Escorial and Arlie House diagnostic criteria: a population-based study, Arch Neurol 57:1171, 2000b.

160. Turner GS, Tjaden K, Weismer G: The influence of speaking rate on vowel space and speech intelligibility for individuals with amyotrophic lateral sclerosis, J Speech Hear Res 38:1001, 1995.

161. Wang YT et al: Alternating motion rate as an index of speech motor disorder in traumatic brain injury, Clin Linguist Phon 17:1, 2003.

161. Turner GS, Weismer G: Characteristics of speaking rate in the dysarthria associated with amyotrophic lateral sclerosis, J Speech Hear Res 36:1158, 1993.

162. Weismer G et al: Acoustic and intelligibility characteristics of sentence production in neurogenic speech disorders, Folia Phoniatr Logop 53:1, 2001.

163. Weismer G et al: Effect of speaking rate manipulations on acoustic and perceptual aspects of the dysarthria in amyotrophic lateral sclerosis, Folia Phoniatr Logop 52:201, 2000.

164. Weismer G et al: Formant trajectory characteristics of males with amyotrophic lateral sclerosis, J Acoust Soc Am 91:1085, 1992.

165. Wenning GK et al: What clinical features are most useful to distinguish definite multiple system atrophy from Parkinson's disease? J Neurol Neurosurg Psychiatry 68:434, 2000.

166. Wenning GK et al: Natural history and survival of 14 patients with corticobasal degeneration confirmed at postmortem examination, J Neurol Neurosurg Psychiatry 64:184, 1998.

167. Williams DB, Windebank AJ: Motor neuron disease (amyotrophic lateral sclerosis), Mayo Clin Proc 66:54, 1991.

168. Windebank AJ: Motor neuron diseases. In Noseworthy JH, editor: Neurological therapeutics: principles and practice, vol 2, New York, 2003, Martin Dunitz.

169. Yorkston KM, Strand EA, Hume J: The relationship between motor function and speech function in amyotrophic lateral sclerosis. In Cannito MP, Yorkston KM, Beukelman DR, editors: Neuromotor speech disorders: nature, assessment, and management, Baltimore 1998, Paul H Brookes.

170. Yorkston KM, Strand EA, Miller RM: Progression of respiratory symptoms in amyotrophic lateral sclerosis: implications for speech function. In Robin DA, Yorkston KM, Beukelman DR, editors: Disorders of motor speech: assessment, treatment, and clinical characterization, Baltimore, 1996, Brookes Publishing Company.

171. Yorkston KM et al: Characteristics of multiple sclerosis as a function of the severity of speech disorders, J Med Speech-Lang Pathol 11:73, 2003.

172. Yorkston KM et al: Management of motor speech disorders in children and adults, ed 2, Austin, Tex, 1999, Pro-Ed.

173. Yorkston KM et al: Speech deterioration in amyotrophic lateral sclerosis: implications for the timing of intervention, J Med Speech-Lang Pathol 1:35, 1993.

174. Yorkston KM et al: The relationship between speech and swallowing disorders in head-injured patients, J Head Trauma Rehabil 4:1, 1989.

175. Young MC: Communication disorders in systemic lupus erythematosus, J Med Speech-Lang Pathol 4:141, 1966.

"This morning I was appalled at my terrible reading aloud a new passage. I had difficulty enunciating most every word. Particularly troublesome were the words 'manipulate' and 'manipulated.' I couldn't seem to get past 'manifested.' Later I tried again and was only barely pronouncing the words correctly. . . . Also, I was full of slurring the sounds of syllables."

(From the written diary of a 72-year-old woman with a progressive apraxia of speech and mild aphasia)

CHAPTER OUTLINE

 I. **Anatomy and basic functions of the motor speech programmer**
   A. Functions of the motor speech programmer
   B. The motor speech programmer network
 II. **Nonspeech, nonoromotor, and nonlinguistic characteristics of patients with apraxia of speech**
III. **Etiologies**
 IV. **Speech pathology**
   A. Terminology and theory
   B. Distribution of etiologies, lesions, and associated deficits in clinical practice
   C. Patient perceptions and complaints
   D. Clinical findings
   E. Acoustic and physiologic findings
 V. **Cases**
 VI. **Summary**

We now turn our attention to a category of motor speech disorders (MSDs) that differs from the dysarthrias. Its designation, *apraxia of speech (AOS)*, distinguishes it from the movement disorders represented by the dysarthrias, as well as from linguistically based speech errors associated with aphasia. The clinical manifestations of AOS are believed to reflect a disturbance in the planning or programming of movements for speech.

Unlike the dysarthrias,* AOS can exist without clinically apparent impairments in the speech muscles for nonspeech tasks. Unlike aphasia, in which there are nearly always multimodality impairments of language, AOS can exist independent of problems with verbal comprehension, reading comprehension, and writing, as well as independent of verbal errors that are unrelated to articulation and prosody. Although AOS often coexists with dysarthria and aphasia, the distinctiveness of its clinical characteristics, its apparent nature as a motor planning or programming disturbance, and its occasional emergence as the only disturbance of communication justify its identification as a unique type of speech disorder. Its distinction from other MSDs is additionally warranted because of its localizing value; it is almost always the result of pathology in the left cerebral hemisphere. To repeat the simple definition provided in Chapter 1, AOS is *a neurologic speech disorder that reflects an impaired capacity to plan or program sensorimotor commands necessary for directing movements that result in phonetically and prosodically normal speech. It can occur in the absence of physiologic disturbances associated with the dysarthrias and in the absence of disturbance in any component of language.*

---

*With the possible exception of speech-induced movement disorders, such as certain dystonia-based hyperkinetic dysarthrias.

AOS is encountered as the primary speech disorder in a large medical practice at a rate comparable to that of several of the major single dysarthria types. Based on data for primary communication disorder diagnoses in the Mayo Clinic Speech Pathology practice, it accounts for 7.6% of all MSDs (see Figure 1-3). It also occurs frequently as a secondary diagnosis in people with left (dominant) hemisphere lesions whose primary communication disorder is aphasia, and it can be a secondary diagnosis in people whose primary diagnosis is dysarthria or some other neurologic communication disorder. Thus AOS is present in far more than 7.6% of people who have communication disorders associated with left hemisphere pathology.

The clinical features of AOS convey the impression that the appropriate message has been formulated but that what should be automatic "decisions" about its physical expression have been inefficiently or poorly organized or controlled, although not because of problems with basic motor abilities. Careful study of AOS can illustrate some of the distinctions between motor speech planning/programming and the neuromuscular execution of speech, and between motor speech planning/programming and the formulation and organization of the linguistic units that are spoken. Such study also highlights the difficulty often encountered in attempts to make such distinctions, both theoretically and clinically.

The concept of AOS has had somewhat of a stormy history since Darley[26,27] introduced it in the 1960s and tied it to problems with the programming of movements for speech. There have been considerable and important debates about its very existence or its underlying nature.* A fundamental problem has been uncertainty about its defining clinical attributes, with subsequent uncertainty about whether clinicians and researchers who claim to have studied the problem have actually been dealing with the same entity. This has introduced considerable "noise" into efforts to better understand the disorder's cognitive, motor, and anatomic bases. However, with refinements in models of language and speech motor control and efforts to fit careful clinical observations

to them, there has in recent years been some honing of the clinical boundaries of the disorder. Rather than dwell too much on historic debate and controversy, an attempt is made here to focus on what at least some clinicians and researchers now propose may be the essential characteristics of AOS and how they fit with notions about speech motor planning/programming. What is presented here seems to make sense at this time. Its staying power depends on future clinical and research efforts.

In this chapter, the location and functions of the motor speech planning/programming network are summarized in broad, general terms. Some of the theoretical and clinical debate about the nature of AOS is reviewed but not dwelled upon. Emphasis is placed on the clinical milieu in which AOS is encountered, its auditory and visible perceptual attributes, relevant acoustic and physiologic data, and some clinical case studies. The distinctions between AOS and dysarthria and aphasia are addressed in some detail in Chapter 15, which focuses on differential diagnosis.

■ ANATOMY AND BASIC FUNCTIONS OF THE MOTOR SPEECH PROGRAMMER

Motor speech control involves the interactive, parallel, and sequential participation of all components of the motor speech system, as well as higher level activities related to conceptualization, language, and motor planning/programming. The motor planning/programming component of these activities is referred to here as the *motor speech programmer (MSP).*

The MSP is a network of interacting structures and pathways rather than a single anatomic structure. It is influenced by sensory feedback, the basal ganglia and cerebellar control circuits, the reticular formation and thalamus, and the limbic system and right hemisphere. From this perspective, motor speech programming involves widespread areas of the central nervous system (CNS). However, for the purpose of understanding the highest levels of speech programming—pathways and structures that specify the patterns and sequences of movements for speech—the *left cerebral hemisphere,* particularly parietal-frontal and related subcortical circuits, can be thought of as the headquarters of the MSP and the locus of lesions that lead to AOS.

Functions of the Motor Speech Programmer

The MSP has a leading role in establishing the plans and programs for achieving the cognitive and linguistic goals of spoken messages. It organizes the motor commands that ultimately result in the

---

*This history is traced with varying degrees of detail in a number of papers, chapters, and books.[33,82,96] Comprehensive, critical reviews that capture current thinking about the nature, clinical characteristics, and management of AOS can be found in McNeil, Robin, and Schmidt,[82] McNeil, Doyle, and Wambaugh,[80] a 2001 Forum in Aphasiology with a lead paper by Varley and Whiteside[124] and commentaries from several investigators, and numerous papers in a recent issue of *Seminars in Speech and Language* edited by McNeil.[75]

production of temporally ordered sounds, syllables, words, and phrases at particular rates and patterns of stress and rhythm.

The left hemisphere functions of the MSP seem to be more strongly tied to the linguistic attributes of speech (phonologic, semantic, syntactic, morphologic, plus linguistic components of prosody) than to its emotional or affective attributes, the latter components perhaps being more strongly influenced by contributions from the limbic system and right hemisphere. The linguistic input to the MSP comes largely from the left hemisphere's perisylvian area, which includes the temporoparietal cortex, posterior portions of the frontal lobe, the insula, and, in less definitive ways, the basal ganglia and thalamus. The anatomic proximity or overlap of these language areas with those of the MSP makes it likely that damage to the perisylvian language zone often results in a cooccurrence of language-related deficits (aphasia) and AOS. In clinical reality, this indeed is often the case.

When speech is the goal, it can be presumed that, once the phonologic representation of a message has been established, the MSP must be activated to organize and activate a plan for its motor execution. This seems to involve a *transformation of the abstract phonemes to a neural code that is compatible with the operations of the motor system*. This neuromotor code presumably specifies the parameters of movement for specific muscles or muscle groups, although McNeil, Robin, and Schmidt[82] point out that "the exact parameters of movement that are programmed and that represent the control variables for the motor programmer are not agreed upon." They suggest, however, that specifications for movement duration and displacement (amplitude), acceleration, deceleration, time to peak velocity, muscle stiffness, and relative timing of speech events are examples of some of the kinematic parameters of movement that might be programmed.

Because much of normal, mature speech is produced quickly and without conscious effort, it is reasonable to assume that the MSP commonly selects, sequences, activates, and controls *preprogrammed movement sequences** that, through learning and practice, can be activated automatically. It is thought that motor plans/programs are established before movement begins, but that they can be modified by peripheral feedback either before the program is readied for movement or during movement execu-

tion.[80,122] All of this permits rapid speech rates and greater allocation of resources to the more conscious formulation and monitoring of the cognitive and linguistic goals of communication. This rapid, direct route for phonetic encoding may occur primarily for frequently used syllables, words, or phrases. For novel syllables or movement patterns (e.g., infrequently or never-before-used multisyllabic or nonsense words), speaking under adverse conditions, or attempting to be particularly precise, it is likely that phonetic encoding is less direct (i.e., less automatic) because the motor patterns need to be freshly computed.[†80] It has been suggested that at least some of the speech characteristics of people with AOS could reflect problems with the access to or use of preprogrammed subroutines and the subsequent need to construct programs anew for each syllable to be uttered (Ziegler, 2002).[80,125,130]

The Motor Speech Programmer Network

The MSP seems to rely heavily on left hemisphere prefrontal, premotor areas, of which *Broca's area* and the *supplementary motor area* may be most important. Broca's area is a candidate area for making important contributions to the specification of simultaneous and sequential speech movements based on input from sensory modalities and areas involved in linguistic formulation. Recall also that premotor areas are linked to the basal ganglia and cerebellar control circuits that have reciprocal connections with the primary motor cortex that puts into effect the motor speech act. Broca's area is often identified as a lesion site in people with AOS.

The supplementary motor area is also involved in the activities of the MSP, although it seems further removed than Broca's area from the actual specification of speech movements. It has connections with the primary motor cortex and Broca's area, the basal ganglia, and the limbic system. It seems tied to cognitive and emotional processes that drive or motivate action and may play an important role in the initiation of propositional speech, as well as in its control. In general, however, it is not a common site of lesions associated with AOS.

The *parietal lobe somatosensory cortex* and the *supramarginal gyrus* are also implicated in the activities of the MSP, probably before initiation of

---

*Other terms that might apply include generalized motor programs; verbal motor memories; engrams; movement gestalts; well-established subroutines; or "macros," to borrow computer terminology.

†Cogent, comprehensive discussions of motor speech planning/programming and its relationship to AOS can be found in several sources (McNeil, Robin, and Schmidt, 1997[22,80,88,122,124] [plus following commentary by several authors]; Ziegler, 2002).[125,130]

movement but, obviously, also during series of movements. These areas may be particularly important in integrating sensory information necessary for skilled motor activity and for transforming sensory information and internal goals into plans and targets for action.[88] The *insula*[*] (Figure 2-16) also may have a specialized role in motor planning/programming for speech, perhaps particularly during speech execution.[88] It recently has been identified as a shared site of damage in people with AOS[31] and sometimes the only site of damage,[90] although AOS can occur without lesions in the insula.[84]

Finally, the basal ganglia, consistent with their known role in motor control, seem active in the activities of the MSP. Lesions of the left basal ganglia have been associated with AOS,[92b] although far from invariably.

In general, conclusions about the presumed anatomy and functions of the MSP are supported by clinical findings. That is, lesions that produce AOS are usually located in the left posterior frontal lobe or parietal lobe, or in the insula or basal ganglia. The speech characteristics of people said to have AOS are distinguishable from those associated with the dysarthrias, and AOS can be evident in people whose speech muscles perform normally for nonspeech activities and who are able to express language through nonspeech channels (e.g., writing). Careful observation and analysis of their speech suggests that something is awry with the planning/ programming of speech movements. This disturbance has come to be called AOS by clinicians and investigators who recognize its distinctiveness, its value in contributing to our understanding of the neurology of speech and the localization of disease, and the unique demands it places on patients and clinicians who try to minimize its effects on communication.

▨ NONSPEECH, NONOROMOTOR, AND NONLINGUISTIC CHARACTERISTICS OF PATIENTS WITH APRAXIA OF SPEECH

Physical speech mechanism findings, oromotor behaviors, and disorders of language that testify to the presence of dominant hemisphere pathology frequently accompany AOS. These characteristics are discussed in the section on speech pathology later in this chapter. Several additional clinical findings commonly accompany AOS. They usually reflect damage to the left frontal or parietal lobe, or to left subcortical pathways and structures associated with the direct and indirect activation pathways.

Many patients have varying degrees of right-sided weakness and spasticity, and some have associated sensory deficits. A Babinski sign and hyperactive stretch reflexes on the right side are also common. A hyperactive gag reflex and pathologic oral reflexes (e.g., suck, snout, jaw jerk) are not commonly present unless there are bilateral upper motor neuron (UMN) lesions, a condition not required for the presence of AOS.

Patients with AOS sometimes, but by no means invariably, have *limb apraxia (LA)*, a disorder also associated with left hemisphere pathology and characterized by deficits in the performance of purposive limb movements that cannot be explained by impairments of strength, mobility, sensation, or coordination. LA usually affects movements in both the right and left limbs, although it is often masked on the right side by hemiparesis or hemiplegia. LA has been more widely accepted in neurology as a distinct clinical entity than has AOS, in spite of approaches to its clinical diagnosis that have been highly variable and subjective. The psychologic, physiologic, and anatomic bases of LA have been addressed extensively in the neurologic literature since before the early part of this century when Liepman[68] presented his historically dominant and widely accepted conceptualization of apraxia.

A comprehensive review of LA is beyond the scope of this chapter.[*] From the theoretical standpoint, it is noteworthy that there are important historical and conceptual similarities and differences between notions of apraxia as it affects the limbs versus speech. Anyone interested in in-depth study of AOS should be familiar with theoretical and clinical issues associated with LA. From the clinical standpoint, it is important to recognize that people with left hemisphere pathology may have difficulty organizing movements of both their right and left extremities, sometimes only on formal testing, but in some cases during activities of daily living. Of special relevance for issues related to communication, LA may interfere with writing as well as with propositional nonverbal communication (such as pantomime and sign language).[†] This is an important consideration for people with severe AOS who may be in need of an augmentative or alternative form of communication.

---

*See Bennett and Netsell[3] for a comprehensive discussion of the possible roles of the insula in speech and language.

*Overviews of theoretical and clinical assessment and diagnostic issues in limb apraxia can be found in a number of sources. For example, brief basic summaries can be found in Brookshire[11] and Mesulam.[86] More detailed reviews and discussion can be found in DeRenzi,[28] Duffy and Duffy,[35,36] Ochipa and Gonzalez Rothi,[91] Roy and Square-Storer,[98] and Square-Storer and Roy.[112]

†Aphasia also is related to difficulty in expressing propositional or symbolic meanings through pantomime and sign language.[38-40]

ETIOLOGIES

Any process that damages dominant hemisphere structures involved in motor speech planning/programming can cause AOS. Because inflammatory and toxic-metabolic diseases usually produce diffuse effects, only rarely are they associated with an obvious AOS.* Demyelinating disorders, such as multiple sclerosis (MS), are not commonly associated with AOS, although the association has been observed.† In contrast, tumors and trauma (especially surgical trauma) are more likely to cause focal unilateral signs. When they affect the left hemisphere, AOS may result.

Stroke is the most common cause of AOS. There is nothing unique about the nature of the vascular disturbances (or any etiology for that matter) that cause AOS, except that they can be and often are localized to the dominant hemisphere's network of structures and pathways that plan and program movements for speech.

Degenerative neurologic diseases, in general, are not commonly associated with AOS. Even conditions in which dysarthria occurs frequently, such as progressive supranuclear palsy (PSP) and multiple system atrophy (MSA), are not usually associated with AOS or other forms of apraxia affecting speech muscles.‡,8,32,44,67 However, it is increasingly recognized that AOS does occur fairly frequently in certain degenerative neurologic conditions and sometimes can be their first sign. For example, although the general clinical literature on corticobasal degeneration (CBD)§ suggests that AOS occurs in less than 5% of reported cases,[66] recent studies that have carefully examined speech and language suggest that it occurs in nearly 40% of cases and is sometimes the first or among the first signs of the disease.[4,45,66] Nonverbal oral apraxia (NVOA) also occurs frequently in CBD,[45,66] and its cooccurrence with AOS has been quite high in some reports.[45]

A few additional degenerative conditions deserve mention, because AOS can be prominent or among their presenting signs. *Creutzfeldt-Jakob disease (CJD),* also designated *subacute spongiform encephalopathy,* is a rapidly progressive, untreatable, degenerative, infectious prion disease. Median age at onset is approximately 60 years, and death usually occurs within 6 months to several years. Its most common clinical features include cognitive decline, ataxia, and myoclonus, but other pyramidal and extrapyramidal signs can be evident.[73] Various dysarthria types may be present, but they have not been well described. Signs and symptoms are rarely unilateral, but a few case reports[64,71,107,129] document that CJD can announce itself focally as aphasia. Review of these reports suggests that at least some of the cases also had AOS.

Primary progressive aphasia (PPA) is characterized by the insidious onset and gradual progression of aphasia without evidence of nonlanguage impairments. It has been associated with a number of degenerative conditions that presumably and predominantly involve the perisylvian region of the left (language dominant) hemisphere,[34,77] at least for an extended period of time. For several years it has been recognized as the prime example of disorders that have been called *asymmetric cortical degenerative syndromes* or *focal cortical atrophy syndromes.*[*,5,15-17] Histopathology is often nonspecific, but specific clinical and pathologic diagnoses with which PPA has been associated include CBD, PSP, amyotrophic lateral sclerosis (ALS), CJD, corticonigral degeneration, and, infrequently, Alzheimer's disease. PPA deserves mention in this context, because a significant proportion of cases said to have PPA may also have had AOS or, possibly, no aphasia at all.[77]

Importantly, several cases of what appears to have been a progressive AOS, without aphasia, have been reported.[12,19,20,48,102,121] A large retrospective report[32] examined data for a group of 70 patients who had a progressive AOS that was the first symptom of degenerative neurologic disease in 81% of the cases and among the first symptoms in an additional 7%. On examination, AOS was isolated in 9% of the cases and occurred with aphasia or dysarthria, or

---

*An example of an uncommon, probable toxic-metabolic cause is the occurrence of AOS as part of a prominent speech disorder that can emerge following orthotopic liver transplantation. It has been estimated that this speech disturbance occurs in approximately 1% of adults undergoing the procedure. Temporary cessation of the drug cyclosporin has been associated with improvement of speech.[10]

†The literature documents cases of MS with aphasia, and several case descriptions suggest that AOS was also present.[30] The author has seen a few cases of MS with AOS, all accompanied by aphasia. AOS has also been reported in a few patients receiving immunosuppressive agents following liver transplantation.[9,41]

‡Exceptions do occur, however. For example, AOS with aphasia has been reported as the first sign of disease in a patient with autopsy-confirmed PSP.[8]

§See Chapter 10 for more information about CBD, including the dysarthrias and other communication disorders that can be associated with it.

---

*Examples of other asymmetric cortical degenerative syndromes include perceptuomotor deficits associated with bilateral (often right greater than left hemisphere) parietal lobe dysfunction and neuropsychiatric disorders associated with frontal lobe dysfunction.

both, in the remaining 91%, but the AOS was the more prominent deficit in 78% of those who also had aphasia and the more prominent deficit in 71% of those who also had dysarthria. Approximately two thirds of the cases received a nonspecific etiologic neurologic diagnosis such as PPA, progressive AOS, asymmetric cortical degeneration, or degenerative CNS disease. However, 28% received neurologic diagnoses tied to conditions with prominent motor manifestations, including CBD (11%), CBD versus PSP (3%), and parkinsonism (6%). Of interest, because it is unexpected, 9% had ALS or motor neuron disease. Thus there is accumulating evidence that AOS can be the first, the only, or the most prominent manifestation of a degenerative neurologic disease. When this is the case, the designation *primary progressive AOS,* or *PPAOS,* seems appropriate.[77]

To summarize, AOS encountered in most clinical settings is usually caused by stroke and sometimes by tumor or trauma. Although uncommon, the insidious development of AOS in the absence of vascular disease, trauma, or tumor may be a presenting or prominent sign of several forms of degenerative CNS disease.

▣ SPEECH PATHOLOGY

Terminology and Theory

Someone once said, "When knowledge is lacking, a name comes to take its place." Different beliefs about the clinical characteristics and nature of AOS, efforts to achieve compatibility with embraced models of language, ego, nationalism, and the politics of academia and medicine have all probably contributed to the abundance of terms that have been applied to the disorder. Some of the terms summarized in Box 11-1 are rarely encountered in clinical practice today; they survive only as vehicles for tracing the history of the disorder. A number of labels are still used in addition to AOS. The most common are speech apraxia and oral verbal apraxia, Broca's aphasia, aphemia, and aphasic phonologic impairment. *Speech apraxia, oral verbal apraxia, and, probably, aphemia* are synonymous with AOS.* Broca's aphasia usually includes, but encompasses more than, AOS. Aphasic phonologic impairment may be confused with, but is different than, AOS.

box 11-1	Terms used in the literature to designate speech disturbances associated with apraxia of speech

Afferent motor aphasia	Peripheral motor aphasia
Anarthria	Phonematic aphasia
Aphemia	Phonetic disintegration
Apraxic dysarthria	Primary verbal apraxia
Articulatory dyspraxia	Pure motor aphasia
Ataxic aphasia	Pure word mutism
Broca's aphasia	Secondary verbal apraxia
Cortical anarthria	Sensorimotor impairment
Cortical dysarthria	Speech apraxia
Efferent motor aphasia	Speech sound muteness
Expressive aphasia	Subcortical motor aphasia
Little Broca's aphasia	Word muteness
Oral verbal apraxia	

The debate about the nature of AOS has traditionally centered on whether or not it is distinguishable from aphasia. The frequent cooccurrence of aphasia with AOS and the overlap of anatomic regions that are crucial to language and motor speech planning/programming help drive this uncertainty. However, there does seem to be general agreement that (1) at least some of the speech sound abnormalities of some aphasic patients are attributable to motor planning/programming rather than linguistic/phonologic deficits, and that (2) a disorder of speech motor planning/programming can result from left cerebral lesions that may or may not also cause difficulties with language. The support for these conclusions comes from studies of people with AOS but normal language in nonspeech modalities, careful clinical perceptual descriptions, and acoustic and physiologic studies, sometimes with comparisons to aphasic and dysarthric speakers.*

It is beyond the scope of this chapter to review the details of the literature on the nature of AOS, particularly its distinction from aphasia. Some basic questions that frequently arise in clinical practice that reflect this debate should be addressed, however, because they bear on differential diagnosis and the use of terminology in clinical practice.

First, *is the term AOS synonymous with Broca's or nonfluent aphasia?* The answer is no. Most definitions of Broca's and nonfluent aphasia do not give

---

*For example, Fox et al.[43] reported a case with aphemia with a small stroke in the left precentral gyrus with undercutting of motor and premotor cortex. There was no aphasia in any modality. The description of speech characteristics was similar to those associated with AOS. The authors concluded: "Our patient's speech apraxia during recovery suggests that aphemia can present as a severe form of apraxia of speech."

---

*It is of interest that questions also have arisen about the distinction between AOS and dysarthria, a distinction that may be as difficult in some respects as that between AOS and aphasia.[79,83,126] Perceptual, acoustic, and physiologic comparisons between AOS and the dysarthrias (particularly ataxic and unilateral UMN dysarthrias) are necessary to sort out these distinctions with greater clarity.

overt recognition to the existence of a motor speech planning/programming deficit.* They do, however, describe patients' speech as slow, labored or effortful, "dysarthric," reduced in phrase length, abnormal in prosody, and having poor "articulatory agility." These characteristics are consistent with those of speakers with AOS. If people with Broca's aphasia truly are *also* aphasic, then grammatical and syntactic errors and problems with word retrieval usually also characterize their speech.

It is reasonable to conclude that people with Broca's or nonfluent aphasia often have an accompanying AOS. In fact, it has been argued that AOS may be an integral part of the syndrome of Broca's aphasia and that its presence may be required for its diagnosis.[78] However, AOS is not synonymous with Broca's aphasia because the aphasic component of the syndrome includes deficits that are not explainable by AOS. They also are not synonymous because AOS can occur without any manifestations of aphasia.

Are all sound level errors made by aphasic patients manifestations of AOS? Again, the answer is no, but with qualifications. This question is motivated by the presence of sound level errors in people with Wernicke's and conduction aphasia.† Their speech, by definition, is usually perceived as fluent, easily produced, and prosodically normal. Many of their sound substitutions, omissions, and additions probably reflect problems at the phonologic level of language. That is, their errors most likely represent inadequate selection or ordering of phonologic units, but with subsequent adequate planning/programming of them for execution by the MSP.

Ease of production and normal prosody appear to be major clues to distinguishing aphasic phonologic errors from those attributable to AOS, although some people with Wernicke's and conduction aphasia make detectable phonetic-level errors.[78] Differences, therefore, may be ones of degree, with motor level deficits predominating in speakers with AOS (and Broca's or nonfluent aphasia), and phonologic deficits, when they are present, predominating in Wernicke's, conduction, and other fluent aphasias.

Are there subtypes of AOS?‡ We do not know. It may be that different patterns of speech disturbance

among people with left hemisphere lesions simply reflect the blurred boundaries between disorders of language and motor planning/programming and between motor planning/programming and motor execution. That is, one "type" of AOS might actually reflect a linguistic phonologic disorder such as that encountered in Wernicke's or conduction aphasia (or an aphasic phonologic disorder plus AOS), and another "type" a dysarthria (or an AOS plus dysarthria). If this is the case, then there may not be types of AOS, only AOS versus aphasia or dysarthria, or AOS plus aphasia or dysarthria. At this time, it thus seems inappropriate to subdivide AOS until the common features of the disorder are better delineated and understood.

At the same time, several theories suggest that breakdowns at different stages of motor planning/programming may lead to different types of apraxia. For example, Rosenbek, Kent, and LaPointe[96] stated, ". . . we might imagine errors in planning to be distinct from errors in serial ordering, which in turn could be distinct from errors in execution or implementation." Square-Storer and Roy[112] stated ". . . several subtypes of apraxia of speech may exist in that several cortical and subcortical sites appear responsible for the programming of spatial and temporal information requisite for normal motor speech production." More recently, on the basis of models postulating that normal speech encoding can be accomplished through different routes (distinct mechanisms, or structures and pathways), it has been suggested that AOS may include a spectrum of disorders in which, for example, different routes might be impaired independently of each other, with subsequent distinctive speech characteristics tied to each damaged route.[22,124] The increasing sophistication of models of speech planning/programming and clarification of their distinction from models of phonologic processing should permit testing of these predictions in people with AOS. If different breakdown patterns are identified, and particularly if they are perceptually salient, then clinically useful subtypes of AOS may be recognized.

At this time, the greatest practical clinical diagnostic challenge relates to the fact that AOS frequently occurs simultaneously with dysarthria and, especially, aphasia. As a result, clinicians and researchers struggle frequently with the interpretation of abnormalities as apraxic versus aphasic or dysarthric. Clinical distinctions between AOS and aphasia and between AOS and dysarthria are addressed in Chapter 15, which covers differential diagnosis.

---

*Representative procedures for identifying Broca's aphasia are included in frequently used tests of aphasia, such as the *Boston Diagnostic Aphasia Examination*[50] and the *Western Aphasia Battery.*[63]

†This is an important issue, because "it is likely that the majority of the literature on AOS, and on phonemic paraphasias as well, is seriously confounded by the observation and quantification of behaviors implicating both praxis and phonologic mechanisms."[80]

‡Discussion of this issue can be found in several sources.[13,70,96,109,112,124]

Etiologies for 155 quasirandomly selected cases with a primary speech pathology diagnosis of AOS at the Mayo Clinic from 1969-1990 ($n = 107$) and 1999-2001 ($n = 48$). Percentage of cases for broad etiologic headings is given in parentheses. Specific etiologies under each heading are ordered from most to least frequent.

Vascular (49%)

Single left hemisphere stroke (41%)
Multiple strokes, including left hemisphere (8%)

Degenerative (26%)

Unspecified degenerative CNS disease (10%)
PPA or AOS, or both (7%)
Alzheimer's disease or dementia (3%)
Other: asymmetric cortical degeneration; CBD; ALS; CBD vs. PSP; CJD; leukoencephalopathy (7%)

Traumatic (15%)

Neurosurgical (14%)
    Tumor resection, aneurysm or AVM repair, hemorrhage evacuation
CHI (1%)

Tumor (Left Hemisphere) (4%)

Other (6%)

AOS of undetermined etiology (3%)
Other: seizure disorder; post liver transplant; multiple causes (2%)

ALS, Amyotrophic lateral sclerosis; *AOS,* apraxia of speech; *AVM,* arteriovenous malformation; *CBD,* corticobasal degeneration; *CHI,* closed head injury; *CJD,* Creutzfeldt-Jakob disease; *CNS,* central nervous system; *PPA,* primary progressive aphasia; *PSP,* progressive supranuclear palsy.

Distribution of Etiologies, Lesions, and Associated Deficits in Clinical Practice

Etiologies

Box 11-2 and Figure 11-1 summarize the etiologies for 155 quasirandomly selected cases seen at the Mayo Clinic with a primary speech pathology diagnosis of AOS.* The cautions expressed in Chapter 4 about generalizing these findings to the general population or all speech pathology practices apply here as well.

The data establish that AOS can result from a number of medical conditions, the distribution of which is quite different from several dysarthria types

*The distribution of etiologies reported here is generally consistent with that reported by Wertz, Rosenbek, and Deal's[128] analysis of etiologies in a group of 176 adults with AOS.

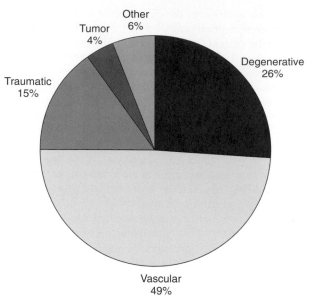

FIGURE 11-1 Distribution of etiologies for 155 quasirandomly selected cases with a primary speech pathology diagnosis of apraxia of speech at the Mayo Clinic from 1969-1990 and 1999-2001 (see Box 11-2 for details).

but somewhat similar to those for spastic and unilateral UMN dysarthria. Approximately half of the cases were accounted for by strokes alone, and 90% of the cases were accounted for by stroke, degenerative, and traumatic etiologies.

Single strokes in the left hemisphere middle cerebral artery distribution accounted for most of the vascular causes. This is consistent with the prominence of stroke as an etiology of focal neurologic signs and the localization of crucial speech planning/ programming functions in the left hemisphere. The remainder of the vascular cases had multiple strokes in which at least one of the lesions was in the left hemisphere.

Twenty-six percent of the cases were degenerative. Ten percent had an unspecified degenerative CNS disease. Seven percent had a diagnosis of PPA or PPAOS. The remaining cases had Alzheimer's disease, a similar dementing condition, or other conditions that frequently included focal or asymmetric findings (e.g., asymmetric cortical degeneration, CBD, CJD). In some cases, AOS was the only or the initial sign of disease, or it was among the most significant deficits at the time of diagnosis. This illustrates that some degenerative neurologic diseases can present as focal disturbances and that AOS can be the first sign of a slowly progressive degenerative neurologic disease.

Surgical trauma was the etiology in 15% of the cases. In most instances, surgery involved the left frontal lobe. One left-handed patient had a right frontal lobe tumor resection and was also aphasic postoperatively; he likely had right hemisphere dominance for speech and language. A few patients had sustained a closed head injury (CHI), further establishing that focal motor speech disturbances can result from such trauma.

Four percent of the patients had a left hemisphere tumor, all including the frontal lobe. In three of these patients, AOS was among the initial neurologic signs. In one patient, AOS was the only clinically apparent evidence of neurologic disease, the tumor being identified on subsequent computed tomography (CT) scan.

Several patients had AOS as the only evidence of neurologic disease, leaving the etiologic diagnosis undetermined. The remaining patients had AOS in association with seizures, liver transplantation, or a combination of disorders.

Lesions

The localization of left hemisphere stroke for people who had CT scans or magnetic resonance imaging (MRI) that identified a lesion was generally consistent with notions about lesion localization in AOS. The frontal lobe was most frequently included in the lesion distribution, though not much more often than the parietal lobe. When only a single lobe was implicated, it was most often the frontal lobe. The temporal lobe was sometimes involved but never alone. The lesion was confined to subcortical structures in some cases.

Associated Deficits*

AOS was among the initial symptoms of neurologic disease in a significant majority of the patients. This is not surprising because of the high proportion of vascular etiologies in which speech-language and motor and sensory deficits usually are present together at onset.

How often was NVOA present? Among 107 patients for whom relevant data were sought, 63% of those for whom observations about NVOA were made had evidence of the disorder. Thus consistent with the literature, there was a frequent but not invariable cooccurrence of AOS and NVOA.

How often was aphasia present? Among the 155 patients for whom observations about aphasia were

made, 72% had evidence of aphasia. Thus it appears that for those in whom AOS is the most prominent speech or language disturbance, accompanying aphasia is often, but not always, present. Although this percentage also suggests that AOS can occur independent of language disturbance, it is inappropriate to conclude that 28% of *all* people with AOS have no aphasia. That is, the sample did not include patients with AOS in whom aphasia was the primary speech-language disturbance.

How often was dysarthria present? Among the 155 patients for whom observations about dysarthria were made, dysarthria was present in 29%. As was the case for aphasia, this figure probably underestimates the percentage of people with AOS who also have dysarthria because the sample did not include patients with AOS in whom dysarthria was the primary speech-language disturbance. When dysarthria type was specified, it was usually unilateral UMN (UUMN) or spastic in type. The fairly frequent cooccurrence of AOS and dysarthria is consistent with the proximity of crucial speech motor planning/programming structures and pathways to cortical and subcortical components of the direct and indirect activation pathways. UUMN dysarthria is the expected dysarthria on this basis, with spastic dysarthria usually occurring in those with lesions in more than just the left hemisphere.

How often was AOS the only neurologic communication disorder (i.e., no dysarthria, aphasia, or nonaphasic cognitive-communication deficits)? Data regarding this were most confidently derived from among the 48 most recently seen of the 155 patients. Among them, AOS was the only apparent communication disorder in four patients, or 8.3%. Of interest, degenerative disease was the etiology in three of the four, raising the possibility that "pure" AOS may be more common in degenerative disease than it is in stroke or trauma. It is important to recognize that the 8.3% figure almost certainly inflates the overall frequency of isolated AOS, because the data are derived only from patients in whom AOS was the primary communication disorder. If all cases with AOS were examined (i.e., including those in whom aphasia or dysarthria were more prominent), this figure, by definition, would have to be lower, probably considerably lower.

Patient Perceptions and Complaints

When AOS occurs without aphasia, individuals often say something like "my speech won't come out right. I know the words I want to say, but they won't come out the right way." Phrases such as "not as fluent as before" and words like "mispronounce" are common descriptors. Complaints nearly always center on articulation and rate and rarely on breathing, phona-

---

*In a comprehensive review of the literature, McNeil, Doyle, and Wambaugh[80] found that 48% to 85% of those with AOS also had NVOA, an average of 81% also had aphasia, and 29% to 47% also had dysarthria.

tion, or resonance. When AOS is mild, patients sometimes note being surprised by errors that intrude into an otherwise fluent narrative. Others report having to speak slowly or carefully in order to prevent errors. Some predict errors on difficult-to-pronounce multisyllabic words, and many recognize errors when they occur and attempt to correct them. The word "stutter" is used occasionally to describe associated dysfluencies, groping for articulatory postures, and attempts at error correction. Many patients say the problem worsens under conditions of stress or fatigue.

Those with isolated AOS do not complain of chewing, swallowing, or drooling difficulties. If such problems are present, they should raise concerns about neuromuscular deficits and an accompanying dysarthria. Patients also deny difficulties with verbal comprehension, reading comprehension, and the linguistic aspects of writing. Because AOS frequently occurs simultaneously with aphasia, however, *all people with suspected AOS should be considered aphasic until comprehensive language assessment proves otherwise.*

Clinical Findings

Nonverbal Oral Mechanism

If dysarthria is not present, the gag reflex and chewing and swallowing functions may be entirely normal, and there may be no pathologic oral reflexes. There need not be any right central lingual or facial weakness. However, it is often the case that the causative lesion is large enough to have damaged corticobulbar pathways. It is thus common to find a right central facial weakness and sometimes right lingual weakness. A UUMN dysarthria may be present and related to such weakness. Any speech deficits attributed to unilateral face or tongue weakness are part of the dysarthria and not the AOS, however.

Because motor planning/programming and control is a *sensori*motor process, it is reasonable to ask if oral sensation (e.g., oral form identification, two-point oral discrimination, mandibular kinesthetic abilities) is impaired. A few studies have addressed this issue, some finding evidence of deficits and a relationship to severity of AOS,[97] and others failing to find such deficits or relationships.[29] Wertz, LaPointe, and Rosenbek[127] concluded from their review of such studies that some people with AOS have oral sensory deficits that may or may not be related to AOS severity. In general, the available data do not support a primary causative role of oral sensory deficits in AOS. Testing for such deficits is not necessary to diagnose AOS.

Nonverbal Oral Apraxia

A substantial proportion of people with AOS exhibit NVOA.* NVOA is an inability to imitate or follow commands to perform volitional movements of speech structures (e.g., cough, blow, click tongue) that cannot be attributed to poor task comprehension or sensory or neuromuscular deficits. The lesions leading to it are in the left hemisphere and tend to include the frontal and central (rolandic) opercula, anterior paraventricular white matter, adjacent portions of the first temporal convolution, anterior portion of the insula, or parietal lobe.[1,118]

Commonly used tasks for detecting NVOA include imitating or following commands to cough, click the tongue, smack the lips, blow, or whistle (see Box 3-1, Chapter 3, for a list of tasks and suggestions for evaluating NVOA).† People with NVOA attempt to respond but do so awkwardly or with off-target responses, effortful groping for correct movements, or inconsistent trial-and-error attempts. Sometimes while trying to perform the act, they simultaneously say the command. For example, asked to cough, a patient may say "cough" and simultaneously attempt to cough. Patients usually are perplexed, frustrated, amused, or embarrassed by these off-target responses and often try to correct themselves but with inconsistent success. Many patients may later cough reflexively, lick their lips, or blow out air in an exhausted sigh after failing to perform the same act on imitation or command.

People with suspected AOS should always be assessed for NVOA because its presence is a sign of left hemisphere pathology, not because it has a necessary causal relationship with AOS. Although AOS and NVOA frequently occur simultaneously, they can be dissociated. The fact that they can occur independently argues against the notion that AOS is simply a reflection of a more fundamental disturbance of nonverbal oral movement, at least in some patients.

Limb, nonverbal oral, other speech-language deficits, and patient complaints that may accompany AOS are summarized in Table 11-1.

---

*Other frequently used terms that are roughly synonymous with NVOA include *oral nonverbal apraxia, buccofacial apraxia, lingual apraxia, oral apraxia,* and *facial apraxia.*

†Volitional coughing, blowing, and whistling are among the most difficult simple tasks, because they require coordination of the breath stream, laryngeal activity, and oral movements.[59] Sequences of nonverbal oral motor movements (e.g., click teeth together and then pucker the lips) are more difficult than single discrete movements,[65,74] but performance can be confounded by verbal comprehension deficits on commanded tasks or by short-term retention difficulties on imitation tasks.

table 11-1	Common limb, nonverbal oral, other speech-language deficits, and patient complaints associated with AOS*

Variable	Findings
Limb	Right hemiparesis or associated sensory deficits, or both
	Babinski sign
	Hyperactive stretch reflexes
	Limb apraxia, usually bilateral
Nonverbal Oral	Right lower face weakness
	Right lingual weakness
	Nonverbal oral apraxia
	Oral sensory deficits
Language & Other Speech Deficits	Aphasia, most often Broca's aphasia when aphasia can be categorized
	Unilateral UMN dysarthria
Patient Complaints	"Speech doesn't come out right"
	Mispronunciation
	Stuttering
	Must speak slowly to prevent errors

AOS, Apraxia of speech; *UMN,* upper motor neuron.
*None of these deficits/complaints are invariably present in people with AOS.

Auditory Processing Skills

There is general consensus that auditory deficits are not present in people with pure AOS and that when they are present in those with AOS and aphasia they do not explain speech errors that are considered apraxic in nature. These conclusions are based on a number of studies of apraxic speakers that have demonstrated adequate perception of stimuli to be produced and, at the least, auditory skills that were superior to speech production skills. In one of the most thorough and convincing investigations of this issue, Square-Storer, Darley, and Sommers[110] concluded that auditory processing abilities can be normal in AOS, and that AOS and aphasia are distinguishable deficits from both motor speech and auditory processing perspectives.

It does appear that apraxic speakers are susceptible to the effects of disrupted auditory feedback, however. For example, delayed auditory feedback (DAF) severely disrupted speech in those with Broca's aphasia, more so than in speakers with any other aphasia type.[18] This effect does not necessarily argue for a causal role for disrupted auditory feedback in AOS, however. That is, it may be that the output deficit (in AOS) "is so fragile that any perturbation of the articulatory system ... seriously affects the quality of their output."[18] It might be argued that apraxic speakers are particularly reliant on adequate auditory feedback to speak as well as they do.

It is reasonable to conclude that AOS can exist in the absence of auditory processing difficulties, but, because AOS usually occurs with aphasia, auditory processing deficits are often present in apraxic speakers. Their presence, however, is not likely to be causally related to their AOS, although such deficits might serve to exacerbate it.

Speech

Tasks placing demands on the sequencing of various sounds and syllables with varying patterns of stress are most likely to elicit the salient and distinguishing features of AOS. Conversational and narrative speech and reading can be revealing for this purpose, particularly if language and reading skills are relatively good and the patient can give more than brief and unelaborated conversational or narrative responses.

Imitative tasks assist the clinical hunt for AOS, because they can contain stimuli that challenge speech planning/programming abilities and because they circumvent demands on word retrieval and other aspects of language formulation. This is important, because aphasia can make assessment of motor speech difficult; it can mask or be difficult to distinguish from AOS.

Speech sequential motion rates (SMRs)* and imitation of complex multisyllabic words and sentences are among the structured tasks most sensitive to AOS. It is not unusual for suspicion of AOS generated during conversation and simple language tasks to blossom into an unequivocal diagnosis after observing attempts to sequence SMRs and repeat words and sentences like "catastrophe," "statistical analysis," and "the municipal judge sentenced the criminal." This does not mean that speakers with AOS have disproportionate difficulty with repetition (in fact, imitation can be superior to spontaneous speech in some respects). It simply means that imitation tasks can be specifically designed to elicit the characteristics of AOS more efficiently than spontaneous speech sampling.

The challenging tasks just described are not always useful for people with marked or severe AOS. For such patients it is more valuable to discover what they are able to do and to contrast that

*Apraxic speakers have relative preservation of speech AMRs, at least when their impairment does not preclude the ability to produce a single syllable accurately. As a group, their AMRs are somewhat slower than normal but faster than for several groups of dysarthric speakers (due to stroke, CHI, and cerebellar disease), although not those with Parkinson's disease.[131]

box 11-3 **Perceptually salient characteristics of apraxia of speech.***

Articulation

Consonant and vowel distortions (imprecise articulation), with consonant distortions usually predominating

Distorted substitutions

Distorted perseverative substitutions (e.g., "nanana"/banana)

Distorted anticipatory substitutions (e.g., "popado"/potato)

Distorted additions

Distorted sound prolongations

Distorted voicing distinctions (blurring of voiced-voiceless boundaries)

Relatively consistent trial–trial articulatory *error location*

Relatively consistent trial–trial *error type*

Rate and Prosody

Slow overall rate regardless of phonemic accuracy, especially for utterances more than one syllable in length

Prolonged but variable vowel duration in multisyllabic words or words in sentences

Prolonged but variable interword intervals regardless of phonemic accuracy

Syllable segregation

Errors of stress assignment, with a tendency to equalize stress across syllables/words

Decreased phonemic accuracy as rate increases

Altered stress occasionally leads to perception of foreign accent in monolingual speakers[†]

Fluency

Successful or unsuccessful attempts to self-correct articulatory errors that cross phonemic boundaries

False articulatory starts and restarts

Effortful visible and audible trial-and-error groping for articulatory postures

Sound and syllable repetitions

Influential Task Variables

Error rates higher for volitional/purposeful versus automatic/reactive utterances, but automatic/reactive utterances often not perceptually normal

Speech SMRs more likely to be abnormal in phonemic accuracy and rate than AMRs

Error rates higher for nonsense syllables/words than meaningful words

Consonant clusters errors more frequent than singleton errors

Initiation of utterances particularly difficult

Errors occur on both imitative and spontaneous speech tasks

Imitation errors generally do not exceed spontaneous speech errors on comparable productions

AMRs, Alternate motion rates; *SMRs,* sequential motion rates.

*A number of these characteristics occur in some dysarthria types (e.g., imprecise articulation, slow rate, distorted voicing distinctions) and aphasia (e.g., attempts to self-correct errors, articulatory groping). It is often the clustering of several characteristics, as well as the absence of other abnormalities, that helps identify speech abnormalities as apraxic, as opposed to dysarthric or aphasic. These distinctions are addressed in Chapter 15.

†See Chapter 13 for a more complete description and discussion of pseudoforeign accent.

with the nature of the tasks in which performance is poor. Thus it may be discovered that a patient who cannot converse intelligibly and cannot perform SMRs or even attempt to imitate multisyllabic words is more adequately able (although often not normally) to count, imitate simple consonant-vowel-consonant (CVC) syllables, sing a familiar tune, and produce speech AMRs because they are highly overlearned, can be produced "automatically," or place minimal or different demands on planning/programming abilities. From this standpoint, examination reflects a search for the threshold at which patients succeed and fail on tasks reflecting a continuum of speech planning/programming demands. For some, the threshold is high and tasks should be difficult; for others, the threshold is low and tasks should be simple. For a few, AOS is so severe that a search for any stimulus that can elicit differentiated speech responses is most appropriate. (Box 3-3 provides a list of tasks and scoring notations that are useful for assessing AOS. A published test, the *Apraxia Battery*

for Adults [ABA-2][23] was also discussed in Chapter 3.)

Modern descriptions of the perceptual characteristics of AOS were born with Darley's clinical observations in the late 1960s[25,26] and an influential study by Johns and Darley.*[58] Since then, the features considered salient to the clinical identification of the disorder have evolved as a product of careful research, refinements in the definition of AOS, and the influence of models of phonology and motor speech planning/programming on the setting of boundaries for the disorder. The salient perceptual characteristics described in Box 11-3 reflect these developments, the author's clinical experience, and the influence of recent papers by McNeil and colleagues[80,82] that have

---

*Those with a serious research interest in AOS should read at least several of the historic, theoretic, or clinical overviews of AOS that have been published over the past few decades.[13,78,80,82,92,96,127]

proposed a list of features that seem to distinguish AOS from aphasic phonemic paraphasias.

The validity of many of the salient speech characteristics summarized in Box 11-3 is supported by the results of acoustic and physiologic studies and perceptual studies using narrow phonetic transcription.* Narrow phonetic transcription has highlighted the presence of vowel errors and the relative pervasiveness of distortions, helping to establish that what are perceived as substitutions† may be the result of, or at least accompanied by, motor/phonetic level distortions. For example, it appears that apraxic speakers produce more consonant distortions than substitutions and that half of their perceived substitutions are also perceived as distortions.[92] This is why many of the substitution, addition, and prolongation characteristics listed in Box 11-3 are characterized as distorted.

The pervasiveness of distortions among the articulatory characteristics listed in Box 11-3 helps distinguish the substitutions, additions, and prolongations associated with AOS from the phonologic errors (phonemic paraphasias) that can occur in aphasia; that is, aphasic phonologic substitutions, additions, and prolongations are not perceptually distorted. In contrast, articulatory distortions are not helpful in distinguishing AOS from dysarthria, although other characteristics are; that is, dysarthria is rarely associated with additions or substitutions.

The rate and prosodic abnormalities listed in Box 11-3 are pervasive problems in AOS‡ and are probably more important than articulatory errors in distinguishing AOS from phonemic paraphasias. That is, abnormalities of rate and prosody are nearly always present in apraxic speakers, even for utterances that are free of perceived substitutions, additions, or omissions, whereas rate and prosody are usually normal within phonemically on-target utterances of aphasic patients who make phonologic errors.[82] However, the rate and prosodic abnormalities of AOS, considered alone, are similar to those in some dysarthria types, such as ataxic, spastic, and unilateral UMN.

The rate and prosodic abnormalities in AOS have several possible explanations, including: (1) they could represent a fundamental feature of AOS, (2) they could be a by-product of a fundamental problem with articulation (e.g., how could rate and prosody possibly be normal in the context of the disorder's characteristic articulatory deficits?), or (3) they could reflect efforts at compensation for a fundamental deficit in articulation. It is probable that all three explanations are valid for many patients, but it is important to recognize that *accumulating evidence suggests that rate and prosodic disturbances are a defining feature of AOS*[82] and not simply (only) secondary to articulation errors or a by-product of compensatory efforts. This is illustrated by the clinical observation that some apraxic speakers who report that they slow their rate to maintain accuracy often fail to normalize their rate when instructed to do so regardless of errors. Admittedly, however, accuracy often suffers when rate can be increased (see Box 11-3).

The abnormal fluency* characteristics associated with AOS may be evident in many patients, but they may also be present in aphasic patients who make phonologic errors,† thus reducing their value in distinguishing AOS from aphasia. Nonetheless, with the possible exception of hypokinetic dysarthria, fluency abnormalities frequently observed in apraxic speakers are uncommon in dysarthric speakers, so they do help distinguish AOS from dysarthria or recognize AOS when it occurs simultaneously with dysarthria. Neurologic fluency disorders are discussed in more detail in Chapter 13.

Apraxic speech performance can be influenced by a number of factors (see Box 11-3), although aphasic speakers are susceptible to many of the same influences. Again, however, such factors are not usually active for dysarthric speakers. For example, AOS

---

*Narrow phonetic transcription is not the only perceptual method for inferring motor-level problems in AOS. For example, a less direct phonologic process analysis of apraxic speakers with Broca's aphasia failed to reveal evidence of phonologic impairment and identified patterns of errors (e.g., prevocalic and postvocalic devoicing) that suggested a motor/phonetic level impairment.[87]

†This may reflect our common "desire" as listeners to perceive meaningful units and ignore signal noise (i.e., distortions), as well as our being primed to look only for phonologic errors by many perceptual studies of AOS that used broad transcription and linguistic phonologic process analyses that were not sensitive to distortions. Another possibility is that some studies that have influenced our thinking may actually have included subjects who had no distortions and were, by today's definition of AOS, not apraxic but rather aphasic and making phonologic errors.

‡The prosodic abnormalities have functional consequences. For example, it has been shown that listeners have difficulty identifying different emotions expressed by apraxic speakers through variations in f_o, duration, and amplitude.[123]

---

*The use of the term *fluency* in this chapter refers to interruptions in the normal flow of speech, such as silent or audible sound-syllable repetition and prolongation (dysfluencies), or groping for articulatory manner or position. It is not used here to refer to abnormalities that are manifestations of language impairment, such as reduced phrase length or agrammatism, characteristics that are often associated with so-called nonfluent aphasia.

†For example, it has been suggested that the notion of effortful trial and error groping as a necessary or differential feature (relative to aphasia) of AOS has not been clearly established.[82]

speakers usually have more difficulty with speech SMRs than AMRs, whereas dysarthric speakers perform about the same on both tasks (or sometimes even better on SMRs than AMRs!). Volitional/propositional utterances generate more abnormalities than automatic/reactive utterances, although the latter often are not entirely normal; dysarthric speakers show no such distinctions.

Not all people with AOS display all of the characteristics summarized in Box 11-3, just as not all people with specific dysarthria types have all of the characteristics that have been reported for their type of dysarthria. The reasons for this are not entirely clear. They probably include natural variability within the disorder, the possible existence of subtypes of AOS, various contaminating effects of concomitant aphasia, variability associated with degree of impairment, or variable methods of description.

Severe Apraxia of Speech

People with mild to moderate AOS probably dominate the database from which much of our clinical descriptions of the disorder are based. Unfortunately, there has been little systematic study of marked to severe (hereafter called severe) AOS. This is probably because people with severe AOS tend to have significant and often severe aphasia that contaminates its study. This is unfortunate because severe AOS probably occurs much more frequently than generally milder pure AOS. It is additionally unfortunate, because the characteristics of severe AOS may not reflect just a greater magnitude of the characteristics that define milder forms.

Box 11-4 summarizes the speech characteristics of people with severe AOS whose speech characteristics depart from those described for less severe forms. The summary is strongly influenced by the astute observations by Rosenbek,[95] who pointed out that speech in severe AOS can be limited to a few meaningful or meaningless utterances on imitation, reading, or spontaneous speech tasks. Even attempts to imitate isolated sounds may be in error and the types of error responses limited. When phonetic repertoire is limited, errors may not approximate the target unless the target happens to resemble sounds or syllables in the repertoire. Automatic speech may not be noticeably better than volitional speech (e.g., a severely impaired patient might produce, slowly and with distortions, "dun, doo, dee, daw, digh," when attempting to count from one to five). Singing a familiar tune may contain the correct number of syllables, with a reasonable approximation of the tune, but contain only a few distorted consonants and a few vowels (e.g., "apee turdee too doo"/"Happy birthday to you"). When only a few different sounds can be produced, errors are highly predictable, sometimes giving the impression that the patient has actually "lost" the representations of movements that generate sounds from their motor repertoire.

The severity continuum for AOS extends to muteness. Most clinicians agree that the inability to phonate *(apraxia of phonation)* in pure AOS is an early and transient problem, usually resolving within a few days, at least when the lesion is confined to Broca's area.[89] It is rare for muteness due to AOS alone to last for more than 2 weeks. In fact, a gratifying aspect of clinical practice is eliciting the first utterances in a mute apraxic patient a few days after a stroke by having him or her count or sing a familiar tune with clinician cuing. Persistence of AOS mutism for more than a few weeks should raise suspicions about a different diagnosis or an additional problem, such as severe aphasia, anarthria, akinetic mutism, or psychogenic mutism. The distinctions among AOS and other forms of mutism are addressed in Chapter 12.

Mute apraxic patients nearly always make attempts to speak on request, with attempts characterized by silent groping attempts to move the jaw, lips, and tongue to articulate, along with gestural and facial expressions of frustration. A severe NVOA is usually present. It is rare that articulation ability significantly exceeds a patient's inability to phonate. That is, apraxia of phonation is nearly always accompanied by severe articulation difficulties.*

---

box **11-4**	**Characteristics of severe apraxia of speech**

Limited repertoire of speech sounds
Speech may be limited to a few meaningful or unintelligible utterances
Imitation of isolated sounds may be in error, and errors limited in variety
Errors may be highly predictable
Automatic speech may not be better than volitional speech
Error responses may approximate target if stimuli are chosen carefully
Muteness may be present but rarely persists for more than 1 to 2 weeks if other speech, language, or cognitive deficits are not present
Usually accompanied by severe aphasia but can occur in the absence of aphasia
Usually accompanied by nonverbal oral apraxia

---

*A case study by Marshall, Gandour, and Windsor[72] represents a dramatic exception. Their patient had a selective impairment of phonation (a laryngeal apraxia) for an extended time and was able to speak normally when using an electrolarynx.

Summary

What features of AOS help distinguish it from the dysarthrias? Among all of the speech abnormalities that may be detected, distorted sound substitutions and additions, segregation of syllables in multisyllabic utterances, decreased phonemic accuracy with increased rate, attempts to correct articulatory errors that cross phonemic boundaries, groping for articulatory postures, greater difficulty on volitional versus automatic speech tasks, and greater difficulty on SMR and multisyllabic word tasks versus AMR and single syllable tasks are the most common distinctive clues to the presence of the disorder. In general, it is usually the clustering of several of these characteristics that help distinguish AOS from the various dysarthria types.

What features of AOS help distinguish it from phonemic paraphasias associated with aphasia? Among all of the speech abnormalities that may be detected, *articulatory distortions, relatively consistent trial–trial phonemic error location and type, slow rate, prolonged interword intervals and syllable segregation,* and *equalized stress and errors in stress assignment* are the most common distinctive clues to the presence of the disorder. Again, it is usually the clustering of several of these characteristics that best help distinguish AOS from aphasic phonologic errors.

Distinctions among the speech features of AOS, the dysarthrias, and aphasic phonologic errors are discussed further in Chapter 15.

Acoustic and Physiologic Findings

Acoustic and physiologic studies have provided confirmation for many of the disorder's perceptual characteristics and have identified additional features that clinicians should attend to perceptually. Equally important, a substantial body of instrumental data supporting the conclusion that AOS is a phonetic disorder of motor planning/programming has accumulated. The following somewhat arbitrary subsections summarize the results of a number of representative acoustic and physiologic studies that have helped to characterize the disorder's clinical features and clarify its general underlying nature. These findings are summarized in Box 11-5.

Voice Onset Time

Voice onset time (VOT) is the duration between the articulatory release of a consonant and the onset of voicing for a following vowel. It is measured acoustically from the onset of the noise burst reflecting stop release to the onset of periodicity in the waveform reflecting the onset of glottal pulsing. Voiced stops are characterized by voicing lead (the onset of voicing before the release of the stop), simultaneous voice onset and stop release, or voice lag (onset of voicing within approximately 20 milliseconds after the stop release). Voice lag of 40 ms or more characterizes voiceless stops. VOT has been used as an acoustic measure of coordination in studies of AOS, because it reflects relative timing between supralaryngeal articulators (e.g., the lips and tongue) and respiratory-laryngeal events that are essential to signaling voicing distinctions. VOT measures have provided valuable insights about motor programming versus phonologic deficits in people with AOS.

Several studies of apraxic speakers indicate *considerable overlap in the distribution of VOT values for voiced and voiceless stops.* VOT values may fall in a range between normal voiced and voiceless values (i.e., between 25 and 40 ms), and have greater than normal variability even when stop productions are perceived as accurate. These abnormalities have also been documented for initial voiced and voiceless fricatives.[2] Although apraxic speakers sometimes produce VOT values that suggest a phonologic error (e.g., a VOT value for a /b/ that clearly falls in the normal VOT range for /p/), the general trend in the data is indicative of a pervasive phonetic rather than phonologic disorder. In fact, VOT values for productions perceived as substitutions tend not to be distributed in a manner consistent with normal productions of the perceived substituted phoneme.

In general, this overlap of VOT values or their greater than normal variability generally indicates that correct phonemes (voiced or voiceless) are selected, but that the timing of articulatory and laryngeal activity is poorly regulated.[6,7,46,53,54,56,103,120] The pervasiveness of VOT abnormalities suggests that AOS is particularly susceptible to phonetic parameters requiring the integration of activities among different speech structures.[2]

Rate

Acoustic and physiologic studies generally support and refine the clinical perception that slow rate is a near-constant perceived abnormality in AOS, and they provide insight into whether slow rate is a core feature of the disorder or a compensatory strategy to maintain articulatory control. Studies have consistently quantified *slow rate*.[49,61,93,103,108,111,125,131] They have also documented excessive *lengthening of consonants*[61,78,126] and *increased vowel duration in syllables, multisyllabic words, word strings, and phrases.* *

---

*References 14, 21, 52, 61, 78, 101, 103, 111, 113, 115, 116.

---

box 11-5

Summary of acoustic and physiologic abnormalities found in studies of AOS. Many of these observations are based on studies of only one or a few speakers, and not all apraxic speakers exhibit these features. Also, these characteristics may not be unique to AOS; some may also be found in other neurologic disorders or nonneurologic conditions.

VOT

Overlap in distribution of VOT values between voiced and voiceless stops and fricatives

Increased variability and abnormal distribution of VOT values, even when perceived as phonemically accurate

Rate

Slow overall rate of speech and underlying movements

Excessive lengthening of consonants and vowels in syllables, multisyllabic words, word strings, and sentences

Increased interword intervals and verbal response times

Reduced ability to adjust speech rate, especially to increase rate—even normally fast rates are sometimes possible

Delayed, deficient, or inconsistent coarticulation among speech structures

Slowed formant trajectories and lengthened steady-state components in diphthongs

Longer and more variable movement durations of lower lip and jaw movements during speech

More frequent velocity changes and increased velocity variability during articulatory movements

Prosody and Stress

Excessive temporal regularity and flattening of intensity envelope (syllable–syllable intensity variability) in phrases and sentences

Reduced f_o contour within sentences

Reduced f_o decline over the course of lengthy sentences

Reduced final word lengthening, relative to non–final words, in sentences

Increased intersyllabic pauses and pause duration within utterances (i.e., syllable segregation)

Uniform syllable durations within utterances, regardless of stress or position within sentences

Equalized stress on stressed and unstressed syllables within utterances

Articulation and Fluency

Failure to achieve complete vocal tract closure for stops (i.e., spirantization)

Abnormal F1 and F2 for vowel production with bite block in place

Misdirected, exaggerated, or "perseverative" formant trajectories

Reduplicated, aborted, "stuttered," or groping articulatory attempts

Variability

Increased variability in onset of coarticulation, formant trajectories (i.e., movement transitions), attainment of vowel targets, and vowel duration

Increased variability in stop gap duration, VOT, and syllable duration

Increased variability in the direction, duration, velocity, peak velocity, and amplitude of jaw, lip, tongue, or velar movements, and the temporal and spatial relationships (coarticulatory patterns) among those structures

Nonspeech Oromotor Control

Instability on measures of nonspeech isometric force and static position control of lips, tongue, and jaw

Difficulty tracking predictable movement patterns with lower lip and jaw movements and modulation of f_o

---

AOS, Apraxia of speech; f_o, fundamental frequency; *F1*, first formant; *F2*, second formant; *VOT*, voice onset time.

Because vowel duration does not carry specific linguistic meaning in many contexts, it is difficult to argue that increased vowel durations reflect an underlying linguistic disorder, especially when findings also indicate that AOS speakers follow certain linguistic rules for vowel duration. For example, like normal speakers, apraxic speakers generally reduce vowel duration in segments as the number of segments in an utterance increases*; for example, the vowel in the syllable "cat" in the word "catapult" is shortened relative to the vowel in the syllable "cat"

produced in isolation.[21,52,115,116] In addition, AOS speakers obey the "vowel shortening rule" to signal the voicing feature for syllable final consonants (i.e., vowels preceding voiceless final consonants are shorter than vowels preceding the voiced cognate).[2,14,37] Thus apraxic speakers vary vowel duration to signal linguistic contrasts even though their vowel durations tend to be longer than in normal speakers.

Acoustic analyses also demonstrate *increased interword intervals,* a finding that supports the perception of syllable segregation. This suggests that apraxic speakers engage in independent (syllable-by-syllable) programming of syllables to a greater extent than normal speakers.[49,61,78,85,113,132] In addition, similar to normal speakers, they decrease interword intervals in sentences relative to interword intervals

---

*This is not always the case. It has been observed that some apraxic speakers actually increase vowel duration in segments as word length increases,[52] a phenomena that could reflect motor planning/programming constraints.

in word strings, but they are less consistent in doing so; this suggests an impaired mechanism for activating and executing motor plans.[113,114] Findings of increased verbal response times in apraxic speakers also support this conclusion.[85,119,125]

It has been difficult to establish if slow rate in AOS is compensatory (i.e., articulatory accuracy may be achieved if rate is "intentionally" slowed) or a primary, fundamental feature of the disorder. However, apraxic speakers are *less efficient in adjusting speech rates,* especially increasing rate, even when they are sometimes able to produce normally fast rates.[83,94,108] These findings suggest a problem with motor control and argue against the notion that all slowed rate in AOS is compensatory. It has also been pointed out that certain temporal parameters in AOS may be artifacts of slow rate, because even normal speakers show some evidence of decomposition or increased variability of relative timing patterns at slow rates when compared to average or fast rates.[78]

Acoustic studies have found evidence of *delayed, deficient,* or *inconsistent coarticulation* among laryngeal, velar, lingual, or labial speech gestures, making it difficult for listeners to predict upcoming articulatory events.[81,132,133] Abnormally *slowed formant trajectories* and *long steady-state portions within diphthongs* have also been identified.[126]

Kinematic measures of lower lip plus jaw movements during word repetition in apraxic speakers have identified normal peak velocity (the maximum speed attained) but *longer and more variable movement durations and more frequent velocity changes and greater velocity variability.*[79] These results suggest that lip movements are not fundamentally slower than normal, even though lip gestures take longer to achieve.* It has been speculated that movements take longer because some are larger (involve greater displacement) or because there are a greater number of aberrations over the course of movement (dysmetrias). It has also been noted that such dysmetrias are not dissimilar to those observed in ataxic dysarthria, although they might be an artifact of slow speaking rate because some normal speakers can look dysmetric when speaking at slow rates.[79]

In summary, speech rate in AOS is generally slower and more variable than normal. Acoustic and physiologic findings generally support a conclusion that these rate aberrations reflect motor or phonetic

level deficits rather than linguistic deficits, especially because apraxic speakers are generally capable of signaling linguistic distinctions that are dependent on rate modifications. Although such studies argue against linguistic explanations for rate deficits, they do raise questions about distinctions between AOS and abnormalities found in certain types of dysarthria, particularly ataxic dysarthria.

Prosody

Prosodic abnormalities are a core and defining feature of AOS. Acoustic data documenting rate abnormalities are strongly predictive and supportive of perceived prosodic abnormalities in most apraxic speakers. A number of additional acoustic studies have addressed prosody and stress abnormalities directly. They also are supportive of perceived abnormalities.

Apraxic speakers tend to show temporal regularity and reduced intensity variation from syllable to syllable within polysyllabic word, phrase, or sentence utterances.[49,61,111,131] This generally means that unstressed syllables are produced with relatively greater duration and intensity than normal, thus blurring their distinction from stressed syllables. This tendency toward temporal and amplitude uniformity seems correlated with the perception of neutralization of stress and dysprosody.[78]

Documentation of *reduced fundamental frequency (f_o) contour in sentences*[100] has confirmed the frequent perception of reduced pitch variability within sentences. Other *abnormalities in regulation of f_o* can also occur. In normally spoken declarative sentences, f_o tends to decline in a linear fashion over the course of an utterance, with the greatest and most rapid decline occurring at the end of the utterance. In addition, the terminal words of declarative sentences tend to be lengthened, also signaling the end of the utterance. Speakers with Broca's aphasia (and, presumably, AOS), while demonstrating a decline in f_o at the end of simple sentences, may not do so over longer utterances. In addition, *duration of final words in utterances are not clearly longer* (and sometimes are shorter) than initial or medial words; this lack of durational distinction might reflect an increase in the length of nonfinal words rather than a shortening of final words.[24] Danly and Shapiro suggested that this occurrence could reflect effortful articulation or difficulty with syntax, reflecting a smaller scope of linguistic or motor planning, or both.

Acoustic studies have also documented *increased intersyllabic pauses within utterances,*[131] suggesting that each syllable is being programmed independently. Acoustic findings of *longer pause time, increased number of pauses within utterances,*

---

*Similarly, apraxic speakers can generate high peak lip velocities when asked to speak rapidly and when a bite block is in place, and their peak lip velocities do not differ between perceptually accurate and inaccurate word productions.[94] However, other kinematic analyses indicate that apraxic speakers may need increased time to reach peak velocity.[76]

stress on each syllable including nonstressed syllables, slower overall rate, shorter phrases, and *uniform syllable durations regardless of stress or sentence position*[49,61] all provide support for the frequent perception of prosodic and stress abnormalities. Taken together, these findings imply a simplification of motor planning/programming in AOS. That is, the perception that each syllable is stressed or produced as a single unit, rather than merged with other syllables and words in a phrase, suggests that *some speakers (must) approach the planning/programming of speech in a syllable-by-syllable manner; normal stress and prosodic flow are lost in the process.*

Articulation and Fluency

Many of the acoustic and physiologic findings already discussed carry an implication that articulation is imprecise, if not inaccurate, in place, manner, and voicing. A few additional findings add to such evidence. They also provide support for perceived dysfluencies in AOS.

Regarding articulatory imprecision, there is acoustic evidence that Broca's aphasic or AOS speakers may *fail to achieve complete vocal tract closure for stops.*[106,126] The resulting noise *(spirantization),* instead of silence reflecting closure, suggests distortion rather than a true fricative for stop substitution.

Imprecision extends to vowels. With a bite block in place, normal speakers are able to achieve normal formant positions for targeted vowels, often at the first glottal pulse of their initial effort. In contrast, speakers with Broca's aphasia (and, presumably, AOS), attempting to produce /i/ with a bite block in place, have abnormally high first formant (F1) and low second formant (F2) values, indicative of undershooting of tongue elevation and fronting.[117] At the least, this suggests that AOS is associated with difficulties in making on-line adjustments for compensatory articulation, including vowels.

Acoustic studies yield evidence of *misdirected formant trajectories* within connected speech. For example, rather than formants following a normal monotonic course, they sometimes initially rise and then fall. Formant trajectories may also be exaggerated (indicative of exaggerated movement), in which the frequency change in a formant transition is greater than normal. Finally, perseverative trajectories, in which formant transitions resemble those in preceding syllables, may occur.[126] Each of these observations imply imprecision or inaccuracy of articulatory movements during speech. Of interest, it has been observed that some of these characteristics are ataxic-like in character, while others might reflect effort at compensation.[126]

A few studies have documented the occurrence of events that support the perception of dysfluencies, aborted articulatory attempts, and attempt at error revision. For example, electromyogram (EMG), kinematic, acoustic, and perceptual studies have documented *reduplicated attempts during the initial segments of words, aborted articulatory attempts, attempts to revise errors, "stuttered" initial consonant segments,* and *added movements and groping.*[47,60,69,111,119,126,130]

Variability

Variability is considered by many to be a hallmark of AOS, at least at less than severe degrees of impairment. Acoustic and kinematic studies have provided considerable evidence of greater than normal variability in AOS. These studies are theoretically important, because abnormal variability has been identified within productions perceived as phonologically accurate, making it difficult to argue that such disturbances are linguistically based.

Several studies of vowel formant trajectories have documented reduced rate but also *greater than normal variability on indices of coarticulation, rate of change,* and *attainment of proper vowel targets.*[83,99,101,103,126,132] Similarly, studies of single syllable, multisyllabic, and phrase productions have generally found greater than normal variability in vowel duration.[14,37,52,103,105,126] Increased variability in stop-gap duration, VOT, duration of consonant-vowel syllables, and between-word duration has also been documented.[103,113]

Abnormal variability, as well as *temporal and spatial dyscoordination* within and among articulators, has been demonstrated through acoustic, kinematic, and EMG measures.[47,115,60] For example, several studies have found marked variability in the height and segmental duration of velar movements across repetitions of the same stimuli, in spite of the fact that a fairly normal pattern of velar movement is maintained; this variability in velar timing can lead to a perception of nasal substitution errors.[54,55,57] *Highly variable coarticulatory patterns* for labial and velar movements during speech, especially for measures of spatial displacement, have also been identified.[60] Similarly, studies of lip and jaw movements have identified *greater than normal variability in peak velocity, velocity changes,* and *relationships between movement amplitude and velocity.*[42,79]

There is also some evidence that nonspeech oromotor movements in people with AOS may not be normal. That is, some apraxic individuals (and some people with ataxic dysarthria) have *greater than normal force and position instability* on measures of nonspeech isometric force and static position control of the lips, tongue, and jaw, although the pattern of instability is not consistent across all structures tested or all AOS subjects tested.[76] Apraxic speakers have also had *difficulty on nonspeech visuomotor tracking tasks* in which lower lip, jaw, and f_o are used to track a visually displayed signal. This difficulty might reflect deficits in retrieving or developing an internal plan for intended movement patterns.[51]

Although not included in this review, it should be noted that some speakers with conduction aphasia and Wernicke's aphasia have displayed acoustic and physiologic abnormalities similar to those found in AOS. Such abnormalities are usually of lesser magnitude than those found in AOS, and they do not argue for linguistic explanations of AOS. They suggest, however, that some degree of motor planning/programming difficulty may be present in people with aphasia who do not display perceptual evidence of AOS.

Cases

CVA causes apraxia

Case 11-1

Lit stroke

A 68-year-old woman awoke one morning unable to speak and with right-sided weakness. Emergency department examination confirmed these deficits and also noted a right central facial weakness.

Speech evaluation the following day demonstrated normal oral movements with the exception of limited tongue excursion to the right. She produced only off-target groping movements of her jaw and lips when asked to clear her throat, click her tongue, blow, or whistle. Her reflexive cough was normal. She produced only awkward, groping, off-target jaw and lip movements when asked to count, sing a familiar tune, or imitate simple sounds or syllables. She could awkwardly produce the vowel "ah" and with effort imitated the vowels /ou/ and /u/. She was able to produce /m/ in isolation but could imitate no other isolated sounds. She achieved correct articulatory place for /f/ but could not simultaneously move air to produce frication. *no aphasia*

Verbal and reading comprehension were normal, even for difficult comprehension tasks. Writing with her preferred right hand was awkward because of weakness, but spelling, word choice, and grammar were normal.

A CT scan 5 days after onset identified a lesion in the left hemisphere at the junction of the posterior frontal and anterior parietal lobes. The neurologic diagnosis was left hemisphere stroke.

Speech therapy was undertaken. At the time of discharge 6 weeks later she was producing most sounds within single syllables, although slowly and with syllable segregation when she attempted to string syllables together. When reassessed 2 months later, she was speaking laboriously in sentences, with moderately slowed rate and segregated syllables, deliberate articulation, and pervasive mild articulatory distortions. When reassessed 2 years later, speech was functional but characterized by moderately slowed rate and occasional perceived articulatory substitutions, especially on multisyllabic words. She had consistent difficulty with /s/, /z/, /l/, and all consonant clusters.

Commentary. (1) Stroke is the most common cause of AOS, and AOS may be the only or most prominent manifestation of stroke. (2) AOS may be characterized by muteness at onset, although people mute from AOS usually attempt to speak. (3) Although AOS usually occurs with aphasia, even severe AOS can exist without any evidence of language impairment. (4) AOS is frequently accompanied by an NVOA. (5) When caused by stroke, AOS tends to improve over time, sometimes dramatically. Prognosis may be best when there is little or no language impairment.

Case 11-2

A 63-year-old man was hospitalized following a left carotid endarterectomy at another institution 6 weeks previously. Postoperative difficulties included speech problems and right hemiparesis. Neurologic examination noted a mild right hemiparesis and "dysarthria from facial weakness and a nonfluent aphasia."

Speech-language evaluation revealed mild difficulty with verbal and reading comprehension and inability to write intelligibly because of right hemiparesis. Speech was telegraphic and characterized by numerous articulatory revisions, hesitancy, and repetitions, as well as reduced loudness, mild hoarseness, and consistent mild articulatory distortions. A right central facial weakness was present.

The clinician concluded that the patient had "an AOS, which is the major variable contributing to his communication disorder; a nonfluent (Broca's-like) aphasia; and a unilateral UMN dysarthria." Speech-language therapy was recommended.

A CT scan and cerebral angiogram the following day identified the presence of a mass in the left frontoparietal region. He underwent surgery for gross total removal of a meningioma. Reassessment 2 days postoperatively indicated that the aphasia had resolved. Mild AOS and unilateral UMN dysarthria remained but were improved. He received therapy for 1 week before his discharge. At the time of discharge, he was able to carry on a conversation without significant difficulty. His AOS was most apparent when he was anxious or attempting to speak at a normal rate. Reassessment by his neurologist several months later suggested that he had continued to improve, but that residual speech difficulty remained.

Commentary. (1) AOS often occurs simultaneously with aphasia and unilateral UMN dysarthria. In this case, all three disorders were present initially, with AOS being the most evident deficit. (2) Etiology of AOS may include vascular disturbances, as well as tumor. In this case, stroke initially appeared to be the etiology, although subsequent identification of a tumor raised the possibility that it was causing the AOS. (3) AOS is associated with a range of severity. In this case, it was relatively mild and improved significantly.

Case 11-3

A 51-year-old woman was admitted to the hospital after several hours of progressive speech and writing difficulty, difficulty counting change, and not knowing how to start her car. Emergency department evaluation revealed a right central facial weakness, disorientation, limb apraxia, and difficulty with verbal expression. Comprehension appeared normal. A cerebral angiogram conducted 4 days later identified occlusion of two ascending frontal-parietal branches of the left middle cerebral artery. A CT scan was negative. A diagnosis of left frontoparietal stroke was made.

Speech-language examination a few days later revealed AOS as her most prominent communication deficit, although aphasia was also present. The AOS was characterized by distorted articulatory substitutions, omissions, groping for articulatory postures, slow rate, and altered prosody. Articulatory difficulties increased with increasing word or utterance length. Speech AMRs were slow, and she had difficulty with SMRs. She had a right central facial weakness and equivocal tongue weakness. The clinician felt she might also have had a unilateral UMN dysarthria.

She had good comprehension for single commands but performed poorly on the challenging comprehension tasks. Linguistically, verbal expression was quite good. She was mildly telegraphic, but the clinician wondered if it reflected compensation for the AOS. She had no difficulty with picture naming, but rapid word retrieval abilities fell outside the normal range. Reading comprehension for sentences and short paragraphs was adequate. Writing was linguistically adequate, but she had some difficulty with letter formation, suggestive of limb apraxia. There was no evidence of NVOA.

The clinician concluded that the patient had moderately severe AOS and mild aphasia. Therapy was recommended. She improved significantly by the time of her discharge a few days later. For example, during a 10-minute conversation she exhibited only three perceived substitutions and one instance of groping for articulatory posture. Slowing of speech rate facilitated articulatory accuracy. She was minimally frustrated by her speech difficulty and confident that she would continue to improve. She decided not to pursue speech therapy after discharge.

Commentary. (1) AOS and aphasia are frequently the initial manifestations of left hemisphere stroke. (2) AOS can be the prominent communication deficit in people with AOS and aphasia. When relatively mild at onset, significant recovery can be expected. (3) AOS can occur without evidence of NVOA.

Case 11-4

An 81-year-old man was admitted to a rehabilitation unit because of speech and limb control difficulties of 2 years' duration, presumably the result of a left hemisphere stroke. A CT scan revealed mild cerebral atrophy but was otherwise normal. An electroencephalogram was suggestive of a left hemisphere lesion. He was referred for speech-language assessment and recommendations.

During initial interview the patient reported that his speech had been deteriorating slowly. Oral mechanism examination revealed a mild right central facial weakness and an NVOA characterized by difficulty voluntarily clicking his tongue and coughing, with associated groping, off-target movements.

He had mild to moderate difficulties comprehending complex spoken or written sentences. He made several self-corrected semantic errors when naming pictures. Conversational speech was slow and characterized by short phrases that were occasionally telegraphic and infrequent semantic errors that he usually corrected. He made numerous spelling errors when writing to dictation. His self-generated written sentences were telegraphic, with self-corrected grammatical errors and some uncorrected spelling errors.

Motor speech evaluation revealed: reduced rate (−2); irregular articulatory breakdowns (1,2); distorted substitutions, with associated groping for articulatory postures; and dysprosody (2,3). Speech AMRs were slow (−1), and SMRs were poorly sequenced. He had considerable difficulty repeating multisyllabic words. Intelligibility was mildly impaired.

The clinician concluded that the patient had a "moderately severe AOS, perhaps with accompanying unilateral UMN dysarthria, both suggestive of left hemisphere posterior frontal dysfunction." He also had a "mild to moderate aphasia affecting all language modalities, although expressive functions were more impaired than receptive. This is also suggestive of left perisylvian, predominantly prerolandic dysfunction." The clinician was concerned about the patient's report of slow progression of symptoms and raised the possibility of a slowly progressive degenerative condition rather than stroke as the etiology for his problems. Subsequently, behavioral neurology consultation concluded that the patient might have an asymmetric cortical degenerative disease such as primary progressive aphasia.

The patient made some equivocal functional gains in speech during his hospital stay. When seen 6 months later for follow-up, he reported that his speech had worsened and said, "I can't read very much . . . words run

together." He was unable to write and had significant difficulty coordinating movements of his right arm. He had had a brief period of speech therapy following his hospital discharge but did not feel it helped. Examination again revealed a significant NVOA. His AOS was similar in character but clearly worse than during initial evaluation. There was little evidence of worsening of his aphasia.

The clinician concluded that he "continues to exhibit a marked AOS that is worse than 6 months ago. He also has a significant NVOA (and upper limb apraxia). His behavior during examination is quite characteristic of people with significant AOS and mild to moderate aphasia. I observed no evidence of behavior which is more typical of patients with generalized cognitive impairment."

Because the patient felt strongly that he would not benefit from speech therapy and because he had benefited minimally from therapy in the past, continued therapy was not pursued. He was advised, however, that therapy might be beneficial if his speech deteriorated to a point where functional verbal communication was difficult. Augmentative means of communication were discussed.

Neuropsychological assessment revealed little evidence of difficulty beyond the speech and language realm. A single photon emission computed tomography (SPECT) scan showed diffusely decreased uptake in the left parietal region and somewhat less decreased uptake in the left frontal region. It was concluded that the patient had an asymmetric degenerative process with the left parietal and left frontal regions being predominantly affected. The patient was not seen again for follow-up, but a phone call to the patient's wife 2 years later established that he was mute and had no functional use of his right upper extremity. His wife believed that his verbal comprehension and use of that his left upper extremity were good.

Commentary. (1) AOS and aphasia can be among the first and, for an extended time, most prominent signs of an asymmetric cortical degenerative process. The nature of the AOS and language disturbance may be indistinguishable from that seen in stroke. (2) AOS sometimes occurs simultaneously with significant LA. LA can make assessment of the linguistic aspects of writing and nonverbal intellectual abilities difficult. (3) Issues related to the management of AOS in people with degenerative disease differ from those for nondegenerative etiologies. These are discussed in the chapters on management.

Case 11-5

A 68-year-old, left-handed man was seen for speech-language assessment 6 weeks following a left hemisphere stroke. MRI showed a small area of increased signal in the left frontal lobe consistent with stroke.

The patient reported that he could produce only a few unintelligible sounds at the time of onset. He felt that his thoughts and the words in his mind were adequate, and he denied difficulty with verbal comprehension. As his speech began to improve, he felt that he had an accent that resembled German; as he continued to improve, it seemed more Norwegian in character. These accents resolved. He did feel that his reading rate had slowed, although he had never been a good reader or speller. He noted that he had always had difficulty in school and "just got by." At the time of examination, he felt that he had recovered to approximately 80% normal and was not having significant frustrations because of his speech difficulty. He denied difficulty with chewing or swallowing.

Oral mechanism examination was normal. There was no evidence of nonverbal oral apraxia. Voice and resonance were normal. Occasional vowel and consonant distortions, with vowel distortions being somewhat more prominent, characterized articulation. Infrequently, he produced distorted substitutions or additions. Overall speech rate was mildly slowed, particularly when he produced multisyllabic words. Speech AMRs were normal, but he had difficulty with SMRs at rapid rates.

Language examination revealed normal verbal comprehension and retention. Conversational language was normal in grammar and syntax, and there was no evidence of phonemic or semantic paraphasias. Confrontation naming ability and rapid word retrieval ability on a word fluency task was reduced. Reading rate was mildly slowed, semantic errors were evident, and he made occasional word reversals. With his preferred left hand, his writing to dictation contained frequent spelling errors, but his own generated sentence was adequate. It was felt that at least a portion of his reading and writing difficulty reflected longstanding problems related to early learning. The clinician concluded that the patient had a mild AOS and, perhaps, mild aphasia.

The patient was pleased with his recovery and stated he was not frustrated with his residual speech difficulties. It was felt that the prognosis for significant further recovery was good. Therapy was not recommended. He was counseled, however, that if his difficulties persisted and became a source of frustration for him, reassessment and consideration of therapy would be appropriate.

Commentary. (1) AOS is frequently caused by stroke in the left posterior frontal lobe, even in left-handed people. (2) AOS can be the dominant communication impairment resulting from stroke, and it can occur with minimal evidence of aphasic language impairment. (3) Prosodic abnormalities associated with AOS sometimes lead to perception of a (pseudo) foreign accent. (4) In general, when lesions are small and language impairment is not significant, prognosis for significant recovery from AOS due to stroke is considered good. (5) Not all patients with AOS require speech therapy. Decisions to recommend therapy need to consider, at the least, patient attitudes, judgments, and desires, as well as examination findings and prognosis.

Case 11-6

A 59-year-old, right-handed man was admitted to the hospital after developing visual difficulties and headache, followed several hours later by the onset of "expressive aphasia." Neurologic examination was normal, with the exception of a "prominent expressive aphasia characterized by hesitant speech with frequent word finding pauses and frequent errors and revisions." He had no obvious difficulties following simple and complex commands. The remainder of his neurologic examination was normal. MRI the day after admission (Figure 11-2) identified an early subacute infarct in the left posterior frontal operculum.

Speech pathology consultation 3 days after onset revealed a normal oral mechanism and no evidence of nonverbal oral apraxia. Language examination revealed normal verbal comprehension and retention. Reading comprehension was also normal, but reading aloud contained occasional semantic errors, mild hesitation, and occasional initial sound prolongations. Expressive language was normal in grammar and syntax, and there were no semantic or phonologic errors. Writing was difficult, with several semantic and spelling errors noted.

Speech was characterized by equivocally strained voice quality, occasional, brief hesitations and initial

Case 11-6—cont'd

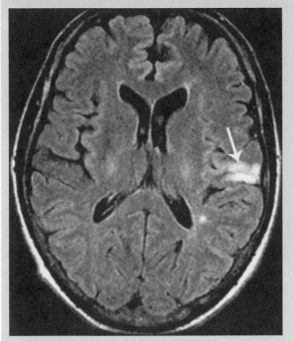

FIGURE 11-2 Magnetic resonance image of a 59-year-old man with mild to moderate apraxia of speech and mild problems with written language (see Case 11-6). The arrow identifies a relatively small lesion in the left posterior frontal operculum.

sound prolongations, and trial-and-error groping for correct place of articulation. These difficulties were more evident during speech SMRs and repetition of multisyllabic words. Intelligibility was normal.

The clinician concluded that the patient had a mild to moderate AOS plus, on the basis of problems with written language, mild aphasia. Therapy was recommended but not started, because the patient underwent a left carotid endarterectomy 2 days later. His speech was described by his surgeon as normal at the time of discharge shortly thereafter. He was not seen for formal speech-language reassessment or therapy postoperatively, however.

Commentary. (1) AOS is frequently associated with lesions in the left posterior frontal lobe. When the lesion is small, the AOS may be isolated or associated with less prominent impairments of language, sometimes confined to expressive modalities. (2) Oral mechanism examination may be entirely normal in people with AOS. (3) Recovery from initially mild AOS following stroke is often quite good (although the true degree of recovery is this case was not formally established).

Case 11-7

A 73-year-old woman was seen for speech-language assessment as part of a workup addressing a 1- to 2-year history of progressive neurologic difficulties, identified elsewhere as parkinsonism.

She described her speech difficulty by saying "I say what I'm gonna say, and I say the opposite," meaning that she made word choice errors and frequently substituted yes/no or vice versa. She denied difficulty with verbal comprehension but admitted to reading difficulty. She was unable to write because of right hand motor difficulties. She and her son agreed that she was able to communicate her basic needs quite adequately, if given enough time.

Oral mechanism examination was essentially normal in size, strength, and symmetry. She had a significant nonverbal oral apraxia, characterized primarily by verbalization or vocalization during orofacial movements she was asked to imitate or perform on command; she also groped for correct postures.

Speech was characterized by strained-harsh-hoarse voice quality (1), articulatory imprecision (1), groping for articulatory postures, occasional variable distortions and distorted substitutions, and difficulty with the sequencing demands of multisyllabic word production. She had some false starts and occasional initial sound/syllable repetitions. Speech AMRs were mildly slow. She was unable to sequence sounds for SMRs.

Language examination revealed mild impairment of verbal comprehension. Delays for word retrieval efforts and occasional semantic errors were apparent during conversation, and she occasionally deleted a function word. Word definitions and proverb explanations were concrete. Oral spelling was poor. She was able to read

Continued

Case 10-7—cont'd

large print words, but semantic and syntactic errors were evident when she read sentence level materials aloud. Her writing was not assessed because of significant limb apraxia and tremulousness.

The clinician concluded that the patient had AOS, NVOA, possibly a mild spastic dysarthria, mild to moderate aphasic language impairment, and some cognitive difficulties that could not clearly be attributable to her aphasia. He stated: "The patient's apraxia of speech, nonverbal oral apraxia, equivocal spastic dysarthria, and aphasia would be very unusual in Parkinson's disease but are not unusual in CBD, in my experience."

Both the patient and her son felt that she was getting along quite well in terms of functional communication in her everyday environment. She did not desire therapy. She and her son were counseled that if she developed increasing communication difficulties, speech-language therapy could be of assistance in developing compensatory strategies to facilitate functional communication.

Subsequent MRI showed marked cerebral atrophy, most prominent in the frontal and parietal lobes bilaterally. SPECT scan showed decreased perfusion in the frontal, parietal, and temporal lobes bilaterally but relatively worse in the left parietal lobe. Neuropsychological assessment confirmed the presence of moderate dementia, with cortical and subcortical features. The final clinical neurologic diagnosis was probable CBD.

Commentary. (1) AOS can occur in association with degenerative neurologic disease, in this case probable CBD. (2) Although it can be the most prominent communication disorder, aphasia, dysarthria, and nonaphasic cognitive deficits can accompany it. The presence of all of these deficits may provide some clues for neurologic diagnosis in people with degenerative neurologic disease. In this case the constellation of difficulties was considered unusual for Parkinson's disease but not unusual for some other degenerative neurologic conditions, such as CBD. (3) Not all patients with neurologic communication disorders desire speech-language therapy, and their lack of desire is often based on a judgment that their functional communication abilities are adequate for their needs. The clinician's responsibility in such cases is to inform the patient and his or her significant others about what therapy might accomplish and to facilitate the provision of such services when desired.

SUMMARY

1. AOS is a motor speech disorder resulting from an impaired capacity to plan or program the sensorimotor commands that direct movements that result in phonetically and prosodically normal speech. Its clinical characteristics are not attributable to the physiologic disturbances that explain the dysarthrias nor to the language processing disturbances that explain aphasia.

2. AOS is nearly always the result of pathology in the left (dominant) cerebral hemisphere. It occurs as the primary speech pathology diagnosis at a rate comparable to that for several of the major single dysarthria types. It is also often a secondary speech pathology diagnosis in people with left hemisphere damage and aphasia.

3. It frequently occurs with other motor and sensory signs of left hemisphere damage, but it can occur as the only evidence of neuropathology. Some people with AOS also have an NVOA and LA, but the three conditions can occur independently.

4. AOS is usually caused by stroke and sometimes by tumor or trauma. It occasionally is the presenting sign of a degenerative CNS disease.

5. AOS can occur in association with dysarthria, most often UUMN dysarthria or spastic dysarthria. Oral sensation may be impaired, but such impairments do not have a clear causal relationship with AOS. People with AOS but no evidence of aphasia generally have normal auditory processing skills.

6. Deviant speech characteristics associated with AOS include a number of abnormalities of articulation, rate, prosody, and fluency. The characteristics that best distinguish it from other motor speech disorders (the dysarthrias) are distorted sound substitutions and additions, decreased phonemic accuracy with increased rate, attempts to correct articulatory errors that cross phonemic boundaries, groping for articulatory postures, greater difficulty on volitional than automatic speech tasks, and greater difficulty on SMR and multisyllabic word tasks than AMR and single syllable tasks. People with severe AOS may have a limited phonetic repertoire, little difference between voluntary and automatic speech utterances, and a highly consistent pattern of perceived speech errors. Articulatory distortions, reduced rate, and various prosodic abnormalities help distinguish AOS from aphasic phonologic errors.

7. A number of acoustic and physiologic studies have provided confirmation for the clinical perceptual characteristics of AOS and have

documented a number of additional acoustic and movement traits that characterize the disorder. In general, they provide strong support for the notion that AOS is a problem of motor speech planning/programming.

References

1. Alexander MP et al: Neuropsychological and neuroanatomical dimensions of ideomotor apraxia, Brain 115:87, 1992.
2. Baum SR et al: Temporal dimensions of consonant and vowel production: an acoustic and CT scan analysis of aphasic speech, Brain Lang 39:33, 1990.
3. Bennett S, Netsell RW: Possible roles of the insula in speech and language processing: directions for research, J Med Speech-Lang Pathol 7:253, 1999.
4. Bergeron C et al: Unusual clinical presentations of cortical basal ganglionic degeneration, Ann Neurol 40:893, 1996.
5. Black SE: Focal cortical atrophy syndromes, Brain Cogn 31:188, 1996.
6. Blumstein SE et al: Production deficits in aphasia: a voice-onset time analysis, Brain Lang 9:153, 1980.
7. Blumstein SE et al: The perception and production of voice onset time in aphasia, Neuropsychologia 15:371, 1977.
8. Boeve B et al: Progressive nonfluent aphasia and subsequent aphasic dementia associated with atypical progressive supranuclear palsy pathology, Eur Neurol 49:72, 2003.
9. Boeve BF et al: Dysarthria and apraxia of speech associated with FK-506 (tacrolimus), Mayo Clin Proc 71:969, 1996.
10. Bronster DJ et al: Loss of speech after orthotopic liver transplantation, Transpl Int 8:234, 1995.
11. Brookshire RH: Introduction to neurogenic communication disorders, ed 6, St Louis, 2003, Mosby.
12. Broussolle E et al: Slowly progressive anarthria with late anterior opercular syndrome: a variant form of frontal cortical atrophy syndromes, J Neurol Sci 144:44, 1996.
13. Buckingham HW: Explanation in apraxia with consequences for the concept of apraxia of speech, Brain Lang 8:202, 1979.
14. Caligiuri MP, Till JA: Acoustical analysis of vowel duration in apraxia of speech: a case study, Folia Phoniatr 35:226, 1983.
15. Caselli RJ: Focal and asymmetric cortical degeneration syndromes, Neurologist 1:1, 1995.
16. Caselli RJ, Jack CR: Asymmetric cortical degeneration syndromes: a proposed clinical classification, Arch Neurol 49:770, 1992.
17. Caselli RJ et al: Asymmetric cortical degenerative syndromes: clinical and radiologic correlations, Neurology 42:1462, 1992.
18. Chapin C, Blumstein SE, Meissner B: Speech production mechanisms in aphasia: a delayed auditory feedback study, Brain Lang 14:106, 1981.
19. Chapman SB et al: Autosomal dominant progressive syndrome of motor-speech loss without dementia, Neurology 49:1298, 1997.
20. Cohen L et al: Pure progressive aphemia, J Neurol Neurosurg Psychiatry 56:923, 1993.
21. Collins M, Rosenbek JC, Wertz RT: Spectrographic analysis of vowel and word duration in apraxia of speech, J Speech Hear Res 26:224, 1983.
22. Croot K: Diagnosis of AOS: definition and criteria. Semin Speech Lang 23:267, 2002.
23. Dabul B: Apraxia battery for adults, ed 2, Austin, Tex, 2000, Pro-Ed.
24. Danly M, Shapiro B: Speech prosody in Broca's aphasia, Brain Lang 16:171, 1982.
25. Darley FL: Aphasia: input and output disturbances in speech and language processing. Presented at the meeting of the American Speech and Hearing Association, Chicago, Ill, 1969.
26. Darley FL: Apraxia of speech: 107 years of terminological confusion. Presented at the meeting of the American Speech and Hearing Association, Denver, Colo, 1968.
27. Darley FL: Lacunae and research approaches to them. In Milliken C, Darley FL, editors: Brain mechanisms underlying speech and language, New York, 1967, Grune & Stratton.
28. De Renzi E: Methods of limb apraxia examination and their bearing on the interpretation of the disorder. In Roy EA, editor: Neuropsychological studies of apraxia and related disorders, New York, 1985, North-Holland.
29. Deutsch SE: Oral form identification as a measure of cortical sensory dysfunction in apraxia of speech and aphasia, J Commun Disord 14:65, 1981.
30. Devere TR, Trotter JL, Cross AH: Acute aphasia in multiple sclerosis, Arch Neurol 57:1207, 2000.
31. Dronkers NF: A new brain region for coordinating speech articulation, Nature 384:159, 1996.
32. Duffy JR: Apraxia of speech in degenerative neurologic disease (in preparation).
33. Duffy JR: Apraxia of speech: historical overview and clinical manifestations of the acquired and developmental forms. In Shriberg LD, Campbell TF, editors: Proceedings of the 2002 Childhood Apraxia of Speech Symposium, Carlsbad, Calif, 2003, The Hendrix Foundation.
34. Duffy JR: Slowly progressive aphasia. In Brookshire RH, editor: Clinical aphasiology, Minneapolis, 1987, BRK Publishers.
35. Duffy JR, Duffy RJ: The assessment of limb apraxia: the limb apraxia test. In GE Hammond, editor: Cerebral control of speech and limb movements, New York, 1990, Elsevier Science.
36. Duffy JR, Duffy RJ: The limb apraxia test: an imitative measure of upper limb apraxia. In Prescott TE, editor: Clinical aphasiology, vol 18, Boston, 1989, College-Hill.
37. Duffy JR, Gawle CA: Apraxic speakers' vowel duration in consonant-vowel-consonant syllables. In Rosenbek C, McNeil MR, Aronson AE, editors: Apraxia of speech: physiology, acoustics, linguistics, management, San Diego, 1984, College-Hill.
38. Duffy, JR, Watt JR, Duffy RJ: Path analysis: a strategy for investigating the multivariate causal relationships in communication disorders, J Speech Hear Res 24:474, 1981.

39. Duffy RJ, Duffy JR: The relationship between pantomime expression and recognition in aphasia: the search for causes. In Hammond GE, editor: Cerebral control of speech and limb movements, New York, 1990, Elsevier Science.

40. Duffy RJ, Duffy JR: Three studies of deficits in pantomime expression and pantomime recognition in aphasia, J Speech Hear Res 24:70, 1981.

41. Eidelman BH et al: Abnormal cerebral blood flow findings in transplant patients with posttransplant apraxia of speech, Transplant Proc 33:2563, 2001.

42. Forrest K et al: Kinematic, electromyographic, and perceptual evaluation of speech apraxia, conduction aphasia, ataxic dysarthria, and normal speech production. In Moore CA, Yorkston KM, Beukelman DR, editors: Dysarthria and apraxia of speech: perspectives on management, Baltimore, 1991, Paul H Brookes.

43. Fox RJ et al: Aphemia: an isolated disorder of articulation, Clin Neurol Neurosurg 103:123, 2001.

44. Frattali C, Duffy JR: Characterizing and assessing speech and language disturbances. In Litvan I, editor: Atypical parkinsonian disorders: clinical and research aspects, Humana Press, (in press).

45. Frattali CM, Sonies BC: Speech and swallowing disturbances in corticobasal degeneration. In Litvan I, Goetz CG, Lang AE, editors: Advances in neurology, corticobasal degeneration and related disorders, vol 82, Philadelphia, 2000, Lippincott Williams & Wilkins.

46. Freeman FJ, Sands ES, Harris KS: Temporal coordination of phonation and articulation in a case of verbal apraxia: a voice onset time study, Brain Lang 6:106, 1978.

47. Fromm D et al: Simultaneous perceptual-physiological method for studying apraxia of speech. In Brookshire RH, editor: Clinical aphasiology: conference proceedings, Minneapolis, 1982, BRK Publishers.

48. Fukui T et al: Primary progressive apraxia in Pick's disease: a clinicopathologic study, Neurology 47:467, 1996.

49. Gandour J, Petty SH: Dysprosody in Broca's aphasia: a case study, Brain Lang 37:232, 1989.

50. Goodglass H, Kaplan E, Barresi B: The Boston diagnostic aphasia examination, ed 3, Philadelphia, 2001, Lippincott Williams & Wilkins.

51. Hageman CF et al: Oral motor tracking in normal and apraxic speakers, Clin Aphasiol 22:219, 1994.

52. Haley KL, Overton HB: Word length and vowel duration in apraxia of speech: the use of relative measures, Brain Lang 79:397, 2001.

53. Hardcastle WJ, Morgan Barry RA, Clark CJ: Articulatory and voicing characteristics of adult dysarthric and verbal dyspraxic speakers: an instrumental study, Br J Disord Commun 20:249, 1985.

54. Itoh M, Sasanuma S: Articulatory movements in apraxia of speech. In Rosenbek C, McNeil MR, Aronson AE, editors: Apraxia of speech: physiology, acoustics, linguistics, management, San Diego, 1984, College-Hill Press.

55. Itoh M, Sasanuma S, Ushijima T: Velar movements during speech in a patient with apraxia of speech, Brain Lang 7:227, 1979.

56. Itoh M et al: Voice onset time characteristics in apraxia of speech, Brain Lang 17:193, 1982.

57. Itoh M et al: Abnormal articulatory dynamics in a patient with apraxia of speech: x-ray microbeam observations, Brain Lang 11:66, 1980.

58. Johns DF, Darley FL: Phonemic variability in apraxia of speech, J Speech Hear Res 13:556, 1970.

59. Johns DF, LaPointe LL: Neurogenic disorders of outputprocessing: apraxia of speech. In Whitaker H, Whitaker HA, editors: Studies in neurolinguistics, vol 1, New York, 1976, Academic Press.

60. Katz W et al: A kinematic analysis of anticipatory coarticulation in the speech of anterior aphasic subjects using electromagnetic articulography, Brain Lang 38:555, 1990.

61. Kent RD, Rosenbek JC: Acoustic patterns of apraxia of speech, J Speech Hear Res 26:231, 1983.

62. Kertesz A: Subcortical lesions and verbal apraxia. In Rosenbek JC, McNeil MR, Aronson AE, editors: Apraxia of speech: physiology, acoustics, linguistics, management, San Diego, 1984, College-Hill.

63. Kertesz A: Western aphasia battery, San Antonio, 1982, Psychological Corporation.

64. Kirk A, Ang LC: Unilateral Creutzfeldt-Jakob disease presenting as rapidly progressive aphasia, Can J Neurol Sci 21:350, 1994.

65. LaPointe LL, Wertz RT: Oral-movement abilities and articulatory characteristics of brain-injured adults, Percept Mot Skills 39:39, 1974.

66. Lehman Blake M et al: Speech and language disorders associated with corticobasal degeneration, J Med Speech-Lang Pathol 11:131, 2003.

67. Leiguarda RC et al: Apraxia in Parkinson's disease, progressive supranuclear palsy, multiple system atrophy and neuroleptic-induced parkinsonism, Brain 120:75, 1997.

68. Liepman H: Das Krankheitsbild der apraxie (moterischen asymbolie) auf grund eines falles von einseitiger apraxie, Monatsschrift fur Psychiatrie und Neurologie 8:15, 1900.

69. Liss JM: Error-revision in the spontaneous speech of apraxic speakers, Brain Lang 62:342, 1998.

70. Luria AR: Higher cortical functions in man, New York, 1980, Basic Books.

71. Mandell AM, Alexander MP, Carpenter S: Creutzfeldt-Jakob disease presenting as isolated aphasia, Neurology 39:55, 1989.

72. Marshall RC, Gandour J, Windsor J: Selective impairment of phonation: a case study, Brain Lang 35:313, 1988.

73. Mastrianni JA: Prion diseases: transmissible spongiform encephalopathies. In Noseworthy JH, editor: Neurological therapeutics: principles and practice, vol 1, New York, 2003, Martin Dunitz.

74. Mateer C, Kumura D: Impairment of nonverbal oral movements in aphasia, Brain Lang 4:262, 1977.

75. McNeil MR, editor: Apraxia of speech: from concept to clinic, Semin Speech Lang 23:4, 2002.

76. McNeil MR, Adams S: A comparison of speech kinematics among apraxic, conduction aphasic, ataxic dysarthric and normal geriatric speakers, Clin Aphasiol 18:279, 1990.

77. McNeil MR, Duffy JR: Primary progressive aphasia. In Chapey R, editor: Language intervention strategies in

aphasia and related disorders, ed 4, Philadelphia, 2001, Lippincott Williams & Wilkins.

78. McNeil MR, Kent RD: Motoric characteristics of adult apraxic and aphasic speakers. In GR Hammond, editor: Cerebral control of speech and limb movements, New York, 1990, North-Holland.

79. McNeil MR, Calguiri M, Rosenbek JC: A comparison of labiomandibular kinematic durations, displacements, velocities, and dysmetrias in apraxic and normal adults. In Prescott TE, editor: Clinical aphasiology, vol 18, Boston, 1989, College-Hill Press.

80. McNeil MR, Doyle PJ, Wambaugh J: Apraxia of speech: a treatable disorder of motor planning and programming. In Nadeau SE, Gonzalez Rothi LJ, Crosson B, editors: Aphasia and language: theory to practice, New York, 2000, Guilford Press.

81. McNeil MR, Hashi M, Southwood H: Acoustically derived perceptual evidence for coarticulatory errors in apraxic and conduction aphasic speech production, Clin Aphasiol 22:203, 1994.

82. McNeil MR, Robin DA, Schmidt RA: Apraxia of speech: definition, differentiation, and treatment. In McNeil MR, editor: Clinical management of sensorimotor speech disorders, New York, 1997, Thieme.

83. McNeil MR et al: Effects of speech rate on the absolute and relative timing of apraxic and conduction aphasic sentence production, Brain Lang 38:135, 1990a.

84. McNeil MR et al: Oral structure nonspeech motor control in normal, dysarthric, aphasic and apraxic speakers: isometric force and static position control, J Speech Hear Res 33:255, 1990b.

85. Mercaitis PA: Some temporal characteristics of imitative speech in non–brain-injured, aphasic, and apraxic adults. Unpublished doctoral dissertation, University of Massachusetts, Amherst, Mass, 1983.

86. Mesulam M-M: Principles of behavioral and cognitive neurology, ed 2, New York, 2000, Oxford University Press.

87. Meuse S, Marquardt TP, Cannito MP: Phonological analysis of apraxia of speech in Broca's aphasia. In Cannito MP, Yorkston KM, Beukelman DR, editors: Neuromotor speech disorders: nature, assessment, and management, Baltimore, 1998, Brookes Publishing.

88. Miller N: The neurological basis of apraxia of speech. Semin Speech Lang 23:223, 2002.

89. Mohr JP: Revision of Broca's aphasia and the syndrome of Broca's area infarction and its implications for aphasia therapy. In Brookshire RH, editor: Proceedings of the conference on clinical aphasiology, Minneapolis, 1980, BRK Publishers.

90. Nagao M et al: Apraxia of speech associated with an infarct in the precentral gyrus of the insula, Neuroradiology 41:356, 1999.

91. Ochipa C, Gonzalez Rothi LJ: Limb apraxia. In Nadeau SE, Gonzalez Rothi LJ, Crosson B, editors: Aphasia and language: theory to practice, New York, 2000, Guilford Press.

92. Odell K et al: Perceptual characteristics of consonant production by apraxic speakers, J Speech Hear Disord 55:345, 1990.

92a. Ozsancak C, Auzou P, Hannequin D: Dysarthria and orofacial apraxia in corticobasal degeneration. Mov Disord 15:905, 2000.

92b. Peach RK, Tonkovich JD: Phonemic characteristics of apraxia of speech resulting from subcortical hemorrhage. J Commun Disord 37:77, 2004.

93. Pellat J et al: Aphemia after a penetrating brain wound: a case study, Brain Lang 40:459, 1991.

94. Robin DA, Bean C, Folkins JW: Lip movement in apraxia of speech, J Speech Hear Res 32:512, 1989.

95. Rosenbek JC: Treating apraxia of speech. In Johns DF, editor: Clinical management of neurogenic communicative disorders, Boston, 1985, Little, Brown & Company.

96. Rosenbek JC, Kent RD, LaPointe LL: Apraxia of speech: an overview and some perspectives (1984). In Rosenbek JC, McNeil MR, Aronson AE, editors: Apraxia of speech: physiology, acoustics, linguistics, management, San Diego, 1984, College-Hill Press.

97. Rosenbek JC, Wertz RT, Darley FL: Oral sensation and perception in apraxia of speech and aphasia, J Speech Hear Disord 16:22, 1973.

98. Roy EA, Square-Storer PA: Evidence for common expressions of apraxia. In Hammond GE, editor: Cerebral control of speech and limb movements, New York, 1990, Elsevier Science.

99. Ryalls JH: An acoustic study of vowel production in aphasia, Brain Lang 29:48, 1986.

100. Ryalls JH: Intonation in Broca's aphasia, Neuropsychologia 20:355, 1982.

101. Ryalls JH: Motor aphasia: acoustic correlates of phonetic disintegration in vowels, Neuropsychologia 19:365, 1981.

102. Sakurai Y et al: Progressive aphemia in a patient with Pick's disease: a neuropsychological and anatomic study, J Neurol Sci 159:156, 1998.

103. Seddoh SAK et al: Speech timing in apraxia of speech versus conduction aphasia, J Speech Hear Res 39:590, 1996.

104. Shankweiler D, Harris KS: An experimental approach to the problem of articulation in aphasia, Cortex 2:277, 1966.

105. Shankweiler D, Harris KS, Taylor ML: Electromyographic studies of articulation in aphasia, Arch Phys Med Rehabil 49:1, 1968.

106. Shinn P, Blumstein SE: Phonetic disintegration in aphasia: acoustic analysis of spectral characteristics for place of articulation, Brain Lang 20:90, 1983.

107. Shuttleworth EC, Yates AJ, Paltan-Ortiz J: Creutzfeldt-Jakob disease presenting as progressive aphasia, J Natl Med Assoc 77:649, 1985.

108. Skenes LL: Durational changes of apraxic speakers, J Commun Disord 20:61, 1987.

109. Square PA, Martin RE, Bose A: Nature and treatment of neuromotor speech disorders in aphasia. In Chapey R, editor: Language intervention strategies in aphasia and related neurogenic communication disorders, Philadelphia, 2001, Lippincott Williams & Wilkins.

110. Square-Storer P, Darley FL, Sommers RK: Nonspeech and speech processing skills in patients with aphasia and apraxia of speech, Brain Lang 33:65, 1988.

111. Square-Storer PA, Apeldoorn S: An acoustic study of apraxia of speech in patients with different lesion loci. In Moore CA, Yorkston KM, Beukelman DR, editors: Dysarthria and apraxia of speech: perspectives on management, Baltimore, 1991, Paul H. Brookes.

112. Square-Storer PA, Roy EA: The apraxias: commonalities and distinctions. In Square-Storer PA, editor: Acquired apraxia of speech in aphasia adults, New York, 1989, Taylor & Francis.

113. Strand EA, McNeil MR: Effects of length and linguistic complexity on temporal acoustic measures in apraxia of speech, J Speech Hear Res 39:1018, 1996.

114. Strand EA, McNeil MR: Evidence for a motor performance deficit versus a misapplied rule system in the temporal organization of utterances in apraxia of speech. In Brookshire RH, editor: Clinical aphasiology, vol 17, Minneapolis, 1987, BRK Publishers.

115. Strauss Hough M, Klich RJ: Lip EMG activity during vowel production in apraxia of speech: phrase context and word length effects, J Speech Hear Res 41:786, 1998.

116. Strauss M, Klich RJ: Word length effects on EMG/vowel duration relationships in apraxic speakers, Folia Phoniatr Logop 53:58, 2001.

117. Sussman H et al: Compensatory articulation in Broca's aphasia, Brain Lang 27:56, 1986.

118. Tognola G, Vignolo LA: Brain lesions associated with oral apraxia in stroke patients: a clinico-neuroradiological investigation with the CT scan, Neuropsychologia, 18:257, 1980.

119. Towne RL, Crary MA: Verbal reaction time patterns in aphasic adults: consideration for apraxia of speech, Brain Lang 35:138, 1988.

120. Tuller B: On categorizing aphasic speech errors, Neuropsychologia 22:547, 1984.

121. Tyrrell PJ et al: Progressive loss of speech output and orofacial apraxia associated with frontal lobe hypometabolism, J Neurol Neurosurg Psychiatry 54:351, 1991.

122. Van Der Merwe A: A theoretical framework for the characterization of pathological speech sensorimotor control. In McNeil MR, editor: Clinical management of sensorimotor speech disorders, New York, 1997, Thieme.

123. Van Putten SM, Walker JP: The production of emotional prosody in varying degrees of severity of apraxia of speech, J Commun Dis 36:77, 2003.

124. Varley R, Whiteside SP: What is the underlying impairment in acquired apraxia of speech? Aphasiology 15:39, 2001.

125. Varley R, Whiteside S, Luff H: Apraxia of speech as a disruption of word-level schemata: some durational evidence, J Med Speech-Lang Pathol 7:127, 1999.

126. Weismer G, Liss JM: Acoustic/perceptual taxonomies of speech production deficits in motor speech disorders. In Moore CA, Yorkston KM, Beukelman DR, editors: Dysarthria and apraxia of speech: perspectives on management, Baltimore, 1991, Paul H Brookes.

127. Wertz RT, LaPointe LL, Rosenbek JC: Apraxia of speech in adults: the disorder and its management, New York, 1984, Grune & Stratton.

128. Wertz RT, Rosenbek JC, Deal JL: A review of 228 cases of apraxia of speech: classification, etiology, and localization. Presented at the meeting of the American Speech and Hearing Association, New York, NY, 1970.

129. Yamanouchi H, Budka H, Bass K: Unilateral Creutzfeld-Jakob disease, Neurology 36:1517, 1986.

130. Ziegler W: Psycholinguistic and motor theories of apraxia of speech. Semin Speech Lang 23:231, 2002.

131. Ziegler W: Task-related factors in oral motor control: speech and oral diadochokinesis in dysarthria and apraxia of speech, Brain Lang 80:556, 2002.

132. Ziegler W, von Cramon D: Disturbed coarticulation in apraxia of speech: acoustic evidence, Brain Lang 29:34, 1986.

133. Ziegler W, von Cramon D: Anticipatory coarticulation in a patient with apraxia of speech, Brain Lang 26:117, 1985.

12 Neurogenic Mutism

"Mutism is like a sphinx—it is both captivating and disquieting. It stares at us defiantly, and we find it difficult to solve its silent riddle."[46]

Y. Lebrun

CHAPTER OUTLINE

I. **Motor speech disorders and mutism**
   A. Anarthria
   B. Locked-in syndrome
   C. Biopercular syndrome
   D. Cerebellar mutism
   E. Apraxia of speech and mutism
II. **Aphasia and mutism**
III. **Nonaphasic cognitive and affective deficits associated with mutism**
   A. Disorders of arousal (coma)
   B. Diffuse impairments of cortical functions
   C. Akinetic mutism
IV. **Etiology specific neurogenic mutism**
   A. Mutism following corpus callosotomy
   B. Speech arrest
   C. Drug-induced mutism
V. **Cases**
VI. **Summary**

Disease can leave its victims conscious and alert but without speech. Sometimes this condition is accompanied by cognitive deficits that make speechlessness an accurate reflection of an affected person's inner state. Sometimes the motor system is so damaged that a normally formulated message cannot be spoken. In the cruelest of circumstances, a cognitively intact person may be "locked in," unable to convey basic thoughts in any conventional way.

Mutism is the absence of speech. Unlike motor speech disorders (MSDs), which by definition are neurologic in origin, mutism has multiple possible causes. It can be deliberate (elected) or a product of subconscious psychiatric disturbances. It can also be organic but nonneurologic, as in some people with profound congenital hearing loss or peripheral structural loss, such as laryngectomy. Mutism can also be caused by neurologic disease, and neurogenic mutism may be congenital or acquired. It can be the result of peripheral nervous system damage or central nervous system (CNS) pathology anywhere from the brainstem to the cortex.

Acquired neurogenic mutism is addressed in this chapter. Congenital neurogenic mutism is not addressed here, nor is muteness associated with deafness or musculoskeletal deficits. Psychogenic mutism is addressed in Chapter 14; it is of special interest because it is sometimes difficult to distinguish from, or is intertwined with, neurogenic mutism.

Neurogenic mutism can take several forms. It can be a product of severe dysarthria, apraxia of speech (AOS), aphasia, or various nonaphasic cognitive and affective conditions. It can also occur under specific medical circumstances (e.g., in association with seizures or after surgical sectioning of the corpus callosum), even though the precise underlying nature of the mutism may be uncertain. Distinctions among these forms of neurogenic mutism can be quite important to differential diagnosis, localization, and management. The definition and clinical manifestations, neurologic substrates, and common etiologies of each of several forms of neurogenic mutism are addressed in the remainder of this chapter. Table 12-1 summarizes types of neurogenic mutism, their neurologic substrates, and common clinical characteristics.

■ MOTOR SPEECH DISORDERS AND MUTISM

Several single dysarthria types, or combinations of them, as well as AOS, can be severe enough to

12-1   Types of neurogenic mutism and their neurologic substrates and distinguishing clinical features

Type	Localization	Primary Clinical Manifestations
Motor Speech Disorders		
Anarthria		
Spastic dysarthria (including LiS)	Bilateral UMN	Oromotor spasticity & weakness, severe dysphagia, pathologic reflexes; quadriplegia if locked-in, but preserved eye movements
Flaccid dysarthria	LMN	Oromotor and/or respiratory weakness paralysis; dysphagia; absent reflexes; atrophy fasciculations
Hypokinetic or hyper-kinetic dysarthria	Basal ganglia control circuit	Oromotor & respiratory rigidity & hypokinesia, or hyperkinetic movement disorder
Cerebellar mutism	Cerebellar control circuit	Transient mutism followed by dysarthria (possibly ataxic in most cases), absence of cranial nerve deficits, difficulty with complex nonspeech oromotor movements, possible AOS
Biopercular syndrome	Lower precentral & postcentral gyri	Minimal voluntary orofacial mobility; hypotonic & weak orofacial muscles; dysphagia; absent gag reflex; relatively preserved cough, yawn, & emotional orofacial responses; ? AOS; ? NVOA
Apraxia of speech	Left hemisphere	Groping efforts to speak, aphonia, normal swallowing & automatic oral movements, NVOA
Aphasia	Left hemisphere	Severe multimodality impairments of language, accompanying AOS & NVOA
Diffuse Cognitive/Affective Deficits		
Arousal	Reticular activating system	Coma, unresponsive or responding only to vigorous stimulation, disturbed sleep-wake cycle
Persistent vegetative state	Cerebral cortex, diffuse	Preserved wake-sleep cycle, no visual tracking or response to stimulation
Apallic state	Cerebral cortex, diffuse	Preserved wake-sleep cycle, may respond to painful stimuli, alterations in tone & posture
Frontal/Limbic System		
Akinetic mutism	Frontal lobes	Preserved motor & sensory ability; seemingly alert but abulic, unresponsive, & apathetic; delayed responses; grasp & snout reflexes
Etiology Specific		
Commissurotomy	Corpus callosum (frontal lobes, SMA?)	Uncertain mechanism (AOS, aphasia, akinetic mutism possible)
Seizure-related speech arrests	Right or left SMA, dominant language cortex	Variable explanations (AOS, aphasia, akinetic mutism, others)
Drug-induced	Uncertain/variable	Uncertain/variable (anarthria, AOS, akinetic mutism possible)

AOS, Apraxia of speech; *LiS,* locked-in syndrome; *LMN,* lower motor neuron; *NVOA,* nonverbal oral apraxia; *SMA,* supplementary motor area; *UMN,* upper motor neuron.

cause mutism. In this section several subcategories of dysarthria associated with mutism are discussed. This includes the generic disorder, anarthria, which captures all forms of dysarthric mutism, but also locked-in syndrome, the biopercular syndrome, and cerebellar mutism. The latter three subcategories are given explicit recognition because they are rare and represent special challenges to differential diagnosis and management or because the nature of the dysarthria (or other underlying deficits) is poorly

understood. Mutism associated with AOS is also discussed.

Anarthria

Definition and Clinical Characteristics

The term *anarthria* refers to *speechlessness due to a severe loss of neuromuscular control over speech.* Although the term is sometimes used to refer to mutism associated with AOS, its use today by speech pathologists and most neurologists is usually reserved for *dysarthria in its most severe form*.

The language and cognitive abilities of anarthric patients may be intact, as may be their emotional drive or desire to communicate, but their neuromuscular system does not permit speech. Thus anarthric individuals do not speak because they cannot speak.

The specific types of dysarthria underlying anarthric muteness can be difficult to establish and technically impossible if differential diagnosis is restricted to distinctions among deviant speech characteristics. However, dysarthria type can be presumed in those with progressive disorders when evaluation before the loss of speech was able to establish it. Inferences about the types of dysarthria also can be made on the basis of confirmatory features and information about etiology and lesion localization. In addition, in many cases the use of the term *anarthria* is not absolute; the label often is used to mean that "for all practical purposes" the patient is mute. Many anarthric individuals can make some visible attempts to speak, and some can produce a few sounds or some voice and even approximate some syllables. These efforts, combined with observations of movement and reflexes during oral mechanism examination and other physical findings (e.g., limb strength, tone, reflexes), permit judgments about the compatibility of the inferred dysarthria type with known etiology and localization. If etiology and localization are unknown, the clinical observations may help to establish them.

In general, flaccid dysarthria alone seldom leads to anarthria because it is unusual for multiple cranial nerves supplying the speech muscles to be involved bilaterally (a near-requirement for anarthria to develop from lower motor neuron [LMN] weakness alone). Flaccid dysarthria associated with myasthenia gravis, Guillain-Barré syndrome, and brainstem tumors affecting multiple cranial nerves bilaterally can lead to mutism, however. It is also unusual for ataxic dysarthria to be so severe that anarthria is the result, although the condition known as "cerebellar mutism" (discussed later in this chapter) may represent an exception. Similarly, hyperkinetic dysarthria, although capable of producing devastating effects on speech intelligibility, only infrequently results in anarthria.

Spastic and hypokinetic dysarthria are the most likely culprits when a single dysarthria type leads to anarthria, with spastic dysarthria probably representing the most frequent cause in vascular diseases. As might be expected, mixed dysarthrias probably account for more cases of anarthria than single types, although this has not been studied systematically. Based on the distribution of types of mixed dysarthrias reviewed in Chapter 10 (see Table 10-3),

it is likely that mixed spastic-flaccid, spastic-ataxic, and spastic-hypokinetic dysarthrias account for many cases of anarthria.

Neurologic Substrates and Etiologies

Bilateral final common pathway (LMN) involvement of speech cranial and respiratory nerves, bilateral direct and indirect activation pathway involvement, and bilateral control circuit pathology may, separately or in combination, lead to anarthria. Combined direct and indirect pathway involvement (as in spastic dysarthria), or basal ganglia control circuit pathology (as in hypokinetic or hyperkinetic dysarthria), are probably more frequently implicated in anarthria than are other components of the motor system.

Table 12-2 summarizes the etiologies and primary speech diagnoses for 30 cases with anarthria, including locked-in syndrome. The cases illustrate, but do not exhaust, what the literature suggests regarding etiology. Stroke was the most frequent etiology. Most strokes were in the brainstem, and a single brainstem

table 12-2 Etiology and type of motor speech disorder for 30 quasirandomly selected cases seen at the Mayo Clinic with a primary speech pathology diagnosis of anarthria, including LiS

Etiology	Speech Diagnosis
Brainstem stroke (9)	LiS, unspecified dysarthria type (6)
	Anarthria, unspecified dysarthria type (2)
	LiS, spastic (1)
Multiple, bilateral strokes (7)	Anarthria, unspecified dysarthria type (4)
	Anarthria, spastic (2)
	Anarthria, spastic + AOS (1)
CHI (5)	Anarthria, unspecified dysarthria type (3)
	Anarthria, spastic (2)
Undetermined CNS degenerative disease (3)	Anarthria, spastic (1)
	Anarthria, unspecified dysarthria + AOS (1)
	Anarthria, unspecified dysarthria (1)
ALS (2)	Anarthria, spastic-flaccid
PSP (1)	Anarthria, spastic-hypokinetic
Brainstem tumor, postsurgical (1)	LiS, flaccid
Anoxic encephalopathy (1)	Anarthria, spastic
MS + multiple strokes (1)	Anarthria, unspecified dysarthria type

ALS, Amyotrophic lateral sclerosis; *AOS,* apraxia of speech; *CHI,* closed head injury; *CNS,* central nervous system; *LiS,* locked-in syndrome; *MS,* multiple sclerosis; *PSP,* progressive supranuclear palsy.

stroke was sufficient to cause anarthria in numerous cases. Multiple strokes leading to anarthria were more widely dispersed, often including cortical or subcortical hemispheric events, but always bilateral; multiple strokes sometimes also included lesions in the brainstem. Closed head injury (CHI) was also a frequent cause, often associated with multifocal and diffuse injuries, frequently including or largely limited to the brainstem. Degenerative CNS disease, sometimes not further specified, but also including amyotrophic lateral sclerosis (ALS), progressive supranuclear palsy (PSP), and multiple sclerosis (MS), led to anarthria in some cases.* Anoxic encephalopathy, as well as multiple cranial nerve injuries associated with a brainstem tumor and subsequent neurosurgery, represented other causes. One individual had MS plus multiple strokes.

Anarthria may also result from severe extrapyramidal diseases (e.g., Parkinson's and Wilson's diseases). A number of other diseases may also be associated with dysarthria and mutism, but the severe cognitive impairments typically associated with them in their later stages make it difficult to determine if muteness is motor or cognitive, or both, in origin (e.g., Alzheimer's disease, Creutzfeldt-Jakob disease, Huntington's chorea, progressive multifocal leukoencephalopathy).

Vogel and von Cramon[86-88] have studied mutism and subsequent dysarthria in individuals with traumatic midbrain injuries. Patients were typically mute for several days to months after regaining consciousness. They had hemiparesis or quadriparesis; limb spasticity or ataxia, or both; and severe limitations of jaw, lip, and tongue mobility. Phonation was apparent only during coughing or gagging. Speech reemerged slowly and was initially characterized by a poorly modulated sound that conveyed affective information such as pain, followed by emergence of a breathy-whispered dysphonia, often high in pitch and poorly modulated, with poor articulation and respiratory control. Dysarthria type was described as mixed spastic-hypokinetic.

Locked-in Syndrome[†]

Definition and Clinical Characteristics

When anarthria is accompanied by total immobility of the body except for vertical eye movements and

blinking, but the individual is sufficiently intact cognitively to communicate with eye movements, the condition is referred to as *locked-in syndrome (LiS)*.*[67] Its distinction from coma is made on the basis of the LiS patient's ability to communicate with eyeblinks, or, in rare cases, by electroencephalogram (EEG) demonstrating normal cortical electrical activity.[6,63] Thus *LiS is a special and dramatic manifestation of anarthria,* one that presents special challenges to diagnosis and management.

Patients with "classical" LiS are mute and usually have a spastic quadriplegia and no craniofacial movements except for upper eyelid and vertical eye movements. Respiratory difficulties are common.[58] LiS is occasionally "incomplete," with remnants of additional voluntary movements such as horizontal gaze or face movement.[63] Rarely, "total" LiS occurs, in which even eye movements are absent. A review of 139 cases found 64% to have classical manifestations, 33% to have incomplete manifestations, and only 2% to have total LiS.[63]

The anarthria of LiS most often reflects severe spastic or mixed spastic-flaccid dysarthria. Typically the patient cannot move the jaw, face, tongue, palate, or vocal folds voluntarily. Dysphagia is severe. Stereotyped chewing and sucking movements or a facial grimace sometimes can be elicited by perioral or noxious stimuli. People with incomplete LiS may produce some face, tongue, jaw, and head or forehead movements.

The outlook for locked-in patients is generally poor, with mortality within the first 4 months after onset approaching 90%; death within the first week after onset usually reflects extension of a brainstem lesion, but pulmonary complications are the most common cause of death overall.[63] Many patients require mechanical ventilatory support and assisted secretion management, and a number need tracheostomy and intubation.

Long-term survival with LiS has improved in recent years. People with nonvascular etiologies tend to show earlier and more complete recovery than those with vascular etiology, and functional recovery in vascular cases is generally quite limited in the first 4 months.[63] However, several independent reports of groups of patients who have survived for more than 5 months (some or many of whom had intensive therapies, including speech therapy) have documented significant motor recovery in approximately 20%, ability to feed orally in 42% to more than 50%, ability to read in 77%, ability to communicate verbally in 28% to 66%, and ability to

---

*It is not uncommon for anarthria to be the end stage of dysarthria (or AOS) in numerous degenerative neurologic diseases (e.g., ALS, multiple system atrophy [MSA], PSP, CBD) that were discussed in Chapter 10.

[†]For a beautifully written and moving personal account of life with locked-in syndrome, read *The Diving Bell and the Butterfly* by Jean-Dominique Bauby.[5]

*LiS is sometimes referred to as the deefferentiated state,[73] ventral pontine syndrome, or bilateral brain pyramidal system syndrome.[21]

communicate with alternative communication devices in approximately 40%.[17,37,47]

Case reports of dramatic improvement in LiS, sometimes over the course of several years, suggest that speech tends to improve later than limb movement.[52,73] Youth and an absence of hypertension or previous stroke may be favorable prognostic signs for such recovery.[52] McGann and Paslawski[53] documented the cases of two highly motivated individuals with LiS who progressed from an eye blink form of communication to the use of computerized communication devices. Importantly, they noted that neither patient was entirely intact cognitively, consistent with what little is known about the cognitive status of people with LiS. This highlights the importance of cognitive and language assessment for LiS.* Most studies emphasize the importance of vigorous physical, dysphagia, and speech-communication therapy for their cases.

Neurologic Substrate and Etiologies

The preservation of consciousness, eye movements, and the ability to communicate in LiS are accounted for by sparing of supranuclear oculomotor pathways and the reticular formation of the pons and midbrain, as well as their connections with relatively intact functions of the cerebral cortex.[6,21]

In the great majority of cases, LiS is caused by vascular occlusion of the basilar artery, affecting the ventral aspect of the pons and severing descending motor pathways to the spinal cord and lower cranial nerves.[46,75] Much less commonly, infarction is in the ventral midbrain or the internal capsule, bilaterally.[21,22] Other etiologies include trauma, central pontine myelinolysis, tumor, encephalitis, MS, and drug toxicity or abuse.*[47,63,65]

Biopercular Syndrome

Definition and Clinical Characteristics

The biopercular syndrome is a rare disorder that can be associated with varying degrees of dysarthria,

---

*It has been shown that P300 event-related potentials (ERPs), which measure electrical activity in the brain during performance of cognitive tasks, are present in at least some people with LiS.[62] ERPs may be particularly useful in demonstrating the integrity of some cognitive functions in individuals who cannot communicate with eye or other volitional movements.

*Trauma may be the second most frequent cause of LiS, at least in those who survive for extended periods. For example, in a survey of 44 members of France's Association of Locked-in Syndrome (ALIS), the LiS was caused by stroke in 86% and by traumatic brain injury (TBI) in 14%.[47]

---

including mutism. It has also been called *flaccid facial diplegia,* the *Foix-Chavany-Marie syndrome,* or the *opercular syndrome.*[46] It is caused by bilateral damage to the lower part of the precentral and postcentral convolutions of the cerebral hemispheres (rolandic operculum).

The syndrome's defining clinical features[16,46,49,91] include the following:

1. Severely reduced voluntary orofacial mobility. Lip, tongue, jaw, and palatal movements are hypotonic, weak, and restricted. The upper face is also often affected, with inability to voluntarily close the eyes or frown. Hypotonicity gives the face a void appearance.
2. Preserved reflexive cough and yawning, preserved automatic and emotional facial and jaw movements, laughing, and crying.
3. The patient is often mute or capable only of minimal, distorted, low-volume speech.
4. Severe dysphagia. Chewing ability is severely limited, and food must often be pushed to the back of the mouth to trigger a swallow, but the pharyngeal phase of swallowing may be normal. The gag reflex is usually absent. There is a high risk of aspiration pneumonia. Percutaneous endoscopic gastrostomy may be required.
5. Limb movements may be preserved. There may be no significant aphasia, and communication through writing may be normal. When the etiology is vascular, the severe dysarthria and dysphagia tend to persist, although facial movement and chewing may show some improvement.

A number of the syndrome's features resemble those encountered in muteness reflecting the anarthria of spastic dysarthria. In fact, it has been called an extreme form of pseudobulbar palsy.[16,91] However, in the biopercular syndrome the speech muscles appear hypotonic rather than spastic, pseudobulbar laughter and crying are not common, and the pharyngeal phase of swallowing may be normal.[46] Of special interest is the apparent dissociation of voluntary and automatic movements. For example, "normal" but stereotypic laughter and crying in appropriate situations have been described, in spite of severe dysphagia and speech limited to an undifferentiated moan.[16]

Neurologic Substrate and Etiologies

Bilateral damage to the rolandic operculum is the apparent cause of the syndrome.[46,49] Stroke is nearly always the etiology. The syndrome frequently occurs after a unilateral opercular lesion from which there may be good recovery, followed by a second stroke on the other side, after which the syndrome emerges. Traumatic, neoplastic, and infectious etiologies are also possible. The syndrome also may emerge as a variant of primary lateral sclerosis or other focal degenerative CNS disease.[13,45,91,92] It can also be present congenitally or in childhood, with several possible etiologies (e.g., in utero events, meningoencephalitis, epilepsy).[23]

The categorization of the biopercular syndrome into a category of MSD is difficult. It almost certainly reflects a severe dysarthria that resembles spastic dysarthria, but the absence of pseudobulbar affect, gag reflex, and pathologic oral reflexes, as well as "preserved" emotional laughter and crying, are atypical for people with spastic dysarthria. The voluntary-automatic dissociation is consistent with a degree of anatomic separation of corticobulbar pathways for voluntary and automatic control of orofacial structures, and it suggests that the lower precentral gyrus is not essential for driving involuntary facial movements.[91] The voluntary-automatic dissociation also raises the possibility that a nonverbal oral apraxia (NVOA), and perhaps AOS, complicate the condition. This author has followed a few individuals who *may* have had the syndrome as the result of degenerative disease. Their speech deficit began as an AOS and NVOA, plus an accompanying dysarthria that was difficult to characterize, but resembled spastic dysarthria because of slow rate, effortful strained voice quality, and prosodic excess.*

It seems reasonable to conclude that the muteness associated with the syndrome represents an anarthria in which the underlying dysarthria type is unclear but perhaps spastic, and in which AOS and NVOA may complicate the clinical picture. Recognition of the syndrome is important because of its localizing value, its clinical distinction from more typical manifestations of anarthria, and the apparently poor prognosis for recovery of functional speech, at least when the etiology is vascular or degenerative.

Cerebellar Mutism

Definition and Clinical Characteristics

An interesting and perplexing form of mutism, usually called *cerebellar mutism* or *mutism of cerebellar origin,* was first recognized by Rekate in 1985.[71] Subsequent reported cases in the literature now number more than 150. It is a unique form of mutism, because it is primarily seen in children, nearly always follows surgery in the posterior fossa, often is delayed in onset after surgery, and is always transient. It is perplexing because its precise

anatomic and physiologic cause and the nature of the mutism itself are poorly understood.

Review of a number of case or case series reports and literature reviews* permits the following summary of the disorder's characteristics:

1. The great majority of cases have had surgery for large midline posterior fossa tumors.† Tumors are in the midline in approximately 90% of cases, and the surgical incision is usually in the vermis. Approximately 8% to 29% of patients undergoing such surgery develop transient mutism, so the problem is not rare in this population. It has been suggested that transient mutism may be the price paid to cure people with cerebellar tumors.[28]

2. The problem is uncommon in adults, probably not simply because posterior fossa tumors are considerably more common in children. The average age range of affected individuals is 6 to 9 years.

3. Preoperatively, mutism is not present and dysarthria usually is not mentioned.

4. Mutism usually does not develop until 1 to 2 days after surgery, with adequate speech usually present before that. The mutism persists from approximately 4 days to 6 months, with an average duration of approximately 4 to 8 weeks.

5. Cranial nerve deficits usually are not apparent. During the period of mutism patients are cognitively alert and without obvious aphasia. Poor oral intake, emotional lability, decreased initiation of voluntary movements, and difficulty performing complex nonspeech oromotor movements have been noted during the mute period; persisting high-level language and cognitive deficits have been documented in a few cases.

6. When speech reemerges, dysarthria is apparent in 80% or more of cases. When type has been specified, it is usually described as ataxic. Long-term follow-up descriptions of speech are limited, but both full recovery and chronic dysarthria have been reported.

Neurologic Substrate and Etiology

Many of the same papers cited earlier have offered explanations for the mutism, but no single explana-

---

*Similar published cases have been described as having "slowly progressive anarthria with late anterior opercular syndrome."[13]

---

*References 15, 19, 25, 26, 29, 31, 33, 39, 40, 50, 55, 60, 61, 68, 80, 82, 84, 85, 89.

†All other causes of transient cerebellar mutism are uncommon and have usually been reported as single case studies. They have included arteriovenous malformation, hemorrhage, stroke, trauma, and viral infection of the cerebellum.

tion has universal acceptance. It may be that multiple explanations are at work within many cases, or different causes are at work among cases. Explanations for the mutism have included the following:

1. Extensive cerebellar damage as a direct result of surgery, especially when the vermis and dentate nuclei are injured.*

2. There is a fairly high incidence of postoperative meningitis or hydrocephalus. Either might explain the delay in onset of mutism, but they usually resolve much faster than the mutism. Some suggest that ischemia caused by manipulation or retraction of the cerebellum is the cause. Others argue that postoperative vasospasm of cerebellar arteries leading to ischemia and edema could cause the mutism and also explain the delay in its onset.

3. Effects of cerebellar/posterior fossa injury on functions elsewhere may also play a role. Some suggest that damage to the dentate nuclei interrupts dentatothalamocortical pathways, thus producing remote effects on supratentorial activities, with subsequent mutism. A few case reports employing single photon emission computed tomography (SPECT) during the mute period have identified reduced perfusion in frontal, temporal, and parietal lobes, and normalization of cortical perfusion after the mutism resolved[34]; however, cortical hypoperfusion during mutism may not always be present.[†55]

It has been argued that incomplete maturation of the complex sensorimotor network that includes the cerebellum, pontine nuclei, thalamus, supplementary motor area, and cortical motor and sensory areas make children more vulnerable to the effects of damage to the cerebellum.[40] This notion receives some indirect support from the fact that mutism following left cerebral hemisphere injury is also much more common in children than adults (see the section on aphasia and mutism).

What is the nature of cerebellar mutism? The facts that dysarthria is frequently evident when speech reemerges and that its type has at least in some cases been described as ataxic certainly support a belief that the mutism is a manifestation of anarthria,

presumably due to severe ataxic dysarthria. Problems with drooling and swallowing and emotional lability are indirectly supportive of a severe dysarthria explanation, although not necessarily ataxic dysarthria.

It is also possible that the mutism represents more than, or something other than, severe ataxic dysarthria, at least in some cases. For example, one of the six cases of Rekate et al.[71] was unable to imitate limb and tongue movements during the mute period, and voice was evident during laughter and crying. Another of their cases could only "whine" when attempting to speak. These behaviors are apraxic-like in character and could implicate motor programming deficits as a mechanism in the muteness (see Case 12-4 later). In fact, observations of difficulty producing complex, voluntary orofacial movements, with recovery of such abilities seeming to precede recovery from mutism,[85] has led some to suggest that the mutism reflects a "loss" of learned activities, or an apraxia.[26] This is a reasonable hypothesis given some of the behavioral characteristics present during the period of mutism, the possibility of remote effects of the posterior fossa event on cortical functions, the "immaturity" in children of the networks responsible for planning/programming speech movements, and the resemblance of a number of deviant speech characteristics of adult-acquired AOS and ataxic dysarthria to each other. It is clear that careful preoperative and postoperative examination and follow-up of a series of cases undergoing surgery for posterior fossa lesions, with special attention to their specific postoperative speech and oral mechanism characteristics, are essential to test these hypotheses.

Finally, there are occasional references to psychologic causes or contributions to the problem.[31] However, such explanations do not explain the obvious dysarthria that usually follows the mutism or the relatively predictable pattern of delayed emergence and limited duration of mutism. There can be little doubt that psychologic factors contribute to the behavior of young children who are coping with the aftermath of neurosurgery, but the current weight of evidence suggests that psychologic contributions are not causally related to the mutism in most cases.

Apraxia of Speech and Mutism

It is not unusual for AOS to be associated with mutism, but it seldom lasts for more than a few days when caused by stroke. Sometimes, however, the mutism persists beyond the acute stage, even in the absence of aphasia or significant dysarthria. There is no clear evidence that the lesions associated with prolonged muteness in AOS, particularly pure AOS, are situated differently than lesions associated with more rapid emergence of speech.

---

*It is known that intended bilateral ablation of the dentate nuclei to treat movement disorders can cause mutism, as can bilateral thalamotomy (damaging cerebellocortical projections).[60]

†SPECT study of two cases with cerebellar mutism of nonsurgical origin (one with cerebellitis, the other with a hemolytic-uremic syndrome) identified diffuse cerebellar hypoperfusion but no supratentorial abnormalities.[55]

Several case studies have documented persistent mutism in association with left hemisphere surgery or stroke,[9,43,51,72] with emergence from mutism usually occurring between 3 and 10 weeks after onset. These patients tend to have an accompanying NVOA. Some are unable to phonate, whisper, hum, or articulate under any circumstance, but some can hum or articulate without phonation during the otherwise mute period. These cases suggest that prolonged muteness in AOS is at least sometimes associated with a disproportionate degree of apraxia affecting phonation.

It has been reported that approximately 3% of people with TBI are mute even though they are not in a persistent vegetative state, locked-in, or akinetically mute.[48] Such cases sometimes have evidence of focal left basal ganglia lesions and tend to have more rapid recovery of consciousness and better overall language and communication outcomes than those with severe diffuse injuries. It is possible that the mutism in those with focal basal ganglia lesions is primarily due to AOS. This is important to recognize because TBI mutism can also be associated with much more severe cognitive, affective, and neuromuscular disorders.

Lebrun[46] had described mutism associated with a "pyramidal hemisyndrome" with unilateral cerebral hemisphere lesion, hemiplegia, and facial weakness. If this occurred only with lesions in the left hemisphere, it could be assumed that it reflected AOS or aphasia. However, he also refers to cases with muteness associated with right hemisphere lesions in the third frontal and first temporal convolutions and the insula, the inner surface of the operculum, and part of the corona radiata (and one case with a lesion in the supplementary motor area). He indicates that such mutism generally remits after a few days, but with residual "dysarthria." Although speculative, it is possible that these cases reflect AOS in individuals with crossed or mixed dominance for motor speech programming (and, possibly, language).

Prolonged mutism in individuals presumed to have AOS of acute onset should raise suspicions about additional influences of dysarthria, aphasia, or psychologic factors on the mutism. For example, some reported cases with prolonged mutism that have been attributed to "buccofacial apraxia"[36] have also had significant dysphagia and bilateral frontal lobe lesions, suggesting that they also may have had significant dysarthria. The mutism in such cases may thus have been due to dysarthria rather than AOS, or to a combination of the two disorders. In general, however, it is important to bear in mind that mutism sometimes persists beyond the acute stage in AOS, even when it is the only manifestation of neurologic disease.

Finally, AOS associated with degenerative neurologic disease can eventually result in mutism, either because of the AOS alone or because of the combined effects of AOS, dysarthria, and language or other cognitive disturbances (see Chapter 11 for discussion of progressive AOS).

◼ APHASIA AND MUTISM

Mutism in the acute period following the onset of aphasia in adulthood is not unusual, but persisting mutism, even in people with global aphasia, is uncommon. In contrast, aphasia (and, probably, AOS) acquired in childhood (e.g., from stroke or trauma) is often associated with a period of mutism.[1,24,38,57] Mutism associated with subcortical lesions leading to aphasia may be more common than when cortical lesions cause aphasia, but it is possible that the mutism in such cases is exacerbated by, or due to, AOS and dysarthria.

Acute lesions in the dominant hemisphere superior premotor area may produce complete muteness for several days and then evolve into so-called *transcortical motor aphasia*, in which spontaneous speech is limited in amount and complexity, but repetition, naming, and reading aloud may be preserved. Emergence from mutism in such cases may be characterized by slowly initiated, brief, unelaborated, and sometimes perseverative verbal responses. Patients may mouth or whisper words before normal phonation emerges, and their prosody may be flat, consistent with their overall affect. It seems that they have difficulty activating speech and communication secondary to damage to frontal lobe activation mechanisms.[2] It is questionable whether the mutism in such cases is due to a language deficit (aphasia) per se. Nonaphasic cognitive deficits associated with frontal lobe pathology, such as akinetic mutism (discussed later), may be a better explanation (and label) for these deficits than transcortical motor aphasia. Of course, some individuals may have aphasia and nonaphasic cognitive communication deficits simultaneously.

In general, persisting mutism in aphasia should raise suspicions about the accuracy of the aphasia diagnosis or the presence of additional problems such as MSDs or nonaphasic cognitive deficits.

◼ NONAPHASIC COGNITIVE AND AFFECTIVE DEFICITS ASSOCIATED WITH MUTISM

Thus far we have discussed mutism secondary to disorders of execution (dysarthrias), a disorder of planning/programming (AOS), and a disorder specifically affecting language (aphasia). In this section, mutism secondary to defects in arousal, affect and drive, cognition, and motor initiation are addressed. There is considerable clinical overlap among such disorders. For example, many patients with mutism associated with defects in affect or drive have significant cognitive deficits, and many with deficits in motor initiation have defects in affect or drive as well as cognition.

Disorders of Arousal (Coma)

Coma is a state of *"unarousable unresponsiveness"* and absence of sleep/wake cycles on EEG. All voluntary behavior is diminished or absent, the eyes remain closed, and there is no evidence of purposeful movement or localizing responses[35]; any observable responses are reflexive. The substrate for coma is typically diffuse bilateral cerebral hemispheric damage or brainstem injury, or both. When the injury is to the brainstem, coma reflects disruption to the reticular activating system (RAS) and its crucial role in arousal and consciousness. Thus the unresponsiveness of coma reflects a failure of the RAS and cortex and the absence of activated functions above the brainstem level. In a sense, the mutism of coma is hardly thought of as a variety of mutism, because speechlessness is expected when a person is neither conscious nor arousable.

Mutism resulting from RAS involvement and decreased arousal can have multiple causes, but TBI and vascular events are probably the most common etiologies encountered in speech pathology practices.

Diffuse Impairments of Cortical Functions

Vegetative State*

Patients in a vegetative state fail to show evidence of viable higher level cerebral function, do not exhibit purposeful behavior, and are unable to interact meaningfully with the environment. Vegetative state generally follows an initial period of coma when caused by TBI, but it can occur without preceding coma in metabolic disorders and severe dementia. It is often associated with severe bilateral cerebral hemispheric pathology with relative preservation of brainstem functions. EEG, computed tomography (CT) scan, or magnetic resonance imaging and measures of cerebral metabolic activity are consistent with gross abnormalities or absence of cortical functioning. Severe TBI, anoxia, drug

toxicity, Wernicke's encephalopathy, Alzheimer's disease, and anencephaly exemplify etiologies capable of producing the widespread cortical dysfunction leading to a vegetative state. Recovery from a vegetative state is considered unlikely when it persists for more than 3 months following nontraumatic injuries and more than 12 months following trauma.[3]

Unlike those in coma, wake-sleep cycles are relatively preserved. When awake, affected people generally do not visually track or respond to normal external stimulation. Motor responses, such as flexion withdrawal or nonspecific patterned movements, may be elicited by noxious stimuli; crying and laughter are sometimes noted, possibly reflecting release of those reflexes.[35] Muteness is thus consistent with a severely reduced level of arousal and cognition.

Apallic State (Coma Vigil)

"Apallism" refers to the absence of the pallium or gray matter of the cortex. Patients in an *apallic state* or *coma vigil* can appear similar to those in a vegetative state, and the difference between the two conditions may be only one of degree. This may explain why the designation is not encountered in many recent discussions of disorders of consciousness (e.g., American Congress of Rehabilitative Medicine, 1995.[3])

Individuals in an apallic state are unresponsive, make few spontaneous movements, and do not generally make reflexive defensive or protective movements, although they do respond to painful stimuli. They occasionally move or shout spontaneously, demonstrating some capacity for movement and vocalization.[46] They may lie with their eyes open and occasionally visually follow the examiner, but eye movements are usually random.[75] They tend to remain in any position in which they are placed, may have prominent sucking and grasping reflexes, and may develop marked alterations in tone and posture, such as rigidity and extrapyramidal hyperkinesia.[59] Their behavior suggests that the bases for feeling, thought, and motivation to act are absent.

The apallic state designation has been used in reference to people with widespread destruction of cortical gray matter. Etiologies include anoxia, carbon monoxide poisoning, degenerative disease (e.g., Creutzfeldt-Jakob disease), meningovascular syphilis, chronic viral encephalitis, and severe TBI.[58,75]

Akinetic Mutism

Definition and Clinical Characteristics

Pathology in the anterior or mesial portions of the frontal lobes may lead to *abulia,* or a lack of

---

*The designations *persistent or permanent vegetative state* are sometimes used when the vegetative state has been present for an extended time (e.g. more than 1 month or 1 year).

initiative or spontaneity in thought, speech, physical action, and affective expression. Abulia in the extreme can cause mutism. This form of mutism therefore reflects a lack of drive or motivation to speak, difficulty initiating and sustaining the cognitive and motor effort required for speech, or an apparent absence of thoughts to be communicated.*

The term for this extreme abulic state is *akinetic mutism (AM)*. It is usually associated with bilateral lesions of the orbito-mesial frontal cortex, portions of the limbic system, and portions of the reticular formation; the behavioral inertia associated with it is caused by disruption in limbic-cortical and reticulo-cortical circuitry.[35] Other terms with anatomic references to a constellation of deficits that can include AM are the *prefrontal syndrome*, the *anterior cerebral artery syndrome*, and the *supplementary motor area (SMA) syndrome*.[81]

AM is a state of muteness and "reluctance" to perform even simple motor activities, in spite of preservation of arousal and alertness, basic motor and sensory abilities, visual tracking ability, and at least some fundamental cognitive abilities. It is important to recognize that AM is not due to neuromuscular difficulties (i.e., anarthria). Akinetically mute patients typically sit with their eyes open, seemingly alert and on the verge of responding to simple requests and questions but basically unresponsive and apathetic. They may follow movement but not truly react to it. They may exhibit vegetative jaw and face movements and may swallow food after it is placed in the mouth, often only after a significant delay.[46]

AM can have gradations of severity. When emerging from the mute state, as in recovery after stroke or trauma, a patient may respond with movement or speech when stimuli are powerful and persistent; such movements are usually simple, brief, and delayed, sometimes for minutes. Speech is *brief, aphonic, whispered* or *reduced in loudness,* and *monotonic,* with articulation and intelligibility appearing more intact than phonation; speech tends to convey an impression of indifference, lethargy, or apathy. Content is *unelaborated*—but not truly telegraphic—and *concrete* and *literal*.[4,46,79] For example, when asked, "Can you tell me the time?" the patient may simply respond "yes." Patients can also seem to be stubbornly refusing to cooperate and sometimes appear to resist the examiner's attempt to open the mouth.[†]

Neurologic Substrate and Etiologies

Two general lesion loci are associated with AM. The first is the mesial (internal) surface of one or both frontal lobes, including the SMA and anterior cingulate gyrus. Involvement of the anterior cingulate region, which is the frontal surface of the limbic system, may be important for the syndrome's emergence,[75] although AM is most often associated with massive frontal lobe damage.[77]

The SMA, its connections to the cingulate gyrus, and its projections to the dorsolateral frontal cortex (including Broca's area), the motor cortex, and the striatum are important to the preparation of movements, particularly internally driven movements, and the activation of motor responses.[44] Damage to the left SMA reduces the drive to speak, sometimes enough to induce mutism. In general, damage to the right SMA also reduces output but does not generally lead to mutism.[2]

Small lesions in the SMA may cause transient muteness, after which articulation may be normal but verbal output is sparse and delayed in initiation. With small lesions, sentence length utterances may emerge within a few weeks.[2] Larger lesions tend to be associated with longer periods of mutism, as well as noticeable apathy, unconcern, and slowness in initiating responses. In such cases, there seems to be an impairment in cingulate cortex and SMA activities that play a role in response activation, as well as in more anterior frontal areas that are involved in organization and executive control.[2]

The second lesion site related to AM is the mesencephalic-diencephalic region, a location where disconnection of thalamic nuclei from ascending RAS impulses is possible. The anatomic distance between the frontal and deeper sites of damage that can lead to AM is explained by the integrated nature of the brainstem-frontal system, in which the brainstem RAS influences states of alertness.[77] Thus severe brainstem pathology may lead to coma or a somnolent akinetic state. Frontal lobe pathology may not be associated with marked somnolence because the RAS is intact, but abulia and lack of drive limit responsiveness and initiative.

AM has multiple possible causes. Infarction of the anterior cerebral arteries or perforating branches of the posterior cerebral artery can cause the frontal lobe and mesencephalic variants of AM, respectively[27,75]; bithalamic stroke has also been associated with AM.[83] Tumor, TBI, encephalitis, vascular malformations, ruptured aneurysms, severe acute hydrocephalus, anoxia, and thalamotomy are additional possible causes.[11,59,79]

ETIOLOGY SPECIFIC NEUROGENIC MUTISM

Neurogenic mutism is sometimes associated with specific events or characteristics, even though the mechanism underlying the mutism is not always clear. Mutism following commissurotomy, speech arrest, and drug-induced mutism are examples of such conditions.

Mutism Following Corpus Callosotomy

Surgical transection of part or all of the corpus callosum is sometimes undertaken to reduce seizure frequency in people with intractable epilepsy that has no single focus and is refractory to pharmacologic management.* Total callosotomy or section of the anterior portion of the corpus callosum can result in mutism or decreased spontaneity of speech for several days to months, occasionally longer.[32,74] For example, a recent study reported transient mutism (4 to 25 days) in 10 of 35 patients who underwent complete or anterior callosotomy.[69] Comprehension and ability to communicate by writing can be spared. Patients tend to go through a period of whispering or hoarseness during recovery, and an NVOA may be present.[8,78]

The mechanism for the muteness is unclear. It is generally not considered the result of the transection per se, however. Mechanical trauma from operative traction, or diaschisis or ischemia affecting the parasagittal cortex, including the SMA, may be significant.[69,70,78] Because the brains of individuals with epilepsy are not normal, it has been speculated that preoperative dominance for speech is bilateral in some individuals. As a result, speech cannot be supported postoperatively because the two hemispheres are disconnected, and a single hemisphere cannot immediately control speech without the help of the other.

The behavioral basis for the mutism is also unclear. Some suggest that "aphemia" (i.e., AOS) is sometimes the explanation,[78] but aphasia and psychologic explanations have also been mentioned.[7] If malfunction of the SMA were the source of difficulty, then difficulty with initiation of speech from motor or cognitive drive mechanism deficits would be implicated.

Callosotomy is also undertaken in individuals undergoing surgical removal of tumors in the third ventricle and pineal region. Sectioning of the anterior, middle, or posterior third of the corpus callosum is undertaken as the chosen route of the surgical approach to such tumors. Mutism is one of the most serious side effects of the procedure, although only rarely does it persist for more than several weeks; children younger than 10 years of age have fewer postoperative deficits, apparently including mutism, than older individuals.[7] Similar to callosotomy for seizure control, the mechanism for the mutism is often uncertain.

Speech Arrest

One of the most common events associated with partial seizures is *speech arrest,* commonly called *ictal speech arrest,* in which speech in progress at the onset of a seizure is halted, even though consciousness is maintained; efforts to speak on such occasions may result only in indistinct sounds.[46] Speech arrest most commonly occurs with frontal lobe seizures, especially when the dominant SMA, superior frontal gyrus, or inferior rolandic areas are involved.[18,20,90] Speech arrest or aphasia may be the only behavioral evidence of seizure activity in some cases.[18]

Although speech arrests are often labeled as "aphasic," the arrest of speech is really not proof of aphasia. Because arrest can originate in the right or left hemisphere SMA, it may be more strongly tied to interference with mechanisms involved in the initiation of motor activity, or its planning/programming (AOS).

Lesions in the SMA, including tumors, can produce sudden speech arrest or uncontrolled vocalization.[42] Speech arrest accompanied by right leg weakness but preserved writing and comprehension has also been observed during migrainous episodes.[41]

Speech arrest can occur during direct electrical stimulation of the cortex in individuals with seizures, most consistently in the temporal–parietal area, Broca's area, and the SMAs of both hemispheres.[64] It can also be observed during cortical mapping in patients undergoing tumor resection in the dominant hemisphere.[56] Stimulation of the ventrolateral thalamus during stereotactic procedures to control movement disorders can also arrest speech.[10] Finally, speech arrest or mutism can be induced temporarily by neurologic tests used to establish hemispheric dominance and investigate localization of speech-language functions. The invasive intracarotid amobarbital procedure, known as *Wada testing,* essentially temporarily anesthetizes a hemisphere and, when it is the language-dominant one, often creates a temporary inability to speak. The more recently developed noninvasive *repetitive transcranial magnetic stimulation (rTMS)* can also induce speech arrest, most often when delivered over the inferior frontal region of the left hemisphere.[30]

---

*The procedure is considered most appropriate for those who suffer recurring injuries from falls during atonic, tonic-clonic, and tonic seizures.[14]

Drug-Induced Mutism

Mutism has been reported as a neurotoxic response to certain immunosuppressive agents (e.g., tacrolimus [FK506], cyclosporine) that are used following liver and heart transplant.[66,76] The exact nature of the mutism is not always clear, although case descriptions have been suggestive of anarthria or AM; positron emission tomography findings in one case suggested that hypometabolism in the cingulate gyrus played a role.[12] Rapid identification of speech loss is considered important, because reduced dose or cessation of the offending drug may reverse the problem.[76]

Cases

Case 12-1

A 65-year-old woman was hospitalized for evaluation of episodes of unsteady gait, facial weakness, and speech difficulty. Following admission she had several transient ischemic attacks and 2 weeks later a stroke. CT scan revealed infarcts in the temporal and occipital lobes, basal ganglia, and cerebellum.

She was seen for speech evaluation 2 weeks later. She was mute but attempted to speak, producing only a grunt with minimal articulatory movements. Her face and tongue were weak. She protruded her tongue slowly and with limited range of movement on request. The palate moved minimally on attempts at phonation and during a gag. Responses on language tasks were noticeably delayed, and verbal and reading comprehension were significantly impaired; responses often were perseverative. These deficits appeared more related to general cognitive impairments than a focal impairment of language.

An attempt was made to establish an augmentative means of communication, but the patient's cognitive impairments precluded success. She was discharged to a nursing home but readmitted for rehabilitation 2 months later. She was still mute but was more responsive nonverbally, answering yes-no questions with head nods or eye blinks, without perseveration. Oral mechanism examination was unchanged. Because of marked visual impairments and inability to use her limbs for pointing or other gestures, head nods and simple eye blinks remained the most viable means of communication.

The clinician concluded that the patient's muteness was primarily due to anarthria resulting from bilateral upper motor neuron involvement.

Commentary. (1) Multiple strokes can lead to mutism due to anarthria. (2) Cognitive deficits frequently accompany anarthric mutism. In combination with visual and limb motor deficits, they may place limits on the sophistication of augmentative means of communication that are possible.

Case 12-2

A 71-year-old woman presented with a 2-year history of decline in gait, speech, and bowel and bladder control. Examination revealed weakness and spasticity in all limbs and the face, with hyperactive reflexes, and positive snout, suck, and jaw jerk reflexes. She was unable to speak and had significant difficulty with chewing and swallowing.

A CT scan revealed generalized cerebral atrophy but no evidence of stroke or tumor. Her neurologic diagnosis was degenerative CNS disease that could not be further specified.

During speech evaluation she confirmed being unable to speak for the past 3 months, following a nearly 2-year gradual decline in speech ability. She answered yes-no questions by raising one or two fingers (she was unable to write secondary to bilateral upper extremity weakness). Her verbal comprehension for simple and complex commands and yes-no questions was quite good, as was sentence level reading comprehension.

Jaw, face, and tongue movements were markedly slowed and restricted in range. The gag reflex was normal. She was unable to cough or clear her throat sharply. She did produce a brief, reflexively phonated sigh and yawn. She was otherwise mute. There was no evidence of NVOA or apraxic-like groping during attempts at speech.

It was concluded that her muteness was due to anarthria stemming from severe spastic dysarthria. She did not remain at the clinic and was referred to a speech pathologist near her home for consideration of alternative communication devices.

Commentary. (1) Anarthria can be the product of degenerative CNS disease. (2) Anarthria can be present without significant cognitive or sensory impairments.

Case 12-3

A 22-year-old man was admitted to the rehabilitation unit for management of deficits stemming from a motor vehicle accident 2.5 years earlier. He had made only minimal progress during previous rehabilitation efforts.

CT scan at the time of admission revealed significant generalized cerebral atrophy, as well as low attenuation changes in the centrum semiovale bilaterally. EEG showed marked, diffuse nonspecific abnormalities. He had occasional seizures.

During speech evaluation, he demonstrated a nearly total disregard for auditory or visual stimuli and showed no evidence of comprehension of any verbal statements made to him. He did not attempt to vocalize, nor did he generate any sound volitionally or reflexively. He occasionally grimaced, made some sucking motions with his mouth, ground his teeth, and lifted his head toward the left, all for no obvious reason. He did not respond to persistent strong auditory, visual, or tactile stimulation during several periods of observation, nor was he observed to do so by other staff.

The clinician concluded that the patient's muteness was due to his severely reduced level of arousal and cognition, although neuromotor impairments could not be ruled out as an additional contributor to his muteness.

During neurologic evaluation he appeared alert but did not respond meaningfully to any stimuli. Some dystonic posturing of the arms and legs was apparent. He did not blink in response to visual threat. He groaned for no apparent reason on a few occasions. The neurologist concluded the patient had a severe encephalopathy and was in a persistent vegetative state.

Efforts to increase responsiveness over a several-week period were unsuccessful. The patient was discharged to a nursing home.

Commentary. (1) Mutism may be associated with diffuse impairment of cortical function, leading to a persistent vegetative or apallic state. (2) CHI is a common cause of this form of mutism.

Case 12-4

A 5-year-old right-handed boy underwent neurosurgery for removal of a large fourth ventricle medulloblastoma. Preoperatively, he had had a history of headaches and ataxic gait but no speech or language difficulty.

On the first postoperative day, he made a few normal-sounding utterances. On the second postoperative day, he became mute.

He was referred for speech assessment 10 days postoperatively because of continued mutism. He was awake, somewhat restless and agitated, but not clearly oppositional. Several times per minute he cried for 1 to 3 seconds, without tears, and for no apparent reason, although this most often followed a verbal request or comment directed to him. He made no attempt to communicate verbally or gesturally, and he made no purposeful movements with his upper extremities, except to scratch his nose and eyes with his right hand. He did not respond to verbal requests to point, answer yes-no questions, or look at objects. Observation a few hours later was similar, although when asked to close his eyes he made some upper face-forehead movements without closing his eyes. They were closed by the examiner and maintained by him, but he did not then open his eyes on command, although he appeared to try. He responded similarly when asked to open and close his mouth, and these activities triggered crying. His jaw and lower face

were not obviously weak. His cry sounded normal. He did not protrude his tongue under any voluntary or involuntary circumstances but did retract it during eating and crying. Sucking was adequate. He had no difficulty swallowing solids or liquids but did occasionally lose liquids and solids out of his mouth, as if their oral handling was uncoordinated. On one occasion he laughed briefly at a humorous comment by the clinician.

Five days later, he was able to protrude his tongue to lick a lollipop; he did this on several trials but with some apparent groping for movement before protrusion. Intermittent crying was still present. He achieved and maintained eye contact more consistently and laughed appropriately on two occasions.

Although his neurologists were suspicious of elective (psychogenic) mutism, the speech pathologist concluded that he had "muteness of undetermined origin. There are several possibilities. Elective mutism is unlikely; it doesn't explain his lack of response to nonspeech demands, and electively mute individuals often communicate adequately nonverbally. It also does not explain the paucity of purposeful limb activity. Conversion mutism is also a possibility, but the same arguments against it apply. If psychogenic explanations are active, strongly suspect there is an additional neurogenic component. Normal

Continued

Case 12-4—cont'd

chewing and swallowing and normal cry argue against a severe spastic or flaccid dysarthria. Could this be a variant of akinetic mutism? Crying, restlessness/agitation, and relatively rapid feeding would be unusual, however. Perhaps more likely is a severe loss of cerebellar control for speech movements or an AOS. Cases of mutism following posterior fossa surgery in children have been reported in the literature."

The patient was discharged from the hospital shortly thereafter. Follow-up phone conversation with his mother indicated that he began to speak 23 days postoperatively. At that time his articulation was reasonably good, but his mother noted that his "accent" was not appropriate and that he was occasionally excessively loud. The excessive loudness had resolved, but the mother felt that the melody of his speech remained impaired.

The patient was seen 4 years later as part of a learning disorders assessment. His receptive and expressive language abilities fell in the low average range. Speech rate was moderately slowed. Excess and equal stress, a voice tremor, and subtle irregular articulatory breakdowns were noted. Speech alternate motion rates were irregular (2,3). The clinician concluded that he had a mild to moderate ataxic dysarthria that did not impair speech intelligibility.

Commentary. (1) Mutism sometimes develops after neurosurgery for posterior fossa tumors in children. It is often called cerebellar mutism. (2) The mechanism for cerebellar mutism is not always clear, but anarthria and motor programming (AOS) deficits deserve consideration; it is probably rarely psychogenic. The emergence of an ataxic dysarthria following the period of mutism suggests that anarthria was, at the least, a significant contributor to mutism in this case.

Case 12-5

A 45-year-old man was admitted to the hospital with a 2-month history of bilateral frontal headaches and more recent left hemiplegia and diffuse neurologic deficits. A CT scan demonstrated bilateral basal ganglia infarcts. A multitude of additional neurologic tests led to a suspicion that he had CNS vasculitis.

During initial speech-language evaluation the patient was unresponsive to any commands for oral volitional movement, with the exception that he slowly protruded his tongue on request after significant delay. He followed some one-step commands and identified some large-print letters accurately, but only after significant delays. There was no spontaneous speech, and he did not respond to attempts to have him count or sing. He made a few unintelligible sounds when attempting to imitate some single syllable words. He wrote his first name after a significant delay. He wrote a few single words to dictation, with significant spelling errors (he had only a seventh grade education).

The clinician stated, "The most impressive features of this exam are: consistent, markedly latent responses; frequently, no responses; nearly all 'errors' are of omission, not commission; reduced amplitude of response; absence of groping or off-target attempts at speech and absence of speech except for a few sounds; drowsy/obtunded appearance, often with failure to achieve eye contact. His general behavior resembles that of abulic or akinetically mute patients but is complicated by his drowsiness/obtundation. There is no convincing evidence of aphasia or apraxia of speech, although they could be masked by his other deficits." Therapy was not recommended at the time.

Examination 1 month later was similar. He was mute but did phonate while yawning. He did not respond to any requests for nonverbal oral movements. He identified a few body parts, pictures, and letters on request after lengthy delays. Again, the clinician concluded that the patient was akinetically mute; dysarthria or AOS could not be ruled out. By the time of his discharge, he was more alert and able to follow some commands, although with delays. He was not seen for further follow-up.

Commentary. (1) Diagnosis of the underlying nature of mutism is often difficult. (2) The patient's marked response latencies to simple concrete tasks and frequent complete unresponsiveness supported the impression of akinetic mutism. The absence of speech or limited speech, particularly in the presence of bilateral basal ganglia infarcts, left open the possibility that the patient was also dysarthric and had an AOS.

Case 12-6

A 51-year-old man was admitted to a rehabilitation unit 2 months after a pontine stroke that left him mute and quadriplegic. He was tracheostomized and fed through a nasogastric tube.

On initial speech evaluation, he was alert and responsive and there was no evidence of aphasia or confusion. His jaw was weak bilaterally, but he was able to partially open, close, and lateralize it. He had a moderate degree of facial weakness but was able to approximate his lips and retract and purse them slowly. He had minimal ability to protrude, retract, lateralize, and elevate his tongue. The palate was immobile, and a gag reflex could not be elicited. He was mute but did attempt to mouth some words and had fairly good jaw and lower face and lip movement during speech attempts.

He was able to answer yes/no questions correctly with head nods or eye blinks. He correctly identified large-print words, letters, and numbers by closing his eyes to stop the examiner's scanning of choices. He could spell words using a combination of head movements and eye blinks as an alphabet board was scanned.

The clinician concluded that the patient was "anarthric, with an incomplete LiS, with some limited ability to move his articulators. Speech would be nonfunctional even if he were not trached." He was considered an excellent candidate for an augmentative system of communication.

For the next month, he communicated with an eye gaze communication system with letters or pictures representing choices. This was slow but effective communication, particularly between him and his wife. He then became able to activate a switch with his right index finger that triggered an electronic scanner on a large alphabet board that also contained some common phrases. He gradually was able to make some lip and tongue movement and to produce weak stop consonants.

Two weeks later he received a speaking trach and was able to phonate quite well, although he tired quickly.

Over the next several weeks he produced some sounds and syllables, although with considerable difficulty synchronizing exhalation and articulation. His trach tube was removed shortly thereafter. Voice quality was breathy, and resonance was hypernasal. Bilateral vocal fold weakness was apparent on laryngeal examination.

Over the next 2 months his speech improved to a point where he was considered 100% intelligible in quiet speaking situations. He was discharged from the hospital shortly thereafter but returned 5 months later for reassessment. His speech at that time was characterized by a breathy-strained voice quality (3), hypernasality (2), and slow rate (−2). There was clear-cut left-sided weakness of the palate and left-sided vocal cord weakness. Speech intelligibility was generally good but considered reduced under adverse conditions.

The patient was seen 2 years later for follow-up. Speech was relatively unchanged. He had mixed spastic-flaccid dysarthria and speech characteristics attributable to respiratory, laryngeal, velopharyngeal, and articulatory impairments. There was also a significant respiratory contribution to his speech difficulties; he had a clavicular pattern of breathing.

Commentary. (1) Incomplete LiS frequently results from brainstem stroke causing quadriplegia, spasticity of cranial nerves supplying bulbar muscles, and LMN cranial nerve impairment. (2) A mixed flaccid-spastic dysarthria is frequently the underlying cause of the anarthria in LiS. (3) Substantial recovery from LiS, although unusual, is possible. (4) Patients who recover from LiS frequently progress from increasingly sophisticated means of alternative communication, to the emergence of some functional speech, to the development of intelligible speech and the discarding of augmentative means of communication. (5) Patients with LiS present special challenges to management and, particularly when considerable recovery occurs, require a number of approaches to treatment.

SUMMARY

1. Mutism, the absence of speech, may have multiple origins, including neurologic disease. When it results from acquired neurologic disease, it may reflect severe dysarthria (anarthria), AOS, aphasia, and various nonaphasic cognitive and affective conditions.

2. Anarthric mutism may reflect various different dysarthria types, lesion loci, and neurologic diseases. It most commonly results from bilateral or diffuse neurologic damage. When a single vascular event causes anarthria, its locus is usually in the brainstem.

3. LiS is characterized by anarthria plus immobility of the body except for vertical eye movements and blinking that allow communication through eye movements. It is usually caused by occlusion of the basilar artery, which affects the ventral aspect of the pons.

4. Anarthria occasionally results from bilateral damage to the lower part of the precentral and postcentral convolutions (biopercular syndrome) and may leave limb movements, language, and cognitive abilities relatively intact. Cerebellar mutism is a rare form of mutism that usually occurs in children following neurosurgery for large midline posterior fossa tumors. The mechanism for the mutism is unclear, although significant dysarthria is usually present when the mutism begins to clear.

5. Mutism associated with AOS is not unusual in the first few days following left hemisphere stroke. Rarely, it persists for several months and is often characterized by disproportionately severe apraxia of phonation.

6. Mutism in the acute period following the onset of aphasia is not unusual, but it usually does not persist. When it does, suspicion should be raised about an accompanying AOS, dysarthria, or nonaphasic cognitive deficits.

7. Mutism may result from cognitive and affective deficits that are distinct from motor speech disorders and aphasia. Severe disorders of arousal stemming from reticular activating system involvement and diffuse impairments of cortical functions can be associated with mutism. Damage to frontal lobe-limbic system structures may lead to akinetic mutism that is usually associated with general unresponsiveness or reluctance to perform simple motor activities, in spite of preserved alertness and basic motor and sensory abilities. Akinetic mutism is strongly associated with deficits reflecting a lack of initiative, as well as impairments in affect, personality, and emotion.

8. Neurogenic mutism may also result from specific neurologic events. For example, mutism following transection of the corpus callosum for control of epilepsy or removal of tumors in deep midline structures is not unusual. Speech arrests during partial seizures are common, typically reflecting involvement of the supplementary motor area or dominant hemisphere language areas.

9. The distinction among different forms of neurogenic mutism can contribute to the localization of neurologic disease, an understanding of the underlying nature of the mutism, and an appreciation of factors that must be considered in its management.

References

1. Alajouanine TH, Lhermitte F: Acquired aphasia in children, Brain 88:653, 1965.
2. Alexander MP, Benson DF, Stuss DT: Frontal lobes and language, Brain Lang 37:656, 1989.
3. American Congress of Rehabilitative Medicine: Recommendations for use of uniform nomenclature pertinent to patients with severe alterations in consciousness, Arch Phys Med Rehabil 76:205, 1995.
4. Aronson AE: Clinical voice disorders, ed 3, New York, 1990, Thieme.
5. Bauby JD: The diving bell and the butterfly, New York, 1997, Alfred A Knopf.
6. Bauer G, Gerstenbrand F, Rumpl E: Varieties of the locked-in syndrome, J Neurol 221:77, 1979.
7. Benes V: Advantages and disadvantages of the transcallosal approach to the III ventricle, Childs Nerv Syst 6:437, 1990.
8. Bogen J, Vogel P: Neurological status in the longterm following complete cerebral commissurotomy. In Michel F, Schott B, editors: Les syndromes de disconnexion calleuse chez l'homme, Lyon, France, 1975, Colloque International de Lyon: Hospital Neurologique.
9. Bone DI: Mutism following left hemisphere infarction, J Neurol Neurosurg Psychiatry 47:1342, 1984.
10. Botez MI, Barbeau A: Role of subcortical structures, and particularly of the thalamus, in the mechanisms of speech and language, Int J Neurol 8:300:1971.
11. Brazis P, Masdeu JC, Biller J: Localization in clinical neurology, ed 4, Philadelphia, 2001, Lippincott Williams & Wilkins.
12. Bronster DJ et al: Tacrolimus-associated mutism after orthotopic liver transplantation, Transplantation 70:979, 2000.
13. Broussolle E et al: Slowly progressive anarthria with late anterior opercular syndrome: a variant form of frontal cortical atrophy syndromes, J Neurol Sci 144:44, 1996.
14. Buchalter JR, Jarrar RG: Therapeutics in pediatric epilepsy, part 2: epilepsy surgery and vagus nerve stimulation, Mayo Clin Proc 78:371, 2003.
15. Cakir Y, Karakisi D, Kocanaogullari O: Cerebellar mutism in an adult: case report, Surg Neurol 41:342, 1994.
16. Cappa SF et al: Speechlessness with occasional vocalizations after bilateral opercular lesions: a case study, Aphasiology 1:35, 1987.
17. Casanova E et al: Locked-in syndrome: improvement in the prognosis after an early intensive multidisciplinary rehabilitation, Arch Phys Med Rehabil 84:862, 2003.
18. Cascino GD et al: Seizure-associated speech arrest in elderly patients, Mayo Clin Proc 66:254, 1991.
19. Catsman-Berrevoets CE et al: Tumor type and size are high risk factors for the syndrome of "cerebellar" mutism and subsequent dysarthria, J Neurol Neurosurg Psychiatry 67:755, 1999.
20. Chee MW, So NK, Dinner DS: Speech and the dominant superior frontal gyrus: correlation of ictal symptoms, EEG, and results of surgical resection, J Clin Neurophysiol 14:226, 1997.
21. Chia LG: Locked-in syndrome with bilateral ventral midbrain infarcts, Neurology 41:445, 1991.
22. Chia LG: Locked-in state with bilateral internal capsule infarcts, Neurology 34:1365, 1984.
23. Christen HJ et al: Foix-Chavany-Marie (anterior operculum) syndrome in childhood: a reappraisal of Worster-Drought syndrome, Dev Med Child Neurol 42:122, 2000.

24. Cooper JA, Flowers CR: Children with a history of acquired aphasia: residual language and academic impairments, J Speech Hear Disord 52:251, 1987.

25. Coplin WM et al: Mutism in an adult following hypertensive cerebellar hemorrhage: nosological discussion and illustrative case, Brain Lang 59:473, 1997.

26. Dailey AT, McKhann GM, Berger MS: The pathophysiology of oral pharyngeal apraxia and mutism following posterior fossa tumor resection in children, J Neurosurg 83:467, 1995.

27. Damasio A: The frontal lobes. In Heilman KM, Valenstein E, editors: Clinical neuropsychology, New York, 1979, Oxford University Press.

28. DiCataldo A et al: Mutism after surgical removal of a cerebellar tumor: two case reports, Pediatr Hematol Oncol 18:117, 2001.

29. Dietze DD, Mickel JP: Cerebellar mutism after posterior fossa surgery, Pediatr Neurosurg 16:25, 1990-91.

30. Epstein CM: Transcranial magnetic stimulation: language function, J Clin Neurophysiol 15:325, 1998.

31. Ferrante L et al: Mutism after posterior fossa surgery in children, report of three cases, J Neurosurg 72:959, 1990.

32. Gazzaniga MS et al: Neurologic perspectives on right hemisphere language following surgical section of the corpus callosum, Semin Neurol 4:126, 1984.

33. Gelabert-González M, Fernández-Villa J: Mutism after posterior fossa surgery. Review of the literature, Clin Neurol Neurosurg 103:111, 2001.

34. Germano A et al: Reversible cerebral perfusion alterations in children with transient mutism after posterior fossa surgery, Childs Nerv Syst 14:114, 1998.

35. Giacino JT: Disorders of consciousness: differential diagnosis and neuropathologic features, Semin Neurol 17:105, 1997.

36. Groswasser Z et al: Mutism associated with buccofacial apraxia and bihemispheric lesions, Brain Lang 34:157, 1988.

37. Haig AJ, Katz RT, Sahgal V: Mortality and complications of the locked-in syndrome, Arch Phys Med Rehabil 68:24, 1987.

38. Hecaen H: Acquired aphasia in children and the ontogenesis of hemispheric functional specialization, Brain Lang 13:114, 1976.

39. Hudson LJ, Murdoch BE, Ozanne AE: Posterior fossa tumors in childhood: associated speech and language disorders post-surgery, Aphasiology 3:1, 1989.

40. Ildan F et al: The evaluation and comparison of cerebellar mutism in children and adults after posterior fossa surgery: report of two adult cases and review of the literature, Acta Neurochir 144:463, 2002.

41. Jenkyn L, Reeves A: Aphemia with hemiplegic migraine, Neurology 29:1317, 1979.

42. Jonas S: The supplementary motor region and speech emission, J Commun Disord 14:349, 1981.

43. Jürgens U, Kirzinger A, von Cramon D: The effects of deep-reaching lesions in the cortical face area on phonation, a combined case report and experimental monkey study, Cortex 18:125, 1982.

44. Krainik A et al: Role of the supplementary motor area in motor deficit following medial frontal lobe surgery, Neurology 57:871, 2001.

45. Lang C et al: Foix-Chavany-Marie syndrome—neurological, neuro-psychological, CT, MRI, and SPECT findings in a case progressive for more than 10 years, Eur Arch Psychiatry Neurol Sci 239:188, 1989.

46. Lebrun Y: Mutism, London, 1990, Whurr Publishers.

47. Leon-Carrion J et al: The locked-in syndrome: a syndrome looking for a therapy, Brain Inj 16:571, 2002.

48. Levin HS et al: Mutism after closed head injury, Arch Neurol 40:601, 1983.

49. Mariani C et al: Bilateral perisylvian softenings: bilateral anterior opercular syndrome (Foix-Chavany-Marie syndrome), J Neurol 223:269, 1980.

50. Marien P, Engelborghs S, DeDeyn P: Cerebellar neurocognition: a new avenue, Acta Neurol Belg 101:96, 2001.

51. Marshall RC, Gandour J, Windsor, J: Selective impairment of phonation: a case study, Brain Lang 35:313, 1988.

52. McCusker EA et al: Recovery from the "locked-in" syndrome, Arch Neurol 39:145, 1982.

53. McGann WM, Paslawski TM: Incomplete locked-in syndrome: two cases with successful communication outcomes, Am J Speech-Lang Pathol 1:32, 1991.

54. Mesulam M-M: Principles of behavioral and cognitive neurology, ed 2, New York, 2000, Oxford University Press.

55. Mewasingh LD et al: Nonsurgical cerebellar mutism (anarthria) in two children, Pediatr Neurol 28:59, 2003.

56. Meyer FB et al: Awake craniotomy for aggressive resection of primary gliomas located in eloquent brain, Mayo Clin Proc 76:677-687, 2001.

57. Miller JF et al: Language behavior in acquired childhood aphasia. In Holland AL, editor: Language disorders in children: recent advances, San Diego, 1984, College-Hill Press.

58. Morariu MA: Locked-in syndrome. In Major neurological syndromes, Springfield, Ill, 1979, Charles C Thomas.

59. Mumenthaler M: Neurology, ed 3, New York, 1990, Thieme.

60. Nagatani K: Mutism after removal of a vermian medulloblastoma: cerebellar mutism, Surg Neurol 36:307, 1991.

61. Nishikawa M et al: Cerebellar mutism after basilar artery occlusion—case report. Neurol Med Chir 38:569, 1998.

62. Onofrj M et al: Event related potentials in patients with locked-in syndrome, J Neurol Neurosurg Psychiatry 63:759, 1997.

63. Patterson JR, Grabois M: Locked-in syndrome: a review of 139 cases, Stroke 17:758, 1986.

64. Penfield W, Roberts L: Speech and brain-mechanisms, Princeton, NJ, 1959, Princeton University Press.

65. Pirzada NA, Ali II: Central pontine myelinolysis, Mayo Clin Proc 76:559, 2001.

66. Pittock SJ et al: OKT3 neurotoxicity presenting as akinetic mutism, Transplantation 75:1058, 2003.

67. Plum F, Posner J: Diagnosis of stupor and coma, Philadelphia, 1966, FA Davis.

68. Pollack IF et al: Mutism and pseudobulbar symptoms after resection of posterior fossa tumors in children: incidence and pathophysiology, Neurosurgery 37:885, 1995.

69. Quattrini A et al: Mutism in 36 patients who underwent callosotomy for drug-resistant epilepsy, J Neurosurg Sci 41:93, 1997.

70. Reeves AG: Corpus callosotomy. In Resor SR, Kutt H, editors: The medical treatment of epilepsy, New York, 1992, Marcel Decker.

71. Rekate HL et al: Muteness of cerebellar origin, Arch Neurol 42:697, 1985.

72. Ruff RL, Arbit E: Aphemia resulting from a left frontal hematoma, Neurology 31:353, 1981.

73. Ruff et al: Long-term survivors of the "locked-in" syndrome: patterns of recovery and potential for rehabilitation, J Neuro Rehabil 1:31, 1987.

74. Sauerwein HC, Lassonde M: Neuropsychological alterations after split-brain surgery, J Neurosurg Sci 41:59, 1997.

75. Segarra JM, Angelo JN: Anatomical determinants of behavioral change. In Benton AL, editor: Behavioral change in cerebrovascular disease, New York, 1970, Harper & Row.

76. Sokol DK et al: Tacrolimus (FK506)-induced mutism after liver transplant, Pediatr Neurol 28:156, 2003.

77. Stuss DT, Benson DF: Neuropsychological studies of the frontal lobes, Psychol Bull 95:3, 1984.

78. Sussman NM et al: Mutism as a consequence of callosotomy, J Neurosurg 59:514, 1983.

79. Trimble MR: Psychopathology of frontal lobe syndromes, Semin Neurol 10:287, 1990.

80. Turgut M: Transient "cerebellar" mutism, Childs Nerv Syst 14:161, 1998.

81. Turkstra LS, Bayles KA: Acquired mutism: physiopathy and assessment, Arch Phys Med Rehabil 73:138, 1992.

82. Vandeinse D, Hornyak JE: Linguistic and cognitive deficits associated with cerebellar mutism, Pediatr Rehabil 1:41, 1997.

83. Van Domburg PH, ten Donkelaar HJ, Notermans SL: Akinetic mutism with bithalamic infarction. Neurophysiological correlates, J Neurol Sci 139:58, 1996.

84. Van Dongen HR, Catsman-Berrevoets CE, Mourik M van: The syndrome of 'cerebellar' mutism and subsequent dysarthria, Neurology 44:2040, 1994.

85. Van Mourik M, van Dongen HR, Catsman-Berrevoets: The many faces of acquired mutism in childhood, Pediatr Neurol 15:352, 1996.

86. Vogel M, von Cramon D: Articulatory recovery after traumatic mutism, Folia Phoniatr Logop 35:294, 1983.

87. Vogel M, von Cramon D: Dysphonia after traumatic midbrain damage: a follow-up study, Folia Phoniatr Logop 34:150, 1982.

88. von Cramon D: Traumatic mutism and the subsequent reorganization of speech functions, Neuropsychologia 19:801, 1981.

89. Wang MC, Winston KR, Breeze RE: Cerebellar mutism associated with a midbrain cavernous malformation. Case report and review of the literature, J Neurosurg 96:607, 2002.

90. Weishmann UC, Niehaus L, Meierkord H: Ictal speech arrest and parasagittal lesions, Eur Neurol 38:123, 1997.

91. Weller M: Anterior opercular cortex lesions cause dissociated lower cranial nerve palsies and anarthria but no aphasia: Foix-Chavany-Marie syndrome and "automatic voluntary dissociation" revisited, J Neurol 240:199, 1993.

92. Weller M, Poremba M, Dichgans J: Opercular syndrome without opercular lesions: Foix-Chavany-Marie syndrome in progressive supranuclear motor system degeneration, Eur Arch Psychiatr Neurol Sci 239:370, 1990.

93. Zeman A: Consciousness, Brain 124:1263, 2001.

13 Other Neurogenic Speech Disturbances

> *"i i i it's dea dealing wi wi with a lo lot of people (2-second pause) . . . who who (2-second pause) . . . ha have a lot of needs."*
>
> *(Self-description of work responsibilities by a man with hypokinetic dysarthria)*

> *"I lack dynamics in my voice, I lack inflection in my voice . . . it doesn't have the dynamicism that I had before my stroke, nor do I have any measurable amount of inflection to make my voice more interesting and more . . . motivating when I talk to people."*
>
> *(Self-description of speech difficulties by a man with aprosodia following a right hemisphere stroke)*

CHAPTER OUTLINE

I. **Other speech disturbances associated with unilateral, bilateral, multifocal, or diffuse central nervous system lesions**
   A. Acquired neurogenic dysfluency or stuttering-like behavior (neurogenic stuttering)
   B. Palilalia
   C. Echolalia
   D. Other cognitive and affective disturbances
III. **Other speech disturbances associated with left hemisphere lesions**
   A. Aphasia—language-related disturbances
   B. Foreign accent syndrome
IV. **Other speech disturbances associated with right hemisphere lesions—aprosodia**
   A. Assessing prosodic production
   B. Definition and clinical characteristics
   C. Associated clinical characteristics and supporting data
   D. Anatomic correlates
   E. Nature of the problem
V. **Cases**
VI. **Summary**

Not all neurogenic speech disturbances are captured under the heading of motor speech disorders (MSDs). This was evident in the previous chapter, which made it clear that neurogenic mutism can reflect disturbances in arousal, drive, motivation, and affect, as well as specific MSDs. Similarly, speaking individuals' verbal output may be aberrant for reasons other than dysarthria and apraxia of speech (AOS). The recognition of these "other" problems as distinct from MSDs is important to understanding the organization of speech, language, and communication in the brain, and it has implications for localization and management. These problems are the focus of this chapter.

The speech disorders discussed here represent a heterogeneous collection of problems that have various close and distant relationships to MSDs. Some are clearly distinct from the dysarthrias and AOS and fall in the realm of cognitive, affective, or language disturbances. Others might be MSDs in their own right but have not been considered so by convention or because their nature is as yet poorly understood. Still others may represent an unusual prominence of a characteristic that is part of an identifiable MSD.

There is no generally accepted way for categorizing these diverse speech disorders. For organizational purposes, they are grouped in this chapter under three broad anatomic headings: (1) those associated with diverse central nervous system (CNS) lesion sites; (2) those usually associated with left hemisphere (LH) abnormalities; and (3) those usually associated with right hemisphere (RH) abnormalities. Deficits under each of these headings are summarized in Table 13-1.

OTHER SPEECH DISTURBANCES ASSOCIATED WITH UNILATERAL, BILATERAL, MULTIFOCAL, OR DIFFFUSE CENTRAL NERVOUS SYSTEM LESIONS

Acquired Neurogenic Dysfluency or Stuttering-Like Behavior (Neurogenic Stuttering)

Definition and Clinical Characteristics

CNS disease occasionally leads to speech disruptions characterized by sound or syllable repetition, prolongation, or hesitation. Sometimes the dysfluencies are the only evident speech abnormality. Sometimes they are embedded within a constellation of symptoms that represent dysarthria, AOS, or aphasia. Also, sometimes they represent a psychologic response to neurologic disease, a condition that is discussed in the next chapter's focus on psychogenic and related nonorganic speech disturbances. Dysfluent speech acquired as a direct result of neurologic disease has been given various labels, including *acquired stuttering, cortical stuttering,* and *neurogenic stuttering.*

The heading used for this section obviously reflects some reservations about the label "stuttering." These reservations stem from a desire to avoid: (1) confusing this disorder with behavioral, etiologic, and theoretical issues associated with idiopathic childhood stuttering; (2) implying that acquired neurogenic dysfluencies represent strong evidence for a neurogenic basis for developmental stuttering; (3) implying that all dysfluencies associated with acquired CNS damage reflect the same underlying disturbance; (4) implying that all acquired stuttering-like behavior is neurogenic—it can also be psychogenic in origin, even in people with neurologic disease.

table 13-1 Designation, lesion loci, and nature of deficits associated with neurogenic speech disturbances that may or may not be explained by dysarthria or apraxia of speech

Designation	Anatomic Locus	Possible Nature of Deficit
Bilateral, Multifocal, or Diffuse		
Neurogenic stuttering	Left hemisphere	Aphasia
		Apraxia of speech
	Basal ganglia	Hypokinetic dysarthria
	Multiple lesion sites (right hemisphere, supplementary motor area, thalamus, midbrain, pons, cerebellum)	Various dysarthria types
		Dysequilibrium of a bilaterally innervated system
Palilalia	Basal ganglia; frontal lobes	? Damaged inhibitory motor circuits
Echolalia	Left hemisphere, diffuse, multifocal; ? basal ganglia central circuit	Preserved input/output with lowered threshold for responding to external stimulation; poor propositional language
Attenuated speech/hypophonia	Frontal lobe, limbic, thalamic	Cognitive-affective; hyperkinesia (e.g., Tourette's)
	Basal ganglia	Hypokinetic dysarthria
Disinhibited vocalization	Diffuse, multifocal	Cognitive-affective
Left Hemisphere		
Aphasia		Nonfluency
		Word retrieval deficits
		Phonologic errors
Pseudoforeign accent		? Motor planning/programming (apraxia of speech)
		? Syntactic deficits (aphasia)
Right Hemisphere		
Aprosodia		? Dysarthria
		? Motor planning/programming
		? Cognitive-affective
		? Other

With these reservations stated, the designation *neurogenic stuttering (NS)* is adopted here in an effort to maintain consistency with its frequent use in the literature, and because it makes explicit the presumed neurologic etiology of the problem. The designation "stuttering" represents a shorthand for "stuttering-like behaviors" that are similar in some but not all respects to the surface features of idiopathic childhood stuttering, the disorder for which the label "stuttering" traditionally has been reserved.*

Whether NS in people with aphasia, AOS, or dysarthria is simply another manifestation of those conditions or represents a concomitant but separate speech disorder may be difficult to determine in individual cases. However, there have been a sufficient number of reported cases without aphasia, AOS, or significant dysarthria to suggest that NS can be a clinically isolated speech disturbance. The characteristics and common associated deficits and etiologies of NS are summarized in Box 13-1.

NS is characterized by repetition, prolongation, or blocking on sounds or syllables in a manner that interrupts the normal rhythm and flow of speech.[53] Sound-syllable repetitions may be the most frequent type of dysfluency, with a majority occurring in the initial position,[114] but the disorder's characteristics are heterogeneous. For example, the dysfluencies of individuals with penetrating head injuries have been described as "like it was 'shot from a gun,'" with intermittent and unpredictable bursts of rapid and unintelligible speech, uncontrolled repetitions or prolongations, and long silences without struggle."[86]

Many descriptions of NS are framed with reference to those associated with idiopathic childhood stuttering. They include the locus of dysfluencies within words and phrases, the kinds of tasks in which dysfluencies are exacerbated or reduced, whether or not there is an adaptation effect (a reduction of dysfluencies with repeated readings), and whether or not there is evidence of anxiety, avoidance, or secondary struggle associated with the dysfluencies. In this context, people with NS have been reported to (1) not necessarily adapt or improve on repeated readings or in response to delayed auditory feedback, choral reading, singing, or other conditions that often reduce developmental stuttering; (2) have dysfluencies that are not restricted to initial syllables; (3) be dysfluent on function words as well as content words; (4) have no consistent differences between spontaneous speech and imitation; and (5) demonstrate annoyance and awareness of dysfluencies but generally not significant anxiety or secondary strug-

---

> ### box 13-1 Neurogenic stuttering—characteristics and commonly associated deficits and etiologies
>
> **Characteristics**
>
> Sound/syllable repetitions, prolongations, and blocking
> May not be restricted to initial syllables
> Can occur within content and function words
> Awareness of dysfluencies but without significant anxiety or secondary struggle behavior
> May not demonstrate an adaptation effect or improvement with choral reading or singing
>
> **Possible Associated Deficits**
>
> Aphasia
> Apraxia of speech
> Dysarthrias (probably hypokinetic more than other types)
>
> **Common Etiologies**
>
> Multiple, but stroke and closed head injury most common
> Also in Parkinson's disease, progressive supranuclear palsy, dementia, seizure disorders, dialysis dementia, tumors, anoxia, bilateral thalamotomy or thalamic stimulation, drug toxicity or abuse

gle beyond mild facial grimacing.* In spite of these differences from developmental stuttering, however, it can be difficult to distinguish developmental stuttering from NS solely on the basis of verbal behavior.[38,139]

Varieties of Neurogenic Stuttering

As is true for MSDs, NS can be associated with a number of etiologies and can be transient or persistent. It can be the predominant or only deficit affecting speech or may occur in association with aphasia, AOS, or dysarthria. Market et al.,[90] in a survey study that identified 81 cases of acquired stuttering, reported that 32% of the cases had aphasia, 12% had dysarthria, and 11% had aphasia and dysarthria (they apparently did not inquire about AOS). The association of NS with or without other speech and language deficits may be the most appropriate way to think of "types" of neurogenic dysfluencies at this time.

Dysfluencies can occur with aphasia, often as a manifestation of word retrieval difficulties or efforts to organize verbal expression or to correct errors. Stuttering-like repetitions have been observed in

---

*With the wisdom of an experienced clinician, Helm-Estabrooks[57] concluded, "It appears that neurogenic 'stuttering' is a distinct speech manifestation, no matter what we choose to call it."

*References 8, 11, 30, 53, 56, 95, 104, 109, 110, 113, 114.

people with Wernicke's, conduction, Broca's, and anomic aphasia, indicating that NS is not associated with any specific aphasia type. This suggests that the inefficiencies in language caused by LH injury can also lead to temporal disorganization in the form of stuttering repetitions.[41]

Rosenbek[113] argued that when dysfluencies are embedded within the numerous manifestations of aphasia, they should not be labeled as stuttering because aphasia is not a necessary condition for NS. In contrast, Lebrun et al.[79] concluded that although NS occurs in the context of aphasia in approximately two thirds of cases, the relationship between the dysfluencies and aphasia might not be causal. Sometimes dysfluencies may be "remarkable" and deserving of special mention as an unusually prominent deficit in aphasia. Consider, for example, the dysfluencies—in the form of word repetitions and fillers—during the following 33-second sample of an aphasic man's attempt to describe peoples' efforts to help him with word retrieval:

> "and uh, and uh, and, and uh, the, the first, the uh nurse, uh um, the nurse, uh would just . . . wait awhile and then and uh sometimes she she would, she would fill in uh, for the the word, and uh and uh and uh and uh and uh, it it got to be uh, to be more and more and more uh more, helpful to get somebody to, to come up with the right word."

Similarly, prominent dysfluencies can also be present in people with AOS.[30,63,112,127] They may reflect efforts to establish or correct articulatory postures for sound or syllable production. Rosenbek[113] suggests that it may be inappropriate to label as stuttering the sound and syllable repetitions and prolongations that reflect attempts to correct articulatory or speech movement errors but also notes that some apraxic speakers may be dysfluent on correctly produced sounds and syllables. Consider the following 30-second sample of a patient's description of his speech and reading difficulties; the sample reflects a combination of his AOS and aphasia:

> "Well, I thing gits uh, git the . . . the words to come, together, the right uhhh, in a sen sen . . . ss . . . ss . . . I yuh . . . wellll . . . I juh juh, hard hard hard time uh make makin' a sen, sens, sentence . . . greading, puh poor uh hard, I have a hard time, rea reading." (Note that several transcribed substitutions are actually distortions, and that distortions are present in some words transcribed as accurate.)

Dysfluencies can also be prominent in dysarthria, especially hypokinetic dysarthria, and they can be a relatively early manifestation of hypokinetic dysarthria in parkinsonism or progressive supranu-

clear palsy (PSP).[55,56] Consider the following relatively rapidly spoken, but broken with pauses, 8-second sample from a man with hypokinetic dysarthria who is describing his work:

> "i i i it's dea dealing wi wi with a lo lot of people (2-second pause) . . . who who (2-second pause) . . . ha have a lot of needs."

Etiologies

NS can have multiple etiologies. In their survey study of acquired stuttering, Market et al.[90] reported an association with traumatic brain injury (TBI) in 38%, stroke in 37%, drugs in 6%, and neurosurgery in 4%. These data confirm impressions from the literature that stroke and TBI are probably the most frequent causes of NS. It should be noted that the onset of NS may be delayed following stroke or TBI,[43,94] although Market et al.[90] reported that most of their survey cases developed dysfluencies within 1 month after onset. Other documented causes of NS include: degenerative diseases such as parkinsonism, PSP, dementia, and even motor neuron disease; seizure disorders; dialysis dementia; metastatic brain tumors; anoxia; and bilateral thalamotomy.* In some reported cases, stuttering was the first or primary sign of disease.

The onset of stuttering-like behavior has also been associated with a wide variety of drugs used to treat an array of disorders such as depression, anxiety, schizophrenia, seizures, Parkinson's disease (PD), and asthma. It is of interest that some of the offending agents have been reported to help developmental stuttering.[26] Drugs include tricyclic antidepressants (e.g., sertraline), antipsychotic agents (e.g., clozapine, risperidone), benzodiazepine derivatives (e.g., Tranxene, Librium), phenothiazines, anticonvulsants (e.g., Dilantin, gabapentin), levodopa, and theophylline.[39,81,85,91,92,103,106,109] These observations implicate a number of neurotransmitter systems, including cholinergic, dopaminergic, noradrenergic, and serotonergic mechanisms, perhaps in an interacting manner. Fortunately, it appears that the stuttering nearly always remits after the offending drug is discontinued.[26]

Also of interest are cases in which developmental stuttering has remitted or reemerged with the onset or progression of neurologic disease. For example, the remission of developmental stuttering has been reported in adults during the course of multiple sclerosis with cerebellar lesions,[95] following bilateral thalamic stroke,[99] following closed head

---

*References 17, 54, 55, 61, 71, 72, 78, 80, 87, 88, 107, 114.

injury (CHI),[58] following seizure,[88] and following neurosurgery for tumor or vascular disturbances in the RH or LH in people with Amytal test–confirmed bilateral language representation.[67] Conversely, the reemergence of developmental stuttering has been reported following LH stroke[50,58,98,114] in association with Parkinson's disease,[128] as an initial complaint in probable Alzheimer's disease,[107] and as an initial symptom in olivopontocerebellar atrophy.[52] Caution must be exercised in these latter cases, however, because the relationship between the developmental stuttering and adult onset of stuttering could have been coincidental.

Anatomic Correlates

The survey study by Market et al.[90] reported that 38% of the cases had LH damage (LHD), 9% RH damage (RHD), 11% subcortical lesions, and 10% bilateral lesions; lesions were not identified in 32% of the cases. This predominance of LHD in NS is consistent with the findings of Yairi, Gintautas, and Avent,[145] who documented three times as many dysfluencies during spontaneous speech in a group with Broca's aphasia and LHD than in a non–brain-injured control group and a group of people with RHD; the control and RHD groups did not differ significantly in the frequency of dysfluencies. It is noteworthy, however, that NS has been reported in several cases with RH lesions without evidence of aphasia or AOS.[8,43,60,75-77,114,131]

The frontal, temporal, and parietal lobes may be involved in people with NS. This is consistent with cortical stimulation studies that have elicited sound and word repetitions from all cortical areas except the occipital lobes.[105] Basal ganglia stroke with subsequent stuttering and the association of NS with parkinsonian syndromes and PSP also implicates the basal ganglia control circuit in the disorder.[31,32,55,56,61] Dysfluencies have also been associated with lesions in the supplementary motor area (SMA), thalamus, midbrain, and pons, and in response to mechanical perturbation of the thalamus during surgery, suggesting that interruption of a corticothalamic feedback circuit might cause dysfluency.[1,5,32,140] In an examination of NS in Vietnam veterans with penetrating head injuries, Ludlow et al.[86] found that lesions in the internal and external capsules, frontal white matter, and striatum were present more often in those with than those without NS. They also reported that cortical speech regions such as Broca's area and the primary motor area were involved in 80% of NS patients, but that the frequency of such lesions was not significantly greater than that for nonstuttering individuals.

Single lesions seem less likely to produce lasting NS than multifocal or diffuse lesions. Helm, Butler, and Benson[53] found that multifocal lesions were most common in their group of 10 NS patients; those with persisting NS had bilateral lesions and those with unilateral lesions tended to have their dysfluencies resolve. NS can be persistent in some patients with unilateral lesions, however.[20,79]

It is also of interest to consider the site of lesion or neural activity that can lead to a cessation of dysfluencies. For example, patients with acquired dysfluencies associated with intractable pain and dyskinesia have experienced alleviation of the stuttering during therapeutic electrical stimulation to the thalamus to relieve the pain and dyskinesias.[6,19] Cooper[37] described an adult with developmental stuttering whose dysfluencies remitted for 6 weeks following a brainstem contusion (see additional references to cases with remission under the discussion of etiologies). These observations, plus those of lesions that induce stuttering, suggest that strategically placed lesions or electrophysiologic abnormalities may generate abnormal neuronal firing patterns in subcortical-cortical circuits that lead to dysfluencies (similar, perhaps, to what occurs in certain movement disorders) and, conversely, that similarly placed lesions or stimulation may interrupt such abnormal firing patterns to permit fluency.

To summarize, NS may occur in the aftermath of lesions in the posterior fossa, subcortical structures, the LH or RH, and frontal white matter of both cerebral hemispheres. The only innocent structures seem to be the occipital lobes and the cranial nerves.[113] NS tends to be more persistent with multifocal or bilateral lesions, but it can occur with single, unilateral lesions. Not infrequently, it may develop in individuals without identifiable lesions, as in certain degenerative diseases, CHI, and drug toxicity.

Nature of the Problem

Why does NS develop? There are a number of possible explanations. As already discussed, when associated with aphasia, dysfluencies may simply be secondary to efforts at word retrieval, verbal formulation, and attempts to revise or correct linguistic errors. When associated with AOS, they may reflect attempts to achieve or correct articulatory movements or perceptual goals. When part of hypokinetic dysarthria, they may represent difficulties with initiation of movements or festination, problems analogous to motor deficits associated with rigidity, bradykinesia, and akinesia.

An explanation is more difficult to come by when dysfluencies are disproportionate to those usually encountered in aphasia, AOS, or dysarthria, or when they occur in the absence of those deficits. In such cases, it may be that the offending pathology—which varies considerably in etiology and localization—disrupts equilibrium in a bilaterally innervated system.[114] The multiplicity of lesion sites associated with NS, and the fact that it can emerge when the left perisylvian language and motor speech programming circuits are spared suggests that "speech rhythm and rate control are not dependent on the left cortical regions traditionally associated with speech and language."[86]

Some additional explanations do not invoke a direct neurologic cause. That is, some patients may become dysfluent in response to the psychologic trauma induced by their other speech or language deficits, or other neurologic deficits, or in response to the general impact of suffering brain injury. In such cases the stuttering-like behavior can be considered psychogenic in origin and must be separated diagnostically from the communication deficits that are direct consequences of brain injury. They may also be managed quite differently. Acquired psychogenic stuttering-like behavior is discussed in the next chapter.

Palilalia

Definition and Clinical Characteristics

Palilalia, sometimes referred to as autoecholalia or pathologic reiterative utterances, is the compulsive repetition of utterances, often in a context of increasing rate and decreasing loudness. Repetitions generally involve words and phrases. Sound and syllable repetitions are usually excluded from definitions of palilalia, although sound and syllable repetitions may be present in palilalic speakers. The characteristics and common associated deficits and etiologies of palilalia are summarized in Box 13-2.

The clinical characteristics of palilalia can be summarized as follows:

- *Word and phrase repetitions,* with *stereotypic prosody,* but often with *progressively reduced loudness and increased rate,* much like the acceleration and reduced loudness associated with hypokinetic dysarthria. However, palilalia can be present in the absence of dysarthria,[23,24] and *increasing rate and reduced loudness over the course of repetitions are not invariably present.*[15,68] Repetitions can be remarkable in frequency; one case study documented up to 52 repetitions during a single occurrence![74]
- Reiterations vary in prevalence across different tasks but tend to occur most often during conversation, narratives, and elicited speech and least often during reading, repetition, and

| box 13-2 | Palilalia—characteristics and commonly associated deficits and etiologies |

Characteristics

Repetitions of words or phrases

Increased rate and decreased loudness with successive repetitions (not invariable)

Most prominent during spontaneous and elicited speech; dysfluencies tend to reduce during reading, repetition, and automatic speech tasks

Most common toward end of utterances but can occur anywhere

Adaptation effect uncommon

Awareness of deficit possible but no anxiety or secondary struggle

Reiterations can be inhibited temporarily, with effort

Associated Deficits

Hypokinetic dysarthria frequent but not invariably present

Variety of deficits that occur with bilateral basal ganglia pathology

Common Etiologies

Parkinson's disease/parkinsonism; Alzheimer's disease and other dementias; progressive supranuclear palsy; CHI; stroke; tumor; multiple sclerosis; Tourette's syndrome; stroke; post thalamotomy; tumor

automatic responses such as counting.[24,27,74]
- Reiterations may occur anywhere within an utterance.[60] They generally occur more often at the end of utterances, but some patients have more reiterations in the beginning than in middle or final sentence segments.[74]
- The locus of reiterations may vary across repeated readings, and adaptation (reduced reiteration) may not occur during repeated readings of the same material.[74]
- Palilalia can occur in the presence of other verbal repetitive behavior, such as echolalia and sound and syllable repetitions.[15]
- Palilalic speakers tend to be aware of their reiterations and are agitated by them.[89] There is no obvious struggle or effort to inhibit them during their course, but reiterations sometimes can be temporarily inhibited with effort and encouragement.[27,141]

Etiologies

Palilalia has been reported in people with postencephalitic parkinsonism, PD, PSP,* Alzheimer's

---

*Palilalia has been reported as an early appearing clinical feature in PSP that helps distinguish it from multiple system atrophy.[134]

disease, Pick's disease, posttraumatic encephalopathy, multiple sclerosis, Tourette's syndrome, traumatic basal ganglia lesions, bilateral cerebral calcinosis, multiple strokes, following stereotactic thalamotomy, and during and after seizures.[2,15,24,27,60,84,133,141,146] Palilalic-like symptoms have also been associated with parasagittal meningiomas in the region of the secondary motor area.[27]

Anatomic Correlates

As a number of the etiologies of palilalia suggest, the disturbance often reflects *bilateral basal ganglia pathology.* This is also consistent with the association of palilalia with hypokinetic dysarthria. Bilateral frontal lobe involvement has also occasionally been implicated,[138] but the justification for this association has been questioned.[27] Palilalia associated with unilateral pathology, which is rarely reported, has also been attributed to degeneration of subcortical structures.[60]

Nature of the Problem

Palilalia is generally considered a problem of speech production—as opposed to a language problem—probably reflecting damage to inhibitory motor circuits that help terminate action.[15,24] It has been likened to the acceleration of gait with progressively smaller steps and the difficulty with terminating movement that may occur in PD,[141] and it has been suggested that it could be induced by abnormal properties or distributions of dopaminergic receptors in the basal ganglia.[2]

Benke and Butterworth[15] point out that palilalia characterized by reiteration of utterances with gradually increasing rate and decreased loudness might reflect an additional level of breakdown in the motor control of speech than palilalia without rate and loudness alterations.* Although both "types" seem to reflect difficulties with termination of action when a word or phrase has been uttered, palilalia with rate and loudness changes also implies malfunctions in maintaining amplitude, rate, and pitch parameters. A useful approach for basic clinical diagnostic purposes may be to distinguish *palilalia without hypokinetic dysarthria* (i.e., without problems maintaining amplitude, rate, and pitch) from *palilalia with hypokinetic dysarthria* (i.e., with problems maintaining amplitude, rate, and pitch control).

Echolalia

Definition and Clinical Characteristics

Echolalia is the *unsolicited repetition of another's utterances.* In its full-blown form, it may be automatic, effortless, compulsive, and parrotlike in quality, without comprehension of meaning. In its less complete form, it is characterized by repetition of all or part of what apparently has been understood. Sometimes an echolalic reply may contain only some of the words in a question or statement, with appropriate grammatical alterations, as if the repetition is serving as an aid to comprehension or production[27,141]; for example, a patient may respond, "Something I like to do is golf" in response to the inquiry, "Tell me something you like to do." Somewhat similar variations can occur in the form of appropriate pronoun changes or spontaneous correction of syntactic errors; a patient may echo "Where am I going?" in response to "Where am you going?" These occurrences are sometimes called *mitigated echolalia.* They demonstrate that echolalia does not always occur in the complete absence of language processing.

Echolalia may extend beyond speech explicitly directed to the patient. For example, *ambient echolalia,* in which portions of speech from television programs or conversations going on around the patient are echoed, have been observed in demented individuals.[42]

Although echolalia is usually associated with relatively good repetition ability and effortless and relatively normal articulation and prosody, its mitigated form can occur in people with dysarthria or AOS and agrammatism or simplified grammatical structure. This *effortful echolalia* is characterized by laborious repetition of portions of statements that precede a self-generated response (mitigated echolalia); affected persons can be aware of the behavior but cannot inhibit it consistently.[51]

Etiologies

Echolalia has been reported in stroke, Pick's disease, Alzheimer's disease and other dementing conditions, corticobasal degeneration (CBD), PSP, Tourette's syndrome, carbon monoxide poisoning, systemic lupus erythematosus, status epilepticus, and when consciousness emerges after coma.[27,45,51,84,96,122,141,148] It is important to note that it can also be evident in people with certain developmental and psychiatric disorders (e.g., autism, pervasive developmental disorder, mental retardation, schizophrenia).

Box 13-3 summarizes the characteristics and common associated deficits and etiologies of echolalia.

---

*Benke and Butterworth[15] provide a useful review of models of speech production that may account for various neurogenic repetitive speech behaviors.

Anatomic Correlates

Echolalia often occurs with diffuse or multifocal cortical pathology, but it can also occur as a sign of LH disease. For example, it may be evident in people with so-called *transcortical sensory* or *motor aphasia* or, more dramatically, mixed transcortical aphasia (*"isolation of the speech area"*). In the latter syndrome, the left perisylvian language area is relatively spared but is surrounded by widespread areas of infarction or degeneration of the anterior and posterior association cortex, as may occur in widespread border zone strokes, medial frontoparietal infarction in the area of the anterior cerebral artery, carbon monoxide poisoning, or dementia.[3,4,27,46,51,122] Lesions in the medial portion of the left frontal lobe have been implicated in effortful echolalia.[51]

Nature of the Problem

Lesions associated with echolalia often preserve basic input and output circuits for spoken language, thus permitting repetition, but they isolate input and output channels from cognitive processes necessary for comprehension and language formulation. It has been suggested that echolalia reflects an inability to propositionize, in combination with a lowered threshold to react to external stimuli.[141] In contrast to palilalia, in which lower-level motor mechanisms appear disinhibited, echolalia seems more strongly tied to higher-level cognitive deficits.

Other Cognitive and Affective Disturbances

Several conditions involve speech characteristics that are not easily captured under the other headings adopted in this chapter. Disturbance of nonlinguistic cognitive and affective functions most likely underlies their clinical manifestations. Behaviorally, they can be divided crudely into disorders that attenuate speech and those that reflect apparent disinhibition of vocalization. Box 13-4 summarizes the characteristics and common associated deficits and etiologies of these disorders.

Attenuation of Speech

Neurogenic mutism, which is discussed in Chapter 12, represents attenuation of speech in the extreme.

---

box 13-4 Cognitive and affective disturbances associated with attenuated or disinhibited speech—characteristics and commonly associated deficits and etiologies

Attenuation of Speech

Characteristics

Reduced loudness and hypophonia
Flattened prosody
Reduced speed of responding
Brief unelaborated responses with reduced complexity of content

Associated Deficits

Cognitive and affective impairments
Dysphonia/aphonia associated with post-intubation, psychogenic, and "inertial" factors

Common Etiologies

Closed head injury common but includes anything that may damage frontal lobes, limbic system, basal ganglia, or thalamus

Disinhibited Vocalization

Characteristics

Involuntary speech or phonation
Inappropriate shouting or laughter
Grunting noises
Verbal and vocal tics
? palilalia, echolalia

Associated Deficits

Diffuse cognitive deficits

Common Etiologies

Alzheimer's disease and other dementing conditions, Tourette's syndrome

---

box 13-3 Echolalia—characteristics and commonly associated deficits and etiologies

Characteristics

Unsolicited repetition of others' utterances
Compulsive, parrotlike quality
Repetition may be complete or partial, sometimes with spontaneous correction of syntax

Associated Deficits

Aphasia
Diffuse cognitive deficits

Common Etiologies

Stroke; carbon monoxide poisoning; Alzheimer's disease; Pick's disease; other dementias; progressive supranuclear palsy; corticobasal degeneration; status epilepticus; schizophrenia; mental retardation; autism/pervasive developmental disorders; Tourette's syndrome

It can reflect anarthria, AOS, or aphasia, but can also be the result of disorders that are not confined to speech or language. Among the cognitive and affective deficits associated with mutism, frontal lobe–limbic system pathology leading to abulia and akinetic mutism is of greatest interest here.

Individuals with abulia and akinetic mutism tend to have extensive frontal lobe damage, although the anterior or mesial portions of the frontal lobes, including the SMA, may be involved most often. Deficits reflect reduced drive, initiative, motivation, and ability to sustain cognitive and motor effort. These translate into apathy, listlessness, unconcern, and slowness in responding, with associated decreased verbal output, facial expression, and gesture.

When damage to frontal activating mechanisms is not severe enough to cause mutism, there often is a constellation of distinctive speech, voice, and language characteristics that seem to reflect attenuation rather than alteration of normal speech output. The term *attenuation* in this context refers to *reduced speed of verbal responding, reduced linguistic and cognitive complexity of content, reduced vocal loudness and completeness of phonation,* and *flattened prosody*. To be more explicit, the patient may be slow to initiate verbal responses and show little or no behavioral evidence of effort during the delay. When responses emerge, they often are *brief, unelaborated,* and *literal*. Rather than inadequacies or errors in language per se, content reflects limited thought, with indifference to its lack of detail or impact on the listener.

It should be noted that reduced loudness (often called *hypophonia*) and flattened prosody can also be associated with damage to subcortical structures that have important connections to cortical frontal and limbic structures. For example, patients with hypokinetic dysarthria due to basal ganglia pathology may have attenuated loudness and prosody as prominent speech characteristics. Additional speech abnormalities and the general clinical milieu in which these attenuations occur tie them to motor rather than cognitive deficits. Taken as isolated symptoms, however, they may be similar to the decreased loudness and prosody associated with the abulic and cognitive deficits associated with cortical frontal-limbic pathology. Similarly, hypophonia and flattened prosody (as well as variable alertness and attention, decreased insight, flat affect, and lack of initiative) are frequently associated with thalamic lesions.*[48,49,65,97] Ignoring other

behaviors that dis-tinguish thalamic from cortical pathology, this constellation of symptoms is similar to the cortical frontal-limbic deficits described earlier.

The phonatory characteristics of these attenuations of speech deserve further mention because the reasons for them can be in doubt. For example, patients with TBI who are abulic and aphonic or dysphonic could be so because of vocal fold edema resulting from intubation/extubation.[83,126,144] It is certainly the case that many patients with TBI have been intubated for varying durations after their injury and that dysphonia can occur after extubation in patients without brain injury.[12,35,66,147] Thus the effects of intubation/extubation must be considered as a source of phonatory abnormality, especially when cognitive abilities and overall affect seem less affected than phonation. At the same time, aphonia/hypophonia following CHI can occur in the absence of vocal fold weakness, dysarthria, or AOS and may resolve quickly with symptomatic therapy.[125] In such cases affective and cognitive deficits might explain the phonatory abnormalities, but Sapir and Aronson[125] discuss two additional possibilities. First, especially when there is a rapid response to symptomatic therapy, the aphonia may represent an acute emotional reaction to the trauma or its physical and psychologic consequences. A second possibility is that there might be an initial vocal fold paralysis (or weakness or edema from intubation) or an apraxia of phonation, with persistence of aphonia after those disorders clear. Such *"inertial aphonia"* can occur in patients who are placed on voice rest following thyroidectomy and then respond rapidly to symptomatic therapy; a similar mechanism could occur following CHI.

Disinhibited Vocalization

Sometimes neurologic disease leads to what appears to be *involuntary vocalization,* a phenomenon that may reflect disinhibition of vocal mechanisms. A prime example is Tourette's syndrome, with its verbal and vocal tics (see Chapter 8). SMA lesions have been associated with involuntary automatic speech and paroxysmal involuntary phonation, more frequently with LH than RH lesions.[64] Severely impaired individuals with Alzheimer's disease may shout and laugh inappropriately,[7] and some patients with PSP and frontotemporal dementias produce involuntary, repetitive grunting, groaning, humming, or lip smacking sounds.[130,135] Cognitively impaired patients with diffuse or multifocal involvement also make brief grunting noises of which they are unaware.

---

*Recall that certain thalamic nuclei have important connections to the frontal lobes, including the SMA.

Finally, inhibitory mechanisms are probably involved in echolalia and perhaps palilalia, as well as some of the dysfluencies that may occur in some forms of neurogenic stuttering. These deficits have been discussed elsewhere in this chapter.

OTHER SPEECH DISTURBANCES ASSOCIATED WITH LEFT HEMISPHERE LESIONS

Aphasia—Language-Related Disturbances

Aphasia is a CNS disturbance of the capacity to interpret and formulate symbols for communicative purposes. It generally affects all modalities of language use (spoken expression, verbal comprehension, reading, writing, and nonverbal propositional communication) but cannot be attributed to global impairments of cognitive functions, confusion, or sensory or motor deficits. Although it has prominent effects on spoken language expression, it is neither an MSD nor, technically, a speech disorder; it is a disorder that affects language.

Aphasia is nearly always the result of damage to the LH perisylvian language zone, which includes the posterior frontal and temporal and parietal cortex. Damage to subcortical structures in the LH, including the basal ganglia and thalamus, can also be associated with aphasia. The LH is dominant for language in approximately 98% of right-handers and 60% to 70% of left-handers. Among left-handers who are not LH-dominant for language are individuals who are either RH-dominant or have mixed language dominance. Stroke is the most common cause of aphasia.

Aphasia is usually most readily apparent in spoken language. In many instances, it is clear that the ability to formulate messages has gone awry and there is little to suggest that the motor aspects of speech are deficient. However, when AOS is also present—which it often is—separating the language problem from the motor speech deficit can be difficult. It is appropriate, therefore, to summarize the common verbal output characteristics of aphasia that can affect phonemic accuracy and prosody. Box 13-5 summarizes the characteristics of aphasia that affect the flow of verbal output, as well as common associated deficits and etiologies.

Grammar and Syntax

Aphasia can affect grammar and syntax. This is most evident in the agrammatic or telegraphic speech of

---

box 13-5   Aphasia—speech characteristics and commonly associated deficits and etiologies*

Characteristics

Grammatical/syntactic: slow rate, altered prosody with tendency to equalize stress, simplified grammar and telegraphic structure

Word retrieval deficits: slow overall rate, interrupted prosodic flow

Phonologic errors: phonemic paraphasias and neologisms, usually in a context of normal prosody

Associated Deficits

Apraxia of speech
Unilateral upper motor neuron dysarthria

Common Etiologies

Stroke most common but can include any process capable of damaging dominant hemisphere language areas

*The characteristics summarized here include only those aphasic deficits that alter the flow of speech.

---

patients with so-called *Broca's or nonfluent* aphasia* who, for example, may say "the fork...eat... meat, potatoes" to describe what one does with a fork. Nonfluent patients' utterances tend to be reduced in length, often with simplified grammar and a relative absence of function words. They are often *produced slowly* with an *abnormal prosodic pattern* that sounds more like a listing of words than the "melodic line" of normally structured sentences. The content of nonfluent utterances reflects the underlying language deficit in many patients, and the abnormal prosody is a natural consequence of the structure of the utterance; that is, prosodic flow is disturbed by the absence of parts of speech that receive varying stress (i.e., sentences containing only nouns and verbs naturally have a pattern of excess and equal stress). In addition, because most patients with Broca's aphasia have an accompanying AOS, it is possible that reduced utterance length and telegraphic content represent an attempt to economize on speech planning/programming demands.

---

*The term *nonfluent* traditionally has been used to refer to the verbal output characteristics of aphasic persons whose speech is characterized by agrammatism and short phrases, and, frequently, prosodic and articulatory characteristics that often reflect AOS. In the context of this book, at least, the term should not be confused with the term *dysfluent*, a designation tied to problems discussed under the heading of neurogenic dysfluency or stuttering-like behavior.

Word Retrieval Deficits

Nearly all aphasic persons have difficulty with word retrieval. This is often characterized by hesitancy and delays that are sometimes silent, but that may also be loaded with fillers such as "um" and "uh" or asides about the problem ("it's a . . . oh I know what it is . . . it's a, a, fork"). Patients may make semantic errors that they may or may not recognize ("It's a knife, no it's not a knife, it's a, oh, it's a fork"). Delays for word retrieval efforts, filled or unfilled, result in a *slowed overall rate* of expression and *interrupted prosodic flow,* giving speech a *halting, hesitant* character. In the absence of AOS, this reduced rate and aborted prosodic flow reflect the underlying language disturbance and not a motor speech problem.

In some patients, word retrieval and other language formulation and expression difficulties are associated with dysfluencies that may have a stuttering-like character (discussed earlier in this chapter).

Phonologic Errors

Some aphasic patients make phonologic errors—called *phonemic* or *literal paraphasias*—which are substitutions, omissions, additions, or transpositions of phonemes in correctly retrieved lexical units (e.g., "religerator" for "refrigerator"). Such errors are usually made by patients who speak grammatically and with relatively normal motor effort and prosody; they are often said to have Wernicke's or conduction aphasia.

Relatively severely affected patients who nonetheless have fluent and prosodically normal speech may produce *neologisms* or words with no currency in the language (e.g., "grundel" for "cigarette," "taidillion" for "pencil"). These phonologically aberrant productions may superficially suggest AOS, but their fluent and effortless production, usually made without awareness or efforts at self-correction, is usually not confused with apraxic errors. The distinction between apraxic and phonologic errors on semantically interpretable words, especially when the patient shows awareness of errors and attempts to self-correct, can be much more difficult (this issue is addressed in Chapters 11 and 15).

To summarize, when aphasia is the only communication disorder, phonation, resonance, and the rate at which individual words and many portions of utterances are produced are usually normal. However, there may be abnormalities in prosodic flow that are by-products of the language formulation problem, with slowed rate and hesitancy associated with word retrieval efforts, correction of semantic errors, and revisions of statements that fail to convey semantic intent. Prosody can also be altered by grammatical and syntactic deficits that omit usually unstressed words (e.g., the, a, of) and disturb prosodic flow. Phonologic errors may suggest articulatory deficits, but distortions of sounds usually are not evident, errors may not be recognized by the speaker, and they occur in utterances that may be produced effortlessly.

Foreign Accent Syndrome

Neurologic disease occasionally yields an unusual disorder whose articulatory and prosodic characteristics are perceived as a foreign accent. This problem is most often referred to as *foreign accent syndrome (FAS).* Because the accents associated with it are not entirely consistent with those of nonnative speakers of specific languages, it is also appropriately called *pseudoforeign accent.**

FAS is rare. Aronson[10] identified 12 published cases from 1907-1978 and added 13 cases from Mayo Clinic files. An additional 16 cases were reported from 1982-2001.[33]

Clinical Characteristics

The clinical characteristics of FAS can be summarized as follows:

1. *FAS is not language specific.* The literature contains reports of native speakers of languages as diverse as British and American English, Czech, French, Norwegian, and Spanish who developed FAS. The accents perceived have been similarly diverse, such as Alsatian, American English, Chinese, Dutch, French, French Canadian, German, Hungarian, Irish, Italian, Norwegian, Polish, Scandinavian, Scottish, Slavic, Spanish, Swedish, and Welsh. The type of accent perceived often differs among listeners or cannot be classified, and true speakers of the perceived language report that the accent is not really that of their language.[9]

2. *There is considerable heterogeneity among the specific speech characteristics* that have been reported, but FAS is commonly *dominated by abnormalities in vowel production and prosody* in comparison to premorbid patterns. These abnormalities, as described in perceptual and acoustic analyses, can be summarized as follows†:

---

*The problem has also been referred to as "dysprosody of pseudoforeign dialect,"[10] and "unlearned foreign accent."[47]

†The summary is based primarily on reports by Aronson[10]; Ardila, Rosselli, and Ardila[9]; Blumstein et al.[22]; Coelho and Robb[33]; Graff-Radford et al.[49]; and Kuroski, Blumstein, and Alexander.[73]

Vowel changes. These may include: diphthongization; distortions and prolongations of vowels; omission of unstressed vowels; insertion of epenthetic vowels between words or at the end of Consonant-vowel-consonant (CVC) syllables (e.g., "dis *uh* boy" for "this boy," "nice*uh*" for "nice"); equalization of vowel duration; vowel shifts (e.g., "feet" for "fit," "soam" for "some," "bock" for "back").

Consonant changes. These may include: alterations in voicing, place, and manner features, leading to perception of substitutions; poor control of voice onset time (VOT), such as long prevoicing of initial stops; slightly off-target consonants (allophonic variations or distortions), such as fronting of alveolar consonants; anomalous consonant production, such as voicing assimilation ("yez I know"); production of full alveolar stops instead of flapping in the medial position, as in "butter" for "budder."

Prosodic changes. These may include several problems with stress, rhythm, and intonation, including: generally altered prosody; failure to reduce unstressed syllables within words; equalized syllabic stress; prolonged intervals; inappropriate pitch patterns; restricted or large fundamental frequency (f_o) excursions; abnormal melodic line, such as uncharacteristic rising pitch contours at the end of simple declaratives; slow rate; reduced fluency; initial consonant blocking; and poor transitions across word boundaries. Some of these features could be independent of abnormalities or differences in segmental or articulatory aspects of speech; others could be secondary to such abnormalities or differences.

Nonspecific changes. Some changes may cross vowel, consonant, and prosodic dimensions, including sound substitutions, nonelided word boundaries, nonnative phonemes, broadening of phonemic boundaries, inconsistency of deviant characteristics, hesitancy, and word searching.

Other motor speech and language deficits can accompany foreign accent syndrome. Many affected patients have right hemiparesis and right central facial weakness. More relevant, many are or have been mildly aphasic, usually with relatively mild verbal output characteristics associated with Broca's aphasia. Aronson[10] observed that 68% of affected cases had their accent embedded in or following dysarthria, aphasia, or AOS. Among his 13 Mayo Clinic patients, 62% had AOS as an antecedent to the perception of an accent.

Etiologies and Anatomic Correlates

Stroke is the presumed etiology in approximately 70% of reported cases, and CHI, 20%. Etiology has

---

box 13-6   Pseudoforeign accent—characteristics and commonly associated deficits and etiologies

Characteristics

Unreliability among listeners regarding the specific accent perceived

Vowels: diphthongization; distortions; prolongations; insertions; omissions when unstressed

Consonants: voice, place, and manner distortions; substitutions; allophonic variations

Prosody: equalized or altered stress; prolonged intervals; inappropriate pitch contours; slow rate; reduced fluency; blocking; poor transitions across word boundaries

Other perceptual attributes: nonnative phonemes; broadening of phonemic boundaries; hesitancy and word searching; grammatical and syntactic errors

Acoustic: poor voice onset time control; abnormal variability; restricted vowel space; poor coarticulation

Associated Deficits

Aphasia
Apraxia of speech
Nonverbal oral apraxia

Common Etiologies

Stroke and closed head injury most common

---

been uncertain in the remaining cases; that is, they have had otherwise negative clinical neurologic examinations and no other unequivocal evidence of neurologic disease.[10,33] This suggests that lesions may be small in some cases or the etiology may not be neurologic.*

In the great majority of cases with stroke, the lesion has been in the *LH*. The lesion site within the LH is often in the motor cortex, premotor area (Broca's area), or striatum.[33,73] A majority of lesions include subcortical areas, and only approximately one quarter have only cortical lesions.[33] Limited data suggest that prognosis for recovery is better if the primary motor cortex is spared and worse if there is involvement of the primary motor and adjacent sensory cortex.[18]

Box 13-6 summarizes the characteristics and common associated deficits and etiologies of pseudoforeign accent.

Nature of the Problem

The underlying nature of FAS is uncertain, although it is clear that affected individuals have not acquired

---

*The etiology of FAS can be psychogenic in some cases, even in the presence of confirmed neurologic disease. This is addressed in Chapter 14.

a "true" foreign accent. Perceptual and acoustic descriptions of vowel distortions, allophonic consonant variations, sound substitutions, initial consonant blocking, equalized stress, prolonged intervals, inappropriate pitch variability, inconsistency of speech characteristics, abnormal tongue retraction during vowel production, abnormal acoustic variability, restricted vowel space, and poor coarticulation have led some to suggest that FAS likely reflects a variant of AOS[10,33] or a problem involving control of complex motor performance.[73] It does seem a reasonable hypothesis that the accent reflects an unusual variant of AOS in which prosodic abnormalities predominate and in which articulatory deficits are relatively confined to distortions of vowels and consonants, with a minimum of perceived frank consonant substitutions and groping for articulatory postures. The addition of syntactic and morphologic errors that may characterize relatively mild Broca's aphasia may also contribute to the perception that the speaker is influenced by a foreign language ("broken English").[9] Why the disorder is so rare is unclear, although isolated "more typical" AOS is itself rare.

What leads to the perception of an accent? It may be that the loss of verbal fluency, a broadening of phonemic boundaries, inadequate suprasegmental features, and agrammatism combine to convey the impression.[9] It may also be that listeners categorize the speech as an accent, because many of the abnormalities fall within the universal features of the world's languages.[22,73] Thus unlike the deviations of articulation and prosody that characterize many of the dysarthrias and AOS, many of the speech abnormalities of FAS do not cross universal boundaries of normal speech production, even though they may cross such boundaries for the affected individual's native/premorbid language; for example, intonational patterns that would be considered pathologic for English can nonetheless be characteristic of other natural languages. This would also explain why the perceived accent usually is not identified reliably; the accent is a generic one, not tied to a particular language.[22,73] The categorical perception of this speech disorder as an accent, therefore, may be similar to the tendency of clinicians to perceive some distorted consonants as substitutions in speakers with AOS.

■ OTHER SPEECH DISTURBANCES ASSOCIATED WITH RIGHT HEMISPHERE LESIONS—APROSODIA

The limbic system plays a crucial role in emotional experience and feelings, but the RH plays a dominant role in recognizing the emotional aspects of information and in producing the affective components of behavior. The perception, comprehension, and production of the prosodic components of speech that are tied to the expression of attitudes, emotion, and emphasis are also lateralized to the RH.[62,100,118] These prosodic functions have been called *extrinsic prosody*[25] and are presumed to require an ability to manipulate speech planning, programming, and monitoring for *pragmatic/social purposes*. This implies an important role for the RH in speech planning and programming and appropriately qualifies the traditional tenet that the LH is dominant for the planning/programming of speech.

In recent years, studies of the processing and production of prosody in people with brain injury have contributed to our understanding of the role of the RH in the comprehension and production of verbal messages. Some have concluded that the RH is specialized for the processing of prosody in the same way that the LH is specialized for the processing of language.[93,115,118] Ross,[115] who coined the term "aprosodia" for the prosodic deficits associated with RHD, has proposed a model that predicts forms of disordered prosody that mirror the classically defined types of aphasia. For example, he discusses motor aprosodia, sensory aprosodia, transcortical motor and sensory aprosodia, and global aprosodia. This model has been criticized[29,62] because of uncertain reliability and validity of methods for assessing aprosodia, questionable validity of the classical notions of aphasia types upon which the model of aprosodia is based, and the relatively small number of patients who have been systematically examined. Nonetheless, clinical observations and formal studies do identify a subgroup of patients with RHD who have unique difficulties with the prosodic aspects of spoken language.

Assessing Prosodic Production

It may help at this point to review the types of tasks that have been used to study prosodic production deficits associated with RHD. A number of these tasks go beyond those commonly used in the assessment of the dysarthrias and AOS.

The most essential observations for the diagnosis of aprosodia are made during conversational and narrative speech, particularly when the patient addresses topics likely to generate a range of affective feelings (e.g., likes and dislikes, relationships, the impact of their illness on lifestyle). It is during these responses that the characteristics of aprosodia may be most evident. It can be argued that if prosodic abnormalities are not apparent during spontaneous conversational interaction that covers a range of affective content, a diagnosis of aprosodic speech is probably not justified.

Beyond conversational speech, many studies have examined *linguistic and affective prosody* at the word, phrase, and sentence levels.* Such tasks may include imitation, reading, and answers to questions in which response content is controlled by picture stimuli or the nature of the questions.

Linguistic or *lexical stress* can be examined by contrasting production of compound words (e.g., greenhouse, whitecaps) with phonetically identical noun phrases (e.g., green house, white caps*). Emphatic stress* may be examined by inducing target stress patterns in responses to questions with prescribed answers (e.g., the word "John" should receive stress in the sentence, "John loves Mary" in response to the question "*Who* loves Mary?"). Production of various sentence forms (e.g., declaratives, interrogatives, imperatives) is another way to examine sentence-level linguistic stress. The examination of *emotional prosody* may employ tasks that require the imitation, reading, or spontaneous production of linguistically neutral or emotional sentences with requested emotions such as happiness, sadness, and anger.

Studies of prosodic production have used perceptual ratings and various acoustic measures. Acoustic studies have examined the f_o, amplitude and durational components of syllables, words, phrases, and sentences that define prosody. Considerable emphasis has been placed on measures of f_o because f_o tends to yield the greatest differences between RHD patients and neurologically normal speakers.[†]

Definition and Clinical Characteristics

Aprosodia can be defined as *a deficit in the interpretation or production of distinctions in the f_o durational or amplitude variations in speech that convey emotional tone, emphasis, and certain linguistic information.* In the context of this chapter, the term aprosodia refers to deficits specifically associated

with RHD, but it should be recognized that *the production of prosody is complex and not localizable to any single area of the brain.* Attenuation of prosodic variations can occur in MSDs (e.g., hypokinetic dysarthria). Other disturbances of prosody (dysprosody) can occur in virtually every type of dysarthria and in AOS. Neurogenic cognitive-affective disorders (e.g., abulia) and psychiatric conditions (e.g., depression) can also be associated with attenuation of prosodic features. The existence of prosodic disturbances among various disorders is no different and no less expected than is the existence of articulatory imprecision in many types of MSDs. This is compatible with the notion that neurologic speech and language disorders "represent graded rather than discrete deficits in the continually evolving transformation of thought into movement that characterizes speech-language production."[25]

The term *dysprosody* is sometimes preferred to the term aprosodia in reference to RHD-related prosodic deficits,[28,123] because the prosodic disturbance does not seem to be characterized by a total absence of prosodic variations. However, the term aprosodia is retained here as a way of identifying a problem that may be uniquely associated with RHD, as well as to avoid confusion with the prosodic deficits (dysprosody) that may be apparent in many of the dysarthrias and in AOS.

In keeping with the purposes of this book, we focus on prosodic *production* deficits associated with RHD. The reader should keep in mind, however, that patients with RHD can also have deficits in the comprehension of prosodic variations. These problems include difficulty identifying and discriminating emotions conveyed by prosody, as well as problems with linguistic prosody that may alter meaning, provide emphatic stress, and convey information about sentence type.[136,137] The nature of these comprehension difficulties is unclear, and the relationship between them and prosodic production difficulties has not been clearly established.

It should also be kept in mind that RHD patients can have various additional cognitive and perceptual impairments that affect communication, and such deficits can be, and often are, more prevalent and handicapping than difficulties with the production of prosody. These problems have been categorized by Myers[101] as nonlinguistic and extralinguistic in character.* Nonlinguistic impairments can, for example, include left-sided neglect, visuoperceptual problems, and attentional deficits. Extralinguistic impairments, which may be at the heart of many RHD communi-

---

*Examples of protocols for assessing prosodic production include those described by Robin, Klouda, and Hug,[111] and Ross, Thompson, and Yenkosky.[118] They include examples of tasks and stimuli, procedures for making perceptual ratings of prosodic adequacy, and identification of acoustic features that can be analyzed to quantify and further characterize prosodic productions.

†Frequently used f_o and durational measures have included: f_o and duration of stressed versus unstressed words (f_o and duration increase in stressed words); f_o pattern over the course of a sentence (it tends to drop over the course of a neutral, declarative sentence); f_o and duration in question forms (f_o tends to rise and duration increases on the last word relative to neutral declarative sentences); and f_o during "happy" versus "sad" expressions (happiness has a higher mean f_o and greater variability than affectively neutral sentences, whereas sadness has a lower mean f_o and flatter contour; sadness is associated with increased sentence duration, and happiness with reduced duration but increased durational variability).[111]

---

*People with LHD and aphasia are not entirely free of nonlinguistic and extralinguistic deficits; for example, some aphasic patients have difficulty with the comprehension and production of prosody.[29,62]

cation problems,[100,101] interfere with the ability to understand and convey intentions, implied meanings, and emotional tone, especially in situations in which verbal and nonverbal cues must be used to assess and convey communicative intents that go beyond the explicit meaning of utterances. As a result, patients with RHD may seem indifferent or flat in affect and may have difficulty interpreting emotions conveyed by facial expression and speech. Problems with the interpretation and production of prosody therefore may be just one of several possible extralinguistic deficits. Unfortunately, the relationship between prosodic deficits—especially prosodic production deficits—and the nonlinguistic and other extralinguistic impairments is unclear. In general, however, *it is possible for prosodic production deficits to be dissociated from other nonlinguistic and extralinguistic deficits;* that is, some patients with significant nonlinguistic and extralinguistic deficits do not have clinically apparent deficits in prosodic expression (that are not explainable by a dysarthria that may be present), and some with significant aprosodia may have no clinical evidence of other nonlinguistic and extralinguistic deficits.

What are the salient perceptual features of aprosodia? Answering this question on the basis of empiric data is difficult because of the highly variable methods and patient selection criteria in studies of patients with RHD. General clinical descriptions provide a starting point, however. Box 13-7 summarizes common complaints, perceptual and acoustic characteristics, and accompanying deficits of RHD patients who have prosodic abnormalities.

It is essential to recognize that *not all patients with RHD have aprosodic speech characteristics.* For example, a recent study of 54 patients with RH lesions due to stroke found that 26% of patients who were evaluated by a speech-language pathologist had aprosodia (30% had deficits in interpersonal interactions); aprosodia tended to cluster together with interpersonal interaction deficits, visuoperceptual deficits, and neglect.[82]

The speech of RHD patients who are said to be aprosodic has been described as: flat; indifferent; computer-like or robotlike; devoid of expression and emotion; monotonous in pitch, loudness, and duration; poorly intoned; and lacking in emphasis. Patients have been described as having little spontaneous prosody, trouble with question forms, and an inability to modulate the voice to convey emotions or express the subtleties of irony and sarcasm.

In spite of the denial of deficits by some people with RHD, it is interesting that *some aprosodic patients spontaneously complain that their voices do not convey the emotions they feel and wish to express.* Some complain of altered pitch, reduced pitch range, reduced loudness, hoarseness, or even a

---

box 13-7 Common patient complaints, perceptual and acoustic characteristics, and accompanying clinical characteristics of RHD patients who are aprosodic. Note that not all RHD patients display all of these characteristics, even if they are judged as aprosodic.

Patient Complaints

Voice does not convey felt emotions
Altered pitch, either lower or higher
Reduced pitch range
Reduced loudness

Perceptual Characteristics

Flattened, robotlike spontaneous prosody
Reduced pitch and loudness variation
Reduced or abnormal intonational range
Reduced affect, expression, and emotion; indifferent
Tendency to equalize stress
Poor expression of irony and sarcasm
Poor projection of voice
Lack of emphasis
Abnormal quality to emotional crying and laughter

Acoustic Characteristics

Less salient and fewer acoustic cues for linguistic stress in narratives
Abnormal amplitude variations in emphasized and non-emphasized sentence final nouns
Reduced linearity and flatter f_o decline in declarative sentences
Poor f_o modulation to distinguish yes-no sentences from other sentence forms
Abnormally high mean f_o in sentences
Restricted f_o modulation for emotional expression during reading
Rapid rate for some speech segments
Reduced acoustic energy in middle- and high-frequency range
Evidence of nasalization
Reduced acoustic contrast in sentences
Failure to achieve stop closure
"Fused" (flat, indistinct syllable chain) prosodic pattern, similar to hypokinetic dysarthria

Accompanying Deficits

Paucity of spontaneous emotional and propositional gestures
Left-sided neglect
Visuoperceptual disturbances
Cognitive-communication deficits
Left central facial weakness
Dysarthria (unilateral UMN)
Left hemiparesis

f_o, Fundamental frequency; *RHD,* right hemisphere damage; *UMN,* upper motor neuron.

strangled feeling.*[124] They may report professional, social, and emotional problems because of these difficulties.[116] These complaints are captured in the following self-description by a man who had an RH stroke and aprosodic speech:

> "I lack dynamics in my voice, I lack inflection in my voice . . . it doesn't have the dynamicism that I had before my stroke, nor do I have any measurable amount of inflection to make my voice more interesting and more . . . motivating when I talk to people . . . and motivate them to my way of thinking, which of course is the way I used my voice my whole career at work."

Findings and issues raised by the results of representative studies that have specifically examined the perceptual characteristics of prosody in people with RHD can be summarized as follows:

1. Based on the work of Benke and Kertesz,[16] RHD patients, as a group, are relatively more impaired in prosody (reduced affective inflection, monotony and tendency to equal stress, and a lack of emphasis and effort), whereas LHD patients have relatively greater articulation deficits and reduced rate.[†] It is not clear if the relatively greater difficulties with prosody in RHD than LHD patients reflect dysarthria or a distinctive disorder of prosody; although some studies of prosodic production in people with RHD have excluded those with dysarthria, others have included them or have failed to note whether or not dysarthria was present. It is quite possible that dysarthria has been a significant contributor to the perceived prosodic abnormalities in some studies.[‡] Any study of prosodic deficits in patients with RH (or LH) lesions needs to account for the possible

contribution of dysarthria to prosodic abnormalities.

2. People with RHD may have trouble producing emphatic and lexical stress, imitating emphatic stress, and imitating or reading interrogative and declarative sentences with appropriate intonation contours. Their prosody during narrative discourse may be abnormal.[28,129,142] They may also have less pitch variation and restricted intonational range when reading or imitating sentences expressing specified emotions.*[129,137] Some of these deficits may be present in people with LHD, but they are generally discounted as attributable to aphasia.[28]

These results suggest that aprosodia may affect linguistic/propositional prosody as well as affective/emotional prosody. This implies that the flat affective prosody of some patients with RHD is not necessarily indicative of depression or unconcern.[115] The results also suggest that aprosodic patients may have a specific deficit in the modulation of prosody that is independent of affective disturbances.[28,129,142]

3. Clinical impressions suggest that prosodic disturbances caused by stroke are usually most evident in the first few days after onset[62] and that they frequently resolve over time, although not always.[93,116] However, recovery from aprosodia has not been studied systematically.

Acoustic Findings

Findings and issues raised by acoustic studies can be summarized as follows:

1. People with RHD produce acoustic linguistic prosodic cues in a manner similar to normal speakers, but they generally use fewer and less salient cues than normal. Their ability to convey stress at the phrase level (e.g., compound nouns vs. noun phrases) and for emphatic stress at the sentence level seems preserved.[13,59] (Emmory, 1987). This suggests that production of linguistic prosody may be spared at the word and noun phrase level.

2. People with RHD may also produce sentence intonational contours that are normal in overall direction and rate of f_o decline for imperatives and interrogatives. Their f_o con-

---

*It may be significant that some of these specific complaints are often heard from dysarthric patients.

†Cancelliere and Kertesz,[29] however, found no significant difference in the frequency of prosodic deficits (receptive or expressive) between groups of patients with RH and LH damage.

‡For example, Ross et al.[119] reported a case of "motor aprosodia" in which the RH lesion was in the posterior two thirds of the anterior limb, the entire genu, and the anterior third of the rostral internal capsule. There was also a smaller, similarly located lesion in the LH that was considered "silent," because the patient had no prior history of right-sided deficits. A moderate left central facial weakness was present. Because unilateral UMN dysarthria often occurs with lesions of the internal capsule and the patient was reportedly "mildly dysarthric," many, most, or all of the deviant prosodic characteristics could have been due to a unilateral UMN dysarthria or even a spastic dysarthria in which the effects of the LH lesion were unmasked by the RH lesion.

---

*On repetition tasks, adequate perception of stimuli is required for adequate performance. Thus poor performance on prosodic repetition tasks could reflect indifference, neglect, or comprehension and discrimination problems[62] rather than a deficit in prosodic production per se.

tours on sentence intonation tasks tend to be less linear and flatter in f_o decline in declarative sentences, and they may have difficulty using f_o to distinguish yes-no sentences from other sentence forms. Behrens[14] suggests that this may reflect problems with the modulation of f_o at the sentence level and that such difficulties may contribute to the impression of speech that is devoid of emotion.

3. Some people with RHD produce greater loudness for unemphasized than emphasized sentence final nouns, a pattern that is the opposite of that observed in normal speakers.[13]

4. During Wada testing in the RH, patients may lose the ability to convey happiness, boredom, anger, and surprise during repetition of semantically neutral sentences. Their spontaneous speech may be flat relative to pre-Wada speech. Statistical analysis suggests that the flattening of prosody is primarily through f_o, not loudness or duration.[120]

5. Some people with RHD may have a basic abnormality in mean pitch level. In their acoustic analysis of f_o mean and variability in read sentences expressing happiness, sadness, anger, and questioning, Colsher, Cooper, and Graff-Radford[36] found that two RHD patients had higher mean f_o and f_o variability relative to controls, but when the data were normalized to control for mean f_o differences, the control speakers had greater variability for most utterances.

6. Some people with RHD have rapid rate in some of their speech segments. For example, some speakers with RHD have shorter than normal durations for both noun phrases and compound nouns, even though they are able to vary duration to distinguish noun phrases from compound nouns.[59]

7. Some RHD patients with prosodic deficits have reduced acoustic energy in the mid- and high-frequency range for vocalic segments and strong low frequency (<500 Hz) energy, probably reflecting nasalization and perhaps inadequate articulation; perceptually, these features translate to monotone, hypernasality, and imprecise articulation. Some speakers also occasionally fail to achieve stop closure, accompanied or characterized by continuous voicing.[69] Kent and Rosenbek[69] describe the overall prosodic pattern as "fused," in which the relief of the syllable chain was flattened or indistinct and consecutive syllables were blurred together into a continuous vocalization, sometimes with a reduction of syllables. Of interest, this prosodic pattern is similar to that encountered in hypokinetic dysarthria,

the dysarthria type most likely to be characterized by a reduction of prosodic contrast. This highlights the possible influence of dysarthria in RH prosodic disturbances, and it suggests that the clinical distinction between aprosodia and hypokinetic dysarthria may be difficult.

8. There is great variability among acoustic parameters within groups of RHD and neurologically normal speakers[13] and considerable overlap between the two groups. For example, some studies have found no differences on sentence repetition between RHD and control speakers in average f_o, f_o range, contour shape, and sentence duration, as well as no differences between patients with anterior or posterior lesions.[124]

Associated Clinical Characteristics and Supporting Data

Nonspeech clinical characteristics that can be present in patients with aprosodia, as well as some clinical findings in brain-injured people that support a role for the RH in prosodic production disorders, can be summarized as follows:

1. Aprosodic patients often have flat nonverbal affect and a paucity of spontaneous emotional and extralinguistic gesturing.[21,115] Despite this, some RHD patients with aprosodic speech may cry in an all-or-none fashion, suggesting that extremes of emotional expression may rely on motor systems that are not identical to RH mechanisms involved in prosody. Observations that the emotional cry and smiling and laughing may seem stilted or feigned in aprosodic patients[116] suggest some overlap in such mechanisms, however.

2. Patients undergoing callosal section may have difficulty repeating different sentence types and sentences expressing different emotions. Some findings suggest that the modulation of f_o may be more disturbed than durational prosodic distinctions.[70] In addition, patients with LHD and mixed transcortical aphasia, although able to repeat propositional speech, may have trouble imitating affective prosody.[132] It is possible in such cases that the left perisylvian area is disconnected from RH structures that mediate affective prosody.

3. The presence of dysarthria and facial weakness in aprosodic patients has already been noted. Dysarthria represents a potential confounding variable in any study of aprosodia in people with RHD.

Anatomic Correlates

The localization of RH lesions that lead to aprosodia has not been well delineated. Evidence suggests that frontal lobe lesions including, but not necessarily limited to, the frontal opercular area (comparable to Broca's area in the LH) are most likely to lead to prosodic production deficits.[40,44,93,115,116,121,129,143] Prosodic difficulties have also been reported in patients with RH subcortical lesions.[16,29,34,120]

Nature of the Problem

The underlying nature of aprosodia is poorly understood. Explanations generally focus on affective and cognitive impairments and the role of motor programming and execution disturbances.

The possible role of underlying affective disturbances is central to the understanding of aprosodic speech. At a basic level, for example, it could be that aprosodic speech reflects decreased arousal or responsiveness or inattention to extralinguistic cues.[100,101] As an emotional disturbance, it could reflect depression, although Ross and Rush[117] reported that aprosodia can persist after depression is effectively treated.*

Although some investigations suggest that dysarthria explains prosodic deficits of some patients,[69,124] some people with RHD have no discernible dysarthria, as it is currently defined. Even when unilateral UMN dysarthria is present, there are some patients whose prominent prosodic abnormalities do not seem explainable by weakness, spasticity, or incoordination. And if, as some studies suggest, the primary acoustic features of aprosodia stem from problems in the modulation of f_o, it would indeed be an unusual "focal" form of dysarthria, unlike any other CNS dysarthria yet described.

Findings that aspects of linguistic prosody are sometimes impaired suggest that prosodic production deficits can exist independent of affective disturbances. The nature of such independence is unclear, however. For example, it may be that limbic system functions that drive the expression of affective prosody are disconnected from speech programming and motor control, effectively leaving speech "emotionless;"[123] or the motor programming of affective and some aspects of linguistic prosody, for which the RH may play a dominant role,[25,100,101] may be disturbed, resulting in prosodic production abnormalities that might be considered a variant of AOS. Thus the disorder could reflect an impaired ability to synthesize or integrate features into a normal prosodic melody, but with relative preservation of linguistic stress and articulation because they reflect segmental (LH) processing. Relatedly, Ryalls, Joanette, and Feldman[124] imply an analogy between efforts to understand prosodic deficits and efforts to distinguish the phonologic and phonetic errors that separate aphasia from AOS when they state, "We cannot be sure whether the patient's problem is one of organizing an emotionally appropriate prosodic contour or one of motor realization of an appropriately organized response." Thus aprosodia could reflect a higher-order deficit in which an appropriate prosodic pattern cannot be "retrieved" and organized or a problem in the motor planning/programming of adequately identified patterns.

It is apparent from studies of prosodic production deficits associated with RHD that results are inconsistent and that clinical impressions of impaired prosody have been difficult to quantify. Some studies find no acoustic evidence of prosodic disturbance at all, even when perceptual judgments suggest abnormalities.[124] Others have found evidence of deficits in affective but not linguistic prosody, and others have found abnormalities in both. To some extent, the inconsistent findings may be attributed to different methods of speech elicitation, differences in perceptual and acoustic measures,* and variability in time after onset of patients studied.[123] Another possibility is that aprosodia simply has not been present in many of the patients studied. That is, group studies have generally tested patients with RHD who are unselected for the presence of aprosodia. Assuming that aprosodic speech is not universally present in RHD[82] and may not be common beyond the acute phase after stroke, group studies probably contain a number of patients without prosodic deficit or whose prosodic deficits are attributable to unilateral UMN dysarthria. If true, the effect would be to wash out the influence of individuals with "true" aprosodia in group statistical comparisons. Efforts to develop a full description and understanding of the characteristics and underpinnings of aprosodia may be more productive if only patients who meet some predefined operational clinical criteria for the diagnosis of the disorder are studied.

---

*Because reduced prosody is encountered in people with major depression without cerebral lesions,[102] aprosodia can be a confounding factor in the diagnosis of depression in people with RHD.[108]

*Perceptual and acoustic measures have focused largely on prosody at the word, phrase, and sentence level. Is it possible that the impression of monotonous and colorless speech in aprosodia derives from the gestalt provided by *discourse extending over a number of sentences,* yielding evidence of a prosodic pattern that is relatively fixed, repetitive and stereotypic, and lacking the variations in pause, rhythm, and inflection that reflect the ebb and flow of emotions and emphasis that emerge over time during communicative interaction?

Cases

Case 13-1

A 63-year-old woman presented with a 7-month history of progressive speech and gait difficulty, problems that were confirmed by neurologic examination. Magnetic resonance imaging (MRI) showed evidence of subcortical demyelinization.

During speech evaluation, she complained that her speech was rapid, that words ran together, and that she occasionally repeated words. Oral mechanism examination was normal, although she had difficulty maintaining a steady tongue posture on protrusion, suggesting either motor impersistence or dyskinesia. Her speech was characterized by rapid rate with acceleration. Articulation was imprecise during periods of rapid speech, and monopitch and monoloudness were present. She also frequently repeated words or short phrases, usually with accelerating rate and decreasing loudness. These repetitions rarely exceeded three times per event. There was no evidence of aphasia. She was uninhibited, occasionally impulsively interrupting the examiner and frequently laughing for no apparent reason.

The clinician concluded that the patient had a "marked hypokinetic dysarthria with palilalia. Conversational intelligibility is approximately 70% to 80%." Speech therapy was recommended, and the patient elected to pursue it closer to her home.

The neurologist concluded that the patient had a subcortical encephalopathy associated with apraxia of gait, ataxia, and an extrapyramidal speech disorder. The cause was undetermined.

Commentary. (1) Palilalia may occur in bilateral subcortical disease affecting the basal ganglia control circuit. When present, it is often associated with hypokinetic dysarthria. (2) Despite its frequent association with hypokinetic dysarthria, etiologies of palilalia are not limited to PD. In this case it was associated with a subcortical degenerative process of undetermined etiology.

Case 13-2

A 72-year-old right-handed man presented with a 6-week history of imbalance, slurred speech, and hearing loss. Neurologic examination revealed normal mental status, marked hearing difficulty, slow speech that did not sound dysarthric, and gait imbalance. Strength was good. The neurologist thought the patient may have had a stroke and that his hearing loss might have been related to a medication he was on for poor circulation. A computed tomography (CT) scan was normal. Audiometric evaluation shortly before his initial neurologic assessment showed a moderate bilateral sensorineural hearing loss.

The patient returned 3 weeks later complaining of loss of appetite, increased dizziness, confusion, and imbalance. On examination, gait had worsened and some jerking in the extremities was apparent. He had bilateral Babinski's signs. He appeared unable to hear but read aloud adequately.

Speech examination 4 days later found the patient unable to comprehend any spoken language, as if he were deaf. Examination was carried out through written instructions. Speech was noticeably slowed in rate, primarily secondary to prolonged vowels that altered prosody in a manner suggestive of a pseudoforeign accent. He had irregular articulatory breakdowns and some difficulty with articulatory sequencing within multisyllabic words. He also had fairly frequent sound, syllable, word, and, occasionally, phrase repetitions without obvious overt struggle. Speech alternate motion rates (AMRs) were equivocally slowed but regular. There was no evidence of aphasia in any language modality.

The clinician concluded: "This is a very unusual speech problem which, I think, reflects multifocal or diffuse impairment. His drawn out speech rate, pseudoforeign accent, and occasional articulatory sequencing difficulties probably reflect an AOS, suggesting dominant hemisphere involvement. He also exhibits a number of stuttering-like behaviors, some of which may be secondary to his AOS, but others which appear almost palilalic in nature, although without hypokinetic elements. Finally, some of his irregular articulatory breakdowns are suggestive of ataxic dysarthria, although these may also be secondary to AOS. There is no evidence of aphasia, nor is he obviously confused or demented. His rapidly progressive hearing loss is very unusual; I don't believe his speech abnormalities can be attributed to his hearing loss, however. Finally, it should be noted that the patient occasionally became oppositional and agitated." Therapy was not recommended because of the rapid progressive nature of the problem and the undetermined diagnosis.

Continued

Case 13-2—cont'd

The patient's condition continued to deteriorate. An electroencephalogram 1 week later was abnormal in a manner strongly suggestive of Creutzfeldt-Jakob disease. MRI was negative.

The patient continued to deteriorate and died 6 weeks later. Autopsy was consistent with the diagnosis of Creutzfeldt-Jakob disease with predominant involvement of the cerebral cortex.

Commentary. (1) A pseudoforeign accent can be perceived in patients with identifiable AOS. (2) Stuttering-like behavior can be associated with AOS, but the nature of the relationship is not always clear. (3) Palilalia may occur in patients with stuttering-like behavior and without clear evidence of hypokinetic dysarthria. (4) Identification of ataxic dysarthria in the presence of AOS may be difficult. (5) FAS, neurogenic stuttering, palilalia, and AOS may occur simultaneously and may be associated with degenerative neurologic disease. It is likely that their cooccurrence reflects diffuse or multifocal pathology. (6) Degenerative neurologic disease may produce multiple, cooccurring motor speech and related speech disorders. (7) Changes in speech may be the first or among the first signs of degenerative neurologic disease, including Creutzfeldt-Jakob disease.

Case 13-3

A 59-year-old right-handed woman was seen for evaluation 2 months following the subacute onset of what outside records described as "aphasia." Neurologic examination was normal with the exception of her speech. A CT scan was normal. She was referred for speech assessment.

She reported that, at onset, "the words just wouldn't come out." She believed she was greatly improved but still had mild difficulty following conversations in noise or with groups of people. She had no complaints about reading or writing.

Oral mechanism examination was normal. Conversational speech and reading aloud were characterized by numerous brief sound prolongations and repetitions, occasional hesitations, and slight delays before word initiation. These dysfluencies were the only evidence of speech abnormality. Performance on various taxing language tasks assessing verbal comprehension and expression, reading, and writing were normal.

The clinician concluded that the patient had "stuttering-like behavior associated with CNS disease.

There are no objective signs of focal aphasic language impairment, although the patient's history and current complaints suggest that aphasia was present and may continue to be present at a subclinical level. Given her history and current speech dysfluencies, her dysfluencies may reflect LH pathology. It should be noted, however, that stuttering following brain damage has been reported with RH or LH lesions, bilateral lesions, and subcortical lesions." The patient had been receiving speech therapy for her dysfluencies. It was recommended that she continue with therapy.

Commentary. (1) Neurogenic stuttering can develop in association with acute neurologic events, such as stroke. Although neurologic examination and CT were normal, by history the patient had been aphasic. (2) Stuttering-like behavior can occur in association with aphasia. In some cases, dysfluencies persist after resolution of clinically apparent language difficulties.

Case 13-4

A 55-year-old man was referred for speech-language assessment following surgery for removal of a recurrent bifrontoparietal parasagittal meningioma. Preoperatively, he had seizures, progressive "mental slowing," and mild right and left lower extremity weakness.

During evaluation, the patient offered no spontaneous speech and was minimally responsive during social interaction. His wife noted that his responses to questions and commands, if he responded, were accurate. During formal testing he followed nearly all simple commands but failed to respond to two-step commands. He read words correctly, named pictures accurately, defined a few words, and answered some questions. All responses were produced with long latencies, and some required prompting. For example, he initially failed to respond within 30 seconds to a request to define the word "island." After being asked, "Is it a kind of building?" he stated, after another 10-second delay, "It's a land mass." His verbal responses were relatively reduced in loudness and flat prosodically. Content was consistently brief and unelab-

orated. He did not write anything on request or spontaneously, even though he adequately grasped a pencil.

The clinician concluded that the patient's behavior was similar to that of patients who are emerging from akinetic mutism and that his difficulties with speech could not be attributed to aphasia, apraxia of speech, or dysarthria but were more likely a manifestation of cognitive and affective disturbances. When discharged from the hospital 3 weeks later, the patient was more verbal and responded more rapidly but continued to have abnormal response latency.

Commentary. (1) Attenuation of speech can occur with bifrontal damage. (2) The speech characteristics of this patient appeared to reflect reduced drive, motivation, initiative, and affect. (3) Clues to the distinction between reduced output secondary to cognitive and affective disturbances versus aphasia were that all of this patient's errors were those of omission rather than commission and that accurate responses emerged if sufficient time was permitted.

Case 13-5

A 24-year-old man was seen for speech-language assessment 12 days following a motorcycle accident. MRI demonstrated an area of hemorrhage in the right frontal lobe, with surrounding edema. Neuropsychological assessment revealed moderate, diffuse cognitive impairment.

Language evaluation found no evidence of aphasia. However, he was slow to respond to all tasks and did not initiate any verbal interaction with the examiner. His performance on more abstract tasks (word definitions and proverb explanations) was adequate linguistically but slowly formulated. His affect was flat.

Moderately reduced loudness, moderately reduced pitch and loudness variability, and mild to moderate breathiness characterized speech. Speech AMRs and sequential motion rates (SMRs) were normal, and articulation was precise. Intelligibility was normal in the quiet setting but reduced in noise because of reduced loudness. His reduced loudness and flat prosody, as well as slowness to initiate speech, were considered his primary communication deficits.

The clinician concluded that the patient's reduced loudness and flat prosody were consistent with frontal or

subcortical injury, or both, associated with CHI and that he had no obvious dysarthria. There was evidence of reduced short-term memory for verbally presented materials and slowness in processing and using complex language, consistent with a nonaphasic, cognitively based communication deficit. There was no evidence of aphasia. His speech normalized within the next month, but his cognitive deficits remained evident, mostly in the form of slowed processing. He was discharged to another facility for continued rehabilitation.

Commentary. (1) Reduced loudness and prosody and delayed initiation of speech are not uncommon in CHI. Such difficulties are consistent with reduced drive, motivation, affect, and general cognitive functioning, and they often reflect impairments in frontal lobe–limbic system functions. (2) The patient's right frontal hemorrhage raises the possibility that his reduced prosody reflected an aprosodia associated with RHD, although he did not have any other lateralizing motor or cognitive deficits. The distinction between RH aprosodia and flattened prosody associated with more widespread neurologic involvement sometimes can be difficult.

Case 13-6

An 81-year-old woman was seen in neurology for evaluation of speech and mental status changes of 2 years' duration. She had a history of a stroke 4 to 5 years previously, after which her speech was "slurred, repetitive, stuttering, and fast." Her speech seemed to have been stable after her stroke, but in the past 2 years she had reduced memory ability and increased confusion. Examination revealed disorientation, difficulty following commands, reduced mental status, and bilateral Babinski's signs and hyperreflexia. A CT scan showed diffuse cerebral atrophy, as well as areas of low attenuation within the centrum semiovale bilaterally, suggestive of demyelinization or multiple strokes.

During speech assessment, her husband reported that her speech had worsened in the past 2 years and that she was talking a great deal more than she had in the past. During language assessment there was no clear evidence of aphasia. She spoke compulsively and made numerous comments that ranged from marginally appropriate to frankly inappropriate. Frequent rapid initial phoneme and word and short phrase repetitions characterized her speech. Articulatory precision was good, as was prosody. Intelligibility was frequently poor secondary to her dysfluencies and rapid speech rate.

The speech diagnosis was "(1) Palilalia characterized by rapid word-phrase repetitions; she also has a number of stuttering-like behaviors, including rapid phoneme repetitions. (2) Hypokinetic-like dysarthria, although this is not a full-blown hypokinetic dysarthria and may be secondary to her palilalia. (3) Cognitive impairments and apparent confusion, but no evidence of focal aphasic language impairment. It should be noted that palilalia is almost always associated with bilateral and/or diffuse dysfunction." The clinician did not believe that the patient would benefit from speech therapy because of her cognitive difficulties. It was suggested that speech therapy should be reconsidered if her cognitive difficulties improved.

Commentary. (1) Palilalia and stuttering-like behavior can occur simultaneously, particularly in the presence of hypokinetic dysarthria. Lesions leading to palilalia (and hypokinetic dysarthria with stuttering-like dysfluencies) are almost always bilateral and subcortical in origin. (2) By history, the patient's "stuttering-like" behavior was present since her stroke but had worsened significantly in recent years. The mechanism for this worsening was unclear in this case, but it is unlikely that her palilalia could be explained by a single unilateral stroke. The neurologist ultimately concluded that the patient had a degenerative CNS disease of undetermined origin.

Case 13-7

A 48-year-old woman was referred for speech-language assessment after admission to a rehabilitation unit 3 weeks following surgery for a right frontotemporal arteriovenous malformation, with subsequent evacuation of an intracerebral hematoma that developed postoperatively. Afterward, she had a marked left hemiparesis and left-sided neglect.

Examination failed to reveal evidence of aphasia. She had considerable difficulty reading; she often read only the right half of printed materials on a page, with accompanying statements that the material did not make sense. When presented with pictured scenes, she consistently ignored information on the left and frequently misinterpreted depicted information. She had a tendency to talk excessively about pictured scenes, frequently labeling objects rather than stating conclusions or interpretations about pictured activities.

Most impressive was the prosodic pattern of her speech. There was no evidence of dysarthria or AOS, and voice quality, resonance, rate, and articulatory precision were normal. Although there was evidence of pitch and loudness variability in her speech, the overall affect conveyed was one of lack of emotion, even when she was discussing emotionally laden information. During the course of a narrative, for example, the intonational pattern of many of her sentences was stereotypic, with little variation as a function of emotional content or salience of information. She was able to place emphatic stress on appropriate words in sentences when answering questions and imitating sentences, but her manner of doing so seemed somewhat artificial and "conscious," almost robotlike. She tended not to reduce pitch and loudness at the end of declarative sentences, often ending them with rising inflection, a pattern that was striking for its frequent occurrence during extended narratives. Finally, the emotions conveyed during a narrative about things that made her happy versus angry was readily apparent in linguistic content but indistinguishable prosodically.

Case 13-7—cont'd

Commentary. (1) Alterations in prosody can occur following RH lesions and in the absence of any recognizable dysarthria or AOS. (2) The aprosodia associated with RH pathology often is accompanied by cognitive impairments and neglect. (3) Aprosodia is not necessarily a complete "flattening" of the prosodic features of speech, as might be heard in hypokinetic dysarthria or the prosody of patients with frontal lobe–limbic system impairments. Rather, it may have a robotlike rhythm and stress pattern, with a recurring repetitive prosodic pattern across many utterances. (4) The aprosodia associated with RHD is not clearly associated with depression. In this patient the emotions expressed prosodically were much less apparent than those conveyed by the content of her language.

SUMMARY

1. Neurologic disease can alter speech in ways that are not attributable to commonly described dysarthrias or apraxia of speech. It is possible that some of these disturbances represent MSDs in their own right or an unusual prominence of a characteristic that may logically be related to a known MSD. Other alterations in speech can be attributed to cognitive, affective, or linguistic disturbances. These heterogeneous problems are sometimes associated with lesions confined to the LH or RH, whereas others may be associated with bilateral, diffuse, or multifocal CNS lesions.

2. Neurogenic stuttering is characterized by various patterns of dysfluency that may occur with or without accompanying aphasia, AOS, or dysarthria. When associated with aphasia, AOS, or dysarthria, the dysfluencies can be part of the language or motor speech disturbance, a response to the language or motor speech disturbance, or relatively independent of the language or motor speech disturbance. Lesion sites associated with neurogenic stuttering are multiple and sometimes not readily apparent, as when dysfluencies develop in response to drugs, metabolic disturbances, or CHI.

3. Palilalia is the compulsive repetition of words and phrases, often in a context of increasing rate and decreasing loudness. It generally reflects bilateral basal ganglia pathology and is frequently but not always associated with hypokinetic dysarthria.

4. Echolalia is the motorically normal, unsolicited repetition of another's utterances. The repetition can be rote or modified in a way that demonstrates some degree of linguistic processing. It usually occurs with diffuse or multifocal cortical pathology in which there is relative sparing of the perisylvian language area, permitting adequate input and output of speech but with limited processing for meaning.

5. Cognitive and affective disturbances can alter the character of speech. Frontal lobe–limbic system pathology may reduce speed of verbal responding, reduce linguistic and cognitive complexity of content, and reduce vocal loudness, completeness of phonation, and prosody. These changes in speech appear to reflect a reduction in drive, initiative, motivation, and sustained cognitive and motor effort. Other cognitive and affective disturbances can lead to disinhibited vocalization or involuntary phonation; inappropriate shouting, laughter, or other noises; or verbal and vocal tics.

6. Aphasia, a disturbance of language, can alter the character of speech. Grammatical and syntactic deficits, word retrieval deficits, and phonologic errors are the primary manifestations of aphasia that alter the rate, fluency, and prosodic flow of verbal expression.

7. A pseudoforeign accent occasionally develops in patients with neurologic disease. The perception of accent seems to reflect an articulatory and prosodic disturbance that is associated with LH pathology and frequently with aphasia or AOS. FAS may represent a variant of AOS.

8. Aprosodia is a disturbance that has been associated with RH dysfunction. Although prosodic disturbances can be associated with various lesion sites, MSDs, and cognitive and affective deficits, evidence suggests that distinctive deficits in prosody can occur with RH lesions. This aprosodic speech pattern is often described as flat, indifferent, devoid of expression and emotion, and computer-like or robotlike. Neither the defining characteristics of the problem nor the nature of the disturbance underlying aprosodia are well understood.

References

1. Abe K, Yokoyama R, Yorifuji S: Repetitive speech disorder resulting from infarcts in the paramedian thalami and midbrain, J Neurol Neurosurg Psychiatry 56:1024, 1993.
2. Ackerman H, Ziegler W, Oertel W: Palilalia as a symptom of L-DOPA induced hyperkinesia, J Neurol Neurosurg Psychiatry 52:805, 1989.
3. Albert ML et al: Clinical aspects of dysphasia, New York, 1981, Springer-Verlag.
4. Alexander MP, Benson DF, Stuss DT: Frontal lobes and language, Brain Lang 37:656, 1989.
5. Andy OJ, Bhatnagar SC: Thalamic-induced stuttering (surgical observations), J Speech Hear Res 34:796, 1991.
6. Andy OJ, Bhatnagar SC: Stuttering acquired from subcortical pathologies and its alleviation from thalamic stimulation, Brain Lang 42:385, 1992.
7. Appell J, Kertesz A, Fisman M: A study of language functioning in Alzheimer patients, Brain Lang 17:73, 1982.
8. Ardila A, Lopez MV: Severe stuttering associated with right hemisphere lesion, Brain Lang 27:239, 1986.
9. Ardila A, Rosselli M, Ardila O: Foreign accent: an aphasic epiphenomenon? Aphasiology 2:493, 1988.
10. Aronson AE: Clinical voice disorders, ed 3, New York, 1990, Thieme.
11. Balasubramanian V et al: Acquired stuttering following right frontal and bilateral pontine lesion: a case study, Brain Cogn 53:185, 2003.
12. Beckford NS et al: Effects of short-term intubation on vocal function, Laryngoscope 100:331, 1990.
13. Behrens SJ: The role of the right hemisphere in the production of linguistic stress, Brain Lang 33:104, 1988.
14. Behrens SJ: Characterizing sentence intonation in a right hemisphere-damaged population, Brain Lang 37:181, 1989.
15. Benke T, Butterworth B: Palilalia and repetitive speech: two case studies, Brain Lang 78:62, 2001.
16. Benke T, Kertesz A: Hemispheric mechanisms of motor speech, Aphasiology 3:627, 1989.
17. Benke TH et al: Repetitive speech phenomena in Parkinson's disease, J Neurol Neurosurg Psychiatry 69:319 2000.
18. Berthier ML et al: Foreign accent syndrome: behavioral and anatomic findings in recovered and non-recovered patients, Aphasiology 5:129, 1991.
19. Bhatnagar S, Andy OJ: Alleviation of acquired stuttering with human centromedian thalamic stimulation, J Neurol Neurosurg Psychiatry 52:1182, 1989.
20. Bijleveld H, Lebrun Y, van Dongen H: A case of acquired stuttering, Folia Phoniatr Logop 46:250, 1994.
21. Blonder L et al: Right hemisphere facial expressivity during natural conversation, Brain Cogn 21:44, 1993.
22. Blumstein SE et al: On the nature of the foreign accent syndrome: a case study, Brain Lang 31:215, 1987.
23. Boller F, Albert M, Denes F: Palilalia, Br J Disord Commun 10:92, 1975.
24. Boller F et al: Familial palilalia, Neurology 23:1117, 1973.
25. Boutsen FR, Christman SS: Prosody in apraxia of speech, Semin Speech Lang 23:245, 2002.
26. Brady JP: Drug-induced stuttering: a review of the literature, J Clin Neuropharmacol 18:50, 1998.
27. Brown JW: Aphasia, apraxia, and agnosia, Springfield, Ill, 1972, Charles C Thomas.
28. Bryan KL: Language prosody and the right hemisphere, Aphasiology 3:285, 1989.
29. Cancelliere AEB, Kertesz A: Lesion localization in acquired deficits of emotional expression and comprehension, Brain Cogn 13:133, 1990.
30. Canter GJ: Observations on neurogenic stuttering: a contribution to differential diagnosis, Br J Disord Commun 6:139, 1971.
31. Carluer L et al: Acquired and persistent stuttering as the main symptom of striatal infarction, Mov Disord 15:343, 2000.
32. Ciabarra AM et al: Subcortical infarction resulting in acquired stuttering, J Neurol Neurosurg Psychiatry 69:546, 2000.
33. Coelho CA, Robb MP: Acoustic analysis of foreign accent syndrome: an examination of three explanatory models, J Med Speech-Lang Pathol 9:227, 2001.
34. Cohen MJ et al: Expressive aprosodia following stroke to the right basal ganglia, Neuropsychology 8:242, 1994.
35. Colice GL, Stukel TA, Dain B: Laryngeal complications of prolonged intubation, Chest 96:877, 1989.
36. Colsher PL, Cooper WE, Graff-Radford N: Intonational variability in the speech of right-hemisphere damaged patients, Brain Lang 32:379, 1987.
37. Cooper E: A brain stem contusion and fluency: Vicky's story, J Fluency Disord 8:269, 1983.
38. Curlee RF: Comments on neurogenic stuttering: an analysis and critique, J Med Speech-Lang Pathol 3:123, 1995.
39. Duggal HS et al: Clozapine-induced stuttering and seizures, Am J Psychiatry 159:315, 2002.
40. Edmondson JA et al: The effect of right-brain damage on acoustical measures of affective prosody in Taiwanese patients, J Phonetics 15:219, 1987.
40a. Emmory KD: The neurological substrates for prosodic aspects of speech, Brain Lang 30:305, 1987.
41. Farmer A: Stuttering repetitions in aphasic and non-aphasic brain-damaged adults, Cortex 11:391, 1975.
42. Fisher CM: Neurologic fragments. I. Clinical observations in demented patients, Neurology 38:1868, 1988.
43. Fleet WS, Heilman KM: Acquired stuttering from a right hemisphere lesion in a right-hander, Neurology 35:1343, 1985.
44. Ghacibeh GA, Heilman KM: Progressive affective aprosodia and prosoplegia, Neurology 60:1192, 2003.
45. Ghika J et al: Environment-driven responses in progressive supranuclear palsy, J Neurol Sci 130:104, 1995.
46. Gonzalez Rothi LJ: Transcortical aphasias. In LaPointe LL, editor: Aphasia and related neurogenic language disorders, New York, 1990, Thieme.
47. Graff-Radford NR, Cooper WE, Colsher PL: An unlearned foreign "accent" in a patient with aphasia, Brain Lang 23:86, 1986.
48. Graff-Radford NR, Damasio AR: Disturbances of speech and language associated with thalamic dysfunction, Semin Neurol 4:162, 1984.

49. Graff-Radford NR et al: Nonhemorrhagic infarction of the thalamus: behavioral, anatomic, and physiologic correlates, Neurology 34:14, 1984.

50. Grant AC et al: Stroke-associated stuttering, Arch Neurol 56:624, 1999.

51. Hadano K, Nakamura H, Hamananka T: Effortful echolalia, Cortex 34:67, 1998.

52. Hartman DE, O'Neill BP: Progressive dysfluency, dysphagia, dysarthria: a case of olivopontocerebellar atrophy. In Yorkston KM, Beukelman DR, editors: Recent advances in clinical dysarthria, Boston, 1989, College-Hill.

53. Helm NA, Butler RB, Benson DF: Acquired stuttering, Neurology 28:1159, 1978.

54. Helm NA, Butler RB, Canter GJ: Neurogenic acquired stuttering, J Fluency Disord 5:267, 1980.

55. Helm-Estabrooks N: Diagnosis and management of neurogenic stuttering in adults. In The atypical stutterer: principles and practices of rehabilitation, St Louis, 1986, Academic Press.

56. Helm-Estabrooks N: Stuttering associated with acquired neurological disorders. In Curlee RF, editor: Stuttering and related disorders of fluency, New York, 1993, Thieme.

57. Helm-Estabrooks N: Comments on neurogenic stuttering: an analysis and critique, J Med Speech-Lang Pathol 3:123, 1995.

58. Helm-Estabrooks N et al: Stuttering: disappearance and reappearance with acquired brain lesions, Neurology 36:1109, 1986.

59. Hird K, Kirsner K: Dysprosody following acquired neurogenic impairment, Brain Lang 45:46, 1993.

60. Horner J, Massey EW: Progressive dysfluency associated with right hemisphere disease, Brain Lang 18:71, 1983.

61. Janati A: Case report: progressive supranuclear palsy: report of a case with torticollis, blepharospasm, and dysfluency, Am J Med Sci 292:391, 1986.

62. Joanette Y, Goulet P, Hannequin D: Right hemisphere and verbal communication, New York, 1990, Springer-Verlag.

63. Johns DF, Darley FL: Phonemic variability in apraxia of speech, J Speech Hear Res 13:556, 1970.

64. Jonas S: The supplementary motor region and speech emission, J Commun Disord 14:349, 1981.

65. Jonas S: The thalamus and aphasia, including transcortical aphasia: a review, J Commun Disord 15:31, 1982.

66. Jones MW et al: Hoarseness after tracheal intubation, Anesthesia 47:213, 1992.

67. Jones RK: Observations on stammering after localized cerebral injury, J Neurol Neurosurg Psychiatry 29:192, 1966.

68. Kent RD, LaPointe LL: Acoustic properties of pathologic reiterative utterances: a case study of palilalia, J Speech Hear Res 25:95, 1982.

69. Kent RD, Rosenbek JC: Prosodic disturbance and neurologic lesion, Brain Lang 15:259, 1982.

70. Klouda GV et al: The role of callosal connections in speech prosody, Brain Lang 35:154, 1988.

71. Kluin KJ et al: Perceptual analysis of speech disorders in progressive supranuclear palsy, Neurology 43:563, 1993.

72. Koller WC: Dysfluency (stuttering) in extrapyramidal disease, Arch Neurol 40:175, 1983.

73. Kurowski KM, Blumstein SE, Alexander M: The foreign accent syndrome: a reconsideration, Brain Lang 54:1, 1996.

74. LaPointe LL, Horner J: Palilalia: a descriptive study of pathological reiterative utterances, J Speech Hear Res 46:34, 1981.

75. Lebrun Y, Bijleveld H, Rousseau JJ: A case of persistent neurogenic stuttering following a missile wound, J Fluency Disord 15:251, 1990.

76. Lebrun Y, Leloux C: Acquired stuttering following right brain damage in dextrals, J Fluency Disord 10:137, 1985.

77. Lebrun Y, Leleux C, Retif J: Neurogenic stuttering, Acta Neurochir 85:103, 1987.

78. Lebrun Y, Retif J, Kaiser G: Acquired stuttering as a forerunner of motor-neuron disease, J Fluency Disord 8:161, 1983.

79. Lebrun Y et al: Acquired stuttering, J Fluency Disord 8:323, 1983.

80. Leder SB: Adult onset of stuttering as a presenting sign in a parkinsonian-like syndrome: a case report, J Commun Disord 29:471, 1996.

81. Lee HJ et al: A case of risperidone-induced stuttering, J Clin Psychopharmacol 21:115, 2001.

82. Lehman Blake et al: Right hemisphere syndrome is in the eye of the beholder, Aphasiology 17:423, 2003.

83. Lesser THJ, Williams RG, Hoddinott C: Laryngographic changes following endotracheal intubation in adults, Br J Disord Commun 21:239, 1986.

84. Linetsky E et al: Echolalia-palilalia as the sole manifestation of nonconvulsive status epilepticus, Neurology 55:733, 2000.

85. Louis ED et al: Speech dysfluency exacerbated by levodopa in Parkinson's disease, Mov Disord 16:562, 2001.

86. Ludlow CL et al: Site of penetrating brain lesions causing chronic acquired stuttering, Ann Neurol 22:60, 1987.

87. Madison DP et al: Communicative and cognitive deterioration in dialysis dementia: two case studies, J Speech Hear Disord 42:238, 1977.

88. Manders E, Bastijns P: Sudden recovery from stuttering after an epileptic attack: a case report, J Fluency Disord 13:421, 1989.

89. Marie P, Levy G: A singular trouble with speech: palilalia (dissociation of voluntary speech and of automatic speech), Le Monde Medical 64:329, 1925.

90. Market KE et al: Acquired stuttering: descriptive data and treatment outcome, J Fluency Disord 15:21, 1990.

91. McCarthy MM: Speech affect of theophylline (letter to the editors), Pediatrics 68:5, 1981.

92. McClean MD, McLean A: Case report of stuttering acquired in association with phenytoin use for post-head-injury seizures, J Fluency Disord 10:241, 1985.

93. Mesulam M-M: Principles of behavioral and cognitive neurology, ed 2, New York, 2000, Oxford University Press.

94. Meyers SC, Hall NE, Aram DM: Fluency and language recovery in a child with a left hemisphere lesion, J Fluency Disord 15:159, 1990.

95. Miller AE: Cessation of stuttering with progressive multiple sclerosis, Neurology 35:1341, 1985.

96. Mimura M et al: Corticobasal degeneration presenting with nonfluent primary progressive aphasia: a clinicopathological study, J Neurol Sci 183:19, 2001.

97. Mohr JP, Watters WC, Duncan GW: Thalamic hemorrhage and aphasia, Brain Lang 2:3, 1975.

98. Mouradian MS, Paslawski T, Shuaib A: Return of stuttering after stroke, Brain Lang 73:120, 2000.

99. Muroi A et al: Cessation of stuttering after bilateral thalamic infarction, Neurology 53:890, 1999.

100. Myers PS: Right hemisphere damage, San Diego, 1999, Singular Publishing Group.

101. Myers PS: Communication disorders associated with right hemisphere brain damage. In Chapey R, editor: Language intervention strategies in aphasia and related neurogenic communication disorders, ed 4, Philadelphia, 2001, Lippincott Williams & Wilkins.

102. Naarding P et al: Aprosodia in major depression, J Neuroling 16:37, 2003.

103. Nurnberg HG, Greenwald B: Stuttering: an unusual side effect of phenothiazines, Am J Psychiatry 138:386, 1981.

104. Peach RK: Acquired neurogenic stuttering, Grand Rounds J Commun Disord 9:177, 1984.

105. Penfield W, Roberts L: Speech and brain mechanisms, Princeton, NJ, 1959, Princeton University Press.

106. Quader S: Dysarthria: an unusual side effect of tricyclic antidepressants, Br Med J 2:97, 1977.

107. Quinn PT, Andrews G: Neurological stuttering—a clinical entity? J Neurol Neurosurg Psychiatry 40:699, 1977.

108. Ramasubbu R, Kennedy SH: Factors complicating the diagnosis of depression in cerebrovascular disease, Part II—neurological deficits and various assessment methods, Can J Psychiatry 39:601, 1994.

109. Rentschler GJ, Driver LE, Callaway EA: The onset of stuttering following drug overdose, J Fluency Disord 9:265, 1984.

110. Ringo CC: Neurogenic stuttering; An analysis and critique, J Med Speech-Lang Pathol 3:111, 1995.

111. Robin DA, Klouda GV, Hug LN: Neurogenic disorders of prosody. In Vogel D, Cannito MP, editors: Treating disordered speech motor control, Austin, Tex, 1991, Pro-Ed.

112. Rosenbek J: Apraxia of speech—relationship to stuttering, J Fluency Disord 5:233, 1980.

113. Rosenbek JC: Stuttering secondary to nervous system damage. In Curlee RF, Perkins WH, editors: Nature and treatment of stuttering: new directions, San Diego, 1984, College-Hill.

114. Rosenbek J et al: Stuttering following brain damage, Brain Lang 6:82, 1978.

115. Ross ED: The aprosodias: functional-anatomic organization of the affective components of language in the right hemisphere, Arch Neurol 38:561, 1981.

116. Ross ED, Mesulam M-M: Dominant language functions of the right hemisphere? Prosody and emotional gesturing, Arch Neurol 36:144, 1979.

117. Ross ED, Rush AJ: Diagnosis and neuroanatomical correlates of depression in brain-damaged patients: implications for a neurology of depression, Arch Gen Neurol 38:1344, 1981.

118. Ross ED, Thompson RD, Yenkosky J: Lateralization of affective prosody in brain and the callosal integration of hemispheric language functions, Brain Lang 56:27, 1997.

119. Ross ED et al: How the brain integrates affective and propositional language into a unified behavioral function: hypothesis based on clinicoanatomic evidence, Arch Neurol 38:745, 1981.

120. Ross ED et al: Acoustic analysis of affective prosody during right-sided Wada test: a within-subjects verification of the right hemisphere's role in language, Brain Lang 33:128, 1988.

121. Ross ED et al: Functional-anatomic correlates of aprosodic deficits in patients with right brain damage, Neurology 50(Suppl 4):A363, 1998.

122. Rubens AB, Kertesz A: The localization of lesions in transcortical aphasias. In Kertesz A, editor: Localization in neuropsychology, New York, 1983, Academic Press.

123. Ryalls JH, Behrens SJ: Review: an overview of changes in fundamental frequency associated with cortical insult, Aphasiology 2:107, 1988.

124. Ryalls J, Joanette Y, Feldman L: An acoustic comparison of normal and right-hemisphere-damaged speech prosody, Cortex 23:685, 1987.

125. Sapir S, Aronson AE: Aphonia after closed head injury: aetiologic considerations, Br J Disord Commun 20:289, 1985.

126. Scholefield JA: Aetiologies of aphonia following closed head injury, Br J Disord Commun 22:167, 1987.

127. Schuell HM, Jenkins JJ, Jiminez-Pabon E: Aphasia in adults, New York, 1964, Harper & Row.

128. Shahed J, Jankovic J: Re-emergence of childhood stuttering in Parkinson's disease; a hypothesis, Mov Disord 16:114, 2001.

129. Shapiro BE, Danley M: The role of the right hemisphere in the control of speech prosody in propositional and affective contexts, Brain Lang 25:19, 1985.

130. Snowden JS et al: Distinct behavioural profiles in frontotemporal dementia and semantic dementia, J Neurol Neurosurg Psychiatry 70:323, 2001.

131. Soroker N et al: Stuttering as a manifestation of right-hemisphere subcortical stroke, Eur Neurol 30:268, 1990.

132. Speedie LJ, Coslett HB, Heilman KM: Repetition of affective prosody in mixed transcortical aphasia, Arch Neurol 41:268, 1984.

133. Stracciari A et al: Development of palilalia after stereotactic thalamotomy in Parkinson's disease, Eur Neurol 33:275, 1993.

134. Testa D et al: Comparison of natural histories of progressive supranuclear palsy and multiple system atrophy, Neurol Sci 22:247, 2001.

135. Thomas M, Jankovic J: Parkinsonism plus disorders. In Noseworthy JH, editor: Neurological therapeutics: principles and practice, vol 1, New York, 2003, Martin Dunitz.

136. Tompkins CA, Flowers CR: Perception of emotional intonation by brain-damaged adults: the influence of task processing levels, J Speech Hear Res 28:527, 1985.

137. Tucker DM, Watson RT, Heilman KM: Discrimination and evocation of affectively intoned speech in patients with right parietal disease, Neurology 27:947, 1977.

138. Valenstein E: Nonlanguage disorders of speech reflect complex neurologic apparatus, Geriatrics 30:117, 1975.

139. Van Borsel J, Tallieu C: Neurogenic stuttering versus developmental stuttering: an observer judgment study, J Commun Disord 34:385, 2001.

140. Van Borsel J, Van Der Made S, Santens P: Thalamic stuttering: a distinct clinical entity, Brain Lang 85:185, 2003.

141. Wallesch C-W: Repetitive verbal behaviour: functional and neurological considerations, Aphasiology 4:133, 1990.

142. Weintraub S, Mesulam M-M, Kramer L: Disturbances in prosody: a right-hemisphere contribution to language, Arch Neurol 38:742, 1981.

143. Williamson JB et al: Quantitative EEG diagnostic confirmation of expressive aprosodia, Appl Neuropsychol 10:176, 2003.

144. Woo P, Kelly G, Kirshner P: Airway complications in the head injured, Laryngoscope 99:725, 1989.

145. Yairi E, Gintautas J, Avent JR: Disfluent speech associated with brain damage, Brain Lang 14:49, 1981.

146. Yankovsky AE, Treves TA: Postictal mixed transcortical aphasia, Seizure 11:278, 2002.

147. Yonick TA et al: Acoustical effects of endotracheal intubation, J Speech Hear Disord 55:427, 1990.

148. Zapor M, Murphy FT, Enzenauer R: Echolalia as a novel manifestation of systemic lupus erythematosus, South Med J 94:70, 2001.

14 Acquired Psychogenic and Related Nonorganic Speech Disorders

> *"It is a real disease but a mental disease."*
>
> *(William James,[32] in reference to hysteria)*
>
> *"Psychological issues may cause, maintain, or be a result of communication disorders."*[40]
>
> G. Mahr

CHAPTER OUTLINE

I. Etiologies
   A. Depression
   B. Schizophrenia
   C. Conversion disorder
   D. Somatization disorder
   E. Stress and stress reactions
   F. Volitional disorders

II. Speech pathology
   A. Distribution of psychogenic and related nonorganic speech disorders in clinical practice
   B. Examination
   C. Speech characteristics associated with specific psychiatric conditions
   D. Psychogenic voice disorders
   E. Psychogenic stuttering-like dysfluency of adult onset (psychogenic stuttering)
   F. Other manifestations of psychogenic and related nonorganic speech disorders
   G. Psychogenic mutism

III. Cases

IV. Summary

Speech is a mirror of personality and emotional state in healthy and ill people. It is particularly sensitive to intrinsic psychologic abnormalities and to the catastrophic, tragic, or even routine physical and emotional traumas that can attach themselves to our lives. The alterations or abnormalities of speech that result from these psychologic states or events may be difficult to distinguish from neurologically based speech disorders.* They are the focus of this chapter.

The following definition, adapted from Aronson's[4] description of psychogenic voice disorders, helps to establish the boundaries of the psychogenic disturbances that are discussed here: *Acquired psychogenic speech disorders represent a wide variety of speech disturbances that result from one or more types of psychologic dysequilibrium, such as anxiety, depression, conversion reaction,*

---

*The evaluation of medically unexplained symptoms is a problem for medicine in general. For example, unexplained physical symptoms in people without relevant organic physical pathology but with relevant psychosocial distress account for approximately 45% of visits to general medical clinics,[68] and approximately 11% of patients seen in certain neurology outpatient clinics have symptoms that are not explained by organic disease.[14] Such problems account for a significant percentage of health care costs, and they can create disability whether or not physical disease is present.[14,34] The fact that our health care system responds more effectively to physical than emotional complaints compounds the problem, because diagnosis often proceeds by first ruling out organic causes rather than concurrently addressing possible psychologic and social causes.[68]

or personality disorders that interfere with volitional control over any component of speech production.

It is noteworthy that not all of the disorders discussed are unambiguously tied to psychiatric disturbance. For this reason, terms such as *functional* and *nonorganic* are often preferred over the designation *psychogenic*. Sometimes when speech is not normal—is in a state of dysequilibrium—there is neither a clear organic/neurologic nor a clear psychiatric explanation for it. For example, in some cases abnormal speech represents a reaction to stress or anxiety but is not obviously linked to any chronic psychiatric disorder (e.g., depression, schizophrenia, somatization disorder). In others, the problem may reflect an intention to deceive (malingering). In still others, it reflects a problem of inertia in which organically based abnormal speech persists after the organic condition has resolved, sometimes for psychologic reasons but sometimes for unexplained reasons or reasons tied to faulty compensation or related "learning" mechanisms. Under these latter circumstances, the label "psychogenic" somehow seems inappropriate. These examples illustrate why the designation *related nonorganic speech disorders* is included in this chapter's title. When appropriate, for the sake of conciseness, the designation *psychogenic/nonorganic speech disorders* is used to refer to psychogenic and related nonorganic speech disorders.

Psychogenic/nonorganic speech disorders are not unusual within a large multidisciplinary medical practice. They accounted for 4.2% of all acquired communication disorders seen in the Mayo Clinic speech pathology practice from 1987-1990 and 1993-2001 (see Figure 1-1). Of relevance to this chapter, many of these patients were referred for speech evaluation as part of a medical workup to determine the cause of their symptoms. Neurologic disease was an etiologic consideration in many cases.

This chapter addresses psychologically based and related nonorganic speech problems that can be difficult to distinguish from those that directly result from neurologic disease. In this context, a few general principles are worth remembering. They include the following:

1. Neurologic and psychogenic/nonorganic disorders can occur simultaneously.*
2. People with neurologic disease can have speech disorders that are psychologic/nonorganic in origin.
3. People with psychologic/nonorganic disorders can have speech disorders that are neurologic in origin.

---

*Anything that disrupts normal brain functions has the potential to cause emotional or cognitive symptoms.[68]

4. It is sometimes difficult to distinguish neurogenic from psychogenic/nonorganic speech disturbances.
5. Psychogenic/nonorganic speech disorders can affect any component of speech.

◼ ETIOLOGIES

Some of the most common etiologies of psychogenic/nonorganic speech disorders are discussed in this section. In general, depression, manic-depression, and schizophrenia lead to logically predictable speech disturbances; in fact, the character of speech may help to define the psychopathology. In contrast, conversion disorders, somatization disorders, responses to life stress, and factitious disorders and malingering have much more unpredictable effects on speech and are a greater challenge to the diagnostic and management efforts of speech pathologists.

Depression

Depression is an affective disorder of mood. Primary or major depression can exist without any nonaffective psychiatric disorder or any serious organic disorder, whereas secondary or minor depression is associated with preexisting organic or psychiatric illness. The lifetime prevalence in the general population for major depression may be as high as 9% in women and 4% in men.[31] It can occur throughout the adult years. There is a presumed precipitating event (e.g., emotional loss, chronic stress) in approximately 25% of cases.[67] Depression frequently presents with physical symptoms.[68]

Depression is accompanied by mania in some people, a condition known as *manic-depression*. Mania is a near-emotional mirror image of depression, with characteristic symptoms including excited mood, euphoria, low frustration tolerance, elevated self-esteem, poor judgment, disorganization, paranoia, little need for sleep, and high energy.[67]

Depressed mood, characterized by sadness and feeling low, hopeless, and gloomy, is the most common characteristic of depression. It, or loss of interest or pleasure, must be present for a diagnosis of major depression, according to the *Diagnostic and Statistical Manual of Mental Disorders (DSM-IV)* of the American Psychiatric Association.*[1] Other symp-

---

*The *DSM-IV*[1] contains criteria for the diagnosis of many categories of mental disorders that are organized under 16 major diagnostic classes (e.g., delirium, dementia, and amnestic and other cognitive disorders; mood disorders; somatoform disorders). It is currently the standard language of communication for mental health professionals in the United States and is widely used in clinical practice, research, and training programs.

toms can include increased or decreased appetite; insomnia or hypersomnia; loss of energy; feelings of worthlessness or guilt; and difficulty with thinking, memory, concentration, or decision making.* Depressed people may also exhibit *psychomotor retardation,* which may be characterized by reduced speech and facial expression, fixed gaze and reduced eye scanning, stooped posture, and slow movement.

Neurologic Disease and Depression

As many as one third of patients with neurologic disease may have severe depression or anxiety.[59] Depression is one of the most common emotional sequelae after traumatic brain injury,[69] and it can occur in almost half of unselected stroke patients.[61] It tends to last longer with cortical lesions than when lesions are elsewhere, but it can be associated with basal ganglia, thalamic, and limbic system lesions.[59,61] It more often occurs with lesions of the left than right hemisphere, and significant depression is more likely with left frontal or basal ganglia lesions.[48-50,61] This has obvious implications for patients with aphasia and apraxia of speech (AOS); in fact, depression is more common in nonfluent aphasic patients than in those with global or fluent aphasia.[47] Depression in aphasic people is not necessarily just a reaction to the aphasia; depression and aphasia can be separate, coexisting outcomes of brain injury. Poststroke depression can be effectively treated with tricyclic antidepressants.[61]

Depression can occur in numerous other neurologic diseases and is common in Parkinson's disease, epilepsy, Alzheimer's disease, multiple sclerosis (MS), and Huntington's disease. There is a 40% to 50% risk of depression in Parkinson's disease, and depression may precede the onset of motor deficits, suggesting that it has a neurophysiologic basis.[60] In the elderly, depression can be mistaken for progressive dementia.

Schizophrenia

Schizophrenia is the most common psychotic disorder.[67] It usually begins in adolescence or early adulthood. It has no pathognomonic features, and its exact nature is unclear. *DSM-IV* criteria for its diagnosis describe characteristic symptoms during the active phase of the illness that include delusions, hallucinations, disorganized speech, grossly disorganized or catatonic behavior, and affective flattening. Affected individuals can also exhibit social isolation or withdrawal; peculiar behavior (talking to self in public); reduced or inappropriate affect; digressive, vague, overelaborated, or metaphoric speech; and odd or bizarre thinking or perceptual experiences.

Several neurologic disorders can produce schizophrenic symptoms. Schizophrenic-like psychoses have been associated with diffuse cerebral injuries and sometimes temporal lobe lesions. A few of the specific conditions that can lead to schizophrenic behavior include closed head injury (CHI), encephalitis, temporal lobe epilepsy, Huntington's chorea, Wilson's disease, and demyelinating disease. The distinction between the psychotic features of schizophrenia and mental disorders induced by substance abuse also can be difficult.[44]

Conversion Disorder

Conversion disorder is a subtype *of somatoform disorders* that involves *physical symptoms without demonstrable organic causes and for which there is at least strong circumstantial evidence of a link between the symptoms and psychologic factors or conflicts.*[72] In conversion disorder there is an actual loss or alteration of volitional muscle control or sensation that represents an unconscious simulation of illness. It appears that the conversion symptom, or the conversion reaction, enables the patient to prevent conscious awareness of emotional conflict or stress that would be intolerable if faced directly. In some cases the symptom has a symbolic relationship to the underlying event or conflict. For example, a person may become aphonic because of conflict over verbally expressing anger at someone who has hurt him or her emotionally. Symptom "choice" can also relate to the person's experience with or conception of illness.[73] In addition to the primary gain of displacing or avoiding mental conflict, conversion reactions can be associated with secondary gain such as sympathy or necessitating a leave of absence from a hated job. Patients are generally unaware of these gains or the relationship of them to their physical symptoms, and they tend to resist psychologic explanations.[59]

Conversion disorder is sometimes called "hysteria" or "hysterical neurosis, conversion type," although hysteria refers to a personality type rather than a conversion response. Immaturity and egocentricity, sometimes characterized by flirtatious, hostile, manipulative, dramatic, and emotionally

---

*Somatoform complaints, such as headache, backache, abdominal pain, fatigue, and weakness are more common presenting symptoms of depression than are low mood and multiple vegetative symptoms.[68]

labile behavior, characterize the hysterical personality. A tendency to develop subjective physical complaints may be present in people with hysterical personalities, but they do not necessarily develop conversion reactions; conversion reactions can occur in any personality type.[4,12]

Characteristics of Affected Individuals

Conversion disorder can occur in people with average or better than average psychologic stability who find themselves in unusually stressful situations. Schizophrenia, various personality disorders (e.g., dependent, histrionic, antisocial, passive-aggressive), and depression in particular are frequently present, however.[10,21,37,51] It is not uncommonly associated with drug abuse and alcoholism, and a history of disturbed sexuality, including sexual abuse and incest, may be present.[26,37] There is a tendency toward lower intelligence or socioeconomic status.[10,26,51] A predisposition within families and various ethnic and social groups suggests a role for hereditary or social and cultural mechanisms.[26,37,51]

Conversion disorders are common in a general hospital population, and 20% to 25% of patients admitted to a general hospital may have had a conversion reaction at one time in their lives.[25,37] Most agree that conversion responses are diagnosed more often in women, although they are frequent in men in combat situations and seem to have been higher in U.S. soldiers in the Vietnam War than in other wars.[12]

Course

Conversion symptoms tend to be abrupt in onset and sometimes remit rapidly. They often emerge on the heels of acute stress or trauma, but they can follow the "true" cause by a prolonged time, suggesting that there may be a latent period until a suitable "face-saving event" occurs that permits the conversion to occur. The history may raise suspicions about previous conversion reactions, with first episodes emerging in adolescence or early adulthood. Patients are generally cooperative with examination but may be indifferent (la belle indifférence) to their symptoms, although it has been noted that indifference is an unreliable indicator of conversion reactions and that some people with a conversion disorder are concerned about their problems.[26,37]

Many conversion symptoms are transient. Persisting symptoms tend to be seen more often in tertiary care settings.[26] The best prognoses for recovery are associated with recent and abrupt onset from an identifiable precipitating event, an absence of major psychiatric or organic illness, and recognition by the patient of a link between negative life events and their physical symptoms.[10,26,37]

Relationship to Neurologic Disease

Conversion symptoms are frequently neurologic in character.[26] Symptoms may include tremor, paresthesia, paraplegia, hemiplegia, lingual weakness, torsion dystonia, seizures,[7,15,21,24,35-37] and a wide variety of speech disturbances. The high incidence of conversion symptoms in people with a history of CHI or other organic injury suggests possible biologic mechanisms for some people with conversion reactions.[51] A history of emotional conflict or personality disorder predating a known neurologic injury may be less common and relevant to diagnosis than in people without known organic neurologic disease.[10]

It is of particular interest that at least some conversion disorders have neurophysiologic correlates. For example, in a recent study of patients with unilateral sensorimotor loss attributed to conversion disorder, single photon emission computed tomography (SPECT) showed consistent hypoactivation in the thalamus and basal ganglia contralateral to the side of deficit, and resolution of the hypoactivation after the symptoms resolved.[70] These results suggest that conversion deficits can be associated with a functional disorder in striatothalamocortical circuits that control sensorimotor function and voluntary motor behavior. The authors point out that the basal ganglia, especially the caudate nucleus, are well situated to modulate motor processes based on emotional and situational cues from the limbic system. It thus appears that conversion disorders characterized by sensorimotor deficits can be associated with abnormal neurophysiology even though the sensorimotor system has not sustained structural damage.

Diagnosis of conversion disorder should not be one of exclusion; a link between symptoms and psychologic factors must be apparent for a confident diagnosis. This is particularly important, because conversion disorders are common in people with neurologic disease and often accompany depression, anxiety, or other psychologic disturbances.[43,51,59] Based on follow-up studies, 15% to 30% of patients with conversion reaction diagnoses actually have organic disease, often neurologic disease. At the same time, however, people without evidence of neurologic disease at initial workup rarely develop identifiable neurologic disease, at least within 6 months after the conversion event.[13] It may be that some neurologic diseases predispose people to conversion reactions or that neurologic disease can be sufficiently subtle, nonspecific, or unusual in its presentation to be mistaken for nonorganic disease.

Neurologic conditions frequently misdiagnosed as conversion disorders include epilepsy, MS, frontal lobe lesions, postconcussion syndrome, encephalitis, dementia, tumor, stroke, and myasthenia gravis (MG).[37,67]

Finally, a factor that complicates the distinction between conversion disorder and organic disease is *somatic compliance*. Somatic compliance is the tendency for nonorganic symptoms to develop in an organ affected by organic disease, such as psychogenic seizures in people with neurologic seizures or psychogenic aphonia in people with vocal fold weakness.[15,58,59]

Somatization Disorder

Somatization disorder is another subtype of somatoform disorder. It is a chronic illness characterized by recurrent, multiple physical complaints and a belief that one is ill.[72] People with the disorder tend to have numerous, dramatic complaints involving multiple organs. They usually insist on and receive multiple tests and treatment and generally fail to be reassured when told there is no evidence of organic disease. They are at risk for drug dependence and complications from unnecessary medications and invasive procedures.

The disorder usually develops before the age of 30 and is more common in women of lower intelligence and socioeconomic status who have interpersonal problems. It tends to run in families and may be accompanied by significant sexual dysfunction and hysterical or antisocial personality traits.[44,63]

Unlike conversion disorders, somatization disorder is not frequently associated with organic illness.[67] It is also distinguished from conversion disorders by the wide variety of complaints within affected individuals and a lack of evidence that symptoms reflect subconscious repression of underlying acute conflict, stress, or anxiety. Patients are rarely indifferent to their symptoms and tend to be highly demanding and manipulative in their efforts to get help. Similar to conversion disorder, complaints may raise suspicion of neurologic disease, and patients are frequently suspected of having MS, MG, or seizures.[15,63]

Stress and Stress Reactions

Stress is a state of bodily or mental tension resulting from factors that alter equilibrium. It is a normal part of life that can invigorate our sense of well-being and accomplishment. Stress comes from many sources, such as working conditions and family and social relationships and events.

Reactions to stress are determined by the degree and chronicity of stress but also by intrinsic personality traits such as flexibility, perfectionism, compulsivity, and ambition. When tension generated by psychologic stress is not appropriately released, it may build to a point where abnormal functioning develops. This can occur in people with or without serious psychiatric disease.

People may be predisposed by personality or physiologic makeup to excessively react to stress through a particular neuromuscular or visceral system. An especially relevant example is the susceptibility of laryngeal muscles to emotional stress, perhaps because of the voice's prominent role in conveying emotional information and its strong links to limbic system influences. Thus the larynx can be a site of neuromuscular tension arising from stress associated with fear, anger, anxiety, or depression.

Stress and other psychologic factors can play a causal role in some organic diseases. When this happens the resulting disorder is called psychosomatic. *Psychosomatic disorders* reflect the effects of psychologic and sociocultural stresses on the "predisposition, onset, course, and response to treatment of some physiological changes and biochemical disorders."[64] This notion of psychologic factors that can affect physical conditions depends on the cooccurrence of factors that include the following:

1. A biologic predisposition to a particular organic disorder
2. A personality vulnerability or a type or degree of stress that a person cannot manage
3. The presence of significant chronic psychosocial stress in the susceptible personality area[64,67]

Psychologic factors can play a role in a number of organic diseases. They include, but are not limited to, cardiovascular (coronary artery disease, hypertension), respiratory (bronchial asthma), gastrointestinal (peptic ulcer, ulcerative colitis), and musculoskeletal (tension headache, low back pain) functions. Some laryngeal pathologies, including vocal cord nodules, polyps, and contact ulcer, may also be linked to such factors.[4,53,54] It thus appears that *the relationship between stress and organic disease can be bidirectional*. Not only can organic pathologies (e.g., neurologic disease) lead to stress and other psychologic sequelae, but stress and other psychologic reactions can play a causal role in the onset and course of organic disease.

Volitional Disorders

Some nonorganic disturbances are under volitional control. They can be difficult to distinguish from neurologic disease and psychiatric disturbances that are not volitional. They can be divided into factitious disorders and malingering.

Factitious Disorders

Individuals with a factitious disorder consciously and deliberately feign physical or psychologic symptoms of disease but do so for uncontrolled, unconscious psychologic reasons that lead them to seek out the role of the patient or sick person.[62,67,72] They are generally loners with personality disorders, often with a history of abuse, trauma, or deprivation. They may report a dramatic history with complaints that may, for example, be neurologic (e.g., seizures, headache, loss of consciousness), abdominal, or dermatologic. They submit to recommended medical tests and procedures, and they are at risk for drug addiction and complications from multiple surgeries.[62,67]

The best-known factitious disorder is *Munchausen's syndrome,* named after a Russian cavalry officer who wandered from town to town telling outlandish war stories. The syndrome is characterized by pathologic lying and extensive travel among cities and hospitals, presenting with a wide variety of factitious illnesses. Factitious disorders can also occur in people whose general behavior is more socially acceptable but who feign or induce illness through, by example, injection of contaminated substances, self-induced bruises, thermometer manipulation, or urinary tract manipulation.[62]

Malingering

Malingering involves the deliberate, voluntary feigning of physical or psychologic symptoms for consciously motivated external purposes (e.g., to avoid work or combat, for financial gain, to evade prosecution). To achieve their goals, malingerers may stage events (e.g., getting hit by a slow-moving car), alter medical tests, take advantage of natural events (e.g., use an accident or injury to maximize compensation), self-inflict injury (e.g., a minor gunshot wound to avoid combat), or invent symptoms that can be neurologic in nature.

Malingering is not considered a mental disorder, but it can be difficult to distinguish it from organic disease and factitious disorders. Among the clinical markers that are useful to its detection are: examination and diagnostic test data incompatible with history and complaints; ill-defined, vague symptoms; overdramatized complaints; uncooperativeness with the workup; resistance to a favorable prognosis; history of recurrent accidents or injury; potential for financial compensation; potential to avoid legal proceedings; requests for addictive

drugs; and antisocial personality traits.[62] Because such traits can also belong to people with organic disease and mental disorders, their diagnostic usefulness is as circumstantial evidence rather than proof. The most important aspects of the workup for such patients are careful, objective assessments and documentation of examination findings and noting their degree of correspondence with known patterns of disease.

■ SPEECH PATHOLOGY

Distribution of Psychogenic and Related Nonorganic Speech Disorders in Clinical Practice

The incidence and prevalence of psychogenic/nonorganic speech disorders in the general population and in medical practice is unknown. Similarly, little is known about the distribution of specific types of psychogenic/nonorganic speech disorders, although some sense of it may be gained by examining their distribution within a speech pathology practice in a large multidisciplinary medical setting. Table 14-1 summarizes the distribution of types of speech disturbance within a group of 215 individuals with psychogenic/nonorganic speech disorders who were

table 14-1	Distribution of psychogenic/nonorganic speech disorders in 215 cases seen for speech pathology evaluation at the Mayo Clinic from 1987-1990

Diagnosis	Percent of Cases
Psychogenic Voice Disorders	80
Aphonia	30
Hoarseness	22
Spasmodic dysphonia	
Adductor	13
Abductor	1
High pitch	6
Ventricular dysphonia	4
Miscellaneous voice problems	3
Inappropriate loudness	<1
Falsetto (excluding mutational falsetto)	<1
Psychogenic/Nonorganic Fluency, Prosodic, & Other Speech Disorders	20
Stuttering	11
Articulation deficits	3
Dysprosody	3
Infantile speech	2
Mutism	<1
Psychotic language	<1

seen over a 4-year period in the Mayo Clinic speech pathology practice.

Approximately 80% of the cases had some type of voice disorder. This high proportion seems consistent with the attention paid to such deficits in the medical and speech pathology literature. Approximately 65% of the voice disorders were characterized by aphonia, hoarseness, or adductor spasmodic dysphonia; aphonia was the most frequent diagnosis in the entire group of 215 cases. Various other voice problems were also present, including high pitch, ventricular dysphonia, abductor spasmodic dysphonia, inappropriate loudness, and falsetto. Approximately 3% had voice abnormalities that did not fit into any easily described category, probably because of their atypical characteristics.

Twenty percent of the cases had problems with fluency, prosody, articulation, or some other aspect of speech that was not isolated to laryngeal function. Stuttering-like behavior represented more than half of the cases in this category. Psychogenic articulation deficits, prosodic abnormalities, and patterns of infantile speech were also encountered. A high proportion of these disorders appeared to reflect conversion disorders or responses to life stresses. Psychogenic mutism and psychotic language were rarely diagnosed, perhaps because only infrequently were such cases difficult to distinguish from neurologic disorders, or because they did not require language or speech therapy.

Examination

The assessment of speech disorders that might be psychogenic/nonorganic in origin should usually include all components of the standard motor speech examination. When a stress-induced speech disorder, conversion disorder, somatization disorder, factitious disorder, or malingering are suspected, several components of the assessment deserve special attention because of their usefulness in distinguishing organic from psychogenic etiology. These relate to the patient's history and to observations of speech during examination.

History

The conditions under which psychogenic/nonorganic speech problems first emerge often differ from those usually associated with neurologic disease. For example, there may have been an associated cold or similar nonneurologic illness shortly before, during, or after onset. The problem may have developed at the time of or shortly after a physically or psychologically traumatic event; with physical trauma, there may or may not have been any loss of consciousness

or injury to the head, face, or neck. When an organic or psychologically significant event cannot be associated with the onset of the speech problem, it is important to review the more distant history for similar evidence. The current deficit may reflect an ongoing pattern of psychologic difficulties or a delayed response to a temporally distant traumatic event. The history following onset is also important because sometimes a problem develops in anticipation of a difficult encounter or illness, such as an anticipated emotional confrontation with a boss or family member, or fear of a life-threatening disease.

When a psychologically significant event is discovered and considered causally related to the speech disorder, it is important to explore if the stress or conflict is currently active or has dissipated. When the triggering event is no longer active, the prognosis for resolution of the speech disorder is usually better than when stress and conflict, or primary or secondary gain issues, remain active.

It is also important to establish if the problem has been constant since onset or if there have been periods of remission, even if brief. Some transient problems can be neurogenic, so the conditions under which exacerbations and remissions occur are also important. Close ties between symptom fluctuation and stressful events or encounters with particular individuals should raise suspicions about psychogenic etiology. Reports of sudden, dramatic deterioration of speech immediately after brief exposure to nonregulated fumes, odors, or environments should raise similar suspicions. The possibility of secondary gain should also be considered (e.g., litigation related to the speech disturbance or its alleged cause; inability to work because of the speech problem, especially if work is described as dissatisfying or stressful).

The clinician should keep in mind that evidence of significant life stress, by itself, does not establish that a speech deficit is psychogenic. Excessive reliance on such evidence can blind one to signs of neurologic or other organic explanations, especially if the patient also believes that his or her difficulty is psychologic. In general, *patients who spontaneously express a belief that their problem is psychologic should heighten suspicions about organic etiology, whereas those who insist on an organic explanation or deny the possibility of a psychologic explanation should heighten suspicions about psychogenic etiology.* Although such suspicions may be unfounded, they help to maintain diagnostic vigilance.

Important Questions

Questions that should be addressed during the examination include the following:

1. *Can the speech disorder be classified neurologically?* Do the speech deficits fit lawful patterns associated with motor speech disorders (MSDs) or other neurogenic speech disturbances? Departures from these lawful patterns may reflect psychogenic etiology or a significant psychogenic or nonorganic contribution to the speech disorder. In people with confirmed neurologic disease, speech symptoms that are incongruent with the known localization, character, and severity of the disease should raise suspicions about psychogenic etiology.

2. *Is the oral mechanism examination consistent with the speech disorder and patterns of abnormalities found in neurologic disease?* In neurologic disease, speech and oral mechanism findings generally have a predictable relationship. Incongruities frequently are evident in psychogenic and related nonorganic disorders. For example, strength testing may reveal weakness that is grossly disproportionate to the severity of the speech deficit. A patient may exhibit *give-way weakness* or no ability to resist movement on strength testing, or his or her efforts may be accompanied by dramatic posturing of oral structures or complaints that the examination is too difficult or uncomfortable to permit compliance.

3. *Is the speech deficit consistent?* Most neurogenic and other organic speech disorders are consistent during examination. Significant fluctuations—especially from normal to grossly abnormal speech—as a function of speech task (e.g., casual conversation versus reading or repetition) or emotional content (e.g., reading versus discussion of personal relationships) are uncommon when the etiology is neurologic. In contrast, some people with psychogenic speech disorders speak much more adequately during conversation than during formal assessment tasks; others regress significantly when sensitive psychosocial issues are addressed. Some patients have grossly irregular speech alternate motion rates (AMRs) in the absence of any irregular articulatory breakdowns during contextual speech or any other evidence of ataxic or hyperkinetic dysarthria, an unusual finding in neurogenic speech disorders.

4. *Is the speech deficit suggestible?* Is there anything that the clinician can do to dramatically improve or worsen the deficit? For example, some patients dramatically worsen if it is suggested that a task is likely to be difficult.

5. *Is the speech deficit susceptible to distractibility?* Neurologic disease usually is not. Psychogenic speech disorders may improve noticeably if the clinician breaks out of the formal examination mode to speak casually with the patient, to clarify points in the history, and so on.

6. *Does speech fatigue in a lawful manner?* With the exception of the flaccid dysarthria associated with MG, MSDs do not fatigue dramatically over the course of examination, even when continuous speaking is required. Some people with psychogenic speech disorders deteriorate dramatically during speech stress testing, especially if MG is a possibility. However, the character of such "fatigue" is often inconsistent with progressive weakness and may actually reflect an increase in musculoskeletal tension. For example, instead of increasing breathiness, short phrases, and hypernasality that lawfully reflect increasing weakness, a patient may develop a strained voice quality with associated orofacial struggle and exaggerated articulation, behaviors associated with increased rather than decreased muscular contraction.

7. *Is the speech deficit reversible?* Unfortunately, motor speech and other neurologic speech disturbances do not completely remit with symptomatic speech therapy. In contrast, it is not unusual for people with psychogenic/nonorganic speech disorders—particularly those with dysphonia, aphonia, or dysfluencies reflecting a conversion disorder or response to life stresses—to respond dramatically to symptomatic treatment during the examination. Sometimes the catharsis of confronting the psychologic dynamic underlying the speech disorder during review of the history is associated with dramatic improvement or resolution of the speech problem. Symptom reversibility rules out neurologic causes for the speech deficit observed during evaluation and confirms the diagnosis as psychogenic or, at least, nonorganic.

Answers to the preceding questions are valuable to diagnostic decision making and to decisions about management and referrals to other medical subspecialists (e.g., neurology, psychiatry). In general, *when examination results are incongruent with expectations for neurogenic or other organic speech deficits, and when the history provides evidence of psychologic factors that are logically related to the disorder, the probability that the speech disorder is psychogenic or nonorganic can be considered high.*

Speech Characteristics Associated with Specific Psychiatric Conditions

Depression and Manic-Depression

The speech characteristics of depressed people often lead to a perception of depression, so there seems to be a close match between underlying mood and speech in the disorder.

Untreated depressed people often have a triad of speech characteristics that includes *reduced stress, monopitch,* and *monoloudness.*[17] Reduced loudness and monoloudness convey an impression of reduced respiratory drive and effort, and flat prosody seems to reflect overall reduced vitality.[17] Speech rate can be reduced[16] but not always.[17] The speech patterns of affected people may represent an index of depression in that both depression and speech patterns improve with antidepressant medication.[16]

It is of special interest that some aspects of the speech of depression are *hypokinetic-like* and suggestive of extrapyramidal system disturbance, an association made more interesting by the common occurrence of depression in Parkinson's disease. This highlights the fact that the speech of depression is sometimes difficult to distinguish from hypokinetic dysarthria. Relatedly, the common occurrence of stroke-related depression, especially in people with left hemisphere lesions, suggests that some prosodic abnormalities associated with nonfluent aphasia, AOS, and perhaps unilateral upper motor neuron (UUMN) dysarthria could reflect the influence of depression, as well as the primary speech or language disturbance in some patients.

In people with manic-depression there can be a dramatic change in speech during the manic phase of the illness. Speech can be *loud* and *pressured* (rapid, as if the drive to speak cannot be controlled), with *vigorous articulation,* a *lively and vital voice, frequent emphasis,* and occasional *word rhyming (clanging).* Ideas may flow freely and be incoherent.[4,67] Manic speech tends not to be confused with dysarthrias or AOS but sometimes resembles Wernicke's aphasia.

Schizophrenia

Schizophrenic speech is not usually mistaken for an MSD. Although schizophrenia does not have a single pathognomonic speech pattern, it does have variations in content and manner of expression that distinguish it from normal. Experienced psychologists and psychiatrists, for example, can distinguish schizophrenic from nonschizophrenic speakers during reading, apparently because they can perceive schizophrenic speakers' slowed rate, dependence, inefficiency, and moodiness.[66]

Schizophrenic people can have exaggerated as well as attenuated speech characteristics that reflect different phases or varieties of the illness. The active phases of the disorder can be associated with *rapidly altering melody and pitch,* with *inappropriate stress patterns* that do not have a clear relationship to ideational content.[4] Speech may contain *verbigeration,* or the stereotypic and seemingly meaningless repetition of words and sentences. Content may contain *loose associations* in which ideas have no apparent relation to one another, and *word salad* in which words have no apparent relationship to one another. In general, content may be *incoherent, illogical, digressive, vague,* or *excessively detailed.* Some patients have a tendency to *pun* and *rhyme words,* and *verbal paraphasias, neologisms,* and *perseveration* can be present. These characteristics can be accompanied by inappropriate affect such as giggling and smiling that are incongruent with verbal content.[28,44]

A number of these "active" speech characteristics are similar to the verbal behaviors associated with Wernicke's aphasia. The similarities can be so striking that the term *schizophasia* has been used to describe the language of some schizophrenic patients.[39] Distinctions between the disorders can be made, however. Comparisons between schizophrenic and aphasic speech[22,28] suggest that schizophrenic speakers (1) have fewer dysfluencies than aphasic speakers; (2) tend to reiterate themes, whereas aphasic speakers reiterate words and phrases; (3) comprehend, read, and write adequately if they attend to the task, whereas aphasic speakers do poorly; (4) make fewer semantic and phonemic errors than aphasic speakers; (5) have good naming and syntax compared with aphasic speakers; (6) tend to be irrelevant whereas aphasic responses are usually relevant; (7) show little awareness of deficits, whereas aphasic speakers (although certainly not all patients with Wernicke's aphasia) show some awareness and frustration. These contrasts are consistent with concepts of aphasia as a language disorder and schizophrenia as a thought disorder, and they are useful to differential diagnosis. In addition, the typical gradual emergence at a relatively young age without evidence of a focal neurologic lesion in schizophrenia, versus the common sudden emergence at a relatively older age with evidence of focal left hemisphere pathology in aphasia, usually helps to distinguish between the two disorders.

During the more chronic phases of schizophrenia, speech and language characteristics may be "negative" or attenuated, with a general decrease in expressiveness and responsiveness. Patients' speech may be *monotonous, weak, flat, colorless,* and *gloomy.*[4] Some patients exhibit *poverty of speech, mutism, increased response latency, reduced ges-*

tures and spontaneous movement, and *poor eye contact.*[44] Such characteristics could be confused with hypokinetic dysarthria or frontal lobe–limbic system cognitive and affective deficits. Again, dissimilarities in onset, course, and neurologic findings between schizophrenia and these other disorders help clarify the diagnosis in most cases.

Psychogenic Voice Disorders

Voice abnormalities probably represent the largest proportion of symptoms of psychogenic/nonorganic speech disturbances. As suggested earlier, this predominance probably reflects the voice's prominent role in the expression of emotion, the links between laryngeal control mechanisms and the limbic system, and the voice's subsequent susceptibility to the effects of stress.

It also seems that some people are *laryngoresponders,*[4] predisposed by personality or physiologic makeup to react through hypercontraction of the laryngeal muscles to minor organic changes in the laryngeal area or to emotional stresses such as fear, anxiety, anger, frustration, and depression.[4,53] Emotional triggers such as acute or chronic stress, family or work discord, poor sex identification, anger, and neurotic life adjustment are common in people with psychogenic voice disorders,[2,5] and people with functional voice disorders without structural laryngeal pathology tend to be introverted or behaviorally inhibited, tense, anxious, and depressed.[54]

In some cases vocal hyperfunction can lead to organic laryngeal pathology such as nodules, polyps, and contact ulcers. Such structural pathologies are not discussed here, however, because they should not be confused with neurologic disease. Of greater interest are voice disturbances that are not associated with structural laryngeal changes.* Such disorders often lead patients on a pilgrimage for diagnosis and treatment, frequently with misdirected efforts to establish an organic explanation. These voice problems include dysphonias associated with excessive musculoskeletal tension in response to life stress, conversion aphonia or dysphonia, some spasmodic dysphonias, iatrogenic and inertial voice disorders, and voice disorders that may develop as secondary responses to other psychogenic symptoms.

---

*See Roy and Bless[53] and Roy, Bless, and Heisey[54] for an excellent theoretical and practical clinical discussion, with supporting data, of personality traits and psychologic factors that contribute to several types of voice disorder. Their explanatory model for functional dysphonias that are not associated with structural pathology is probably also relevant to other psychogenic speech disorders, particularly psychogenic stuttering.

Musculoskeletal Tension Disorders

Prolonged hypercontraction of laryngeal muscles in response to psychologic stress is often associated with elevation of the larynx and hyoid bone and with pain and discomfort in response to digital palpation in the area because of muscular soreness.* Hoarseness, strained-breathiness, alterations in pitch, and *aphonia* may result despite an absence of laryngeal lesions. Such difficulties can develop without serious psychopathology in people under considerable psychologic stress, particularly those who also must talk under demanding or stressful situations. These dysphonias usually are not mistaken for neurologic disease, and patients are often most concerned about structural laryngeal pathology. Ruling out structural pathology[†] and identifying the presence of musculoskeletal tension and the underlying sources of psychologic stress usually lead to accurate diagnosis and recommendations for management.

Conversion Aphonia

Aphonia is listed in many psychiatric texts as a common conversion symptom. Conversion aphonia can occur in the absence of laryngeal pathology; is usually linked to stress, anxiety, depression, or conflict; and serves as a vehicle for avoiding underlying psychologic conflict. It may also have symbolic significance, such as reflecting an inability to confront verbally a person who has hurt the patient in some way.[4]

Patients with conversion aphonia whisper involuntarily. The whisper may be *pure, harsh,* or *sharp,* sometimes with *high-pitched squeaky* traces of phonation and sometimes with *traces of normal phonation.* The sharpness of the whisper and its strained and high-pitch components are different from the weak, breathy, and hoarse quality associ-

---

*Clear descriptions of the examination of laryngeal musculoskeletal tension and methods for relieving such tension during diagnostic assessment and management of psychogenic voice disorders can be found in Aronson[4] and Roy, Ford, and Bless.[55]

†Although videostroboscopy is invaluable in the identification and understanding of numerous organic laryngeal disorders, some data suggest it may not be a reliable or useful index of nonorganic or functional voice disorders (Schneider, Wendler, and Scidner, 2002). This illustrates the importance of more fundamental skills for the clinical diagnosis of nonorganic (and organic) speech disorders. It is understandable that many clinicians are seduced by the sophistication; "objectivity"; frequent usefulness; and, often, reimbursability of instrumental assessments, but unfortunate when it dulls the human interactive skills and ability to synthesize information from various sources to arrive at meaningful diagnoses and recommendations for management.

ated with vocal fold weakness or paralysis. *The cough is usually sharp,* another clue to the capacity for vocal fold adduction. Excessive musculoskeletal tension can be detected as a narrowing of the thyrohyoid space during digital examination, as well as patients' frequent pain or discomfort response during that examination.

The onset of the aphonia is often sudden and associated with a cold or flu in which the aphonia persists after the physical illness subsides. Patients may complain of pain in the neck, throat, or chest. The history often reveals acute or chronic emotional stress and evidence of primary or secondary gain from the symptom. A history of previous episodes of voice loss or other possible conversion symptoms may be present. Some patients are indifferent to the aphonia and unimpressed by the rapid return of their voice with symptomatic treatment. Others are concerned and then pleased when the voice returns with symptomatic treatment. Still others may not focus much on their improved voice when it returns, because they are focused on their discovery during discussion with the clinician of the underlying psychologic reason for their conversion reaction.

Conversion aphonia is commonly investigated as a manifestation of neurologic disease. MG and MS are among the most common neurologic diseases being investigated in people referred to speech pathologists for assessment of conversion aphonia.

Conversion Dysphonia

Conversion disorder can also manifest as dysphonia characterized by hoarseness with or without a strained component, high-pitched falsetto pitch breaks, breathiness, intermittent whispering, and a wide variety of other abnormal voice characteristics. People with conversion dysphonia are not fundamentally different from those with conversion aphonia or muteness in history, personality, or clinical criteria for conversion disorder diagnosis.[5] Aronson[4] also notes that among such patients, "few have incapacitating psychiatric disturbances. In many ways, they have adjusted to their anxiety and depression."

Psychogenic Spasmodic Dysphonia

Neurogenic spasmodic dysphonia and general demographic characteristics associated with all forms of spasmodic dysphonia were discussed in Chapter 8. Despite the growing tendency for higher proportions of spasmodic dysphonias to be diagnosed as neurogenic, some are clearly psychogenic in origin,[56] sometimes reflecting conversion disorder or a more general response to life stresses.

The diagnosis of psychogenic spasmodic dysphonia can be difficult to make, although symptom reversibility in some patients confirms the diagnosis as psychogenic. The common emergence of tremor and dystonia as the basis for spasmodic dysphonia in some patients with histories of prominent acute or chronic psychologic stress raises questions about spasmodic dysphonia as a psychosomatic disorder in some patients with neurogenic or idiopathic spasmodic dysphonia.

Psychogenic spasmodic dysphonia can be adductor or abductor in form. The adductor form is characterized by a continuous or intermittent strained, jerky, grunting, squeezed, groaning, and effortful quality. The abductor form has continuous or intermittent breathy or aphonic segments. Their vocal characteristics can be highly similar to those of neurogenic dysphonia, although underlying voice tremor or evidence of laryngeal dystonia should not be encountered in psychogenic etiologies unless a combination of causes is present. Careful history and examination can help identify probable etiology, although it is not unusual for etiology to remain uncertain. It should be noted that the prolonged persistence of spasmodic dysphonia (e.g., more than a year) is expected when etiology is neurogenic but is less common when conversion response or reaction to life stresses are responsible, especially when the psychogenic triggers have ceased to exist or vary in their presence or intensity. The history and personality traits associated with psychogenic spasmodic dysphonia can be quite similar to those of patients with psychogenic aphonia, dysphonia, and muteness.

Iatrogenic Voice Disorders

An iatrogenic disorder is one *induced by the actions of the clinician* and is dependent on suggestibility and other psychologic characteristics of affected patients. For example, carotid endarterectomy carries some risk for vocal fold paralysis, and patients are typically informed of this risk when they must decide whether to consent to surgery; a suggestible patient may develop a postoperative psychogenic dysphonia in response to the "suggestion" that it might occur. On a deeper psychologic level, a psychogenic voice disorder may represent unconscious hostility toward the surgeon following laryngeal surgery.[4] Finally, patients who are placed on voice rest—often unnecessarily or inappropriately as a treatment for vocal abuse, musculoskeletal tension dysphonia, or other psychogenic/nonorganic dysphonias—may develop a fear of speaking, with subsequent dysphonia or aphonia because of the suggestion that to speak would be harmful.

Inertial Aphonia or Dysphonia

Patients with voice disorders of neurogenic origin, secondary to laryngeal pathology, or in response to psychologic factors or a recommendation for voice rest, sometimes develop an *inertial aphonia or dysphonia.** In these cases, patients "seem to lose their sense or feel for volitional phonation . . . some sort of loss of recall, memory, or even praxis for normal voice production."[4] Such inertial factors might explain the persistence of aphonia in some head-injured patients.[57] *They might also explain the persistence of conversion or nonconversion psychogenic voice disorders after the triggering psychologic events have resolved.*

Dysphonias as Secondary Responses to Other Psychogenic Symptoms

Physical manifestations of psychologic difficulties, particularly those that involve the airway, can have indirect effects on the voice. For example, chronic coughing or throat clearing linked to psychologic factors can result in dysphonia secondary to vocal fold trauma.

A problem—in some cases a very important problem—that can contribute to or exacerbate psychogenic/nonorganic voice disorders is *hypervigilance* or *spectatoring,* in which a normally automatic function becomes abnormal because of the intrusion of conscious attention.[40] Hypervigilance can result in excessive attention to normal somatic stimuli in which, for example, a fleeting sensation of muscle tightness or irritation is magnified in meaning, because the person has become a "spectator" of a function that does not and should not require vigilant attention. If this abnormal attention persists, it can interfere with normal automatic control or lead to maladaptive movements to avoid the abnormal sensation. This phenomenon is probably also active in some people with psychogenic speech disorders other than dysphonias, especially perhaps in those with psychogenic stuttering. The notion of hypervigilance/spectatoring can be useful during therapy by helping some patients understand that the ultimate goal is to pay less attention to speech and work less in order to improve (see Chapter 20, which addresses management of psychogenic/nonorganic speech disorders).

Dysphonia can also develop in association with *paradoxical vocal fold motion* (also known as *vocal cord dysfunction, functional stridor, paroxysmal vocal cord movement/motion, paroxysmal vocal cord dysfunction, or episodic paroxysmal laryngospasm*). The disorder is typically characterized by paradoxical adduction of the vocal folds during inspiration with subsequent inhalatory stridor, high-pitched wheezing, cough, shortness of breath, and chest tightness. It is often mistaken for asthma and frequently occurs simultaneously with asthma. Affected individuals tend to be females in their teens to 30s. The problem is most often assumed to be nonorganic, but emotional conflict or psychiatric disturbances often are not uncovered.[42] Upper airway hypersensitivity is implicated in some cases.[3,42] Most relevant in the context of this book, neurologic causes,* such as laryngeal dystonia, can sometimes be the culprit.[42]

Psychogenic Stuttering-Like Dysfluency of Adult Onset (Psychogenic Stuttering)

That stuttering can emerge in adulthood as a manifestation of psychologic difficulties has been recognized for many years. In 1922, for example, Henry Head[30] observed that stuttering was one of the possible manifestations of hysteria. Only in recent years has the disorder received much attention in the speech pathology literature, however.†

Acquired neurogenic stuttering was discussed in Chapter 13. The reservations expressed there about using the term *stuttering* to refer to adult-acquired dysfluencies hold here. The term is also retained here to maintain consistency with much of the literature and to highlight the difficulties that can arise when attempting to establish etiology of acquired stuttering as neurogenic or psychogenic. The designation *psychogenic stuttering (PS)* is used to refer to stuttering-like behavior that emerges in adulthood and is psychogenic in origin.

PS is not nearly as common as are psychogenic voice disorders, but it is almost certainly more frequently mistaken as a sign of central nervous system (CNS) disease than are psychogenic voice disorders. Although uncommon, a number of PS cases have been reported. Most illustrate the need to establish

---

*The influence of somatic compliance may be important in such cases. For example, Hartman, Daily, and Morin[29] discussed a case with a psychogenic voice disorder that cooccurred or evolved along with signs of a unilateral superior laryngeal nerve paresis in which the psychogenic component reflected either a conversion reaction or a musculoskeletal tension disorder. Voice therapy relieved the nonorganic component of the problem.

*For example, wheezing and stridor have also been reported in a person with a posterior fossa subarachnoid cyst that presumably caused the symptoms by compressing the brainstem. The symptoms resolved following surgical treatment.[45]

†Readers with a specific interest in psychogenic stuttering should read Baumgartner's[8] comprehensive overview of the concept, clinical characteristics, evaluation, differential diagnosis, and management of the disorder.

etiology as neurogenic or psychogenic because many have occurred in the presence of confirmed CNS disease or symptoms that raised the possibility of CNS disease.

Baumgartner and Duffy[9] summarized the characteristics of 49 people with PS in the absence of neurologic disease and 20 people with PS in the presence of neurologic disease. Because their series is the largest reported to date, their findings serve as the primary vehicle for summarizing the features of PS. Relevant demographic characteristics of the two groups are summarized in Table 14-2. There were no substantial differences between the two groups in education or age at onset. Approximately as many men as women were affected, a noticeable difference from the predominance of women in those with psychogenic aphonia. Educational level approximated the national average. Age at onset was younger than the average age of onset for many neurologic disorders of adult onset. Approximately half of the patients had their speech problem for more than 3

months at the time of evaluation, and more than 25% had been affected for more than 1 year. Thus PS can be more than a transient problem.

For those who had formal psychiatric assessment, the most common diagnosis was conversion disorder, followed by depression, anxiety neurosis, and hysterical neurosis. Some patients had personality or adjustment disorders, and some were dealing with drug dependence or posttraumatic difficulties. There were no clear differences in the distribution of psychiatric diagnoses between those with or without neurologic disease. These diagnoses, plus combat neurosis, are consistent with those reported in the literature.[11,18,23,41,52,71]

The specific chronic or acute life stresses that emerge in the histories of patients with PS include: marital discord or divorce; coping with family tragedies, illnesses, or deaths; inability to manage work responsibilities; anger and loss of self-esteem from unemployment; physical disability; accumulation of psychologically traumatic childhood experi-

table 14-2	Characteristics of individuals with psychogenic stuttering with or without evidence of neurologic disease	
	Without Neurologic Disease (n = 49)	**With Neurologic Disease (n = 20)**
Male : female	26:23	9:11
Education (M & SD in years)*	12.6 (3.7)	12.6 (2.7)
Age at onset		
M	46.3	45.2
SD	13.7	13.0
Range	19-79	26-67
Duration of disorder at time of assessment*		
1-90 days	50%	53%
91-365 days	24%	16%
> 1 year	26%	32%
Psychiatric diagnoses[†]	Conversion reaction (40%)	Conversion reaction (60%)
	Depression or reactive depression (35%)	Hysterical neurosis (60%)
	Anxiety neurosis (25%)	Depression (40%)
	Personality disorder (15%)	Personality disorder (20%)
	Posttraumatic neurosis (5%)	
	Adjustment disorder (5%)	
	Drug dependence (5%)	
	Unspecified (5%)	
Response to sx therapy[‡]		
Normal	48%	45%
Near-normal	29%	18%
Some improvement	19%	18%
No change	5%	18%

Modified from Baumgartner J, Duffy JR: Psychogenic stuttering in adults with and without neurologic disease, *J Med Speech-Lang Pathol* 5:75, 1997.
M, Mean; *SD*, standard deviation.
*Data not recorded for all patients.
[†]Only 20 patients in the group without neurologic disease and 5 patients in the group with neurologic disease had psychiatric evaluations. Some patients received more than one psychiatric diagnosis.
[‡]Therapy provided in one or two sessions, often including initial diagnostic encounter. Results of treatment are based on responses of the 43% of patients without neurologic disease and the 55% of patients with neurologic diseases who were treated.

ences; dissatisfaction with work but conflict over change; unjust accusations of wrongdoing; religious differences with offspring; and emotional responses to an accident.[6,23,52]

Roth, Aronson, and Davis[52] reported that their patients with PS were similar to those with psychogenic mutism, aphonia, or dysphonia. They tended to be emotionally immature and neurotic, and some had a history of multiple conversion symptoms. A common theme was struggle over expressing anger, fear, or remorse in conventional ways or a breakdown in communication with an important person. The authors observed that voice problems are rarely switched for stuttering and that stuttering, unlike voice problems, rarely develops in the aftermath of an upper respiratory infection. They also noted that both PS and psychogenic voice disorders tend to be highly responsive to symptomatic therapy and disclosure of conflict.

More than 80% of Baumgartner's and Duffy's cases without neurologic disease had nonspeech complaints of a possible neurologic nature, including weakness or incoordination, fatigue, sensory difficulties, seizures, and cognitive difficulties, but none had neurologic disease confirmed. Those with identifiable neurologic disease most often had degenerative disease, convulsive disorder, traumatic brain injury, or stroke.* Lesion sites included the right and left cerebral hemispheres and the brainstem and cerebellum. Approximately three quarters of the patients with neurologic disease had no associated dysarthria, AOS, or aphasia. Twenty percent had a dysarthria, and a few had equivocal evidence of aphasia (10%) or AOS (5%).

More than 60% of the patients in both of Baumgartner and Duffy's groups who received symptomatic therapy improved to normal or near-normal within one or two sessions, change dramatic and lasting enough to rule out neurologic etiology.† This observation highlights the diagnostic value of attempts to modify dysfluencies (and other speech disturbances) within the diagnostic setting when psychogenic etiology is suspected.

Box 14-1 summarizes the characteristics of dysfluencies and other speech-related behaviors that

---

*Several case studies help confirm that PS may be associated with neurologic disease, including epilepsy,[6,20,65] stroke,[11] and anoxic encephalopathy.[65] Others conclude that a neurologic event (e.g., migraine attack) directly caused stuttering (e.g., Perino et al.[46]), although psychogenic versus neurogenic influences on stuttering can be ambiguous.

†Some patients require a longer period of treatment to make major gains. For example, Brookshire[11] reported marked improvement after 21 therapy sessions in a patient whose probable PS developed after a stroke that produced speech and language problems and dyskinesias.

---

box 14-1

Characteristics of dysfluencies associated with psychogenic stuttering in people without evidence of neurologic disease. Percentage of cases in which characteristics were observed is given in parentheses.

Dysfluencies

Sound or syllable repetitions (80%)
Prolongations (27%)
Hesitations (27%)
Word repetitions (20%)
Blocking (18%)
Tense pauses (14%)
Phrase repetitions (8%)
Interjections (2%)

Associated Behaviors

Secondary struggle (e.g., facial grimacing) (53%)
"Bizarre" struggle (12%)
Telegraphic speech (10%)
Slow rate (10%)
Fast rate (4%)

Factors Influencing Dysfluencies

Unvarying (33%)
Situationally specific (28%)
Conversation more fluent than reading (13%)
No adaptation effect (10%)
Adaptation effect (5%)
Intermittent/unpredictably present (3%)
Fluctuation by time of day (3%)
Reading more fluent than conversation (2%)

Based on data from Baumgartner J, Duffy JR: Psychogenic stuttering in adults with and without neurologic disease, *J Med Speech-Lang Pathol* 5:75, 1997.

---

were present in Baumgartner's and Duffy's[9] cases. They are representative of those described in the literature. The dysfluencies themselves are similar to those described for developmental stuttering, with *sound and syllable repetitions* occurring most frequently. *Struggle behavior* in the form of facial grimacing or bizarre face, neck, or limb shaking or tremulous movements were common. *Rate abnormalities* during periods of fluency were present in some patients. In addition, 10% of the cases had *telegraphic syntax/grammar* that superficially resembled that encountered in nonfluent or Broca's aphasia, a characteristic that could fuel suspicions of neurologic etiology; in most instances, however, such telegraphic expressions had an infantile structure and prosody that should not be mistaken for aphasia or AOS. It is important to keep in mind that *there is no single profile of speech characteristics that define PS;*[8] there is considerable heterogeneity among people with the disorder.

PS dysfluencies, in contrast to those of developmental stuttering, often are not reduced by choral reading, masking, delayed auditory feedback, singing, or mimed speaking.[19] Relatedly, an increase in dysfluency with simplification of the speech task is considered strongly suggestive of psychogenicity.[8] Although it has been suggested that secondary struggle behavior or concern about stuttering is often absent in people with PS,[19] Baumgartner and Duffy[9] reported some form of struggle in more than half of their patients, with many expressing distress over the problem. They also observed that variables that influenced the presence and severity of PS had highly variable effects across patients within their groups. For example, some had speech that was unvarying under any observed circumstance, including adaptation, whereas others varied according to task, environment, or time of day. In some patients, the near-absence of any variability in dysfluency was considered incompatible with neurologic etiology (see Case 14-3 at the end of this chapter), whereas in others the situational specificity or seemingly random presence or absence of dysfluencies was considered incompatible with neurologic etiology. It seems that too little is known at this time to establish a single diagnostic rule about adaptation, choral speaking, singing, responses to masking, and other circumstances. It could be that such variables have no diagnostically predictable or meaningful relationship with PS.

Other Manifestations of Psychogenic and Related Nonorganic Speech Disorders

The data in Table 14-1 suggest that most psychogenic/nonorganic speech disturbances are reflected in abnormalities of voice or fluency. Although rarely reported in the literature, they also can be manifest as disturbances in articulation, resonance, and prosody. It is also noteworthy that psychogenic speech disturbances can have multiple effects on speech, in which voice, fluency, articulation, resonance, and prosody can all be affected in the same individual.

It is not always clear why some speech disorders take these less conventional routes of expression. The existence of varieties of psychogenic speech disorders raises questions about the symbolic differences among voice abnormalities versus stuttering versus disorders of resonance, articulation, or prosody. In cases of physical trauma, somatic compliance may be important; for example, a neck injury may lead to dysphonia, whereas oral surgery may lead to an articulation problem (malingering or true

organic explanations deserve serious consideration in such cases). In other cases the symptom may reflect the affected individual's experiences or ideas about the effects of illness on speech.

Psychogenic articulation, resonance, and prosodic abnormalities most often seem to be associated with physical trauma to speech structures or with conversion or somatization disorders, rather than a "simple" response to life stress. In some cases malingering may be suspected, especially if litigation is pending.

Articulation Disorders

Acquired articulation disturbances can have a psychogenic basis. Most psychogenic articulation difficulties need to be distinguished from oral structure abnormalities or flaccid or hyperkinetic dysarthria.

The speech problems may develop following traumatic injury to oral structures, such as occurs during oral surgery. In this case they can be accompanied by oral sensory complaints. When they represent a conversion disorder, the articulation problem is not usually subtle. The errors can be quite consistent and isolated to specific sounds, often the most frequent persistent developmental articulation errors or those portrayed negatively in the media (/r/, /l/, /s/). Sometimes the errors are bizarre and associated with unusual tongue posturing, such as speaking with the tongue consistently elevated and retracted. The consistency of errors can suggest lingual weakness and raise suspicions about flaccid dysarthria, but when the deficit is dramatic and limited to only a few sounds, and especially when there are no associated chewing, swallowing, or saliva control difficulties, true weakness can be ruled out. When abnormal posturing of articulators is responsible for the articulation problem, a movement disorder (hyperkinetic dysarthria) must be considered. When problems are subtle, differential diagnosis can be difficult.*

Resonance Disorders

Although rare, acquired hypernasality can be psychogenic in origin. Psychogenic hypernasality can be a symptom of conversion reaction or may reflect the effects of speech lacking in vigor as the result of poor self-image.[4] Oral or sinus surgery seems to serve as a trigger for a conversion reaction in some cases.

---

*The challenges presented by such cases are illustrated by the "atypical dysarthria" reported in a person ultimately diagnosed with Munchausen's syndrome, in whom MS was initially suspected partly because of a nonorganic speech pattern that contained pervasive glottal stop substitutions.[33]

Malingering must be considered if litigation is involved.

Psychogenic hypernasality can be difficult to distinguish from oral or nasal structural defects and flaccid dysarthria. Psychogenic hyponasality is rare but should be given consideration in cases without evidence of nasal obstruction.*

Prosodic Disturbances

Prosody may be disturbed on a psychogenic basis in ways that are quite different from the prosodic attenuations or exaggerations that are associated with depression, mania, and schizophrenia and in ways that are not simply secondary to psychogenic voice or stuttering disorders. Abnormal resonance and articulation may accompany the prosodic abnormalities. In most instances they are associated with conversion or somatization disorders; in some cases malingering is suspected. The abnormal prosody can be highly variable. It may have a *deaflike quality* or convey the impression of accent, not dissimilar to the *pseudoforeign accent* that may be associated with neurologic disease. These disturbances of prosody are often associated with suspicions about neurologic rather than peripheral structural disease.

Infantile Speech

Speech sometimes regresses to an infantile pattern. The perception of infantile speech is created by a

---

*An unusual problem, known as *patulous eustachian tube*, can lead to hyponasality that is misinterpreted as psychogenic in origin. This syndrome is characterized by a roaring sound and sense of fullness in the ears; hyponasality; depression, anxiety, and preoccupation with the problem; and disappearance of the problem when lying down. The cause of the symptoms is patency of the eustachian tube because of loss of tissue mass around its orifice or a change in velopharyngeal muscle tone. Causes include significant weight or tissue fluid loss, nasopharyngeal radiation, and estrogen hormones. The reason for hyponasality is probably protective; palatal closure prevents voice and other airway noise from reaching the open eustachian tube and producing excessive loudness. The symptom disappears when reclining because of venous engorgement of the area around the opening of the tube, helping to close it off.[4]

---

combination of prosodic, voice, resonance, and articulatory alterations that usually include an *increase in pitch, exaggerated inflectional patterns,* and *production of common developmental articulation errors* (e.g., lisping, w/r or w/l substitutions). These are usually accompanied by nonvocal affective behaviors that convey an impression of childlike behavior (e.g., demure gestures and wide-eyed, childish smiling). Infantile speech sometimes develops in adults suspected of having neurologic disease, especially when it is accompanied by other deficits in volitional motor control (e.g., walking, dressing). It seems to serve the purpose of avoiding interactions on the adult plane.[4] It can reflect a conversion disorder, hysterical personality disorder, or other psychopathology.

Psychogenic Mutism

Mutism can be psychogenic or neurogenic in origin (see Chapter 12). It can occur in schizophrenia, severe depression, and other severe psychiatric conditions. It can also be a sign of conversion disorder and can be mistaken for neurologic disease when it is. People with conversion mutism are similar to those with conversion aphonia and dysphonia in their personality traits, histories, and meeting of criteria for conversion disorder diagnosis.[5]

Patients with psychogenic mutism either make *no attempt to speak,* or they *mouth words without voice or whispering.* They usually do not have chewing, swallowing, or drooling difficulties. Their cough is normal, establishing the capacity for vocal fold adduction. They often initiate writing to communicate their thoughts and answer questions and may show no distress at their inability to speak. *They may exhibit other abnormalities in speech as they emerge from their mute state.* For example, Aronson[4] discussed a case in which telegraphic speech and stuttering-like blocking was present as the transition during symptomatic therapy was made from mutism to normal speech. Finally, it is important to remember that organic mutism following an acute neurologic insult, such as CHI, may persist on a psychogenic basis after the neurologic barriers to speech have resolved.[38]

Cases

Case 14-1

A 31-year-old woman came to the clinic with a 4-month history of voice difficulty, pharyngitis, and pain with swallowing. Examination by an internist was normal with the exception that her voice was a "barely audible whisper." Subsequent assessment of thyroid function was normal, as were all other tests during a complete physical examination. She was referred for ear, nose, and throat (ENT) and neurologic evaluations, both of which were normal. ENT examination raised suspicions about spasmodic dysphonia.

During speech evaluation the patient reported losing her voice following an upper respiratory infection. She had seen six different physicians about the problem and had been placed on antibiotics and given flu shots. She had several thyroid investigations, all failing to explain or remediate her aphonia.

Psychosocial history revealed that she had been working for a large department store for approximately a year. Three months before the onset of her voice problem, she was transferred from a personnel office to an automotive department, at which time she lost her voice for approximately a week. She was unhappy with the new job and was promised that she could eventually return to personnel. She subsequently discovered that this would not be the case but was not told so directly by her supervisor. Shortly thereafter she lost her voice again. She had been out of work since that time because of her inability to speak. She planned to go back to work when her voice returned.

The patient lived with her parents and a younger brother. She had a relationship with a man but felt he was pushing her too hard toward marriage. Her parents thought she could do better than her current boyfriend. She admitted to uncertainty about whether to continue the relationship.

Her voice was completely aphonic, but her whisper was strong. All other aspects of speech and oral mechanism examination were normal. She experienced pain with minimal digital pressure in the thyrohyoid space. Symptomatic voice therapy was undertaken. Within 40 minutes her voice returned to normal. She was able to speak without effort for the next hour, including in the presence of her mother and uncle, who had accompanied her to the clinic.

The clinician subsequently, and privately, told the patient there was no current physical restriction to her speaking normally, even if her initial aphonia might have been triggered by organic illness. The role of stress, con-flict, and other emotional factors in the maintenance of her aphonia were discussed, as was the importance of confronting issues that could be producing conflict. At this time, she admitted that she did not like her job and wanted to quit and strike out on her own. She admitted that she had never confronted her employer about being "double crossed" regarding her transfer to a more acceptable job. She declined to pursue psychiatric assessment. She was asked to write to the clinician about her voice in 1 month, and she agreed.

The clinician concluded that the patient had a "psychogenic aphonia, resolved with symptomatic therapy. The exact mechanism for her aphonia is not entirely clear, but work-related and perhaps family and personal relationship issues are probably involved."

A month later the clinician received a letter from the patient stating that her voice had remained normal. She also stated, "I took care of the important things we discussed. I went back to my place of employment to confront my boss in personnel. I was asked to stay on, but I made my final decision and said no. Now I'm looking for another job. Also, I ended a relationship that I thought was causing a lot of stress. I feel I'm more capable of handling stress now due to your interest in me. Thank you for your encouragement in dealing with my symptoms. It was a great help and opened my eyes."

Commentary. (1) Psychogenic aphonia frequently develops on the heels of an upper respiratory infection. (2) The psychosocial history can reveal significant stress, anxiety, or conflict; it is often essential to understanding the mechanism underlying the speech disorder. (3) Psychogenic aphonia often leads to multiple medical examinations and recommendations for the treatment of a presumed organic cause; this often serves to reinforce the notion that the problem is organic. (4) Symptomatic therapy, combined with discussion of psychosocial issues, often results in rapid return of normal voice. (5) Patients with psychogenic voice disorders may decline psychiatric assessment; frequently it is not essential. This patient apparently did quite well, at least in the short term, after her voice returned to normal. (6) Effective management of psychogenic voice disorders often must be multidisciplinary. Speech evaluation and management was crucial in this case, but it might not have been successful if the patient had not been reassured by other medical subspecialists about the absence of serious organic illness.

Cases 14-2

A 50-year-old woman who was a medical science writer came to the clinic with a 10-month history of fatigue and 8-month history of severe pain in her right shoulder and the fingers of her right hand; evaluation elsewhere suggested a brachial plexus neuropathy of unknown cause. Three months after onset of her initial symptoms she developed a voice problem following a flulike illness. Neurologic evaluation suggested a spasmodic dysphonia or "neurologic amyotrophy" of undetermined etiology. An immunologist suspected a viral infection and told her it would take a long time for her nerves to regenerate. One month before coming to the clinic she developed increasing shortness of breath, a tremorlike disorder of breathing, and an unsteady gait.

The internist who first saw her at the clinic noted the striking dysphonia and "tremorous loss of organized muscle activity in the muscles of breathing." There was no evidence of airway compromise. His impression was that the patient had a neurologic disorder, most likely on a degenerative or inflammatory basis. Subsequent neurologic examination identified mild weakness in her right arm and shoulder and evidence of an old right radiculopathy. There was no evidence of a peripheral neuropathy or defect in neuromuscular transmission. Magnetic resonance imaging (MRI) of the head and cervical spine and additional x-rays and laboratory studies were negative. The neurologist noted her voice difficulty and irregularities in breathing and felt that the patient had an indeterminate CNS disease. A second neurologist evaluated the patient and felt that there was evidence of laryngeal myoclonus or dystonia and maybe respiratory myoclonus, perhaps on an autoimmune basis. Multiple laboratory tests failed to reveal evidence of autoimmune disease. Botox injection for her voice problem was recommended.

Before Botox injection, the patient was seen for speech evaluation. She stated that her voice difficulty was accompanied by shortness of breath, a rushing sound in her ears, and a need to maintain conscious awareness of swallowing because her throat felt full. Her voice worsened under conditions of stress and fatigue.

During speech, and occasionally at rest, there were coarse, somewhat jerky side-to-side tremorlike movements of her head and occasional myoclonic-like jerking of her arms. Her breathing was paradoxical and jerky, and inspiratory and expiratory cycles tended to be short, especially during speech. There was considerable neck tension during speaking. She engaged in some effortful and dramatic groping when attempting to puff her cheeks. The thyrohyoid space was markedly narrowed, and she experienced considerable pain with minimal pressure in that area. Her speech was characterized by a continuous marked strained, tight, spasmodic voice quality with mildly reduced loudness. Phrase length was variable secondary to the dysphonia and abnormal breathing. She could not sustain a vowel for more than 4 seconds. Her attempts to produce speech AMRs were accompanied by significant orofacial struggle.

The clinician suspected a psychogenic component to the voice problem. Symptomatic therapy was undertaken, and the patient's voice returned to normal within approximately 15 minutes and was maintained for the next 45 minutes without noticeable effort on her part. As her voice improved, her breathing pattern normalized and her coarse head tremor/shakiness subsided. The myoclonic jerking of her arms and torso persisted but were reduced in frequency. The patient was extremely pleased with the improvement of her voice. The scheduled Botox injection was canceled.

The patient was perplexed at her dramatic improvement. When her psychosocial history was discussed, she revealed that she had been under considerable stress because of her difficult-to-manage adolescent son, who had problems with the law and drug abuse. She was urged to complete her medical workup and return in several days to evaluate her progress. Five days later, she reported that her voice had remained normal. She was also reevaluated by her neurologist, who stated, "I am left to conclude that her movement disorder(s) were not due to primary organic etiology. Her response to voice therapy is obviously very gratifying." The final neurologic diagnosis was that she had had a brachial plexus injury but no evidence of other neurologic disease. Follow-up assessment was recommended.

She returned 6 months later. She had had no recurrence in voice difficulty but still had ongoing shoulder pain. Family stresses persisted, but she, her husband, and son were in counseling. The possible causes of her spasmodic dysphonia were discussed, and the meaning of the "nonorganic" or "psychologic" origins of her problem was clarified. She was told that her problem might best be viewed as a learned response to her neck/shoulder pain and to a viral illness that was present at the time her voice difficulty began. It was suggested that her physical response to her organic illnesses became habituated and that therapy was effective, because it helped put her physical manner of speaking into a more normal mode. The possible role of psychologic stress in producing her disorder was also discussed. She was urged to contact the clinician if she had any further questions or difficulties. Nine months later she called the clinician to indicate that she maintained her normal voice in spite of an occasional sensation of tightness in her neck, often associated with stress. Her mother had died recently, so she was grieving and now responsible for her father's care. Her son continued to have difficulty. She had not developed any breathing difficulty or abnormal movements in her torso or arms.

Case 14-2—cont'd

Commentary. (1) Adductor spasmodic dysphonia can be psychogenic in origin. (2) Psychogenic voice disorders can develop in association with neurologic disease (brachial plexus injury in this case), as well as respiratory or upper airway problems. (3) Psychogenic voice disorders can be misinterpreted as neurologic in origin. The voice problem may be associated with other nonorganic disorders of movement, such as the abnormal patterns of breathing and jerkiness in the limbs noted in this patient. (4) Symptomatic therapy can lead to the rapid resolution of psychogenic voice disorders, with obvious benefits to the patient and with clear implications for diagnosis. (5) Successful treatment of psychogenic voice

disorders can put an end to treatment recommendations based on an assumption of organic illness (Botox injection was planned in this case). This eliminates the risks and expense associated with an invasive procedure, as well as reinforcement of the patient's belief that the problem is organic. (6) The exact mechanism for psychogenic voice disorders is not always apparent. In this case the patient's brachial plexus injury, the suggestion to her about the possible serious nature of her voice and breathing difficulty, and perhaps issues related to family stress may have combined to set the stage for her nonorganic movement disorders.

Case 14-3

A 38-year-old man presented to the emergency department with a 3-day history of swelling and pain on the left side of his face. He had also been "stuttering" since his discharge from a local hospital 3 months earlier, when he was first worked up for pain, headache, and right extremity tremor. The admitting resident was suspicious of primary CNS disease. Neurologic consultation identified the presence of speech abnormality, right extremity tremor, and gait difficulty but raised suspicions that at least some of his problems might be nonorganic.

Subsequent neurologic tests were negative with the exception that an electromyogram demonstrated a mild right ulnar neuropathy at the elbow. Speech and psychiatric evaluations were requested.

During speech evaluation, the patient reported some fluctuation of his stuttering since onset but no return to normal. Speech therapy at his local hospital resulted in no improvement. The oral mechanism was normal with the exception of what appeared to be give-way weakness during testing of lower face strength. His conversational speech, reading, and repetition were characterized by remarkable dysfluencies in which he repeated each phoneme of each word four to six times. Mild facial grimacing, eye closing, and neck extension accompanied repetitions. He did not adapt during repeated readings of the same material. A prolonged vowel was produced in a staccato/repetitive manner consistent with the speech repetitions. Speech AMRs were irregular and slow but followed the same pattern of his conversational dysfluencies. His conversational speech was telegraphic, often characterized by omissions of articles, pronouns, prepositions, and so on. He admitted to doing this intentionally in order to economize physical effort.

During 40 minutes of symptomatic speech therapy, he could prolong a vowel normally and initiate some simple single words without repetitions. During 1 hour of therapy the following day, the clinician could alter the patient's abnormal pattern from one of multiple sound/syllable repetitions to one of exaggerated prolongation of all syllables produced. He returned to his presenting speech pattern whenever he stopped concentrating on the new pattern of speech, however. The prolonged time it took the patient to produce any utterances precluded a review of psychosocial history; it was assumed that this would be addressed during his scheduled psychiatric consultation.

The clinician concluded that the patient had "stuttering-like behavior of adult onset, almost certainly psychogenic in origin. His repetitions do not reflect palilalia, nor are they consistent with typical manifestations of neurogenic stuttering. His repetitions are remarkably consistent; this is highly unusual, even in developmental stuttering, and would be very rare in neurogenic stuttering." The clinician reassured the patient that his problem might improve spontaneously or with therapy. The patient self-mockingly referred to the problem as being "all in my head." He appeared indifferent to the severity of his speech difficulty, the efforts made to help him improve, and the explanation given to him about the nonneurologic nature of his deficit.

Psychiatric evaluation the following day noted his bizarre speech. The psychiatrist found no evidence of prior psychiatric disease and stated, "The only finding of note is his consistency of denial of *ever* experiencing or knowing distressful emotions such as fear, anxiety, anger,

Continued

Case 14-3—cont'd

or sadness, and constantly minimizing the effects of trying to keep up with three jobs and raising three children." (The patient was divorced.) The patient admitted to chronic tiredness but denied any awareness or need to give into it or change his patterns. His affect was described as inappropriately indifferent. The psychiatrist felt that the findings supported a diagnosis of conversion disorder. Psychotherapy was not recommended because the patient had so little awareness of his emotions. Continued speech and physical therapy were suggested. The patient chose to return home to pursue those treatments. He was not heard from again.

Commentary. (1) Stuttering-like dysfluencies can develop in adulthood. They can be psychogenic in origin but often present in a context suggestive of neurologic disease. (2) The nature of the patient's dysfluencies and their remarkable consistency seemed incompatible with dysfluencies encountered in neurogenic stuttering. Although symptomatic therapy did not improve speech, it did alter it. These observations led to a conclusion that the stuttering was psychogenic. (3) Psychogenic speech disorders often develop at about the same time as other physical deficits that seem to represent organic disease. (4) The diagnosis of conversion disorder, in the absence of rapid resolution of symptoms, is often based on circumstantial evidence. Multidisciplinary evaluations can increase confidence in the diagnosis, however.

Case 14-4

A 44-year-old man came to the clinic with a 15-month history of tremor in his arms and hands, severe headaches, and speech difficulty, problems for which his local physicians were unable to establish a cause.

He had developed sudden onset of numbness and weakness on the left side of his body 15 months previously. This was accompanied by sudden hearing impairment on the left and "stuttering and slurring." Angiogram and MRI scan were normal at the time of onset. His symptoms resolved over several days, with some persistence of mild numbness in the left hand and arm. A week later a tremor developed in his left upper extremity, and he was unable to return to work as an insurance agent. He had been out of work for a year. For several months he had had some visual spells and headaches and "halting speech."

Neurologic examination observed a tremor, noted that there were "few hard findings," and raised suspicion about nonorganic causes. Subsequent MRI scan, however, showed evidence of an old small hemorrhage in the right brainstem, which might have been responsible for his initial deficits.

During speech evaluation the patient described his speech as "stuttering" with slow rate and poor enunciation. He denied difficulty with language. He denied a childhood history of speech or language problems, although he had a brother who stuttered as a child.

AMRs of the tongue, lip, and jaw were produced with hesitation and struggle. Frequent repetition and prolongation of initial phonemes and sometimes the initial phoneme of the second syllable of a multisyllabic word characterized his speech. Orofacial tension and eye closing accompanied these dysfluencies. He was slow to initiate speech, and overall rate was moderately reduced. Prosody was flat, as was his overall affect, with the exception of an occasional sudden smile or laugh. His head nodding in response to yes-no questions was hesitant and jerky. Speech AMRs were markedly irregular and hesitant but not in a manner consistent with ataxia or hyperkinetic dysarthria. His conversational language was telegraphic but not like that typically heard in Broca's aphasia.

During 30 minutes of symptomatic therapy that focused on adoption of a prolonged and somewhat singsong prosody, fluency improved markedly; by the end of the session speech was approximately 90% normal with only infrequent hesitancies or repetitions. As fluency improved, facial animation also improved. The patient was seen again the following day. He had maintained his speech improvement and described it as "97% normal." The clinician agreed.

The clinician concluded: "His speech difficulty is best characterized as stuttering of psychogenic origin. Its presentation was inconsistent with neurogenic stuttering, and its resolution during a brief period of behavior modification does not occur in neurogenic stuttering. We did not explore the possible origin of this problem, but I explained to the patient that whatever event tipped him into his speech problem was no longer active. I also explained that his speech gains could be maintained and that further improvement could be expected, perhaps in a short period of time." The patient accepted this explanation, although somewhat blandly, and expressed confidence that his speech gains would be maintained.

When he was seen for psychiatric consultation 4 days later, his speech was normal. The psychiatrist established that a number of his symptoms had developed shortly after becoming extremely angry during a confrontation

Case 14-4—cont'd

with a claims adjustor at the insurance company where he worked. History also established a difficult childhood, an early failed marriage to a repeatedly unfaithful woman, rejection by a church of his attempts to become a minister, remarriage to a person with significant visual and hearing deficits necessitating fairly constant assistance from him, and frustrations in his and his spouse's attempts to adopt a disabled child. The psychiatrist described the patient as intense and tense, rigid, and only superficially insightful. Affect was generally flat. He hesitated to call the patient's problems a conversion reaction but did feel that he was amplifying his symptoms. He offered the patient inpatient treatment that would include physical and speech therapy, if necessary, as well as psychotherapy. The patient opted to return home, however.

Commentary. (1) Psychogenic speech disorders can occur in individuals with neurologic disease. This patient's brainstem hemorrhage probably explained some of his early symptoms but did not explain his speech deficit. (2) Symptomatic therapy for psychogenic stuttering can result in rapid improvement of speech. It can also help confirm the diagnosis as psychogenic and facilitate psychiatric evaluation. (3) Patients who develop psychogenic speech disorders can have what appears to be a single triggering event, but their histories often contain evidence of multiple life stresses. (4) Psychogenic stuttering is sometimes accompanied by a nonfluent pattern of speech that may superficially resemble Broca's aphasia. Of interest, the patient's telegraphic speech resolved as his dysfluencies resolved.

Case 14-5

A 45-year-old woman was seen at the clinic for evaluation of a 2-year history of leg weakness and speech difficulty. She initially had used a wheelchair but had graduated to a walker and then a cane. MRI of the head and spine was normal.

Neurologic evaluation revealed a bizarre flailing and lurching gait. She would not stand alone and would not stand without touching something with both hands. There was no evidence that her ability to control her center of gravity was impaired, and her ability to remain upright despite her bizarre movements suggested excellent balance. She gave way during muscle testing, but there was no evidence of loss of muscle bulk. The neurologist felt that her gait disorder was "hysterical" in nature. The remainder of the neurologic workup was normal.

During speech evaluation the patient denied any change or difficulty with speech. She admitted that when she answered the phone, people would ask if they could talk to her mother. There was marked give-way weakness on strength testing of the jaw, face, and tongue, and bizarre strugglelike behavior when she was asked to perform oral volitional movements. There was no evidence of weakness, spasticity, incoordination, or movement disorder during physical examination.

Speech was high in pitch; infantile in prosody, grammar, and content; and frequently accompanied by dysfluencies that included hesitancies and some phrase and word repetitions, with accompanying facial grimacing and eye closing. Eye contact was nearly nonexistent, and her nonverbal behavior was floridly infantile. A brief attempt was made to modify her voice and speech pattern. No change occurred.

The clinician concluded that she had a "psychogenic infantile speech pattern characterized by elevated pitch, immature prosody, and some grammatical variations that are infantile. I hear no evidence to suggest the presence of a dysarthria or AOS or other neurogenic motor speech disturbance." The clinician felt that the patient's denial of speech change or difficulty precluded the likelihood that she would benefit from speech therapy.

Psychiatric examination failed to find evidence of a depressive, psychotic, or chemical dependency disorder. Her father had died when she was 3 months old, and the patient had always been sickly. She had lost two infants between her living children's births. Her mother had been neurotically overprotective, and it appeared that her husband was doing the same. She appeared to the psychiatrist to be "totally regressed," unable to walk and speaking in a childlike manner. A probable conversion disorder was diagnosed, and inpatient psychiatric therapy was recommended. The patient refused, returned home, and was lost to follow-up.

Commentary. (1) Infantile speech can develop as a symptom of conversion disorder. (2) Conversion disorder can occur in a context suggestive of neurologic disease. (3) Symptomatic therapy for psychogenetic speech disorders is not always recommended. At the least, the patient must be aware of and express some concern about his or her speech difficulty, an attitude not present in this case. (4) Oral mechanism examination is often helpful to diagnosis of psychogenic speech disorders. In this case the deficits observed were disproportionate to anything that would be predicted by the patient's speech pattern.

Case 14-6

A 26-year-old man was seen at the clinic for evaluation of low back pain, leg numbness, and dysarthria. His problem began 2 months earlier, following a fall while leaving a restaurant. There was no loss of consciousness, but he had immediate onset of severe low back pain that required hospitalization for several weeks. His pain improved, but 1 week after hospital discharge he became unable to walk because of cramps in his legs. He also developed "slurred" speech that could not be understood. He stated, "The tongue would curl up inside my mouth, and I couldn't control it." This had improved somewhat.

After a complete neurologic examination and appropriate laboratory tests, the neurologist concluded, "Neither the story nor the examination would support a diagnosis of a radiculopathy, peripheral nerve lesion, or spinal cord lesion. The distribution of his pain did not conform to any known organic neurologic condition." The neurologist referred the patient for speech evaluation.

During speech evaluation the patient revealed that he had two children through an earlier marriage, divorced 2 years ago, remarried a year ago, and recently had another child approximately 1 month after the onset of his speech problem. He had owned a used car dealership for approximately 6 months but had to close it down since his illness. Of interest, he reported that his father once ran a used car dealership but had to close his business 13 years ago after suffering "crushed vertebrae" in an automobile accident. His father fully recovered and was able to begin another business.

During oral mechanism examination the tongue was held in an elevated posture with some spontaneous variable movements at rest, usually characterized by further retraction or lateralized movements. With prodding he could move his tongue forward and protrude it. He could also lateralize, elevate, and point his tongue toward his chin. Tongue strength was normal. He was able to swallow water without difficulty.

His speech was characterized by numerous articulatory distortions secondary to his retracted and elevated tongue posture. Anterior lingual fricatives and affricates were fairly consistently omitted or slighted, and lingual alveolar stops and nasals were palatized. His abnormal tongue posturing noticeably altered oral resonance. Speech AMRs were normal. During conversation there were secondary struggle behaviors in the form of eye closing, mild facial grimacing, and neck extension.

An attempt was made to modify his tongue posture. With great effort he could produce some anterior lingual stops and nasals and reduce some of his secondary struggle behaviors. He was unimpressed with his ability to change these behaviors but did admit that they represented improvement. He stated that he felt his speech had been improving and that he did not need speech therapy.

The clinician concluded that the patient had a "probable psychogenic articulation disorder which, at this point in time, seems resistant to symptomatic therapy. Although there is a possibility that his abnormal tongue posturing represents a hyperkinetic-like dysarthria (lingual dyskinesia), I have never seen it take this specific form. The absence of chewing or swallowing difficulty in the presence of lingual retraction and elevation is quite unusual in organic disturbance." The patient was told that his speech problem might represent a psychologic reaction to his recent medical difficulties or other undefined problems. He was told that his speech problem did not fit any commonly recognized neurologic speech deficit, and that his pattern of slow, steady improvement was reason for optimism about continued recovery. He was told that he might benefit from symptomatic speech therapy if improvement ceased or regression occurred.

The speech pathologist and the patient's neurologist recommended psychiatric consultation, but the patient declined. He was lost to follow-up, but 2 years later the neurologist and speech pathologist were called to give depositions related to a suit the patient had filed against the owner of the restaurant where he had fallen.

Commentary. (1) Psychogenic speech disorders can affect articulation. (2) Psychogenic speech disturbances can begin following a physical injury. (3) Psychosocial history occasionally reveals a "model" for nonorganic physical deficits. The similarity of the patient's difficulties to his father's was, at the least, an interesting coincidence and perhaps of diagnostic significance. (4) Psychogenic speech disturbances occasionally occur in people who are considering or are involved in litigation related to their physical or speech difficulties. In some cases this can raise concerns about malingering or represent a vehicle for secondary gain in conversion disorder.

Case 14-7

A 31-year-old woman was admitted to the emergency department with right-sided weakness and mutism. Initial impression was that she had had a stroke. Neurologic examination the following day, however, suggested the presence of give-way weakness of the right extremities, raising suspicions of a nonorganic component to her deficits. Subsequent computed tomography scan was normal. She was referred for speech evaluation.

During the initial part of the evaluation she was virtually mute, with occasional high-pitched grunting. She appreciated the humor in jokes, and she followed complex commands without error. She communicated normally through writing. When pushed to speak, she ultimately produced some broken syllables with much associated facial grimacing. Symptomatic treatment was undertaken, and within 45 minutes her speech had returned to normal. The clinician concluded that her speech deficit was psychogenic.

Subsequent evaluation in psychiatry, conducted with the help of family members, indicated that she had significant problems with impulse control and longstanding difficulties with low self-esteem and conflict with her mother. She had attempted suicide at age 18.

She received a psychiatric diagnosis of conversion disorder and probable borderline personality disorder.

During subsequent inpatient psychiatric treatment, her right-sided weakness resolved and her mood improved. When discharge was discussed, she became hostile and depressed and reported suicidal ideation. She was transferred to a closed psychiatric unit, where she had what were described as temper tantrums with shouting and striking out at others. She was eventually transferred to outpatient treatment in her hometown.

Commentary. (1) Conversion disorder can present as muteness that can be accompanied by other physical deficits suggestive of focal neurologic impairment. In this case it initially appeared that the patient had suffered a left hemisphere stroke, with right-sided weakness and muteness due to aphasia or AOS. (2) Symptomatic speech therapy can lead to rapid speech improvement, helping to rule out organic pathology as the primary explanation for muteness. (3) In some people, conversion disorder seems to occur as a relatively isolated event. In others, it may represent a symptom of more serious and long-standing psychologic difficulties.

Case 14-8

A 56-year-old woman presented to the clinic with a 7-month history of jerks involving multiple areas of her body, plus several episodes of blurred vision and hoarseness. There was no obvious precipitating event. Neurologic examination noted intermittent jerks of the head and trunk, and sometimes both lower extremities, some of which were lightninglike and appeared characteristic of organic myoclonus. Physiologic evaluation detected occasional jerks that were typical of organic myoclonus, although the level of the nervous system involvement could not be determined. Depakote was prescribed.

She returned 6 months later, noting that her myoclonus had resolved after she saw a chiropractor who had manipulated "a bad nerve behind my ear." However, for the past month she had had difficulty with her speech, leading her to talk incoherently and in "gibberish." The problem was currently constant, leading her to quit her job and seek disability. She had also developed head shaking that was present on a nearly constant basis, and during the past 3 weeks she had begun to "pass out" five to six times per day.

Neurologic examination was difficult because of her speech abnormalities. She did have a spell in which she

became hypotonic, unresponsive, and seemingly unaware of her surroundings. A nonorganic disorder was suspected, and she was referred for speech pathology and psychiatric evaluation.

The psychiatric examination was of questionable validity because of her speech problems. The patient was polite and superficially cooperative in that she allowed her husband to answer questions and attempted to answer some herself by writing, shaking her head yes or no, and holding up her fingers to indicate numbers. The psychiatrist concluded that the patient probably had issues, "such as fear of abandonment in this four-time married woman with a four-time married husband." She noted that the patient and her husband were angry with multiple physicians who had told them the illness was "in their heads." They were also angry about the denial of disability. The psychiatrist concluded that she likely had a somatoform disorder that could not be more specifically diagnosed.

Speech-language assessment was conducted the following day. The patient's husband noted that for quite some time the patient had to communicate solely with

Continued

Case 14-8—cont'd

gestures, pantomimes, and writing because her speech was unintelligible. She did not have any difficulties with chewing or swallowing. On language examination, she performed normally on all verbal and reading comprehension measures. Her writing was laborious, but her penmanship was good. She wrote words and dictated sentences without errors. She wrote intelligible responses rapidly and accurately to a number of questions.

She verbalized on a nearly constant basis with normal voice quality, resonance, and rate. Her prosodic pattern conveyed the impression of an Oriental and sometimes Lakota Sioux accent. Most of her syllables took a consonant-vowel form. Her speech was relatively devoid of fricatives and affricates. Attempts to imitate single vowels and consonants were often off target and almost always accompanied by struggle and effort. Her speech AMRs were regular and only mildly slowed. Oral mechanism examination was essentially normal. Her constant speaking ceased only when she was following complex verbal commands or writing and during a few intervals when she "passed out" or closed her eyes and let her chin slump to her chest, only to be revived by a light slap on the cheek by her husband or later by the clinician.

During approximately 20 minutes of symptomatic therapy, including some gentle laryngeal massage and manipulation, the patient began to produce intelligible speech, initially only imitatively but then during reading and conversation. Her speech continued to improve during the remainder of the session, although it remained mildly slow and halting; her pseudoforeign accent had disappeared, however. She was reassured that whatever had caused her speech disturbance was probably no longer active, because with her hard work she had made dramatic improvement in a short time. Symptomatic speech therapy was recommended if she noted any lasting regression, but the clinician expressed optimism that she could continue to improve spontaneously. The patient expressed concern about what might happen if she became increasingly stressed. The clinician told her

that this was an important concern but that the improvement she had made during the session established the capacity for normal speech.

She subsequently had an electroencephalogram that was normal, including during an episode of unresponsiveness. MRI was negative. The neurologist noted that the patient's speech was substantially different than it was when she presented a week earlier, and that it was now intelligible, although not entirely normal. The patient was reassured that the examination did not reveal any organic neurologic disorder, such as stroke, infection, or a neurodegenerative process. The neurologist expressed optimism that she could improve with a rehabilitation approach. She was referred to a facility closer to home, where a comprehensive program of physical rehabilitation could be undertaken. The patient and her husband refused a recommendation that she be seen for psychiatric care. The neurologist concluded that the patient had speech and gait disorders and spells of nonorganic etiology.

Commentary. (1) Psychogenic speech disorders can be accompanied by other symptoms that suggest neurologic disease. This patient's initial presentation was suggestive of organic myoclonus. (2) Pseudoforeign accent and other prosodic abnormalities, as well as unintelligible speech, can characterize psychogenic speech disturbances. (3) Symptomatic speech therapy can produce significant improvement in a relatively short period of time. Even when speech does not return to completely normal, symptomatic therapy can produce sufficient changes to establish the diagnosis as nonorganic. (4) Symptomatic speech therapy can result in dramatic improvement, even when issues of secondary gain (disability in this case) remain active and other physical symptoms persist. (5) Significant speech deficits can make psychiatric evaluation difficult. The improvement in the patient's speech would have permitted a more adequate psychiatric evaluation, although the patient refused.

SUMMARY

1. Speech can be altered in various ways by psychologic disturbances. Such disorders are not unusual within large multidisciplinary medical practices. Of importance, they can be similar to and difficult to distinguish from organic disease, including neurologic disease and its associated MSDs. Psychogenic/nonorganic and neurogenic speech disorders can also occur simultaneously.

2. Depression, manic-depression, and schizophrenia tend to be associated with logically predictable speech characteristics, and such characteristics may actually help identify the psychopathology. It is important to keep in mind that depression occurs frequently in neurologic disease and that the language of schizophrenic patients may be difficult to distinguish from some characteristics of aphasia.

3. Speech disorders that reflect responses to life stress, conversion, or somatization disorders or factitious disorders or malingering are most often manifest as changes in voice, fluency, or prosody. Voice disorders probably represent the

largest category of psychogenic speech disturbances, and most are characterized by aphonia, hoarseness, or spasmodic dysphonia. Stuttering-like behavior probably represents the next largest category of psychogenic speech disturbance. Articulation and prosodic deficits, infantile speech, and mutism can also reflect psychologic disorders.

4. Psychogenic and related nonorganic speech disorders frequently present in a manner that raises suspicions about neurologic disease. The distinction between the two etiologies can be difficult to make. Details of the history, as well as observations made during clinical evaluation, are important to diagnosis. The degree to which a speech disturbance can be classified neurologically, consistency of oral mechanism and speech findings, the degree to which the speech deficit is suggestible and distractible, patterns of fatigue of speech, and reversibility of the speech deficit are particularly important in identifying the presence of a psychogenic or nonorganic speech disorder.

5. Symptomatic therapy for suspected psychogenic or nonorganic speech disorders can result in rapid and dramatic speech improvement. Such symptom reversibility helps to rule out neurologic causes and confirm the diagnosis as psychogenic or nonorganic. This establishes the value of symptomatic therapy during diagnostic assessment. The absence of an immediate response to symptomatic therapy, however, does not rule out psychogenic/nonorganic etiology.

6. Because psychogenic/nonorganic speech disturbances can occur in people with neurologic disease, it is important to recognize the lawful manifestations of neurogenic MSDs and features of speech production that are incompatible with neurologic disease. The ability to make such distinctions is facilitated by clinical experience with large numbers and wide varieties of MSDs, as well as familiarity with the varieties of speech disturbances that can occur secondary to psychologic or nonorganic disturbances. Distinguishing between neurogenic and psychogenic/nonorganic speech disorders not only has implications for the diagnosis and management of the speech disorders themselves, but it can contribute importantly to the diagnosis of neurologic and nonneurologic disorders in general.

References

1. American Psychiatric Association: Diagnostic and statistical manual of mental disorders, ed 4, Washington, DC, 1994, American Psychiatric Association.

2. Anderson K, Schalén L: Etiology and treatment of psychogenic voice disorder: results of a follow-up study of thirty patients, J Voice 12:96, 1998.

3. Andrianopoulis MV, Gallivan GJ, Gallivan KH: PVCM, PVCD, EPL, and irritable larynx syndrome: what are we talking about and how do we treat it? J Voice 14:607, 2000.

4. Aronson AE: Clinical voice disorders, New York, 1990, Thieme.

5. Aronson AE, Peterson HW, Litin EM: Psychiatric symptomatology in functional dysphonia and aphonia, J Speech Hear Disord 31:115, 1966.

6. Attanasio JS: A case of late-onset or acquired stuttering in adult life, J Fluency Disord 12:287, 1987.

7. Baker JHE, Silver JR: Hysterical paraplegia, J Neurol Neurosurg Psychiatry 50:375, 1987.

8. Baumgartner J: Acquired psychogenic stuttering. In Curlee RF, editor: Stuttering and related disorders of fluency, New York, 1999, Thieme.

9. Baumgartner J, Duffy JR: Psychogenic stuttering in adults with and without neurologic disease, J Med Speech-Lang Pathol 5:75, 1997.

10. Binzer M, Andersen PM, Kullgren G: Clinical characteristics of patients with motor disability due to conversion disorder: prospective control group study, J Neurol Neurosurg Psychiatry 63:83, 1997.

11. Brookshire RH: A dramatic response to behavior modification by a patient with rapid onset of dysfluent speech. In Helm-Estabrooks N, Aten JL, editors: Difficult diagnoses in communication disorders, Boston, 1989, College-Hill Press.

12. Carden NL, Schramel DJ: Observations of conversion reactions seen in troops involved in the Viet Nam conflict, Am J Psychiatry 123:21, 1966.

13. Carson AJ et al: Do medically unexplained symptoms matter? A prospective cohort study of 300 new referrals to neurology outpatient clinics, J Neurol Neurosurg Psychiatry 69:207, 2000a.

14. Carson AJ et al: Neurological disease, emotional disorder, and disability: they are related: a study of 300 consecutive new referrals to a neurology outpatient department, J Neurol Neurosurg Psychiatry 68:202, 2000b.

15. Chabolla DR et al: Psychogenic nonepileptic seizures, Mayo Clin Proc 71:493, 1996.

16. Darby J, Hollien H: Vocal and speech patterns of depressive patients, Folia Phoniatr 29:279, 1977.

17. Darby JK, Simmons N, Berger PA: Speech and voice parameters of depression: a pilot study, J Commun Disord 17:75, 1984.

18. Deal JL: Sudden onset of stuttering: a case report, J Speech Hear Disord 47:301, 1982.

19. Deal J, Cannito MP: Acquired neurogenic dysfluency. In Vogel D, Cannito MP, editors: Treating disordered speech motor control, Austin, Tex, 1991, Pro-Ed.

20. Deal JL, Doro JM: Episodic hysterical stuttering, J Speech Hear Disord 52:299, 1987.

21. Deuschl G et al: Diagnostic and pathophysiological aspects of psychogenic tremors, Mov Disord 13:294, 1998.

22. DiSimoni FG, Darley FL, Aronson AE: Patterns of dysfunction in schizophrenic patients on an aphasia battery, J Speech Hear Disord 42:498, 1977.

23. Duffy JR: A puzzling case of adult onset stuttering. In Helm-Estabrooks N, Aten JL, editors: Difficult diagnoses in communication disorders, Boston, 1989, College-Hill Press.

24. Fahn S, Williams DT: Psychogenic dystonia, Adv Neurol 50:431-455, 1988.

25. Folks DG, Ford CV, Regan WM: Conversion symptoms in a general hospital, Psychosomatics 25:285, 1984.

26. Ford CV, Folks DG: Conversion disorders: an overview, Psychosomatics 26:371, 1985.

27. Freeman RL et al: The neurology of depression: cognitive and behavioral deficits with focal findings in depression and resolution after electroconvulsive therapy, Arch Neurol 42:289, 1985.

28. Gerson SN, Benson DF, Frazier SH: Diagnosis: schizophrenia versus posterior aphasia, Am J Psychiatry 134:9, 1977.

29. Hartman DE, Daily WW, Morin KN: A case of superior laryngeal nerve paresis and psychogenic dysphonia, J Speech Hear Disord 54:526, 1990.

30. Head H: An address on the diagnosis of hysteria, BMJ 1:827, 1922.

31. Hirschfeld RMA, Goodwin FK: Mood disorders. In Talbott JA, Hales RE, Yudofsky SC: Textbook of psychiatry, Washington, DC, 1988, American Psychiatric Press.

32. James W: On exceptional mental states: the 1896 Lowell lectures, New York, 1896, Scribner's Sons.

33. Kallen D, Marshall RC, Casey DE: Atypical dysarthria in Munchausen syndrome, Br J Disord Commun 21:377, 1986.

34. Katon WJ, Walker EA: Medically unexplained symptoms in primary care, J Clin Psychiatry 59(suppl 20):15, 1998.

35. Keane JR: Wrong-way deviation of the tongue with hysterical hemiparesis, Neurology 36:1406, 1986.

36. Koller W et al: Psychogenic tremors, Neurology 39:1094, 1989.

37. Lazare A: Current concepts in psychiatry: conversion symptoms, N Engl J Med 305:745, 1981.

38. Lebrun Y: Mutism, London, 1990, Whurr.

39. Lecours AR, Vanier-Clement M: Schizophasia and jargonaphasia, Brain Lang 3:516, 1976.

40. Mahr G: Psychogenic communication disorders. In Johnson AF, Jacobson BH, editors: Medical speech-language pathology: a practitioners guide, New York, 1998, Thieme.

41. Mahr G, Leith W: Psychogenic stuttering of adult onset, J Speech Hear Res 35:283, 1992.

42. Mathers-Schmidt BA: Paradoxical vocal fold motion: a tutorial on a complex disorder and the speech-language pathologist's role, Am J Speech-Lang Pathol 10:111, 2001.

43. Merskey H: Conversion symptoms revised, Semin Neurol 10:221, 1990.

44. Nicholi AM Jr: The New Harvard Guide to Psychiatry, Cambridge, England, 1988, The Belknap Press of Harvard University Press.

45. Patton H et al: Paradoxical vocal cord syndrome with surgical cure, South Med J 80:256, 1987.

46. Perino M, Famularo G, Tarroni P: Acquired transient stuttering during a migraine attack, Headache 40:170, 2000.

47. Robinson RG, Benson DF: Depression in aphasic patients: frequency, severity, and clinical-pathological correlations, Brain Lang 14:282, 1981.

48. Robinson RG, Lipsey JR, Price TR: Diagnosis and clinical management of post-stroke depression, Psychosomatics 26:769, 1985.

49. Robinson RG et al: Mood disorders in stroke patients: importance of location of lesion, Brain 107:81, 1984a.

50. Robinson RG et al: A two-year longitudinal study of post-stroke mood disorders: dynamic changes in associated variables over the first six months of follow-up, Stroke 15:510, 1984b.

51. Ron MA: Somatization and conversion disorders. In Fogel BS, Schiffer RB, editors: Neuropsychiatry, Philadelphia, 1996, Williams & Wilkins.

52. Roth CR, Aronson AE, Davis LJ: Clinical studies in psychogenic stuttering of adult onset, J Speech Hear Disord 54:634, 1989.

53. Roy N, Bless DM: Personality traits and psychological factors in voice pathology: a foundation for future research, J Speech Lang Hear Res 43:737, 2000.

54. Roy N, Bless DM, Heisey D: Personality and voice disorders: a superfactor trait analysis, J Speech Lang Hear Res 43:749, 2000.

55. Roy N, Ford CN, Bless DM: Muscle tension dysphonia and spasmodic dysphonia: the role of manual laryngeal tension reduction in diagnosis and management, Ann Otol Rhinol Laryngol 105:851, 1996.

56. Sapir S: Psychogenic spasmodic dysphonia, J Voice 9:270, 1995.

57. Sapir S, Aronson AE: Aphonia after closed head injury: aetiologic considerations, Br J Disord Commun 20:289, 1985.

58. Sapir S, Aronson AE: Coexisting psychogenic and neurogenic dysphonia: a source of diagnostic confusion, Br J Disord Commun 22:73, 1987.

59. Sapir S, Aronson AE: The relationship between psychopathology and speech and language disorders in neurologic patients, J Speech Hear Disord 55:503, 1990.

60. Schiffer RB: Depressive syndromes associated with diseases of the central nervous system, Semin Neurol 10:239, 1990.

60a. Schneider B, Wendler J, Seidner W: The relevance of stroboscopy in functional dysphonias, Folia Phoniatr Logop, 54:44, 2002.

61. Starkstein SE, Robinson RG: Depression following cerebrovascular lesions, Semin Neurol 10:247, 1990.

62. Stoudemire GA: Somatoform disorders, factitious disorders, and malingering. In Talbott JA, Hales RE, Yudofsky SC, editors: Textbook of psychiatry, Washington, DC, 1988, American Psychiatric Press.

63. Teitelbaum ML, McHugh PR: Psychiatric conditions presenting as neurologic disease. In Johnson RT, editor: Current therapy in neurologic disease, vol 3, Philadelphia, 1990, BC Decker.

64. Thompson TL: Psychosomatic disorders. In Talbott JA, Hales RE, Yudofsky SC, editors: Textbook of psychiatry, Washington, DC, 1988, American Psychiatric Press.

65. Tippett DC, Siebens AA: Distinguishing psychogenic from neurogenic dysfluency when neurologic and psychologic factors coexist, J Fluency Disord 16:3, 1991.

66. Todt EH, Howell RJ: *Vocal cues as indices of schizophrenia,* J Speech Hear Res 23:517, 1980.

67. Tomb DA: *Psychiatry for the house officer,* Baltimore, 1981, Williams & Wilkins.

68. Tucker GJ et al: *Psychological impact of neurological diseases,* Continuum 3:95, 1997.

69. Uomoto JM: *Evaluation of neuropsychological status after traumatic brain injury.* In Beukelman DR, Yorkston KM, editors: *Communication disorders following traumatic brain injury: management of cognitive, language, and motor impairments,* Austin, Tex, 1991, Pro-Ed.

70. Vuileumier P et al: *Functional neuroanatomical correlates of hysterical sensorimotor loss,* Brain 124:1077, 2001.

71. Wallen V: *Primary stuttering in a 28-year-old adult,* J Speech Hear Disord 26:393, 1961.

72. Williams JBW: *Psychiatric classification.* In Talbott JA, Hales RE, Yudofsky SC, editors: *Textbook of psychiatry,* Washington, DC, 1988, American Psychiatric Press.

73. Ziegler FJ, Imboden JB: *Contemporary conversion reactions: II a conceptual model,* Arch Gen Psychiatry 6:37, 1962.

15 Differential Diagnosis

"The act of clinical diagnosis is classification for a purpose: an effort to recognize the class or group to which a patient's illness belongs so that, based on our prior experience with that class, the subsequent clinical acts we can afford to carry out, and the patient is willing to follow, will maximize the patient's health."[8]

D.L. Sackett et al.

CHAPTER OUTLINE

   I. General guidelines for differential diagnosis
 II. Distinguishing among the dysarthrias
    A. Anatomy and vascular distribution
    B. Etiology
    C. Oral mechanism findings
    D. Speech characteristics
 III. Distinguishing dysarthrias from apraxia of speech
    A. Anatomy and vascular distribution
    B. Etiology
    C. Oral mechanism findings
    D. Speech characteristics
 IV. Distinguishing motor speech disorders from aphasia
    A. Dysarthria versus aphasia
    B. Apraxia of speech versus aphasia
 V. Distinguishing among forms of neurogenic mutism
    A. Anarthria
    B. Apraxia of speech
    C. Aphasia
    D. Cognitive-affective disturbances
 VI. Distinguishing motor speech disorders from other neurogenic speech disorders
    A. Neurogenic stuttering
    B. Palilalia
    C. Echolalia
    D. Cognitive and affective disturbances (abulia)
    E. Aprosodia
 VII. Distinguishing neurogenic from psychogenic speech disorders
    A. Depression
    B. Schizophrenia
    C. Conversion disorders and responses to life stress

VIII. Cases
 IX. Summary

Is a speech disorder present? If so, is it neurogenic? If so, what is its type? What are the implications of the type of neurogenic speech disorder for lesion localization? To answer these and related questions, the meaning of speech signs and symptoms must be understood. Meaning in this case derives from the application of a knowledge base and clinical skill to the clinical problem.

Sometimes examination findings are unambiguous and have only one possible interpretation. More often there are several possible interpretations, and diagnosis can be expressed only as an ordering of those possibilities. *The process of narrowing possibilities and reaching conclusions about the nature of a deficit is known as differential diagnosis.*

This chapter addresses differential diagnosis by summarizing the distinctive clinical characteristics of the primary speech disorders that have been discussed in previous chapters. It also highlights the similarities and differences among the speech disorders that are clinically most difficult to distinguish from one another.

■ GENERAL GUIDELINES FOR DIFFERENTIAL DIAGNOSIS

A few guidelines should be kept in mind in the context of the diagnostic process. They help focus the clinician's thinking and serve as a guide to communicating with referring professionals who have an interest in the diagnosis.

1. *Speech examination should always lead to an attempt at diagnosis.* Establishing the meaning

of clinical observations is essential, especially when diagnosis is the primary purpose of examination. This is often ignored by clinicians who view their only role as that of therapist. However, even when the primary goal of examination is to address management issues, the nature of the problem should be established as clearly as possible, because we usually treat more adequately what we understand than what we do not understand.

2. *When the results of examination cannot go beyond description, the reasons why should be stated explicitly.* Sometimes a diagnosis cannot be made. This can happen when abnormalities are subtle, atypical, or combine in ways that are incompatible with known patterns of deficit in neurologic disease. It can also occur when a patient does not or cannot cooperate with the simplest aspects of examination. When these circumstances occur, they should be stated as reasons for inability to establish a diagnosis.

   Even under difficult assessment circumstances, or with equivocal or atypical findings, some valuable interpretations sometimes can be made. For example, if the purpose of examination is to establish if a patient has dysarthria versus a psychogenic speech disorder, enough information may be obtained to conclude that a dysarthria is present, even if its type cannot be specified. Conversely, enough speech might be produced to establish that a dysarthria is not present, even though formal examination is not possible. In still other cases, it may be possible to state what the problem is not. For example, a clinician might determine that a patient has an indeterminate motor speech disorder (MSD), but that it is not hypokinetic or hyperkinetic dysarthria; such a narrowing of diagnostic possibilities would imply that the source of the speech deficit is probably not in the basal ganglia control circuit.

3. *The clinician should not state a diagnosis when one cannot be determined.* To offer a diagnosis when evidence for it is lacking can be misleading at best and dangerous at worst. There are numerous instances in which the best diagnosis is an undetermined one. In fact, knowing that a speech diagnosis cannot be made can be helpful. For example, a diagnosis of "diagnosis undetermined" may help eliminate diseases in which the presence and nature of an MSD should be predictable, or it may help confirm suspicions that neurologic disease is not present. Relatedly, it may be appropriate and helpful to express a degree of confidence in a diagnosis through qualifiers such as "unambiguous," "probable," "possible," or "equivocal."

4. *Speech diagnosis should be related to the suspected or known neurologic diagnosis or lesion localization.* Referring neurologists usually have, at the least, suspicions about lesion localization and etiology. Therefore it is appropriate to address whether the speech diagnosis is consistent with such suspicions. If it is not, it may raise questions about the neurologic diagnosis or suggest that there is an additional lesion or disease process at work.

5. *Different speech disturbances can occur simultaneously.* Although a single diagnosis is parsimonious, it is not always correct. Disease does not always respect the divisions we impose on the nervous system. As a result, some neurologic diseases lead to combinations of dysarthria types, apraxia of speech (AOS), and other neurogenic speech disturbances. In addition, the presence of one neurologic disease does not preclude the presence of another, so different neurogenic speech disorders can occur simultaneously as a result of cooccurring neurologic diseases. Finally, neurogenic speech disorders can occur simultaneously with nonneurologic but organic speech disorders or with psychogenic speech disturbances. Therefore it is important to recognize that *diagnosis does not end when a single disorder is recognized.* The clinician must establish that the recognized disorder can explain all of the deviant speech characteristics that are present. If it cannot, the presence of additional disorders should be considered.

6. *Examination sometimes leads to a conclusion that speech is normal.* A conclusion that speech is normal is not unusual when baseline assessment of speech and language is sought (1) as part of routine screening of speech (e.g., screening all patients admitted to a rehabilitation unit), (2) for individuals with neurologic disease frequently associated with speech deficits (e.g., amyotrophic lateral sclerosis [ALS]), or (3) when a medical procedure carries risk for speech deficits (e.g., baseline assessments of patients who will undergo temporal lobectomy for control of seizure disorders, thalamotomy or deep brain stimulation for control of movement disorders).

   A diagnosis of normal speech sometimes requires explanation. Referral for speech evaluation is often based on someone's suspicion or complaint that speech is abnormal in some way, and the concern must be addressed. Possible explanations include, but are not limited to, the following:

   a. *Speech may have changed but is still in the normal range.* This is not uncommon in the early stages of some diseases; the patient hears or feels that speech has changed, but the change is insufficient to be perceived by others or detected on physical examination or by other tests. If the patient can provide a good history and description of the changes perceived, however, a list of diagnostic possibilities can sometimes be formulated.

  b. *A change has occurred outside the motor system.* For example, some depressed individuals report that speaking is effortful or abnormal. This may reflect the effect of their mood on their energy level for speech, their focus on physical manifestations rather than psychologic explanations for the depression, or the effect of other factors not directly related to motor speech.

  c. *Speech is normal, but psychologic factors have triggered a perception of abnormality by the patient.* For example, fear of a disease associated with speech difficulty might be triggered by the presence of the disease and speech difficulty in a loved one or by exposure to someone with a threatening communicable disease.

  d. *Speech is normal, but a physically (or psychologically) traumatic event has generated a complaint of speech change.* This can occur in people involved in litigation who may have something to gain from the presence of speech difficulty (malingering or conversion disorder).

  e. *The referring individual has misidentified a longstanding "developmental" speech abnormality (e.g., distortion of /r/ or /l/) as a sign of new neurologic disease.*

7. *Fixing a diagnostic label is convenient shorthand for communicating information.* A diagnostic label can be misleading or of no value if it is applied without thinking of its implications, without explanation to people who may not know its meaning, or to impart an air of knowledge when knowledge is lacking. However, if the meaning of the label is clear to the user, if clinical evidence supports its use, and if its meaning and implications are made clear in communication of findings, a label can convey information concisely and precisely. To experienced clinicians, a label can convey a gestalt of speech characteristics. To neurologists familiar with the neurologic correlates of MSDs, the label has implications for lesion localization. Also, in some instances, the label may generate predictions about likely management approaches. For example, a diagnosis of hypokinetic dysarthria may suggest that treatment

will likely focus on increasing vocal loudness or reducing speech rate. All such implications may be tentative, but in the hands of clinicians who have a common understanding of diagnostic labels they promote effective, efficient communication.

▨ DISTINGUISHING AMONG THE DYSARTHRIAS

There is considerable overlap among the speech characteristics that are present across dysarthria types. For example, imprecise articulation can be present in any of the dysarthrias. This means that although identification of imprecise articulation may help identify the *presence* of dysarthria, it is not consistently useful in *distinguishing among types* of dysarthria. There are a number of speech characteristics, oral mechanism findings, etiologies, and lesion loci for which there are varying degrees of overlap among the dysarthrias. There also are some speech characteristics and patterns of deficit that are relatively unique and allow distinctions among them. Because the dysarthrias are a predominant focus of this book, it is appropriate to summarize here the commonalities and distinctions among them.

Anatomy and Vascular Distribution

When the anatomic localization or vascular source of a lesion is known, certain predictions can be made about expected MSDs. This information may aid (or bias) differential diagnosis and help guide judgments about the compatibility of the speech diagnosis with localization.

Table 15-1 summarizes the associations between each of the dysarthrias and the gross anatomic levels of the nervous system and their major vascular supply. Although there is considerable anatomic and vascular overlap across dysarthria types, certain distinctions are apparent. They can be summarized as follows:

1. Flaccid and ataxic dysarthria are not associated with supratentorial lesions or with lesions in the distribution of the anterior, middle, or posterior cerebral arteries.

2. Hypokinetic dysarthria is associated only with supratentorial (subcortical) lesions. Posterior fossa lesions and lesions in the distribution of the vertebrobasilar system may cause any type of dysarthria, except hypokinetic.

3. Only flaccid dysarthria is associated with lesions at the spinal and peripheral levels of the nervous system and their associated vascular supply.

| table 15-1 | Distinctions among MSDs as a function of major anatomic levels of the nervous system and vascular supply* |

Anatomic Level	Vascular Supply	Flaccid	Spastic	Ataxic	Dysarthria Hypokinetic	Hyperkinetic	Unilateral UMN	AOS
Supratentorial (cerebral hemispheres, basal ganglia, thalamus)	Carotid system (major cerebral arteries & their branches)	-	+	-	+	+	+	+†
Posterior Fossa (pons, medulla, midbrain, cerebellum)	Vertebrobasilar system (vertebral & basilar arteries & their branches)	+	+	+	–	+	+	–
Spinal	Spinal arteries	+	–	–	–	–	–	–
Peripheral	Branches of major extremity vessels	+	–	–	–	–	–	–

+, Lesions may produce disorder; –, lesions do not produce disorder; AOS, apraxia of speech; MSDs, motor speech disorders; UMN, upper motor neuron.
See Tables 2-1 and 2-2 for a detailed summary of the relationships among MSDs and anatomic levels, the skeleton and meninges, and the ventricular and vascular components of the nervous system.
†*Left (dominant) hemisphere only.*

Etiology

When etiology is known, expectations also arise about the type of MSDs that could be present. This can aid (or bias) differential diagnosis and guide judgments about the compatibility of the speech diagnosis with the known or suspected etiology.

Table 15-2 summarizes the types of MSDs encountered with various neurologic conditions. The table makes clear that there is much overlap among dysarthria types as a function of etiology, but there are also some clear distinctions. These similarities and differences can be summarized as follows:

1. Vascular disease can cause virtually any type of dysarthria. It is a frequent cause of spastic and unilateral upper motor neuron (UUMN) dysarthria and a common cause of ataxic dysarthria. It can cause flaccid and hyperkinetic dysarthria, though not frequently. Nonhemorrhagic stroke is the most frequent vascular cause of dysarthrias.

2. Degenerative disease can cause any type of dysarthria. It is a frequent cause of spastic, ataxic, and hypokinetic dysarthria and a common cause of flaccid dysarthria. It can cause hyperkinetic and UUMN dysarthria, though not frequently. Among the degenerative diseases, ALS is a frequent cause of flaccid and spastic dysarthria but not usually any other dysarthria type; thus the presence of another dysarthria type in someone with a diagnosis of ALS should raise suspicions about an additional disease or questions about the ALS diagnosis. Similarly, Parkinson's disease is associated only with hypokinetic dysarthria, and certain degenerative cerebellar diseases only with ataxic dysarthria. The presence of other dysarthria types in those conditions should raise similar doubts about etiology.

3. Traumatic brain injury can cause any type of dysarthria. In closed head injury, spastic dysarthria probably occurs more frequently than other types, but any type can be encountered. Penetrating head injuries rarely cause flaccid dysarthria but can cause any central nervous system (CNS) dysarthria. In contrast, skull fracture and neck trauma can cause flaccid dysarthria but not usually other types of dysarthria.

4. Surgical trauma can cause any type of dysarthria, with the possible exception of hypokinetic dysarthria. Ear, nose, and throat and cardiac/chest surgeries are exclusively associated with flaccid dysarthria. Neurosurgery can result in CNS dysarthrias and is also a possible cause of flaccid dysarthria.

5. Toxic and metabolic disturbances rarely cause flaccid or UUMN dysarthria but are possible causes of other dysarthria types. Toxic/metabolic disturbances, especially those associated with drug abuse and toxic effects

table 15-2 Distinctions among MSDs as a function of etiology*

Etiology	Flaccid	Spastic	Ataxic	Dysarthria Hypokinetic	Hyperkinetic	Unilateral UMN	AOS
Vascular	+	++	+	+	+	++	++
Aneurysm rupture	−	+	+	+	−	+	+
Anoxia, cardiac arrest	−	+	+	+	−	−	−
Hypoxic encephalopathy	−	+	+	+	+	−	−
Intracranial arteritis	−	+	+	−	−	+	+
Stroke, hemorrhagic	+	+	+	+	+	+	+
Stroke, nonhemorrhagic	+	++	+	+	+	++	++
Degenerative Disease	++	++	++	++	+	+	+
ALS/motor neuron disease	++	++	−	−	−	−	−
Alzheimer's disease	−	−	−	+	−	−	+
Cerebellar & brainstem degeneration	−	+	+	−	−	−	−
Corticobasal degeneration	−	+	+	+	+	−	+
Dystonia musculorum deformans	−	−	−	−	+	−	−
Familial basal ganglia calcification	−	−	−	+	+	−	−
Friedreich's ataxia	−	+	+	−	−	−	−
Hereditary cerebellar disease	−	−	+	−	−	−	−
Hereditary cerebral calcinosis	−	−	+	−	−	−	−
Hereditary degenerative CNS disease	−	+	+	+	+	+	+
Huntington's chorea	−	−	−	+	+	−	−
Kennedy's disease	+	−	−	−	−	−	−
Leukoencephalopathy	−	+	+	−	−	−	+
Lewy body disease	−	−	−	+	−	−	−
Multiple system atrophy	+	+	+	+	+	−	−
Olivopontocerebellar atrophy	+	+	+	+	−	−	−
Parkinson's disease	−	−	−	++	−	−	−
Parkinsonism	−	−	−	++	−	−	−
Pick's disease	−	−	−	+	−	−	−
Primary generalized dystonia	−	−	−	−	+	−	−
Primary lateral sclerosis	−	+	−	−	−	−	−
Primary progressive aphasia	−	−	−	−	−	+	+
Progressive bulbar palsy	+	+	−	−	−	−	−
Progressive supranuclear palsy	−	+	+	+	−	−	−
Shy-Drager syndrome	+	+	+	+	−	−	−
Spinal muscle atrophies	+	−	−	−	−	−	−
Spinocerebellar ataxias	−	+	+	+	−	−	−
Striatonigral degeneration	−	+	+	+	+	−	−
Traumatic	+	+	+	+	+	+	+
CHI	+	+	+	+	+	+	+
Neck trauma	+	−	−	−	−	−	−
Penetrating head injury	−	+	+	+	+	+	+
Skull fracture	+	−	−	−	−	−	−
Surgical Trauma	++	+	+	−	−	+	+
Chest/cardiac	+	−	−	−	−	−	−
ENT	++	−	−	−	−	−	−
Neurosurgical	+	+	+	−	+	+	+
Neoplastic	+	+	+	+	−	+	+
Paraneoplastic syndrome	−	+	+	−	−	−	−
Primary or metastatic	+	+	+	+	+	+	+
Toxic/Metabolic	−	+	+	+	++	−	−
Botulism	+	−	−	−	−	−	−
Carbon monoxide poisoning	−	+	+	+	−	−	−
Central pontine myelinolysis	−	+	+	+	+	−	−
Dialysis encephalopathy	−	+	+	−	+	−	−
Drug toxicity/abuse	+	+	+	+	+	−	+
Heavy metal or chemical toxicity	−	−	−	+	+	−	−
Hepatic encephalopathy	−	+	+	−	+	−	−

Continued

table 15-2 Distinctions among MSDs as a function of etiology*—cont'd

Etiology	Flaccid	Spastic	Ataxic	Dysarthria Hypokinetic	Hyperkinetic	Unilateral UMN	AOS
Toxic/Metabolic—cont'd							
Hepatocerebral degeneration	–	+	+	+	+	–	–
Hypoparathyroidism	+	+	–	+	+	–	–
Hypothyroidism	–	–	+	–	–	–	–
Hypoxic encephalopathy	–	–	–	+	+	–	–
Inborn errors of metabolism	–	–	–	+	+	–	–
Liver failure	–	–	–	+	–	–	–
Wilson's disease	–	+	+	+	+	–	–
Infectious	+	+	+	+	+	–	+
AIDS	+	+	+	–	–	–	–
CNS tuberculosis	–	–	+	+	–	–	–
Creutzfeldt-Jacob disease	+	+	+	+	+	+	+
Herpes zoster	+	–	–	–	–	–	–
Infectious encephalopathy	–	+	+	+	+	–	–
Inflammatory	–	+	+	–	–	–	+
Encephalitis	–	+	+	+	–	–	+
Meningitis	+	+	+	–	–	–	–
Multifocal leukoencephalopathy	–	+	+	+	–	–	–
Demyelinating Disease	+	+	+	–	+	+	+
Chronic demyelinating polyneuritis	+	–	–	–	–	–	–
Guillain-Barré	+	–	+	–	–	–	–
Multiple sclerosis	+	+	+	+	+	+	+
Anatomic Malformation	+	+	+	–	–	–	–
Arnold-Chiari	+	+	+	–	–	–	–
Syringobulbia	+	+	+	–	–	–	–
Syringomyelia	+	–	–	–	–	–	–
Neuromuscular Junction Disease	+	–	–	–	–	–	–
Botulism	+	–	–	–	–	–	–
Lambert-Eaton syndrome	+	–	–	–	–	–	–
Myasthenia gravis	+	–	–	–	–	–	–
Muscle Disease	+	–	–	–	–	–	–
Muscular dystrophy	+	–	–	–	–	–	–
Myopathy	+	–	–	–	–	–	–
Myotonic dystrophy	+	–	–	–	–	–	–
Polymyositis	+	–	–	–	–	–	–
Other	+	+	+	+	+	+	+
Chorea gravidarum	–	–	–	–	+	–	–
Hydrocephalus	–	+	+	+	–	–	–
Meige's syndrome	–	–	–	–	+	–	–
Myoclonic epilepsy	–	–	–	–	+	–	–
Radiation necrosis	+	–	+	+	–	+	–
Seizure disorder	–	–	–	–	–	–	+
Tourette's syndrome	–	–	–	–	+	–	–
Undetermined Cause (Idiopathic)	+	+	+	+	++	+	+

++, Very frequent cause; +, possible cause; –, rare, never, or uncertain cause; AIDS, acquired immunodeficiency syndrome; ALS, amyotrophic lateral sclerosis; AOS, apraxia of speech; CHI, closed head injury; CNS, central nervous system; ENT, ear, nose, and throat; MSDs, motor speech disorders; UMN, upper motor neuron.
This table is based primarily on reviews of Mayo Clinic cases in Chapters 4 through 12 but supplemented by published data when applicable. Mixed dysarthrias are not included in the table, but any etiology associated with more than a single dysarthria type can be assumed capable of causing a mixed dysarthria containing the individual types listed.

of prescribed medication, cause hyperkinetic or ataxic dysarthria more than any other type.

6. Infectious and inflammatory conditions are possible but not common causes of dysarthrias. Because their effects are diffuse or have multiple possible foci, they generally do not lead to distinctive expectations regarding dysarthria type. Examples of exceptions include botulism, herpes zoster, and polio (flaccid dysarthria); hypothyroidism (ataxic dysarthria); and Sydenham's chorea (hyperkinetic dysarthria).

7. Demyelinating diseases can cause any type of dysarthria but rarely hypokinetic dysarthria. Guillain-Barré syndrome is associated with flaccid and, rarely, ataxic dysarthria but not other dysarthria types. Multiple sclerosis probably causes ataxic dysarthria more frequently than any other dysarthria type.

8. Anatomic malformations such as Arnold-Chiari, syringobulbia, and syringomyelia are more frequently associated with flaccid dysarthria than any other dysarthria type. Because Arnold-Chiari malformation and syringobulbia can affect posterior fossa structures, however, they may also be associated with spastic or ataxic dysarthria.

9. Neuromuscular junction disorders, muscle disease, and neuropathies are, by definition, disorders of peripheral nerves. As a result, they are exclusively associated with flaccid dysarthria.

10. The "other" conditions listed in Table 15-2 are not common causes of dysarthrias, but some of them are associated with only one dysarthria type.

11. Any type of dysarthria can be present in the absence of an established neurologic diagnosis. The etiology is undetermined frequently in hyperkinetic dysarthria and often in spastic and ataxic dysarthria.

Oral Mechanism Findings

Table 15-3 summarizes oral mechanism findings associated with various MSDs. There is considerable overlap, but some findings are much more common in some MSDs than others; some findings are unusual or should not be present in other MSD types.

The presence or absence of certain oral mechanism findings is not a requirement for any MSD diagnosis. They are confirmatory signs only. That is, they may support a diagnosis but are not diagnostic by themselves. The major distinguishing features of oral mechanism findings can be summarized as follows.

Flaccid Dysarthria

Atrophy and fasciculations in speech muscles are frequently but not invariably present in flaccid dysarthria, but they are not expected in any other MSD. Hypotonia and a hypoactive gag reflex are encountered more commonly in flaccid dysarthria than in any other MSD. Rapid deterioration in the strength of speech muscles during nonspeech tasks is distinctive of myasthenia gravis, but should not be encountered in any other flaccid dysarthria or in any other MSD. Nasal regurgitation is a possible finding in flaccid dysarthria but is uncommon in other MSDs.

Spastic Dysarthria

Pathologic oral reflexes, a hyperactive gag reflex, and pseudobulbar affect are common and more frequently found in spastic dysarthria than in any other MSD. Dysphagia and drooling are probably more common in people with spastic dysarthria than any other MSD, but they are not distinctive of spastic dysarthria.

Ataxic Dysarthria

A normal oral mechanism examination is not uncommon in speakers with ataxic dysarthria. However, their jaw, face, and lingual nonspeech movements are frequently dysmetric, an observation not commonly made in other MSDs.

Hypokinetic Dysarthria

Facial masking, tremulousness of orofacial structures, and reduced range of movement on nonspeech alternate motion rate (AMR) tasks is common in hypokinetic dysarthria. Such abnormalities are uncommon in other MSDs.

Hyperkinetic Dysarthria

A number of oral mechanism abnormalities may be apparent at rest, during nonspeech sustained postures or movement, and during speech. Quick or slow patterned or unpatterned adventitious movements are strong confirmatory signs of hyperkinetic dysarthria. It should be kept in mind, however, that some hyperkinesias occur only during speech and that the absence of hyperkinesias at rest or during nonspeech tasks does not preclude a diagnosis of hyperkinetic dysarthria. The presence of abnormal, involuntary movements in the orofacial muscles (with the exception of fasciculations, synkinesis, and myokymia in some speakers with flaccid dysarthria) are uncommon in other MSDs.

table 15-3   Distinguishing oral mechanism findings among motor speech disorders

Physical Findings	Flaccid	Spastic	Ataxic	Dysarthria Hypokinetic	Hyperkinetic	Unilateral UMN	AOS
Hypoactive gag	+	−	−	−	−	−	−
Hypotonia	+	−	+	−	−	−	−
Atrophy	++	−	−	−	−	−	−
Facial myokymia	++	−	−	−	−	−	−
Fasciculations	++	−	−	−	−	−	−
Rapid deterioration & recovery with rest	++	−	−	−	−	−	−
Synkinesis (eye blink/lower face)	++	−	−	−	−	−	−
Nasal regurgitation	++	−	−	−	−	−	−
Unilateral palatal weakness	++	−	−	−	−	−	−
Dysphagia	+	+	−	+	+	+	−
Drooling	+	+	−	+	−	+	−
Hyperactive gag	−	++	−	−	−	−	−
Sucking reflex	−	++	−	−	−	−	−
Snout reflex	−	++	−	−	−	−	−
Jaw jerk reflex	−	++	−	−	−	−	−
Pseudobulbar affect	−	++	−	−	−	−	−
Dysmetric jaw, face, tongue AMRs	−	−	++	−	−	−	−
Masked facies	−	−	−	++	−	−	−
Tremulous jaw, lips, tongue	−	−	−	++	−	−	−
Reduced range of motion on AMR tasks	−	+	−	++	−	−	−
Head tremor	−	−	+	+	+	−	−
Involuntary head, jaw, face, tongue, palate, respiratory movements during sustained postures or during movement	−	−	−	−	++	−	−
Sensory "tricks"	−	−	−	−	++	−	−
Relatively sustained head deviation (torticollis)	−	−	−	−	++	−	−
Myoclonus of palate, pharynx, larynx, lips, nares, tongue, or respiratory muscles	−	−	−	−	++	−	−
Multiple motor tics	−	−	−	−	++	−	−
Jaw, lip, tongue, pharyngeal, or palatal tremor	−	−	−	−	++	−	−
Facial grimacing during speech	−	−	−	−	++	−	−
Unilateral lower face weakness	−	−	−	−	−	++	+
Unilateral lingual weakness without atrophy/fasciculation	+	−	−	−	−	+	+
Nonverbal oral apraxia	−	−	−	−	−	+	++

+, May be present but not generally distinguishing; ++, distinguishing when present; −, not usually present; AMRs, alternate motion rates; AOS, apraxia of speech; UMN, upper motor neuron.

Unilateral Upper Motor Neuron Dysarthria

Unilateral right or left central facial or lingual weakness without atrophy or fasciculations is a common finding. Such a unilateral finding is unusual in other dysarthria types, although flaccid dysarthria can also be associated with unilateral facial and lingual weakness.

Speech Characteristics

Distinctions among the dysarthrias are made primarily on the basis of perceived deviant speech characteristics. Experienced clinicians probably arrive at a diagnosis through perception of a gestalt of speech abnormalities, rather than a simple listing of deviant characteristics. However, the gestalt is created by the cooccurrence of individual characteristics whose presence should be documented in support of the diagnosis. Table 15-4 lists the speech characteristics that are most helpful in distinguishing among the dysarthrias (and AOS). The list is not as exhaustive as those provided in each chapter on the individual dysarthrias, because only characteristics that are helpful in distinguishing among the dysarthrias are included. The distinctive characteristics of each single dysarthria type and its relationship to other dysarthria types are summarized as follows.

Flaccid Dysarthria

Phonatory and resonatory abnormalities are the most common distinguishing features of flaccid dysarthria. Continuous breathiness, diplophonia, audible inspiration, and short phrases—reflecting vocal fold or laryngeal-respiratory weakness—may be prominent when the vagus nerve is involved. They are uncommon or less pronounced in other dysarthria types. Laryngeal stridor can occur in hyperkinetic dysarthria, but it is usually accompanied by other obvious hyperkinesias. Short phrases can be present in spastic and hyperkinetic dysarthria, but they are generally not accompanied by continuous breathiness or other evidence of vocal fold weakness. Breathiness can occur in hypokinetic dysarthria and can be difficult to distinguish from the breathiness of flaccid dysarthria, although diplophonia and hoarseness in flaccid dysarthria may aid the distinction between the two types. Although hypernasality may occur in other dysarthria types—especially spastic and hypokinetic—it is usually most pronounced in flaccid dysarthria. Audible nasal emission and nasal snorting are uncommon in other dysarthria types. Finally, flaccid dysarthria is the only MSD in which rapid deterioration of speech can occur during continuous speaking (with recovery with rest), as in myasthenia gravis.

Spastic Dysarthria

A combination of slow rate, slow and regular speech AMRs, and a strained voice quality represent the "classic" speech pattern of spastic dysarthria. The cooccurrence of these three characteristics is unexpected in other dysarthria types. Strained voice quality can occur in hyperkinetic dysarthria (e.g., adductor spasmodic dysphonia) but is generally not associated with significant slowing of AMRs in a regular manner or a dramatic slowing of speech rate. Slow rate is not uncommon in other dysarthria types but usually is not also accompanied by strained voice quality. Slow rate and excess and equal stress can make spastic dysarthria difficult to distinguish from

ataxic dysarthria, but ataxic dysarthria is not associated with strained-strangled voice quality.

Ataxic Dysarthria

Irregular articulatory breakdowns during connected speech, irregular speech AMRs, and dysprosody are the primary distinctive features of ataxic dysarthria. These features can also be present in hyperkinetic and UUMN dysarthrias. However, adventitious movements of the jaw, face, or tongue—abnormalities not present in ataxic dysarthria—often accompany hyperkinetic dysarthria. UUMN dysarthria sometimes has ataxic-like irregular articulatory breakdowns; in such cases, the presence of unilateral lower facial weakness and lingual weakness may aid conclusions about dysarthria type, because isolated ataxic dysarthria usually is not associated with asymmetric facial or lingual weakness.

Hypokinetic Dysarthria

The classic constellation of speech characteristics associated with hypokinetic dysarthria include monopitch, monoloudness, reduced stress and loudness, a tendency toward rapid or accelerated rate, and rapid and blurred speech AMRs. Hypokinetic dysarthria is the only dysarthria in which rapid or accelerated rate may occur, and it is rapid rate that is most useful in differential diagnosis. It should be noted, however, that rapid or accelerated rate is not invariably present in hypokinetic dysarthria. Finally, although repeated phonemes and palilalia are not always present in hypokinetic dysarthria, their presence is distinctively associated with hypokinetic dysarthria.

Hyperkinetic Dysarthria

Hyperkinetic dysarthria can be manifest in multiple ways. Of all of the dysarthria types, it is probably the one in which visual observation during speech helps to define the disorder, because involuntary movements of the jaw, face, and tongue during speech so obviously explain many of its deviant auditory perceptual characteristics.

Speech abnormalities such as tremor or palatopharyngolaryngeal myoclonus distinguish hyperkinetic dysarthria from other types by their regularity. Unpredictable and variable speech abnormalities, such as chorea and dystonia, distinguish hyperkinetic dysarthria from other types by their capacity to unpredictably interrupt the flow of speech in nonstereotypic ways. Hyperkinetic dysarthria is the only dysarthria in which abnormal

Dimensions	Flaccid	Spastic	Ataxic	Dysarthria Hypokinetic	Hyperkinetic	Unilateral UMN	AOS
Hypernasality	++	+	–	+	+	–	–
Breathiness (continuous)	++	–	–	+	–	–	–
Diplophonia	++	–	–	–	–	–	–
Nasal emission (audible)	++	–	–	–	–	–	–
Audible inspiration (stridor)	++	–	–	–	+	–	–
Short phrases	++	+	–	–	+	–	–
Rapid deterioration & recovery with rest	++	–	–	–	–	–	–
Speaking on inhalation	++	–	–	–	–	–	–
Harshness	–	++	–	–	+	–	–
Low pitch	–	++	–	–	+	–	–
Slow rate	–	++	+	–	+	+	+
Strained-strangled quality	–	++	–	–	+	–	–
Pitch breaks	+	++	–	–	–	–	–
Slow & regular AMRs	–	++	–	–	–	–	–
Excess & equal stress	–	+	++	–	–	–	+
Irregular articulatory breakdowns	–	–	++	–	+	+	+
Irregular AMRs	–	–	++	–	++	+	–
Distorted vowels	–	–	++	–	++	–	+
Excess loudness variation	–	–	++	–	++	–	–
Prolonged phonemes	–	–	++	–	+	–	+
Telescoping of syllables	–	–	++	–	–	–	+
Monopitch	+	+	–	++	+	–	+
Reduced stress	–	–	–	++	–	–	–
Monoloudness	+	+	–	++	–	–	+
Reduced loudness	+	–	–	++	–	+	–
Inappropriate silences	–	–	–	++	+	–	–
Short rushes of speech	–	–	–	++	–	–	–
Variable rate	–	–	–	++	+	–	–
Increased rate in segments	–	–	–	++	–	–	–
Increased overall rate	–	–	–	++	–	–	–
Rapid, "blurred" AMRs	–	–	–	++	–	–	–
Repeated phonemes	–	–	–	++	–	–	+
Palilalia	–	–	–	++	–	–	–
Prolonged intervals	–	–	–	–	++	–	+
Sudden forced inspiration/expiration	–	–	–	–	++	–	–
Voice stoppages/arrests	–	–	–	–	++	–	–
Transient breathiness	–	–	–	–	++	–	–
Voice tremor	–	–	–	–	++	–	–
Myoclonic vowel prolongation	–	–	–	–	++	–	–
Intermittent hypernasality	–	–	–	–	++	–	–
Slow & irregular AMRs	–	–	+	–	++	–	–
Marked deterioration with increased rate	–	–	–	–	++	–	–
Inappropriate vocal noises	–	–	–	–	++	–	–
Echolalia	–	–	–	+	+	–	–
Coprolalia	–	–	–	–	++	–	–
Intermittent strained voice/arrests	–	–	–	–	++	–	–
Intermittent breathy/aphonic segments	–	+	–	–	++	–	–
Poorly sequenced SMRs	–	–	–	–	–	–	++
Articulatory groping	–	–	–	–	–	–	++
Distorted substitutions	–	–	–	–	–	–	++
Attempts at self-correction	–	–	–	–	–	–	++
Regressive articulatory errors	–	–	–	–	–	–	++
Reiterative articulatory errors	–	–	–	–	–	–	++
Metathetic articulatory errors	–	–	–	–	–	–	++
Articulatory additions/complications	–	–	–	–	–	–	++
Automatic > volitional speech	–	–	–	–	–	–	++
Inconsistent articulatory errors	–	–	+	–	+	–	++
Increased errors with increased length	–	–	–	–	–	–	++

+, May or may not be present but is not distinguishing by itself; ++, prominent or distinguishing, or both, (but not necessarily always present); –, never or uncommon and not distinguishing; AMRs, alternate motion rates; AOS, apraxia of speech; SMRs, sequential motion rates; UMN, upper motor neuron.

noises can interrupt speech or be produced when the patient is not speaking.

Hyperkinetic dysarthria is probably most frequently difficult to distinguish from spastic and ataxic dysarthria. The strained voice quality of spastic dysarthria may occur in hyperkinetic dysarthria, but hyperkinetic dysarthria can affect isolated speech valves, an unusual occurrence in spastic dysarthria. Variability of breakdowns can make hyperkinetic and ataxic dysarthria sound similar, but the presence of involuntary movements in hyperkinetic dysarthria generally helps to distinguish it from ataxic dysarthria.

Unilateral Upper Motor Neuron Dysarthria

UUMN dysarthria is distinguished from other dysarthria types more by its mildness and somewhat nebulous or mixed speech characteristics than by any distinctive characteristics of its own. It is probably most easily confused with flaccid, spastic, or ataxic dysarthria because of the predominance of imprecise articulation and the occasional presence of strained voice quality or irregular articulatory breakdowns. The fact that it is rarely accompanied by resonance or voice abnormalities and never associated with atrophy or fasciculations can help distinguish it from flaccid dysarthria. There is a tendency for AMRs in UUMN dysarthria to be regular, despite the occurrence of irregular articulatory breakdowns during contextual speech; this may help distinguish it from ataxic dysarthria, in which speech AMRs are usually irregular.

▣ DISTINGUISHING DYSARTHRIAS FROM APRAXIA OF SPEECH

Distinguishing between dysarthrias and AOS usually is not as difficult as distinguishing among the dysarthrias. Difficulties arise most often when attempting to differentiate AOS from ataxic dysarthria or when attempting to establish if both AOS and a dysarthria are simultaneously present. In the latter case, the separation of apraxic from UUMN dysarthric characteristics often must be made. The following subsections summarize the localization, etiologic, oral mechanism, and speech characteristics of AOS and dysarthria that best distinguish between them.

Anatomy and Vascular Distribution

Anatomically, AOS is a supratentorial disorder. It is nearly always associated with left hemisphere pathology, except in cases with right hemisphere or mixed language dominance. In contrast, dysarthrias can arise from supratentorial, posterior fossa, spinal, or peripheral lesions. Similarly, with vascular etiologies AOS is caused by carotid system lesions, usually in the distribution of the left middle cerebral artery, whereas dysarthrias can be associated with lesions in a much wider vascular distribution (see Table 15-1).

In terms of gross localization, therefore, AOS is most like spastic, hypokinetic, hyperkinetic, and UUMN dysarthria. In dysarthria, supratentorial lesions are more often subcortical than cortical, whereas lesions leading to AOS are probably more often cortical than subcortical. Of the supratentorial dysarthrias, UUMN dysarthria is the most difficult to distinguish from AOS.

Etiology

Table 15-2 summarizes etiologies associated with AOS and dysarthria in a manner that identifies etiologic similarities and distinctions among them. AOS is most often associated with nonhemorrhagic stroke, which can cause virtually any type of dysarthria. Similar to the dysarthrias, AOS can be caused by degenerative disease, although, as indicated in Table 15-2, there is no single degenerative disease that commonly causes AOS. There is also a large number of degenerative diseases that are never or only rarely associated with AOS, even though they frequently cause dysarthria. For example, patients whose only neurologic disorder is Parkinson's disease, multiple system atrophy, or spinocerebellar degeneration would not be expected to have AOS.

Similar to nearly all dysarthria types, traumatic injuries, neurosurgery, and tumors can produce AOS, although AOS is expected only when the lesion is in the left (dominant) hemisphere. In contrast to several dysarthria types, AOS is unusual in toxic/metabolic and infectious disorders, and it generally develops in inflammatory and demyelinating disorders only when they produce dominant hemisphere effects. Like all dysarthria types, except flaccid dysarthria, AOS does not occur in conditions with exclusive effects on the peripheral nervous system, such as neuromuscular junction disease and muscle disease.

Oral Mechanism Findings

Table 15-3 summarizes distinctive oral mechanism findings among the dysarthrias and AOS. It establishes that AOS can be present without any abnormal oral mechanism findings, an unusual occurrence for dysarthria (with the possible exceptions of ataxic and hyperkinetic dysarthria). AOS is often associated with right central facial weakness and somewhat less frequently with right lingual weakness, both of which occur frequently in UUMN dysarthria, but there is no causal relationship between such weakness and AOS when they do occur simultaneously. The one positive oral mechanism finding in AOS that is useful in differential diagnosis is the presence of nonverbal oral apraxia (NVOA), because NVOA is uncommon in dysarthria and has no obvious causal relationship with any dysarthria when the conditions occur together. Thus with the exception of NVOA, when any other characteristics noted in Table 15-3 are found in a patient with AOS, they probably represent incidental findings or raise the possibility of additional speech disorders.

Speech Characteristics

The distinction between AOS and dysarthria is dependent on the identification and interpretation of deviant speech characteristics. Table 15-4 makes it clear that AOS and some dysarthria types share several deviant characteristics. Differential diagnosis hinges mostly on the recognition of deviant speech characteristics found in AOS that are not present in dysarthrias.

General Distinctions

Some general distinctions between the dysarthrias and AOS include the following:

1. The speech and oral mechanism examinations usually make it apparent that the deviant characteristics of dysarthria are secondary to neuromuscular alterations, particularly those related to strength, tone, range, and steadiness of movement. Such alterations are not obvious in AOS or, when they are, do not explain its deviant characteristics.

2. In most dysarthrias, all components of speech—respiration, phonation, resonance, articulation, and prosody—can be affected. AOS is predominantly an articulatory and prosodic disorder.

3. Dysarthria is infrequently associated with aphasia. AOS is often associated with aphasia.

4. In dysarthria, deviant speech characteristics are generally consistent across utterances and are relatively uninfluenced by the degree of automaticity of the utterance, stimulus modality (e.g., spontaneous, reading, imitation), or linguistic variables. In AOS, errors across repetition of identical utterances may be variable, automatic speech may be somewhat better than propositional speech, and error rate may be influenced by variables such as word length and frequency of occurrence, meaningfulness, and stimulus modality.

5. The predominant articulatory abnormalities in dysarthrias are usually related to distortions or simplification of speech gestures. Distortions also are common in AOS, but perceived substitutions as well as additions, repetitions, prolongations, or complications of targeted sounds can also occur. Variable dysfluencies are probably more common in AOS than in dysarthria.

6. Dysarthric speakers rarely grope for correct articulatory postures or attempt to correct errors. Trial-and-error groping and attempts at self-correction are common in AOS.

Some Specific Distinctions

Perusal of Table 15-4 shows that AOS shares a number of deviant speech characteristics with spastic, hyperkinetic, and ataxic dysarthria. Because of this, the distinctions between these dysarthrias and AOS deserve attention.

1. Although they share a number of common features, AOS is usually not difficult to distinguish from spastic dysarthria. The deviant features of spastic dysarthria are usually highly predictable and consistent, regardless of stimulus or utterance conditions or characteristics. AOS is typically less predictable along several stimulus and response parameters. Spastic dysarthria is classically associated with a strained-harsh dysphonia and frequently with hypernasality, neither of which is usually present in AOS. Oral mechanism findings are also distinguishing. People with spastic dysarthria frequently have dysphagia, drooling, and pseudobulbar affect, as well as pathologic or hyperactive oromotor reflexes. The oral mechanism examination in speakers with AOS can be entirely normal or demonstrate only unrelated abnormalities. Aphasia occurs simultaneously more frequently with AOS than dysarthria.

2. Although hyperkinetic dysarthria can be predominantly an articulatory or prosodic problem, similar to AOS, the distinction between the two disorders usually is not difficult. The presence of visible involuntary movements in hyperkinetic dysarthria is common, whereas such movements are not present in AOS. Hyperkinetic dysarthria is generally not influenced by stimulus or response parameters, but AOS can be.

3. Ataxic dysarthria and AOS can be difficult to distinguish. This is not unexpected, given the cerebellum's role in motor control and coordination and the irregular nature of articula-

tory breakdowns and predominance of articulatory and prosodic abnormalities in ataxic dysarthria. AOS shares these features. In addition, oral mechanism examination in patients with ataxic dysarthria and AOS may be normal. The most helpful distinguishing speech characteristics between the two disorders are as follows: (1) speech AMRs are usually irregular in ataxic dysarthria but regular in AOS; (2) the sequencing of speech SMRs is usually normal in ataxic dysarthria but often abnormal in AOS; (3) irregular articulatory breakdowns and *variable* prosodic abnormalities are often more pervasive in ataxic dysarthria than in AOS; (4) automatic speech is no better than propositional speech in ataxic dysarthria, but a mismatch between them may exist in AOS; (5) ataxic speakers rarely grope for articulatory postures and do not usually attempt to correct articulatory errors, whereas many speakers with AOS do; and (6) perceived substitutions are not nearly as frequent in ataxic dysarthria as in AOS.

4. Although UUMN dysarthria and AOS do not share a large number of deviant features, they often occur together with left hemisphere lesions. In such cases, especially when UUMN dysarthria has ataxic-like features, it can be difficult to attribute specific errors/characteristics to one versus the other disorder. In most instances, such distinctions are not important to lesion localization (both problems may be localized to the left hemisphere). Relative to management, if the disorders coexist, the AOS is usually the focus of treatment.

▓ DISTINGUISHING MOTOR SPEECH DISORDERS FROM APHASIA

Dysarthria versus Aphasia

Distinguishing dysarthria from aphasia is not difficult. Distinctions between the two categories of disorder on anatomic, vascular, and etiologic grounds are the same as those that distinguish AOS from the dysarthrias. With the exception of right central facial weakness and sometimes right lingual weakness and NVOA, the aphasic patient's oral mechanism examination can be entirely normal. The language difficulties of aphasic patients are nearly always evident in their verbal and reading comprehension and writing, as well as in their verbal expression. In contrast, speakers with dysarthria alone do not have deficits in any input or output modality beyond speech, and their speech is linguistically normal. Their complaints regarding communication center

on speech production and not on word retrieval or language formulation or interpretation.

Even when dysarthria and aphasia occur simultaneously, it is generally not difficult to distinguish speech distortions associated with neuromuscular deficits from verbal deficits associated with inefficiencies and errors in language formulation and expression. However, when dysarthria reduces intelligibility, it can be difficult to establish if unintelligible content reflects only the dysarthria or is also a function of aphasic deficits. Delays during speech or attempts to revise utterances, however, may signal the presence of language difficulties. When these traits are not apparent, careful assessment of verbal and reading comprehension and writing can usually establish if aphasia is present. When aphasic difficulties are evident in other modalities, it can be assumed that language deficits are also present in spoken language.

Apraxia of Speech versus Aphasia

Distinguishing AOS from aphasia can be difficult for several reasons. First, there are no significant differences between the two disorders in their gross anatomic and vascular characteristics or in their etiology. Second, although aphasia frequently occurs in the absence of AOS, it is uncommon for AOS to be present in the absence of aphasia; the cooccurrence of the two disorders can make distinguishing between them difficult. Third, aphasic patients may make sound errors that are presumably linguistic (phonologic) in nature, whereas apraxic patients make sound errors that presumably reflect motor planning/programming problems. These two types of errors can be difficult to distinguish from one another, and they present the biggest challenge to differential diagnosis. Finally, patients with a prominent AOS and a less severe aphasia may nonetheless make some sound errors that are aphasic in nature, and patients with prominent aphasia and less severe or no apparent AOS may nonetheless make some sound errors that are apraxic in nature.

McNeil, Robin, and Schmidt[6] rightly state that "it is unlikely that a 'checklist' method of features can be developed that will allow the differential diagnosis of AOS . . . It is the behaviors that occur in particular clusters, likely influenced by severity, that allow the differential identification of AOS." This is true for the diagnosis of any MSD, but in order to build some sense of the members of distinguishing clusters, a listing of contrasts can be helpful. Table 15-5 summarizes the attributes of AOS and aphasia that may help to distinguish them. The following points clarify those distinctions.
1. Although AOS is usually accompanied by aphasia, AOS can occur independently of

table 15-5 Similarities and distinctions between AOS and aphasia		
	AOS	**Aphasia**
Localization	Left hemisphere, middle cerebral artery	Left hemisphere, middle cerebral artery
	Frontal > temporoparietal	Temporoparietal > frontal
Etiology	Stroke predominant	Stroke predominant
Accompanying Deficits	Aphasia frequent, often Broca's	AOS may or may not be present
	NVOA present > absent	NVOA less often present
	Right hemiparesis common	Right hemiparesis less common
Speech/Language	UUMN dysarthria probably common	UUMN dysarthria less common
	Nonspeech language modalities intact	Nonspeech language modalities impaired
	Need not mask detection of aphasia	May mask detection of AOS
	When aphasic, usually nonfluent in character	Fluent or nonfluent verbal output
	Prosody abnormal	Prosody normal
	Distortions frequent	Distortions infrequent
	Articulatory hesitancy & groping	Articulation effortless
	Often attempt to correct articulatory errors	Frequently unaware of articulatory errors
	Errors approximate target	Errors further from target
	Errors influenced by articulatory complexity	Errors less affected by complexity

AOS, Apraxia of speech; NVOA, nonverbal oral apraxia; UUMN, unilateral upper motor neuron.

aphasia. When AOS is "pure," there is no difficulty with verbal or reading comprehension, and the linguistic aspects of writing can be normal. In contrast, and by definition, aphasia is a multimodality disorder of language.

2. Aphasic verbal deficits can be severe enough to mask the presence of AOS, in that a sufficient and valid speech sample for AOS diagnosis might not be obtainable. AOS need not mask identification of aphasia, however. Even if AOS is severe enough to produce muteness, careful assessment of other language modalities can establish if language deficits are present. If AOS is isolated, performance in other language modalities is normal. If aphasia is present, careful examination can detect language deficits in other modalities.

3. When AOS and aphasia occur simultaneously and the AOS is moderately severe or worse, the patient's profile of difficulty across language modalities is disproportionately severe in the verbal output modality. This is often apparent during casual observation and may also be apparent in response profiles across language modalities on standard aphasia examinations. For example, patients with AOS or AOS plus aphasia often have poorer percentile scores on the verbal subtests of the *Porch Index of Communicative Ability (PICA)*[7] than in any other modality tested. In addition, the multimodality scoring scale used in the PICA often shows a disproportionate number of "4-7-14" responses on verbal subtests, scores that reflect a predom-

inance of unintelligible, close approximation or distorted speech responses, a pattern uncommon in aphasic patients who do not have an accompanying AOS.

4. Patients with AOS alone or AOS plus aphasia often have distinctive profiles on other standard aphasia tests, usually falling into one of the "nonfluent" categories of aphasia. On the *Boston Diagnostic Aphasia Examination*[4] and the *Western Aphasia Battery*,[5] they often are classified as having Broca's aphasia and are rarely classified as having one of the so-called transcortical aphasias or fluent aphasias such as Wernicke's or anomic aphasia. On the *Minnesota Test for the Differential Diagnosis of Aphasia*,[9] aphasic patients with AOS often are classified as having *aphasia with sensorimotor impairment*.

5. AOS with or without aphasia is probably more commonly associated with UUMN dysarthria than is aphasia without AOS. This probably reflects the tighter alignment of the neuromuscular execution system with motor speech planning/programming mechanisms than with the language mechanism. Similarly, although AOS and aphasia are usually accompanied by right-sided motor findings, the association between right hemiparesis and AOS is probably stronger than that between such deficits and aphasia.

6. In general, AOS is more often associated with posterior frontal or insular lesions than lesions in the temporal or parietal lobes, whereas

aphasia without AOS tends to be associated with temporal or temporoparietal lesions.

7. Because phonologic errors can be frequent in aphasia, especially in Wernicke's and conduction aphasia, it is the distinction between them and AOS that is most difficult. Careful consideration of these distinctions by McNeil, Robin, and Schmidt*[6] plus prior contributions by a number of investigators[1,2,3,10,12] provide helpful clues in this regard. They include the following:

a. Patients with AOS have articulation and fairly pervasive prosodic disturbances, including slow rate, difficulty increasing rate, segregated syllables, and increased interword intervals. Wernicke's and other fluent aphasic speakers usually have normal rate and prosody for phonemically on-target utterances. Even when substitutions are perceived in AOS, they are usually also distorted and produced in a context of slow rate and sometimes articulatory hesitancy or effort. Distortions can lead to a perception that non-English phonemes have been produced. In contrast, aphasic phonologic errors are usually perceived as well articulated (nondistorted) English phonemes, even when hesitancy or effort accompanies them.

b. Apraxic speakers often recognize and attempt to self-correct their articulatory errors. Phonologic errors are more likely (although certainly not always) to go unnoticed by aphasic patients without AOS.

c. Apraxic errors are more consistent in location and type and generally closer to the articulatory target than phonologic errors. For example, the word "banana" may be produced slowly and with distortion and effort as "bamama" by an apraxic speaker but as "streeble" by a speaker with Wernicke's aphasia; repeated attempts generally would be less variable in the apraxic than the aphasic speaker.

8. Treatment that facilitates language production in aphasia is not effective for AOS, and treatment that facilitates speech production in AOS is not effective for aphasia (management of AOS is discussed in Chapter 18).

---

*McNeil, Robin, and Schmidt[6] provide a detailed contrast among the prosodic, phonologic, kinematic, and related features of AOS and phonemic paraphasias. Their critical discussion of these distinctions calls into question the differential diagnostic value of some speech characteristics previously associated with AOS. For the most part, the distinctions addressed here are compatible with those proposed by McNeil, Robin, and Schmidt.

■ DISTINGUISHING AMONG FORMS OF NEUROGENIC MUTISM

Distinguishing among different forms of neurogenic mutism can be difficult, but a number of nonverbal communicative behaviors and other observations often permit such distinctions. Table 15-6 summarizes major distinguishing features among anarthric, AOS, aphasic, and cognitive-affective forms of mutism. Etiology is not of particular value to differential diagnosis, except that conditions that have diffuse or multifocal effects are more likely to be associated with mutism associated with cognitive/affective disturbances than with anarthria, AOS, or aphasia. Conversely, conditions that produce focal disturbances, such as stroke, are more likely to produce mutism associated with motor speech or language disturbances.

The following subsections summarize the clues that help distinguish among the forms of neurogenic mutism.

Anarthria

Anarthric patients usually have significant and obvious neuromuscular deficits in the bulbar muscles that help explain the basis for their mutism. Dysphagia, drooling, pseudobulbar affect, and pathologic oromotor reflexes associated with anarthria may not be present at all in apraxic and aphasic mutism and may be absent or less pronounced in mutism that reflects cognitive/affective disturbances. Similarly, quadriplegia or evidence of weakness, spasticity, rigidity, and movement disorders in the limbs (and bulbar muscles) may be prominent in anarthric patients and absent or less evident in other forms of mutism.

Anarthria is occasionally present without significant limb motor deficits. This can lead to its misdiagnosis as aphasia, AOS, or even psychogenic mutism. However, the significant dysphagia and other oromotor abnormalities associated with anarthria help clarify diagnosis because anarthric mutism in the absence of nonspeech oromotor abnormalities rarely, if ever, occurs.

Anarthric patients can be normally alert and responsive even if their alertness and ability to respond is evident only in eye movements (as in locked-in syndrome). Their responses may be initiated fairly rapidly, in contrast to slower response initiation in other forms of mutism, such as akinetic mutism. Finally, when anarthric patients attempt speech, their slowness and restricted range of articulatory movements and their reduced loudness and strained-groaning-effortful phonatory quality help establish the neuromuscular basis of their disorder.

table 15-6 Distinctions among major types of mutism

	Motor Speech		Language	Cognitive/Affective	
	Anarthria	**AOS**	**Aphasia**	**Decreased Arousal/ Diffuse Cortical Dysfunction**	**Akinetic Mutism**
Etiology (Most Common)	Stroke, CHI	Stroke	Stroke	CHI, anoxia, infectious, inflammatory	Stroke, tumor, CHI
Localization	Bilateral UMN Bilateral LMN Basal ganglia Cerebellum	Left hemisphere	Left hemisphere	Reticular activating system	Frontal lobes/limbic system
Mechanism	Neuromuscular (dysarthria)	Motor programming	Language	Arousal Cognitive	Drive, initiative Cognitive
Accompanying Deficits	Dysphagia Quadriparesis Weakness Spasticity Rigidity Hyperkinesias Pathologic reflexes	Aphasia NVOA Hemiparesis	Multimodality language deficits AOS NVOA Hemiparesis	Coma Unresponsiveness Altered tone/posture Pathologic reflexes	Abulia Delayed responses Unresponsiveness Apathy Pathologic reflexes
Retained Capacities	Alert Responsive in other modalities	Alert Responsive & accurate in other language modalities Normal chew/ swallow	Alert Responsive but inaccurate in other language modalities Normal chew/ swallow	Minimal	Alert Normal but slow chew & swallow
Speech & Vocal Characteristics When Present	Severe dysarthria with severely reduced intelligibility	Limited sound repertoire, few meaningful or nonmeaningful utterances	Automatic social utterances Stereotypic recurrent utterances	Vocalization (cry, groan, shout)	Delayed, unelaborated, concrete responses Aphonic, whispered, reduced in loudness, monotonous

AOS, Apraxia of speech; CHI, closed head injury; LMN, lower motor neuron; NVOA, nonverbal oral apraxia; UMN, upper motor neuron.

Apraxia of Speech

Apraxic mutism, in contrast to anarthria, can be associated with a normal oral mechanism examination or evidence only of right lingual or central facial weakness. Reflexive facial movements, such as yawning, smiling, and crying are normal, and there may be no significant drooling or dysphagia. The reflexive cough may be normal and may actually contain traces of normal sounding phonation, an unusual finding in anarthria.

Mute apraxic patients attempt to perform nonverbal oromotor tasks; if NVOA is present, responses may be off target and reflect groping or efforts at self-correction, but range and rate of movement during such attempts may be normal. Right hemiplegia may or may not be present. Limb apraxia in both upper extremities may be evident. NVOA and limb apraxia are not commonly encountered in cognitive/affective forms of mutism, although they may be present in mute aphasic patients. In contrast to aphasic and mute patients with cognitive/affective disturbances, the performance of mute apraxic patients in other language modalities may be initiated and completed rapidly and accurately. As a general rule, however, muteness due to AOS is nearly always accompanied by some degree of aphasia, so difficulty in other language modalities is often evident.

Mute apraxic patients usually attempt to speak and display frustration at their inability to do so, in contrast to the indifference that is common in muteness associated with cognitive-affective disturbances. Finally, the mute apraxic patient may occasionally curse when frustrated or respond reflexively with a "hi" or "bye," or few notes of a song in unison singing, even when he or she is otherwise mute.

Aphasia

The mute aphasic patient may be much like the mute apraxic patient on oral mechanism examination and during reflexive oromotor responses, except that he or she may not follow verbal directions for such examination as readily because of verbal comprehension deficits. Their aphasia is almost always severe when mutism is present, so they perform poorly on measures of verbal and reading comprehension and writing. Similar to apraxic patients and in contrast to many people with nonaphasic cognitive/affective disturbances (e.g., akinetic mutism), they may respond emotionally to their deficits and other events.

Cognitive-Affective Disturbances

Mutism associated with cognitive-affective disturbances can be attributed to decreased arousal, alertness, drive, or initiative, as well as to higher-level cognitive deficits. When the reticular activating system is impaired, the muteness may be associated with coma or hypoarousal or to complete lack of alertness, eye contact, or responsiveness. These states are dissimilar to those of anarthric or mute apraxic or aphasic patients.

When muteness is associated with frontal lobe/limbic system deficits, as in akinetic mutism, the patient may be awake and seemingly alert, and eye contact may be achieved. The patient may eat

slowly and retain food in the mouth, unchewed or simply never swallowed, but swallowing may be adequate once the pharyngeal phase is initiated.

If the akinetically mute patient is responsive, responses are typically delayed, with the delay characterized by apathetic silence or lack of evidence of effort, in contrast to anarthric or mute aphasic or apraxic individuals, who usually attempt to speak. Unresponsiveness or delayed responses are as evident nonverbally and in other language modalities as they are in the failure to speak; such traits are unusual in other forms of neurogenic mutism. When such patients do speak, speech emerges after lengthy delays; is brief and unelaborated; and is whispered, aphonic, or markedly reduced in loudness and prosodically flat. In contrast, articulation may be normal, although sometimes with reduced range of articulatory movement. Such phonatory characteristics, in the presence of good articulation, are much less common in individuals emerging from anarthria, AOS, and aphasia.

▪ DISTINGUISHING MOTOR SPEECH DISORDERS FROM OTHER NEUROGENIC SPEECH DISORDERS

Chapter 13 addressed several neurogenic speech disturbances that bear various relationships to dysarthrias and AOS. Aphasia was discussed at that time, and its distinction from MSDs has already been addressed in this chapter. Distinctions between other neurogenic speech disturbances and MSDs are now addressed. A number of them are summarized in Tables 15-7 and 15-8.

table 15-7	Distinctions among dysfluencies associated with neurogenic stuttering, palilalia, motor speech disorders, and aphasia				
	Neurogenic Stuttering	**Palilalia**	**Dysarthria**	**AOS**	**Aphasia**
Localization	CNS motor system (multiple loci) Often bilateral, when persistent	Bilateral basal Ganglia	CNS motor system (multiple loci)	Left hemisphere	Left hemisphere
Mechanism	Unknown (? Dysequilibrium)	? motor disinhibition	Neuromuscular	Motor programming	Language
Speech Characteristics	Sound/syllable/word dysfluencies only or dysfluencies disproportionate or not explainable by coexisting motor speech or aphasic disorder	Reiterative word and phrase repetition only Frequently associated with hypokinetic dysarthria	Sound/syllable/ word dysfluencies consistent with characteristics of dysarthria, plus dysarthria	Sound/syllable/ word dysfluencies consistent with characteristics of AOS, plus AOS	Sound/ syllable/word dysfluencies consistent with language deficit, plus language deficits

AOS, Apraxia of speech; CNS, central nervous system.

| table 15-8 | Distinctions among abulia, aprosodia, hypokinetic and unilateral UMN dysarthrias, and depression |

	Abulia	Aprosodia	Unilateral UMN Dysarthria	Hypokinetic Dysarthria	Depression
Localization	Frontal/limbic system (bilateral)	Right hemisphere	Upper motor neuron	Basal ganglia control circuit	No structural lesion
Mechanism	Cognitive-affective	Uncertain	Weakness/? incoordination	Rigidity, bradykinesia, hypokinesia	Mood disorder
Speech/Language					
Prosody	Reduced (flat, emotionless, apathetic)	Reduced (flat, indifferent, robotlike, stereotypic)	Normal or dysprosodic	Reduced (flat, monopitch, monoloudness)	Reduced (flat, monopitch, monoloudness)
Loudness	Reduced/ hypophonic	Normal	Normal or mildly reduced	Reduced/ hypophonic	Reduced
Articulation	Normal	Normal	Impaired	Impaired	Normal
Rate	Normal or slow	Normal	Normal or mildly slow	Normal, slow, or fast	Slow or normal
Dysfluencies	No	No	No	Sometimes	No
Response latency	Slow	Normal	Normal	Slow or normal	Slow or normal
Content	Brief, unelaborated, concrete	Normal linguistic structure & complexity	Normal linguistic structure & complexity	Normal linguistic structure & complexity	Unelaborated but normal linguistically
Complaints	None	Speech does not convey emotion	Speech imprecise	Speech imprecise & loudness reduced	No speech complaints

UMN, Upper motor neuron.

Neurogenic Stuttering

The line distinguishing neurogenic stuttering from the dysarthrias and AOS can be drawn in several places because neurogenic dysfluencies are so heterogeneous in their behavioral and neuroanatomic underpinnings. When significant dysfluencies are present, the challenge is to decide if they are a component of dysarthria, AOS, or aphasia, or if they represent a separate, independent disorder. This decision has implications for localization and behavioral management. The distinctions among the various neurogenic speech disorders associated with dysfluencies are summarized in Table 15-7.

Dysarthria and Neurogenic Stuttering

Dysfluencies can occur in dysarthria, probably more frequently in hypokinetic dysarthria than in any other type. They should not be encountered in flaccid dysarthria, however, and when they are it should be assumed that there is either a CNS-based dysfunc-

tion in addition to the lower motor neuron (LMN) lesion or lesions causing the flaccid dysarthria, or that the dysfluencies are maladaptively compensatory or psychogenic in origin.

Dysfluencies associated with hypokinetic dysarthria tend to occur at the beginning of phrases and are characterized by rapid and sometimes blurred initial sound or syllable repetitions. They are consistent with the rapid or accelerated rate and reduced range of articulatory movement that characterize the gestalt of hypokinetic dysarthria and should be considered one of the defining characteristics of the hypokinetic dysarthria rather than a separate disorder. When dysfluencies are a prominent feature of a hypokinetic dysarthria, it is appropriate to describe the speech disorder as a "hypokinetic dysarthria with prominent dysfluencies." This designation implies that a single rather than two speech disorders are present and that a single lesion or disease process involving the basal ganglia is responsible. Highlighting the dysfluencies in the dysarthria diagnosis may signal a need to address them specifically in management efforts.

Apraxia of Speech and Neurogenic Stuttering

Hesitations, repetitions, and prolongations of sounds and syllables can occur in AOS. These dysfluencies may reflect efforts to establish or revise articulatory targets or movements and may be linked to the searching, groping, off-target efforts of many apraxic speakers. When they reflect compensatory efforts to correct sound or movement errors, they are best considered as characteristics of AOS and not as a separate disorder. When they are a prominent characteristic of AOS, it is appropriate to describe the disorder as "AOS with prominent dysfluencies," a designation indicating that a single rather than two speech disorders are present and that a single lesion or disease process in the left hemisphere is probably responsible. Highlighting the dysfluencies in the diagnosis may signal a need to address them specifically during management.

Aphasia and Neurogenic Stuttering

Dysfluencies can occur in aphasia as a manifestation of word retrieval difficulties or efforts to correct linguistic errors or organize verbal expression. They may be characterized by fillers ("um," "well uh"); hesitations and prolongations; and sound, syllable, word, and even short phrase repetitions. When dysfluencies are part of the numerous manifestations of aphasic verbal impairments, they should not be singled out as a distinct, separate disorder. When they are prominent, they should be highlighted in the diagnosis as "aphasia whose verbal output characteristics include prominent dysfluencies," a designation that implies that the aphasia and dysfluencies share the same etiology and left hemisphere localization. Highlighting the prominence of dysfluencies suggests that they may deserve attention during therapy.

Neurogenic Stuttering as a Distinct Diagnosis

When dysfluencies are the only evident speech abnormality or when their characteristics are not compatible with a cooccurring dysarthria, AOS, or aphasia, and when psychogenic explanations for them can be ruled out, they deserve a designation as neurogenic stuttering. The diagnosis of neurogenic stuttering as a distinct entity is more than an academic exercise because it implies the presence of neurologic disease when there may be no other such evidence and may broaden the possible etiologies and anatomic loci of the neuropathology to numerous areas of the nervous system if it is not consistent with dysfluencies associated with AOS, aphasia, or a single type of dysarthria. Relative to management, it identifies a disorder for which intervention may be appropriate.

Palilalia

The differential diagnosis of palilalia is not difficult, because the behaviors that define it—compulsive repetition of one's own words and phrases—has little behavioral overlap with MSDs and other neurogenic speech disturbances (see Table 15-7).

The stereotypic prosody, progressively increased rate and decreased loudness, the sometimes numerous repetitions, and the definitional limitation of palilalia to word and phrase repetition (as opposed to sound or syllable repetitions) help distinguish it from dysfluencies associated with AOS, aphasia, and neurogenic stuttering. In addition, when apraxic and aphasic speakers repeat words or phrases, they are often accompanied by obvious efforts to articulate or express specific meanings, as well as slowed rate and attempts at self-correction. Palilalic speakers tend to speak rapidly and without effort, and they show no obvious attempts to inhibit their repetitions.

Palilalia often occurs with hypokinetic dysarthria, though not invariably. Both disorders usually reflect bilateral basal ganglia pathology. The typical dysfluencies associated with hypokinetic dysarthria involve sound and syllable repetitions, and the repetitions tend to occur at the beginning of utterances or phrases; palilalic repetitions tend to occur at the end of utterances. When word and phrase repetitions occur frequently with hypokinetic dysarthria, it is appropriate to identify the presence of both hypokinetic dysarthria and palilalia.

Echolalia

There is minimal overlap between echolalia and motor speech and other neurogenic speech disorders. Echolalic utterances are motorically normal, so they should not be confused with dysarthria or AOS. In contrast to palilalia, echolalia involves the repetition of others' utterances and not one's own utterances, and it generally does not involve multiple, uninterrupted repetitions.* Because echolalia is motorically precise and does not involve sound or syllable dysfluencies, it should not be confused with neurogenic stuttering. Although it can occur with aphasia (and diffuse cognitive deficits), it is not simply a manifestation of aphasia because it is usually associated with diffuse or multifocal lesions that extend beyond the perisylvian language zone.

Cognitive and Affective Disturbances (Abulia)

Cognitive and affective disturbances can lead to mutism (already discussed). At lesser degrees of

---

*Palilalia and echolalia can occur simultaneously, however.

severity, they can alter speech in ways that resemble MSDs, especially hypokinetic dysarthria.

When damage to frontal lobe activating mechanisms leads to abulia, speech initiation may be delayed and then characterized by reduced loudness, hypophonia, and flattened prosody. These characteristics are also encountered in hypokinetic dysarthria. Two general observations can help distinguish abulic speech from hypokinetic dysarthria. First, the content of the abulic patient's speech is usually brief, unelaborated, and concrete, and the delay in initiating an utterance is unaccompanied by behavioral evidence of effort. In contrast, speech content in those with hypokinetic dysarthria may be normal in length and linguistic and cognitive complexity, and delays in initiating speech may contain evidence of physical effort to initiate speech. Second, the abulic patient's speech rate is slow or normal and does not accelerate, and articulation is precise and without dysfluency. Hypokinetic dysarthria can be associated with rapid or accelerated rate, speech AMRs can be rapid or blurred, and articulation can be imprecise and sometimes dysfluent (see Table 15-8 for summary).

Aprosodia

Aprosodia associated with right hemisphere lesions can be difficult to distinguish from dysarthria and from the speech characteristics of patients with attenuated speech associated with abulia or frontal/limbic pathology. Because aprosodia is not well understood or described, only a few guidelines can be offered for differential diagnosis (see Table 15-8 for summary).

Aprosodia versus Dysarthria

UUMN dysarthria can result from right hemisphere lesions and may explain speech abnormalities without invoking a separate disorder of aprosodia as an explanation for them (see Chapter 13 for a discussion of some of these issues). In addition, the prosodic deficits of patients with hypokinetic dysarthria can resemble those of aprosodic patients with right hemisphere lesions. However, these dysarthrias can often be distinguished from aprosodia on the basis of some of their predominant speech characteristics. Such distinctions include the following:
1. Aprosodia is characterized by flat, indifferent, or stereotypic prosodic patterns, without obvious distortions, irregular articulatory breakdowns, or reductions in loudness or rate. UUMN dysarthria is primarily an articulatory disorder characterized by imprecise consonants and sometimes by irregular artic-

ulatory breakdowns; prosodic deficits, if present, may be more dysprosodic than aprosodic and tied to articulatory imprecision or breakdown. Both prosody and articulation are impaired in hypokinetic dysarthria, loudness may be reduced, and rate is sometimes increased.
2. The aprosodic speaker may be noticeably deficient in his or her ability to produce correct intonational patterns on imitation or in conversation or affective prosodic tasks. The speaker with UUMN dysarthria may approximate such intonational patterns fairly well.
3. The aprosodic speaker may convey linguistic stress adequately but express affective prosody poorly. The prosodic patterns of people with UUMN or hypokinetic dysarthria generally do not vary as a function of linguistic or affective stimulus or response parameters.
4. Aprosodic patients may complain about their inability to convey felt emotions but rarely complain about articulatory imprecision. UUMN and hypokinetic dysarthric speakers may have the opposite pattern of complaints.

Aprosodia versus Abulia

The flattened prosody of aprosodia can be similar to that of abulic patients with frontal/limbic pathology. The distinction between the two disorders may be made more on the basis of content and general behavior than the speech characteristics themselves, although speech distinctions may also exist. These distinctions may include the following:
1. Aprosodic patients generally have normal response latency and normally long (sometimes excessively long) narrative responses, in contrast to the delayed, unelaborated, and concrete responses of the abulic patient.
2. Aprosodic patients may be quite responsive nonverbally (except when neglect interferes), in contrast to abulic patients, who can be as slow and impoverished in their nonverbal as in their verbal behavior.
3. Aprosodic patients may state that they feel emotions, and their linguistic content may reflect such emotions. In contrast, the abulic patient's apathy, indifference, and impoverished thought are often as evident in the content of their speech as they are in their tone.
4. Aprosodic patients may have normal loudness and are not usually hypophonic. Their prosodic pattern may be stereotypic but not unvarying in loudness, duration, or pitch and

not suggestive of apathy. In contrast, abulic patients' speech is often reduced in loudness or hypophonic, and prosody may sound truly apathetic.

▣ DISTINGUISHING NEUROGENIC FROM PSYCHOGENIC SPEECH DISORDERS

Distinguishing neurogenic from psychogenic speech disorders is important but sometimes difficult. The distinction is important because it can send medical diagnostic and management efforts down a neurologic versus a psychiatric pathway. The distinction can be difficult, because the speech characteristics associated with neurogenic and psychogenic disorders can be quite similar and because neurogenic and psychogenic speech disorders can occur simultaneously.

Psychogenic speech disorders were addressed in Chapter 14. A number of clues useful to differential diagnosis were reviewed in that chapter, and the reader should refer to it for details that are not repeated here. In this section, an attempt is made to summarize the distinctions between the characteristics of some of the more common psychiatric disturbances and the MSDs with which they can be confused. Psychogenic speech disturbances associated with conversion disorders and life stresses are emphasized, because they are the problems that challenge differential diagnosis most frequently in speech pathology practices.

Depression

Because the speech of depressed people tends to be characterized by monopitch, monoloudness, and reduced stress and loudness, it may raise suspicions about hypokinetic dysarthria. The distinction can be complicated further by the common occurrence of depression in Parkinson's disease.

In addition to nonspeech physical findings on neurologic examination (e.g., resting tremor) that help distinguish Parkinson's disease from depression, there are some clues in speech that distinguish the speech of depression from that of hypokinetic dysarthria. Some of them are similar to those that help distinguish among abulia, aprosodia, and dysarthria (see Table 15-8). The distinctions include the following:

1. Depressed individuals' contextual speech and speech AMRs tend to be slow or normal in rate. Hypokinetic dysarthria may be associated with rapid or accelerated speech and AMRs.
2. The speech of depression reflects attenuations in loudness and prosody, but articulatory precision is not generally affected;

hypokinetic dysarthria can be characterized by significant articulatory imprecision. In addition, voice quality is generally adequate in depressed people, whereas dysphonia, breathy, or aphonic quality is often present in hypokinetic dysarthria.
3. The facial expression of depressed people conveys sadness, whereas hypokinetic speakers may appear expressionless or devoid of emotion. Saliva accumulation; drooling; dysphagia; and jaw, lip, and tongue tremulousness are common in hypokinetic dysarthria but generally are not present in depression.

Schizophrenia

Schizophrenic speech is not difficult to distinguish from MSDs. It may, however, be difficult to distinguish from that of individuals with Wernicke's aphasia (see Chapter 14).

Conversion Disorders and Responses to Life Stress

People with psychogenic speech disorders that reflect conversion reactions (or other somatoform disorders) or responses to life stress present to medical speech pathologists who work closely with neurologists or otorhinolaryngologists. Many of them have been on a long medical journey in search of an organic explanation for their speech disorder, and many report being dismissed by physicians with an explanation that "there's nothing wrong with you" or "it's all in your head." Some of these patients have undetected neurologic disease, but many do not. The diagnosis often becomes evident during careful review of the history of the speech disorder and psychosocial issues, examination of speech, and behavioral efforts to modify the speech disorder.

History

Points about the history that may be of value to distinguishing psychogenic from neurogenic disturbances were addressed in Chapter 14. In general, the following contrasts between the histories of people with psychogenic versus neurogenic speech disorders are useful in differential diagnosis (see Table 15-9 for summary).

Relative to people with neurogenic speech disorders are the following:

1. The onset of psychogenic speech disorders is more frequently associated with a cold or nonneurologic illness or a physically (but nonneurologic) or psychologically traumatic event.

table 15-9	Distinctions between psychogenic (conversion and stress-related) speech disorders and neurogenic speech disorders

	Relative to Neurogenic Speech Disorders, Conversion and Stress-Related Speech Disorders Tend To Be Associated with …
History	Nonneurologic illness or nonneurologic physical trauma at onset
	Prior history of unexplained speech or other physical deficits
	Ongoing psychologic stress/conflict unrelated to speech or other physical symptoms
	Evidence of primary or secondary gain
	Denial of possibility that psychologic factors may be playing a role
	Unexplained fluctuations in presence and severity of symptoms or fluctuations as a function of situational emotional content
	Indifference to the speech disturbance
Examination	Speech characteristics that do not fit known patterns of neurogenic speech disorders
	Inconsistencies between speech characteristics and oral mechanism examination findings
	Variability in severity or specific speech characteristics as a function of task or emotional content
	Improvement or worsening of symptoms as a function of clinician suggestion
	Improvement of speech when distracted
	A pattern of speech fatigue inconsistent with common patterns of speech changes with physical fatigue
	Significant, sometimes rapid improvement in speech with symptomatic therapy

2. Psychogenic speech disorders are more frequently associated with a prior history of unexplained speech disturbance or other physical deficits of unexplained origin.

3. Psychogenic speech disorders are more frequently associated with ongoing psychologic stress or conflict, unrelated to those in response to the individual's speech or other physical symptoms. People with neurogenic speech disturbances are more likely to complain of stress generated by their speech and other physical symptoms.

4. Psychogenic speech disorders are more frequently associated with evidence of "gain" from the speech disorder, such as avoidance of confrontation or leave of absence from a hated job requiring normal speech).

5. People with psychogenic speech disorders are more likely to deny the experience of stress, anxiety, or conflict and more likely to deny the possibility that their speech problem may be related to such psychologic states.

6. Unexplained fluctuations in the presence or severity of the speech disorder, especially as a function of stress and anxiety in specific situations, are more likely in psychogenic speech disorders.

7. Indifference to the speech disturbance is more likely in psychogenic speech disorders. It is important to distinguish indifference from stoicism and denial, however, because many people dealing with organic disease respond in a stoic manner. Denial of speech difficulty caused by neurologic disease is not unusual when the problem is mild or before a neurologic diagnosis has been made.

Examination Observations

Chapter 14 summarized important questions that should be addressed during the examination of individuals with suspected psychogenic speech disorders. Their purpose is to determine if the disorder follows the lawful patterns of speech deficits and oral mechanism examination findings that exist for motor speech and other neurogenic speech disorders. Table 15-9 summarizes the answers to these questions as they relate to differential diagnosis. They apply to the differential diagnosis of psychogenic voice disorders, psychogenic stuttering and mutism, and other psychogenic speech disturbances that affect articulation, resonance, or prosody. The reader is referred to Chapter 14 for descriptions of the specific characteristics of these psychogenic disturbances and some additional clues that help distinguish them from neurogenic speech disorders.

It is particularly noteworthy that neurogenic and psychogenic speech disturbances can and do occur together and that distinguishing between them can be difficult. It is not unusual, for example, to conclude that a patient has both a neurogenic and a psychogenic speech disorder, the psychogenic disorder representing a response to the neurologic disease or one or more of its outward signs. It is also possible for psychogenic and neurogenic speech disorders to coexist as independent, unrelated entities. Missing the coexistence of these disorders can have serious consequences for medical diagnosis, as well as for medical and behavioral management.

Cases

A total of 73 cases were reviewed at the end of Chapters 4 through 14. Each illustrated the history, clinical findings, and diagnostic interpretations and conclusions drawn from the examination of people with specific MSDs, related neurogenic speech disorders, or psychogenic speech disorders. The diagnosis in many of the cases was fairly straightforward, in keeping with the intent to illustrate unambiguously the specific disorders discussed in each chapter. However, approximately two thirds of the cases illustrated problems in differential diagnosis, either during medical workups before speech pathology assessment or during the speech evaluation itself. The reader might want to reread these cases at this time, because they illustrate that diagnosis can be straightforward or tentative or uncertain. The following list organizes in a general way some of the more diagnostically challenging cases that were presented in Chapters 4 through 14:

Distinguishing among the dysarthrias: Cases 4-2, 4-4, 4-5, 5-1 through 5-3, 6-6, 7-3, 8-3, 8-4, 8-6, 8-7, 10-1, 10-5, 10-8, 10-9, and 11-4.

Distinguishing among motor speech disorders and other neurogenic speech disorders: Cases 5-2, 7-1, 11-7, 12-1 through 12-5, 13-3, and 13-5 through 13-7.

Recognizing the presence of more than one neurogenic speech disorder: Cases 9-6, 11-2 through 11-7, 13-1, 13-2, and 13-6.

Distinguishing neurogenic from nonneurogenic or psychogenic speech disorders: Cases 4-1, 5-2, 6-6, 8-6, 9-5, 10-3, 10-5, and 14-1 through 14-8.

SUMMARY

1. Differential diagnosis is the process of narrowing diagnostic possibilities and reaching conclusions about the nature of a deficit. It requires the application of knowledge and clinical skill to a specific clinical problem.

2. Speech examination should always lead to an attempt at diagnosis. If a diagnosis is not possible, the reasons why should be stated. A specific diagnosis should never be stated if one cannot be determined.

3. Diagnosis of a neurogenic speech disorder should be related to the suspected or known neurologic diagnosis or lesion localization. This may help confirm or modify neurologic diagnosis and localization.

4. Different speech disturbances can occur simultaneously, so multiple diagnoses are possible in any given patient. At the same time, referral for speech examination does not guarantee abnormal findings. A diagnosis of normal speech is among the diagnostic possibilities in many cases.

5. Although the fixing of a diagnostic label carries certain risks, it is convenient shorthand for communicating information concisely and precisely.

6. Distinguishing among the dysarthrias can be difficult, because there is considerable overlap among their characteristics and because various combinations of them can be present within individuals. However, the dysarthrias differ in their anatomic and vascular localization, etiologic distributions, oral mechanism findings, and speech characteristics. Although many deviant speech characteristics are associated with several major types of dysarthria, diagnosis is often derived from the recognition of only a few deviant characteristics that are distinctive of a given dysarthria type.

7. When a distinction between dysarthria and AOS must be made, distinguishing AOS from ataxic or UUMN dysarthria is usually most difficult. Diagnosis usually depends on recognizing deviant speech characteristics commonly associated with AOS that are uncommon in the dysarthrias.

8. The distinction between dysarthrias and aphasia is usually not difficult, but distinguishing AOS from aphasia can be. Although there are some differences between AOS and aphasia in their sound level error characteristics, the distinction between the two disorders must often rely on confirmatory evidence from oral mechanism and language examinations, the prosodic features of speech, and patients' responses to their articulatory difficulties.

9. Distinguishing among various forms of neurogenic mutism generally relies on nonverbal communicative behaviors and other nonspeech observations. The constellation of deficits that accompany mutism and identification of retained capacities are most useful to diagnosis.

10. The diagnosis of neurogenic stuttering depends on recognizing dysfluencies and their relationship to any cooccurring dysarthria, AOS, or aphasia, because stuttering-like behavior may occur in all of those conditions. In contrast, the

characteristics of palilalia and echolalia are quite distinctive, and it is usually not difficult to distinguish between them and the repetitions that can be associated with the dysarthrias, AOS, and aphasia.

11. Distinguishing among the prosodic deficits associated with cognitive and affective disturbances, aprosodia associated with right hemisphere lesions, and certain dysarthria types can be difficult. Certain speech characteristics and the clinical milieu in which they occur are helpful in distinguishing among them, however.

12. Distinguishing neurogenic from psychogenic speech disorders is important, because the distinction can have a substantial impact on overall medical diagnosis and medical and behavioral management. People for whom this distinction is important require a careful psychosocial history and speech examination, each of which can provide important clues to differential diagnosis. The rapid and dramatic improvement of speech during examination of some individuals can confirm a diagnosis of psychogenic speech disorder, even in those with suspected or confirmed neurologic disease.

References

1. Burns MS, Canter GJ: *Phonemic behavior of aphasic patients with posterior cerebral lesions, Brain Lang 4:492, 1977.*

2. Canter GJ, Trost JE, Burns MS: *Contrasting speech patterns in apraxia of speech and phonemic paraphasia, Brain Lang 24:204, 1985.*

3. Darley FL: *Aphasia, Philadelphia, 1982, WB Saunders.*

4. Goodglass H, Kaplan E: *The Boston diagnostic aphasia examination, Philadelphia, 1983, Lea & Febiger.*

5. Kertesz A: *Western aphasia battery, New York, 1982, Grune & Stratton.*

6. McNeil MR, Robin DA, Schmidt RA: *Apraxia of speech: definition, differentiation, and treatment. In McNeil MR, editor: Clinical management of sensorimotor speech disorders, New York, 1997, Thieme.*

7. Porch BE: *Porch index of communicative ability, Palo Alto, Calif, 1981, Consulting Psychologists Press.*

8. Sackett DL et al: *Clinical epidemiology: a basic science for clinical medicine, Boston, 1991, Little, Brown & Company.*

9. Schuell HM: *Minnesota test for differential diagnosis of aphasia, Minneapolis, 1972, University of Minnesota Press.*

10. Trost JE, Canter GJ: *Apraxia of speech in patients with Broca's aphasia: a study of phoneme production accuracy and error patterns, Brain Lang 1:63, 1974.*

11. Wertz RT: *Neuropathologies of speech and language: an introduction to patient management. In Johns DF, editor: Clinical management of neurogenic communicative disorders, Boston, 1985, Little, Brown & Company.*

12. Wertz RT, LaPointe LL, Rosenbek JC: *Apraxia of speech in adults: the disorder and its management, Orlando, Fla, 1984, Grune & Stratton.*

Management

16 Managing Motor Speech Disorders: General Principles

> *"The brain is not a structurally static organ . . . but instead is a dynamic system that continuously changes in structure and function . . . The discovery that central nervous system plasticity after injury can be directed toward functional improvement . . . has opened up a new dimension in the care of the neurologically impaired patient."* [22]
>
> A. Drubach, M. Makley, and M.L. Dodd

CHAPTER OUTLINE

I. **Management issues and decisions**
   A. The territory
   B. Management goals
   C. Factors influencing management decisions
   D. Focus of treatment
   E. Duration of treatment and its termination
II. **Approaches to management**
   A. Medical intervention
   B. Prosthetic management
   C. Behavioral management
   D. Augmentative and alternative communication
   E. Counseling and support
III. **Rationale, principles, and guidelines for behavioral management**
   A. The brain is not a static organ
   B. Neural adaptation occurs with muscle use
   C. The organization of the cortex in adult animals is not fixed
   D. The nervous system is capable of recovery and reorganization after injury
   E. Motor reorganization after injury requires use
   F. Medical and speech diagnoses are relevant to management
   G. Management should start early, but not always
   H. Baseline data are necessary for establishing goals and measuring change
   I. Increasing physiologic support often should be the initial focus of treatment
   J. Compensation requires that speech production become conscious
   K. Principles of motor learning should influence the structure of speech-oriented treatment
   L. Organization of sessions

IV. **Treatment efficacy**
V. **Summary**

It is fair to state that more time and effort has been expended to describe and understand motor speech disorders (MSDs) than to establish effective methods for managing them. This state of affairs reflects the natural history of efforts to "solve" any medical or neurologic problem. A problem's defining clinical features first must be identified so that it can be recognized reliably. Then it must be studied in various ways so that an understanding of its nature begins to emerge. As these efforts evolve, management strategies emerge, usually slowly and crudely at first, and then, if things go well, with sustained momentum. Thus *the development of effective treatments and management strategies typically lags behind problem description and understanding.* When a goal of management is to change behavior, this lag also reflects some substantial challenges to acquiring evidence that establishes treatment effects. It is relatively simple to identify methods that should help, or that seem to help, but it is an altogether different matter to establish that a treatment has earned a scientific seal of approval.

Currently, a wide variety of techniques and strategies are used to treat and manage MSDs. Some are linked to scientific evidence that supports their use. Others have good face validity but only anecdotal endorsement. Others are no more than reasonable ideas that require testing, and still others enjoy popularity for reasons no stronger than tradition or fervent advocacy. In general, however, there is sufficient support for concluding that *the communication difficulties of many people with MSDs can be managed in beneficial ways.* It is also the case that no single approach is effective for all people with MSDs.[87]

The management of MSDs and related neurogenic and psychogenic speech disturbances is addressed in the remaining chapters of this book. In this chapter the broad issues involved in managing MSDs, the primary avenues for their treatment, and principles for their behavioral management are emphasized. Chapters 17 and 18 discuss specific approaches to managing the dysarthrias and apraxia of speech (AOS), respectively. Chapter 19 addresses the management of other neurogenic speech disturbances. Chapter 20 provides a broad overview of the principles and behavioral strategies for managing psychogenic and related nonorganic speech disorders.

■ MANAGEMENT ISSUES AND DECISIONS

The Territory

There are three reasons for thinking about *communication* rather than speech when considering the management of MSDs:

1. It places the ultimate goal where it belongs—on the ability to transmit thoughts and feelings to others. During most interpersonal communication, this usually occurs through speech and various extralinguistic, nonverbal cues. However, various additional channels exist, including writing and deliberate gesturing. Some people with severe MSDs may need to shift the degree to which they use different channels to convey information. For example, they may need to repeat statements or answer questions that clarify their intended meaning, supplement speech by pointing to the first letter of each spoken word on an alphabet board, or write or type portions of messages.
2. A focus on communication broadens the goals of management. Rather than focusing only on speech, it recognizes that actions other than speech can improve the accuracy and efficiency of communication.
3. It broadens the criteria by which the effectiveness of treatment is judged. A focus on communication influences management planning, prognosis, counseling of patients and those in their environment, decisions about whether or not direct treatment is appropriate, the conduct of management activities, and the point at which formal therapy might be terminated.

Management Goals

The primary goal of management is to *maximize the effectiveness, efficiency, and naturalness of communication.*[59,87] Achieving this goal requires efforts that can take one or more of several directions.[80] For people with mild MSDs, treatment might emphasize efficiency and naturalness of speech; for those with moderate MSDs, it might focus on intelligibility and efficiency; for those with severe MSDs, it might emphasize effective and efficient alternative means of communication. The key words that represent these directions are *restore, compensate,* and *adjust.* Their meanings are discussed next.

Restore Lost Function

This effort aims to reduce impairment. Its likelihood of success is influenced by the etiology and course of the causal disease and by the type and severity of the MSD. For example, a person with a mild to moderate unilateral upper motor neuron (UMN) dysarthria due to a single, unilateral stroke 2 days before initial speech assessment has a reasonably good chance of near-complete return of normal speech on the basis of physiologic recovery alone. A person with an isolated, idiopathic unilateral vocal fold paralysis might achieve full or near-complete recovery of voice as a result of natural nerve recovery/regeneration or thyroplasty surgery. People with reduced physiologic support for speech, such as respiratory, laryngeal, or lingual weakness, may benefit from efforts to increase muscle strength, power, or endurance to meet the physiologic demands of speech.

It is crucial that clinicians and patients realize that reducing speech impairment through behavioral therapy is not a realistic goal for many patients and that full restoration of normal speech through therapy alone is not a realistic goal in most cases. However, some degree of recovery occurs for many patients and may be enhanced with treatment, especially when etiology is an acute vascular or traumatic event or other etiology in which full or partial physiologic recovery can be expected.

Promote the Use of Residual Function (Compensate)

Knowing that full restoration of normal speech will probably not occur should lead to efforts to compensate for lost abilities. Compensation can take many forms but is exemplified by modifications of rate and prosody; the use of prosthetic devices to amplify voice, reduce nasal airflow, or pace the rate of speech; augmentation of speech during verbal efforts (e.g., gestures, referring to a list of words to indicate a change in topic); using alternative means of communication (e.g., alphabet board, computer-based systems); or modifying the physical environment or behavior of people within it in ways that enhance intelligibility, comprehensibility, or efficiency.

Reduce the Need for Lost Function (Adjust)

For those who earn their living by speaking (e.g., teacher, lawyer, broadcaster), an MSD could mean the end of a career. For others, it might require a reorganization of their work environment or responsibilities or a change in lifestyle, such as restricting verbal interactions to individuals or small groups. Depending on the course of the underlying disease, the prognosis for speech recovery, and the severity of the speech disorder, these adjustments could be temporary or permanent. For those with degenerative disease, planning for the progressive loss of speech may be necessary. Management has an important role to play in these adjustments, its primary goal being to maximize speech and communication functions so that the need to reorganize other life activities can be minimized.

Factors Influencing Management Decisions

Unfortunately, many people with MSDs are never referred for management because of ignorance about what can be done to help them. It is also unfortunate that some people receive treatment when they should not or are treated longer than necessary. There are no firm rules for deciding whether treatment should be pursued, but the decision should be based on a good deal more than receipt of a referral to evaluate or treat someone. One general assumption that can be made is that *not all people with MSDs are candidates for therapy*. The decision to treat or not treat should be based on consideration of the factors discussed next.

Medical Diagnosis and Prognosis

Did the underlying neurologic disease develop acutely or subacutely or is it now chronic? Is its predicted course one of complete resolution or improvement with eventual plateauing, or will it be chronic and stable, exacerbating-remitting, or progressive? Is there a medical treatment for the disease that can resolve or significantly improve speech, and will such treatment take place soon and with subsequent rapid benefits? Answers to questions like these help decide whether or not to begin treatment, or when treatment should be reconsidered if it is deferred. The following scenarios illustrate how decisions about treatment can vary as a function of neurologic diagnosis and prognosis:

1. Patients seen for assessment shortly after stroke, who are not yet neurologically stable and whose stamina and alertness are fluctuating, but who have only mild or moderate speech impairment and adequate intelligibility, are probably not treatment candidates. Assuming that their stamina and alertness improve, the prognosis for significant spontaneous improvement of speech is quite good. If they fail to improve or deteriorate neurologically, it is not likely that they would be interested or concerned about speech intervention or benefit from it if it were provided. In general—and ignoring a number of other influential factors—the best decision in such cases is to not recommend therapy or to recommend reassessment when the patient's physical status and alertness have stabilized.

2. Providing speech treatment before planned medical treatment is rarely justified. For example, patients who are about to undergo neurosurgery related to the underlying cause of their MSD (e.g., tumor removal, carotid endarterectomy) should have speech management decisions deferred until after surgery. In such cases, if necessary, augmentative or alternative means of communication should be provided before surgery, but if speech is functional for the person's communication needs at the time, full assessment and reconsideration of management is best done postoperatively.

3. Patients with degenerative neurologic disease and MSDs that are expected to worsen can nonetheless benefit from efforts to help maintain intelligibility and prepare for augmentative or alternative communication. Patients with significant MSDs who have had strokes and are still in the spontaneous phase of recovery also may be good treatment candidates. Patients whose physiologic recovery from stroke or traumatic brain injury has probably plateaued may similarly benefit from management.

Disability and Societal Limitation*

The diagnosis of MSDs relies on detecting impairment or loss of function stemming from nervous

---

*See Yorkston et al.[87] for a discussion of MSDs from a chronic disease perspective. They provide an excellent discussion of the parameters of pathophysiology, impairment, functional limitation, disability, and societal limitation, and the relationships among them. Here, the author has chosen to simplify the discussion by collapsing these parameters under notions of impairment, disability, and societal limitations (handicap), because they seem to capture the concepts most critical to management decision making and execution.

system pathophysiology. Although the nature of the impairment often influences the specific focus of therapy, *the mere presence of impairment has little to do with a decision to recommend behavioral treatment.* That decision depends on assessment of disability and societal limitation.[87] Disability reflects the degree of inability to speak and communicate normally in social and physical settings because of the speech impairment. It can be assessed through measures such as intelligibility, comprehensibility, rate, loudness, and articulatory precision. *Societal limitation,* often called *handicap,* relates to the ability to accomplish a role in a social context that, in the absence of handicap, would be played in the future. Societal limitation or handicap is determined by impairment; disability; the patient's communication needs; and societal attitudes, barriers, or policies.[87]

Impairment, disability, and societal limitation are not always correlated. For example, mild, isolated hypernasality caused by velopharyngeal weakness (impairment) might not reduce speech intelligibility (disability) but could represent a major handicap to a media broadcaster. A marked spastic dysarthria (impairment) with subsequent significantly reduced intelligibility (disability) might not be a great limitation or handicap to a shy and reclusive retired person who never placed great value on social or verbal interaction.

Estimates of disability and handicap also may vary among patients, their significant others, and the clinician. For example, some patients with speech and cognitive impairments minimize or are oblivious to the degree to which their family does not understand them, but their family is constantly frustrated with how hard they must work to understand the patient. Some patients with uncompromising personal standards or difficulty adjusting to their impairment or disability view themselves as unable to perform prior roles (such as leading a meeting), even though their impairment and disability are mild and their listeners find little reason for them not to continue to play those roles.

It is important that a clinician's discussions with patients and their significant others make clear the distinctions among impairment, disability, and handicap when discussing management issues and goals. *In general, ongoing intervention is not recommended if there is negligible disability and no limitation or handicap associated with an MSD.* Obviously, when the causal disease is degenerative, the passage of time may lead to a need for intervention.

Environment and Communication Partners

Management decisions must consider the environments in which patients speak and the people to whom they speak. The problems encountered in noisy, poorly lit, bustling places in which listeners may not know the patient or may have disabilities themselves are quite different from those faced in quiet, familiar settings in which listeners are cognitively and sensorily intact, familiar with the patient, care about them, and are sensitive to their disability. Such considerations play a role in determining not only the need for management but also the needs to be addressed during management. The environment and traits of communication partners can have a significant impact on prognosis for benefiting from management as well as on specific treatment goals and approaches. This is a major reason why treatment planning so often involves partnerships among the clinician, patient, and their families or significant others.[85a]

Motivation and Needs

Therapy is carried out *by* or *with* the affected person, not provided *to them* or *for them.*[19] Thus speech rehabilitation planning and efforts should always involve the patient and often should involve the patient's significant others. In this context it is essential to address the patient's motivation and need for verbal communication because *the need to communicate may be the most important determinant to a decision to provide treatment.*[54] Specific needs are determined by many factors, including, but almost certainly not limited to: age; educational level; premorbid personality, intelligence, and lifestyle; personal goals; coexisting motor, sensory, and cognitive deficits; general health issues; and living environment.

It is surprising how frequently a clinician's initial estimates of disability and handicap do not match those of the patient. Many elderly patients, for example, are accepting of their impairment and disability, do not feel particularly handicapped, and deny a need or desire for intervention. To say that they are unmotivated is pejorative or misguided in many cases. Their judgment is simply based on standards that differ from those of the clinician; this is often borne out by patients' significant others, who may be in full agreement with them. The clinician's responsibility in such cases is to explain what therapy might accomplish if undertaken and to respect patients' wishes if they decline the offer.

When a patient is truly unmotivated because of depression, cognitive impairments, or other more pressing personal concerns, direct intervention should not be recommended. Counseling of the patient and significant others may be undertaken instead, with an option to reassess direct management options if motivation changes.

Associated Problems

Most people with MSDs have other neurologic deficits. *Limb motor deficits* are common, but if speech is not so impaired that augmentative or alternative means of communication are required, they may not have a big impact on speech management. Such deficits do influence the priorities of patients, however; some with functional verbal abilities are much more concerned about their mobility and ability to manage their basic physical needs than they are about their speech.

Cognitive deficits can significantly influence the conduct of management, and they frequently accompany all of the central nervous system (CNS)–based dysarthrias. For example, across the cases reviewed for etiology of each dysarthria type (except flaccid dysarthria) in previous chapters, the prevalence of cognitive deficits ranged from approximately 15% to 70%. Such deficits vary widely in severity. They often include problems with attention, memory, learning, insight, planning, and motivation. In addition, some patients with MSDs, particularly AOS and unilateral UMN (UUMD) or spastic dysarthria, may be *aphasic* and have significant difficulties in all language modalities.

The presence of nonaphasic cognitive or aphasic language deficits can have various influences on communication and efforts to improve it. When they are pronounced, they can magnify the speech disability and handicap, strongly influence communication needs and motivation to speak, and have a major negative influence on the potential to benefit from therapy for the MSD. They may require that an MSD take a low priority in rehabilitation efforts or a decision not to address the MSD at all. In general, *if accompanying cognitive deficits preclude attention, drive, or motivation to communicate or result in speech that has no functional communicative value, then the MSD should not be treated directly.*

The Health Care System

Managing MSDs can be costly, and cost must be weighed in management decisions. It is clear that the health care systems in many countries, in their financial motivation to do less instead of more (or, more positively, to redefine quality in terms of value rather than quantity), have had a significant impact on patterns of clinical practice and patient care. Such changes have placed great value on evidence of treatment effectiveness and efficiency of care. In addition, there has been a shift to an objective standard of decision making in which external templates override clinicians' and patients' autonomy in management decisions.[68] Clinicians, patients, and their families are faced with decisions about what can be done to help and how quickly it can be accomplished. Actually, such issues are at the foundation of excellence in clinical practice and should be addressed independent of cost or reimbursement considerations. Nonetheless, the recommendations of clinicians and the desires of their patients are not always congruent with the health care system's templates for management. It is thus likely that some treatment decisions are influenced by factors beyond the clinician-patient relationship. The practical challenge to clinicians is to maintain quality while increasing effectiveness and efficiency. The more fundamental challenge to clinicians and researchers is to acquire evidence that establishes the efficacy, effectiveness, and efficiency of approaches to treating and managing MSDs. This is addressed in the section on treatment efficacy at the end of this chapter.

Focus of Treatment

In general, the component of speech that should be treated is the one from which the greatest functional benefit will be derived most rapidly or that will provide the greatest support for improvement in other aspects of speech. For example, improved respiratory support or vocal loudness might improve intelligibility rapidly and also allow subsequent improvements in articulation to have a more obvious additional impact on intelligibility. These issues are addressed in detail when specific approaches to treatment are discussed.

Duration of Treatment and Its Termination

For how long should treatment be provided? The obvious answer is *for as long as is necessary to accomplish its goals but for as short a time as possible.* This must be qualified by recognition that the shortest time possible may nonetheless require intensive and protracted treatment.

In general, *no management program should begin without a plan about when it will end.* The clinician and patient should have in mind how long it will take to achieve goals, with an understanding that revision is possible along the way. This temporal plan helps some patients decide if they wish to pursue treatment in the first place. Many, for example, are willing to commit to therapy when told that goals are likely to be reached within a short time. For others, it may assist their need to know how long it will take before they are "on their own" and able to communicate independently.

Duration of treatment is influenced by many factors. Etiology, the predicted course of the causal disease, the severity of deficits, the specific goals of management, efficacy or outcome data for similar patient characteristics and treatment approaches, patients' motivation and communication needs, the duration of hospitalization, the ability to travel for outpatient services, and health care coverage all have an impact on the duration of treatment.

When management goals are reached or plateauing occurs, or when patients decide for other reasons that they do not wish further treatment, then treatment should end. After treatment ends, however, it may be appropriate to periodically reassess speech and communication abilities and needs. For example, patients who plateau during therapy but might improve further if new potential emerges or if their environment or needs change should be reassessed periodically to address such changes. Patients with degenerative disease whose speech problems are likely to worsen, but who currently are functioning optimally, may be discharged with prescheduled reassessment or the option for reassessment when change takes place.* Whenever reassessment takes place, the clinician and patient should address the options for future management and what each of them can be expected to accomplish.

◼ APPROACHES TO MANAGEMENT

There is no single approach to treating MSDs. This reflects the significant differences that exist among MSDs in pathophysiology, severity, and specific abnormal speech characteristics, as well as multiple additional factors that influence management decisions (e.g., etiology, prognosis, disability, societal limitations, environment, communication needs).

Approaches to management can be conceptualized in several ways. Here we will parse them into five distinguishable but frequently overlapping and sometimes inseparable areas of effort. They include *medical intervention, prosthetic management, behavioral management, alternative and augmentative communication,* and *counseling and support.* The goal within each of these areas is to improve communication, preferably by directly improving intelligibility, efficiency, and naturalness of speech, but sometimes by other means. A broad overview of each areas follows. Specific methods are discussed in Chapters 17 and 18.

Medical Intervention

Medical management includes pharmacologic and surgical interventions that can directly or indirectly

affect speech. In general, medical management should always precede or be provided concurrently with other management approaches because it may maximize physiologic functioning and have a rapid or dramatic effect on speech.

Medical interventions that are specifically directed at improving speech require collaboration between the medical speech pathologist and otolaryngologist, plastic surgeon, or neurologist. The primary responsibility of the medical speech pathologist in such cases is to carefully assess speech and establish (1) the need for medical or surgical intervention, (2) the likelihood that the patient will benefit from such intervention, (3) the specific benefits to be derived, (4) what the intervention will not accomplish for speech, (5) the need for postprocedure behavioral management and the provision of such management, and (6) clear communication of all of this information to the medical subspecialist and patient. An understanding of the medical risks and costs of such procedures is important so that the decision to refer for such management can weigh risks and costs against expected benefits.

Pharmacologic Management

Pharmacologic management is almost always directed at relieving symptoms, but sometimes it effectively "cures" the underlying disorder. Such approaches are directed to the underlying disease process (e.g., infection) rather than designed to improve speech per se. Thus neurologic disease that can be treated pharmacologically may improve speech in the process. Because some drugs improve some symptoms but not others, improvement in a patient's general condition may not always be matched by improvement in speech. Examples of drugs with indirect effects on speech include antibiotics for the treatment of CNS infection, steroids to treat the inflammatory effects of disease, and anticonvulsants to control seizures.

Some neurologic diseases commonly associated with dysarthrias are effectively managed but not cured by drugs, and the benefits sometimes include improved speech. Dopaminergic agents for Parkinson's disease (PD), Mestinon for myasthenia gravis, dietary modifications and chelating agents for Wilson's disease, and various drugs that may control movement disorders* are examples of such drugs. Injection of botulinum toxin (Botox) into certain laryngeal muscles for the treatment of spasmodic

---

*For example, Yorkston et al.[88] indicate that they follow individuals with amyotrophic lateral sclerosis (ALS) at 2-week to 4-month intervals, depending on their needs and rate of disease progression.

*Some medications have side effects that may worsen or alter the character of a dysarthria. For example, a significant proportion of people with PD and hypokinetic dysarthria develop dyskinesias (including hyperkinetic dysarthria) at some time during their treatment with levodopa.[60]

dysphonia or into the jaw, face, or neck muscles to treat orofacial dystonias or spasmodic torticollis is a prime example of the use of a substance for the sole purpose of altering the functions of specific muscles and sometimes for the sole purpose of improving speech.

Before beginning behavioral management, the clinician should know if the patient is taking medication for the neurologic problem, if there are plans to initiate such treatment, or if drug therapy has been tried and abandoned. Behavioral management should be delayed until drug therapy that might improve speech is started, because such therapy may make behavioral management unnecessary or change its focus. The exceptions are patients whose speech disorder necessitates the use of *augmentative and alternative communication (AAC)*. Provision of AAC strategies and devices (usually "low tech") should always be undertaken to permit functional communication until medication might have its desired effect on speech. Fluctuations in speech that occur over the course of a medication cycle as, for example, may be the case for patients taking medication for PD are important to establish; behavioral management might be directed only to problems that emerge at a particular time during the drug cycle.

Surgical Management

Surgery to manage neurologic disease may have direct and indirect effects on speech. Neurosurgery for aneurysms, hydrocephalus, tumors, seizures, and occluded arteries are examples of procedures directed to the causes of neurologic deficits rather than the deficits themselves. In some cases, surgery may resolve signs and symptoms. In others, there may be improvement but not resolution, stabilization but not improvement, deterioration, or the development of new deficits. In still others, such as tumor resection, gains may only be temporary.

Some surgeries are performed for the sole purpose of improving speech. Prime examples are *pharyngeal flap* or *sphincter pharyngoplasty* procedures to improve velopharyngeal function for speech and *thyroplasty* for vocal fold paralysis or weakness.

Prosthetic Management

A number of mechanical and electronic prosthetic or assistive devices are available to improve speech. Some may be temporary, used only until physiologic recovery or the effects of behavioral management allow them to be discarded. Others may be permanent because disability or handicap would be increased without them.

Some prosthetic devices directly modify what happens in the vocal tract during speech and help to promote perceptual normalcy. For example, a *palatal lift prosthesis* or *nasopharyngeal obturator* may facilitate velopharyngeal closure during speech, with resultant reduced hypernasality and increased intraoral pressure for pressure consonants; a bite block positioned between the upper and lower teeth may inhibit mandibular hyperkinesia.

Other prosthetic devices modify speech after it is produced. For example, *voice amplifiers* can increase vocal loudness in speakers whose primary speech difficulty is reduced loudness or inability to increase loudness to overcome noise, distance, or reduced hearing acuity in listeners.

Some prostheses are designed to modify the manner of speech production rather than simply support normal production or modify the speech signal. These devices may actually alter rate or prosody in the direction of abnormality in order to improve intelligibility. Examples include *pacing boards, metronomes,* and *delayed auditory feedback (DAF),* all of which slow speech rate and increase syllabic stress. Certain biofeedback devices may indicate to the patient when speech is failing to meet certain preset standards. For example, a *vocal intensity monitoring device* might provide an audible, visible, or vibratory signal when loudness falls below a preset level that is necessary to maintain intelligibility.

Finally, prosthetic devices are available to augment speech or serve as alternatives to speech. They are actually a tool of behavioral management, but their distinction from other prosthetic devices and other behavioral approaches to management justifies thinking about them as a separate approach to management. AAC, as mentioned earlier, includes *picture, letter,* and *word boards* and more sophisticated *computerized devices* with multiple control and output options, sometimes including *synthesized speech* or the computerized recognition of speech. When limb movements are insufficient to conventionally activate AAC devices, various assistive devices are available, including *light pointers* that may be worn on the head or *switches* that may be placed on any part of the body under volitional control. In the future, muscle-independent interfaces between the brain and computers may open additional possibilities for communication for locked-in or severely motorically impaired individuals.[43]

Decision making about the need for and benefits to be derived from prosthetic management is similar to that for medical/surgical intervention. Implementation is often multidisciplinary, frequently requiring the skills of prosthodontists, occupational and physical therapists, rehabilitation engineers, educators, and others. When heavy reliance on AAC is required, it is often essential to involve a speech pathologist with subspecialty expertise in that area, at least on a consultative basis. Also, obviously, the affected person must be centrally involved in such decision making. Without minimizing the increasingly significant contribution that prosthetic interventions, including AAC, can make to communication ability, Kent[40] has noted that "innovations in biotechnology are not necessarily welcome to those who are expected to be their beneficiaries . . . some patients reject the sheer idea of such intervention."

Behavioral Management

Behavioral management includes all intervention efforts that are neither medical nor prosthetic. As already stated, medical, prosthetic, and behavioral interventions are not mutually exclusive, and some patients require all approaches. Behavioral management is almost certainly provided to a larger proportion of people with MSDs than is medical or prosthetic management.

Behavioral management has a wide variety of goals and can take many forms. Its primary goal, however, is to *maximize communication* by whatever means produces the most effective and natural results. For many patients, this involves a direct attack on speech. For others, it requires a combination of speech and AAC strategies or the sole use of avenues other than speech for communication.

The goals of behavioral management can be accomplished in numerous ways, including improving physiologic support for speech, modifying speech through compensatory speaking strategies, developing AAC, and controlling the environment and communicative interactions.[59,87] These approaches can be divided into *speech-oriented approaches* and *communication-oriented approaches*.

Speech-oriented approaches work to restore or modify impaired communication by *altering speech*. In contrast, communication-oriented approaches work to improve communication by altering speaking strategies, the behavior of listeners, or the environment in which communication occurs. Their methods improve communication by *modifying aspects of the communicative interaction*. Treatment of mild impairments tends to be speech oriented, whereas treatment of severe impairments tends to be communication oriented. Both approaches may be employed at all severity levels, however.

Speech-Oriented Approaches

Speech-oriented treatment focuses primarily on *improving speech intelligibility* and secondarily on *improving efficiency and naturalness* of communication. These goals are shared with communication-oriented approaches, but the MSD itself is the focus of speech-oriented approaches. These goals are accomplished (1) by *reducing impairment* by increasing physiologic support for speech or (2) through *compensation* by making maximum use of residual physiologic support.[59,87] Both approaches require motor learning and effort.

Although efforts to reduce impairment and assist compensation for impairment are both appropriate, it seems that clinicians' efforts are more frequently directed toward compensation. The reasons for this are partly dependent on neurologic diagnosis, severity of impairment, time after onset, prognosis, and motivation. Another reason is the likelihood that compensation can be achieved more rapidly than reduction of impairment, a particularly desirable goal in acute hospital and inpatient rehabilitation settings that stress reduced length of stay and, consequently, rapid achievement of functional goals (primary outcome measures). This emphasis on compensation may be entirely justified in many instances, but it may be shortsighted in others when potential to reduce impairment exists. In fact, it has been suggested that *focus on compensation may actually limit activity-dependent neural reorganization that is necessary to the reduction of specific impairment*.[19] The potential for behavioral treatment to reduce impairment is discussed later in the section on principles and guidelines.

Treatments to reduce impairment by increasing physiologic support attempt to remediate the deficits in posture, strength, and tone that underlie the speech disorder. Such approaches can include speaking activities, but they can also be *indirect*[8] or conducted independent of speech. Indirect activities may include sensory stimulation, strengthening exercises, the modification of muscle tone, altering posture and positioning, and improving respiratory capacity and efficiency. For some patients these indirect efforts are among the first goals of treatment, and medical and prosthetic management may be important components of them.[59]

Making maximum use of residual physiologic support is characterized as a *behavioral compensation method* because it focuses directly on modifying respiration, phonation, resonance, articulation, or prosody in order to compensate for residual impairment; these compensations can also include medical and prosthetic management. This approach assumes that some patients are more disabled by their speech impairment than need be because they are not making maximum use of their residual physiologic capacity. Some patients fail to compensate spontaneously because they lack the knowledge to do so, wish to persist in speaking as they did in the past, have difficulty doing consciously what was once a subconscious process, have cognitive deficits that limit their capacity to learn and employ new strategies, or are anxious, depressed, or unmotivated.[59] Some of these traits limit progress or preclude treatment, but others can be overcome during treatment.

Compensatory approaches also focus on improving *efficiency* and *naturalness. Efficiency means increasing rate of communication without sacrificing intelligibility or comprehensibility.** This can be done by manipulating speech directly, by adopting certain augmentative strategies, by altering language content or style, by manipulating the environment, or by developing strategies for efficiently handling breakdowns in intelligibility or comprehensibility when they occur.

Improving *naturalness* involves attention to prosody. Working on prosody may be important at all severity levels because prosody contributes to the identification of speech segments and provides clues to meaning. Rate, rhythm, intonation, and stress carry important syntactic information and substantially increase the amount of redundancy in the speech signal. Thus efforts to increase naturalness can improve intelligibility.

In their efforts to speak more adequately, or in response to physiologic limitations or abnormalities, some patients develop *maladaptive behaviors* or persist in using an adaptive strategy long after it is necessary or helpful. For example, some patients with vocal fold paralysis or respiratory weakness speak on inhalation in order to normalize phrase length; others use phrase lengths that are shorter than necessary or longer than can be physiologically supported. Such behaviors can substantially affect intelligibility, efficiency, or naturalness of speech. Their elimination sometimes results in dramatic speech improvement.

Communication-Oriented Approaches

Communication-oriented treatment can improve communication even when speech itself does not improve. It includes various modifications ranging from altering the number of listeners, the amount of noise, speaker-listener distance, and eye contact to informing new listeners about the speech problem, its cause, and the speaker's preferred method of communicating. It also includes identification of the most effective strategies for repairing breakdowns in communication; for example, repeating utterances, rephrasing, spelling, writing, or answering clarifying questions.

Communication strategies may change from one speaking environment to another or from one listener to another. They often require negotiation, practice,

and demonstration (proof) that one strategy works better than another. The patient must manage some of these environmental manipulations and speaking strategies, but others are the primary responsibility of listeners.

Augmentative and Alternative Communication

An MSD can severely limit the degree to which speech and the gestures that normally accompany it transmit messages intelligibly and efficiently. The affected person may need to augment or substitute other means of communication for speech, either temporarily or permanently. As mentioned earlier, the area of clinical practice that focuses on meeting these needs is known as AAC. Activities associated with AAC are part of behavioral management strategies but also include prosthetic management because they often rely on the use of aids—physical objects or devices—for the transmission or receipt of messages. These activities lead to the development of an AAC *system* that is an "integrated group of components, including the symbols, aids, strategies, and techniques used by individuals to enhance communication."[3]

The development and refinement of AAC in recent years has been dramatic. It has had a significant impact on many people with MSDs, including people with locked-in syndrome.[72] AAC is considered a subspecialty area of practice within the profession of speech-language pathology. It holds Special Interest Division (Division 12, Augmentative and Alternative Communication) status within the American Speech-Language-Hearing Association.

The tools of AAC are heterogeneous. They include: (1) gestural communication that may not require the use of any additional physical aid, such as eye gaze, facial, head, and hand gestures, and body postures; (2) various symbols beyond the spoken word, such as pictures, photos, icons, printed words and letters, objects, signs/pantomime, Braille, and Morse code; and (3) various aids to facilitate message transmission, such as communication books or boards, a wide array of mechanical and electronic devices, and computer-based systems with output options including synthesized speech.* Speech recognition devices also have potential for AAC.[21,74]

The use of AAC in the management of MSDs can be highly variable across and even within individuals.

---

*Recall the discussion of intelligibility, comprehensibility, and efficiency (ICE) in Chapter 3.

*Synthesized speech is improving at a rapid rate, but it continues to have some disadvantages when compared to natural speech. For example, it has less acoustic redundancy and suprasegmental information, and phonetic cues are sometimes misleading.[37]

For those whose expected disease and speech course is one of improvement, AAC may be relied on heavily before improvement begins and then faded as improvement occurs.* For people with degenerative disease, there may be no need for AAC early, but total reliance on it may be necessary in the later stages; for example, for people with ALS, it may be appropriate to begin to explore AAC options when speech rate slows and intelligibility becomes inconsistent in adverse speaking situations.[51,88] Thus *staging of management,* which can be thought of as doing the right things for people at the right time,[83] is appropriate in many cases. How to time this staging can be challenging, but guidelines are emerging for some degenerative disorders, particularly ALS. For example, speaking rate is correlated with intelligibility and also seems to be an important predictor of subsequent performance in people with ALS.[5,88] Data suggest that when speaking rate drops below 100 wpm, a significant decline in intelligibility can be anticipated.[4] Thus as patients' rate is reduced to 90 to 125 words per minute, or when intelligibility becomes inconsistent in adverse listening situations,[4,88] AAC evaluation should be pursued.†

For those with chronic and stable disorders, AAC strategies may remain constant, although changes in technology may permit refinements over time. For example, voice recognition devices may play an increasingly important role for some speakers with chronic disease who are poorly intelligible but capable of some variety in speech production.

The decision to use AAC strategies is based on careful assessment of speech and communication abilities and needs, prognosis, and the individual's potential to benefit from them. Use of AAC may be minimal for many patients; for example, a person may use an alphabet board to identify the first letter of each word he or she says because it improves intelligibility, and he or she may drop that strategy as soon as intelligibility is adequate without it. In contrast, patients with locked-in syndrome may rely entirely on alternatives to speech, using eye gaze, forehead, or other volitional movements to identify symbols or trigger switches that transmit messages.

It is beyond the scope of this book to provide a comprehensive review of AAC systems and techniques. Chapter 17 discusses a few low-technology augmentative strategies that are useful for people with dysarthrias. Several excellent, clinically relevant overviews and in-depth discussions of AAC are available.[6,7,87] They are valuable resources for clinicians who work with patients in need of a range of AAC systems.

Counseling and Support

Behavioral management includes important counseling and supportive roles. There is usually a need to provide information about why certain aspects of speech are not normal and may not ever be normal, what can be done to remediate the underlying impairment or compensate for it, what kind of efforts it will take, and the likely outcome of those efforts. For people with degenerative disease, counseling may include discussion about what may happen to speech over the course of the disease and what can be done to maintain intelligibility and communicative effectiveness as deterioration takes place. Obviously, the prognosis will determine the degree to which such information will generate feelings of optimism or hope for improvement, a need to accept permanent limitations, or a need to prepare for a loss of the ability to communicate easily and naturally.

These responsibilities require knowledge, confidence, experience, sensitivity, and empathy. Sensitivity and empathy are especially difficult-to-quantify traits. They tend to be intrinsic traits of many clinicians, but they can be difficult to maintain in a health care environment that increasingly bases its rewards on efficiency and quantifiable results. Clinicians who provide this form of care—improving or maintaining communication—often must struggle against a "body shop" mentality of care and keep in mind that their patients may not ever have known anyone with their particular problem, that they are *living with and not just working with* their problems, and that they are interested in success and not just the probability of success in their treatment. Overt sensitivity to their bewilderment, grieving, and sometimes outrage at their predicament can help forge a strong therapeutic alliance, one that can facilitate the more technical aspects of care. There is no formula for developing or maintaining these traits,* except perhaps to remember that, as is true for many encounters in health care, *the manner in which care*

---

*Some case reports illustrate the value of periodically readdressing severely impaired patients' potential for developing functional speech after an effective alternative means of communication has been established.[1,39] This is particularly important when onset is acute and recovery with plateauing seems to have occurred, as in stroke or traumatic brain injury.

†Clinicians sometimes express concern about whether people with ALS will accept the need for AAC. A recent study of 50 people with ALS established that 96% accepted AAC technology, and no person who used AAC later discontinued use of it.[4]

*See Kent[40] for some valuable insights and references about the contributions of memoirs to our understanding of the perspectives of people with communication disorders. See *The Healer's Art*[13]

is provided may be as important from the patient's perspective as the actual outcome of efforts to improve their speech or communication.

Appendix A lists a number of information resources for both clinicians and patients. Many of them provide information and assistance to people with specific diseases that can cause MSDs. Some are more specific to communication disorders, whereas others are more generic sources of information about neurologic disease and research.

RATIONALE, PRINCIPLES, AND GUIDELINES FOR BEHAVIORAL MANAGEMENT

Before addressing principles and guidelines, a basic rationale for behavioral management must be established, especially as it relates to speech-oriented approaches. A number of facts about motor skill learning and nervous system plasticity provide a rationale for predicting that behavioral management aimed at reducing speech impairment or improving the physiologic capacity for speech in people with MSDs is possible.* These are covered next.

The Brain Is Not a Static Organ

Its structure and function can be altered as a function of intracellular changes, changes in intercellular and synaptic interconnections, biochemical or genetic level modifications and, most relevant in this context, behavioral training.[19,22]

Neural Adaptation Occurs with Muscle Use

Adaptive changes in the nervous system—a process known as *neural adaptation* or *plasticity*—result from muscle use and changes in patterns of behavior.[22,32,48] Neural adaptation can permit an increase in the firing rate of motor units or the recruitment of previously underused motor units, with a subsequent increase in strength and power and better coordinated activation of muscle groups. Thus "acting upon the environment by means of motor activity is one of the most powerful drives of cortical reorganization"[22] in normal skill acquisition and following

neurologic injury. The notion of *motor plasticity* recognizes a two-way interaction in which repeated motor performance influences cortical reorganization, with subsequently improved motor performance. In recent years, a number of studies of nonimpaired and impaired individuals have demonstrated the effect of motor practice on motor system reorganization. For example, the cortical representation for the reading finger in proficient Braille readers is larger than the representation of other fingers, and as people become skilled at finger exercise on a piano, the size of the cortical representation of the hand increases.[34] Thus motor activity has the capacity to influence the organization of motor areas of the brain.

The Organization of the Cortex in Adult Animals Is Not Fixed

Although plasticity is more evident in the young, within certain limits the adult cortex can be modified or reorganized by experience, learning, and demands for use, presumably because of synaptic plasticity. Under some circumstances, and to varying degrees, such plasticity can occur at all levels of the nervous system, not just the cerebral cortex.[19,12]

The Nervous System Is Capable of Recovery and Reorganization After Injury

Some of the recovery of function that occurs reflects natural physiologic responses that may be independent of volitional behavior, such as resolution of edema, certain synaptic changes, or recruitment of other areas of the brain to perform certain functions, all of which can occur within hours of injury; genetic factors may also influence aspects of plasticity.[19,22] Other changes are more related to sensorimotor and cognitive activity. For example, functional magnetic resonance imaging (fMRI) evidence suggests that reorganization within the CNS occurs in patients who have recovered from hemiparesis caused by cortical stroke; findings suggest increased activity in a larger region of motor cortex than is normally activated, as well as increased activity in sensorimotor cortex in the unaffected hemisphere, ipsilateral premotor cortex, and the contralateral cerebellar hemisphere.[16] Evidence from studies of ALS also suggests that partial compensation between functionally related motor areas might help optimize function if the primary motor pathway is unavailable. For example, fMRI findings from a finger flexion motor learning task identified activation patterns in ALS patients that were distinctly different from healthy controls, mostly shifted anteriorly to

---

for a sensitive examination of the "human elements" that play a role in the relationship between patient and physician. The issues it addresses apply to all health professionals whose responsibilities include personal interactions with patients.

*See the overview articles by Drubach, Mackley, and Dodd[22] and Gonzalez-Rothi[32] for excellent summaries of the neurophysiologic bases of rehabilitation.

encompass the premotor gyrus, supplementary motor area (SMA), pre-SMA, contralateral inferior area 6, and bilateral parietal area 40; the findings suggested that degeneration of first and second order neurons led to increased activity in motor areas usually involved in initiation and planning of movement.[42] Finally, it also appears that after lesions in the peripheral nervous system (PNS), areas of cortex that receive sensory information from the damaged structures, or that influence motor activity of those structures, are taken over by body representations adjacent to the cortical representation of the damaged body part; thus sensory and motor cortex reorganize themselves following peripheral deafferentiation.[34] These observations suggest that cortical reorganization can occur in response to both PNS and CNS lesions affecting motor functions. Assuming replication of these findings, it is reasonable to predict that similar reorganization is possible in the speech sensorimotor system of people with MSDs.

Motor Reorganization after Injury Requires Use

There is evidence that the motor cortex can be reorganized after lesions but that it requires use, particularly voluntary use, of the weakened body part. For example, limb motor training consisting of voluntary movements leads to greater performance improvement and greater activation and reorganization of the motor cortex than does passive or externally manipulated movements; this argues for a crucial role of volitional drive in motor learning and rehabilitation of neuromotor impairments.[48] Additional evidence for this comes from positive findings in studies of *constraint-induced movement therapy* that has forced the use of the hemiplegic limb in people with chronic stroke.[19,22,32,34] These observations provide circumstantial support for the notion that recovery of speech in people with MSDs, at least when they have a nonprogressive disease, requires speaking, and probably lots of it. It is also increasingly recognized that certain pharmacologic agents can positively or negatively influence recovery of motor functions,* and that the most positive results occur when some agents are combined with behavioral rehabilitation. The potential of pharmacologic agents to "prime" the brain to benefit from behavioral intervention is an exciting prospect and suggests a need for increased interaction among physicians and rehabilitation subspecialties,[22] including speech-language pathology.

---

*For example, dextroamphetamine may enhance recovery of motor functions, whereas agents such as phenytoin, clonidine, neuroleptics, and benzodiazepines have restricted gains in some experiments.[19,56]

With these supporting rationale in mind, some general principles and guidelines can be applied to the organization and conduct of behavioral management. They relate to decisions about when to start treatment, influences on treatment planning, baseline data, the focus of treatment, principles of motor learning, and the organization and format of treatment sessions. Many of them derive from consideration of factors that have already been discussed. Some of them are more relevant to the management of dysarthrias than to AOS; the differences are apparent in Chapters 17 and 18.

Medical and Speech Diagnoses Are Relevant to Management

It is generally true that the better we understand a problem the better we are able to manage it. Thus, medical and speech diagnoses contribute to decisions about how to focus management.

Medical Diagnosis

Many medical diseases have a known course and therefore have prognostic implications for speech. Some diseases are associated with an identifiable pathophysiology that explains many or most features of the speech disorder; when this is the case, it can help set broad management goals. If a disease is confined to a single part of the motor system or a single pathophysiologic process (e.g., weakness), it tells us in a general way what goals and tasks are or are not likely to be relevant to efforts to improve speech. For example, knowing a patient has a *rapidly* progressing degenerative disease makes it unlikely that efforts to restore physiologic function should be part of the management program and makes maintenance rather than improvement of speech a legitimate goal. Similarly, efforts to increase strength would be counterproductive for those with flaccid dysarthria due to myasthenia gravis; that is, strengthening exercises would induce weakness rather than increase strength.

Speech Diagnosis

Optimal treatment derives from fitting our understanding of the determinants of abnormal speech patterns to available treatments.[53] The diagnosis of a specific dysarthria type or AOS implies a specific underlying neurophysiologic deficit. Diagnosis in this sense has meaning for treatment directed at improving speech. For example, because flaccid dysarthria is the result of weakness and reduced muscle tone, treatment efforts might attempt to increase strength. Because ataxic dysarthria reflects incoordination, treatment might focus on facilitating coordination or compensating for incoordination;

efforts to improve strength would be misdirected. In Chapter 17, treatment approaches that may be particularly relevant to specific dysarthria types are discussed. Similarly, distinguishing dysarthrias from AOS is crucial, because AOS requires a different approach to management; this is apparent in Chapter 18.

Despite its value, MSD type does not establish the focus of management completely. Identifying specific deviant speech characteristics, their relationship to each subsystem of speech production, and their relationship to each other is also necessary. Relating speech characteristics to dysfunction in various muscle groups helps determine the component of the speech system that should receive attention. For example, reduced loudness is usually linked to deficits at the respiratory or laryngeal level and hypernasality to deficits at the velopharyngeal level.

Speech impairments should also be related to each other, because *a hierarchical organization of symptoms can enhance treatment efficiency*. In this context, a hierarchy refers to hypotheses about causal relationships among speech characteristics or the degree to which a deviant speech characteristic at one level of the mechanism may lead to the emergence of a deviant speech characteristic(s) at other levels. For example, imprecise articulation may result from rapid rate, short phrases may result from breathiness stemming from laryngeal weakness, and so on.

The ability to establish hierarchies of symptoms can help determine where to begin treatment.[59] In general, treatment should begin as close to the bottom of the hierarchy—as close to the source or cause—as possible, because change at that level is most likely to have the biggest effect on intelligibility. For example, establishing that imprecise articulation is secondary to nasal emission caused by velopharyngeal weakness may lead to management of velopharyngeal function, with resultant reduction in hypernasality, nasal emission, and articulatory imprecision. Establishing that short phrases and reduced loudness are linked to reduced respiratory support and not to laryngeal weakness may lead to efforts to improve respiratory support, with resultant increases in loudness and phrase length.

The preceding examples suggest that the bottom of the hierarchy also tends to be related to the vertical level of the speech system. That is, focus on a vertically lower level of the speech system tends to have an impact on upstream events to a greater degree than focus on upstream events influences events downstream. Thus initial focus on respiration—when it can be related to speech symptoms—could yield more immediate and dramatic change than would focus at higher levels of the system. Of course, if physiologic support cannot be improved at a lower level, then treatment should move to compensation at that level or to a higher level. This tendency does not always hold, however. A more appropriate general rule for focusing treatment is that *treatment should begin with whatever component will have the most beneficial effect on other components*. In general, "effect" refers to the impact of treatment on intelligibility.[80]

Identifying features that are readily modified with minimal instruction is also useful in establishing the initial focus of treatment. For example, what happens if the patient slows his or her rate, attempts to speak more forcefully, inhales more deeply before speaking, or speaks with his or her nares occluded? For some patients, immediate improvement is apparent in response to such simple instructions. Such improvement may not guarantee long-term gains, but what changes with minimal effort may be easiest to change habitually.

Management Should Start Early, but Not Always

For problems in the acute stage of illness or afterward, behavioral management generally should not begin until the patient is medically stable (i.e., not in medical danger, physical distress or pain, or otherwise limited in attention or responsiveness). In acute hospital settings, it also usually should not begin until medical management is complete or under way, unless medical management is delayed for a prolonged time. For some patients with intelligible speech, achieving stability relative to other physical disabilities and limitations may take precedence over speech therapy.

With the preceding qualifications in mind, it is generally agreed that early treatment* is desirable. For example, it appears that the success of stroke rehabilitation, in the broad sense, seems more strongly related to early intervention and intensity of intervention than it is to the duration of intervention.[†44,55]

---

*Unfortunately, there is no universally accepted definition of what constitutes "early" treatment. However, given the qualifications expressed earlier, it is almost certainly the case that initiating impairment-oriented therapy within days of an acute event is "too early" for many patients. In general, initiation of structured behavioral treatment for an MSD within 2 to 4 weeks after onset would probably be considered "early" by many clinicians and researchers.

†Because early intervention may be preferred over deferred intervention, this does not mean that treatment cannot be effective if delayed. For example, people in the chronic phase of stroke can increase hamstring strength when they engage in low-intensity treadmill exercise.[71] More relevant are case reports that demonstrate functional speech gains in people who receive therapy in the chronic phase of their illness.[1,39]

Although no data clearly establish that early treatment is better than deferred treatment for MSDs, there is face validity to the notions that early intervention may help slow deterioration of speech in degenerative diseases and that it may prevent the development of maladaptive speaking strategies in disorders that will improve or become chronic.[18,59] When factors such as efficiency of management and the desirability of bringing individuals to a maximum level of function as soon as possible are also considered, *early treatment is usually preferable to deferred treatment*.

Baseline Data Are Necessary for Establishing Goals and Measuring Change

Before behavioral management begins, the clinician should have baseline data that are relevant to the ultimate goals of treatment and to the specific tasks that will be the initial focus of therapy. Diagnosis and an inventory of deviant speech characteristics are generally insufficient as baseline data for measuring change during treatment. Diagnosis is independent of severity of impairment, disability, or societal limitation, and ratings of deviant speech characteristics on a severity scale have an uncertain relationship to more direct measures of disability and handicap.

Baseline data should include quantitative ratings or more specific measures of word and sentence intelligibility and efficiency of communication (see Chapter 3). These measures, as well as approaches that emphasize functional communication or the ability to communicate specific information or communicate in specific contexts,[38] can serve as the standard for measuring change, for judging the effectiveness of treatment, and for decision making about altering or terminating treatment.*

---

*The Motor Speech component of the Functional Communication Measures (FCMs), a series of severity scales developed by the American Speech-Language-Hearing Association (ASHA), is an example of a measure that rates speech on a seven-point scale of functional abilities, ranging from attempts to speak that cannot be understood at any time by familiar and unfamiliar listeners (1) to successful independent ability to participate in various situations without limitations imposed by speech (7). This FCM for motor speech abilities could be used as a crude index of functional change during treatment but not as a measure of impairment level change. FCMs also contribute to ASHA's National Outcome Measurement System (NOMS), a database intended to establish national benchmarks that can be used for various purposes, including quality improvement, predictions about expected outcome, and negotiations with third-party payers (additional information about FCMs and NOMS can be retrieved from *http://professional.asha.org/resources/noms/treatment_outcomes.cfm*). The intelligibility rating scale for MSDs presented in Chapter 3 (Table 3-4) is an example of a (nonstandardized) scale that can be used to index changes in intelligibility during the course of treatment.

Although difficult to quantify, it is important to inventory patients' communicative needs and goals,* their motivation to improve, their daily speaking environment, communication strategies they and their listeners find useful, and characteristics of their listeners. The potential influence of cognitive and sensory or motor deficits on prognosis and treatment activities must also be considered.

Finally, it is important to obtain baseline data on specific treatment tasks. For example, if the goal is to increase respiratory control by learning to generate 5 cm of water pressure for 5 seconds by blowing through a straw into a glass, it makes sense to establish the degree to which the patient can do this before treatment. This is important, because it allows measured progress to be task specific and because it allows progress on the task to be related to the overall goals of improving intelligibility and efficiency. It should be recognized, however, that *progress on a specific task might not and need not always lead to a temporally concurrent change in intelligibility or efficiency*. It is possible that small amounts of progress on a number of different tasks aimed at different levels of the speech system must add together before changes in intelligibility or efficiency become apparent; case reports illustrate this possibility.[52,69]

Increasing Physiologic Support Often Should Be the Initial Focus of Treatment

Treatment should usually begin by improving functions that support speech.[59] Thus modifying posture and increasing strength, speed, range, and muscle tone, if relevant to speech deficits, should be attended to first to ensure maximum physiologic capacity for speech. When this is achieved, then efforts at compensation can be made through prosthetic and other forms of behavioral management.

Compensation Requires That Speech Production Become Conscious

Darley, Aronson, and Brown[18] included the notion of *purposeful activity* among their basic principles of treatment. They stressed the need to make speech highly conscious, recognizing that doing so requires a major shift in the speaker's orientation to the speech act, one in which being heard and understood takes precedence over quick and emotive expression. Conscious control requires constant monitoring and self-criticism, at least during early stages of therapy,

---

*Yorkston, Bombardier, and Hammen[84] have presented and discussed a 100-item questionnaire that is useful for gathering information about patients' perspectives on their disability and handicap.

as well as recognition by the clinician and patient that maximum effort rarely can be maintained constantly.

Principles of Motor Learning Should Influence the Structure of Speech-Oriented Treatment

The patient's understanding of the management process is important, but simply knowing that something is necessary seldom leads to persisting improvement. Physical and cognitive "work" are essential.

Steps in motor learning can be broken down into *cognitive, associative,* and *autonomous or automatic stages.*[25,58] The cognitive stage includes understanding the nature of the problem, knowing why it is necessary to do certain things to achieve a goal, and learning the procedures that are to be followed. In the context of behavioral management, this includes understanding what it will take for speech to improve (e.g., understanding that rate must be slowed to improve intelligibility) and understanding the procedures required to achieve that improvement.

The associative stage includes the transition from conscious to more automatic control through trial and error, with feedback being especially important to learning what does and does not work. It is unclear if people with MSDs can ever get beyond the associative stage of learning, but the goal of behavioral management should be to bring the patient at least to the associative stage.

During the autonomous or automatic stage, a skill can be performed quickly, with little conscious effort. Feedback is less crucial and, if truly automatic, performance is possible even when the person is involved in another task.

The structure and organization of therapy can benefit from what is known about the acquisition of motor skills in normal individuals. The following points represent some "principles" that seem most relevant in this regard. The reader is cautioned that the validity of some of these principles for treating MSDs has yet to be established. In fact, the validity of some principles of motor learning in nonimpaired people is not firmly established. Schmidt and Bjork,[65] in a comprehensive and compelling discussion of commonly accepted principles of training, argue that "certain conceptualizations about how and when to practice are at best incomplete, and at worst incorrect." Of particular relevance, they said manipulations that facilitate performance during training sometimes can be detrimental in the long run and manipulations that degrade speed of acquisition during training can actually facilitate long-term carryover. At the least, these issues indicate that the effectiveness of a technique must be assessed by measures of long-term retention and generalization, as well as its more immediate effects on the rate and degree of skill acquisition during therapy tasks. Put another way, *clinicians should not assume that techniques that maximize performance during therapy necessarily facilitate the ultimate goal of treatment—long-term retention of improved performance within a variety of natural communicative contexts.*

Improving Speech Requires Speaking

People with MSDs must speak to improve their speech. This is self-evident but must be kept in mind considering the natural tendency to talk less when impairment makes speaking difficult, triggers a change in self-concept, or generates negative reactions from listeners. In nonimpaired individuals, disuse leads to muscle atrophy and less capacity for exercise (increased muscle fatigue), and gains derived from exercise are lost when exercise ceases; in people who are ill and confined to bed, deconditioning can occur independent of the underlying disease.[15] The importance of speech "exercise" is probably greatest during the recovery or improvement phase of therapy because it is generally agreed that less activity is necessary to maintain a skill once it has been achieved.[62] It is likely that speaking in order to maintain speech is more important for people with MSDs than it is for nonimpaired speakers.

It is possible that mental practice—imagining the performance of the task—can contribute to motor learning. In general, however, *mental practice is more effective than no practice but is less effective than physical practice.*[58] Thus a judicious mixture of mental and physical practice may reduce the amount of physical practice needed to achieve a given level of performance. The contribution of mental practice to improvement of MSDs is largely unexplored. It may have greater potential relevance to the management of AOS than dysarthria.

Drill Is Essential

Drill is the systematic practice of specially selected and ordered exercises.[59] Drill implies repetitiveness and tedium, but most patients do not mind it if tasks are selected in ways that lead to progress.

Multiple opportunities for practice are probably important, and therapy to improve speech, at least during its early stages, should be frequent (e.g., twice daily),[59] including periods of practice beyond formal treatment sessions.[87] The immediate effects of *brief periods of practice distributed over time may be better than lengthy periods of massed practice.*[70,81] This may be particularly true for MSDs, in which fatigue with extended periods of speaking is often a problem.* This suggests that drill be conducted for short periods of time, but frequently. *Alternating drill with short periods of rest or nondrill activities may help combat the effects of fatigue.*[27]

In this context it should be noted that fatigue does not seem to be an essential component of strength training. Data from healthy individuals undergoing isotonic strength training suggest that although high fatigue exercise results in faster strength gains than low fatigue exercise, both forms of exercise produce similar final outcomes.[26] In addition, light resistance exercise can safely increase strength in people with UMN disease and diseases affecting the motor unit.[17,19]

Instruction

Most patients do not improve simply by talking. They often need some instruction and demonstration about what to do. For example, instructing dysarthric speakers to be "more forceful" results in increased intraoral pressure during speech.[35] The ability to alter speech with instruction is generally thought to be a positive prognostic sign, but this assumption has not been tested formally and may not be correct. That is, *the momentary accessibility of a response during practice is quite different from the retention of that response once practice has ended.*[64]

Self-Learning

Although instruction can set the stage for learning, there is evidence that discovery learning, in which the individual determines how best to achieve goals, may lead to better retention and generalization than learning that is highly prompted.[70,81] Thus a balance must be struck between clinician-provided instruction and allowing patients to learn on their own. The best strategy may be to set a general goal (e.g., slow rate) and then allow the patient to discover how best to accomplish it, providing instruction only when he or she is unsuccessful after repeated efforts. Instruction generally should be faded as soon as possible, perhaps even if it slows the rate of improvement on a therapy task; that is, slower progress without instruction may lead to better long-term carryover.[65]

Feedback

Knowledge of results (feedback) is crucial to motor learning, especially in its early stages.[58,70] Feedback can be provided by the clinician (or other people) or be instrumental.

Clinician-provided feedback is most appropriate when the immediate goal is intelligibility or some aspect of performance for which other feedback is not available. It appears that the more specific listener feedback is, the more likely it is to influence subsequent responses. For example, dysarthric speakers are more likely to modify voice onset time in response to feedback in which the type and locus of errors are specified than when feedback simply indicates that a message is not understood.[77] The long-term effects of such feedback during therapy, however, are unknown.

Feedback provided during group therapy by other individuals with dysarthria has been reported by some patients as more potent and "appreciated" than clinician-provided feedback by some patients.[75] Reviewing audiotapes or videotapes can also demonstrate to patients the effects of adopting certain strategies for speaking and repairing communication breakdowns. It is also useful to show the patient evidence of progress over time (e.g., improvement of intelligibility scores). Such feedback is motivating and psychologically reinforcing, and it can be useful when discussing the continuation, modification, or termination of treatment.

Instrumental feedback or *biofeedback** can be useful when a specific motor behavior or acoustic result is the focus of treatment. Effective feedback instruments range from simple to sophisticated. A mirror can provide information about range of jaw movement, a hand on the abdomen can provide feedback about range of inspiratory or expiratory effort, a volume unit meter can indicate volume, an acoustic display can pace or reflect rate or stress or loudness, an electromyogram may signal excessive or insufficient muscle contraction, and so on. The precision and immediacy of instrumental feedback can facilitate online adjustments in speech. Such feedback is more directly linked to motor behavior than is the more "cognitive" nature of feedback about completed performance. Some data suggest that visual biofeedback may be most effective for people with a relatively poor response to initial training (i.e., are not stimulable during initial attempts to alter motor behavior), and perhaps not helpful for people who are highly stimulable.[78]

It is generally accepted that immediate, accurate, and frequent feedback (including biofeedback) facil-

---

*Fatigue is common in people with neurologic disease. For example, even 2 years following stroke, nearly 40% of survivors report always or often feeling tired. Even when age is controlled for, fatigue is often a significant problem.[30]

*Biofeedback involves transforming physiologic information about a variable of interest into a format that facilitates regulation or control over the physiologic variable. It is based on an assumption that immediate and accurate information about the variable facilitates motor learning.[76]

itates performance when a skill is being acquired. However, data on motor and verbal learning suggest that *frequent feedback during acquisition may actually degrade performance on long-term retention and generalization.*[64,65] It may be that frequent feedback becomes part of the task so that performance is degraded later when feedback is removed or altered. Another possibility is that external feedback might block processing of kinesthetic feedback, leading to less effective error-detection when external feedback is removed.[64,65] There is some limited evidence that this applies to speech motor learning. That is, retention of learned slower-than-normal speech rate is better when summary feedback is provided after every five trials than when it is provided after every trial.[2] Thus *less frequent feedback or feedback provided in summary form may have better long-term effects than frequent, immediate feedback.*

Beyond the basic principles of feedback just discussed, variables such as age, cognitive ability, and motivation can and should also influence decisions about the nature and frequency of feedback during therapy.[87]

Specificity of Training

A general principle of strength training is that neural and functional changes in strength are greatest for the trained movement. For example, it has been shown that velocity of nonspeech movements during training is correlated with the degree to which strength is improved for the goal task; thus low-velocity training increases strength for low-velocity but not high-velocity movements, and vice versa.[46] This is consistent with differences within the CNS motor system for the control of quick versus slower aspects of volitional movements (i.e., the direct versus indirect activation pathways). This specificity of training effect suggests that *training should be as specific as possible to the movement patterns, range of motion, velocity, and muscle contraction type and force of the ultimate goals to which training is directed.*[14,31,46] This has considerable face validity as applied to MSDs.

Treatment tasks should be relevant to speech, and movements practiced should be representative of those needed for speech, even when they are nonspeech in nature. There are (limited) data for dysarthric speakers that suggest that practice on nonspeech oral movement tasks may not lead to any improvement in speech.[66]

In general, treatment should not begin with any skill below the most advanced skill that can be demonstrated during assessment.[53] This means that, for many and perhaps most patients, speech and not nonspeech tasks should be the focus of treatment activities. Relatedly, treatment should focus on

changing motor abilities only as far as is necessary to achieve the goals of treatment.[87] For example, working on respiratory support beyond what is necessary for normal phrase length and loudness is generally unnecessary or inappropriate.

Consistent Practice and Variable Practice

Consistent practice refers to repetitive practice on an unvarying task before moving to the next level; this is often called *blocked practice.* An unvarying task can be defined in a number of ways. It might involve repetitive production of a single sound, sounds with the same manner of production (stops), single syllable words, three-word sentences with stress on the first syllable, and so on. *Variable (or random) practice* involves the same number of trials as blocked practice, but with randomization of tasks so that the same task is not practiced on successive trials. For example, one might focus on slowing rate on a randomly ordered set of single and multisyllabic words and sentences or focus on stress by producing sentences of varying length with stress placed at various locations within the sentence.

Variability of responses is frequently not allowed early in motor learning.[58] This reduction in "degrees of freedom" promotes consistency of response by limiting what must be attended to and controlled. It also appears that when a series of responses is produced over and over again as quickly as possible, speed is higher when responses are identical over repetitions than when they vary. This suggests that consistent practice may facilitate speed and, perhaps, automaticity of responses. It should be kept in mind, however, that this kind of drill is a poor representation of natural speaking conditions.

Increasing task variability during practice tends to depress performance during training— relative to consistent practice—but it tends to lead to better retention and generalization to different contexts.*[63-65] This may happen because an *average* representation of experience is more readily developed with variable practice, possibly because trial-to-trial changes in task demands require processing that provides information about the relationships that should exist among tasks components.[64,65] In addition, efficiency and naturalness tend to increase with practice, perhaps more so when degrees of freedom are allowed to vary and more than a single stereotyped response is permitted to achieve the same or variable

---

*However, when practice is minimal, blocked practice produces better retention than random practice.[64] This might be relevant to the structure of treatment tasks for patients who have frequent, extended therapy versus infrequent, short-term therapy.

motor goals.[58] There is evidence that this principle applies to people with motor deficits following stroke. For example, random practice seems to be more effective than blocked practice in promoting retention of learned functional upper limb motor skills in people with unilateral stroke.[36] Data regarding speech learning are sparse, but it has been shown that random practice or practice on multiple tasks leads to better retention than blocked practice in normal speakers learning to produce slower than normal speech rates.*[2] In addition, blocked practice does not lead to retention of novel nonsense words produced in a carrier phrase in healthy speakers and speakers with PD.[67] It is quite possible that there are motor learning principles common to the acquisition and retention of both speech and limb motor skills.[2]

These notions suggest that consistent practice may be most effective early in motor learning or when impairment is severe and the capacity to vary responses is limited. Variable practice may be more valuable in promoting generalization and naturalness and when recovery is sufficient to require that new responses be distinguished from preceding responses. This is especially relevant to the unique character of speech and language—the production of novel utterances that have not been practiced previously.

Increasing Strength

Little is known about optimal strategies for increasing force, power, or endurance in the oral muscles. Even less is known about the necessity and effectiveness of attempts to do so within the context of managing MSDs.[†] As a result, efforts to develop strength as part of MSD management remain controversial. In general, nonspeech strengthening exercises are probably appropriate only for people with

---

*Variable training for speech may be defined by more than the dynamics of the specific movements that are trained. For example, in normal-speaking children and adults, lower lip movements during production of six-syllable phrases are more stable when spoken in isolation than when embedded in sentences of high and low syntactic complexity.[49]

[†]A tutorial by Clark[14] provides an excellent overview of principles of strength training and other neuromuscular treatments as they might apply to speech and swallowing disorders. She points out that many nonspeech neuromuscular techniques for improving speech do not seem to have a solid theoretic basis, that they fail to address specificity of training or principles of strength training, that there is a general lack of empiric support for their use, and that their selection for use in any given patient must be tied to specific underlying neuromuscular impairments and disease processes.

weakness* sufficient to cause speech disability who are willing to invest the time and effort required of a strengthening program and in whom there are no contraindications to strengthening exercise. In general, high-intensity exercise is contraindicated for people with degenerative neurologic disease (e.g., ALS) who have severe and rapidly progressing weakness due to lower motor neuron involvement.[27] It has been noted that when all of these factors are considered, the number of people for whom speech strengthening exercise is appropriate is probably relatively small.[87] Even when appropriate, such exercise is likely to complement rather than replace activities that focus directly on speech.[14]

It is generally felt that, even when appropriate, strengthening exercises should not be excessively emphasized. However, efforts to increase strength may have positive effects in some patients, especially when physiologic support for speech is significantly compromised. A few observations about strength training in normal individuals may help clinical decisions about strength training for dysarthric speakers (*strength training is not appropriate for AOS*).

1. *Strength can be increased only by overloading muscle in some way.* Strength increases when muscle mass (the size and number of muscle fibers) is increased or when neural control (the recruitment and firing rates of motor units) increases. These increases can be achieved by low-resistance/high-repetition exercise or by high-resistance/low-repetition exercise. Because growth of muscle may depend on the tension developed within muscle with exercise, low-repetition/high-resistance exercise may be better for muscle growth.[31]

2. *Exercise can be isometric or isotonic.* Isometric exercise involves exertion against stationary resistance, whereas isotonic exercise requires movement of the structure to be strengthened. Isotonic exercise may be preferable for speech, because it comes closer to meeting specificity of training principles and requires agility and range of movement, both of which may be more important to speech than strength. It has been suggested that patients move from isometric to isotonic

---

*It has been shown that strength training (for 6 weeks) can increase limb strength in children with spastic cerebral palsy and results in improved capacity to walk faster.[17] At least in the limbs, therefore, CNS-based weakness, in a context of spasticity, can be modified by training. This raises the possibility that appropriately conducted strength training in people with spastic dysarthria might have an impact on speech; there is no evidence of such an effect at this time, however.

exercise as soon as short sequences of simple movements are possible.[8]

3. *Strengthening requires repetition.* Rosenbek and LaPointe[59] recommend sets of 5 to 10 repetitions with rest between sets, with approximately 1 to 2 minutes devoted to each muscle group. Although exercise at maximal levels (true weight training) should not exceed two to three times per week, more frequent training at less than maximal levels is justifiable.[31] To be effective, muscle activity should be greater than that required by normal nontreatment activities, but probably not so great that exhaustion occurs.[59] Striking this balance means that training at submaximal but greater-than-average levels of effort probably can occur daily.

4. *Once strengthening has been achieved, less activity is needed to maintain strength.* When strength is sufficient to support demands for speech, strengthening exercises can probably be discontinued in favor of activities that are speech specific; that is, speaking may be sufficient at that point to maintain strength for speaking.

5. *If maximum strength is required on some treatment tasks, it is not for the purpose of having the patient use maximum strength or effort all of the time.* Ultimately, speaking should demand less than maximum effort, because maximum effort can rarely be maintained for extended periods.[59,80]

Speed-Accuracy Tradeoff

Emphasizing speed tends to reduce accuracy, whereas emphasizing accuracy reduces speed.[70,81] This effect has been demonstrated on a speech learning task in speakers with PD.[67] Thus the early stages of treatment for most patients with MSDs may emphasize speed *or* accuracy but not both.

Accuracy should be emphasized initially for most patients because of its impact on intelligibility. In fact, accuracy is achieved initially by many patients through a reduction of speech rate. Increasing speed tends to be addressed only when acceptable intelligibility is achieved. Increases in rate must be constantly weighed against the possible trade-off with intelligibility.

Organization of Sessions

Frequency

The optimal frequency and duration of treatment for rehabilitation in general is unknown, but it is gener-

ally believed that greater intensity leads to better ultimate performance.[19] Thus as a general rule, treatment sessions should be frequent, especially early in the course of treatment. Many clinicians suggest two sessions daily, which is quite possible in most rehabilitation settings. When only one formal session is possible, practice at home should be required, preferably frequently but only for short periods. After formal therapy has ended, short periods of practice on a daily basis to maintain communication skills are often important.[87]

Task Ordering

How should treatment tasks be sequenced within sessions? Little is known about this for MSD management, but clues are available from the aphasia treatment literature.

Studies of aphasic patients suggest that easy tasks should precede difficult ones and treatment sessions should start with easy familiar tasks, proceed to novel or more difficult tasks, and end with tasks that ensure success.[9-11,29,59] In addition, within treatment sessions some time should be spent on activities that focus on maximizing the ability to communicate; that is, even if most tasks are nonspeech in nature, some time should always be devoted to the ultimate goal, the improvement of communication.

Error Rates

In aphasia therapy it is often recommended that error rates be kept low because high error rates tend to promote failure and may induce fatigue and reduce learning. Working on a given task in which performance is 60% to 80% correct and immediate is felt to be a good starting point, because success is achieved frequently but effort must be exerted to succeed.[8] When 90% or more of responses are completely adequate (e.g., accurate and immediate and without self-corrected errors), task difficulty should be increased. It is also reasonable in some cases to train beyond a criterion of 90% (require maintenance of criterion over several sessions), because overlearning may lead to better retention.[70,81]

It is not known if this approach to minimizing error rates during therapy maximizes retention or generalization for aphasic patients, but some argument can be made for permitting more errors (or making tasks more difficult) during acquisition phases of treatment, at least for people with MSDs. This derives from studies of motor learning that suggest *challenges that slow the rate of improvement during acquisition of a skill may actually result in improved posttraining performance.*[64]

Fatigue*

Physical exercise before language therapy negatively affects the performance of aphasic patients, especially on speaking and writing tasks.[50] It is reasonable to assume that such effects exist for people with MSDs, especially because the focus of their treatment is motoric. This suggests that therapy may be most productive early in the day or before or at least not immediately after physical or occupational therapy or other vigorous exercise. Relatedly, therapy may be most successful when benefits from drugs designed to manage the underlying disease are at a point of peak benefit.

Individual versus Group Therapy

There are no data to establish the advantages of individual versus group treatment for MSDs. Clinicians generally prefer individual therapy, especially early in the course of treatment. The advantages of individual work include the ease of focusing on specific aspects of performance, the opportunity to obtain a maximum number of responses, and the opportunity to alter treatment activities quickly as a function of response adequacy. Most of what is known about treatment efficacy for MSDs comes from the study of individual treatment.

Group therapy for MSDs has received little study. A recent systematic review of evidence regarding the behavioral management of respiratory/phonatory dysfunction in dysarthria concluded that there currently is insufficient evidence to confirm the effectiveness of group treatment for that purpose.[†85] Nonetheless, it has been observed that group therapy may be desirable for patients with milder degrees of disability and for those who are ready to work on carryover of skills and strategies learned during individual work.[75] This is especially true if family members or other caregivers are group members, because the group can engage in communication-oriented activities in which all members of the interaction have an opportunity to practice their own responsibilities. Group sessions that include several patients provide an opportunity for carryover, a chance for patients to observe the strategies used by others that they must also use, and an opportunity to receive feedback from peers. It is also an opportunity to share common experiences, frustrations, and successes.

■ TREATMENT EFFICACY

We do not know nearly as much about the effectiveness of treatment as we should, although evidence of treatment efficacy and effectiveness has increased substantially during the past decade. This lack of knowledge is not unusual. For example, it has been estimated that data from controlled trials to support the efficacy of *medical* intervention, in general, is available for only approximately 15% of interventions.[23,47] In contrast, disinformation from advertising, vested interests, and poor science is available to support almost anything.[47] The long-range goal should be for the management of MSDs to be conducted with universally firm evidence of efficacy, that ineffective and inefficient treatments will be recognized and discarded, and that new treatments will be embraced because of factual rather than factitious information about their efficacy.

There is a general sense among clinicians that treatments for dysarthria and AOS help patients to speak more intelligibly or communicate more efficiently and that treatment benefits can extend even to people with chronic or degenerative conditions.[53,54] These beliefs come from clinical experience and anecdotal reports, a fairly substantial number of well-controlled (and uncontrolled) case studies or reports, studies of aggregated cases, and some group studies that document gains in response to various treatment approaches for various dysarthria types and AOS.

In general, more is known about the effectiveness of surgical, pharmacologic, and prosthetic treatments for MSDs than about their behavioral management. Several reasons probably explain this. Effective medical and prosthetic approaches tend to have immediate and more rapidly dramatic effects on speech; their results are, therefore, more readily apparent and easier to measure. When they do not work, the outcome is known more rapidly, the reason for their failure may be apparent, and subsequent modifications or new treatments can be pursued. Behavioral management takes time, experimental control is often difficult to achieve, the precise reasons for success or failure often are not readily apparent, effects are not always dramatic or stable, and replication of results can be difficult. Nonetheless, a substantial number of case studies of behavioral management suggest treatment efficacy.

---

*Fatigue is an adaptive response to sustained activity. Mechanisms that produce it can involve all elements of the motor system, from CNS formulation and drive to contractile elements of muscle. An important component of fatigue is "sense of effort," or the perception of the amount of effort necessary to exert force and, eventually, an inability to produce desired force. Fatigue is influenced by motivation; degree of force, intensity and duration; speed of contraction; and movement strategies.[24]

†One study has reported that group treatment for individuals with PD and their spouses resulted in gains in some aspects of speech production and use of strategies to enhance communication in some patients, but generalization beyond treatment was not assessed.[73]

There are few group treatment studies in the literature on behavioral management of MSDs. Perhaps more significant is a dearth of data on the merits of various treatment approaches in comparison to each other.[53] Kent[41] has suggested that, for the present, it may be sufficient to know that a procedure works. He implies, however, that we should be making greater efforts to determine the efficiency of various procedures, the degree of benefit derived from them, whether one treatment approach is better than another, and whether some approaches are better for some patients than for others.

When reviewing published treatment studies, clinicians, researchers, and editors are disinclined to publish negative results. This is unfortunate, because the scientific purpose of treatment studies is to establish *if* a treatment is effective, not to prove that a treatment *is* effective. *It is as important to establish what does not work and who will not benefit from treatment as it is to establish what does work and who does benefit.*

Evidence-Based Practice and Practice Guidelines

The past decade has seen enormous development of the concepts of *evidence-based practice (EBP)* and *practice guidelines,* which are aids to clinical decision making that emphasize evidence of efficacy and effectiveness. The goal of these tools is to assist decisions about the most appropriate, effective, and cost-effective methods of care[86] by using the literature to aid the choice of assessment and treatment methods, as well as identify information about prognosis and cost-effectiveness.[82]

EBP emphasizes available data as a basis for informed clinical decision making for individual patients. It deemphasizes subjectivity or judgments based on intuition and unsystematic clinical impression as the only means for decision making[28] because nondatabased clinical judgments and uncontrolled clinical outcomes are not optimally sound approaches for evaluating treatment effects.*[33,79] However, *EBP is not meant to replace clinical experience because "not even the best of large-scale or randomized clinical trials can take the place of well-sharpened clinical judgment, made on a patient-by-patient basis."*[28] That is, even the best evidence is unlikely to account for all of the variables that affect clinical decisions for individual patients. Thus good

clinicians should use both their individual expertise and experience as well as identify the best available scientific evidence when confronted with specific clinical questions.[20,61] The ability to remain up-to-date is facilitated by practice guidelines and increasingly available rapid access to large literature databases, such as Medline, PsycINFO, and CINAHL, which make it possible for clinicians to regularly update information from thousands of journals. EBP has a secondary advantage of identifying gaps in clinical knowledge[83] that require further study. Many such gaps exist for MSDs.

Dollaghan[20] summarized the value of EBP by noting that it "offers us a framework by which we can systematically improve our efforts to be better clinicians, colleagues, advocates, and investigators—not by ignoring clinical experience and patient preferences but rather by considering these against a background of the highest quality scientific evidence that can be found." The charge to researchers, therefore, is to develop the evidence. The charge to clinicians is to use it appropriately.

Practice guidelines are explicit statements that can assist clinicians and patients in decision making about the care of specific problems. Panels of experts who review research evidence and consensus opinion develop them. Ideally, they are logical, specific, clearly stated, and practical, and ultimately they improve both equality (by reducing variability of care) and quality of service. Unlike *standards* (accepted management approaches based on a high degree of certainty) or *options* (approaches for which there is little clinical certainty), guidelines are rigorously developed outlines—but not rigid rules—for clinical conduct based on evidence that exceeds mere clinical opinion and for which there is moderate certainty that the value of particular clinical strategies exceeds their risks to a degree that make them worth providing.[83,86]

EBP and practice guidelines are now influencing most areas of health care,* including speech-language pathology,[28,82] and they have begun to have an impact on decisions about payment for certain services provided to people with MSDs.[86] Several subcommittees of the Academy of Neurologic Communication Disorders and Sciences (ANCDS)† are developing practice guidelines for MSDs and a number of other neurologic communication disorders that will become valuable resources for practicing clinicians and students in training. A number of

---

*Gruber et al.[33] and Wertz[79] provide a useful review and discussion of the importance of empirical evidence for evaluating treatment and why clinical judgment alone is not an optimally sound basis on which to evaluate treatment effects. They also address sources of bias that threaten the validity of outcome-based research.

*For an example of how EBP and practice guidelines have influenced clinical practice in neurology and the prevention and care of stroke, see Ringel and Hughes.[57]

†These efforts have also been supported by ASHA and the Department of Veterans Affairs (DVA).

publications are now available that address EBP and practice guidelines as they apply to communication disorders in general and MSDs specifically. Relevant references are listed in Appendix B, along with a number of more generic sources of information about EBP and practice guidelines.

Chapters 17 and 18 discuss specific treatment approaches for the dysarthrias and AOS, respectively. Reference will be made within those chapters to specific practice guidelines and published findings that can contribute to EBP.

SUMMARY

1. The goal of management of MSDs is to improve communication. This may involve an exclusive emphasis on improving speech intelligibility, efficiency, and naturalness, but it may also include the development of augmentative or alternative means of communication.

2. Management may focus on restoring, compensating, or adjusting to impaired speech functions. The degree to which management emphasizes restoration, compensation, and adjustment depends on many factors. Many patients engage in efforts to achieve all of these goals.

3. Not all people with MSDs are candidates for treatment. A decision to treat and selection of management strategies are influenced by numerous factors, including medical diagnosis and prognosis; disability and societal limitation; the environment in which communication will occur and the characteristics of the patient's communication partners; the patient's motivation and needs for communication; and the presence and nature of additional problems that may affect communication, such as memory and learning impairments and other sensory and motor deficits. Ongoing changes in the health care system also influence management decisions.

4. Treatment should be provided for as long as necessary to achieve treatment goals, but it should be accomplished in as short a time and in as cost-effective a manner as possible. Management should not begin without a plan for when it will end. It should be terminated when goals are reached, when plateauing has occurred, or when the patient decides he or she does not want further management. Follow-up reassessment is appropriate in many cases.

5. Management of MSDs may be medical, prosthetic, or behavioral. Medical management includes pharmacologic and surgical interventions, some of which may be conducted for the sole purpose of improving speech and others

intended to treat the general effects of the causal condition. Prosthetic management includes a number of mechanical and electronic devices; some improve speech and intelligibility, whereas others augment or substitute for verbal communication.

6. Behavioral intervention can be speech oriented or communication oriented. Speech-oriented approaches focus on improving intelligibility, efficiency, and naturalness of spoken communication by reducing or compensating for underlying impairment. Communication-oriented approaches emphasize environmental modifications and strategies for interacting and repairing breakdowns in communication when they occur. AAC systems represent a wide variety of nonspeech symbols, aids, strategies, and techniques that enhance communication. AAC is an important temporary or permanent part of management for many patients with MSDs.

7. Management includes important counseling and supportive roles for the clinician. These roles can be as important as efforts to improve speech and communication in some cases.

8. Universal prescriptions for managing MSDs are not possible, but some general principles can be applied to many patients. They include recognizing the relevance of medical and speech diagnoses to management, the advantages of starting management early in many cases, the need to acquire baseline data to set goals and measure change, and the value of increasing physiologic support early in treatment. Actual treatment activities must recognize the patient's need to make speech a conscious activity; the importance of principles of motor learning in the organization of treatment tasks; the importance of drill; the value of instruction, self-learning, and feedback; and the value of consistent and variable practice. When strength training is appropriate, principles of strength training should be employed.

9. Treatment should generally occur frequently, with sessions organized to move from easy to more difficult tasks, and end with success. Treatment sessions are likely to be most effective when fatigue is minimal. Individual and group therapy may be appropriate, but data that establish the relative advantages of each approach are unavailable.

10. Efficacy data for MSDs come mostly from individual case studies, aggregated case reports, and a small number of group studies. In general, they support a conclusion that management of MSDs is efficacious. Little is known about the relative merits of different approaches to treatment or

the specific disorders and other patient characteristics for which they are most effective. This state of knowledge may not be substantially different from what we understand about the effectiveness of medical interventions in general, especially interventions that focus on the modification of voluntary behaviors. Increased efforts to improve our understanding of the effectiveness of management for MSDs is essential if the quality and efficiency of management is to improve. In this regard, the development of practice guidelines and the framework provided by the concept of EBP are likely to reduce variability and improve quality of care because of their emphasis on evidence to support the use of particular treatment approaches.

References

1. Abkarian GG, Dworkin JP: Treating severe motor speech disorders: give speech a chance, J Med Speech-Lang Pathol 1:285, 1993.
2. Adams SG, Page AD: Effects of selected practice and feedback variables on speech motor learning, J Med Speech-Lang Pathol 8:215, 2000.
3. American Speech-Language-Hearing Association: Report: augmentative and alternative communication, ASHA 33(suppl 5):9, 1991.
4. Ball LJ, Beukelman DR, Pattee G: AAC clinical decision making for persons with ALS, ASHA SID 12 (Augmentative and Alternative Communication) Newsletter, vol 11, pp 7-12, April 2002.
5. Ball LJ, Beukelman DR, Pattee GL: Timing of speech deterioration in people with amyotrophic lateral sclerosis, J Med Speech-Lang Pathol 10:231, 2002.
6. Beukelman D, Mirenda P: Augmentative and alternative communication: management of severe communication disorders in children and adults, Baltimore, 1992, Paul H Brockes.
7. Beukelman DR, Yorkston KM, Reichle J, editors: Augmentative and alternative communication for adults with acquired communication disorders, New York, 2000, Paul H Brookes Publishing.
8. Brookshire RH: Introduction to neurogenic communication disorders, ed 6, St Louis, 2003, Mosby.
9. Brookshire RH: Effects of task difficulty on sentence comprehension performance of aphasic subjects, J Commun Disord 9:167, 1976.
10. Brookshire RH: Effects of task difficulty on the naming performance of aphasic subjects, J Speech Hear Res 15:551, 1972.
11. Brookshire RH: Effects of trial time and inter-trial interval on naming by aphasic subjects, J Commun Disord 3:289, 1971.
12. Buonomano D, Merzenich M: Cortical plasticity: from synapses to maps, Annu Rev Neurosci 21:385, 1998.
13. Cassell EJ: The healer's art, Cambridge, Mass, 1985, MIT Press.
14. Clark HM: Neuromuscular treatments for speech and swallowing: a tutorial, Am J Speech-Lang Pathol 12:400, 2003.
15. Convertino VA, Bloomfield SA, Greenleaf JE: An overview of the issues: physiological effect of bed rest and restricted physical activity, Med Sci Sports Exerc 29:187, 1997.
16. Cramer S et al: A functional MRI study of subjects recovered from hemiparetic stroke, Stroke 28:2518, 1997.
17. Damiano D, Abel M: Functional outcomes of strength training in spastic cerebral palsy, Arch Phys Med Rehabil 79:119, 1998.
18. Darley FL, Aronson AE, Brown JR: Motor speech disorders, Philadelphia, 1975, WB Saunders.
19. Dobkin BH, Thompson AJ: Principles of neurological rehabilitation. In Bradley WG et al, editors: Neurology in clinical practice: principles of diagnosis and management, vol 1, ed 3, Boston, 2000, Butterworth-Heinemann.
20. Dollaghan C: Evidence-based practice: myths and realities, ASHA Leader 9:5, 2004.
21. Doyle PC et al: Dysarthric speech: a comparison of computerized speech recognition and listener intelligibility, J Rehabil Res Dev 34:309, 1997.
22. Drubach A, Makley M, Dodd ML: Manipulation of central nervous system plasticity: a new dimension in the care of neurologically impaired patients, Mayo Clin Proc 79:796, 2004.
23. Eddy DM: Medicine, money and mathematics, Bull Am Coll Surg 77:36, 1992.
24. Enoka RM, Stuart DG: Neurobiology of muscle fatigue, J Appl Physiol 72:1631, 1992.
25. Fitts PM: Perceptual motor skill learning. In AW Melton, editor: Categories of human learning, New York, 1964, Academic Press.
26. Folland JP et al: Fatigue is not a necessary stimulus for strength during resistance training, Br J Sports Med 36:370, 2002.
27. Fowler WM: Consensus conference summary: role of physical activity and exercise training in neuromuscular diseases, Am J Phys Med Rehabil 81:S187, 2002.
28. Frattali C, Worrall LE: Evidence-based practice: applying science to the art of clinical care, J Med Speech-Lang Pathol 9:ix, 2001.
29. Gardner B, Brookshire RH: Effects of unisensory and multisensory presentation of stimuli upon naming by aphasic patients, Lang Speech 15:342, 1972.
30. Glader EL, Stegmayr B, Asplund K: Poststroke fatigue: a 2-year follow-up study of stroke patients in Sweden, Stroke 33:1327, 2002.
31. Gonyea WJ, Sale D: Physiology of weight-lifting exercise, Arch Phys Med Rehabil 63:235, 1982.
32. Gonzlez-Rothi LJ: Neurophysiologic basis of rehabilitation, J Med Speech-Lang Pathol 9:117, 2001
33. Gruber FA et al: Approaches to speech-language intervention and the true believer, J Med Speech-Lang Pathol 11:95, 2003.
34. Hallett M: Brain plasticity and recovery from hemiplegia, J Med Speech-Lang Pathol 9:107, 2001.
35. Hammen VL, Yorkston KM: Effect of instruction on selected aerodynamic parameters in subjects with dysarthria and control subjects. In Till JA, Yorkston KM, Beukelman DR, editors: Motor speech disorders: advances in assessment and treatment, Baltimore, 1994, Paul H Brookes.
36. Hanlon R: Motor learning following unilateral stroke, Arch Phys Med Rehabil 77:811, 1996.

37. Higginbotham DJ et al: Discourse comprehension of synthetic speech across three augmentative and alternative communication (AAC) output methods, J Speech Hear Res 38:889, 1995.

38. Hustad KC, Beukelman DR, Yorkston KM: Functional outcome assessment in dysarthria, Semin Speech Lang 19:291, 1998.

39. Keatley A, Wirz S: Is 20 years too long?: improving intelligibility in long-standing dysarthria—a single case treatment study, Eur J Disord Commun 29:183, 1994.

40. Kent RD: Insights from memoirs of illness and disability, ASHA 40:22, 1998.

41. Kent RD: The clinical science of motor speech disorders: a personal assessment. In Till JA, Yorkston KM, Beukelman DR, editors: Motor speech disorders: advances in assessment and treatment, Baltimore, 1994, Paul H Brookes.

42. Konrad C et al: Pattern of cortical reorganization in amyotrophic lateral sclerosis: a functional magnetic resonance imaging study, Exp Brain Res 143:51, 2002.

43. Kubler A et al: Brain-computer communication: unlocking the locked in, Psychol Bull 127:358, 2001.

44. Kwakkel G et al: Effects of intensity of rehabilitation after stroke, Stroke 28:1550, 1997.

45. LaPointe LL: Base-10 programmed stimulation: task specification, scoring, and plotting performance in aphasia therapy, J Speech Hear Disord 42:90, 1977.

46. Liss JM, Kuehn DP, Hinkle KP: Direct training of velopharyngeal musculature, J Med Speech-Lang Pathol 2:243, 1994.

47. Little JM: Communication and the humanities: the nature of the nexus, Mayo Clin Proc 68:921, 1993.

48. Lotze M et al: Motor learning elicited by voluntary drive, Brain 126:866, 2003.

49. Maner KJ, Smith A, Grayson L: Influences of utterance length and complexity on speech motor performance in children and adults, J Speech Lang Hear Res 43:560, 2000.

50. Marshall RC, King PS: Effects of fatigue produced in isokinetic exercise on the communication ability of aphasic adults, J Speech Hear Res 16:222, 1973.

51. Mathy P, Yorkston KM, Gutmann ML: AAC for individuals with amyotrophic lateral sclerosis. In Beukelman DR, Yorkston KM, Reichle J, editors: Augmentative and alternative communication for adults with acquired communication disorders, New York, 2000, Paul H Brookes.

52. McHenry MA, Wilson RL, Minton JT: Management of multiple physiologic system deficits following traumatic brain injury, J Med Speech-Lang Pathol 2:59, 1994.

53. Netsell R: A neurobiologic view of the dysarthrias. In McNeil MR, Rosenbek JC, Aronson AE, editors: The dysarthrias: physiology, acoustics, perception, management, San Diego, 1984, College-Hill Press.

54. Netsell R, Rosenbek J: Treating the dysarthrias. Speech and language evaluation in neurology: adult disorders, New York, 1985, Grune & Stratton.

55. Ottenbacher KJ, Jannell S: The results of clinical trials in stroke rehabilitation research, Arch Neurol 50:37, 1993.

56. Reding M, Solomon B, Borucki S: Effect of dextroamphetamine on motor recovery after stroke, Neurology 45(suppl 4):A222, 1995.

57. Ringel SP, Hughes RL: Evidence-based medicine, critical pathways, practice guidelines, and managed care. Reflections on the prevention and care of stroke, Arch Neurol 53:867, 1996.

58. Rosenbaum DA: Human motor control, San Diego, 1991, Academic Press.

59. Rosenbek JC, LaPointe LL: The dysarthrias: description, diagnosis, and treatment. In Johns DF, editor: Clinical management of neurogenic communication disorders, Boston, 1985, Little, Brown, & Company.

60. Rosenfield DB: Pharmacologic approaches to speech motor disorders. In Vogel D, Cannito MP, editors: Treating disordered speech motor control, Austin, Tex, 1991, Pro-Ed.

61. Sackett DL et al: Evidence-based medicine, New York, 1997, Churchill Livingstone.

62. Saxon K: Exercise physiology and vocal rehabilitation, Miniseminar presented at the Annual Convention of the American Speech-Language-Hearing Association, Anaheim, Calif, November 1993.

63. Schmidt RA: Frequent augmented feedback can degrade learning: evidence and interpretations. In Stelmach GE, Requin J, editors: Tutorials in motor neuroscience, Dordrecht, The Netherlands, 1991, Kluwer.

64. Schmidt RA, Bjork RA: New conceptualizations of practice: common principles in three paradigms suggest new concepts for training. In Robin DA, Yorkston KM, Beukelman DR, editors: Disorders of motor speech: assessment, treatment, and clinical, Baltimore, 1996, Brookes Publishing.

65. Schmidt RA, Bjork RA: New conceptualizations in practice: common principles in three paradigms suggest new concepts for training, Psychol Sci 3:207, 1992.

66. Schulz, Dingwall O, Ludlow CL: Speech and oral motor learning in individuals with cerebellar atrophy, J Speech Lang Hear Res 42:1157, 1999.

67. Schulz GM et al: Speech motor learning in Parkinson disease, J Med Speech-Lang Pathol 8:243, 2000.

68. Siegler M: Falling off the pedestal: what is happening to the traditional doctor-patient relationship? Mayo Clinic Proc 68:461, 1993.

69. Simpson MB, Till JA, Goff AM: Long-term treatment of severe dysarthria: a case study, J Speech Hear Disord 43:433, 1988.

70. Singer RN: Motor learning and human performance: an application to motor skills and movement behaviors, New York, 1980, Macmillan.

71. Smith GV et al: Task-oriented exercise improves hamstring strength and spastic reflexes in chronic stroke patients, Stroke 30:2112, 1999.

72. Soderholm S, Meinander M, Alaranta H: Augmentative and alternative communication methods in locked-in syndrome, J Rehabil Med 33:235, 2001.

73. Sullivan MD, Brune PJ, Beukelman DR: Maintenance of speech changes following group treatment for hypokinetic dysarthria of Parkinson's disease. In Robin DA, Yorkston KM, Beukelman DR, editors: Disorders of motor speech: assessment, treatment, and clinical characterization, Baltimore, 1996, Brookes Publishing.

74. Sy BK, Horowitz DM: A statistical causal model for the assessment of dysarthric speech and the utility of com-

puter-based speech recognition, IEEE Trans Biomed Eng 40:1282, 1993.

75. *Thomas JE, Keith RL: Group therapy for dysarthric speakers. Paper presented at the American Speech-Language-Hearing Association Convention, St Louis, Mo, 1989.*

76. *Thompson-Ward EC, Murdoch BE, Stokes PD: Biofeedback rehabilitation of speech breathing for an individual with dysarthria, J Med Speech-Lang Pathol 5:277, 1997.*

77. *Till JA, Toye AR: Acoustic and phonetic effects of two types of verbal feedback in dysarthric subjects, J Speech Hear Disord 53:449, 1988.*

78. *Volin RA: A relationship between stimulability and the efficacy of visual biofeedback in the training of a respiratory control task, Am J Speech-Lang Pathol 7:81, 1998.*

79. *Wertz RT: Approaches to speech-language intervention and the true believer: a response, J Med Speech-Lang Pathol 11:105, 2003.*

80. *Wertz RT: Neuropathologies of speech and language: an introduction to patient management. In Johns DF, editor: Clinical management of neurogenic communicative disorders, Boston, 1985, Little, Brown & Company*

81. *Wertz RT, LaPointe LL, Rosenbek, JC: Apraxia of speech in adults: the disorders and its management, New York, 1984, Grune & Stratton.*

82. *Worrall LE, Bennett S: Evidence-based practice: barriers and facilitators for speech-language pathologists, J Med Speech-Lang Pathol 9:xi, 2001.*

83. *Yorkston KM, Beukelman DR: Decision making in AAC intervention. In DR Beukelman, KR Yorkston, Reichle J, editors: Augmentative and alternative communication for adults with acquired neurologic disorders, Baltimore, 2000, Paul H Brookes.*

84. *Yorkston KM, Bombardier C, Hammen VL: Dysarthria from the viewpoint of individuals with dysarthria. In Till JA, Yorkston KM, Beukelman DR, editors: Motor speech disorders: advances in assessment and treatment, Baltimore, 1994, Paul H Brookes.*

85. *Yorkston KM, Spencer KA, Duffy JR: Behavioral management of respiratory/phonatory dysfunction from dysarthria: a systematic review of the evidence, J Med Speech-Lang Pathol 11:xiii, 2003.*

85a. *Yorkston KM, Strand EA, Kennedy MRT: Comprehensibility of dysarthric speech: implications for assessment and treatment planning, Amer J Speech-Lang Pathol 5:55, 1996*

86. *Yorkston KM et al: Evidence-based practice guidelines: application to the field of speech-language pathology, J Med Speech-Lang Pathol 9:243, 2001.*

87. *Yorkston KM et al: Management of motor speech disorders in children and adults, ed 2, Austin, Tex, 1999, Pro-Ed.*

88. *Yorkston KM et al: Speech deterioration in amyotrophic lateral sclerosis: implications for the timing of intervention, J Med Speech-Lang Pathol 1:35, 1993.*

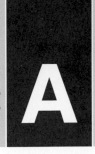

Academy of Neurologic Communication Disorders and Sciences
PO Box 26532
Minneapolis, MN 55426
Tel: (952) 920-0484; Fax: (952) 920-6098
www.ancds.duq.edu

ALS Association
27001 Agoura Road, Suite 150
Calabasas Hills, CA 91301
Tel: (818) 880-9007
www.alsa.org

American Brain Tumor Association
2720 River Road
Des Plaines, IL 60018
Tel: (800) 886-2282; Fax (847) 827-9918
www.abta.org

American Epilepsy Society
342 North Main Street
West Hartford, CT 06117-2507
Tel: (860) 586-7505
www.aesnet.org

American Heart Association
National Center
7272 Greenville Avenue
Dallas, TX 75231
Tel: (800) 242-8721
www.americanheart.org

American Speech-Language-Hearing Association
10801 Rockville Pike
Rockville, MD 20852
Tel: (800) 498-2071
www.asha.org

American Stroke Association
National Center
7272 Greenville Avenue
Dallas, TX 75231
Tel: (888) 478-7653
www.strokeassociation.org

Brain Injury Association of America
8201 Greensboro Dr., Suite 611
McLean, VA 22102
Tel: (703) 761-0750
www.biausa.org

Epilepsy Foundation
4351 Garden City Drive
Landover, MD 20785-7223
Tel: (800) 332-1000
www.epilepsyfoundation.org

Huntington's Disease Society of America
158 West 29th Street, 7th Floor
New York, NY 10001-5300
Tel: (800) 345-4372; Fax: (212) 239-3430
www.hdsa.org

Multiple Sclerosis International Federation
www.msif.org

National Aphasia Association
29 John St., Suite 1103
New York, NY 10038
Tel: (212) 267-2814; Fax: (212) 267-2812
www.aphasia.org

National Ataxia Foundation
750 Twelve Oaks Center
15500 Wayzata Boulevard
Wayzata, MN 55931
Tel: (612) 473-7666; Fax: (612) 473-9892
www.nwwin.com/houston/mall-a/ataxia.htm

National Center for the Dissemination of Disability Research
211 East Seventh Street, Room 400
Austin, TX 78701-3253
Tel: (800) 266-1832 or (512) 476-6861; Fax (512) 476-2286)
www.ncddr.org

National Council on Patient Information and Education
4915 Saint Elmo Ave., Suite 505
Bethesda, MD 20814-6082
Tel: (301) 656-8565; Fax: (301) 656-4464
www.talkaboutrx.org

National Institute on Deafness and Other Communication Disorders
31 Center Drive, MSC 2320
Bethesda, MD 20892-2320
www.nidcd.nih.gov

The National Parkinson Foundation, Inc.
Bob Hope Parkinson Research Center
1501 NW 9th Avenue
Bob Hope Road
Miami, FL 33136-1494
Tel: (305) 547-6666 or (800) 327-4545; Fax: (305) 243-4403
www.parkinson.org

National Stroke Association
9707 E. Easter Lane
Englewood, CO 80112
Tel: (303) 649-9299; Fax: (303) 649-1328
http://199.239.30.192/NationalStroke/default.htm

Office of Disability Employment Policy
U.S. Department of Labor
Frances Perkins Building
200 Constitution Avenue, NW
Washington, DC 20210
Tel: (866) 633-7365; Fax: (202) 693-7888
www.dol.gov

Office of Rare Disease
National Institute of Health
6100 Executive Boulevard, 3B-01
Bethesda, MD 20892-7518
Tel: (301) 402-4336; Fax: (301) 480-9655
http://rarediseases.info.nih.gov

Office of Special Education and Rehabilitative Services
U.S. Department of Education
400 Maryland Avenue, SW
Washington, DC 20202
Tel: (800) 872-5327; Fax: (202) 401-0689
www.ed.gov/about/contacts/gen

Rehabilitation Engineering & Assistive Technology Society of North America
1700 N. Moore Street, Suite 1540
Arlington, VA 22209-1903
Tel: (703) 524-6686; Fax: (703) 524-6630
www.resna.org

Shy-Drager Syndrome Support Group
Dorothy Trainor-Kingsbury
1607 SE Silver Avenue
Albuquerque, NM 87106
Tel: (505) 243-5118

Society for Neuroscience
11 Dupont Circle, NW
Suite 500
Washington, DC 20036
Tel: (202) 462-6688
http://web.sfn.org

The Society for PSP
Woodholme Medical Building, Suite 515
1838 Greene Tree Road
Baltimore, MD 21208
Tel: (410) 486-3330 or (800) 457-4777; Fax: (410) 486-4283
www.psp.org

Tourette Syndrome Association, Inc.
42-40 Bell Boulevard
Bayside, NY 11361
Tel: (718) 224-2999
www.tsa-usa.org

United Cerebral Palsy
1660 L Street, NW, Suite 700
Washington, DC 20036
Tel: (800) 872-5827 or (202) 776-0406; Fax: (202) 776-0414
www.ucp.org

United Leukodystrophy Foundation
2304 Highland Drive
Sycamore, IL 60178
Tel: (800) 728-5483; Fax: (815) 895-2432
www.ulf.org

The Wilson's Disease Association International
1802 Brookside Drive
Wooster, OH 44691
Tel: (330) 264-1450 or (800) 399-0266; Fax: (509) 757-6418
www.wilsonsdisease.org

Practice Guidelines and Evidence-Based Practice Information Sources

Publications and related sources of information relevant to evidence-based practice guidelines for speech-language pathology, with emphasis on MSDs, include the following:

Academy of Neurologic Communication Disorders and Sciences: *Evidence-based practice guidelines for the management of communication disorders in neurologically impaired individuals,* retrieved Sept. 17, 2004, from *http://www.ancds.duq. edu/guidelines.html.*

American Speech-Language Hearing Association: *Evidence-based practice,* retrieved Sept. 17, 2004, from *www.asha.org/members/slp/topics/ebp.*

Duffy JR, Yorkston KM: Medical interventions for spasmodic dysphonia and some related conditions: a systematic review, *J Med Speech-Lang Pathol* 11:ix, 2003.

Duffy JR et al: *Medical interventions for spasmodic dysphonia and some related conditions: a systematic review (technical report 2),* Minneapolis, 2001, Academy of Neurologic Communication Disorders and Sciences.

Frattali C et al.: Development of evidence-based practice guidelines: committee update, *J Med Speech-Lang Pathol* 11:ix, 2003.

Hanson EK, Yorkston KM, Beukelman DR: Speech supplementation techniques for dysarthria: a systematic review, *J Med Speech-Lang Pathol* 12:ix, 2004.

Spencer KA, Yorkston KM, Duffy JR: Behavioral management of respiratory/phonatory dysfunction from dysarthria: a flowchart for guidance in clinical decision-making, *J Med Speech-Lang Pathol* 11:xxxix, 2003.

Spencer KA et al: *Practice guidelines for dysarthria: evidence for the behavioral management of the respiratory/phonatory system (technical report 3),* Minneapolis, 2002, Academy of Neurologic Communication Disorders and Sciences.

Threats T: Evidence-based practice research using a WHO framework, *J Med Speech-Lang Pathol* 10:17, 2002.

Yorkston KM et al: *Practice guidelines for dysarthria: evidence for the effectiveness of management of velopharyngeal function (technical report 1),* Academy of Neurologic Communication Disorders and Sciences, retrieved Sept. 17, 2004, from *www.ancds.duq.edu/guidelines.html.*

Yorkston KM et al: Evidence-based medicine and practice guidelines: application to the field of speech-language pathology, *J Med Speech-Lang Pathol* 9:243, 2001a.

Yorkston KM, Hanson E, Beukelman D: *Speech supplementation techniques for dysarthria: a systematic review (technical report 4),* Minneapolis, 2003, Academy of Neurologic Communication Disorders and Sciences.

Yorkston KM, Spencer KA, Duffy JR: Behavioral management of respiratory/phonatory dysfunction from dysarthria: a systematic review of the evidence, *J Med Speech-Lang Pathol* 11:xiii, 2003.

Yorkston KM et al: Evidence-based practice guidelines for dysarthria: Management of velopharyngeal dysfunction, *J Med Speech-Lang Pathol* 9:257, 2001.

Evidence-based practice: general sources of information

Muir Gray JA: *Evidence-based healthcare. How to make policy and management decisions,* New York, 1997, Churchill Livingstone.

Sackett DL et al: *Evidence-based medicine,* New York, 1997, Churchill Livingstone.

The following websites represent resources for information relevant to evidence-based practice in health care (as provided by Dollaghan, 2004):

- Agency for Healthcare Research and Quality: *www.ahrq.gov.*

- *British Medical Journal: http://bmj.com/collections.*

- The Centre for Evidence-Based Medicine, University of Toronto Health Network: *www.cebm.utoronto.ca.*

- Cochrane Library:
  www.update-software.com/cochrane.

- Ebell MH, Department of Family Practice, Michigan State University:
  www.poems.msu.edu/InfoMastery.

- Oxford Centre for Evidence-Based Medicine:
  www.cebm.net.

- National Guideline Clearinghouse:
  www.guideline.gov.

- PubMed: *www.ncbi.nlm.nih.gov.*

Additional web-based sources of information for clinicians, researchers, and consumers include the following:

- National Institutes of Health (NIH): *www.nih.gov.* A good resource for health information, including health resources, clinical trials and other studies, health hotlines, and drug information. Also provides information about NIH grants and funding opportunities.

- National Institute on Deafness and Other Communication Disorders (NIDCD): *www.nidcd.nih.gov.* An institute within the NIH. The website provides health information and information about ongoing research and grant funding opportunities specific to various voice, speech, and language disorders. It is linked to health resources that include free publications and a combined health information database that includes book, articles, and patient education materials.

- Medline Plus: *www.nlm.nih.gov/medlineplus.* A service of the U.S. National Library of Medicine and the NIH. It is a consumer-oriented resource for a large number of health topics, drug information, and other resources, including health organizations.

17

Managing the Dysarthrias

"There is both scientific and clinical evidence that individuals with dysarthria benefit from the services of speech-language pathologists."[236]

K.M Yorkston

CHAPTER OUTLINE

I. Speaker-oriented treatment
   A. Respiration
   B. Phonation—medical treatments
   C. Phonation—prosthetic management
   D. Phonation—behavioral management
   E. Resonance
   F. Articulation
   G. Rate
   H. Prosody and naturalness

III. Speaker-oriented treatment for specific dysarthria types
   A. Flaccid dysarthrias
   B. Spastic dysarthria
   C. Ataxic dysarthria
   D. Hypokinetic dysarthria
   E. Hyperkinetic dysarthrias
   F. Unilateral upper motor neuron dysarthria
   G. Mixed dysarthrias

IV. Communication-oriented treatment
   A. Speaker strategies
   B. Listener strategies
   C. Interaction strategies

V. Summary

It has been said, "There is no special treatment for the dysarthric disturbance of speech."[150] It is unclear if this was meant to imply that treatment for dysarthria is homogeneous and provided without regard for severity or the specific nature of the speech disturbance, or that nothing can be done to help dysarthric speakers. Neither implication is true, however. There are numerous ways in which clinicians manage dysarthria, and much of the diversity is a function of type and severity of the disorder. Also, although efficacy data are limited, there are data that document the effectiveness of several approaches to management,[236] even for people with severe dysarthria or anarthria.[30]

This chapter addresses the management of people with dysarthria.* It is assumed that the reader has read Chapter 16 and is aware of the basic issues and general approaches to managing motor speech disorders (MSDs). It is also assumed that the reader has an appreciation of the general principles and guidelines for the behavioral management of MSDs, because most of them are directly applicable to the dysarthrias.

This chapter first addresses speaker-oriented approaches to intervention. Medical, prosthetic, and behavioral interventions directed at modifying respiration; phonation; resonance; articulation; and the rate, prosody, and naturalness of dysarthric speech are the focus of this first section. Next, the degree to which specific speaker-oriented management strategies apply to each of the dysarthria types is addressed. It makes clear that treatment does not vary only as a function of severity, that not all available management approaches are appropriate for all dysarthria types, and that some approaches may be contraindicated for some dysarthria types. It also illustrates the value of differential diagnosis to management; that is, because diagnosis implies an understanding of underlying pathophysiology, it helps determine to some extent the most relevant approaches to treatment.

The last section of the chapter focuses on communication-oriented approaches. Such approaches are relatively independent of dysarthria type and are more strongly tied to individuals' communication needs and desires and to the degree of their disability.

The parsing of approaches to management under various headings is not meant to imply that different approaches are mutually exclusive. In fact, it is likely

---

*Many of the broad issues, concepts, and techniques that are discussed here, although based on the efforts of many clinicians and researchers, have been strongly influenced by the contributions of Yorkston, Beukelman, and Bell[240] and Rosenbek and LaPointe.[182]

that multiple approaches to managing dysarthria are appropriate and necessary for many dysarthric speakers.*

Evidence for the effectiveness of the approaches discussed here is addressed when relevant data are available. The availability or lack of such data should help guide the enthusiasm or caution with which these approaches should be embraced. Note that a distinction must be made between evidence-based support (at least one study reporting a positive outcome for at least one dysarthric person) and expert opinion (support based on the experience of experts but without published data-based evidence).

SPEAKER-ORIENTED TREATMENT

Respiration

Darley, Aronson, and Brown (DAB)[43] felt that respiration usually does not require attention in treatment, because respiratory demands for speech are not great and because improving function at the phonatory, resonatory, and articulatory valves generally promotes efficient use of the airstream. Even the presence of abnormal respiratory function does not necessarily mean that respiration is not adequate for speech. Some people with significant respiratory compromise do quite well during speech, whereas some with less impairment breathe atypically and sometimes maladaptively during speech. In general, *if a patient has adequate loudness and demonstrates flexible breath patterning during speech, then respiration does not require attention.*[245]

Many dysarthric speakers do not need to attend specifically to respiration. However, even dysarthric speakers who do not have significant general respiratory compromise tend to have reduced words per breath group, less variability in breath group length, and occasionally take breaths at nonsyntactic boundaries[85]; such characteristics can negatively influence perceived naturalness[†] of speech and possibly reduce

intelligibility. In addition, poor respiration may affect other speech functions, especially phonation. Thus attention to speech breathing may be necessary to maximize consistent respiratory support for speech and to ensure appropriate breath group lengths and variability for speech. At the least, *treatment planning should explicitly address the possible need to attend to respiration.** When the need exists, management efforts are primarily behavioral and prosthetic.[†]

Increasing Respiratory Support

Respiration may not require attention as long as steady subglottal air pressure of 5 to 10 cm of water can be sustained for 5 seconds.[164] Work to increase respiratory support may be necessary or appropriate if 5 cm of water pressure on speech or speechlike tasks cannot be generated, if consistent air pressure cannot be sustained for 5 seconds, if respiratory pressure cannot support phonation, or if more than one word per breath group cannot be produced during speech.[245]

Nonspeech respiratory exercises are probably unnecessary and inappropriate when speech exercise can accomplish the treatment goal. However, some patients who are unable to generate subglottal air pressure sufficient to support phonation may need to work on respiration in isolation before they can engage in speech tasks.[210]

Nonspeech tasks that may improve respiratory support and subglottal air pressure include blowing into a water glass manometer (see Figure 3-5) with a goal of sustaining 5 cm of pressure for 5 seconds ("5 for 5").[‡100,129,163] An air pressure transducer with a target cursor and responses displayed on an oscilloscope or computer screen can be used for the same purpose; these can provide more easily seen and monitored feedback about performance.

A related speech task is *maximum vowel prolongation,* with duration and loudness goals. Feedback

---

*A report of treatment that focused on increased respiratory support, contrastive stress, and verbal repair strategies for seven patients with ataxic or mixed ataxic-spastic dysarthria associated with multiple sclerosis (MS),[93] as well as a report describing the management of dysarthria in a patient with traumatic brain injury (TBI) who required a palatal lift prosthesis and rate reduction strategies (among a number of strategies)[142] are good illustrations of the use of a combination of well-reasoned management techniques.

[†]Breath patterning (or words per breath group) is a crucial aspect of naturalness, because it is the foundation on which intonation and stress patterns (prosody) are based.[245] Normal speakers take more than 70% of their breaths at primary syntactic boundaries (e.g., at the end of sentences) and only a few within phrases or clauses. Dysarthric speakers may take less than half of their breaths at primary syntactic boundaries.[85]

*For a detailed guide to evaluation and a flowchart that aids clinical management decision making, see the Academy of Neurologic Communication Disorders and Sciences (ANCDS)-sponsored publication regarding the behavioral management or respiratory/phonatory dysfunction associated with dysarthria.[210]

[†]Detailed description and discussion of specific treatment techniques and procedures for managing respiratory function in dysarthria can be found in Dworkin,[54] Rosenbek and LaPointe,[182] and Yorkston et al.[245] For a comprehensive review of speech breathing abnormalities in children with cerebral palsy and related strategies to address muscle weakness and incoordination and body positioning issues, see Solomon and Charron.[207]

[‡]Yorkston et al.[245] describe a modification of the water glass manometer device and the use of a custom mouthpiece or full face mask for use by patients who cannot seal their lips around the straw/tube because of facial weakness.

can be provided by the clinician, a tape recorder's volume unit (VU) meter, or a Visipitch or similar acoustic feedback device. Practice exhaling at a steady rate for several seconds, sometimes with glottal frication and eventually with voicing, may help promote respiratory control.[157] Steady vocal output for 5 seconds would be the goal of such activities, followed by producing several syllables on one exhalation.

Linebaugh's[129] concept of the *optimal breath group* has special relevance for speech respiratory control. An optimal breath group is *the number of syllables that a patient can produce comfortably on one breath*. Establishing this can help teach patients to keep utterances within the optimal breath group and establish a baseline against which attempts can be made to increase breath group length. Contextual speech tasks may include gradually *increasing the length of phrases and sentences* that can be uttered in a single breath group without significant decreases in loudness or acceleration of rate.

Pushing, pulling, and *bearing down* during speech or nonspeech tasks may help to increase respiratory drive for speech. *Controlled exhalation tasks,* in which a uniform stream of air is exhaled slowly over time, may help increase respiratory capacity and enhance control of exhalation for speech.

In a study that may be relevant to managing respiratory weakness in dysarthria, Cerny, Panzarells, and Stathopoulis[31] examined the effects of an *expiratory muscle conditioning* program in 10 children with speech impairments (ranging from 8 to 14 years old), "soft voice" and "low muscle tone," but without specific neurologic diagnoses such as cerebral palsy or muscular dystrophy. Subjects wore a facemask for 15 minutes per day, 5 days a week, for 6 weeks to condition the expiratory muscles. The mask covered the mouth and nose and required active inhalation to overcome a threshold resistance provided by a spring-loaded valve in the expiratory port of the mask. Expiratory strength increased by 30% within 2 weeks and by 69% by 6 weeks, and it remained 44% better at 3 weeks after treatment. Sound pressure level during comfortable speech improved 18% by 6 weeks and remained 11% better at 3 weeks after conditioning.

Posture can be important for maintaining adequate physiologic support for respiration. Patients who need to make *postural adjustments* for speech may benefit from beds, wheelchairs, or chairs with backs that can be adjusted to maximize intelligibility and efficiency during conversation.[245] Sometimes, simply encouraging and reinforcing a patient to sit upright improves respiratory support.

The need for postural adjustments is often determined by the nature of the neuromuscular impairment. In general, patients with greater expiratory than inspiratory weakness for speech do better in the supine than sitting position because of its stabilizing effects, and because gravity and abdominal contents may help push the diaphragm into the thoracic cavity and assist expiration.[164] This effect has been observed in some people with TBI, MS, and spinal cord injury.[245] In contrast, patients with amyotrophic lateral sclerosis (ALS) and lung disease tend to do more poorly in the supine position because of their significant inspiratory problems; they do better in the upright position, because gravity helps lower the diaphragm into the abdomen on inspiration.[171,245]

Prosthetic Assistance

Prostheses that provide postural support during respiration or help control expiration can be useful during speech. *Abdominal trussing (binders or corsets)* can enhance posture, support weak abdominal muscles, and improve respiratory support and air flow with reduced effort, especially for people with spinal cord injuries who may have intact diaphragmatic function but weak expiratory muscles.[8,182,240] Positive effects of abdominal trussing on utterance duration, syllables per utterance, and pausing at appropriate locations have been demonstrated in patients with C5-C6 spinal cord injury and weakness or paralysis of abdominal muscles.[233] Slight to substantial speech improvement after abdominal binding has also been reported in patients with high cervical cord injuries and phrenic nerve pacers.[102] *Medical approval and supervision is important when binding is used, because it can restrict inspiration and increase the risk of pneumonia.*[182] The duration of each period of use generally should be limited.

Leaning into a flat surface during expiration or using an *expiratory board* or *paddle* mounted on a wheelchair and swung into position at the abdominal level may help increase respiratory force for speech.[182] Unfortunately, the people who may most need such assistance often lack sufficient trunk strength or balance to use it well.[245] Some patients with adequate arm strength can push in on the abdomen with their hands during expiration and obtain similar assistance.

Behavioral Compensation

Some patients simply need to practice *inhaling more deeply* or *using more force when exhaling* during speech.[84,144] Working to inhale more deeply may take advantage of elastic recoil forces of the lungs during expiration in weak patients. Working to increase inspiratory range can be tied to attempts to sustain isolated sounds for 5 seconds while keeping intensity and quality constant.[182]

If unchecked during exhalation, the higher expiratory pressures permitted by inhaling more deeply—either intentionally, involuntarily, or mal-adaptively—may lead to excessive loudness bursts, rapid air wastage, and no functional improvement in speech. In this regard, it may be important to use *inspiratory checking,* which is the use of inspiratory muscles to "check" or control exhalatory forces to maintain steady subglottal pressure.[160,165] The key instruction for this is to "take a deep breath and *let it out slowly when speaking.*" "Deep breath" with this technique means inhalation to approximately 50% of inspiratory capacity. Netsell[160] reported a dramatic increase in syllables per breath group and intelligibility in a patient who was able to follow this instruction.

Some patients initiate speech at inappropriately variable points in the respiratory cycle and need to learn to be more consistent in inspiratory control.* Similarly, some patients need to terminate speech earlier in the expiratory cycle if they speak at low lung volume levels that are insufficient to sustain adequate loudness or voice quality.[245] For example, patients with Parkinson's disease (PD) and chest wall rigidity may find it easier to use short phrases per breath group rather than long phrases during which loudness may decrease or excessive energy be expended.[208]

Sometimes, patients adopt maladaptive compensatory breathing strategies. For example, they may produce only one word per breath group when, in fact, they have respiratory support for lengthier breath groups. A clue to this maladaptive strategy is the ability to sustain a vowel significantly longer than syllable level breath groups. This faulty strategy often is easily overcome by pointing it out to the patient and providing an opportunity to practice more appropriate respiratory patterns. A useful practice strategy for increasing breath group length and variability is to read paragraphs in which respiratory breaks are marked, with progression to marked conversational scripts, and eventually to noncued conversation and narrative tasks.[245]

There are also some compensatory techniques of breathing for speech that can be used by people with flaccid paralysis of the ribcage, diaphragm, and abdomen.[101] One is known as *neck breathing,* in which the sternocleidomastoid, scaleni, and trapezius muscles of the neck are used to bring about to-and-fro displacement of the rib cage for inspiration. Another, known as *glossopharyngeal breathing* (or "frog breathing"), is a self-generated positive-pressure strategy in which the larynx and upper airway structures are used to pump small volumes of air into the lungs in a stepwise fashion. A case report[101] has documented that one patient used these strategies well enough to be judged normal in intelligibility, despite respiratory weakness sufficient to put him at ventilatory risk and require breathing assistance much of the time. His voice quality was mildly strained, fricative duration was shortened, and stops were sometimes substituted for fricatives; all of these characteristics probably reflected compensatory efforts to decrease rate of airflow and improve expiratory efficiency. The authors pointed out that such compensatory breathing patterns may be adopted automatically; their subject spontaneously adopted neck breathing and was taught glossopharyngeal breathing.

People who have impaired bulbar muscle function, as well as respiratory weakness, may not have the strength or coordination for respiratory compensations; thus their benefit may be limited to patients with isolated respiratory impairment. Also, because of the prolonged inspiratory phase of breathing required for neck and glossopharyngeal breathing, the clinician should consult a physician knowledgeable about pulmonary function to get medical clearance for use of these respiratory compensations.

Instrumental Biofeedback

Biofeedback has been used specifically to improve respiratory control (i.e., independent or relatively independent of phonation) in some dysarthric speakers. In a single-subject multiple baseline design study[218] a dysarthric patient with a right hemisphere lesion who had significant impairment in speech respiratory support was provided with visual feedback about the movement, excursion, and coordination of the chest wall muscles during speech and nonspeech tasks, with and without simultaneous feedback about the onset, control, and offset of phonation. Both feedback conditions led to altered aspects of respiratory function, including increased excursion of the abdominal muscles and improved lung volumes. Biofeedback about coordination between phonation and chest wall movements also helped improve coordination and phonation times. Using an A-B-A-B single-subject experimental design to compare the effects of visual biofeedback about ribcage circumference during speech and nonspeech tasks to the effects of traditional behavioral techniques (e.g., understand movements of respiratory muscles, establish optimal posture and subglottic air pressure), Murdoch et al.[156] demonstrated similar positive results from visual biofeedback for a child with chronic dysarthria following a severe TBI. The biofeedback condition was superior to the traditional therapy techniques. An additional study that pro-

---

*Normal speakers generally inhale to approximately 60% of their lung volume. It has been suggested that dysarthric speakers aim for a target inspiratory level at 60% or more of their lung volume.[245]

vided visual biofeedback about vital capacity enhanced inspiratory volume and respiratory support for speech in a single dysarthric speaker.[202]

A systematic review of the evidence as part of ANCDS' efforts to establish practice guidelines concluded that biofeedback can be effective in changing physiologically measured variables related to respiratory/phonatory problems associated with dysarthria, but noted that changes in specific aspects of speech production and communication participation have not yet been clearly established.[242] There are also insufficient data to identify dysarthric speaker characteristics that predict potential to benefit from kinematic respiratory feedback. However, a study of normal speakers who learned a respiratory rate control task either with postresponse verbal feedback or visual biofeedback concluded that visual biofeedback may be most appropriate for speakers with a poor response to initial training (i.e., not very stimulable) and least appropriate for those with a good initial response.[229]

Approaches for modifying respiration for speech from the perspective of available evidence compiled from an ANCDS-sponsored practice guidelines development effort can be summarized as follows[210]:

1. Regarding nonspeech tasks, there is evidence-based support for the effectiveness of breathing against resistance (e.g., water manometer, resistive mask), pushing or pulling techniques, and biofeedback from chest wall movement. There is support from expert opinion, but not evidence-based support, for the effectiveness of maximum inhalation and exhalation tasks, controlled exhalation tasks, breathing against resistance through pursed lips, and using visual feedback about air pressure or sustained phonation. There is no evidence to support the effectiveness of several techniques that have sometimes been recommended, including blowing exercises (e.g., balloons, bubbles), applying pressure or vibration to respiratory structures (e.g., diaphragm, ribs), applying ice to the diaphragm, or electrical stimulation.

2. Regarding postural adjustments, there is support from expert opinion, but not evidence-based support, for adopting an upright posture for people with inspiratory problems and a supine position or other adaptive seating system for people with expiratory difficulties.

3. Regarding prosthetic assistance, there is evidence-based support for abdominal trussing. There is support from expert opinion, but not evidence-based support, for pushing in on the abdomen with the hands during expiration.

4. Regarding speech tasks geared to modify respiration for speech, there is evidence-based support for biofeedback regarding air pressure levels. There is support from expert opinion, but not evidence-based support, for modifying inhalatory and exhalatory patterns, as well as for inspiratory checking.

Phonation—Medical Treatments

Several medical interventions are available to improve phonatory function. Many are appropriate for only certain types of dysarthria, a fact that is pointed out when treatment for specific dysarthria types is addressed later.

Laryngeal Framework and Related Laryngeal Surgeries

Medialization laryngoplasty, or *type I thyroplasty,* is a type of *phonosurgery* or *laryngeal framework surgery* that attempts to improve phonation in people with vocal fold paralysis or weakness and sometimes in people with vocal fold bowing. It involves placing cartilaginous or alloplastic implant material between the thyroid cartilage and inner thyroid perichondrium at the level of the vocal fold on the involved side, in effect displacing the paralyzed fold medially and facilitating vocal fold approximation—particularly anterior approximation—during phonation.[108,119,120] The procedure is reversible, so medialization can be undone if vocal fold function returns. People with unilateral paralysis who undergo the procedure may obtain good improvement in pitch, loudness, and intonation; they are generally satisfied with the results, although breathiness, harshness, and vocal fatigue may persist.[79,113] Another procedure, *arytenoid adduction surgery,* repositions the paralyzed vocal fold by manipulating the arytenoid cartilage, without the lateral compression induced by type I thyroplasty[81]; it also facilitates vocal fold adduction.*

Surgical procedures also have been developed for managing spasmodic dysphonia (SD). *Recurrent laryngeal nerve resection* induces unilateral vocal fold paralysis and, in effect, prevents hyperadduction and reduces laryngospasm in adductor SD (ADSD). Until approximately 15 years ago it was the preferred method for managing ADSD of neurogenic origin,

---

*Twelfth nerve–recurrent laryngeal nerve (RLN) anastomosis has been used to reinnervate the RLN in nine patients with unilateral vocal fold paralysis.[168] The procedure generally resulted in good voice quality and improvement in preoperative aspiration, but it must undergo more thorough investigation before it can be considered an effective treatment for vocal fold paralysis.

because it resulted in significant improvement for many patients. However, recurrence of signs and symptoms within 3 years is common, apparently because of increased hyperadduction of the nonparalyzed fold, ventricular folds, or supraglottic pharyngeal constrictors[6]; when recurrence occurs, laser thinning of the paralyzed fold is reportedly effective for some patients.[53] The procedure in most settings has now been replaced by botulinum toxin injection (see later).

More recently developed procedures for ADSD include *recurrent laryngeal nerve avulsion,* in which the distal portion of the recurrent laryngeal nerve is removed up to its insertion into laryngeal muscle with the intent of limiting functional regrowth of nerve; selective *laryngeal adductor denervation-reinnervation,* in which the recurrent laryngeal nerve is denervated bilaterally with reinnervation of the nerves' distal portions with branches of the ansa cervicalis nerve; and a thyroplasty procedure involving lateralization of the vocal folds (midline lateralization thyroplasty) in order to reduce hyperadduction of the vocal folds. Positive outcomes for a limited number of patients have been reported for these procedures but without long-term follow-up data. Regarding abductor spasmodic dysphonia (ABSD), medialization thyroplasty may have potential for managing it,[119] but data are limited. An ANCDS-sponsored practice guidelines review of medical interventions for spasmodic dysphonia[53] concluded that data for these surgical procedures are currently insufficient to recommend them as routine treatments for SD.

Autologous Fat, Collagen, and Teflon Injection

Injection of Teflon into the submucosal tissue of a paralyzed vocal fold has previously been a popular procedure for managing vocal fold paralysis. Injected into the middle third of the fold, it increases bulk and narrows the glottis. It is generally not used until approximately 1 year after onset because removal of Teflon is not possible without compromising normal vocal fold anatomy. Its value is questionable for vocal fold bowing or when neurologic involvement goes beyond the recurrent laryngeal nerve.[119] McFarlane et al.[141] found that the results of behavioral voice treatment were superior to Teflon injection on preinjection and postinjection comparisons across several perceptual voice parameters. They suggested that voice therapy may be justified while waiting for spontaneous recovery from vocal fold paralysis when the patient has a competent cough and no problems with aspiration.

Collagen may be used for the same purpose as Teflon and may be preferable to it; it is structurally similar to natural collagen in the vocal folds and is

subject to only limited absorption. It has been documented to reduce aspiration and airflow, improve glottal efficiency and intensity, and generally improve the dysphonia associated with vocal fold paralysis.[63,178]

More recently, autologous fat, harvested from the abdomen, has been used as an alternative substance for augmenting vocal fold function for unilateral vocal fold paralysis. Some reports suggest that it results in significant short- and long-term voice improvement when the glottal gap is small, there is no aspiration, no involvement of the superior laryngeal nerve, and no other cranial neuropathy.[94] Other reports point out that resorption of the injected fat makes it difficult to predict long-term outcome.[124,140] The frequent resorption of fat may make the procedure an appropriate method for temporary vocal fold medialization when return of vocal fold function is expected.[201]

Botulinum Toxin Injection

Unilateral or bilateral injection of botulinum toxin type A (Botox) into the thyroarytenoid muscle has become the preferred method for treating neurogenic ADSD and idiopathic ADSD that resists behavioral management. Patients whose ADSD is associated with voice tremor benefit from the treatment but less dramatically than those with underlying dystonia.[98,231] The toxin blocks the release of acetylcholine (ACh) from presynaptic nerve endings, in effect denervating some of the thyroarytenoid muscle fibers. Because the vocal folds are not completely paralyzed, they can be approximated, but with less than the degree of hyperadduction before injection. The effect occurs 24 to 72 hours after injection and lasts for 3 to 4 months, with return of symptoms occurring because new nerve sprouts develop and reinnervate the muscle. Unilateral or bilateral injections can be successful, but bilateral injection is generally preferred. The injection can be given to individuals with failed recurrent laryngeal nerve resection.

Side effects occur in a significant percentage of patients and include transient breathiness and mild dysphagia for fluids, which may last for days to weeks. The course of improvement and eventual regression is variable, with maximum gains generally occurring 5 to 10 weeks after injection and average onset of decline approximately 3 to 4 months after injection.[6,7,234] As a group, patients are pleased with the results, often rating the reduction of physical effort for speech as more beneficial than the actual improvement in voice.[7] Intelligibility improves in people with severe ADSD and reduced intelligibility before injection.[13] The ANCDS-sponsored practice guidelines comprehensive review of medical interventions for SD[53] concluded that the

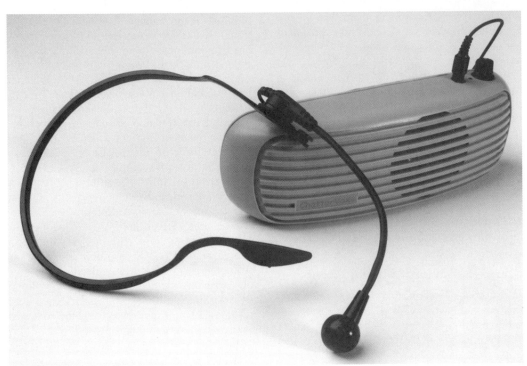

FIGURE 17-1 Portable amplification system with speaker and microphone. (Courtesy Ted Simons, Enhanced Listening Technology Systems, Inc.)

weight of evidence indicates that injection results in substantial positive benefits on indices of impairment, activity limitations, and participation in a significant percentage of patients.

Injection of Botox into the thyroarytenoid or posterior cricoarytenoid muscles, or both muscle groups, has also been successful for patients with ABSD. However, in comparison to results for patients with ADSD, effectiveness is less pronounced and occurs in a smaller percentage of patients.*[53]

Pharmacologic Management

Some medications occasionally contribute to the management of phonatory impairments. They are generally directed at specific dysarthria types. They are discussed later in the section on management of specific dysarthria types.

Phonation—Prosthetic Management

Patients with inadequate loudness but adequate articulation who have responded suboptimally to behavioral interventions to improve loudness may benefit from a *portable amplification system* (Figure 17-1) in which a speaker is located on the body, chair, or bed, or in which the voice is transmitted by frequency modulation signal to a speaker at a distance. Amplifiers vary in quality and cost; some patients seem to do well with a relatively inexpensive device, whereas others require a high-quality and more costly system.* Outcomes from the use of amplification devices with appropriately selected speakers have generally been positive, with gains in intelligibility and reduced activity limitation.[242]

Although this kind of voice amplifier is preferable in most instances, some patients who are aphonic, severely breathy, or lacking sufficient respiratory support for speech, but who have good articulation skills, may benefit from the use of an *artificial*

*A single case report has documented that voice quality and intelligibility improved in an adult with dysarthria secondary to cerebral palsy following laryngeal Botox injection.[125] Considerable additional research would be necessary before laryngeal Botox injection could be considered safe and effective for managing spastic dysarthria, however.

*The use of a sophisticated device that amplifies and clarifies speech using a proximity microphone and an automated speech processing system (The Speech Enhancer) by two speakers with PD and hypokinetic dysarthria resulted in improved intelligibility in various environmental settings. Its effect was superior to no amplification and a comparison amplification device.[28]

larynx. Patients with movement disorders or significant neck weakness may benefit from *neck braces* or *cervical collars* that stabilize the head and neck during speech.[182]

A *vocal intensity controller* can provide feedback about excessive or inadequate loudness. This can be accomplished with a loudness monitoring device that samples vocal intensity from a throat microphone and provides feedback if intensity is below (or above) a predetermined threshold. The successful use of such a device in speaking situations outside the clinical setting has been documented in a dysarthric patient with mild to moderate PD.[186] An example of a simple feedback device for increasing loudness is the VU meter on an audio recorder, adjusted by the clinician to set goals for loudness.

Phonation—Behavioral Management

The primary goal of behavioral work on phonation usually is to increase utterance length per breath group and to obtain loudness levels that are sufficient for the social context.

Patients with unilateral or bilateral vocal fold weakness or paralysis may benefit from *effort closure techniques.* These include grunting and controlled coughing, pushing, lifting, and pulling.[6,182,240] These effortful movements presumably maximize vocal fold adduction and may ultimately improve vocal fold strength. Patients with vocal fold weakness may also benefit from learning to *initiate phonation at the beginning of exhalation,* a strategy that can reduce air wastage and fatigue and possibly increase loudness and phrase length.

Some patients improve quality and loudness by *turning the head* to the left or right when speaking, or by *lateral digital manipulation* of the thyroid cartilage; such postures may increase tension within the weak vocal fold and facilitate glottal closure.[6,141] However, such mechanical manipulation is cosmetically undesirable and not likely to lead to any true improvement in vocal fold adduction.[182] In general, head turning and digital displacement should be considered compensatory, perhaps reserved only for when there is a clear situational demand for increased loudness.

Behavioral treatment of voice quality often is not undertaken because it is so difficult to modify and may not contribute greatly to improving intelligibility. However, some suggest that strained voice quality can be decreased if pitch is increased, the head is rotated back, and speech is initiated at high lung volume (i.e., after a deep breath). In a case report of a patient who benefited from initiating speech at high lung volume, it was felt that the lower diaphragm position associated with increased lung volume induced passive vocal fold abduction by tugging on the trachea.[206] Others suggest that traditional relaxation exercise and laryngeal massage used for nonneurologic, hyperfunctional voice disorders may also be of help in some dysarthric speakers with strained voices,[182] but, in general, any improvement usually seems transient or inconsistent. Patients with vocal fold hyperadduction may also benefit from learning to initiate phonation with a breathy onset or sigh in order to avoid stenosis.[43] Evidence suggests that lowering of pitch results in a reduction of tremor amplitude,[51] but it is not known if lowering (or otherwise altering) pitch is a viable way of managing the voice problems of people with significant organic voice tremor.

The Lee Silverman Voice Treatment (LSVT) program, involving vigorous vocal exercise for people with PD, is, in many respects, a voice-strengthening program. It is discussed in the section on speaker-oriented treatment for hypokinetic dysarthria. Additional behavioral phonatory treatment tasks are addressed in the discussion on improving intonation and prosody.

Resonance

Managing velopharyngeal inadequacy is important for some dysarthric speakers.* Excessive nasal airflow can result in air wastage during speech and place extra demands on marginally adequate respiratory and laryngeal functions; the result can be reduced breath groups and increased pauses for inhalation.[165] Damping effects of the nasal cavity can also reduce loudness, and nasal emission may reduce the perceptual distinctiveness of consonants requiring intraoral pressure.

A crude but often effective way of determining the impact of velopharyngeal inadequacy on speech intelligibility, loudness, phrase length, and articulatory precision is to compare speech with the nares occluded (by fingers or a nose clip) versus unoccluded, or with the patient in the upright versus supine position (patients with marked palatal weakness may be aided by the effect of gravity on palatal position in the supine position). Marked improvement under facilitated conditions may signal the need to focus on velopharyngeal function early in management.

---

*Clinicians who treat dysarthric people who have significant problems with velopharyngeal function for speech are urged to read a recent evidence-based practice guidelines publication that reviews evidence for surgical, prosthetic, and behavioral interventions for velopharyngeal problems associated with dysarthria.[244] A flowchart and additional information are useful to clinical decision making about managing velopharyngeal problems.

Surgical Management

Pharyngeal flap surgery (usually a superiorly based flap) is the preferred method for managing velopharyngeal incompetence in people with repaired palatal clefts. On occasion, dysarthric speakers with velopharyngeal incompetence also benefit from a superiorly based pharyngeal flap, sometimes even after behavioral and prosthetic management have failed.[110] However, the relatively infrequent use of the procedure for dysarthric speakers has generally produced results that are less favorable than prosthetic management.[76,92,95,147] Teflon injection into the posterior pharyngeal wall has been used to manage velopharyngeal inadequacy in some dysarthric speakers,[127] but the procedure has not been well investigated and is infrequently used. The current status of these surgical interventions is best summarized in a recent evidence-based practice guidelines publication that concluded there is insufficient evidence to permit recommendations about surgical interventions (including pharyngeal flaps, pharyngeal implants, and Teflon injection) for velopharyngeal dysfunction in dysarthria.[244]

Prosthetic Management

The *palatal lift prosthesis* is probably the most frequently studied intervention for managing velopharyngeal dysfunction in dysarthria, and it is the most frequently used individually fabricated prosthetic device employed for managing dysarthria in general. The published evidence-based practice guidelines for managing velopharyngeal function in dysarthria concluded that palatal lift treatment is an effective treatment for selected individuals with dysarthria.[244]

A palatal lift consists of a palatal portion that is attached to the teeth and a lift portion that extends posteriorly to lift the palate in the direction of velopharyngeal closure (Figure 17-2). Fitting it requires adequate dentition to retain the device.* Some patients must first adapt to wearing only the palatal portion, with the lift built in stages until adaptation and maximum benefit occur.

The best candidates for palatal lifts are those (1) with significant velopharyngeal weakness (usually flaccid dysarthria) whose deficits at other levels of the speech system are minimal or would be minimized by more adequate velopharyngeal closure, (2) who have evidence of lateral pharyngeal wall movement during speech, (3) whose deficits are stable or not rapidly worsening, (4) who have sufficient sup-

porting dentition, (5) who do not have significant spasticity or a hyperactive gag reflex, (6) who are motivated to improve speech and willing to tolerate the time to fit and adapt to the device, and (7) who are able to insert and remove the lift without assistance. The fundamental question the clinician must address is whether a patient's intelligibility or efficiency will improve significantly if velopharyngeal closure can be provided by a palatal lift. Patients whose respiratory, phonatory, and articulatory abilities are significantly impaired may not derive functional benefit. In contrast, some patients who wear a palatal lift eventually develop improved palatal function for speech without the prosthesis, perhaps through stimulation of neuromuscular responses by the lift and the successful exercise provided by it.[57,110] Attributes that are favorable and unfavorable for the success of palatal lift prostheses in people with progressive versus static or improving disorders are summarized in Table 17-1.

Problems encountered in palatal lift fitting and use include inadequate retention of the lift because of poor dental support; hyperactive gag responses that are unresponsive to desensitization or appliance modification; a spastic or stiff palate that does not tolerate the lift; and lack of cooperation, lack of acceptance, or unrealistic expectations.*[57,182,244]

The effectiveness of palatal lift prostheses—as indicated by increased intelligibility, decreased hypernasality, and improved articulation—has been reported for patients with flaccid (most often), spastic, and mixed flaccid-spastic dysarthrias. Etiologies in these successful cases have been quite variable, but stroke, TBI, ALS, and cerebral palsy are the most frequently reported causes.[185,244]

Some "minor" prosthetic devices can sometimes be quite helpful for some patients, especially those who could benefit from but, for various reasons, are not candidates for a palatal lift. For example, intelligibility sometimes improves noticeably by wearing a *nose clip* (or simply manually occluding the nares during speech); although this is not usually done on a constant basis, it may represent an effective strategy for improving intelligibility when a statement has not been understood. The fabrication and use of a relatively visually unobtrusive *nasal obturator* that can be inserted into the nares for the purpose of occluding nasal airflow during speech has facilitated

---

*Lifts have been successfully fitted to an upper denture in edentulous patients by attaching the lift portion to a maxillary retainer or existing dentures with wire connectors instead of the traditionally used solid acrylic material.[8a]

---

*Problems with fitting a lift can sometimes be overcome. For example, a patient who had considerable difficulty tolerating a lift was helped dramatically by applying a topical anesthetic (lidocaine [Xylocaine] gel) to the surface of the lift to reduce sensation. The patient was then able to retain the lift, with benefits to speech, for several hours at a time, and the gel was reapplied as part of cleaning and reinsertion procedures.[19]

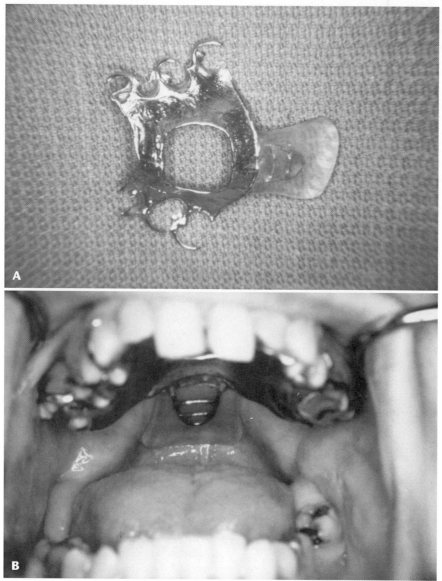

FIGURE 17-2 Palatal lift prosthesis. **A,** Palatal portion with fasteners and extended lift portion; **B,** in place.

speech improvement in a person with flaccid dysarthria resulting from TBI.[213]

Behavioral Management

Behavioral management of velopharyngeal function and resonance has historically generated mixed opinions and results. Most conclusions are derived from expert opinion rather than evidence, but it is generally felt that dysarthric people with severe and chronic velopharyngeal impairment do not benefit from behavioral intervention[245] and that prosthetic or surgical intervention should be considered in such cases.

Behavioral approaches can be grouped under four general headings based on a recent evidence-based practice guidelines review.[244] They can be summarized as follows:

1. *Modifying the pattern of speaking.* These techniques do not focus directly on velopharyngeal function but rather work to influence it by having speakers use increased effort, reduce rate,* or overarticulate. Overarticulation can be cued by demonstration—cuing to open the mouth more during speech or,

*Reduced hypernasality has been reported in some dysarthric speakers when their speaking rate was reduced.[238]

table 17-1	Attributes that are favorable and unfavorable for benefiting from a palatal lift prosthesis			
	Progressive Disorders		**Stable or Improving Disorders**	
Variable	**Favorable**	**Unfavorable**	**Favorable**	**Unfavorable**
Pathophysiology	Flaccid	Severe spasticity	Flaccid	Severe spasticity
Rate of Change	Slow	Rapid	Stable or slow gains	Rapid gains
Respiratory/ Phonatory Function	Adequate	Poor	Adequate or improving	Poor
Articulation	Adequate	Poor	Adequate or improving	Poor
Resonance Change with Occlusion	Yes	Absent or minimal	Yes	Absent or minimal
Pressure Sounds vs. Others	Pressure sounds less adequate than others	No or minimal difference	Pressure sounds less adequate than others	No or minimal difference
Ability to Inhibit Gag	Yes	No	Yes	No
Swallowing & Saliva Management	Adequate	Reduced	Adequate	Reduced
Dentition	Adequate	Poor	Adequate	Poor
Cognition	Intact	Reduced	Intact	Reduced
Manual Dexterity	Can insert/manage lift	Cannot insert/manage lift	Can insert/manage lift	Cannot insert/manage lift
Goals for Speech	Important to maintain functional speech	Decreased speech function acceptable	Improved speech is critical	Decreased speech function acceptable

Modified from Academy of Neurologic Communication Disorders and Sciences guidelines; Yorkston KM et al: Evidence-based practice guidelines for dysarthria: management of velopharyngeal function, *J Med Speech-Lang Pathol* 9:257, 2001.

simply, to speak more precisely. These approaches are most likely helpful when velopharyngeal problems do not significantly outweigh problems at other levels of the speech system. Modifications in speaking strategies that might improve resonance and reduce nasal air flow include exaggerated jaw movement to increase oral opening during speech; increasing loudness; and reducing the duration of stops, fricatives, and affricates to reduce demands for sustained intraoral pressure. Speaking in the supine position may facilitate velopharyngeal closure in some speakers, but there should be no expectation that adopting this posture will eventually lead to better velopharyngeal function in the upright position.

2. *Resistance treatment during speech.* Continuous positive airway pressure (CPAP)—frequently used for people with obstructive sleep apnea*—delivers positive airflow into the nasal cavities through a hose and nasal

mask assembly. In recent years it has been used in the treatment of palatal inadequacy and weakness, including in a small number of dysarthric speakers.[121,122,132] It essentially involves challenging the velopharyngeal muscles during speech to overcome positive airway pressure to achieve velopharyngeal closure. Success in treatment of two dysarthric speakers with TBI has been reported, one of which resulted in a significant and lasting reduction in hypernasality and allowed a palatal lift to be discarded.[122] It is felt that this strength training (i.e., exercise against resistance) of the velopharyngeal muscles helps to modify the degree and timing of velopharyngeal closure and that its success may reflect careful subject selection and the specificity of the training to speech.[132]

3. *Feedback.* Some speakers may benefit from feedback from a mirror, nasal-flow transducer, nasoendoscope, or any other simple or sophisticated device that can provide feedback during efforts to decrease hypernasality and nasal airflow during speech.

4. *Techniques focused on nonspeech velopharyngeal movement.* Nonspeech activities to

---

*CPAP has also been used successfully to temporarily treat severe inspiratory stridor associated with myasthenia gravis in a patient in whom stridor was the first symptom of the disease.[221]

improve speech have a certain appeal because of their direct physical attack on muscles and the hope that such physical manipulations will alter function. Unfortunately, *techniques focusing on velopharyngeal structures or nonspeech movements of the velopharyngeal mechanism for the purpose of improving speech are generally not effective.* An evidence-based practice guidelines report[244] concluded that evidence and expert opinion suggest that pushing exercise, nonspeech strengthening exercise (e.g., blowing, sucking), tasks to control and modify the breath stream (e.g., blowing bubbles, cotton balls, whistles), and inhibition or facilitation techniques (e.g., icing, stroking, brushing, pressure to muscle insertion points) are not effective for improving velopharyngeal function for speech. Without future data-based evidence to the contrary, their use for managing velopharyngeal impairment in dysarthria cannot be justified.

Articulation

A behavioral focus on articulation has traditionally been viewed as a major part of dysarthria treatment for many patients. This is probably less frequently the case for many patients today, especially if efforts to improve articulation by slowing rate and modifying prosody are placed outside the realm of articulation activities. Although the goal of many treatment efforts is to improve the accuracy and precision of sound production, it is often accomplished by focusing on functions other than those directly related to place and manner of articulation. For example, articulation sometimes improves when respiratory support is optimized.[245]

Surgical Management

Neural anastomosis is occasionally pursued to restore function to a nerve. In dysarthric patients, this most often involves attempts to restore function to the facial nerve for both cosmetic and functional purposes (e.g., smiling and other aspects of facial expression), although not to improve speech. The anastomosis usually involves connecting a branch of the twelfth nerve to the damaged seventh nerve. The hypoglossal-facial anastomosis sometimes leads to facial synkinesis during speech, a result that might be socially embarrassing and interfere with articulation.[148] The procedure is usually pursued in people with normal hypoglossal function and no clear evidence of dysarthria because some degree of lingual weakness usually develops after surgery.[42,87,136,237] Yorkston[237] reported worsening of dysarthria plus

difficulty with the oral phase of swallowing and saliva control postoperatively, but with eventual improvement to preoperative baseline, in a patient with relatively mild dysarthria and lingual impairment. She recommended that such surgery be pursued with caution for patients more involved than the case she reported and that presurgical counseling clearly review the risks to speech and swallowing.

Botox injection, in addition to its usefulness in treating SD, also can be an effective treatment for hemifacial spasm, spasmodic torticollis, oral mandibular dystonia, lingual protrusion dystonia, and jaw tremor.[20,32,53,109,116,222] To the extent that the injection decreases abnormal movement in these disorders, it should decrease any associated hyperkinetic dysarthria. Positive results in this regard have been reported for patients with oromandibular tremor or dystonia who have had injections into the genioglossus, styloglossus, pterygoid, masseter, temporalis, digastric, or risorius muscles; acoustic analyses have documented improvements in word and sentence duration, reduction of inappropriate silences, and reduction of tremor amplitude.[116,193] A systematic review of the evidence as part of practice guideline development efforts[53] led to a conclusion that Botox injections have potential as an effective treatment for lingual protrusion dystonia and orofacial and mandibular dystonias that impair speech.

Pharmacologic Management

General clinical impressions are that drugs that facilitate or improve movement in the extremities often do not have a significant impact on the bulbar speech muscles. To date, the use of pharmacologic agents that might improve articulation or other aspects of speech are primarily tied to hypokinetic, hyperkinetic, and spastic dysarthrias. Unfortunately, for the most part the impact of such drugs on articulation has received little formal investigation. Effects of specific drugs on specific dysarthria types are addressed in the section on speaker-oriented treatments for specific dysarthria types.

Prosthetic Management

Prostheses to aid articulation are limited.* A *bite block* is a small piece of material (acrylic, putty) that is custom fitted to be held between the lateral upper and lower teeth.[54,161] Speaking with a bite block in place may help patients whose jaw control is dis-

---

*A number of oral and oropharyngeal handheld prostheses designed for use as "oral musculature exercisers" have been described.[128] However, there is no evidence documenting their applicability to or effectiveness for treating dysarthria.

proportionately impaired relative to other articulators, and it has been noted anecdotally to be helpful in patients with hypokinetic, hyperkinetic, and spastic dysarthrias.[161]

A bite block may be of particular use to patients with jaw opening dystonia who are often able —temporarily, at least—to inhibit jaw opening by clenching the teeth or biting on an object during speech; its effectiveness for this purpose has been documented.[55,56] Its usefulness is intuitively contraindicated for flaccid dysarthria because jaw movement may be necessary to compensate for weakness in other articulators. However, a bite block could be used to "force" increased lip and tongue movement during therapy activities by taking jaw movement out of the speech loop and removing its capacity to compensate for weak or otherwise reduced lip and tongue movements.[129,164]

Behavioral Management

Behavioral management of articulation includes strength training, relaxation, stretching, biofeedback, and traditional articulation methods. Patients requiring focus on articulation almost always receive traditional treatments, whereas other techniques are probably less universally applied.

1. *Strengthening.* The use of *strength training* to improve articulation is controversial, primarily because of limited data about its effectiveness. It is certainly possible to engage in activities that might increase strength in the articulators. The jaw can be opened, closed, lateralized, and pushed forward against resistance; the lips can be rounded, spread, puffed, and closed isometrically with or without clinician-provided resistance; the tongue can be protruded and lateralized against resistance or pushed against the alveolus, cheeks, or a tongue blade, and so on. Patients with marked weakness or limited movement may simply be asked to perform movements without external resistance; for example, exercise that requires attempts at rapid tongue movements, rather than resistance-based exercise, may generate sufficient force to increase strength.[81] Nonspeech exercise can be done with instrumentation designed to measure force and strength, especially when it is capable of providing feedback about results.*

   Expert opinion suggests that strengthening exercises are probably only appropriate for a

small number of patients.[245] That strengthening exercise may be unnecessary for many patients is supported by the facts that the tongue and lips use only 10% to 30% of their maximum forces for speech, and the jaw only 2%, and that up to one third of motor nerve fibers can be lost before functional impairments are encountered.[9,44] Data from patients with ALS suggest that weakness is not directly related to intelligibility, possibly because many orofacial muscles can trade off or compensate for weakness and only low levels of force are required for speech.[44] In addition, at least for patients with neuromuscular diseases such as ALS, there is consensus that high-intensity exercise, in general, should be avoided based on animal studies suggesting that reduced strength could be the result.[65]

There are also some logical arguments and relevant data that support a role for strengthening exercise in some dysarthric people. They include the fact that *strength training can be directed at variables other than increasing tension and force.* For example, it could be focused on improving endurance or speed of movement.[33] Endurance training aimed at improving the ability to sustain articulatory force (including less than maximum force) over increasing periods of time could make sense for some of the many dysarthric patients who complain of fatigue when speaking; such exercise is usually conducted at low levels of resistance. Speed training aimed at increasing power or the speed at which articulatory force can be produced could be a legitimate goal for patients with slow speech rates who do not have rapidly degenerative disease; power can be increased by increasing rate without increasing force.[33] There is also support for light resistance exercise or "fitness training" for the limbs in people with upper motor neuron (UMN) and lower motor neuron diseases and extrapyramidal diseases.[46,41] There is consensus that moderate-intensity exercise, in general, can lead to modest increases in strength if disease progression is slow.[65] Limited non–experimentally controlled data suggest that regular orofacial and articulation exercises can contribute to treating dysarthria following stroke.[180]

In general, nonspeech strengthening exercises should be used only after establishing that weakness is present and clearly related to speech impairment and disability and that there are no contraindications to exercise

---

*The Iowa Oral Pressure Instrument (IOPI) (described in a footnote in Chapter 3) is an example of an instrument that provides quantified feedback about lingual force and fatigue.

(e.g., vigorous nonspeech exercise is generally contraindicated in rapidly degenerative disease and myasthenia gravis). If a clinician and patient commit to improving strength during nonspeech activities, the effort should be concerted; for example, exercises done in 5 sets of 10 repetitions each, 3 to 5 times per session, with 5 to 10 exercise periods per day.[129]

Articulator strength training is most logically relevant to people with nonprogressive flaccid dysarthria because weakness is the primary underlying impairment that contributes to the articulation deficits. It should be noted, however, that weakness is also present in many patients with UMN lesions, and the speed with which muscles can be activated is reduced in many patients with bradykinesia and basal ganglia disease (e.g., PD). As a result, strengthening exercise for the articulators might be appropriate for some patients with unilateral UMN (UUMN) dysarthria, spastic dysarthria, and hypokinetic dysarthria. Strength training for people with ataxic or hyperkinetic dysarthria cannot be supported on the basis of the physiologic deficits that are presumed to explain those disorders.

2. *Relaxation.* Some clinicians suggest that *relaxation exercises* may improve muscle tone in patients with spasticity or rigidity. For example, shaking the head and jaw to create lateral movements of the jaw when open may help loosen jaw movements for speech; chewing movements to promote relaxation may help decrease mild muscle hypertonus in the jaw and tongue.[182] The problem with such exercises is that the movements necessary to accomplish them (jaw shaking) are often as impaired as those they are designed to improve (jaw movement for speech). Focus on speech movements rather than relaxation of speech structures seems most appropriate for most patients.[182]

3. *Stretching.* The notion of slow stretching is one of the foundations for inhibiting the stretch reflex and reducing motion-sensitive symptoms of spasticity in the limbs. It is generally recommended that stretching in the limbs be slow, steady, continuous, prolonged, and directional, with avoidance of sudden changes in force or direction because they can stimulate muscle spindle activity and promote spasticity.

Stretching exercise is felt to prevent joint and muscle contractions and also modulate spasticity.[46,145] For example, there is evidence

that passive range of movement with terminal stretch applied to finger flexion muscles temporarily improves control of finger extension movement in patients with spastic hemiparesis, perhaps by improving joint mobility[27]; stretching exercise can also improve range of motion of voluntary hip adduction.[166] Range of limb motion exercises that are not vigorous or fatiguing are also recommended for patients with ALS, to stretch unaffected muscles and prevent joint stiffness and muscle contraction.[204]

These findings for the limbs raise the possibility that stretching exercise involving slow movement of articulators beyond their typical range of motion may have some effect on increasing range of motion and decreasing the effects of spasticity on speech. Sustained maximum jaw opening; tongue protrusion, retraction, or lateralization; and lip retraction, pursing, and puffing are examples of such activities. Because stretch of articulators is necessarily voluntary and not passive, it might also contribute to increasing strength. Stretching may be most applicable for those with spasticity and rigidity; the possible strengthening effect of stretch might help some patients with weakness. *There is neither positive nor negative evidence regarding the effect of stretching exercise on speech.* Because the lips and tongue do not exhibit the typical pattern of stretch reflexes, however, stretching them for the purpose of reducing spasticity may not be beneficial.[33]

4. *Instrumental biofeedback.** Some limited data (i.e., from only a few subjects) suggest that hypertonicity (e.g., dystonia) and spasticity in articulatory muscles can be modified by *biofeedback.* For example, biofeedback from the upper lip has been used with some success in a few individuals with parkinsonism to modify lip stiffness and retraction and to permit improved bilabial productions under some conditions.[88,162] Electromyogram (EMG) biofeedback provided during nonspeech activity has successfully reduced hemifacial spasm with overflow to the tongue and larynx during speech, resulting in marked speech improvement that was maintained following treatment,[187] and it has

---

*The use of biofeedback to treat disorders of increased muscle tone is generally identified as a complement to stretching programs. By itself, its effectiveness is considered modest, perhaps improving performance during training but not necessarily when feedback guidance stops.[46]

helped an individual with spastic dysarthria to reduce tension and facilitate restoration of voluntary mandibular control, with subsequent reduction of drooling and improved speech intelligibility.[159]

Electropalatography (EPG) has provided new insights into the nature of lingual movement abnormalities in dysarthric speakers,[74,77,78,155] and it has potential as a feedback tool for tongue movements during speech. A single case report of a child with congenital suprabulbar paresis and severe dysarthria has documented the application (but not necessarily the effectiveness) of EPG in providing feedback about speech and nonspeech movements of the tongue.[152]

In general, it appears that instrumental biofeedback can be used in the management of articulation deficits in well-selected individuals with dysarthria. The data to date are sparse, however, and its general efficacy cannot be considered established.

5. *Traditional approaches.* Rosenbek and LaPointe[182] emphasized the importance of traditional methods of articulation therapy for dysarthric speakers. These include (1) *integral stimulation* (watch and listen imitation tasks); (2) *phonetic placement* (e.g., hands-on assistance in attaining targets and movements, pictured illustrations of articulatory targets); and (3) *phonetic derivation* (using an intact nonspeech gesture to establish a target, such as blowing to facilitate production of /u/). These techniques remain the foundation of many efforts to modify articulation.

Articulation work often emphasizes the *exaggeration of consonants* to prevent their slighting and improve precision, especially in the medial and final position of syllables.[43,164] Instruction to increase effort and slow rate may facilitate efforts at exaggeration. Although some patients need to work on sounds in isolation before they can integrate them into syllables and words, it is generally agreed that articulatory drills should emphasize movements and syllables and not simply fixed positions.[182]

Some patients need to learn compensatory articulatory movements. They may include, for example, use of the tongue blade instead of the tongue tip when the tongue is markedly weak, or lingual-dental contact instead of bilabial closure when lip weakness or hypertonicity is significant. Patients with poor laryngeal control who are unable to adjust voice onset time to distinguish voiced from voiceless consonants may learn to release final consonants or shorten vowels preceding final consonants to signal voiceless consonants.

A careful inventory of articulatory errors that contribute to decreased intelligibility is important to ordering of stimuli in treatment. In general, stops and nasals are easier than fricatives and affricates, especially when respiratory support is decreased. When the palate is weak, nasals, vowels, and glides are generally easier than consonants requiring intraoral pressure. Phonetic environment also must be considered in stimulus selection. For example, producing lingual alveolar consonants is generally facilitated in high-vowel environments as opposed to environments in which the jaw is relatively open or the tongue retracted. Finally, even the demands of syntactic complexity may influence motor outcome on tasks aimed to improve articulation.[137]

Working on *minimal contrasts* may be particularly helpful in achieving control over consonants, especially when moving from a single syllable to longer productions (e.g., contrasting productions of "pay-may," "pie-bye," "chew-shoe," "stop-top"). It is important during such *contrastive drill tasks* that the patient know that the purpose is to make the distinction between the minimal contrasts as clear as possible. Such tasks can involve contrasts between consonants or vowels and can be used with word, phrase, or sentence stimuli in order to increase or decrease difficulty.* In general, meaningful stimuli are preferred over nonsense syllables, although this can be limited when working on minimal contrasts at the syllable level.

Intelligibility drills can be useful during work on articulation, rate, and prosody.[245] These drills involve *referential tasks* in which the clinician-listener is naive to the target produced by the patient. The materials can be randomized word lists, sentences, pictures to be described, and so on. The listeners' task is to tell the speaker what they heard. These drills are useful, because they (1) promote discovery learning—the patient does not receive instruction but rather discovers how to make his or her speech intelligible; (2) focus on the primary goal of treatment, which is improved intelligibility; (3) can be adjusted to ensure success—that is, even markedly impaired speakers can be given materials that result in a high but not perfect degree of intelligibility; (4) they promote the development of speaker and listener strategies to repair breakdowns in intelligibility.

Rate

Rate may be the most powerful single, behaviorally modifiable variable for improving intelligibility.[241]

---

*Keith and Thomas's[112] Speech Practice Manual contains various stimulus materials that are designed for contrastive drill and related articulation tasks.

Rate modification, most often rate reduction, is used with many dysarthric speakers because it frequently facilitates articulatory precision and intelligibility by allowing time for a full range of movement (reduces undershooting), increased time for coordination, and improved linguistic phrasing. There is also evidence that it reduces spatiotemporal variability of speech movements in dysarthric speakers.[143] It can bring speech rate to within the normal range in speakers with hypokinetic dysarthria who speak at abnormally rapid rates.[82] Reducing rate may also be easier to achieve than other motor goals given the physiologic limitations imposed by many dysarthrias, and it can give listeners extra time to process the degraded speech signal.[83,245] Computerized insertion of brief (160 ms) pauses between words in sentences can improve intelligibility by approximately 5% in dysarthric speakers.[80]

Rate reduction is not a panacea for management—functionally meaningful generalization often requires intensive and extended training,[245] and it does not always improve intelligibility.* For example, the perceptual integrity of consonants and vowels can deteriorate at extremely slow rates,[224] and not all speakers with ALS achieve improved intelligibility if instructed to speak more slowly than their habitual rate.[225] Thus if intelligibility is not impaired or if reducing rate does not improve intelligibility, it should not be used because it reduces efficiency and naturalness.

There are many ways to achieve reduced rate. Some employ prosthetic devices, whereas others use more natural methods. Some impose rigid rate reductions while sacrificing prosody and naturalness, whereas others do not. In normal adults, it appears that self-determined methods of slowing rate are perceived as more natural than externally imposed strategies.[134]

Rate reduction often uses *pause time* as much as reduced articulatory rate to achieve its desired effects. *Pauses,* which occupy as much as 30% to 50% of the time during reading and spontaneous speech,[75,97,245] are important to variations in speech rate and are probably particularly important to modifying rate in dysarthria.[182,245] Pauses carry considerable information about syntactic boundaries and meaningful units, and they are more modifiable than the duration of actual speech production. When normal speakers increase rate, they do so mostly by reducing pause time.[245] It has also been shown that dysarthric speakers who repeat a statement that has not been understood tend to slow rate by increasing interword intervals, and that intelligibility benefits most when the repair strategy has been modeled for them.[115] This suggests that work on rate using natural (nonprosthetic) methods may be enhanced if the clinician adopts the rate strategy in his or her own speech during interactive practice.

Prosthetic Management

Several prosthetic devices may aid rate reduction. Among the most useful for well-selected patients (mostly with hypokinetic dysarthria) is *delayed auditory feedback (DAF).* DAF is an instrumental procedure in which the rate at which an individual's speech is fed back (through earphones) to him or her is delayed by varying intervals that can be set by the clinician or patient (Figure 17-3). The effect of the delay is to slow speech rate and, presumably, increase articulation time and accuracy. DAF requires little training; the speaker must attend to the feedback, but other learning is unnecessary, and its effect is usually rapidly apparent. It may be effective when other rate control techniques fail and may have temporary value in demonstrating to patients that slowing speech rate has positive effects on intelligibility.[182] Effective delays generally range from 50 to 150 ms.

It is felt that "rigid rate control" techniques such as DAF should be used when techniques that more adequately preserve prosody and naturalness are ineffective.[245] DAF does tend to disrupt naturalness, may be cosmetically unacceptable to some speakers, and adaptation to its effects may occur. It may not be effective in conversations in which utterances are short, so it may not be appropriate for patients who are only capable of or choose only to make statements that are brief and unelaborated.

Several reports and reviews have documented the success of DAF for patients with hypokinetic dysarthria.[3,38,48,89,90,210,240] Improvement was usually achieved rapidly and dramatically, and it lasted for months to years. Weaning from DAF while maintaining benefits generally has not been possible. Benefits have included marked reductions in speech rate, increased loudness, reduced phonetic errors, increased acoustic distinctiveness, increased amplitude of lip and jaw movements, and improved intelligibility. The benefits for several reported cases were maintained outside the clinical setting, with obvious functional and social benefits in several cases. However, not all patients, and perhaps only a small percentage of patients with hypokinetic dysarthria associated with PD, achieve reduced rate from DAF.[38] In addition, even when DAF reduces

---

*There are few published studies of failed treatments, but one by Marshall and Karow[138] is instructive. Their efforts to modify rate failed in a person with a TBI and rapid speech. The authors discussed motivation, minimal disability but the presence of cognitive deficits, and limited treatment time as possible explanations. Treatment failures, examined carefully, can be as instructive to future treatment efforts as treatment successes.

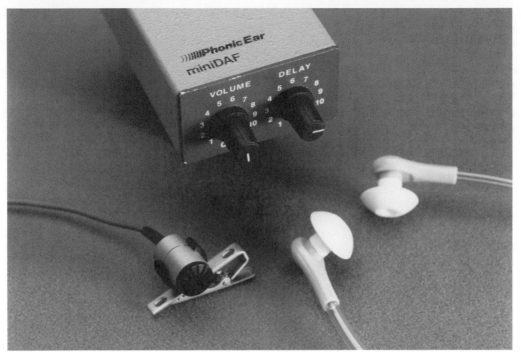

FIGURE 17-3 Delayed auditory feedback unit. (Courtesy Phonic Ear.)

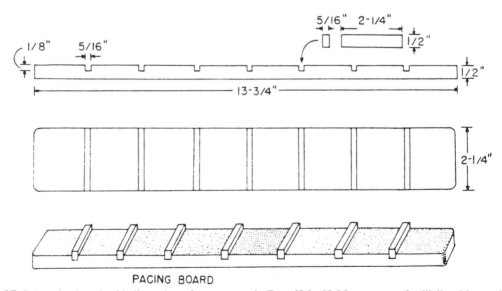

PACING BOARD

FIGURE 17-4 A pacing board, with dimensions, for rate control. (From Helm N: Management of palilalia with a pacing board, *J Speech Hear Disord* 44:350, 1979).

rate in speakers with PD, it may not improve intelligibility and may reduce fluency.[39]

Pacing devices can be useful in modifying rate. A *pacing board* (Figure 17-4), initially described by Helm,[96] requires the patient to point sequentially to each slot on a board as each word or syllable is produced. This promotes rate reduction and a syllable-by-syllable approach to speaking. It seems particularly appropriate for some people with hypokinetic dysarthria whose rate is rapid or accelerated or speakers with low baseline intelligibility.[170] The effectiveness of pacing board use has been documented in speakers with PD and hypokinetic dysarthria and palilalia, as well as in speakers with mixed spastic-ataxic dysarthria from TBI.[96,170] Other pacing devices such as auditory or visual metronomes can produce similar results.[170]

Alphabet board supplementation[16] is a rate control technique that can be an ideal transition from augmented to unaugmented communication (or vice versa) for some patients, or a lasting aid to people with stable deficits. It requires the speaker to *point to the first letter of each spoken word* on an alphabet board (Figure 17-5). Although rate is reduced substantially (to approximately a maximum of 40 words per minute) in comparison to nonsupplemented speech, case reports have documented some impressive results, including increased intelligibility (from approximately 5% to 70%) over nonsupplemented speech, up to a fourfold faster rate of communication than when the entire word is spelled out, and improved perception of articulatory accuracy.[36,91,105,107,239] The effect seems attributable to a combination of rate reduction and the information provided by the first letter of each word. The disadvantages of the technique are the slow rate, loss of eye contact and related cosmetic distortions, reduced naturalness (e.g., disrupted breath groups), and possible eventual adaptation to the technique.[245] For many patients, however, the gains in intelligibility outweigh the disadvantages. A systematic review of the literature on speech supplementation techniques as part of ANCDS' efforts to develop practice guidelines[91] has concluded that the technique can be effective for speakers with dysarthria that interferes with communication in natural settings who have adequate cognitive and pragmatic skills and the motor capacity to generate the cues.

Nonprosthetic Rate Reduction Strategies

Nonprosthetic strategies for decreasing rate include the following:

1. *Hand or finger tapping* in pace with syllable production. It should be noted, however, that many parkinsonian patients accelerate their hand tapping, as well as their speech rate, and that ataxic patients may be uncoordinated in tapping. Some patients can speak in a syllable-by-syllable fashion simply by being told to do so, although they may need considerable practice to make the strategy habitual.

2. Using *visual feedback* from a computer screen or storage oscilloscope to pace rate. For example, decreased rate and increased intelligibility were the result in a case study that provided oscilloscopic feedback to an ataxic speaker who was asked to speak at a rate that would "fill the screen" during reading tasks; the oscilloscopic display was set to modify rate.[14] Increased pause time, a strategy adopted spontaneously by the speaker, probably contributed to improvement. An advantage of a technique like this is that it allows for discovery learning regarding the best strategy for slowing rate.[245]

3. *Rhythmic cueing*[238] is a technique in which the clinician points to words in a written passage in a rhythmic fashion, giving more time to prominent words and pauses at syntactic boundaries. The effectiveness of the technique has been documented for a person with Friedreich's ataxia.[240] It may be that

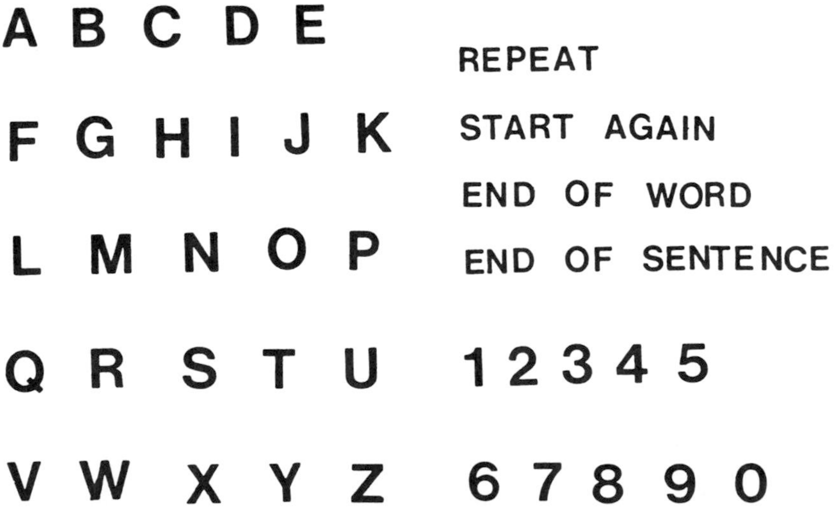

A B C D E   REPEAT

F G H I J K   START AGAIN

    END OF WORD

L M N O P   END OF SENTENCE

Q R S T U   1 2 3 4 5

V W X Y Z   6 7 8 9 0

FIGURE 17-5 Alphabet board for alternative or augmentative communication. Note that board layout can be organized in a variety of ways to best meet specific patient needs. (From Yorkston KM, Beukelman D, Bell K: *Clinical management of dysarthric speakers,* San Diego, 1988, College-Hill Press.)

external pacing of rate is more effective when "metered," in which each word is given equal time, as opposed to "rhythmic," in which timing patterns more closely simulate natural speech. For example, it has been demonstrated that ataxic and hypokinetic speakers' intelligibility improves during reading to a greater extent when pacing is metered than when it is rhythmic. Of interest, ratings of naturalness are not worse at paced rates than at unpaced speech rates, although metered rates are associated with poorer ratings of naturalness than rhythmic rates.[246] These findings highlight the tradeoffs that must be made between intelligibility and naturalness when rate is modified. The rhythmic cuing approach has been computerized,[17] with the capacity to set and vary the target rate. This permits selection of a precise rate and allows independent practice. Computerized rate pacing has been shown to slow rate in dysarthric speakers.[83,86,217]

4. *Backdoor approaches.*[245] These are techniques or programs that are not explicitly intended to reduce rate but that often result in rate reduction, with positive effects on intelligibility. Examples include activities geared to increase loudness, alter pitch variability, alter word and sentence stress patterns, or alter phrasing or breath patterning.

Prosody and Naturalness

Work on prosody can be appropriate at all severity levels, with potential benefits to intelligibility when impairment is severe* and benefits to naturalness when impairment is mild.[169,245] Some clinicians believe that working on stress should be an early part of treatment and that it can begin once respiration and articulation are sufficient to support connected utterances.[182] The goal of this work is to maximize the naturalness of prosodic patterns.

Naturalness reflects the overall adequacy of prosody.[245] When it is compromised by prosodic abnormalities, it is often perceived as monotonous or unpredictably variable. Prosodic features may

be out of sync with syntactic structures, such as when inhalation does not occur at natural syntactic boundaries. Pitch, loudness, and durational characteristics that signal stress may send contradictory messages when variations in each do not occur simultaneously in ways that naturally signal stress. Yorkston et al.[245] suggest that when intelligibility falls within an acceptable range (more than 90%), working to achieve naturalness, with a slight tradeoff with intelligibility, may be justified.

Acoustic analysis may be helpful in managing prosodic deficits. Displaying f_o, intensity, and durational contours of words and phrases can provide information about how a speaker is signaling stress and also about the source of perceived unnaturalness.[240] It can also serve as a feedback device during management. Some empiric support for this comes from a study of three dysarthric speakers who were provided oscilloscopic feedback about intensity, duration, and intraoral pressure; gains in rate and prosody were generally superior to those derived from auditory perceptual feedback alone.[25]

The following strategies may be useful in modifying prosody and increasing naturalness.

1. Working at the level of the *breath group*—the prosodic pattern during a single exhalation—is important because the breath group is a basic unit of prosody. In normal speakers, a breath group is more dependent on syntax than physiologic requirements of respiration. The duration of the breath group in speech is highly variable as a function of syntax, sometimes less than 2 seconds and as long as 8 seconds.[62] In addition, when asked to increase speech rate, normal speakers usually reduce pauses and only minimally increase articulation rate. In contrast, dysarthric speakers may pause more frequently because of physiologic limitations; subsequently, their breath groups may be short and not associated with syntactic boundaries.[12] This suggests that some patients may need to work to increase breath control (respiratory and phonatory control) to extend breath groups, a goal that requires increasing physiologic capacity or more adequately using available capacity.

   Physiologic limitations can reduce breath group length. Some speakers need to learn to *chunk utterances into natural syntactic units,* within the limits of their physiologic capacity. That is, speakers capable of only four to five words per breath group may learn to use pauses at logical syntactic boundaries within the limited breath group, removing one potential source of confusion to listeners.

---

*Indirect evidence supports this assertion. For example, flattening fundamental frequency (f_o) is known to reduce intelligibility in dysarthric speakers.[22] Less direct support derives from the role of prosody in natural language learning in children. Adults speak differently to children than to other adults, and many of the differences are prosodic. The "enhanced" prosody helps children "crack the language code."[11] Unfortunately, the converse often happens in MSDs. When prosody is "broken," breaking the language code can become challenging for listeners.

2. Rosenbek and LaPointe[182] emphasize the value of *contrastive stress tasks.* These can use scripted responses in which segmental information does not vary, but stress patterns do (stress patterns mark the prominence of syllables or words within an utterance). For example, the core response, "John loves Mary" may be produced in response to questions like "Does John love Mary?" "Does John hate Mary?" and "Does John love Jane?" Similar tasks can be used to practice intonation for questions versus statement forms ("John loves Mary" versus "John loves Mary?") or expressions of mood ("John loves Mary" with happy versus sad versus surprised affect). Obviously, vocabulary, syntax, and length need not be as stereotyped as these examples. Working on contrastive stress has resulted in improved ratings of naturalness and speech precision when included as part of a behavioral management program for individuals with MS and ataxic or mixed spastic-ataxic dysarthria.[93]

3. *Referential tasks,* in which the patient reads randomized phrases or sentences containing prespecified stress targets that are unknown to a listener, may help promote discovery learning of ways to signal stress, as well as a way to evaluate the effectiveness of actively taught stress strategies. That is, if the listener can identify the targeted stressed word, the patient has succeeded.

   Some patients can signal stress by modifying pitch, loudness, or duration but cannot use all parameters at the same time. Some use one parameter better than any other. Baseline tasks in which the patient is required to stress specified words and phrases may help identify the feature spontaneously used to signal stress; that feature may then become the focus of stress drills.

   The manner in which naturalness is impaired can vary both within and across dysarthria types, so a single effective trategy for modifying stress probably does not exist.[130,247] However, it has been observed that ataxic speakers are often encouraged to prolong syllables and insert pauses at appropriate times to signal stress. The strategy seems easier than pitch and loudness variations, and exaggerating duration seems to be perceived as less bizarre than exaggerating pitch or loudness.[240,247] Pitch and loudness variation sometimes spontaneously become more natural when durational adjustments are used effectively.

4. Some patients benefit from work *across breath groups.* A case report[12] discussed a patient with a monotonous stress pattern and slow rate who signaled stress within breath groups adequately, but who inhaled on 93% of his pauses during reading (compared with approximately 65% for normal speakers). He was physiologically more capable, however, because although his mean breath group length was approximately five words, he could produce 25 words on a single breath when counting. Treatment focused on increasing the frequency of pauses without inhalation and increasing the number of words per breath group. Materials consisted of reading sentences and paragraphs marked for pauses and inhalation, with gradual fading of cues. The speaker accomplished the treatment goals and developed greater variability in words per breath group. This led to reduced perception of monopitch, suggesting that breath groups of equal length may contribute to perceptions of monopitch. The case illustrates the value of obtaining information on both habitual and maximum performance as a way of identifying problems and potential for benefiting from treatment.

5. Working on prosody may have beneficial effects on rate control. For example, it has been shown that working on loudness and pitch variation, as well as word and stress patterns, can reduce speaking rate even when rate is not a focus of treatment.[203]

6. It is often advised that the sequence of therapy activities should begin with highly structured tasks and then transition gradually to spontaneous speech, perhaps through the use of short dialogues or scripts of conversation. It may be important for patients to critique their own production.[245] Audiotape and videotape review may be useful in this regard.

▪ SPEAKER-ORIENTED TREATMENT FOR SPECIFIC DYSARTHRIA TYPES

A number of treatment approaches are applicable to almost any dysarthria type. The applicability of others varies according to dysarthria type, either as a function of the underlying pathophysiology or the predominance of particular speech characteristics. As a result, some speaker-oriented treatments are appropriate for only certain dysarthria types or are likely to be used much more frequently for some dysarthria types than others. Some treatment approaches are inappropriate for some dysarthria types.

The purpose of this section is to highlight speaker-oriented approaches that are used exclusively or predominantly—or that may be contraindicated—with certain dysarthria types. Table 17-2 summarizes behavioral, prosthetic, medical/surgical, and pharmacologic techniques that are particularly useful, frequently used, or logically relevant to the management of specific dysarthria types, as well as those techniques that are contraindicated or of uncertain usefulness for particular dysarthria types.

Flaccid Dysarthrias

Because flaccid dysarthrias are caused by weakness, their unique treatments tend to be designed to increase strength or compensate for weakness. These include treatments aimed at the respiratory, phonatory, resonatory, and articulatory components of speech. If lower motor neuron innervation to specific muscles is completely lost, exercise to strengthen those muscles is doomed to failure.[81] Speaker-oriented treatments in such cases is necessarily compensatory rather than restorative.

Patients with respiratory weakness may benefit from efforts to increase physiologic support for speech breathing. Thus activities designed to increase subglottal air pressure on nonspeech tasks, increase maximum vowel duration, increase loudness, increase breath group duration and words per breath group, and establish maximum breath groups for speech are often appropriate. Pushing/pulling exercises to increase respiratory support and drive, postural adjustments, prosthetic aids (e.g., abdominal trussing), and compensatory efforts such as deep inhalation, controlled exhalation, inspiratory checking, and increased force are more likely to be applied to people with flaccid dysarthria than other dysarthria types. Patients with relatively isolated, severe respiratory weakness are probably the only dysarthric speakers who might be taught to use neck breathing or glossopharyngeal breathing for speech.

Patients with adductor vocal fold weakness or paralysis may be candidates for medialization laryngoplasty; arytenoid adduction surgery; or autologous fat, collagen, or Teflon injection, procedures more appropriate for flaccid dysarthria than any other dysarthria type. Some patients with reduced loudness that is not likely to be helped by medical/surgical interventions or behavioral efforts to increase loudness can benefit from voice amplifiers on a temporary or permanent basis. Effort closure exercises may be appropriate for patients with vocal fold weakness or paralysis, and, in fact, such behavioral approaches to improving vocal fold function for speech often precede surgical intervention or make it unnecessary.

More frequently than any other dysarthria type, flaccid dysarthric speakers have management attention focused on resonance and velopharyngeal function.[244] They are the best candidates for palatal lift prostheses and pharyngeal flap surgery. They also are the group most likely to benefit from postural adjustments or nares occlusion to prevent excessive nasal flow during speech. Velopharyngeal strengthening exercises, particularly CPAP, are more likely to be effective for flaccid than other dysarthria types.

Patients with paralysis of the facial nerve are the only dysarthric patients likely to have facial nerve anastomosis surgery and subsequently receive EMG feedback training to improve facial movement. Flaccid dysarthrias associated with lingual and lip weakness may benefit from the use of a bite block during treatment designed to increase tongue or lip movement for speech, but a bite block would never be a permanent prosthesis for flaccid dysarthria. Strength training of the jaw, face, and tongue to improve articulation has the greatest face validity for people with flaccid dysarthria, but efficacy is uncertain.

Behavioral speech treatment is contraindicated for people with flaccid dysarthria resulting from myasthenia gravis. Such patients are managed most effectively surgically (thymectomy) or pharmacologically (e.g., pyridostigmine bromide [Mestinon], adrenal corticosteroids). The best that can be done for speech beyond medical treatments is to teach conservation of strength by limiting speaking to durations that do not produce significant fatigue. Most patients with myasthenia gravis do this on their own.

Spastic Dysarthria

Some techniques that are appropriate for flaccid dysarthria are contraindicated for spastic dysarthria because they might increase rather than decrease deficits. For example, pushing, pulling, and other effort closure techniques to enhance vocal fold adduction are usually contraindicated because hyperadduction is generally already a problem for the spastic speaker. Surgical procedures to medialize the vocal folds (medialization laryngoplasty and Teflon/collagen injection) would be contraindicated for the same reasons. Antispasticity medications such as chlordiazepoxide (Librium), diazepam (Valium), dantrolene (Dantrium), baclofen (Lioresal), and tizanidine are sometimes effective in decreasing limb spasticity,[1,46,145] but their effects on articulation are uncertain at best, and side effects such as weakness may be undesirable for speech. It has been suggested that Dantrium may reduce strained voice in some patients with spastic dysarthria.[54]

Speakers with spastic dysarthria may benefit from relaxation exercises more than those with other dysarthria types, but whether such relaxation actually facilitates speech is a matter of conjecture. Sim-

Approach	Flaccid	Spastic	Ataxic	Hypokinetic	Hyperkinetic	Unilateral UMN
Behavioral	+	+	+	+	+	+
Respiration	+	+	+	+	+	−
"5 for 5" respiratory tasks	+	+	+	+	−	−
Pushing/pulling exercise	++	−	−	−	−	−
Postural adjustments	+	+	−	−	+	−
Manual push on abdomen	+	−	−	+	−	−
Neck breathing	++	−	−	−	−	−
Glossopharyngeal breathing	++	−	−	−	−	−
Expiratory muscle conditioning	++	−	−	−	−	−
Inspiratory checking	++	−	+	+	−	−
Maximum vowel prolongation	+	+	+	+	−	−
Inhale more deeply before speech	+	+	−	+	−	−
Speak at onset of exhalation	+	+	+	+	−	−
Terminate speech earlier during exhalatory cycle	+	+	+	+	−	−
Optimal breath group	+	+	+	+	−	−
Increase phrase length	+	+	+	+	−	−
Shorten fricative duration	+	−	−	−	−	−
Shorten phrases	+	+	+	+	−	−
Phonation	+	+	−	+	+	−
Turn head during speech	++	−	−	−	−	−
Lateralize thyroid cartilage	++	−	−	−	−	−
Effort closure techniques	++	−	−	++	−	−
Abrupt glottal attack	++	−	−	++	−	−
Intense, high-level phonatory effort	++	−	−	++	−	−
LSVT	+	−	−	++	−	−
Speak at onset of exhalation	+	+	+	+	−	−
Head back, increase pitch, deep breath	−	+	−	−	−	−
Relaxation, massage	−	+	−	−	+	−
Breathy onset	−	++	−	−	++	−
Continuous voicing of consonants	−	−	−	−	++	−
Optimal breath group	+	+	+	+	−	−
Resonance	+	+	−	+	−	−
CPAP	++	−	−	−	−	−
Supine positioning	++	−	−	−	−	−
Occlude nares	+	+	−	−	−	−
Exaggerate jaw movement	+	−	−	+	−	−
Increase loudness	+	+	−	+	−	−
Reduce pressure consonant duration	++	−	−	−	−	−
Reduce rate	+	+	+	+	+	+
Articulation	+	+	+	+	+	+
Strengthening exercises	++	−	−	−	−	+
Conservation of strength	+	+	−	−	−	−
Stretching	+	++	−	+	−	−
Relaxation exercise	−	+	−	−	+	−
Alternative place/manner/voicing strategies	++	+	−	−	−	−
Biofeedback	+	+	+	+	+	+
Sensory tricks	−	−	−	−	++	−
Exaggerate consonants	+	+	+	+	−	+
Integral stimulation	+	+	+	+	−	+
Phonetic placement	+	+	+	+	−	+
Phonetic derivation	+	+	+	+	−	+
Minimal contrasts	+	+	+	+	−	+
Intelligibility drills	+	+	+	+	+	+
Referential tasks	+	+	+	+	+	+
Rate	+	+	+	+	+	+
Rate modification	+	+	+	+	+	+
Hand/finger tapping	+	+	+	+	−	+
Rhythmic or metered cueing	−	−	+	+	−	+
Visual/auditory feedback	+	+	+	+	+	+
Modify pauses	+	+	+	+	−	+
Identify first letter on alphabet board	+	+	+	+	+	+
Prosody & Naturalness	+	+	+	+	+	+
Breath group duration	+	+	+	+	+	+
Modify syllable duration & pause time	+	+	+	+	+	−

table 17-2 Speaker-oriented treatments and techniques and their relationship to various dysarthria types—cont'd

Approach	Flaccid	Spastic	Ataxic	Hypokinetic	Hyperkinetic	Unilateral UMN
Across breath group tasks	+	+	+	+	−	−
Chunk by syntactic units	+	+	+	+	−	−
Contrastive stress tasks	+	+	+	+	+	+
Referential stress tasks	+	+	+	+	+	+
Prosthetic	+	+	+	+	+	−
Abdominal binders/corsets	++	−	−	−	−	−
Expiratory board/paddle	++	−	−	+	−	−
Vocal intensity controller	+	+	−	+	−	−
Vocal amplifier	+	+	−	+	+	−
Artificial larynges	++	−	−	−	−	−
Palatal lift	++	+	−	−	−	−
DAF	−	−	−	++	−	−
Pacing board	−	−	−	++	−	−
Metronome	−	−	−	++	−	−
Bite block	+	−	−	−	++	−
Nose clip/nasal obturator	+	+	−	−	−	−
Neck brace/cervical collar	+	−	+	−	+	−
Medical/Surgical	+	+	−	+	+	−
Medialization laryngoplasty	++	−	−	+	−	−
Arytenoid adduction	++	−	−	−	−	−
Fat/collagen/Teflon injection	++	−	−	+	−	−
Pharyngeal flap	++	+	−	−	−	−
Neural anastomoses	++	−	−	−	+	−
Recurrent laryngeal nerve resection, avulsion, denervation-innervation	−	−	−	−	++	−
Botox injection	−	−	−	−	++	−
Midline lateralization thyroplasty	−	−	−	−	++	−
Pallidotomy*	−	−	−	+	+	−
Thalamotomy*	−	−	−	+	+	−
Deep brain stimulation*	−	−	−	+	+	−
Pharmacologic†	+	+	+	+	+	−
Artane (trihexyphenidyl)	−	−	−	−	+	−
Clonidine	−	−	−	−	+	−
Clozaril (clozapine)	−	−	−	−	+	−
Dantrium (dantrolene)	−	+	−	−	−	−
Deprenyl (selegiline)	−	−	−	+	−	−
Diamox (acetazolamide)	−	−	+	−	−	−
Elavil (amitriptyline)	−	+	−	−	−	−
Fluphenazine	−	−	−	−	+	−
Guanfacine	−	−	−	−	+	−
Haldol (haloperidol)	−	−	−	−	+	−
Inderal (propranolol)	−	−	−	−	+	−
Klonopin (clonazepam)	−	−	−	+	+	−
L-Dopa (levodopa)	−	−	−	++	−	−
Librium (chlordiazepoxide)	−	+	−	−	−	−
Lioresal (baclofen)	−	+	−	−	+	−
Lithane, Eskalith (lithium)	−	−	−	−	+	−
Mestinon (pyridostigmine bromide)	++	−	−	−	−	−
Mysoline (primidone)	−	−	−	−	+	−
Neptazane (methazolamide)	−	−	−	−	+	−
Olanzapine	−	−	−	−	+	−
Pimozide	−	−	−	−	+	−
Reserpine	−	−	−	−	+	−
Risperdal (risperidone)	−	−	−	−	+	−
Sinemet (carbidopa-levodopa)	−	−	−	++	+	−
Tegretol (carbamazepine)	−	−	−	−	+	−
Tizanidine	−	+	−	−	−	−
Valium (diazepam)	−	+	−	−	−	−
Xanax (alprazolam)	−	−	−	−	+	−

+, May be appropriate; ++, uniquely appropriate but not necessarily for all patients; −, rarely necessary, uncertain, or contraindicated; CPAP, continuous positive airway pressure; *DAF,* delayed auditory feedback; *LSVT,* Lee Silverman Voice Treatment; *UMN,* upper motor neuron.

*Not used specifically to improve speech and may have no effect on speech; may result in speech improvement or impairment in some cases.

†No pharmacologic agent is specifically designed to improve speech. Many of these agents may relieve neurologic motor deficits in nonbulbar muscles but have no effect on speech. Most of the listed agents do not have documented consistent beneficial effects on motor speech disorders, and some may negatively affect speech.

ilarly, stretching exercise of the articulators has some face validity for speakers with spastic dysarthria but has not been investigated.

The management of pseudobulbar affect (pathologic crying and laughter) deserves mention because it occurs more commonly in spastic than in any other dysarthria type and can interfere significantly with verbal communication. In patients for whom pseudobulbar affect is a significant problem, low doses of amitriptyline may be effective in relieving the behavior. For example, dramatic improvement of pathologic laughter and crying in response to the drug has been reported in a small double-blind crossover study comparing amitriptyline (Elavil) with placebo in people with multiple sclerosis.[192] It is also possible for the problem to respond to behavior modification techniques in some patients.[8,21] For example, Brookshire[21] described a man whose crying was so frequent that it precluded speech therapy because he would cry whenever asked to repeat or speak more clearly. A program was developed in which head turning that usually preceded crying was modified and eliminated by verbal reinforcement of incompatible behavior. Crying was greatly reduced and intelligible speech was achieved with subsequent therapy. This suggests that some aspects of this apparently involuntary behavior may be under voluntary control, at least in some patients. Working to modify such behavior when medication is ineffective or inappropriate seems justified when it is pervasive enough to consistently interfere with speech or therapy activities. For some patients with spastic dysarthria, treating the laughter and crying may be the first goal of treatment.

Ataxic Dysarthria

Efforts to increase physiologic support by increasing muscle strength or reducing muscle tone are generally unnecessary for ataxic speakers, and there is no compelling evidence to support their effectiveness for the disorder.*[26] Similarly, surgical or prosthetic efforts to improve phonation or resonance are unnecessary because they are not relevant to the motor problems of ataxic speakers. Pharmacologic treatments for cerebellar ataxia, in general, have not been successful, but clonazepam (Klonopin) or propranolol (Inderal) may relieve voice tremor in some

cases.[26] Acetazolamide (Diamox) may be effective in treating episodic ataxia.[61]

In general, the focus of management activities for ataxic dysarthria is behavioral, with activities centered on improving or compensating for problems related to motor control and coordination. The potential to improve and not simply compensate receives some support from studies that demonstrate motor skill learning in ataxic people, especially at slow rates,[223] including for speech and oral movements.[194]

Although some patients benefit from isolated work on respiratory control, particularly controlled exhalation over time,[157,182] most of the focus is generally on *modifying rate and prosody* to improve intelligibility and, when possible, further modifying rate and prosody to improve naturalness. For example, several clinicians explicitly note that ataxic speakers may benefit from using durational adjustments as their primary method of signaling stress.[245,247] Several studies of ataxic speakers have reported improved intelligibility or naturalness with behavioral techniques that emphasized rate, loudness, or pitch control.[14,25,203,241,246]

Hypokinetic Dysarthria

In some respects, the treatment of hypokinetic dysarthria (at least its voice characteristics) resembles that for flaccid dysarthria, but the overlap is far from complete. There are also some behavioral treatment approaches that have been developed specifically for hypokinetic dysarthria.

Surgical Interventions

Some hypokinetic speakers have a prominent dysphonia that may be related to bowing or weakness of the vocal folds. When severe and the prominent manifestation of the dysarthria, medialization laryngoplasty or Teflon/collagen injection may result in improved voice.

A number of surgical interventions have been developed to relieve the movement disorders associated with PD and related conditions. They include *thalamotomy, pallidotomy,* and *deep brain stimulation (DBS).* None are intended to improve speech, and, in general, each procedure carries some risk for speech impairment. Sometimes, however, improvement in speech occurs. The following paragraphs summarize these surgical interventions and their reported effects on speech. It is noteworthy that many studies of speech outcome following thalamotomy, pallidotomy, and DBS have been perceptually based and not rigorously conducted.

1. *Pallidotomy.* Pallidotomy involves placing a lesion in the posteroventral portion (globus pallidus interna [Gpi]) of the globus pallidus

*A single-subject study[189] has reported improved phonatory and articulatory functions following LSVT for a person with ataxic dysarthria from thiamine deficiency. LSVT involves a rigorous and vigorous program of vocal exercise aimed at improving vocal loudness; it is discussed in the next section. The treatment may have been effective because the patient had a weak and breathy voice, characteristics that are not usually prominent in ataxic dysarthria.

to abolish tremor, including parkinsonian tremor, or akinesia and postural instability. The best candidates are healthy, cognitively normal individuals with asymmetric idiopathic PD who have levodopa responses characterized by motor fluctuations and bothersome dyskinesias. Speech problems are a known possible side effect of the procedure, especially when done bilaterally.[200] However, the effects on speech are quite variable across patients. Unilateral pallidotomy has been associated with improvement on some phonatory and articulatory measures in some but not all patients,[196] and some studies report a low frequency (≈3%) of complications.[99] Some patients undergoing bilateral pallidotomy (whose intelligibility is normal preoperatively) make improvements in force control of the perioral structures and may report that moving their lips during speech is easier, their face feels more relaxed, and eating and drinking are easier.[10] In contrast, a study of 57 consecutive patients who underwent unilateral pallidotomy that resulted in significant improvement in motor functions found that speech intelligibility was typically preserved but declined to a mild degree in approximately one third of patients[226]; reduced intelligibility has been reported by others as well.[215] Bilateral pallidotomy has also been associated with observable worsening of preexisting dysarthria, hypophonia, and drooling and dysphagia in some patients, although sometimes without "significant functional consequences."[73,197] It is possible that preoperative speech status has some impact on surgical outcomes for speech. For example, one study of vocal intensity in 25 patients with PD who underwent unilateral pallidotomy found that mildly dysarthric patients preoperatively had significantly greater increases in postoperative sound pressure level (SPL) than moderately or severely dysarthric patients who actually had reduced SPL postoperatively.[195]

2. *Thalamotomy.* In thalamotomy, a lesion is placed in the ventrolateral nucleus of the thalamus with the intent of reducing severe parkinsonian, cerebellar, or essential tremors that have not responded well to pharmacologic treatments. Recognized side effects, especially when lesions are placed bilaterally, include persistent severe dysarthria and neuropsychological deficits.[103,200] Following unilateral thalamotomy, major persisting speech deficits are rare, but there may be a mild worsening of preexisting dysarthria or the emergence of mild dysarthria in approximately half of patients, with a majority eventually returning to their preoperative baseline.[4,114]

3. *DBS.* The goal of DBS, in general, is to treat the same problems targeted by thalamotomy and pallidotomy by reducing activity in overactive brain structures through inhibition of neuronal firing or facilitation of inhibitory interneurons. Stimulating the Gpi or subthalamic nucleus seems to offer broader control of parkinsonian problems than thalamic DBS. Stimulators are implanted in the thalamus, globus pallidus, or subthalamic nucleus, with a pulse generator placed in the chest wall (similar to a cardiac pacemaker) that can be activated by a handheld magnet and programmed for stimulation parameters by an external computer.[200] The results of DBS regarding speech and oromotor functions have been described in detail for pallidal DBS, and they are variable, ranging from no effect to benefits to undesired side effects. Positive results have included relief of painful oromandibular dystonia; improved willingness to speak; reduced vocal strain; increased intelligibility, pitch, and loudness; and reduced tremulousness. Undesirable effects have included marked hypophonia.[139,209]

Pharmacologic Treatments

Dopamine agonist medications such as carbidopa-levodopa (Sinemet), levodopa, and selegiline (Deprenyl) are sometimes associated with general improvements in speech for patients with PD and hypokinetic dysarthria, but not consistently, and often to a lesser degree than improvements in nonspeech motor functions.[2,149,179,212,230,235] Some studies suggest that lip function improves during speech and nonspeech tasks following levodopa treatment.[23]

Clonazepam (Klonopin) may be effective for treating hypokinetic dysarthria in some patients. For example, 9 of 11 parkinsonian patients in a double-blind study with the drug had sufficient functional improvement of speech (mostly in rate and pause characteristics and consonant precision) that they decided to continue the drug after completion of the study.[18] A number of other drugs can be effective in treating PD, but their effects on speech have received little attention.

It is important to keep in mind that *the effects of parkinsonian medications, including on speech, can fluctuate as a function of the drug cycle.* For example, variability across patients and fluctuation in improvements in the velocity and amplitude of lip movements over a 2- to 3-hour period have been documented in some people taking Sinemet.[24] Thus positive effects of these drugs on speech can be variable within the drug cycle, heterogeneous across patients, and not necessarily systematically predictable within patients.[126] In addition, during the course of the disease a high percentage of patients develop hyperkinesia during treatment with levodopa, with fluctuations over the course of the drug cycle. It is possible, therefore, to encounter patients whose hypokinetic dysarthria improves but then evolves to a hyperkinetic or mixed hypokinetic-hyperkinetic dysarthria and then returns to baseline within a single dosage period.

Behavioral Management

Many hypokinetic speakers with rapid or accelerated rate are prime candidates for rate control efforts, at least partially because articulatory hypokinesia may be reduced at slower speaking rates.[24] Rigid rate control approaches may be necessary for many patients, and several reports document the success of devices such as DAF and pacing boards.[3,89,90,96] Similarly, the reduced loudness associated with hypokinetic dysarthria may respond favorably to vocal intensity monitors and feedback devices[186] or to voice amplifiers when loudness cannot be improved behaviorally and other aspects of speech production are relatively preserved. The tendency for some people with hypokinetic dysarthria to sit in a hunched-forward position can reduce the depth of inspiration. Loudness in such individuals can be facilitated by having them adopt a more optimal posture.[245]

In the past, behavioral therapy for people with PD has been viewed with pessimism,[191] the common opinion being that the dysarthria might respond favorably within treatment sessions but that little carryover is ever achieved. This is indeed the case for some patients, but recent evidence suggests that intensive, focused treatment can be beneficial and lasting for others. Some of these treatments appear to improve physiologic functions for speech. They are usually intensive (e.g., 6 to 9 hours over 6 weeks; 10 hours over 2 weeks; 35 to 40 hours over 2 weeks) and tend to include work on prosody and loudness, as well as rate control and articulation.[111,151,181,198,199] Carryover for 3 to 6 months after treatment has been noted in some studies, although gains are not always completely maintained. Investigators usually note the importance of follow-up activities after the initial intensive treatment program.

Although strength is not usually thought of as significantly impaired in PD, bradykinesia (a common problem in PD) affects the speed with which muscles can be activated, and strength is related to the way in which muscles are activated and the speed of movement. It has been demonstrated that withdrawal of antiparkinsonian medication can lead to muscle weakness because of reduced agonist muscle activation and reduced rate of force generation. Such findings suggest that exercise programs to increase muscle strength and power may be beneficial,[34] and there is evidence that physical therapy or a general program of physical exercise can improve motor performance in people with PD.[64,167] Exercise also seems to have some value for speech, as attested to by the studies of speech therapy referred to in the preceding paragraph and in the following section.

Lee Silverman Voice Treatment*

As mentioned earlier, LSVT is a promising program for patients with PD. Its development was based on the hypothesis that reduced drive to respiratory and laryngeal muscles underlies the reduced vocal loudness and prosodically flat speech so often associated with PD. LSVT focuses on the voice and attempts to modify laryngeal pathophysiology through exercise designed to increase loudness and decrease breathiness.

LSVT deserves attention here for two reasons. First, its emphasis on high effort, multiple repetitions, and intensity embodies principles of motor learning.[67] For that reason, it may serve as a general model for the structure of impairment-focused behavioral therapies for many MSDs. Second, the programmatic nature of the research on which LSVT is based is exemplary and uncommon among behavioral treatments for MSDs, and the evidence for its effectiveness is good in comparison to other impairment-oriented treatments. Researchers and clinicians interested in developing new treatments or examining existing ones can benefit from a careful review of the programmatic development of evidence regarding efficacy of LSVT.

The distinctive characteristics of LSVT are its (1) *intensity* (four times per week for 1 month), (2) requirement for *energetic, high levels of physical effort* to increase vocal loudness and vocal fold adduction, (3) exclusive *focus on respiratory-phonatory effort* (i.e., not resonance, articulation, rate, or prosody), and (4) focus on *increasing sensory awareness of loudness and effort*. Exercise includes vowel, word, phrase, sentence, and conversation production tasks.

A systematic review of the evidence as part of practice guideline development efforts by ANCDS concluded that *there is good evidence of immediate*

---

*See Fox et al.[67] for an excellent overview of the rationale for LSVT and a summary of results of related treatment studies.

posttreatment improvement and some evidence of long-term maintenance of effect with LSVT.[242] Positive outcomes have been documented at the impairment level by a range of acoustic, aerodynamic, and kinematic and related physiologic measures. Perceptual measures and family and self-reports have also documented the positive impact of intervention in some studies.

More specifically, the most pertinent studies of LSVT can be summarized as follows:

1. Treatment outcomes using perceptual ratings of loudness, voice quality, and intelligibility have demonstrated posttreatment improvement.[35,67,174,216,232]

2. Treatment outcomes using acoustic, aerodynamic, electromyographic, and kinematic measures have documented improved maximum vowel duration, SPL, mean f_o, maximum range of f_o, subglottic air pressure, vocal fold adduction, phonatory stability, and thyroarytenoid muscle activity variability.[50,67,174,216,232] Pretreatment compensatory supraglottic hyperadduction is reduced in some cases.[35] Respiratory kinematics do not necessarily improve following treatment.[104]

3. Maintenance of gains on various outcome measures have been evident at 6, 12, and 24 months after treatment in some patients.[67,173,232]

4. In some studies, including controlled, randomized, prospective studies, laryngoscopy and various acoustic, aerodynamic, and perceptual measures have demonstrated superiority of LSVT to treatment of comparable intensity and duration that focused on respiratory function only.[172,173,175,177,205]

5. Some studies demonstrate changes beyond phonatory-respiratory functions. For example, some data suggest that the amplitude, coordination, endurance, or stability of motor activity in the orofacial system occurs, as reflected in measures of formant transition duration, lip kinematics, vowel space, spatiotemporal variability, and tongue pressure and endurance.[49,50,67,216,232] Some data suggest improvements in swallowing function.[58] It is possible that LSVT results in an increase in amplitude of movement in the speech motor system, in general, and may therefore simplify treatment for many patients, particularly those with cognitive deficits who do better when the explicit focus of treatment is on a single rather than multiple goals.[67] Some findings suggest that the spatial and temporal organization associated with speaking loudly in patients with PD resembles that of normal speech, a factor that may contribute to the success of LSVT.[117]

6. Positron emission tomography (PET) data before versus after LSVT identify posttreatment changes in activation patterns suggestive of improved automaticity of speech motor actions.[131]

7. Some findings suggest that LSVT may be helpful in patients with conditions other than PD, such as stroke, TBI, and MS, and with dysarthria types other than hypokinetic.[67,190] At this point, however, clinicians should be cautious when considering LSVT for disorders other than PD,[67] and particularly for dysarthria types other than hypokinetic.

Variables that predict LSVT treatment success have not yet been clearly defined,[67] and the percentage of patients with PD-associated hypokinetic dysarthria who are likely to benefit from LSVT has not yet been established. It does appear that lack of motivation and depression may be important variables that limit the success of the treatment in some patients.[176] The data to date support the efficacy of this intensive voice therapy for at least some patients with PD. The general principles of motor learning and intensity of treatment upon which LSVT is based may be applicable to the management of MSDs other than hypokinetic dysarthria.

Hyperkinetic Dysarthrias

The effective management approaches for hyperkinetic dysarthria are primarily surgical and pharmacologic. The underlying pathophysiology of hyperkinetic dysarthria logically predicts this, because the abnormal movements that cause the speech disturbance are not under voluntary control. Fortunately, there are an increasing number of nonbehavioral treatments available that do provide relief for the speech deficits associated with some of the hyperkinetic dysarthrias.

Pallidotomy, thalamotomy, and DBS are used to manage tremor, dyskinesia, and dystonia, and improvement in dysarthria associated with such movement disorders is occasionally observed (see the discussion of these neurosurgical procedures in the previous section on hypokinetic dysarthria). Such procedures are not employed with the intent of treating hyperkinetic dysarthrias, however.*

As already discussed, Botox injection is the preferred method for managing spasmodic dysphonias,

---

*One study[214] has reported the effect of bilateral thalamic DBS on voice tremor in seven patients who had the surgery explicitly to manage the voice tremor. Improvement was noted. Without considerable further study, however, DBS cannot be considered a primary treatment for voice tremor.

particularly ADSD. A systematic review of the literature has also concluded that Botox injection is frequently effective in managing jaw opening and jaw closing mandibular dystonias and that it is potentially effective in managing lingual dystonias that cause involuntary tongue protrusion.[53] Injection of Botox into the tensor veli Palatini muscle has also been used to treat palatal myoclonus.[227]

Medication is only occasionally helpful in the management of movement disorders that cause hyperkinetic dysarthria, and positive effects, at best, are usually only modest. Regarding tremor, agents that can help essential tremor in the limbs, such as Inderal, primidone (Mysoline), carbamazepine (Tegretol), baclofen (Lioresal), and combinations of trihexyphenidyl (Artane) and lithium are noted to only infrequently help head or voice tremor.[118,184] Methazolamide (Neptazane) is reportedly effective in relieving essential tremor, particularly head or voice tremor, in some patients.[153] Small amounts of alcohol frequently decrease the amplitude of essential voice tremor,[118] although its use obviously must be judicious and limited to appropriate social situations. A recent review of the available evidence concluded that pharmacologic management for essential voice tremor cannot at this time be considered a primary treatment for most individuals with the disorder.[53]

For movement disorders other than tremor, Artane has been used with significant benefit to speech in a patient with laryngeal and respiratory dystonia.[135] Lioresal, combinations of Artane and lithium, and alprazolam (Xanax) are said to occasionally reduce symptoms of oromandibular dystonia and spasmodic dysphonia.[184] Intramuscular injection of diluted lidocaine and alcohol has reduced the severity of otherwise drug-resistant oromandibular dystonia in some patients,[248] but its specific effects on speech have not been reported. Lioresal, reserpine, and haloperidol (Haldol) may have some minimal effects on chorea-induced dysarthria.[184] Choreiform movements are sometimes decreased with reserpine, Haldol, or Lioresal. Medications to suppress tics in Tourette's syndrome and other tic disorders include alpha agonists such as clonidine and guanfacine or neuroleptics that act as dopamine receptor antagonists such as haloperidol, clozapine, olanzapine, risperidone, fluphenazine, and pimozide.[123] Some patients with palatal myoclonus have benefited from clonazepam, carbamazepine, or trihexyphenidyl.[68]

A few behavioral and prosthetic approaches may help some patients with certain types of hyperkinetic dysarthria, although most of them provide only temporary and less than optimal relief. They include the following:

1. Some patients with mandibular dystonias or other hyperkinesias affecting jaw movement benefit from the use of a bite block (or pipe or other socially acceptable device held in the mouth), which may inhibit or limit adventitious jaw movements during speech, with resultant improvement in articulation and rate.[55,56]

2. Some patients with focal dystonias of the jaw, tongue, or face spontaneously discover sensory tricks (postural adjustments) that inhibit adventitious movements and facilitate speech. It is usually worth exploring for such sensory tricks in patients who have not discovered them on their own. If discovered tricks are socially acceptable, they may provide relief and improvement of speech, at least under some circumstances. Unfortunately, they are rarely maximal or lasting solutions.

3. Patients with the hyperkinetic dysarthria of action myoclonus often discover on their own that speech improves if rate is slowed. When they do not, actively taught rate reduction strategies can be beneficial.

4. Some patients with ADSD benefit from increasing vocal pitch or adopting a breathy onset of phonation. Similarly, some patients with ABSD may reduce the abductor spasm by adopting a hard glottal onset of phonation and voicing voiceless consonants. This reduces requirements for vocal fold abduction, which may trigger the abductor spasms.[6] These strategies are most often beneficial when the disorder is mild and when demands for excellent speech are not great. Unfortunately, they rarely become automatized. For most patients it is also difficult to maintain such compensatory strategies, the benefits are less than optimally acceptable, and they are often lost if the disorder progresses. A recent review of available evidence as part of efforts to develop practice guidelines for the management of spasmodic dysphonia[53] concluded that "neither expert opinion nor experimental studies support the effectiveness of behavioral treatment alone for SD." It is possible, however, that voice therapy for ADSD may be more effective when it follows successful treatment with Botox injection. That is, one study with a small number of subjects who were not randomly assigned to treatment groups[158] found that speakers with ADSD who received both Botox treatment and behavioral voice therapy improved phonation, as measured by increased airflow rate and acoustic measures of variability and perturbation, and that those changes persisted for longer periods compared to subjects who

received Botox treatment alone. This deserves further investigation.

A few reports on limited numbers of patients have examined the effects of biofeedback, chiropractic manipulation, and stimulation of the vagus or recurrent laryngeal nerves on ADSD. None of these techniques can be considered established effective treatments for the disorder.[53]

5. Case reports of the effectiveness of EMG feedback in modifying lip dystonia and hemifacial spasm have already been noted. The limited number of such reports warrants caution in assuming the technique can provide significant benefit to most patients in a cost-effective and efficient manner that significantly alters intelligibility and efficiency of speech. Biofeedback for treating movement disorders deserves continued study, but its use should not be considered an accepted, common treatment for orofacial movement disorders at this time.

Unilateral Upper Motor Neuron Dysarthria

There have been no formal reports of treatment for UUMN dysarthria, although Duffy and Folger's[52] retrospective study noted that therapy was recommended for a substantial number of patients who had the disorder and that many improved over the course of treatment. Because the disorder is usually relatively mild, patients with it are not generally candidates for medical or prosthetic management to explicitly manage the speech deficit. Behavioral approaches usually focus on rate, prosody, and articulation, and compensation may receive more emphasis than efforts to restore physiologic support. Some patients seem to benefit from mirror work to monitor drooling or squirreling of food in the cheek on the weak side.* Efforts to strengthen the unilateral face and tongue weakness that often accompany the disorder might be justified, although most clinicians probably focus more directly on speech than nonspeech oromotor exercise. Specific efforts to address impairment might vary as a function of specific speech deficits and whether they seem to be explained by a predominance of UMN weakness, spasticity, or incoordination. When the lesion causing the disorder is cortical, management often focuses primarily on the aphasia or cognitive-communication deficits associated with right hemisphere lesions that are often present.

---

*The author is indebted to his colleague Jack Thomas for this observation.

Mixed Dysarthrias

Patients with mixed dysarthrias may benefit from treatments that are appropriate for any of the component types that are present. However, the presence of a particular dysarthria type may contraindicate the use of some approaches or significantly reduce the likelihood that a particular approach will be helpful. In general, mixed dysarthrias are managed behaviorally, rather than prosthetically, surgically, or pharmacologically. A few studies illustrate possible exceptions to this rule.

A palatal lift prosthesis can be effective for some patients with mixed flaccid-spastic dysarthria associated with ALS. For example, one retrospective study reported reduced hypernasality and reduced effort to speak in more than 80% of 25 patients with ALS who were thought to be good lift candidates, with approximately 75% of the patients deriving moderate benefit for 6 months.[60]

Low-dose amitriptyline has reportedly reduced severe motor dysfunction including dysarthria in some people with progressive supranuclear palsy.[59] Dysarthria type was not specified, but it was possibly mixed.

One report has documented resolution of dysarthria in two individuals with MS following treatment with extracranial application of brief AC pulsed electromagnetic fields, known as *weak electromagnetic field stimulation*.[188] Dysarthria type was not specified, but reference was made to lesions of the cerebellum and its outflow tracts, implying that, at the least, dysarthria type included ataxia. It was suggested that the improvement was the result of changes in cerebellar neurotransmitter functions.

▨ COMMUNICATION-ORIENTED TREATMENT

What can be done to enhance communication between dysarthric speakers and their listeners when intelligibility or efficiency are reduced and direct medical, prosthetic, and behavioral approaches to restoring or compensating for speech deficits have failed, have had their desired effect, are in progress, or must be deferred? Solutions are to be found in the adoption of strategies that often improve the comprehensibility of messages rather than the intelligibility of speech. They are based on the fact that a good deal more than the acoustic attributes of speech determine whether a message is understood. These strategies are *independent of dysarthria type*. They are strongly dependent on degree of disability and handicap, accompanying deficits, the environment in which communication occurs, and the dysarthric person's communication

table 17-3	Summary of communication-oriented management strategies
Speaker Strategies	Prepare listeners with alerting signals (get the listeners' attention)
	Convey how communication should take place
	Set the context and identify the topic
	Modify sentence content, structure, and length
	Gestures may help
	Monitor listener comprehension
	Alphabet board supplementation
Listener Strategies	Maintain eye contact
	Listen attentively and actively, and work at comprehension
	Modify the physical environment
	Maximize hearing and visual acuity
Interaction Strategies	Time important interactions
	Select a conducive speaking environment
	Maintain eye contact between listener and speaker
	Identify breakdowns and establish methods for feedback
	Repair breakdowns
	Establish what works best when

partners.* Many of these strategies can be implemented by patients alone, their listeners alone, or by cooperation between speakers and listeners. Sometimes a single strategy can have a major impact, but in many cases small gains derived from each of a number of strategies determine improvement. These strategies are summarized in Table 17-3.†

Speaker Strategies

Dysarthric speakers can do numerous things to increase the predictability and comprehensibility of their speech. The best candidates for using such

---

*See Yorkston et al.'s[245] *Communicative Effectiveness Survey,* a clinically useful rating form that provides insight into speakers' and listeners' judgments of communicative effectiveness in various social situations.

†See Yorkston, Strand, and Kennedy[243] for a useful checklist to summarize recommendations about strategies to improve comprehensibility derived from careful clinical evaluation and consultation with dysarthric speakers and their listeners.

---

strategies are those with moderate to severe dysarthria who do not have language or other cognitive problems that would preclude learning and generalization of the strategies.[243] They include the following measures.

Prepare Listeners with Alerting Signals

Having the attention of listeners before initiating speech can enhance intelligibility and comprehensibility. Such signals can be vocal or verbal (e.g., saying the listener's name, "excuse me") or nonverbal (e.g., a hand gesture, achieving eye contact).

Convey How Communication Should Occur

This is especially important for speakers who use augmentative means of communication. This ground rule may be conveyed to novel listeners at the outset of an interaction. It may state that the speaker has a neurologic impairment that makes speaking difficult and that communication will be easiest if, for example, the speaker points to the first letter of each word as the word is spoken. The speaker may instruct the listener to repeat each word or utterance as soon as it is completed in order to confirm comprehension, to wait until a sentence is completed before asking for clarification, to ask for clarification as soon as something is misunderstood, to be sure to watch the patient, and so on. These directions can be mounted on a lap board or presented on a card.

Set the Context and Identify the Topic

The availability of semantic or contextual information (e.g., topic cues, such as a specific activity or things to buy in a grocery store) can enhance word and sentence intelligibility in severely dysarthric speakers[29,71] and may contribute to more positive listener attitudes toward the speaker when it does.[106] The effect can be pronounced for single word utterances, with nearly 30% to fivefold increases in intelligibility with contextual cues reported by some investigators.[47,241] Such cues can also significantly influence sentence intelligibility,[69,71] especially when combined with alphabet supplementation cues.[105]

Context can be set by indicating the semantic context or topic of conversation through speech or nonverbally (e.g., from a topic list on a word board, in writing). Semantic cues allow predictions to be made about content before the specific message is initiated. Signaling a shift in topic during conversation can also be valuable and can be accomplished by announcing the new topic or, more simply, using an agreed-upon gesture to signal a desire to change topics; this can also be done in writing or with an alphabet board that lists topics or the phrase "shift topic."[245] Gains in intelligibility vary from negligible to approximately 50% but average approximately 11%, with the largest gains occurring for speakers in the midrange of severity.[91] A systematic review of the literature[91] concluded that the technique can be effective for speakers with dysarthria that interferes with communication in natural settings and who have adequate cognitive and pragmatic skills and the motor capacity to generate the cues.

Modify Sentence Content, Structure, and Length

Some dysarthric speakers improve intelligibility by increasing redundancy or elaboration in their utterances. Others may need to be more concise, simplifying or limiting content and length to the essentials of the message.[228] This may be especially relevant when answering questions. For example, learning to say "coffee" when asked if one would like coffee or tea is far more efficient than saying "I've had too much coffee already today, but I suppose one more cup won't hurt." Normal speakers can afford to elaborate and explain simple things, whereas many dysarthric speakers cannot. Some speakers may need to modify their use of idiomatic expressions and metaphors and focus on more literal meanings,[228] and many of them adopt such changes automatically. Others may have difficulty, especially when such changes represent a major alteration in style and projection of personality or when cognitive deficits are present. A compromise for such individuals may be to reserve style shifts to situations in which communication has broken down.

Adjusting length can also improve intelligibility. It appears that speakers with severely reduced intelligibility are more intelligible on words than sentences but that less severely impaired speakers are more intelligible in sentences than words.[47,239] It is likely that listeners benefit from redundancy within sentences when word intelligibility reaches a critical threshold. Telegraphic structures should probably be avoided, but sentence structure that is simple and predictable (e.g., active rather than passive sentences) is more likely to be easily understood.[245]

Gestures May Help

The use of gestures can enhance comprehensibility. Such gestures can include pointing to objects or locations, using props, or using natural gestures or pantomime.[245] At a basic level, simple gestures can help signal turn taking in conversation; for example, leaning forward or raising a hand can indicate a desire to speak or to continue speaking.[245]

In some people with severe dysarthria the use of gestures, along with high message predictability and contextual cues, facilitates verbal message understanding.[69,71,91] Other findings suggest that natural gestures and iconic gestures (e.g., "stop" signaled by a stop gesture) alter temporal patterns of speech, may increase rate, and may reduce interword intervals in dysarthric speakers.[70,72,91] These gestures might improve naturalness of speech, but effects on comprehensibility are less certain. *The facilitory effect of gestures may depend on the naturalness of the gestures (including their motoric normalcy), a trait that may not be present in many dysarthric patients with poor head control or limb motor deficits.* It has been shown, for example, that distorting natural head movements during speech can reduce syllable identification.[154]

Monitor Listener Comprehension

This can be done by maintaining eye contact with listeners and asking if the message has been understood, particularly with listeners who are reluctant to admit they have not understood. In general, the more rapidly a failure to comprehend is perceived, the more efficiently repairs can be made.

Alphabet Board Supplementation

This has already been addressed within the discussion of speaker-oriented treatment for rate. The technique can significantly improve comprehensibility and enhance listeners' attitudes toward the dysarthric speaker.[106] Its use should be introduced to novel listeners, so they know to watch the speaker as well as the letter board. The speaker must control these interactions; using control phrases on the letter board may be helpful in this regard (e.g., "end of word," "end of sentence," "start again") (see Figure 17-5). When hand function is inefficient or inadequate for pointing, augmentative devices such as a head-mounted light pointer can be used for letter identification.[245]

Listener Strategies

Listeners can do many things to enhance speaker intelligibility, comprehensibility, and efficiency. Some of these can only be accomplished by the listener, whereas others can be undertaken by the speaker as well. Because many dysarthric speakers are disabled in ways other than speech, listeners/caregivers may need to take responsibility for many environmental modifications that can facilitate communication. Following are suggested strategies.

Maintain Eye Contact

Listeners can derive important information by maintaining eye contact with the speaker. This is clearly the case when people listen to normal speakers. For example, natural gestures of the head during normal speech enhance message understandability, perhaps partly because they tend to correlate with f_o and loudness.[154] Seeing a speaker's face enhances the perception of normal speech in noise, and experience with such cues can make them more effective.[183] Sentence understandability can also improve with visual-auditory information, as opposed to auditory alone, in some dysarthric speakers.[72]

Listen Attentively and Actively, and Work at Comprehension

Not all listeners bring the same skills to their interaction with dysarthric speakers. In general, for example, young adult listeners comprehend severely dysarthric speech better than do elderly listeners[146] and speech clinicians do better than nonclinicians.[37,40] A highly familiar listener (e.g., a spouse) can be superior to unfamiliar listeners when dysarthria is moderately severe.[45]

It is likely that most listeners need to attend to dysarthric speakers more vigilantly than they do to normal speakers. They may need to consciously (overtly or covertly) confirm their understanding or lack thereof in an ongoing way, because the normal expectation that redundancy during discourse eventually will clarify meaning may not hold. Repeating or clarifying far downstream may be inefficient and time consuming at best or abort the communicative attempt at worst. When listeners recognize that they are not comprehending a message, it is often appropriate to initiate a response that will repair a breakdown in intelligibility rapidly.

Counseling of significant others often must stress these points, as well as the possibility that practice and "work" at listening can improve comprehension. It has been shown that listeners who are familiarized with dysarthric speech—even with relatively brief exposures—produce higher intelligibility scores than those who are not familiarized,[133,211,220] and it has been suggested that familiarization procedures may be a useful intervention strategy in some cases.[45,220] For some listeners such procedures may involve active training and practice, with tangible evidence of its value demonstrated to them. This may be particularly worthwhile when the dysarthric speaker has a progressive disease and his or her significant others are cognitively intact, have adequate hearing, and are committed to communicating with the dysarthric speaker but who demonstrate much less adequate comprehension than does the clinician or other listeners.

Modify the Physical Environment

Modifying the physical environment can enhance intelligibility and comprehensibility.[15] These modifications may include *reducing sources of noise* or *increasing signal-noise ratio* (e.g., turning off or muting the TV or radio, closing windows, using rugs and drapes to dampen noise, speaking away from fans or air conditioners); *avoiding noisy dark settings* (e.g., crowded, poorly lit restaurants) when communication is essential; and *limiting distance from the speaker*.

Maximize Listener Hearing and Visual Acuity

Listeners who have hearing aids and glasses should wear them, or their possible need for such sensory aids should be investigated.

Interaction Strategies

Speakers and listeners can do many things together to facilitate comprehensibility and improve efficiency. Sometimes these strategies need to be negotiated to accommodate the needs, desires, and assets and liabilities of the speakers and listeners. *The strategies often need to be trained and practiced.* Some relate to maximizing comprehensibility and efficiency on the first attempt. Many relate to *breakdown resolution strategies* to establish comprehensibility when a message is not understood. Communication diaries about the environment, context, speaking task, and listeners—kept by dysarthric individuals or significant others—can help identify barriers to communication in natural settings and circumstances that lead to breakdowns in intelligibility or comprehensibility.[245] Then strategies can be developed to reduce the barriers or repair communication breakdowns when they occur.

Time Important Interactions

When the adequacy of speech is significantly influenced by fatigue or stress, as it often is, scheduling important interactions at times when those variables are likely to be minimal can maximize intelligibility, comprehensibility, or efficiency.

Select a Conducive Speaking Environment

Minimizing noise, distractibility, or poor lighting can maximize communicative effectiveness. It can also help reduce fatigue and stress and their effects on speech that can occur in poor speaking environments.

Maintain Eye Contact between Listener and Speaker

The exception to this is when certain augmentative strategies are used. For example, when the speaker supplements speech with a letter or word board or other augmentative device, the listener should look at the letter board and listen to speech.

Identify Breakdowns and Establish Methods for Feedback

The first thing that must be done to repair a breakdown in intelligibility or comprehensibility is to identify that a breakdown has occurred. Some speakers prefer to complete an utterance without interruption, whereas others desire feedback as soon as a listener does not understand something. However, *listener feedback often is most effectively used if it is specific and immediate*. For example, aspects of speech production are more effectively changed when feedback identifies the locus and type of error than when it is general (e.g., "Pardon me?"), as long as the speaker has the capacity to correct the error.[219] This suggests that the more precise feedback is about when and where errors occur, the more likely that repetition or revision will be effective. This precision may be specific to the location of a word, but it may take other forms. For example, a listener who has grasped little or nothing may ask the speaker to identify the topic (who or what is being talked about), or may summarize what he or she has understood and establish what is missing ("I know you're going somewhere tomorrow, but I don't know where").

For patients with frequent breakdowns in intelligibility, a strategy called *shadowing*[245] can help to localize the problem. It requires the listener to repeat each word, phrase, or sentence immediately after it is produced by the speaker. If alphabet supplementation is being used, each word should be repeated. The strategy allows the speaker to confirm accuracy of interpretation or to know precisely where the breakdown occurred.

Many speakers spontaneously improve speech when informed that intelligibility has broken down, but some do not. Listeners who know what speakers are capable of doing with help may be able to provide explicit cues about what is likely to work (e.g., slow down, use one word at a time, tap it out, speak louder, take a deep breath, give the first letter).* That such explicit feedback will be given can

be established as a general rule of interaction that is negotiated between listener and speaker. This is particularly useful for speakers who are unable to use their maximum capacity all of the time because of physiologic or cognitive limitations, but who can use it when cued. When communication partners are familiar with each other, a simple gesture may be sufficient to trigger the need to increase effort or adopt a specific compensatory strategy. Finally, when a first repair attempt fails, a strategy with guaranteed success should then be used (e.g., spelling).

Referential communication tasks during treatment are valuable for establishing feedback strategies because they allow patients and their listeners to discover what works best and provide an opportunity to practice feedback and repair strategies. Review of videotapes of communicative interaction also can be a valuable source of feedback about the effectiveness of communicative strategies.

Repair Breakdowns

When speakers are interrupted with a general indication that comprehensibility has broken down, their spontaneous adjustments often include total repetition, partial repetition of a phrase, partial repetition with elaboration, or total repetition with elaboration.[5] However, following identification, a predetermined plan for repair can improve efficiency and predictability. For example, the speaker and listener may agree that the statement will be repeated (the logical first step) a single time, with other methods to follow if the repetition fails.[243] The other methods could include rephrasing or use of synonyms, spelling problem words, alphabet supplementation, or writing. The selection and ordering of such options are influenced by dysarthria severity and previously established successful repair strategies. A given speaker may need to vary his or her use of strategies across different listeners and contexts.[245]

Establish What Works Best When

Combinations of communication strategies are often appropriate. For example, speech may be quite adequate when exchanging social greetings and may represent the most rapid and efficient means of doing so. The same speaker, however, may need to spell

---

*During treatment sessions, some patients respond favorably when the clinician consistently uses the manner of speaking the patient is being asked to adopt during conversational interaction or during repairs. This provides a natural model and can pace the interaction in a way that promotes more consistent patient

responses. Thus for example, the clinician may speak slowly, increase pause duration, tap his or her hand with each syllable spoken, and take a deep breath at phrase boundaries. An alternative is for the clinician or listener to model the technique during their verbal feedback that represents what the speaker should do to repair a breakdown (The author is indebted to his colleague Jack Thomas for this suggestion).

out more elaborated or novel messages or use a letter or word board to introduce new topics.

Communication strategies may also vary considerably across listeners. Speech without augmentation is most often possible with familiar listeners, whereas augmentative strategies are often necessary with novel listeners or under adverse speaking conditions.

SUMMARY

1. Various speaker-oriented and communication-oriented approaches are used to manage the dysarthrias. Although evidence of their efficacy is relatively limited, a substantial number of reports document the effectiveness of a number of management approaches and techniques.

2. Speaker-oriented approaches may focus on restoration or compensation for impairments in respiration, phonation, resonance, articulation, rate, and prosody. A number of medical/surgical, prosthetic, and behavioral approaches are available for improving respiratory, phonatory, resonatory, and articulatory functions for speech. Prosthetic and behavioral management approaches are generally used to improve rate and prosody.

3. Many techniques used in speaker-oriented treatments can be applied to patients with various dysarthria types. However, some approaches and techniques are much more useful for some dysarthria types than others, some are useful for only a single dysarthria type, and some are contraindicated for use with some types. Differences in management across dysarthria types exist for medical/surgical, prosthetic, and behavioral approaches.

4. Communication-oriented approaches to treatment include a number of strategies that can be adopted by speakers and listeners. Although such approaches do not result in modification of speech production per se, they can contribute substantially to improving comprehensibility of messages and the efficiency with which they are transmitted. Communication-oriented approaches to treatment are independent of dysarthria type, but they are strongly dependent on degree of disability and handicap, the presence and severity of deficits that may accompany MSDs, the environment in which communication takes place, and the characteristics of dysarthric individuals' communication partners.

References

1. Abbruzzese G: The medical management of spasticity, Eur J Neurol 9:30, 2002.
2. Adams SG: Hypokinetic dysarthria in Parkinson's disease. In McNeil MR, editor: Clinical management of sensorimotor speech disorders, New York, 1997, Thieme.
3. Adams SG: Accelerating speech in a case of hypokinetic dysarthria: descriptions and treatment. In Till JA, Yorkston KM, Beukelman DR, editors: Motor speech disorders: advances in assessment and treatment, Baltimore, 1994, Paul H Brookes.
4. Andrianopoulos MV, Duffy JR, Kelly PJ: The effects on speech of ventral lateral thalamotomy for treatment of movement disorders. Unpublished manuscript.
5. Ansel BM et al: The frequency of verbal and acoustic adjustments used by cerebral palsied dysarthric adults when faced with communicative failure. In Berry W, editor: Clinical dysarthria, Boston, 1983, College-Hill Press.
6. Aronson AE: Clinical voice disorders, New York, 1990, Thieme.
7. Aronson AE et al: Botulinum toxin injection for adductor spastic dysphonia: patient self-ratings of voice and phonatory effort after three successive injections, Laryngoscope 103:683, 1993.
8. Aten JL: Treatment of spastic dysarthria. In Perkins WH, editor: Current therapy of communication disorders: dysarthria and apraxia, New York, 1983, Thieme-Stratton.
8a. Aten JL: Efficacy of modified palatal lifts for improved regonance. In McNeil MR, Rosenbek J, Aronson AE, editors: The dysarthrias: physiology, acoustics, perception, management. Austin, Tex, 1984, Pro-Ed.
9. Barlow SM, Abbs JH: Force transducers for the evaluation of labial, lingual, and mandibular function in dysarthria, J Speech Hear Res 26:616, 1983.
10. Barlow SM et al: The effects of posteroventral pallidotomy on force and speech aerodynamic in Parkinson's disease. In Cannito MP, Yorkston KM, Beukelman DR, editors: Neuromotor speech disorders: nature, assessment, and management, Baltimore, 1998, Brookes Publishing.
11. Bedore LM, Leonard LB: Prosodic and syntactic bootstrapping and their clinical applications, Am J Speech-Lang Pathol 4:66, 1995.
12. Bellaire K, Yorkston KM, Beukelman DR: Modification of breath patterning to increase naturalness of a mildly dysarthric speaker, J Commun Disord 19:271, 1986.
13. Bender BK et al: Speech intelligibility in severe adductor spasmodic dysphonia, J Speech Hear Res 47:21, 2004.
14. Berry W, Goshorn E: Immediate visual feedback in the treatment of ataxic dysarthria: a case study. In Berry W, editor: Clinical dysarthria, Boston, 1983, College-Hill Press.
15. Berry WR, Sanders SB: Environmental education: the universal management approach for adults with dysarthria. In Berry WR, editor: Clinical dysarthria, Boston, 1983, College-Hill Press.
16. Beukelman DR, Yorkston K: A communication system for the severely dysarthric speaker with an intact language system, J Speech Hear Disord 42:265, 1977.
17. Beukelman DR, Yorkston KM, Tice RL: Pacer/tally rate measurement software, Lincoln, Neb, 1997, Tice Technology Services.

18. Biary N, Pimental PA, Langenberg PW: A double-blind trial of clonazepam in the treatment of parkinsonian dysarthria, Neurology 38:255, 1988.

19. Brand HA, Matsko TA, Avart HN: Speech prosthesis retention problems in dysarthria: case report, Arch Phys Med Rehabil 69:213, 1988.

20. Brin MF et al: Localized injections of botulinum toxin for the treatment of focal dystonia and hemifacial spasm, Mov Disord 2:237, 1987.

21. Brookshire RH: Control of "involuntary" crying behavior emitted by a multiple sclerosis patient, J Commun Disord 3:171, 1970.

22. Bunton K et al: The effects of flattening fundamental frequency contours on sentence intelligibility in speakers with dysarthria, Clin Linguist Phon 15:181, 2001.

23. Cahill LM et al: Effect of oral levodopa treatment on articulatory function in Parkinson's disease: preliminary results, Motor Control, 2:161, 1998.

24. Caligiuri MP: Short-term fluctuations in orofacial motor control in Parkinson's disease. In Yorkston KM, Beukelman DR, editors: Recent advances in clinical dysarthria, Boston, 1989, College-Hill.

25. Caligiuri MP, Murry T: The use of visual feedback to enhance prosodic control in dysarthria. In Berry W, editor: Clinical dysarthria, Boston, 1983, College-Hill Press.

26. Cannito MP, Marquardt TP: Ataxic dysarthria. In MR McNeil, editor: Clinical management of sensorimotor speech disorders, New York, 1997, Thieme.

27. Carey J: Manual stretch: effect on finger movement control and force control in stroke subjects with spastic extrinsic finger flexion muscles, Arch Phys Med Rehabil 71:888, 1990.

28. Cariski D, Rosenbek J: Clinical note: the effectiveness of the speech enhancer, J Med Speech-Lang Pathol 7:315, 1999.

29. Carter CR et al: Effects of semantic and syntactic context on actual and estimated sentence intelligibility of dysarthric speakers. In Robin DA, Yorkston KM, Beukelman DR, editors: Disorders of motor speech: assessment, treatment, and clinical characterization, Baltimore, 1996, Brookes Publishing.

30. Casanova E et al: Locked-in syndrome: improvement in the prognosis after an early intensive multidisciplinary rehabilitation, Arch Phys Med Rehabil 84:862, 2003.

31. Cerny FJ, Panzarella KJ, Stathopoulis E: Expiratory muscle conditioning in hypotonic children with low vocal intensity levels, J Med Speech-Lang Pathol 5:141, 1997.

32. Charles P et al: Tongue protrusion dystonia: treatment with botulinum toxin, South Med J 90:522, 1997.

33. Clark HM: Neuromuscular treatments for speech and swallowing: a tutorial, Am J Speech-Lang Pathol 12:400, 2003.

34. Corcos DM et al: Strength in Parkinson's disease: relationship to rate of force generation and clinical status, Ann Neurol 39:79, 1996.

35. Countryman S et al: Supraglottal hyperadduction in an individual with Parkinson disease: a clinical treatment note, Am J Speech-Lang Pathol 6:74, 1997.

36. Crow E, Enderby P: The effects of an alphabet chart on the speaking rate and intelligibility of speakers with dysarthria. In Yorkston KM, Beukelman DR, editors: Recent advances in clinical dysarthria, Austin, Tex, 1989, Pro-Ed.

37. Dagenais PA, Garcia JM, Watts CR: Acceptability and intelligibility of mildly dysarthric speech by different listeners. In Cannito MP, Yorkston KM, Beukelman DR, editors: Neuromotor speech disorders: nature, assessment, and management, Baltimore, 1998, Brookes Publishing.

38. Dagenais PA, Southwood MH, Lee TL: Rate reduction methods for improving speech intelligibility of dysarthric speakers with Parkinson's disease, J Med Speech-Lang Pathol 6:143, 1998.

39. Dagenais PA, Southwood MH, Mallonee KO: Assessing processing skills in speakers with Parkinson's disease using delayed auditory feedback, J Med Speech-Lang Pathol 7:297, 1999.

40. Dagenais, PA et al: Intelligibility and acceptability of moderately dysarthric speech by three types of listeners, J Med Speech-Lang Pathol 7:91, 1999.

41. Damiano D, Abel M: Functional outcomes of strength training in spastic cerebral palsy, Arch Phys Med Rehabil 79:119, 1998.

42. Daniel R, Guitar B: EMG feedback and recovery of facial and speech gestures following neural anastomosis, J Speech Hear Disord 43:9, 1978.

43. Darley FL, Aronson AE, Brown JR: Motor speech disorders, Philadelphia, 1975, WB Saunders.

44. DePaul R, Brooks B: Multiple orofacial indices in amyotrophic lateral sclerosis, J Speech Hear Res 36:1158, 1993.

45. DePaul R, Kent RD: A longitudinal case study of ALS: effects of listener familiarity and proficiency on intelligibility judgments, Am J Speech-Lang Pathol 9:230, 2000.

46. Dobkin BH, Thompson AJ: Principles of neurological rehabilitation. In Bradley WG et al, editors: Neurology in clinical practice: principles of diagnosis and management, vol 1, ed 3, Boston, 2000, Butterworth-Heinemann.

47. Dongilli PA: Semantic context and speech intelligibility. In Till JA, Yorkston KM, Beukelman DR, editors: Motor speech disorders: advances in assessment and treatment, Baltimore, 1994, Paul H Brookes.

48. Downie AW, Low JM, Lindsay DD: Speech disorders in parkinsonism. Usefulness of delayed auditory feedback in selected cases, Br J Disord Commun 16:135, 1981.

49. Dromey C: Articulatory kinematics in patients with Parkinson disease using different speech treatment approaches, J Med Speech-Lang Pathol 8:155, 2000.

50. Dromey C, Ramig LO, Johnson AB: Phonatory and articulatory changes associated with increased vocal intensity in Parkinson disease: a case study, J Speech Hear Res 38:751, 1995.

51. Dromey C, Warrick P, Irish J: The influence of pitch and loudness changes on the acoustics of vocal tremor, J Speech Lang Hear Res 45:879, 2002.

52. Duffy JR, Folger WN: Dysarthria associated with unilateral central nervous system lesions: a retrospective study, J Med Speech-Lang Pathol 4:57, 1996.

53. Duffy JR, Yorkston KM: Medical interventions for spasmodic dysphonia and some related conditions: a sys-

tematic review, J Med Speech-Lang Pathol 11:ix, 2003.

54. Dworkin JP: Motor speech disorders: a treatment guide, St Louis, 1991, Mosby.

55. Dworkin JP: Bite-block therapy for oromandibular dystonia. In Cannito MP, Yorkston KM, Beukelman DR, editors: Neuromotor speech disorders: nature, assessment, and management, Baltimore, 1998, Brookes Publishing.

56. Dworkin JP: Bite-block therapy for oromandibular dystonia, J Med Speech-Lang Pathol 4:47, 1996.

57. Dworkin JP, Johns DF: Management of velopharyngeal incompetence in dysarthria: a historical review, Clin Otolaryngol 5:61, 1980.

58. El Sharkawi et al: Swallowing and voice effects of Lee Silverman voice treatment (LSVT): a pilot study, J Neurol Neurosurg Psychiatry 72:331, 2002.

59. Engel PA: Treatment of progressive supranuclear palsy with amitriptyline: therapeutic and toxic effects, J Am Geriatr Soc 44:1072 1996.

60. Esposito SJ, Mitsumoto H, Shanks M: Use of palatal lift and palatal augmentation prostheses to improve dysarthria in patients with amyotrophic lateral sclerosis: a case series, J Prosthetic Dentistry 83:90, 2000.

61. Evidente VG et al: Hereditary ataxias, Mayo Clin Proc 75:475, 2000.

62. Fonagy I, Magdics K: Speech of utterance in phrases of different lengths, Lang Speech 3:179, 1960.

63. Ford CN, Bless DM: A preliminary study of injectable collagen in human vocal fold augmentation, Otolaryngol Head Neck Surg 94:104, 1986.

64. Formisano R et al: Rehabilitation and Parkinson's disease, Scand J Rehabil Med 24:157, 1992.

65. Fowler WM: Consensus conference summary: role of physical activity and exercise training in neuromuscular diseases, Am J Phys Med Rehabil 81:S187, 2002.

66. Fox CM, Ramig LO: Vocal sound pressure level and self-perception of speech and voice in men and women with idiopathic Parkinson disease, Am J Speech-Language Pathol 6:85, 1997.

67. Fox CM et al: Current perspectives on the Lee Silverman Voice Treatment (LSVT) for individuals with idiopathic Parkinson disease, Am J Speech-Lang Pathol 11:111, 2002.

68. Frucht SJ: Myoclonus. In Noseworthy JH, editor: Neurological therapeutics: principles and practice, vol 1, New York, 2003, Martin Dunitz.

69. Garcia JM, Cannito MP: Influence of verbal and nonverbal contexts on the sentence intelligibility of a speaker with dysarthria, J Speech Hear Res 39:750, 1996.

70. Garcia JM, Cobb DS: The effects of gesturing on speech intelligibility and rate in ALS dysarthria: a case study, J Med Speech-Lang Pathol 8:353, 2000.

71. Garcia JM, Dagenais PA: Dysarthric sentence intelligibility: contribution of iconic gestures and message predictiveness, J Speech Lang Hear Res 40:1282, 1998.

72. Garcia JM, Dagenais PA, Cannito MP: Intelligibility and acoustic differences in dysarthric speech related to use of natural gestures. In Cannito MP, Yorkston KM, Beukelman DR, editors: Neuromotor speech disorders: nature, assessment, and management, Baltimore, 1998, Brookes Publishing.

73. Ghika J et al: Bilateral contemporaneous posteroventral pallidotomy for the treatment of Parkinson's disease: neuropsychological and neurological side effects. Report of four cases and review of the literature, J Neurosurg 91:313, 1999.

74. Gibbon F et al: Q2: A procedure for profiling impaired speech motor control of the tongue using electropalatography, J Med Speech-Lang Pathol 8:239, 2000.

75. Goldman-Eisler F: The significance of changes in the rate of articulation, Lang Speech 4:171, 1961.

76. Gonzalez JB, Aronson AE: Palatal lift prosthesis for treatment of anatomic and neurologic palatopharyngeal insufficiency, Cleft Palate J 7:91, 1970.

77. Goozée JV, Murdoch BE, Theodoros DG: Electropalatographic assessment of tongue-to-palate contacts exhibited in dysarthria following traumatic brain injury: spatial characteristics, J Med Speech-Lang Pathol 11:115, 2003.

78. Goozée JV, Murdoch BE, Theodoros DG: Electropalatographic assessment of articulatory timing characteristics in dysarthria following traumatic brain injury, J Med Speech-Lang Pathol 7:209, 1999.

79. Gray S et al: Vocal evaluation of thyroplasty surgery in the treatment of unilateral vocal cord paralysis, NCVS Status and Progress Report 1:87, 1991.

80. Gutek JM, Rochet AP: Effects of insertion of interword pauses on the intelligibility of dysarthric speech. In Robin DA, Yorkston KM, Beukelman DR, editors: Disorders of motor speech: assessment, treatment, and clinical characterization, Baltimore, 1996, Brookes Publishing.

81. Hageman C: Flaccid dysarthria. In MR McNeil, editor: Clinical management of sensorimotor speech disorders, New York, 1997, Thieme.

82. Hammen VL, Yorkston KM: Speech and pause characteristics following speech rate reduction in hypokinetic dysarthria, J Commun Disord 29:429, 1996.

83. Hammen VL, Torp JN: Effects of speaking rate reduction on segmental characteristics: a preliminary analysis, J Med Speech-Lang Pathol 7:97, 1999.

84. Hammen VL, Yorkston KM: Effect of instruction on selected aerodynamic parameters in subjects with dysarthria and control subjects. In Till JA, Yorkston KM, Beukelman DR, editors: Motor speech disorders: advances in assessment and treatment, Baltimore, 1994a, Paul H Brookes.

85. Hammen VL, Yorkston KM: Respiratory patterning and variability in dysarthric speech, J Med Speech-Lang Pathol 2:253, 1994b.

86. Hammen VL, Yorkston KM, Minifie FD: Effects of temporal alterations on speech intelligibility in parkinsonian dysarthria, J Speech Hear Res 37:244, 1994.

87. Hammerschlag PE et al: Hypoglossal-facial nerve anastomosis and electromyographic feedback rehabilitation, Laryngoscope 97:705, 1987.

88. Hand CR, Burns M, Ireland E: Treatment of hypertonicity in muscles of lip retraction, Biofeedback Self-Regul 4:171, 1979.

89. Hansen WR, Metter EJ: DAF as instrumental treatment for dysarthria in progressive supranuclear palsy: a case report, J Speech Hear Disord 45:268, 1980.

90. Hanson W, Metter E: DAF speech rate modification in Parkinson's disease: a report of two cases. In Berry W,

editor: *Clinical dysarthria,* Boston, 1983, College-Hill Press.

91. Hanson EK, Yorkston KM, Beukelman DR: Speech supplementation techniques for dysarthria: a systematic review, *J Med Speech-Lang Pathol* 12:ix, 2004.

92. Hardy JC et al: Surgical management of palatal paresis and speech problems in cerebral palsy: a preliminary report, *J Speech Hear Disord* 26:320, 1961.

93. Hartelius L, Wising C, Nord L: Speech modification in dysarthria associated with multiple sclerosis: an intervention based on vocal efficiency, contrastive stress, and verbal repair strategies, *J Med Speech-Lang Pathol* 5:113, 1997.

94. Havas TE, Priestley KJ: Autologous fat injection laryngoplasty for unilateral vocal fold paralysis, *ANZ J Surg* 73:938, 2003.

95. Heller JC et al: Velopharyngeal insufficiency in patients with neurologic, emotional, and mental disorders, *J Speech Hear Disord* 39:350, 1974.

96. Helm N: Management of palilalia with a pacing board, *J Speech Hear Disord* 44:350, 1979.

97. Henderson A, Goldman-Eisler F, Skarbek A: Sequential temporal patterns in spontaneous speech, *Lang Speech* 9:207, 1966.

98. Hertegrad S, Granqvist S, Lindestad P: Botulinum toxin injections for essential voice tremor, *Ann Otol Rhinol Laryngol* 109:204, 2000.

99. Higuchi Y, Iacono RP: Surgical complications in patients with Parkinson's disease after posteroventral pallidotomy, *Neurosurgery* 52:558, 2003.

100. Hixon TJ, Hawley JL, Wilson KJ: An around-the-house device for the clinical determination of respiratory driving pressure: a note on making the simple even simpler, *J Speech Hear Dis* 47:413, 1982.

101. Hixon TJ, Putnam A, Sharpe J: Speech production with flaccid paralysis of the rib cage, diaphragm, and abdomen, *J Speech Hear Disord* 48:315, 1983.

102. Hoit JD, Banzett RB, Brown R: Binding the abdomen can improve speech in men with phrenic nerve pacers, *Am J Speech-Lang Pathol* 11:71, 2002.

103. Hubble JP: Essential tremor: diagnosis and treatment. In Adler CH, Ahlskog JE, editors: *Parkinson's disease and movement disorders: diagnosis and treatment guidelines for the practicing physician,* Totowa, NJ, 2000, Humana Press.

104. Huber JE et al: Respiratory function and variability in individuals with Parkinson disease: pre- and post-Lee Silverman Voice Treatment, *J Med Speech-Lang Pathol* 11:185, 2003.

105. Hustad KC, Beukelman DR: Effects of linguistic cues and stimulus cohesion on intelligibility of severely dysarthric speech, *J Speech Lang Hear Res* 44:497, 2001.

106. Hustad KC, Gearhart KJ: Listener attitudes toward individuals with cerebral palsy who use speech supplementation strategies, *Am J Speech-Lang Pathol* 13:168, 2004.

107. Hustad KC, Jones T, Dailey S: Implementing speech supplementation strategies: effects on intelligibility and speech rate of individuals with chronic severe dysarthria, *J Speech Lang Hear Res* 46:462, 2003.

108. Isshiki N, Okamura H, Ishikawa T: Thyroplasty type 1 (lateral compression) for dysphonia due to vocal cord paralysis or atrophy, *Acta Otolaryngol* 80:465, 1975.

109. Jankovic J: Blepharospasm and oromandibular-laryngeal-cervical dystonia: a controlled trial of botulinum A toxin therapy. In Fahn S, editor: *Advances in neurology, vol 50, dystonia 2,* New York, 1989, Raven Press.

110. Johns DF: Surgical and prosthetic management of neurogenic velopharyngeal incompetency in dysarthria. In Johns DF, editor: *Clinical management of neurogenic communication disorders,* New York, 1985, Little, Brown.

111. Johnson JA, Pring TR: Speech therapy and Parkinson's disease: a review and further data, *Br J Disord Commun* 25:183, 1990.

112. Keith RL, Thomas JE: *Speech practice material for dysarthria, apraxia, and disorders of articulation,* Toronto, 1989, BC Decker.

113. Kelchner LN et al: Etiology, pathophysiology, treatment choices, and voice results for unilateral adductor vocal fold paralysis: a 3-year retrospective, *J Voice* 13:592, 1999.

114. Kelly PJ et al: Computer-assisted stereotactic ventralis lateralis thalamotomy with microelectrode recording control in patients with Parkinson's disease, *Mayo Clin Proc* 62:655, 1987.

115. Kennedy MRT, Strand EA, Yorkston KM: Selected acoustic changes in the verbal repairs of dysarthric speakers, *J Med Speech-Lang Pathol* 2:263, 1994.

116. Kent RD et al: Severe essential vocal and oromandibular tremor: a case report, *Phonoscope* 1:237, 1998.

117. Kleinow J, Smith A, Ramig LO: Speech motor stability in IPD: Effects of rate and loudness manipulations, *J Speech Lang Hear Res* 44:1041, 2001.

118. Koller W, Graner D, Mlcoch A: Essential voice tremor: treatment with propranolol, *Neurology* 35:106, 1985.

119. Koufman JA: Laryngoplastic phonosurgery. In Johnson JT, editor: *Instructional courses American Academy of Otolaryngology—Head and Neck Surgery,* St Louis, 1988, Mosby.

120. Koufman JA: Laryngoplasty for vocal cord medialization: an alternative to Teflon, *Laryngoscope* 96:726, 1986.

121. Kuehn DP: The development of a new technique for treating hypernasality: CPAP, *Am J Speech-Lang Pathol* 6:5, 1997.

122. Kuehn DP, Wachtel JM: CPAP therapy for treating hypernasality following closed head injury. In Till JA, Yorkston KM, Beukelman DR, editors: *Motor speech disorders: advances in assessment and treatment,* Baltimore, 1994, Paul H Brookes.

123. Kurlan R: Tourette's syndrome and tic disorders. In Noseworthy JH, editor: *Neurological therapeutics: principles and practice, vol 2,* New York, 2003, Martin Dunitz.

124. Laccourreye O et al: Intracordal injection of autologous fat in patients with unilateral laryngeal nerve paralysis: long-term results from the patient's perspective, *Laryngoscope* 113:541, 2003.

125. Lapco PE et al: Laryngeal botulinum toxin A for spastic dysarthria associated with cerebral palsy; a case study, *J Med Speech-Lang Pathol* 7:63, 1999.

126. Larson KK, Ramig, LO, Scherer RC: Acoustic and glottographic voice analysis during drug-related fluctuations in Parkinson disease, *J Med Speech-Lang Pathol* 2:227, 1994.

127. Lewy RB, Cole R, Wepman J: *Teflon injection in the correction of velopharyngeal insufficiency*, Ann Otol Rhinol Laryngol 74:874, 1965.

128. Light J: *A review of oral and oropharyngeal prostheses to facilitate speech and swallowing*, Am J Speech-Lang Pathol 4:15, 1995.

129. Linebaugh CW: *Treatment of flaccid dysarthria*. In Perkins WH, editor: *Current therapy of communication disorders: dysarthria and apraxia*, New York, 1983, Thieme-Stratton.

130. Linebaugh CW, Wolfe VE: *Relationships between articulation rate, intelligibility, and naturalness in spastic and ataxic speakers*. In McNeil MR, Rosenbek JC, Aronson AE, editors: *The dysarthrias: physiology, acoustics, perception, and management*, San Diego, 1984, College-Hill.

131. Liotti M et al: *Hypophonia in Parkinson disease: neural correlates of voice treatment revealed by PET*, Neurology 60:432, 2003.

132. Liss JM, Kuehn DP, Hinkle KP: *Direct training of velopharyngeal musculature*, J Med Speech-Lang Pathol 2:243, 1994.

133. Liss JM et al: *The effects of familiarization on intelligibility and lexical segmentation in hypokinetic and ataxic dysarthria*, J Acoust Soc Am 112:3022, 2002.

134. Logan KJ et al: *Speaking slowly: Effects of four self-guided training approaches on adults' speech rate and naturalness*, Am J Speech-Lang Pathol 11:163, 2002.

135. Ludlow CL, Sedora SE, Fujita M: *Inspiratory speech with respiratory dystonia*. In Helm-Estabrooks N, Aten JL, editors: *Difficult diagnoses in communication disorders*, Boston, 1989, College-Hill.

136. Magliulo G, D'Amico, Forino M: *Results and complications of facial reanimation following cerebellopontine angle surgery*, Eur Arch Otorhinolaryngol 258:45, 2001.

137. Maner KJ, Smith A, Grayson L: *Influences of utterance length and complexity on speech motor performance in children and adults*, J Speech Lang Hear Res 43:560, 2000.

138. Marshall RC and Karow CM: *Retrospective examination of failed rate-control intervention. Am J Speech Lang Pathol 11:3, 2002.

139. Maruska KG et al: *Sentence production in Parkinson disease treated with deep brain stimulation and medication*, J Med Speech-Lang Pathol 8:265, 2000.

140. McCulloch TM et al: *Long-term follow-up of fat injection laryngoplasty for unilateral vocal cord paralysis*, Laryngoscope 112(7 Pt 1):1235, 2002.

141. McFarlane SC et al: *Unilateral vocal fold paralysis: perceived vocal quality following three methods of treatment*, Am J Speech-Lang Pathol 1:45, 1991.

142. McHenry M, Wilson R: *The challenge of unintelligible speech following traumatic brain injury*, Brain Injury 8:363, 1994.

143. McHenry MA: *The effect of pacing strategies on the variability of speech movement sequences in dysarthria*, J Speech Lang Hear Res 46:702, 2003.

144. McHenry MA, Wilson RL, Minton JT: *Management of multiple physiologic system deficits following traumatic brain injury*, J Med Speech-Lang Pathol 2:59, 1994.

145. Merritt JL: *Management of spasticity in spinal cord injury*, Mayo Clin Proc 56:614, 1981.

146. Mertz-Garcia J, Hayden M: *Young and older listener understanding of a person with severe dysarthria*, J Med Speech-Lang Pathol 7:109, 1999.

147. Minami RT et al: *Velopharyngeal incompetency without overt cleft palate*, Plast Reconstr Surg 55:573, 1975.

148. Mingrino S, Zuccarello M: *Anastomosis of the facial nerve with accessory or hypoglossal nerves*. In Samii M, Janetta PJ, editors: *The cranial nerves: anatomy, pathology, pathophysiology, diagnosis, treatment*, New York, 1981, Springer-Verlag.

149. Mlcoch AG: *Diagnosis and treatment of parkinsonian dysarthria*. In Koller WC, editor: *Handbook of Parkinson's disease*, New York, 1992, Marcel Decker.

150. Mohr JP: *Disorders of speech and language*. In Wilson JD et al, editors: *Hanson's principles of internal medicine*, ed 12, New York, 1991, McGraw-Hill.

151. Moore CA, Scudder RR: *Coordination of jaw muscle activity in parkinsonian movement: description and response to traditional treatment*. In Yorkston KM, Beukelman DR, editors: *Recent advances in clinical dysarthria*, Boston, 1989, College-Hill Press.

152. MorganBarry RA: *EPG treatment of a child with the Worster-Drought syndrome*, Eur J Disord Commun 30:256, 1995.

153. Muenter MD et al: *Treatment of essential tremor with methazolamide*, Mayo Clinic Proc 66:991, 1991.

154. Munhall KG et al: *Visual prosody and speech intelligibility*, Psychol Sci 15:133, 2004.

155. Murdoch BE, Gardiner F, Theodoros DG: *Electropalatographic assessment of articulatory dysfunction in multiple sclerosis: a case study*, J Med Speech-Lang Pathol 8:359, 2000.

156. Murdoch BE et al: *Real-time continuous visual biofeedback in the treatment of speech breathing disorders following childhood traumatic brain injury: report of one case*, Pediatr Rehabil 3:5, 1999.

157. Murry T: *The production of stress in three types of dysarthric speech*. In Berry WR, editor: *Clinical dysarthria*, San Diego, 1983, College-Hill Press.

158. Murry T, Woodson G: *Combined-modality treatment of adductor spasmodic dysphonia with botulinum toxin and voice therapy*, J Voice 9:460, 1995.

159. Nemec RE, Cohen K: *EMG biofeedback in the modification of hypertonia in spastic dysarthria: a case report*, Arch Phys Med Rehabil 65:103, 1984.

160. Netsell R: *Inspiratory checking in therapy for individuals with speech breathing dysfunction*, Presentation at American Speech-Language-Hearing Association Annual Convention San Antonio, Tex, 1992.

161. Netsell R: *Construction and use of a bite-block for use in evaluation and treatment of speech disorders*, J Speech Hear Disord 50:103, 1985.

162. Netsell R, Cleeland CS: *Modification of lip hypertonia in dysarthria using EMG feedback*, J Speech Hear Disord 38:131, 1973.

163. Netsell R, Hixon JT: *A noninvasive method of clinically estimating subglottal air pressure*, J Speech Hear Disord 43:326, 1978.

164. Netsell R, Rosenbek J: Treating the dysarthrias. Speech and language evaluation in neurology: adult disorders, New York, 1985, Grune & Stratton.

165. Netsell RW: Speech rehabilitation for individuals with unintelligible speech and dysarthria: the respiratory and velopharyngeal systems, J Med Speech-Lang Pathol 6:107, 1998.

166. Odéen IN: Reduction of muscular hypertonus by long-term muscle strength, Scand J Rehab Med 13:93, 1981.

167. Palmer S et al: Exercise therapy for Parkinson's disease, Arch Phys Med Rehabil 67:741, 1986.

168. Paniello RC: Laryngeal reinnervation with the hypoglossal nerve: II. Clinical evaluation and early patient experience, Laryngoscope 110:739, 2000.

169. Patel R: Prosodic control in severe dysarthria: preserved ability to mark the questions-statement contrast, J Speech Lang Hear Res 45:858, 2002.

170. Pilon MA, McIntosh KW, Thaut MH: Auditory vs visual speech timing cues as external rate control to enhance verbal intelligibility in mixed spastic-ataxic dysarthric speakers: a pilot study, Brain Inj 12:793, 1998.

171. Putnam AHB, Hixon TJ: Respiratory kinematics in speakers with motor neuron disease. In McNeil M, Rosenbek J, Aronson AE, editors: The dysarthrias, San Diego, 1984, College-Hill Press.

172. Ramig L et al: Changes in vocal loudness following intensive voice treatment (LSVT) in individuals with Parkinson disease: a comparison with untreated patients and normal age-matched controls, Mov Disord 16:79, 2001a.

173. Ramig L et al: Intensive voice treatment (LSVT) for individuals with Parkinson's disease: a two year follow up, J Neurol Neurosurg Psychiatry 71:493, 2001b.

174. Ramig LO: Voice treatment for patients with Parkinson's disease: development of an approach and preliminary efficacy data, J Med Speech-Lang Pathol 2:191, 1994.

175. Ramig LO, Dromey C: Aerodynamic mechanisms underlying treatment-related changes in vocal intensity in patients with Parkinson disease, J Speech Hear Res 39:798, 1996.

176. Ramig LO, Horii Y, Bonitati C: The efficacy of voice therapy for patients with Parkinson's disease, NCVS Status and Progress Report 1:61, 1991.

177. Ramig LO et al: Comparison of two forms of intensive speech treatment for Parkinson disease, J Speech Hear Res 38:1232, 1995.

178. Remacle M et al: Initial long-term results of collagen injection for vocal and laryngeal rehabilitation, Arch Otorhinol 246:403, 1989.

179. Rigrodsky S, Morrison EB: Speech changes in parkinsonism during L-Dopa therapy: preliminary findings, J Geriat Soc 18:142, 1970.

180. Robertson S: The efficacy of oro-facial and articulation exercises in dysarthria following stroke, Int J Lang Commun Disord 36(suppl):292, 2001.

181. Robertson SJ, Thompson F: Speech therapy in Parkinson's disease: a study of the efficacy and long-term effects of intensive treatment, Br J Disord Commun 19:213, 1984.

182. Rosenbek JC, LaPointe LL: The dysarthrias: description, diagnosis, and treatment. In Johns DF, editor: Clinical management of neurogenic communication disorders, Boston, 1985, Little, Brown, & Company.

183. Rosenblum LD, Johnson JA, Saldana HM: Point-light facial displays enhance comprehension of speech in noise, J Speech Hear Res 39:1159, 1996.

184. Rosenfield DB: Pharmacologic approaches to speech motor disorders. In Vogel D, Cannito MP, editors: Treating disordered speech motor control, Austin, Tex, 1991, Pro-Ed.

185. Roth CR, Poburka BJ, Workinger MS: The effect of a palatal lift prosthesis on speech intelligibility in amyotrophic lateral sclerosis: a case study, J Med Speech-Lang Pathol 8:365, 2000.

186. Rubow R, Swift E: A microcomputer-based wearable biofeedback device to improve transfer of treatment in parkinsonian dysarthria, J Speech Hear Disord 50:178, 1985.

187. Rubow RT et al: Reduction of hemifacial spasm and dysarthria following EMG biofeedback, J Speech Hear Disord 49:26, 1984.

188. Sandyk R: Resolution of dysarthria in multiple sclerosis by treatment with weak electromagnetic fields, Int J Neurosci 83:81, 1995.

189. Sapir S et al: Effects of intensive voice treatment (the Lee Silverman Voice Treatment [LSVT]) on ataxic dysarthria: a case study, Am J Speech-Lang Pathol 12:387, 2003.

190. Sapir S et al: Effects of intensive phonatory-respiratory treatment (LSVT) on voice in two individuals with multiple sclerosis, J Med Speech-Lang Pathol 9:141, 2001.

191. Sarno MT: Speech impairment in Parkinson's disease, Arch Phys Med Rehabil 49:269, 1968.

192. Schiffer RB, Herndon RM, Rudick RA: Treatment of pathologic laughing and weeping with amitriptyline, N Engl J Med 312:1480, 1985.

193. Schulz GM, Ludlow CL: Botulinum treatment for orolingual-mandibular dystonia: speech effects. In Moore CA, Yorkston KM, Beukelman DR, editors: Dysarthria and apraxia of speech: perspectives on management, Baltimore, 1991, Paul H Brookes.

194. Schulz GM, Dingwall WO, Ludlow CL: Speech and oral motor learning in individuals with cerebellar atrophy, J Speech Lang Hear Res 42:1157, 1999.

195. Schulz GM, Greer M, Freidman W: Changes in vocal intensity in Parkinson's disease following pallidotomy, J Voice 14:589, 2000.

196. Schulz GM et al: Voice and speech characteristics of persons with Parkinson's disease pre- and post-pallidotomy surgery: preliminary findings, J Speech Lang Hear Res 42:1176, 1999.

197. Scott R et al: Neuropsychological, neurological and functional outcome following pallidotomy for Parkinson's disease: a consecutive series of eight simultaneous bilateral and twelve unilateral procedures, Brain 121:659, 1998.

198. Scott S, Caird FI: Speech therapy for Parkinson's disease, J Neurol Neurosurg Psychiatry 46:140, 1983.

199. Scott S, Caird FI: Speech therapy for patients with Parkinson's disease, BMJ 283:1088, 1981.

200. Shannon KM: Surgical treatment of Parkinson's disease. In Adler CH, Ahlskog JE, editors: Parkinson's disease

and movement disorders: diagnosis and treatment guidelines for the practicing physician, Totowa, NJ, 2000, Humana Press.

201. Shindo ML, Zaretsky LS, Rice DH: Autologous fat injection for unilateral vocal fold paralysis, Ann Otol Rhinol Laryngol 105:602, 1996.

202. Simpson MB, Till JA, Goff AM: Long-term treatment of severe dysarthria: a case study, J Speech Hear Disord 53:433, 1988.

203. Simmons N: Acoustic analysis of ataxic dysarthria: an approach to monitoring treatment. In Berry W, editor: Clinical dysarthria, San Diego, 1983, College-Hill Press.

204. Sinaki M: Physical therapy and rehabilitation techniques for patients with amyotrophic lateral sclerosis. In Cosi V et al, editors: Amyotrophic lateral sclerosis, New York, 1987, Plenum Publishing.

205. Smith ME et al: Intensive voice treatment in Parkinson disease: Laryngostroboscopic findings, J Voice 9:453, 1995.

206. Smitheran J, Hixon T: A clinical method for estimating laryngeal airway resistance during vowel production, J Speech Hear Disord 46:138, 1981.

207. Solomon NP, Charron S: Speech breathing in able-bodied children and children with cerebral palsy: a review of the literature and implications for clinical intervention, Am J Speech-Lang Pathol 7:61, 1998.

208. Solomon NP, Hixon TJ: Speech breathing in Parkinson's disease, J Speech Hear Res 36:294, 1993.

209. Solomon NP et al: Effects of pallidal stimulation on speech in three men with severe Parkinson's disease, Am J Speech-Lang Pathol 9:241, 2000.

210. Spencer, KA, Yorkston KM, Duffy JR: Behavioral management of respiratory/phonatory dysfunction from dysarthria: a flowchart for guidance in clinical decision making, J Med Speech-Lang Pathol 11:xxxix, 2003.

211. Spitzer SM et al: Exploration of familiarization effects in the perception of hypokinetic and ataxic dysarthric speech, J Med Speech-Lang Pathol 8:285, 2000.

212. Stewart C et al: Speech dysfunction in early Parkinson's disease, Mov Disord 10:562, 1995.

213. Stewart DS, Rieger WJ: A device for the management of velopharyngeal incompetence, J Med Speech-Lang Pathol 2:149, 1994.

214. Taha J, Janszen M, Favre J: Thalamic deep brain stimulation for the treatment of head, voice, and bilateral limb tremor, J Neurosurg 91:68, 1999.

215. Theodoros DG et al: The impact of pallidotomy on motor speech function in Parkinson disease, J Med Speech-Lang Pathol 8:315, 2000.

216. Theodoros DG et al: The effects of the Lee Silverman Voice Treatment program on motor speech function in Parkinson disease following thalamotomy and pallidotomy surgery: a case study, J Med Speech-Lang Pathol 7:157, 1999.

217. Thomas-Stonell N, Leeper HA, Young P: Evaluation of a computer-based program for training speech rate with children and adolescents with dysarthria, J Med Speech-Lang Pathol 9:17, 2001.

218. Thompson-Ward EC, Murdoch BE, Stokes PD: Biofeedback rehabilitation of speech breathing for an individual with dysarthria, J Med Speech-Lang Pathol 5:277, 1997.

219. Till JA, Toye AR: Acoustic phonetic effects of two types of verbal feedback in dysarthric speakers, J Speech Hear Disord 53:449, 1988.

220. Tjaden K, Liss JM: The influence of familiarity on judgments of treated speech, Am J Speech-Lang Pathol 4:39, 1995.

221. Todisco T et al: Myasthenic inspiratory vocal cord dysfunction: efficacy of nasal continuous positive airway pressure treatment, Respiration 67:94, 2000.

222. Tolosa E, Marti MJ, Kulisevsky J: Botulinum toxin injection therapy for hemifacial spasm. In Jankovic J, Tolosa E, editors: Advances in neurology, vol 49, facial dyskinesias, New York, 1988, Raven Press.

223. Topka H et al: Motor skill learning in patients with cerebellar degeneration, J Neurol Sci 158:164, 1998.

224. Turner GS, Weismer G: Characteristics of speaking rate in the dysarthria associated with amyotrophic lateral sclerosis, J Speech Hear Res 36:1134, 1993.

225. Turner GS, Tjaden K, Weismer G: The influence of speaking rate on vowel space and speech intelligibility for individuals with amyotrophic lateral sclerosis, J Speech Hear Res 38:1001, 1995.

226. Uitti RJ et al: Unilateral pallidotomy for Parkinson's disease: speech, motor, and neuropsychological outcome measures, Parkinsonism Relat Disord 6:133, 2000.

227. Varney SM et al: Palatal myoclonus: treatment with Clostridium botulinum toxin injection, Otolaryngol Head Neck Surg 114:317, 1996.

228. Vogel D, Miller L: A top-down approach to treatment of dysarthric speech. In Vogel D, Cannito MP, editors: Treating disordered speech motor control: for clinicians, by clinicians, Austin, Tex, 1991, Pro-Ed.

229. Volin RA: A relationship between stimulability and the efficacy of visual biofeedback in the training of a respiratory control task, Am J Speech-Lang Pathol 7:81, 1998.

230. Wang E et al: An instrumental analysis of laryngeal responses to apomorphine stimulation in Parkinson disease, J Med Speech-Lang Pathol 8:175, 2000.

231. Wang N, Lu C: Botulinum Toxin management of adductor spasmodic dysphonia with vocal tremor, J Med Speech-Lang Pathol 12:1, 2004.

232. Ward EC et al: Changes in maximum capacity tongue function following the Lee Silverman voice treatment program, J Med Speech-Lang Pathol 8:331, 2000.

233. Watson PJ, Hixon TJ: Effects of abdominal trussing on breathing and speech in men with cervical spinal cord injury, J Speech Lang Hear Res 44:751, 2001.

234. Whurr R et al: The use of botulinum toxin in the treatment of adductor spasmodic dysphonia, J Neurol Neurosurg Psychiatry 56:526, 1993.

235. Wolfe VI et al: Speech changes in Parkinson's disease during treatment with L-Dopa, J Commun Disord 8:271, 1975.

236. Yorkston KM: Treatment efficacy: dysarthria, J Speech Hear Res 39:S46, 1996.

237. Yorkston KM: Facial anastomosis in a dysarthric speaker. In Helm-Estabrooks N, Aten JL, editors: Diffi-

cult diagnoses in adult communication disorders, Boston, 1989, College-Hill.

238. *Yorkston KM, Beukelman DR: Ataxic dysarthria: treatment sequences based on intelligibility and prosodic considerations, J Speech Hear Disord 46:398, 1981.*

239. *Yorkston KM, Beukelman DR: A comparison of techniques for measuring intelligibility of dysarthric speech, J Commun Disord 11:499, 1978.*

240. *Yorkston KM, Beukelman D, Bell K: Clinical management of dysarthric speakers, San Diego, 1988, College-Hill Press.*

241. *Yorkston KM, Dowden PA, Beukelman DR: Intelligibility measurement as a tool in the clinical management of dysarthric speakers. In Kent RD, editor: Intelligibility in speech disorders, Philadelphia, 1992, John Benjamins Publishing.*

242. *Yorkston KM, Spencer KA, Duffy JR: Behavioral management of respiratory/phonatory dysfunction from dysarthria: a systematic review of the evidence, J Med Speech-Lang Pathol 11:xiii, 2003.*

243. *Yorkston KM, Strand EA, Kennedy MRT: Comprehensibility of dysarthric speech: implications for assessment and treatment planning, Am J Speech-Lang Pathol 5:55, 1996.*

244. *Yorkston KM et al: Evidence-based practice guidelines for dysarthria: management of velopharyngeal function, J Med Speech-Lang Pathol 9:257, 2001.*

245. *Yorkston KM et al: Management of motor speech disorders in children and adults, ed 2, Austin, Tex, 1999, Pro-Ed.*

246. *Yorkston KM et al: The effect of rate control on the intelligibility and naturalness of dysarthric speech, J Speech Hear Disord 55:550, 1990.*

247. *Yorkston KM et al: Assessment of stress patterning. In McNeil MR, Rosenbek JC, Aronson AE, editors: The dysarthrias: physiology, acoustics, perception, management, San Diego, 1984, College-Hill Press.*

248. *Yoshida K et al: Muscle afferent block for the treatment of oromandibular dystonia, Mov Disord 13:699, 1998.*

"There is some limited evidence from well-conducted small-sample and single-subject studies to support the general efficacy of treatment for apraxia of speech. However, additional systematic research is needed . . . that will more directly address questions as to which facilitative techniques are most effective for achieving specific outcomes in specific patients."[40]

M.R. McNeil, P.J. Doyle, and J. Wambaugh

CHAPTER OUTLINE

I. General perspectives
   A. Management territory and goals
   B. Factors influencing management decisions
   C. Focus, duration, and termination of treatment
II. Approaches to management
   A. Medical intervention
   B. Prosthetic management and augmentative and alternative communication
   C. Behavioral management
III. Principles and guidelines for behavioral management
   A. Baseline data and stimulus selection and ordering
   B. Physiologic support
   C. Principles of motor learning
IV. Behavioral management approaches
   A. The eight-step (integral stimulation) continuum for treating apraxia of speech
   B. Sound production treatment
   C. Prompts for restructuring oral muscular phonetic targets
   D. Melodic intonation therapy
   E. Biofeedback
   F. Additional approaches and techniques
   G. Efficacy
V. Summary

Similar to management of the dysarthrias, the management of apraxia of speech (AOS) has received less attention than efforts to describe and understand its nature. This is understandable, especially given the history of debate over the very existence of AOS as a unique speech disorder and ongoing uncertainty about its underlying nature. Despite this, a number of methods for treating AOS have been developed during the past several decades. These approaches have been based on careful observation and study of the unique clinical characteristics of the disorder, the behavioral conditions under which it worsens or improves, and an assumption that it reflects a disturbance of motor speech planning or programming.

This chapter provides an overview of methods used to improve speech and communication in people with AOS. Management issues and decisions, approaches to management, and principles and guidelines for behavioral treatment that are applicable to motor speech disorders (MSDs) in general are reviewed briefly, with emphasis on factors that are especially relevant to AOS. Specific treatment approaches are then discussed.

◼ GENERAL PERSPECTIVES

It first may be helpful to revisit some of the general issues and decisions involved in managing MSDs. This will help establish the degree to which the management of AOS corresponds to or is different from the management of dysarthrias. It is clear that the two types of MSDs share many things relative to management. Most of the important differences lie in specific treatment techniques and their purposes.

Management Territory and Goals

The primary goal of managing AOS is to maximize the effectiveness, efficiency, and naturalness of communication. The reasons for this are identical to those discussed in Chapter 16 for MSDs in general. Similarly, management focuses on restoring or compensating for impaired functions, as well as adjusting to the loss of normal speech or modifying the need for it. The only difference between managing dysarthrias and AOS along these lines is the nature of speaker-oriented activities that attempt to restore lost functions. For dysarthrias, an attempt is made to improve physiologic support for adequately planned and programmed speech. For AOS, treatment focuses on (1) reestablishing plans or programs or (2) improving the ability to select or activate them or set the parameters (e.g., duration, force) for speech movements in a given context[29] that will then be executed by an "intact" neuromuscular apparatus.

Factors Influencing Management Decisions

The general factors that influence management decisions for dysarthria and AOS are identical. The rule that not all people with MSDs are candidates for treatment applies equally to AOS and dysarthrias, and the factors that influence decisions to treat or not are highly similar.

The influence of aphasia on decisions about treatment for AOS deserves special mention. Aphasia is present in a high proportion of those with AOS by virtue of the overlap of lesion sites that are associated with the two disorders. In fact, it has been observed that there have been no treatment studies of AOS in which aphasia (or dysarthria) was not also present.[40]

Aphasia influences treatment in at least three important ways. First, because it affects language functions in all modalities, it can reduce a patient's ability to comprehend spoken and written stimuli during treatment. Second, because aphasia affects verbal expression, it can be difficult to distinguish aphasic from apraxic errors during AOS treatment activities. Third, and most important to decisions about whether or not to treat the AOS, the aphasia may be so severe that verbal communication would not be functional even if motor speech ability was intact. When deciding whether to focus some pro-

portion of treatment efforts on AOS in a patient with aphasia, the clinician must ask, "How well would this person be able to communicate if he or she did not have AOS?" If the answer is that communication would not be functional because of the aphasia (or nonaphasic cognitive-communication deficits), then treatment of AOS should not be undertaken or should be deferred until language (or other cognitive abilities) is sufficient to generate adequate verbal messages. This judgment can be difficult to make and often must rely on careful assessment of verbal and reading comprehension, writing or typing, or other nonverbal means of communication (e.g., pantomime, signing).

The reader is cautioned that the specific approaches to treatment discussed later in this chapter do not, in general, explicitly address the influence of aphasia and nonaphasic cognitive deficits on AOS treatment. To do so would detract from the goal of understanding AOS treatment, but it admittedly highlights the pervasive inability of textbook information to adequately capture clinical reality. The defense, of course, is that all of the variations in people's behaviors and problems cannot be captured concisely in print (at least this writer does not know how to do so). If the "theme" and principles of treatment can be understood, however, they can be adapted to the realities of clinical practice by the experienced, thoughtful, and creative clinician.

Focus, Duration, and Termination of Treatment

Treatment for AOS should focus on tasks that provide the greatest functional benefit most rapidly or that provide the best foundation for improvement over the course of treatment. The general issues surrounding the duration of treatment and its termination that were discussed in Chapter 16 also apply to the management of AOS.

Just as is the case for dysarthrias, management for people with AOS due to degenerative disease is often appropriate. It is generally felt that people with progressive AOS, particularly those without major language or other cognitive impairments, should begin treatment early and be followed regularly to appropriately stage management (e.g., efforts to improve speech, maintain comprehensibility, establish augmentative and alternative communication [AAC]).*[39] The primary goal of such treatment is to enhance communication, not to reverse or prevent

---

*Many proactive strategies for managing primary progressive aphasia that are discussed in detail by Rogers, King, and Alarcon[48] apply to patients with progressive AOS.

decline. There are no convincing efficacy data, but descriptive case studies of patients with progressive AOS and nonfluent aphasia have reported temporary improvement in several speech production tasks and conversation[21] or have demonstrated the staging of treatment from focus on facilitating communication in traditional modalities to the use of AAC technology.[43]

◼ APPROACHES TO MANAGEMENT

The parsing of management approaches into medical, prosthetic, and behavioral categories begins to shape some of the distinctions that exist between dysarthria and AOS management. In contrast to managing dysarthria—for which there are numerous medical, prosthetic, and behavioral treatments— managing AOS is primarily a behavioral enterprise.

Medical Intervention

There are no medical interventions specifically designed to improve AOS for which there is strong evidence of efficacy. Pharmacologic intervention may be used for people with AOS to treat the underlying etiology or prevent further impairment (e.g., antibiotics for infection, anticoagulants to prevent stroke, anticonvulsants to prevent seizures) and may, indirectly, result in speech improvement or prevent deterioration.

A few studies have examined the use of dextroamphetamine or the dopamine agonist, bromocriptine, in the treatment of aphasia, including Broca's aphasia or nonfluent aphasia,[2,4,36,43,76] which are frequently accompanied by AOS. The results have been encouraging enough to warrant continued study (particularly for dextroamphetamine), but the depth of investigations thus far is insufficient to recommend routine use of either drug in aphasia treatment. The degree to which such studies have implications for treating AOS is unknown, but examining the effects of various drugs that may influence speech initiation, planning, and programming appears warranted. Just as Bachman and Albert[3] suggest that "certain features of aphasia may be amenable to pharmacologic manipulation," the same *may* be true for AOS. As yet, however, there are no convincing data that establish this is the case.

Similar to dysarthria, AOS may improve following surgery to manage the underlying neurologic disease (e.g., aneurysm repair, endarterectomy, tumor resection), but such surgeries are not designed to manage AOS per se. No surgical procedures are designed specifically to improve AOS, and surgeries available for managing the dysarthrias (e.g., pharyngeal flap, Teflon/collagen injection, and thyroplasty) are not appropriate for managing AOS.

Prosthetic Management and Augmentative and Alternative Communication

The use of mechanical and prosthetic devices is appropriate for some people with AOS, but generally far less frequently than for dysarthric individuals. Their use is nearly always temporary and primarily intended to stimulate improved speech without the prosthesis.

Prostheses that modify vocal tract events during speech (e.g., a palatal lift) or modify the acoustic signal after it is produced (e.g., a voice amplifier) are rarely appropriate because AOS usually is not characterized by deviations in resonance or loudness that are consistent or pervasive enough to be aided by a relevant prosthesis. There are occasional exceptions, however. For example, Marshall, Gandour, and Windsor[38] described a patient who was unable to phonate or articulate normally because of an apraxia of phonation, but who was able to articulate normally when using an electrolarynx. This suggests that an electrolarynx may be worth a trial for persistently mute apraxic patients[58] who are not responsive to traditional treatment approaches, or for the occasional patient whose apraxia affects phonation to a much greater degree than articulation.

In conjunction with other behavioral management techniques, some apraxic patients can benefit from prostheses that assist rate reduction or the pacing of word production, but not always. For example, Shane and Darley[56] failed to find a beneficial effect of a metronome on articulatory accuracy in apraxic speakers. They speculated that external cues for pacing and setting the rate of speech might be less effective than self-generated ones, such as finger tapping or a pacing board. It is important to note, however, that their investigation examined the immediate effect of the metronome, not its effect over the course of treatment. This distinction may be important because metronome use to pace speech and oromotor control tasks during treatment has been successful in some cases.[18,19,60,79] These contrasting findings demonstrate that *variables that do or do not affect performance on a single nontreatment trial do not necessarily establish that those variables will or will not influence the acquisition, maintenance, or generalization of learning during systematic treatment.*

Delayed auditory feedback (DAF), despite its established benefits for some dysarthric patients, does not seem to be a viable prosthetic aide or form of instrumental feedback for AOS. In fact, it has actually been found to disrupt speech in patients with Broca's aphasia.[10] It may be that although apraxic speakers may benefit from enhanced feedback or instrumental pacing, they cannot tolerate any distortion of feedback, such as that associated with DAF. At this time, no data suggest that DAF is beneficial for patients with AOS.

A pacing board may help apraxic speakers to slow rate and produce words and phrases in a syllable-by-syllable fashion to facilitate articulatory accuracy. However, stress and rhythm may also require attention when a pacing board is used, because board use tends to promote stereotypic prosody.[86]

Various prostheses used as part of AAC systems are as appropriate for patients with AOS as for those with dysarthria. These tools of behavioral intervention (e.g., pictures, letter and word boards, electronic and computerized devices) can be useful for some patients with AOS, although the degree of accompanying aphasia may preclude or place limits on the sophistication of linguistic messages that can be communicated through them. Several studies have documented the success of AAC strategies (e.g., Amerind sign language, Blissymbols, HandiVoice) for people with AOS, occasionally with some carryover of treatment effects to improved verbal communication.[15,30,45,59] In general, as is true for people with dysarthria, some people with AOS accept AAC and have success with it, whereas others reject it or have limited success,[32] especially when a significant degree of aphasia is present.

Behavioral Management

Behavioral intervention is at the heart of managing AOS. It is unlikely that any pharmacologic treatment or prosthetic management that might be appropriate would be beneficial without concomitant behavioral intervention, and behavioral intervention alone is most often used.

Like the management of dysarthria, behavioral approaches can be speaker oriented or communication oriented. Communication-oriented approaches—those efforts at improving communication in the absence of changes in speech—are as applicable to AOS as they are to dysarthria. The strategies, although individually determined and often influenced by accompanying aphasia, are identical to those that may be used for dysarthric patients. The reader should consult Chapters 16 and 17 for an overview of communication-oriented approaches. They are not discussed further in this chapter.

Speaker-oriented approaches—those that seek to improve speech itself—aim for improved intelligibility, efficiency, and naturalness of communication. Their goals are achieved through efforts to improve the planning or programming of speech or to compensate for residual inadequacies in the planning or programming of speech. In most instances, treatment focuses on speech itself. Sometimes it is directed to nonspeech oromotor tasks to improve the ability to plan or program nonspeech oromotor movements as a necessary precursor to similar gains for speech.

Because AOS is predominantly a disorder of articulation and prosody, impairment-level behavioral treatment focuses on articulation and prosody. Focus on resonance is rarely appropriate or necessary, and work on respiration and phonation is rarely undertaken for any but the most severely impaired patients.

There are additional ways to parse speaker-oriented treatment approaches to AOS. For example, they are often classified as to whether they address articulatory movements for speech at the sound or syllable level or the sequencing of sounds in longer utterances.[40] They can also be divided into approaches that focus on articulatory kinematic aspects of speech (e.g., articulation cues, modeling, minimal contrasts); the rate or prosodic features of speech (e.g., pacing tasks, metronome, finger tapping); performance of articulatory gestures with biofeedback (e.g., electropalatography [EPG]); and reorganization of speech using manual gestures.[5] All of these categories are addressed subsequently, even if they are not given subheading status.

Most of the remainder of this chapter focuses on speaker-oriented approaches to AOS management. We begin with a review of principles and guidelines for behavioral management that are especially important to managing AOS. Specific treatment approaches are then addressed.

▮ PRINCIPLES AND GUIDELINES FOR BEHAVIORAL MANAGEMENT

Many of the principles and guidelines for managing MSDs that were discussed in Chapter 16 apply without qualification to the management of AOS. They do not require repeating here. A few points deserve minor qualification or emphasis, and others deserve special recognition.

Management should generally start early, as it should for dysarthria. It should be noted, however, that recommending treatment is not precluded by extended time after onset, especially for patients who have not received any treatment or whose treatment has not focused on their AOS. Several single-case or small-group studies have established treatment benefits in patients with AOS who were in the chronic stage after stroke.[14,19,60,72] For patients with degenerative disease, treatment usually focuses on efforts to maintain speech, develop compensatory strategies for maintaining intelligibility or comprehensibility, and address current or future needs for AAC.

Baseline Data and Stimulus Selection and Ordering

Obtaining general measures of intelligibility and efficiency of communication, establishing the presence and degree of associated deficits, and obtaining an inventory of the patient's communication needs and goals, motivation, speaking environment and communication partners, difficult and easy communication situations, and their perception of others' reaction to their problem are as important to planning AOS treatment as they are for dysarthria. Beyond these things, *it is essential that a careful inventory of the nature of articulatory errors and accurate articulatory responses be acquired,* as well as information on factors that influence the accuracy and adequacy of speech. This is because successful responses during treatment tasks often are highly dependent on the selection and ordering of treatment stimuli.[44,49] Tasks for assessing motor speech programming capacity (see Table 3-6), published tests for the diagnosis of AOS, tasks for assessing nonverbal oral movement control and sequencing (see Table 3-2), and, possibly, the Word Intelligibility Test,[28] can provide a useful database in this regard, although patient idiosyncrasies often require a more individually tailored inventory. In general, it is important to establish the degree to which a patient's errors correspond to the "typical" articulatory and prosodic characteristics of AOS and the variables that influence error frequency. For example, based on averages, the following "typical" patterns may be helpful to ordering stimuli in treatment:

- Automatic/reactive speech is easier than volitional purposive speech.
- Oral/nasal distinctions are easier than voicing distinctions, which are easier than manner distinctions, which are easier than place distinctions.
- Bilabial and lingual/alveolar places of articulation are easier than other places of articulation.
- Consonant singletons are easier than clusters.
- High-frequency words are easier than low-frequency words, and meaningful words are easier than nonsense words. It may also be relevant to consider syllable frequency and the frequency of consonant patterns (the sequencing of consecutive consonants within and across consecutive syllables).[44]
- Single syllable words are easier than multisyllabic words, and words are easier than phrases or sentences.
- Combined visual and auditory stimulation (watch and listen) lead to more accurate responses than auditory or visual stimulation alone.
- Production of stressed words is easier than production of unstressed words.

These examples illustrate but a few of the variables that should be addressed when acquiring baseline information. They are invaluable to the initial selection and ordering of treatment stimuli. However, the identification of variables that establish that some stimuli are more easily produced than others does not necessarily mean that the easiest stimuli should always be the initial target of treatment. That is, although stimulability often determines initial target selection, it should be recognized that *working on less stimulable (more difficult) targets may promote better generalization even if initial acquisition is more difficult.* Thus working on the more difficult component of contrasting stimuli (low-frequency words or nonsense syllables instead of high-frequency, real words), assuming they can be produced at all, may yield greater generalization to untrained stimuli, including easier stimuli.[44]

Physiologic Support

Treatment for AOS does not require efforts to improve posture or increase strength, speed, range, and tone; that is, it does not require efforts to increase physiologic support for speech.[68,86] Nonetheless, is it relevant to ask if nonspeech oromotor movements should be targeted in treatment? Because there does not seem to be any consistent, reliable relationship between speech and nonspeech abilities in people with AOS, using speech stimuli as targets is usually more appropriate than nonspeech stimuli, especially when the patient demonstrates some capacity for speech. However, when AOS is so severe that sounds or sound segments cannot be produced, work on nonspeech postures or movement sequences may be appropriate because treatment should begin at a level at which some success can occur. When used, nonspeech oromotor practice should always involve movement targets or patterns that closely approximate speech gestures (e.g., lip rounding, tongue elevation to the alveolar ridge, deep inhalation or prolonged exhalation). These tasks would be used under the untested assumption that development of such control will pave the way for improved programming of speech movements.

Principles of Motor Learning

Principles of motor learning are highly relevant to AOS treatment, and they are embedded within the treatment principles for virtually all of the specific approaches to treating the disorder. The following paragraphs summarize the principles that seem most relevant to AOS.

Drill

Every specific behavioral treatment approach for AOS emphasizes drill. The need for intensive and systematic drill is consistent with general principles of motor learning and the possibility that, for some patients, their disorder represents more than inefficiency in speech planning or programming. A substantial number of apraxic speakers actually seem to have "lost" some of the "preprogrammed subroutines" for movement sequences that make normal speech so automatic and effortless. Thus Darley, Aronson, and Brown (DAB)[13] observed that apraxic speakers seem to have "forgotten" how to perform speech movements, and Wertz, LaPointe, and Rosenbek[86] indicated that AOS treatment is "the structured *relearning* of skilled speech movements." As articulated by Rosenbek et al.,[52] an essential principle of treatment for AOS is that *systematic intensive and extensive drill is necessary to regain or learn lost speech skills.* Drill becomes systematic when target responses are based on careful selection and ordering of stimuli that ensure success at each step of the treatment program. Drill is intensive and extensive when as many responses as possible occur during each of frequent treatment sessions.

Self-Learning and Instruction

As early as possible in treatment, patients should be urged to monitor their speech, search for correct targets, and self-correct errors.[52,86] Self-learning is possible for many apraxic speakers, especially if their impairment is not severe, and what they learn on their own might not be improved upon by clinician instruction. Clinicians can often help by identifying the productive self-cueing strategies used by patients and then helping them to use them consciously in various situations.[46]

Apraxic speakers, particularly those whose treatment must begin at the sound, syllable, or word level, may need help in knowing how to produce speech movements. Sometimes this takes the form of simple *watch and listen imitation tasks* in which the clinician shows what is to be done. Sometimes, more explicit instruction or explanation is necessary. Techniques of *phonetic placement* and *phonetic derivation* are often essential for teaching sound production, as are instructions and cues for *modifying rate and stress*. In addition, instruction is a necessary component of some of the highly structured treatment programs discussed later. In all instances, *instruction should be faded as soon as learning has occurred.*

Feedback

Knowledge of results is considered a general principle of AOS treatment.[86] Many apraxic patients can judge the accuracy of their responses reliably and accurately, and they should be encouraged at the outset to do so, with efforts at self-correction when they judge responses as inadequate. Clinician-provided feedback is also reinforcing and encouraging. It may be especially important when working on nonspeech tasks, on speech tasks in which targets are noncategorical (such as tasks emphasizing stress or rate), or when intelligibility is the immediate goal.

Instrumental biofeedback and other forms of feedback may also be useful. The use of a mirror may help some patients develop a strong visual image of correct movement or targets,[49,52] although some patients do not benefit or are confused by such feedback. The use of electromyography (EMG) and EPG biofeedback and vibrotactile stimulation for some patients[41,53] is discussed in the section on specific behavioral management approaches.*

It is noteworthy that the *retention and transfer (generalization) of learning are enhanced if feedback is not constant* (provided on approximately 30% to 60% of trials). In addition, studies of limb motor learning suggest that *feedback is more effective if it is provided 3 to 4 seconds after a response and if a 3- to 4-second delay is present between the feedback and the next stimulus.*[29] These delays, although reducing the total number of responses obtainable in a given session, provide uninterrupted time for the speaker to retain the sensory aspects of the movement and self-evaluate and understand adequate versus inadequate responses.[40,55]

Specificity of Training

In general, when a patient has fairly frequent success at the word or phrase level, it is neither necessary nor appropriate to focus on nonspeech, sound-level, or syllable production tasks. Words and phrases are motivating and more meaningful and specific to the ultimate goal of treatment than are their precursors. However, some patients cannot produce words or syllables, and some cannot even produce a few sounds. When AOS is marked or severe and initial attempts to improve speech have failed, focusing on syllable, sound, or even nonspeech tasks may be necessary; in addition, some patients may respond more adequately on syllable-level tasks when syllables are meaningless. Thus learning to plan, program, execute, evaluate, and self-correct nonverbal oral movements, sounds in isolation, and meaningless syllables may be necessary precursors to meaningful speech for some patients.

Some clinicians place emphasis on sound and nonsense syllable mastery, including their rapid

---

*The caveats about the value of feedback discussed in Chapter 16 should be considered in the conduct of treatment for AOS.

repetition, before moving to meaningful speech,[12] and others recommend the inclusion of nonspeech oromotor planning activities as part of a recommended sequence of activities for AOS.[17] It should be noted, however, that some data indicate that nonspeech oromotor and speech alternate motion rate (AMR) tasks do not necessarily generalize to speech tasks.[19]

For mute apraxic patients, vegetative actions such as grunting, coughing, laughing, and singing may need to be reflexively elicited and then shaped toward volitional control as a precursor to voluntary or automatic speech production.[58] *The purpose of nonspeech tasks is not to increase strength or other parameters of physiologic support for speech but to improve the planning or programming of volitional oral movements.*

Consistent and Variable Practice

The use of consistent practice is part of many treatment approaches. For example, clinical researchers often use multiple trials of multiple repetitions of words, phrases, nonsense syllables, or nonspeech oromotor movements in treatment, sometimes without intervening stimuli.[12,19,52,73] These consistent practice efforts usually eventually give way to variable practice in which the patient is required to program more elements into responses, with syllable-to-syllable or response-to-response variability. Thus for example, repetition of a syllable ("see") may merge into phonetic contrast tasks in which variability of responses must be produced, either with minimal (e.g., sue-zoo), intermediate (sue-moo), or greater contrasts (e.g., tomato-tornado).

Consistent and variable practice can also include contrastive stress tasks in which stereotypic stress patterns in sentences of identical length and structure ("*John* likes Mary," "*Mary* likes John") give way to stress tasks with variable stress placement in phrases of varying length and structure ("John *likes* Mary," "Mary likes to *sing* in church").

There is some evidence from a few patients with AOS that variable practice, in which target sounds or syllables are presented randomly, is more effective in facilitating acquisition and retention of learned targets than consistent (blocked) practice.[29] This is compatible with the general principle of motor learning that random practice is more effective than blocked practice in facilitating retention and transfer of motor skills, probably because it forces retrieval and organization of a response on every trial, a challenge that is not present or is minimized in blocked practice. Although blocked practice may be necessary in the early stages of treatment for patients with marked or severe AOS, this principle and these findings suggest that *variable practice*

probably should be used as soon as progress can be demonstrated in response to it.

Speed-Accuracy Tradeoffs

The speed-accuracy tradeoff applies to AOS treatment, with reduced rate nearly always emphasized early in treatment, giving way to attempts to increase speed as accuracy increases.* Rate reduction can take several forms. Markedly impaired patients may need to be silent before responding in order to have their response "in mind," and for all but the most automatic utterances, a slow, deliberate pattern of speech may be necessary to achieve accuracy.[86] This may take the form of a syllable-by-syllable approach to production, or a conscious prolongation of vocalic nuclei.[60]

The value of rate reduction may derive from a different source for apraxic than dysarthric speakers. For example, normal speakers' rate and movement velocity profiles suggest that alterations in rate are associated with changes in motor control strategies.[1] Rapid rate seems to involve "unitary" movements that may be predominantly preprogrammed, whereas slow rates appear composed of multiple submovements that may be influenced by feedback mechanisms. For many apraxic speakers who seem to have lost—or lost access to—preprogrammed subroutines, rate reduction may facilitate feedback and the "relearning" of the submovements necessary for accurate speech.

Once accurate articulation is achieved during treatment, increased rate should be pursued. This can be done within AMR-like tasks at the syllable, word, or phrase level, within contrastive stress tasks at the phrase level, during sentence and paragraph reading tasks, and so on.

Although never formally assessed for efficacy, divided attention tasks may be useful for mildly impaired patients in order to assess and challenge the degree to which speech programming is approaching an automatic stage of learning. For example, how well can a patient maintain normal phrase rate when asked to recall a picture, letter, color, and so on presented before or during their production? Such tasks might also serve as a final criterion step before moving to another level of response difficulty in treatment. For example, when a patient can produce multisyllabic words accurately, he or she might then be required to produce them in the context of a divided attention task, being allowed to move to the phrase level of production only when he or she can

---

*Some apraxic speakers sometimes do better when they speak rapidly, without making conscious efforts to "think" about how they are producing speech.

maintain acceptable accuracy of multisyllabic words during the divided attention task.

◼ BEHAVIORAL MANAGEMENT APPROACHES

A number of specific speaker-oriented approaches for managing AOS have been developed, for which there are single-subject design data, case study, and anecdotal reports of effectiveness. Many of these approaches are more similar than different from one another and are distinguished primarily by the nature of stimuli used to elicit speech. *They all share an emphasis on careful stimulus selection, an orderly progression of treatment tasks, and the use of intensive and systematic drill.*

Imitation is an integral part of most treatment programs,[86] especially during treatment's early stages. There are several reasons for this. First, imitation requires volitional responses to clearly established targets whose parameters can be carefully selected to ensure an appropriate level of challenge and success. Second, stimuli to be imitated provide a "map" for programming the response (e.g., auditory and visual cues) that is facilitory for many patients. Third, it is efficient, because it simplifies drill, facilitates obtaining a maximum number of responses, reduces demand for cognitive and linguistic processing, and bypasses some of the language deficits that affect comprehension and formulation in the many patients who are also aphasic. Most programs also include steps that move beyond imitation to spontaneous speech; they recognize that imitation is less specific to the training goal than normal interactive communication and that achieving neuromotor control for imitation may not carry over to spontaneous speech.[50]

Most speaker-oriented behavioral treatment approaches employ the concepts of *intersystemic* or *intrasystemic reorganization.* Both concepts recognize that behavioral treatment for AOS requires some kind of reorganization of the way in which planning or programming for speech is accomplished.

Intrasystemic reorganization[49,86] refers to attempts to improve performance by emphasizing a more primitive or automatic level of function *or* a higher level of control. Making speech more volitional or conscious (e.g., through imitation) is an example of higher-level control. Eliciting automatic responses such as counting, singing, or automatic social phrases are examples of more primitive intrasystemic activities. *Phonetic placement* and *phonetic derivation* techniques (used easily in imitation tasks) probably combine both higher-level and lower-level functions. For example, using tongue protrusion to help shape production of "th" uses a simple, lower-level movement in a highly volitional way to derive correct placement for a sound. Phonetic placement and derivation techniques are useful for many patients but may be ineffective for those with a significant accompanying nonverbal oral apraxia.

Intersystemic reorganization refers to the use of nonspeech activity to facilitate speech. Its use receives some support from studies of limb movement. For example, the *"magnet effect"* refers to the tendency for the tempo of one movement to influence the tempo of another, with the sustaining of a mutual phase relationship; simultaneous movements (such as of the right and left arm or limb movement and speech) generally can be performed accurately as long as there is a harmonic relationship between them. Neurophysiologically, the programming of a particular activity in the brain may "spread out" in cerebral space and affect other movements that are being programmed. Interference occurs when simultaneous movements are not compatible.[74]

Gestural reorganization[35,49,51,86] is a prime example of an attempt to use nonspeech movements to facilitate speech. It may include strategies such as hand or finger tapping, foot tapping, head movements, or the use of a pacing board to facilitate rate reduction and rhythm and stress patterns. In patients whose gestural control of such activities is better than speech, the dominance of the gesture is intended to help organize the control of speech. The pairing of a gesture with speech has been shown to facilitate sound production acquisition and generalization to untrained exemplars within speech imitation tasks.[47]

In the following subsections, several specific treatment approaches are reviewed. We begin with the "eight-step continuum" of Rosenbek and colleagues because it has been for some time a prototypic model for treating AOS, one that can be applied across many severity levels. It possesses—by design—considerable flexibility. If its "theme" is understood, the clinician will know how to think about the components of treatment, although perhaps not the specific sequencing of treatment steps. Following that discussion, several other approaches or programs are reviewed. The acronyms associated with several of them should not be construed as automatically providing them with greater status or evidence of efficacy than other approaches and techniques that have not been formally titled. They deserve attention either because they have been fairly well described and studied or because they focus on a particular method of stimulation or response requirements. Finally, a number of additional useful techniques for facilitating speech production are reviewed.

The Eight-Step (Integral Stimulation) Continuum for Treating Apraxia of Speech

Rosenbek and colleagues, in their article "A Treatment for Apraxia of Speech in Adults,"[52] described an eight-step task continuum that they had found effective for teaching words, phrases, or sentences to three severely impaired patients. The themes and general principles of treatment they addressed are reflected in many other treatment approaches in use today, and reports of outcomes using their method were among the first to address the effectiveness of AOS treatment.[40] Notable was their emphasis on the importance of *task continua* to ensure high levels of success, the importance *of intensive and extensive drill,* the need to work on *meaningful and useful communication* as soon as possible, and the importance of *self-correction.* They also recognized the importance of selecting and ordering stimuli on the basis of the pattern of observed phonetic breakdowns. Also, fundamental to their program, they stressed the importance of *integral stimulation** (watch, listen, say it with me) in the early steps of treatment, with gradual fading of auditory and visual cues. The overall theme of their program is one in which stimulus prompts are initially maximal and gradually faded, and response requirements are gradually increased. A brief summary of the eight steps follows. Each step may use stimuli at the syllable, word, phrase, or sentence level.

Step 1—*Integral stimulation* in which the clinician presents a target stimulus that the patient then imitates while watching and listening to the clinician's simultaneous production.

Step 2—Same as step 1, but the patient's response is delayed and the clinician mimes the response (without sound) during the patient's response; that is, the simultaneous auditory cue is faded.

Step 3—Integral stimulation followed by imitation without any simultaneous cues from the clinician.

Step 4—Integral stimulation with several successive productions without any intervening stimuli and without simultaneous cues.

Step 5—Written stimuli are presented without auditory or visual cues, followed by patient production while looking at the written stimuli.

Step 6—Written stimuli, with delayed production following removal of the written stimuli.

Step 7—A response is elicited with an appropriate question. For example, instead of imitating "I'd like a cup of coffee," the patient is asked to respond with that phrase to the query, "Would you like anything?"

Step 8—The response is elicited in an appropriate role-playing situation.

The authors point out that not all patients need to go through all steps and that some steps can be bypassed because they are particularly difficult. In addition, phonetic derivation and placement techniques should be employed when integral stimulation fails. Subsequent modifications of stimulus presentation, program steps, and criteria for progressing from one step to another have yielded improvements in speech.[14]

Sound Production Treatment

Sound Production Treatment (SPT) is a relatively recently developed and refined treatment that focuses on improving accuracy of spatial targeting and timing of articulation at the segmental and syllable level. Developed by Wambaugh and colleagues, it deserves recognition for its programmatic experimental documentation of the acquisition, generalization, and maintenance of its treatment effects.[77,81-83] *Efficacy data are more adequate for SPT than any other treatment for AOS.*

SPT relies on strategies common to many AOS treatments, including repetition, integral stimulation, modeling, and phonetic placement cues and feedback to facilitate consonant production. Its most unique characteristic is its frequent (although not exclusive) emphasis on *minimal contrasts.* In fact, SPT is sometimes referred to *as minimal contrast treatment.*[83] The minimal contrast tasks used in SPT involve the production of words or phrases in which target contrasts are minimally different (e.g., shock-sock; conical-comical). It is believed that the use of minimal contrast pairs provides a context for practicing and refining the movement patterns necessary to distinguish among minimally different sounds and that such practice is important when errors are due to a movement programming disorder.[82] The stimuli used in treatment are determined by a given patient's unique error patterns. The targets of treatment are sounds.

An example of the basic steps in the treatment hierarchy can be summarized as follows, based on those described by Wambaugh[77]:

Step 1—Produce a target word or phrase in a minimal pair context (or alone) following a verbal model.

Step 2—Repeat step 1 but with a written cue, such as a written letter representing the target sound.

Step 3—Produce the target word only (i.e., not a phrase) with integral stimulation (up to three attempts allowed).

**Watch and listen strategies are not always best. Some patients respond more adequately when they only listen or only read stimuli than when they watch and listen to the clinician's model or listen and read a target word.[31]

Step 4—Produce the target word only with placement cues and modeling from the clinician.

Step 5—Produce the target sound in isolation with a model from the clinician.

Step 6—Next item.

Verbal feedback is provided after each step. The minimal contrast step is sometimes emphasized strongly across several steps of the program,[83] but it may be eliminated for more complex word or sentence stimuli when contextually appropriate contrasting words cannot be identified. Other variations in the steps of the program have been described, with differences determined by the properties of target stimuli and unique patient characteristics. SPT is thus quite flexible, but its theme of orderly progression, minimal contrasts, integral stimulation, modeling, phonetic placement cues, and feedback are constant.

Further study is clearly necessary to continue documenting efficacy and effectiveness, but SPT can be considered "a partially established" treatment for AOS.[78] Positive results—to varying degrees within and across subjects—have been reported in several single-subject design studies for acquisition of trained sounds, generalization to untrained exemplars of trained sounds, generalization across sounds, and stimulus generalization (i.e., the use of trained targets in untrained contexts, such as in sentences when only words were targeted).[77,81-83] Maintenance of gains following cessation of treatment, although usually not complete and sometimes quite limited, has been reported.[81,82] Declines following cessation of treatment for a given sound have sometimes reflected overgeneralization of the next targeted sound to the previously treated sound.[81] Thus it may be important to focus on multiple sound targets simultaneously to increase variability during treatment (i.e., variable practice versus consistent practice); the positive effects on acquisition and generalization during simultaneous treatment of multiple sounds have been demonstrated.[80] If sequencing of sounds treated instead of concurrent treatment is pursued, it is probably best if the next-targeted sounds do not share features with previously treated sounds.[81]

Prompts for Restructuring Oral Muscular Phonetic Targets

The prompts for restructuring oral muscular phonetic targets (PROMPT) approach to treatment was initially developed by Chumpelik[11] for children with developmental AOS, but it has subsequently been applied to adults.[6,20,66,67] Its distinctive feature is its use of tactile cues to provide touch pressure, kinesthetic, and proprioceptive cues to facilitate speech production. In this sense, the clinician acts as an "external programmer" for speech, providing intersystemic cues for spatial and temporal aspects of speech production.[71] The tactile-kinesthetic input used in PROMPT is typically paired with auditory and visual stimulation.[69]

PROMPT uses highly structured finger placements on the patient's face and neck to signal articulatory target positions as well as cues about other movement characteristics such as manner of articulation, degree of jaw movement, and syllable and segment duration. For example, the thumb placed on the side of the nose may signal a requirement for nasality while, at the same time, another finger signals place of production, such as bilabial contact; the duration of the cues signals sound duration. By chaining together a series of PROMPT cues, movements between phonemes may be facilitated. Square-Storer and Hayden[71] indicate that "extensive training and practice are required in order to competently and efficiently administer this form of treatment." This fact has limited the replication of PROMPT treatment effects by other clinician researchers.[40]

It is likely that patients with chronic, severe AOS whose spontaneous verbal output is limited, and for whom traditional methods of treatment have failed, are the most appropriate patients for this approach.[71] Improvements in speech in response to PROMPT have been reported for a small number of patients.[6,20,66,67,71] Among the few well-controlled single-subject design studies, one has documented good acquisition and maintenance of target words, although without generalization to untrained words,[20] and another has documented improved production of imperative and active declarative sentences with generalization to untrained sentences of the same type.[6] In general, the positive results from these studies reported by different investigators support a cautious conclusion that PROMPT can be considered a "partly established" treatment for AOS.[78]

Melodic Intonation Therapy

Melodic intonation therapy (MIT) is a formal treatment program originally intended for patients with severe nonfluent aphasia.[61,62] It has been used by some clinicians to treat AOS, with proponents of MIT recognizing that such use is appropriate.[63] Its distinctive feature is its reliance on singing and a variant of it in which intoned utterances are based on the melody, rhythm, and patterns of stress in a spoken model provided to the patient. Unlike many other approaches, it does not target sound accuracy explicitly. However, its systematic, structured approach and many of its general principles are similar to approaches that do emphasize articulation at the sound and segment level (e.g., SPT, the eight-step integral stimulation approach).

Repetition forms the core of MIT, although its use is faded during progression through the program. Other principles include the use of various high-probability utterances with semantic value to the patient; working at levels that ensure a high degree of success; the use of verbal and gestural cues (but avoidance of picture or written cues, which are considered distracting); and frequent treatment sessions. Because it uses a departure from the normal speaking mode, it has been recommended that concurrent speech treatments not be used during MIT.[64]

Good candidates for MIT have been described fairly carefully. They include those with good verbal comprehension, preserved self-criticism, a paucity of spontaneous verbal output, and nonfluent speech characteristics, including distorted, pause-filled utterances with attempts at self-correction of articulation errors (some patients may have stereotyped, perseverative utterances). Good candidates have a "typical" Broca's aphasia language profile and often a significant nonverbal oral apraxia. Stated criteria for candidacy suggest that patients will usually (perhaps always) have AOS—as it has been defined in this book—that is more severe than any aphasia that may be present. Some clinicians suggest that MIT may be appropriate for those who fail to respond to more traditional integral stimulation or eight-step approaches.[70]

MIT begins with the gradual teaching of prese-lected (but flexible) hand-tapping rhythms, eventually with simultaneous humming, in unison with the clinician, with gradual fading of the clinician's model. When these basics are acquired, meaningful linguistic material is added. Eventually, clinician cues and patient hand tapping are faded and imitation gives way to the patient answering questions. The singing employed avoids the use of familiar tunes but emphasizes exaggerated pitch, tempo, and rhythm, with tempo lengthened and pitch varied to create a lyrical melodic pattern, as well as rhythm and stress exaggerated for the purpose of emphasis.* When this singing style can be used for the accurate repetition of verbal materials, it is modified to "sprechgesang," or "spoken song," a prosodic pattern lying between singing and speech.† Some

clinicians have successfully modified MIT to meet the special needs of their patients.[16,37]

It has been estimated that approximately 75% of carefully selected patients can benefit from MIT.[65] However, responses to the program have been reported for only approximately 20 patients and the associated studies generally have not been well controlled.[40] Because the best candidates probably have a marked to severe AOS and relatively mild aphasia, it is probable that only a small segment of the aphasic and AOS population can benefit from MIT. It probably should be used only when more traditional approaches have failed, at least partly because methods that focus only on rhythm may be less efficient than other approaches.[86] However, there are no controlled experimental data that document MIT effectiveness relative to other AOS treatments.[8] It is possible that MIT can provide some patients with imitation skills that prepare them to subsequently benefit from other treatment techniques.[75]

Biofeedback

Some forms of instrumental biofeedback have facilitated improvement in a small number of apraxic speakers. *EMG biofeedback* from the frontalis muscle to facilitate muscle relaxation has led to improvement in four apraxic patients.[41] *Vibrotactile stimulation* to the right index finger of an apraxic speaker during a clinician's verbal model has resulted in improved single-word imitative production that was greater than improvement in response to auditory cues alone.[53] The investigators suggested that the vibrotactile stimuli provided an organizational framework for the sequencing of speech movements and represented an example of gestural or intersystemic reorganization.

More recently, *electromagnetic articulography (EMA)* has been used to provide visual feedback about tongue position to treat a lingual sound production error and nonspeech lingual movements in a patient with Broca's aphasia and AOS. Kinematic and auditory perceptual data revealed improvements in response to the visual feedback and no changes in response to a foil treatment for nonspeech and, to a lesser extent, speech tasks,[26] suggesting that visual feedback about tongue position can contribute to the management of nonspeech oral and speech motor behavior. EPG has reportedly provided valuable visual feedback about lingual nonspeech and speech movements during treatment of a patient with chronic, severe AOS. The EPG feedback reduced certain errors and clarified aspects of oral movement dynamics that could not have been obtained by auditory perceptual methods alone.[25]

The evidence regarding instrumental biofeedback for treating AOS is limited. In general, it suggests

---

*A study using a melody-based intervention that emphasized the tonal and rhythmic attributes of target utterances for two subjects with nonfluent aphasia found that exercises that emphasized rhythm led to substantial gains, whereas exercises that emphasized tonal aspects did not.[7] This raises the possibility that the rhythmic aspects of MIT may be more important to inducing change than the program's tonal aspects.

†Sparks[63] and Sparks and Deck[64,65] have provided detailed descriptions of the MIT program.

that biofeedback may have potential as a useful adjunct (not a primary method) for treating some of the articulatory deficits of some patients with AOS. At this time, however, it cannot be considered an established method for treating the disorder.

Additional Approaches and Techniques

The general concepts of intersystemic and intrasystemic reorganization and gestural reorganization, the usefulness of imitation and phonetic placement and derivation techniques, and the themes conveyed by integral stimulation, SPT, PROMPT, and MIT approaches capture the scope and essence of behavioral management for AOS. The following subsections discuss some additional approaches and specific techniques that can also be useful in management. They are not exhaustive but do help to round out the management theme for the disorder.

Techniques for the Speechless Apraxic Patient

When AOS is characterized by muteness or extremely limited or unreliable ability to vocalize—whether or not aphasia is present—there are some techniques that often can get speech going. In general, it is best to begin with techniques that elicit meaningful speech, rather than focusing on nonverbal activities. The following techniques will often elicit vocalization and, sometimes, intelligible words and phrases, even in patients who have been mute.

1. *Automatic speech tasks* such as counting or saying the days of the week may elicit speech when all other volitional attempts to speak fail. When this is effective, patients are sometimes also able to recite portions of overlearned poems, pledges, nursery rhymes, or prayers.
2. Apraxic patients without severe aphasia may be able to complete predictable *carrier phrases* (e.g., "I'd like a cup of _____;" "The American flag is red, white, and _____").
3. *Singing.* Some patients can sing familiar songs ("Happy Birthday," "Jingle Bells"), sometimes only the tune without intelligible words, but sometimes with reasonable approximation of the lyrics, even when they cannot vocalize under other conditions. Sometimes this ability to sing familiar tunes can be used as a primary mode of treatment to facilitate production of communicative words and phrases.[27]
4. When phonation cannot be elicited with automatic speech tasks, but the mouth is opened in an attempt to speak, a quick *push on the abdomen* at the onset of exhalation may

trigger vocal fold closure and phonation and provide a foundation for voluntary phonation. Similarly, if a reflexive yawn or cough can be induced, phonation may emerge with it or be shaped from it. Some patients can produce a vowel when the clinician's hand is placed on the larynx and they are asked to say "ah"; pressure or lowering of the thyroid cartilage sometimes facilitates phonation.

5. As already noted, an *artificial larynx* may facilitate articulation (or phonation) in some mute apraxic patients.[38]
6. *Pairing a highly used symbolic gesture with its associated sound or word* may elicit vocalization or facilitate accuracy of word imitation in severely impaired patients who are otherwise not capable of speech.[47] For example, waving "hi" or "bye" (especially in appropriate context), or encouraging the patient to use the gesture themselves, may elicit the appropriate verbal response. Other social questions can also help trigger automatic responses ("How are you?" leading to "okay" or "fine"). Placing the index finger to the lip to say "sh" may elicit the sound, blowing out a match may be shaped to a phonated vowel, and so on.

Patients who remain mute or unable to produce intelligible syllables may need to work on nonspeech oromotor movements with the same degree of drill and systematic progression that characterize speech tasks. For example, with a bite block in place, activities such as raising and lowering the tongue repetitively to the beat of a metronome have helped to develop oromotor control in an apraxic patient.[19] A number of additional nonspeech oromotor planning exercises for the tongue, lips, jaw, and respiration have also been described.[17]

Techniques at the Volitional Sound, Syllable, and Word Level

For patients whose AOS has them working at the volitional sound, syllable, or single-word level, phonetic placement and derivation techniques and gestural reorganization may be helpful. A number of useful general techniques can be employed at this stage to supplement integral stimulation and other treatment programs.

Some clinicians stress the importance, for some patients, of working at the sound or meaningless syllable level of production. Wertz, LaPointe, and Rosenbek[86] note that some patients do better if meaning is removed from treatment tasks, and DAB[13] recognized the need for some patients to work on isolated sounds, which could then be shaped to syllables and words. For example, humming "m" could give way to the addition of a vowel to form "ma," which then would be repeated multiple times. This might be followed by the addition of various vowels and then consonant-vowel-consonant (CVC) syllables ("mom") and then two-word phrases ("my mom"), and so on. Dabul and Bollier[12] emphasized the importance of sound mastery and then the rapid repetition of nonmeaningful syllables as building blocks for meaningful speech. They presented data for two chronic patients with AOS who benefited from such a program. Dworkin[17] describes a number of vowel and syllable exercises that are useful for drill work at this level.

The *key word technique*[86] is used by many clinicians. The technique takes words that are uttered accurately and automatically and requires the patient to repeat them frequently in order to establish voluntary control. The patient may also be asked to answer questions with the word, read the word, and so on. Then the initial sound of the word, for example, is used to build new utterances. For example, patients who can say "fine" in response to "how are you?" may be asked to repeat "fine" multiple times after the clinician and then attempt words such as "fire," five," and "fight."

Cueing strategies are particularly relevant for sound, syllable, and word level activities, with phonetic derivation and placement being especially useful cues. At the word level, there seems to be a hierarchy of cues that are effective, although they usually need to be individually determined.[46] In addition to biofeedback, cues that facilitate accurate responses at the word level may include word imitation (watch and listen), sentence completion, first sound of the target word, the printed target word, description of function, and presentation of associated words.[13,33,34,46,86] Rau and Golper[46] emphasize the importance of developing cueing hierarchies on an individual basis, use of the most minimal cue that elicits an adequate response, and the value of teaching patients to self-cue rather than rely on clinician-provided cues.

Some response parameters that can be used at the syllable and word level (and beyond) that may facilitate or challenge response adequacy include prolongation of initial consonants, prolongation of vowels and syllables, clinician-imposed or patient-imposed delays before responding, rehearsal before responding, and immediate responding.[9,84] Similar to cueing strategies, the value of these response parameter modifications must be individually determined.

Multiple Input Phoneme Therapy

Multiple input phoneme therapy (MIPT) is a treatment approach that is designed for severely aphasic and apraxic patients whose repetition abilities are severely impaired and whose verbalizations are characterized by repetitive verbal stereotypies.[72,73] Its purpose is to shape from the perseverative verbal stereotypies a variety of utterances that may eventually be used volitionally.

MIPT initially requires reducing the struggle to speak voluntarily with resultant involuntary stereotypic responses (e.g., the patient may say only "two-two-two" with varying inflections). The first step is to identify the most frequently occurring stereotypic utterance, which becomes the initial target of treatment (a key word). The patient then watches the clinician slowly produce the target 8 to 10 times, emphasizing the initial phoneme, with the patient tapping simultaneously with the ipsilesional arm. The patient then joins the clinician in several repetitions of the utterance. Following this, the clinician fades voice but continues to mouth the utterance and tap as the patient repeats the target. These steps are then repeated for other stereotypic utterances. When complete, new single-syllable words are created, using the same initial phoneme of the stereotypy (e.g., "two" may become "tie," "toe," "tune," "tulip," and so on). Targets are then broadened to all phonemes and then clusters, multisyllabic words, phrases, and short sentences. Eventually, repetition is faded, and written cues, picture naming, and assisted phrase productions elicit responses.

Stevens[73] described MIPT such that it conveyed the theme of the approach quite adequately. Data regarding efficacy are limited, and new data have not been reported in the past 15 years. One paper reported five patients whose verbal stereotypies were decreased and whose verbal expressive abilities increased during MIPT.[72] Another report summarized a Veterans Administration pilot project in which five patients receiving 50 sessions of MIPT improved from pretreatment to posttreatment in comparison to five patients who received "traditional procedures" for aphasia and apraxia and who failed to improve from pretreatment to posttreatment. Improvement occurred on standard aphasia tests, including spoken communication tasks.[73]

Voluntary Control of Involuntary Utterances

Voluntary control of involuntary utterances (VCIU) was developed as a method for modifying the speech of aphasic patients with moderately intact comprehension and nonfluent speech who were not responsive to integral stimulation approaches or MIT.[22] Its target population and general theme are similar to that of MIPT, although its specific methods are different. For example, VCIU relies on visual (written)-verbal input in its initial steps, whereas MIPT relies on auditory-verbal input.

The approach begins by identifying any real words that the patient has uttered in any context (e.g., socially, imitatively), even if it was inaccurate or inappropriate for that context. The words are then written on a card for oral reading. If a word is read correctly, it is retained; if it is replaced by another word when read (e.g., the written word "dog" is read as "cat"), the original stimulus is discarded and the "voluntary" response is retained. For patients with a limited repertoire of utterances, the clinician also may present written words he or she thinks the patient may be able to read; Helm-Estabrooks[23] suggests that emotionally laden words (e.g., "love," "die," "damn") are particularly successful. Other likely candidates tend to be short consonant-vowel or CVC, high-frequency words with simple initial consonants (e.g., "no," "bye," "good"). These strategies are used to build a list of written words the patient can read voluntarily. The next step is to have the patient produce the words in a confrontation or responsive naming mode. Thus a picture of a "dog" may be presented with a request that it be named. For a nonpicturable word such as "bad," the patient may be asked, "What is the opposite of good?" Success at this level is followed by conversational activities that elicit target words. New words uttered during any of these steps are added to the list of utterances that receive attention.

One attractive aspect of VCIU is its reliance on the patient's spontaneous utterances to establish the stimuli for treatment, thus facilitating a high level of success, even for severely impaired patients. For this reason, the technique may help to "get speech going" for apraxic patients with severely limited verbal output.

Data supporting the usefulness of the technique are anecdotal, limited, and decades old. Anecdotal reports have discussed three patients who developed more than 250 voluntary utterances, improved performance on a standard aphasia test, and apparently made carryover gains to daily activities,[22] as well as two patients who improved spontaneous speech and functional communication.[23]

Techniques at the Multiple Syllable Utterance Level

Phonetic contrast, rate control, stress, and prosody become important when patients begin to move beyond the single-syllable response level and, as has been discussed, may be important components of integral stimulation programs and MIT. In general, focus on rhythm, stress, and intonation should be concurrent with work on articulation when targets go beyond the single-syllable level.[42]

Practice in the use of *phonetic contrasts* may be important for some patients in order to establish articulatory control across syllables. Such contrasts may be identical to those used in SPT, reflecting minimal differences in voicing ("bye-pie"), place ("key-tea"), and manner ("to-chew"), vowels ("toe-to"), singletons versus clusters ("sing-sting"), and so on.[13,51,68]

Rate modification plays a significant role at the multisyllabic word, phrase, or sentence level. A pacing board, metronome, hand/finger tapping, and other intersystemic gestural rate control strategies may be helpful, as well as slowing rate without cues from other modalities. For example, the simple use of "finger counting," in which a finger is held up for each word uttered, helped improve the adequacy of speech in an aphasic and severely apraxic patient who had plateaued after receiving many different treatment approaches.[57] Improved articulation has been reported in two patients who were instructed to prolong the vowel in each syllable and stretch out words in each phrase.[60] Positive effects of metronome use, sometimes in combination with hand tapping, to pace speech and oromotor control tasks during treatment have been reported.[18,19,60,79] These techniques probably help to provide a temporal basis for organizing sequences of speech movements.[40]

Many clinicians note the *powerful facilitory effects of stress and rhythm on articulation* in AOS treatment.[24,51,68,86] *Contrastive stress tasks,* with or without accompanying gestural cues for stress, such as those described in Chapter 17, are applicable to patients with AOS, both because they slow rate and because they take advantage of the facilitory effects of rhythm on speech. For some patients, these rate and rhythm efforts are so powerful that they allow them to succeed at the multisyllabic word or phrase level even when they have done poorly at the sound, syllable, and word level.* Written stimuli can be useful at the sentence level when the patient moves beyond imitation, with targeted stressed words highlighted in the text. Frequently used phrases such as "Time to go" and "How are you?" may be useful in stabilizing stress, pause, and intonation skills.[24]

For mildly impaired patients, treatment generally abandons imitation tasks and emphasizes spontaneous conversational interaction, with the patient bearing responsibility for self-cueing and monitoring. Tasks may include putting target words into sentences, answering open-ended questions, and generating narratives about picture stimuli, articles, movies, and so on.

---

*Wertz, LaPointe, and Rosenbek[86] provide a detailed description of the construction of contrastive stress tasks that includes imitation, question-and-answer dialogue with stress on a target word, and more complex utterances with different locations for target words or multiple stressed target words.

Efficacy

The preceding discussion of treatment referred to a number of case reports and single-subject experimental design studies that reported the results of various programs and techniques for managing AOS. Almost all AOS treatment studies report positive outcomes and there seems to be a general consensus, based on the available data and expert opinion, that treatment of AOS, especially when aphasia is not present or prominent, is effective. Rosenbek[51] estimated that "about 90% of those patients with an apraxia more severe than their aphasia regained some functional communication" and that the prognosis for recovery of functional communication in such patients is excellent with treatment. This enthusiasm is tempered by Brookshire's[8] opinion that only a small proportion of patients with AOS whose problems remain severe 3 months after onset of stroke will regain functional communication; most such patients have significant aphasic language impairment.

Prospective group studies of treated and untreated patients with AOS have not been reported.[40] However, Wertz,[85] discussing the efficacy of treatment for aphasic patients who also had AOS in a Veterans Administration Cooperative Study on aphasia therapy, noted that 14 of 19 patients with AOS in the study improved and that 4 of 5 who did not improve had received group treatment with no direct manipulation of their AOS. These data represent circumstantial evidence that treatment of aphasic patients with AOS is beneficial, and that AOS responds better to treatment that directly attacks it, rather than to general language stimulation provided within group settings.

A good deal more must be learned about the efficacy and effectiveness of treatment for AOS. It seems particularly important to establish the relative value of the various approaches that have been developed so that treatment may be provided in the most efficient and beneficial ways. For example, if EMG and EPG feedback and vibrotactile stimulation are proven effective for a larger number of patients than thus far demonstrated, do they contribute to management outcome and efficiency beyond that provided by behavioral treatments that do not rely on such feedback? Is MIT more effective than integral stimulation approaches, such as SPT, for some patients with AOS; if so, for which patients? Are nonspeech oromotor exercises necessary precursors to the development of adequate speech in severely impaired patients with AOS, or should treatment be deferred for such patients until potential emerges for benefiting from direct work on speech? Which principles of motor learning are applicable to and have the most powerful influence on the management of AOS? The answers to these questions and many more like them will not be obtained quickly or without difficulty, but they will influence the evolution of approaches to treating the disorder.

SUMMARY

1. Treatment of AOS and treatment of the dysarthrias are similar in many ways but not identical. Differences in treatment between these two categories of MSDs derive mostly from differences in their underlying nature.

2. The cooccurrence of aphasia with AOS often has an important bearing on AOS treatment. Aphasia can affect a patient's comprehension during treatment activities, complicate interpretation of speech errors, and limit gains in functional speaking abilities. For some patients, the severity of an accompanying aphasia may preclude treatment of AOS.

3. There are no surgical or pharmacologic interventions with clearly demonstrated efficacy for managing AOS. Prostheses for modifying the vocal tract or the acoustic signal, such as palatal lifts and vocal amplifiers, are generally not appropriate for people with AOS. Rate control devices, biofeedback, and AAC prostheses are applicable to AOS treatment.

4. Communication-oriented approaches to treatment are appropriate for people with AOS and are generally identical to those used in the management of the dysarthria.

5. Speaker-oriented behavioral approaches to AOS focus primarily on articulation and prosody. A careful inventory of articulatory characteristics and factors that influence the accuracy and adequacy of speech are essential to systematic treatment planning. Occasionally, the initial focus of treatment may be on activities that promote nonspeech oromotor control.

6. Systematic, intensive, and extensive drill is an essential component of all speaker-oriented behavioral approaches to AOS. Principles of motor learning related to self-learning, instruction, feedback, specificity of training, consistent and variable practice, and speed-accuracy tradeoffs are important to the conduct of AOS treatment.

7. Several specific speaker-oriented approaches have been developed for AOS. They share an emphasis on careful stimulus selection, orderly progression of treatment tasks, and the use of intensive and systematic drill. Most also employ intersystemic and intrasystemic reorganization concepts in their techniques. A number of less-structured or less-studied techniques that are not tied to any specific treatment program are

recognized by experienced clinicians as effective for facilitating speech at various points along the AOS severity continuum.

8. Efficacy data and clinical impression suggest that various programs and techniques can be effective in managing AOS, especially when aphasia is not present or prominent. Little is known about the comparative effectiveness and efficiency of the various approaches and techniques, however.

References

1. Adams SG, Weismer G, Kent RD: Speaking rate and speech movement velocity profiles, J Speech Hear Res 36:41, 1993.
2. Albert ML et al: Pharmacotherapy of aphasia, Neurology 38:877, 1988.
3. Bachman DL, Albert ML: The pharmacotherapy of aphasia: historical perspective and directions for future research, Aphasiology 4:407, 1990.
4. Bachman DL, Morgan A: The role of pharmacotherapy in the treatment of aphasia: preliminary results, Aphasiology 2:225, 1988.
5. Ballard KJ: Response generalization in apraxia of speech treatments: taking another look, J Commun Disord 34:3, 2001.
6. Bose A et al: Effects of PROMPT therapy on speech motor function in a person with aphasia, Aphasiology 15:767, 2001.
7. Boucher V et al: Variable efficacy of rhythm and tone in melody-based interventions: implications for the assumption of a right-hemisphere facilitation in non-fluent aphasia, Aphasiology 15:131, 2001.
8. Brookshire RH: An introduction to neurogenic communication disorders, ed 4, St Louis, 1992, Mosby.
9. Bugbee JK, Nichols AC: Rehearsal as a self-correction strategy for patients with apraxia of speech. In Brookshire RH, editor: Clinical aphasiology: conference proceedings, Minneapolis, 1980, BRK Publishers.
10. Chapin C et al: Speech production mechanisms in aphasia: a delayed auditory feedback study, Brain Lang 14:106, 1981.
11. Chumpelik (Hayden) D: The PROMPT system of therapy. In Aram D, editor: Semin Speech Lang 5:139, 1984.
12. Dabul B, Bollier B: Therapeutic approaches to apraxia, J Speech Hear Disord 41:268, 1976.
13. Darley FL, Aronson AE, Brown JR: Motor speech disorders, Philadelphia, 1975, WB Saunders.
14. Deal J, Florance C: Modification of the eight-step continuum for treatment of apraxia of speech in adults, J Speech Hear Disord 43:89, 1978.
15. Dowden PA, Marshall RC, Tompkins CA: Amerind sign as a communicative facilitator for aphasic and apractic patients. In Brookshire RH, editor: Clinical aphasiology: conference proceedings, Minneapolis, 1981, BRK Publishers.
16. Dunham MJ, Newhoff M: Melodic intonation therapy: rewriting the song. In Brookshire RH, editor: Clinical aphasiology: conference proceedings, Minneapolis, 1979, BRK Publishers.
17. Dworkin JP: Motor speech disorders: a treatment guide, St Louis, 1991, Mosby.
18. Dworkin JP, Abkarian GG: Treatment of phonation in a patient with apraxia and dysarthria secondary to severe closed head injury, J Med Speech-Lang Pathol 4:105, 1996.
19. Dworkin JP, Abkarian CG, Johns DF: Apraxia of speech: the effectiveness of a treatment regimen, J Speech Hear Disord 53:280, 1988.
20. Freed DB, Marshall RC, Frazier KE: Long-term effectiveness of PROMPT treatment in a severely apractic-aphasic speaker, Aphasiology 11:365, 1997.
21. Hart RP, Beach WA, Taylor JR: A case of progressive apraxia of speech and nonfluent aphasia, Aphasiology 11:73, 1997.
22. Helm NA, Barresi B: Voluntary control of involuntary utterances: a treatment approach for severe aphasia. In Brookshire R, editor: Clinical aphasiology: conference proceedings, Minneapolis, 1980, BRK Publishers.
23. Helm-Estabrooks N: Treatment of subcortical aphasia. In Perkins W, editor: Language handicaps in adults, New York, 1983, Thieme-Stratton.
24. Horner J: Treatment of Broca's aphasia. In Perkins WH, editor: Language handicaps in adults, New York, 1983, Thieme-Stratton.
25. Howard S, Varley R: Using electropalatography to treat severe acquired apraxia of speech, Eur J Disord Commun 30:246, 1995.
26. Katz WF, Bharawaj SV, Carstens B: Electromagnetic articulography treatment for an adult with Broca's aphasia and apraxia of speech, J Speech Lang Hear Res 42:1355, 1999.
27. Keith RL, Aronson AE: Singing as therapy for apraxia of speech and aphasia: report of a case, Brain Lang 2:483, 1975.
28. Kent RD et al: Toward phonetic intelligibility testing in dysarthria, J Speech Hear Disord 54:482, 1989.
29. Knock TR et al: Influence of order of stimulus presentation on speech motor learning: a principled approach to treatment for apraxia of speech, Aphasiology 14:653, 2000.
30. Lane VW, Samples JM: Facilitating communication skills in adult apraxics: application of Blissymbols in a group setting, J Commun Disord 14:157, 1981.
31. LaPointe LL, Horner L: Repeated trials of words by patients with neurogenic phonological selection-sequencing impairment (apraxia of speech). In Brookshire RH, editor: Clinical aphasiology: conference proceedings, Portland, Ore, 1976, BRK Publishers.
32. Lasker JP, Bedrosian JL: Acceptance of AAC by adults with acquired disorders. In Beukelman DR, Yorkston KM, Reichle J, editors: Augmentative and alternative communication for adults with acquired neurologic communication disorders, Baltimore, 2000, Paul H Brooks.
33. Linebaugh C, Lehner L: Cueing hierarchies and word retrieval: a therapy program. In Brookshire RH, editor: Clinical aphasiology: conference proceedings, Minneapolis, 1977, BRK Publishers.
34. Love R, Webb WG: The efficacy of cueing techniques in Broca's aphasia, J Speech Hear Disord 42:170, 1977.
35. Luria AR: Traumatic aphasia, The Hague, 1970, Mouton.
36. MacLennon DL et al: The effects of bromocriptine on speech and language function in a man with transcortical motor aphasia. In Prescott TE, editor: Clinical aphasiology, vol 20, Austin, Tex, 1991, Pro-Ed.

37. Marshall N, Holtzapple P: Melodic intonation therapy: variations on a theme. In Brookshire RH, editor: Clinical aphasiology: conference proceedings, Minneapolis, 1976, BRK Publishers.

38. Marshall RC, Gandour J, Windsor J: Selective impairment of phonation: a case study, Brain Lang 35:313, 1988.

39. McNeil MR, Duffy JR: Primary progressive aphasia. In Chapey R, editor: Language intervention strategies in aphasia and related disorders, ed 4, Philadelphia, 2001, Lippincott Williams & Wilkins.

40. McNeil MR, Doyle PJ, Wambaugh J: Apraxia of speech: a treatable disorder of motor planning and programming. In Nadeau SE, Gonzalez Rothi LJ, Crosson B, editors: Aphasia and language: theory to practice, New York, 2000, Guilford Press.

41. McNeil MR, Prescott, TE, Lemme ML: An application of electromyographic feedback to aphasia/apraxia treatment. In Brookshire RH, editor: Clinical aphasiology: conference proceedings, Minneapolis, 1976, BRK Publishers.

42. McNeil, MR, Robin DA, Schmidt RA: Apraxia of speech: definition, differentiation, and treatment. In McNeil MR, editor: Clinical management of sensorimotor speech disorders, New York, 1997, Thieme.

43. Murray LL: Longitudinal treatment of primary progressive aphasia: a case study, Aphasiology 12:651, 1998.

44. Odell KH: Considerations in target selection in apraxia of speech treatment, Semin Speech Lang 23:309, 2002.

45. Rabidoux PC, Florence CL, McCauslin LS: The use of the HandiVoice in the treatment of a severely apractic patient. In Brookshire R, editor: Clinical aphasiology: conference proceedings, Minneapolis, 1980, BRK Publishers.

46. Rau MT, Golper LA: Cueing strategies. In Square-Storer P, editor: Acquired apraxia of speech in aphasic adults, Philadelphia, 1989, Taylor & Francis.

47. Raymer AM, Thompson CK: Effects of verbal plus gestural treatment in a patient with aphasia and severe apraxia of speech. In Prescott TE, editor: Clinical aphasiology, 20:285, Austin, Tex, 1991, Pro-Ed.

48. Rogers MA, King JM, Alarcon NB: Proactive management of primary progressive aphasia. In Beukelman DR, Yorkston KM, Reichle J, editors: Augmentative and alternative communication for adults with acquired neurologic communication disorders, Baltimore, 2000, Paul H Brookes.

49. Rosenbek JC: Treating apraxia of speech. In Johns DF, editor: Clinical management of neurogenic communicative disorders, Boston, 1985, Little, Brown & Company.

50. Rosenbek JC: Advances in the evaluation and treatment of speech apraxia. In Rose FC, editor: Advances in neurology, vol 42: progress in aphasiology, New York, 1984, Raven Press.

51. Rosenbek JC: Treatment for apraxia of speech in adults. In Perkins WH, editor: Dysarthria and apraxia, New York, 1983, Thieme-Stratton.

52. Rosenbek JC et al: A treatment for apraxia of speech in adults, J Speech Hear Disord 38:462, 1973.

53. Rubow RT et al: Vibrotactile stimulation for intersystemic reorganization in the treatment of apraxia of speech, Arch Phys Med Rehabil 63:150, 1982.

54. Sabe L, Leiguarda R, Starkstein S: An open-label trial of bromocriptine in nonfluent aphasia, Neurology 42:1637, 1992.

55. Schmidt RA, Bjork RA: Motor control and learning: a behavioral emphasis, ed 3, Champaign Ill, 1992, Human Kinetics.

56. Shane H, Darley FL: The effect of auditory rhythmic stimulation on articulatory accuracy in apraxia of speech, Cortex 14:444, 1978.

57. Simmons NN: Finger counting as an intersystemic reorganizer in apraxia of speech. In Brookshire RH, editor: Clinical aphasiology: conference proceedings, Minneapolis, 1978, BRK Publishers.

58. Simpson MB, Clark AR: Clinical management of apractic mutism. In Square-Storer P: Acquired apraxia of speech in aphasic adults, London, 1989, Taylor & Francis.

59. Skelly M et al: American Indian sign (Amerind) as a facilitation of verbalization for the oral verbal apraxia, J Speech Hear Disord 39:445, 1974.

60. Southwood H: The use of prolonged speech in the treatment of apraxia of speech. In Brookshire R, editor: Clinical aphasiology: conference proceedings, Minneapolis, 1987, BRK Publishers.

61. Sparks R, Holland A: Method: melodic intonation therapy, J Speech Hear Disord 41:287, 1976.

62. Sparks R, Helm N, Albert M: Aphasia rehabilitation resulting from melodic intonation therapy, Cortex 10:303, 1974.

63. Sparks RW: Melodic intonation therapy. In Chapey R, editor: Language intervention strategies in aphasia and related neurogenic communication disorders, Philadelphia, 2001, Lippincott Williams & Wilkins.

64. Sparks RW, Deck JW: Melodic intonation therapy. In Chapey R, editor: Language intervention strategies in adult aphasia, Baltimore, 1994, Williams & Wilkins.

65. Sparks RW, Deck JW: Melodic intonation therapy. In Chapey R, editor: Language intervention strategies in adult aphasia, Baltimore, 1986, Williams & Wilkins.

66. Square P, Chumpelik (Hayden) D, Adams S: Efficacy of the PROMPT system of therapy for the treatment of acquired apraxia of speech. In Brookshire R, editor: Clinical aphasiology: conference proceedings, Minneapolis, 1985, BRK Publishers.

67. Square P et al: Efficacy of the PROMPT system of therapy for the treatment for the apraxia of speech: a follow-up investigation. In Brookshire R, editor: Clinical aphasiology: conference proceedings, Minneapolis, 1986, BRK Publishers.

68. Square PA, Martin RE: The nature and treatment of neuromotor speech disorders in aphasia. In Chapey R, editor: Language intervention strategies in adult aphasia, Baltimore, 1994, Williams & Wilkins.

69. Square PA, Martin RE, Bose A: Nature and treatment of neuromotor speech disorders in aphasia. In Chapey R, editor: Language intervention strategies in aphasia and related neurogenic communication disorders, Philadelphia, 2001, Lippincott Williams & Wilkins.

70. Square-Storer PA: Traditional therapies for apraxia of speech—reviewed and rationalized. In Square-Storer P, editor: Acquired apraxia of speech in aphasic adults, London, 1989, Lawrence Erlbaum.

71. Square-Storer PA, Hayden (Chumpelik) D: PROMPT treatment. In Square-Storer P, editor: Acquired apraxia of

speech in aphasic adults, London, 1989, Lawrence Erlbaum.

72. Stevens E, Glaser L: *Multiple input phoneme therapy in the treatment of severe expressive aphasia. In Brookshire RH, editor: Clinical aphasiology: conference proceedings, Minneapolis, 1983, BRK Publishers.*

73. Stevens ER: *Multiple input phoneme therapy. In Square-Storer P, editor: Acquired apraxia of speech in aphasic adults, Philadelphia, 1989, Taylor & Francis.*

74. Swinnen S, Walter CB, Shapiro DC: *The coordination of limb movements with different kinematic patterns, Brain Cogn 8:326, 1988.*

75. Tonkovich JC, Peach RK: *What to treat: apraxia of speech, aphasia, or both. In Square-Storer P, editor: Acquired apraxia of speech in aphasic adults, London, 1989, Lawrence Erlbaum.*

76. Walker-Batson D et al: *A double-blind, placebo-controlled study of the use of amphetamine in the treatment of aphasia, Stroke 32:2093, 2001.*

77. Wambaugh JL: *Stimulus generalization effects of sound production treatment for apraxia of speech, J Med Speech-Lang Pathol 12:77, 2004.*

78. Wambaugh JL: *A summary of treatments for apraxia of speech and review of replicated approaches, Semin Speech Lang 23:293, 2002.*

79. Wambaugh JL, Martinez AL: *Effects of rate and rhythm control treatment on consonant production accuracy in apraxia of speech, Aphasiology 14:851, 2000.*

80. Wambaugh JL, West JE, Doyle PJ: *Treatment for apraxia of speech: effects of targeting sound groups, Aphasiology 12:731, 1998.*

81. Wambaugh JL et al: *Sound production treatment for apraxia of speech: overgeneralization and maintenance effects, Aphasiology 13:821, 1999.*

82. Wambaugh JL et al: *Effects of treatment for sound errors in apraxia of speech and aphasia, J Speech Lang Hear Res 41:725, 1998.*

83. Wambaugh JL et al: *A minimal contrast treatment for apraxia of speech, Clin Aphasiol 24:97, 1996.*

84. Warren RL: *Rehearsal for naming in apraxia of speech. In Brookshire RH, editor: Clinical aphasiology: conference proceedings, Minneapolis, 1977, BRK Publishers.*

85. Wertz RT: *Response to treatment in patients with apraxia of speech. In Rosenbek J, McNeil M, Aronson A, editors: Apraxia of speech: physiology, acoustics, linguistics, management, San Diego, 1984, College-Hill Press.*

86. Wertz RT, LaPointe LL, Rosenbek JC: *Apraxia of speech in adults: the disorder and its management, New York, 1984, Grune & Stratton.*

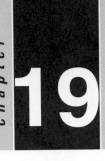
19 Management of Other Neurogenic Speech Disturbances

"SAAND (stuttering associated with acquired neurological disorders) is not a unitary disorder, nor is it typically unidimensional. It is, therefore, difficult to predict how well a specific patient will respond to therapeutic intervention."[23]

N. Helm-Estabrooks

"There currently are no data available on . . . when and for whom the methods might be most facilitatory."[29]

(Meyers discussing treatment of aprosodia associated with right hemisphere lesions)

CHAPTER OUTLINE

   I. Neurogenic stuttering
    A. Medical management
    B. Behavioral management
  II. Palilalia
 III. Echolalia
 IV. Cognitive and affective disturbances
  V. Aphasia
 VI. Pseudoforeign accent
 VII. Aprosodia
VIII. Summary

Neurogenic speech disturbances that are not traditionally categorized under the headings of dysarthria or apraxia of speech (AOS) may or may not be legitimate targets for management. When they are a reflection of, or are embedded within, a larger constellation of affective, cognitive, or linguistic deficits, their direct treatment may be inappropriate or unnecessary. When they are the only or primary impairment or when they represent a major source of disability or activity limitation, their direct treatment may be appropriate and necessary.

Management of the "other neurogenic speech disturbances" that were discussed in Chapter 13 is the subject of this chapter. The emphasis is on speech production deficits and not the affective, cognitive, or linguistic disturbances that may underlie the

speech characteristics of a number of these problems. To do otherwise would go considerably beyond the scope of this book. Thus for example, the management of word retrieval and phonologic errors in people with aphasia is not addressed, because such difficulties reflect language disturbances and not speech deficits per se.

Little is known about the behavioral management of these speech problems. Our lack of knowledge extends beyond a paucity of efficacy data and includes a relative lack of even anecdotal suggestions or expert opinion about best treatments in some instances. For some of these problems, this probably partly reflects low incidence and limited understanding of their nature. For others, it reflects the fact that treatments are usually directed at cognitive deficits underlying the surface speech abnormalities rather than the speech abnormalities themselves.

▣ NEUROGENIC STUTTERING

As noted in Chapter 13, neurogenic stuttering (NS) is a heterogeneous disorder that may exist as a separate entity or be embedded within a constellation of abnormalities that represent dysarthria, AOS, or aphasia. When the dysfluencies are manifestations of a dysarthria or AOS, and when their prominence is not disproportionate to other manifestations of those motor speech disorders (MSDs), management will probably be consistent with the principles and techniques generally used to treat the dysarthria or AOS.

These have already been discussed in Chapters 16 to 18 and are not repeated here. When dysfluencies are prominent, predominant, or disabling, they may require attention and may benefit from some of the strategies that seem to be effective in managing NS.

NS can be mild, transient, and resolve spontaneously following stroke in many patients.[24,33,36,38] This implies that supportive reassurance that fluency will improve spontaneously may be the most appropriate management strategy early after onset and that such reassurance may reduce anxiety that could inhibit improvement. The problem, of course, is uncertainty about the prognosis in specific cases. It seems reasonable to introduce direct treatment if the problem persists for more than a few days to a week after onset, especially if NS is the only or the most disabling communication problem.

Strategies for managing NS center on medical intervention and behavioral treatment. Behavioral treatment includes rate-reduction strategies, self-monitoring, and other techniques, several of which are used in the treatment of developmental stuttering.

Medical Management

As noted in Chapter 13, the onset of NS has been associated with the use of many pharmacologic agents, particularly those used to treat depression, anxiety, schizophrenia, seizures, Parkinson's disease (PD), and asthma. These agents include tricyclic antidepressants (e.g., sertraline, fluoxetine, tranylcypromine), antipsychotic agents (e.g., clozapine, risperidone), benzodiazepine derivatives (e.g., Tranxene, Librium), phenothiazines, anticonvulsants (e.g., Dilantin), levodopa, and theophylline. Fortunately, among many case reports of drug-induced stuttering, it appears that *dysfluencies nearly always remit or significantly improve after the offending drug is discontinued.*[10a] For example, one case report noted a reduction in stuttering in a woman with a seizure disorder following a traumatic brain injury (TBI) when Dilantin and phenobarbital were instituted; the seizures and stuttering returned but diminished again when the regimen was changed to Dilantin and Tegretol.[7] In another case, stuttering began after Dilantin was introduced to control post-traumatic seizures. Dysfluencies decreased after discontinuing Dilantin and substituting Tegretol.[28]

When dysfluencies are drug induced, they usually emerge within a few weeks of starting the drug and remit within several days after discontinuation. Preexisting brain pathology (e.g., seizures) may be a predisposing factor in affected individuals.[6,17,46] It has been suggested that the onset of stuttering in patients taking clozapine should prompt investigation for a seizure disorder.[46]

In some cases, a drug may effectively treat NS. For example, Paroxetine, a serotonin selective reuptake inhibitor antidepressant, has reportedly resulted in resolution of NS in three individuals with brain injuries.[43]

Dysfluencies that occur in people with PD (and hypokinetic dysarthria) may vary as a function of dopaminergic drug levels. One study noted an increase in dysfluencies during the levodopa "on" state in comparison to the "off" state in a man with PD plus a history of developmental stuttering.[3] Another study, however, failed to find differences in the percentage of dysfluencies in a group of nine patients whose speech was assessed before taking medication (when dopamine levels were presumably low) and after taking medication (when dopamine levels were presumably high).[20]

These limited observations suggest that drugs may play a role in causing or in reducing symptoms of NS. It seems reasonable to address their possible causal role in those who take them and then develop NS and to address the possibility of modifying drug regimens to control or reduce dysfluencies. Such issues should be addressed and any changes in drug regimen stabilized before introducing behavioral treatment in most cases.

Technologic medical advances may have implications for the nonpharmacologic treatment of NS. For example, acquired dysfluencies have remitted during therapeutic electrical stimulation to the thalamus to relieve pain and dyskinesias.[5,9] A dramatic reduction in stuttering has been reported in a man with parkinsonism following regular treatments with transcranial alternating current–pulsed electromagnetic fields (EMFs); the speech disorder returned when regular EMF treatments were temporarily discontinued.[41] The patient's speech had also improved to some degree after sertraline was added to his dopaminergic medications, prompting a belief that speech improved in response to the EMFs because they facilitated serotonergic transmission, perhaps in part through an interaction with the sertraline.

Behavioral management for NS should probably be deferred if neurosurgery is pending. For example, a case report has documented stuttering and right-sided motor and sensory problems that developed in association with vascular problems and then remitted following a left carotid endarterectomy.[15] It is possible that surgery had palliative effects on the stuttering by improving cerebral blood flow and perhaps restoring equilibrium to the motor system.[36]

Behavioral Management

Some clinical experts suggest that treatment of NS tends to be successful,[12] but others are not so optimistic.[36] A survey of clinicians who had encountered acquired stuttering that was not considered part of aphasia or an MSD found that treatment outcome was rated favorably for 82% of treated cases.[26] However, such anecdotal reports are weak evidence of treatment effectiveness, because they are uncontrolled for the effects of spontaneous recovery and other influences on outcome.

In general, behavioral treatment strategies focus on rate reduction, self-monitoring, and other techniques that are frequently associated with the management of developmental stuttering.

Rate-Reduction Strategies

Techniques designed to decrease rate to reduce dysfluencies are commonly used by clinicians[26] and have been used in nearly all reports of successful management of NS. The rate-reduction techniques seem no different than those already described for managing MSDs. For example, a program of syllable-timed speech that slowed rate to 50 words per minute was associated with fluent speech after six treatment sessions in a patient with NS following a right hemisphere stroke[38]; however, there could be no certainty that the improvement was attributable to the treatment because spontaneous recovery alone could have led to the same outcome.

Some and perhaps many people with NS have difficulty maintaining slow rate without assistance, but may benefit from self-pacing strategies such as a pacing board or finger counting or tapping.*[24] Delayed auditory feedback (DAF) may also be effective,[16,27] especially when dysfluencies are associated with the accelerated or rapid rate of hypokinetic dysarthria, but it may be counterproductive or disruptive for patients with AOS or aphasia. It is possible that many of the other rate-reduction strategies discussed in Chapter 17 are applicable to the behavioral management of NS.

Self-Monitoring

Whitney and Goldstein[47] reported a dramatic decrease in dysfluencies in three patients with mild aphasia who were trained to self-monitor their dysfluencies. Dysfluencies included audible pauses ("uh," "well"); word or phrase break-offs or revisions ("Water is bein' thrown/comin' off"); and part-word ("Di-dishes"), word, or phrase repetitions. Their approach may be applicable to patients whose

NS or dysfluencies are strongly tied to aphasic verbal language deficits, and it is possible that they can be applied to other types of NS as well. The training they used can be summarized as follows: (1) a baseline transcription of the patients' dysfluencies was read to them while the clinician identified each dysfluency (target behavior); (2) the patient listened and identified each target behavior, with feedback from the clinician about accuracy; (3) the patient self-monitored dysfluencies (by pressing a counter) during picture description tasks, with similar feedback from the clinician; and (4) independent self-monitoring without clinician feedback. Using a multiple-baseline, single-subject experimental design, the authors documented dramatic decreases in dysfluencies, with generalization to nontreatment tasks. Of interest, the actual accuracy of self-monitoring was low during treatment, so accurate monitoring did not seem crucial to the program's success. Although rate was slowed by the technique, communication was more efficient and was rated positively by patients and unfamiliar listeners because utterances were not interrupted by dysfluencies. It was concluded that self-monitoring seemed to provide a "delay strategy," presumably for word retrieval efforts, even though delay was not actively taught. The authors also noted that one patient had AOS that may have explained some of his dysfluencies and that the delay strategy may have aided speech programming. The simplicity, efficiency, and effectiveness of this approach make it a viable way to manage the dysfluencies of mildly aphasic people, and perhaps apraxic patients, and it probably justifies examining its effectiveness for other types of NS as well.

Other Approaches

An anecdotal report has indicated that biofeedback and relaxation treatment were successful for a patient with moderately severe NS associated with multiple strokes.[24] Electrodes were placed over the masseter muscle, with subsequent visual and auditory feedback to reduce masseter muscle tension. A 4-month, twice-weekly program of biofeedback, speech therapy, and home practice reduced the dysfluencies to a "mild" degree by the time of discharge.

"Traditional" approaches for managing developmental stuttering have been applied to NS, with anecdotal reports of success.[26] For example, miming, singing, and reading may be used therapeutically to facilitate fluency in some patients.[18] Therapy focused on easy-onset phonation and desensitization to decrease anxiety was successful in reducing dysfluencies in a 7-year-old whose dysfluencies emerged during recovery from aphasia secondary to a left hemisphere stroke.[29] An intensive 1-week treatment

---

*Helm and Butler[22] reported a case whose severe NS as a result of multiple strokes did not respond to a pacing board approach but did improve when transcutaneous nerve stimulation was applied to the left hand during speech.

program for 8 hours per day that included several traditional techniques helped a patient whose stuttering was associated with a TBI.*[40]

PALILALIA

The word and phrase repetitions that characterize palilalia may not be a prominent component of the constellation of problems that affect communication in some people with the disorder. For example, occasional word and phrase repetitions may be produced by patients with hypokinetic dysarthria, but their reduced loudness, accelerated rate, and imprecise articulation may be much more pervasive, obvious, disabling, and disruptive to intelligibility. In such cases the dysarthria should be treated first, with a good possibility that palilalia will be decreased by the approaches used to manage other aspects of the dysarthria. When palilalia occurs in people with significant cognitive impairments, deficits in attention, motivation, and memory make it unlikely that efforts to reduce the palilalia will be successful.

When prominent, pervasive, or disabling, and when the patient's cognitive abilities are sufficiently intact to allow him or her to cooperate and learn, attempts to reduce the reiterative utterances are necessary and justified. Unfortunately, little is known about how to treat palilalia or the effectiveness of such treatment. In general, it is probably most appropriate to rely on principles and techniques that are appropriate for managing hypokinetic dysarthria and NS, as well as careful analysis of conditions that increase or decrease the palilalia. With this in mind, the following principles and techniques may be useful:

1. Some medications can exacerbate or reduce palilalia. In patients on medication for PD, determining if palilalia fluctuates over the drug cycle is important. Institution of drug treatment may decrease palilalia and eliminate the need for behavioral management. If palilalia occurs during peak dose levels of antiparkinsonism medication and associated hyperkinesias, modification in dosage may reduce it.[1] Other drugs may help reduce palilalia in some cases. One case report noted a reduction after administration of chlorpromazine (Thorazine) in a patient with chorea and evidence of bilateral basal ganglia, cortical, and cerebellar lesions, with worsening when the medication was withheld.[10] Another report noted improvement in response to trazodone in a patient with vascular dementia.[44]
2. Because palilalia and hypokinetic dysarthria frequently occur simultaneously, approaches

to managing hypokinetic dysarthria may reduce palilalia without attention to the palilalia per se or may be effective in direct efforts to decrease palilalia. Rate-reduction techniques seem particularly applicable.[25] Helm's[21] initial description of a pacing board for a patient with parkinsonism was designed primarily to modify palilalia. Helm's report represents the only reported behavioral treatment for palilalia. Her patient had not been responsive to verbal instruction, hand tapping, or a metronome to reduce rate, but his use of the board resulted in a syllable-by-syllable pattern "with no palilalia," which he was able to use—with reminders—during conversation. The use of DAF, hand or finger tapping, rhythmic cueing, and alphabet board supplementation, because they slow rate and have some reported success for people with hypokinetic dysarthria, are other possible treatment techniques. Self-monitoring treatment, similar to that described by Whitney and Goldstein[47] for dysfluencies associated with aphasia (previous section), may also be worthy of investigation.

3. Careful analysis of the speaking modes in which palilalia is most and least frequent may assist the ordering of treatment tasks. For example, reading and repetition tend to be associated with fewer reiterations than conversation, narratives, and elicited speech, suggesting that treatment efforts for patients with such profiles might profitably begin with repetition or reading and then progress to elicited or narrative speech tasks.

ECHOLALIA

The unsolicited repetition or partial repetition of others' utterances that characterize echolalia is typically normal motorically and associated with diffuse or multifocal cortical pathology and severe aphasia or generalized impairments of cognition. The associated language and other cognitive deficits represent the true barriers to the formulation and expression of speech. In a sense, echolalia in such patients represents a residual, relatively intact ability, even though its expression in most circumstances is inappropriate. When behavioral management is appropriate for such patients and echolalia is pervasive, it may be necessary to inhibit or reduce the echolalia before the underlying language and other cognitive deficits can be addressed. However, methods for doing so have not been described, and the outcome of behavioral treatment for the communication impairments of patients with pervasive echolalia has not been reported.

---

*The description of this case raises the possibility that the stuttering was psychogenic.

◼ COGNITIVE AND AFFECTIVE DISTURBANCES

The management of attenuations of speech that derive from cognitive and affective disturbances are not addressed in detail here because the fundamental problem in such disturbances is not one of speech per se. Behavioral management of the underlying cognitive and affective deficits usually does not focus on the motor aspects of speech production. Improvement in the underlying cognitive and affective impairments is usually reflected in increased speed of verbal responding and increased loudness and more normal voice quality and prosody.

Because of the hypothesized role of impaired dopaminergic transmission in some people with akinetic mutism, dopaminergic pharmacologic treatment, in combination with appropriate stimulation, may be of benefit in some cases.[19,30] For example, administration of bromocriptine or a combination of carbidopa/levodopa and pergolide has reportedly improved signs of akinetic mutism in a small number of cases.[2,39]

In Chapter 13 the similarity between the hypophonia and reduced loudness associated with frontal lobe–limbic system pathology and the hypokinetic dysarthria due to basal ganglia pathology was discussed. This association raises the possibility that some of the vocal "exercise" programs described in Chapter 17 for managing hypokinetic dysarthria might benefit patients with hypophonia associated with abulia, perhaps as part of treatment efforts to increase their general levels of effort and drive. Although speculative, attempts to modify vocal production may also be justified on the basis of Sapir and Aronson's[42] report of two patients with posttraumatic aphonia (with no vocal fold pathology or MSD) who regained normal phonation (but not normal prosody) after a session of symptomatic therapy using techniques applied to people with conversion aphonia. Sapir and Aronson suggested that the persisting aphonia might have been due to an emotional response to trauma or to "inertial aphonia" that persisted beyond the effects of the initial organic cause of the aphonia (e.g., vocal fold weakness or paralysis, effects of intubation, apraxia of phonation). At the least, their observations suggest that a trial of behavioral efforts to improve loudness and phonation may be justified in patients with frontal lobe pathology and hypophonia or aphonia, particularly when onset is acute and the degree of speech attenuation is disproportionate to other cognitive or affective deficits.

◼ APHASIA

Aphasia can have prominent effects on spoken language. Grammatical and syntactic errors, delays, hesitancy, dysfluencies, word retrieval errors, a lack of substantive words, and phonologic errors are but a few of its manifestations in verbal expression. These difficulties affect the form, content, rate, prosody, and fluency of speech, but they result from underlying language deficits and not abnormalities in motor speech planning, programming, or execution. Their management is directed at the inefficiencies in language and not the physical production of speech.

When significant AOS accompanies aphasia, management of the AOS may complicate the management of aphasia (and vice versa), take precedence over it, be conducted concurrently with it, or be deferred because of it. *It is essential to recognize that the management of aphasia and AOS (and dysarthria) are quite different from each other and that treatment of one disorder cannot be expected to remediate deficits in the other.*

The literature on the management of aphasia is extensive, considerably larger than that for MSDs. Discussion of aphasia management is beyond the scope of this book, although management of dysfluencies associated with it was discussed in the section on NS. It is noteworthy that aphasia and efforts to treat and manage it can have a substantial influence on the management of patients with MSDs.*

◼ PSEUDOFOREIGN ACCENT

The rare and unusual disorder of pseudoforeign accent associated with neurologic disease has been described in a limited number of case reports. No published report has discussed its behavioral management. The disorder may resolve fairly rapidly in some patients[8] and, therefore, may not require behavioral management. However, too little is known about the problem to predict who will and will not recover from it. It is also apparent that some affected people find the problem to be socially handicapping even when it does not affect speech intelligibility.

The frequent association of pseudoforeign accent with aphasia and AOS, the possibility that the perception of accent is conveyed by grammatical and syntactic deficits attributable to aphasia, and articulatory and prosodic errors associated with a variant of AOS suggest that the "accent" may be managed at least partially during traditional treatment activities for aphasia and AOS. It may be quite appropriate to adapt principles and techniques for managing AOS (see Chapter 18) to efforts to modify the voice, place and manner distortions, substitutions, and allophonic variations in consonant production that

---

*Some texts that address the manifestations and management of aphasia include: Brookshire[11]; Chapey[13]; Davis[14]; and Rosenbek, LaPointe, and Wertz.[37]

contribute to the perception of accent. Similarly, and perhaps more importantly, a greater than average amount of attention may need to focus on vowel "errors" that convey accent, extending in some cases to vowel articulation drill activities.

The crucial role of prosody in conveying accent suggests that treatment of pseudoforeign accent may require special attention to the techniques for improving prosody, stress, rhythm, and naturalness that were discussed for the management of dysarthria and AOS in Chapters 17 and 18, respectively. When such techniques are exhausted—or in conjunction with them—materials that are used for reducing foreign accent in neurologically normal, nonnative English speakers may be useful.

◼ APROSODIA

As discussed in Chapter 13, the aprosodia associated with right hemisphere damage (RHD) is not well understood, and its relationship to other perceptual and cognitive disturbances that may affect communication in people with right hemisphere lesions has not been clearly established. This lack of understanding, as well as uncertainty about the prevalence of significant, lasting, and unique prosodic deficits in people with RHD, suggests that information about management of aprosodia is limited. Indeed, this is the case.

Myers,[32] recognizing the existence of problems producing emotional prosody and linguistic stress in RHD patients, nonetheless stated that prosodic deficits are not generally considered a high treatment priority because they often are not the most prominent deficits affecting communication. She has also noted that little is known about when and for whom behavioral interventions for aprosodia are most beneficial.[31]

When someone with RHD has significant deficits in prosodic production that are isolated or disproportionately severe in comparison to other communication deficits, when those deficits persist beyond the acute phase of the causative illness, and when the individual or significant others are aware of and concerned about the problem, direct treatment should be considered. At the least, patients and their significant others may benefit from counseling about the nature of the problem as a consequence of RHD.[31] For example, knowing that the lack of emotion conveyed by prosody does not reflect an absence of true emotional feeling and that "tone of voice" cannot be relied upon to convey emotions may minimize misinterpretations about affective state and may prompt the patient and others to rely more heavily on linguistic content rather than intonation as an index of feelings. In this context, it may be useful to focus on

verbal language strategies that explicitly identify emotional states (e.g., stating aprosodically, "My arm is not getting any better" may sound like a simple statement of fact when, in fact, the intent was to convey that "I'm upset and feeling down that my arm is not getting any better"). Similarly, family members may learn to ask, "How do you feel about that?" or "Does that make you happy/sad?" when a statement or topic is likely to be associated with strong emotions. This may be particularly helpful when aprosodic speakers are not aware that their emotional state is not adequately conveyed by their prosodic patterns.

Several studies have reported the results of explicit impairment-focused treatments for aprosodia. A single case report has documented improvement in prosodic expression for a woman with aprosodia secondary to TBI.[45] Twenty-four sessions of treatment, conducted over a 2-month period, consisted of tasks requiring imitation of a target pitch with accompanying visual feedback from a Visi-Pitch device and modeling an affective tone of voice or facial expression, with instruction about how to improve imitation. Prosodic imitation and production both improved. Anderson and colleagues[4] reported the case of a man with aprosodia associated with right hemisphere stroke who received treatment using three strategies: prosody repetition, a cognitive-linguistic self-cuing strategy, and a facial expression cross-cuing strategy. The most powerful treatment was the prosody repetition treatment.

The most convincing study, because of its use of a single-subject ABAB design, is that of Rosenbek and colleagues,[38a] who used two treatments for three people with expressive aprosodia from right hemisphere stroke. One treatment was imitative, and the other was cognitive-linguistic (both are well described in the report, which should be consulted for details). The imitative treatment involved a hierarchy of six steps, starting with (1) the clinician modeling a sentence using a target emotional tone of voice, followed by unison clinician-patient production, and ending with (6) the clinician asking a question requiring a patient response using a target emotional tone as the patient imagines that he or she is speaking to a family member. The cognitive-linguistic treatment also involved a six-step hierarchy, starting with (1) providing the patient with a written description of the characteristics of a specific emotional tone of voice (e.g., "loud," "harsh," "fast rate") that the patient reads aloud and then restates in his or her own words to ensure comprehension, proceeding to (2) matching written and then pictured facial emotions (e.g., happy, sad) to the descriptions of emotional tone of voice. Eventually the patient reaches (6) production of sentences containing a targeted emotional tone without the written descriptions of emotional tone of voice, the written emotion, or the pictured emotional cue. Data analysis indicated that both treatments resulted in modest to substantial improvement for all three patients, although there was no generalization to an untreated emotion. The results of this study are encouraging and justify further study of both treatments.

Many of the techniques emphasizing prosody that are used for treating dysarthrias and AOS—discussed in Chapters 17 and 18—may be useful. For example, some clinicians emphasize the use of contrastive stress tasks using emotional (e.g., happy vs. sad) or linguistic stress as the basis for contrasts, recognizing that linguistic stress might be emphasized initially because of the probability that it is less impaired than emotional prosody.[35] Imitation of a clinician's model (similar to those employed in the treatment studies just discussed), in combination with instrumental feedback about pitch, duration, and loudness, may be useful in the early steps of a treatment program.[31,35] Instrumental analysis may also help determine if problems with pitch, loudness, or duration lie at the heart of the disturbance and establish which of those parameters is most easily modified by the patient in a direction that facilitates prosodic accuracy.

Providing contextual support when working on prosodic tasks can make them less artificial.[31] For example, using short story scripts that lead to an emphatic or emotional final statement can set the mood and provide the verbal content, leaving the patient with the goal of adequately conveying, through prosody, the appropriate emotion or emphasis to end the script. Such tasks can be done imitatively, following a clinician's model, or can be based solely on the written script. Embedding requirements for emphasis or emotional prosody within a script, with target words or phrases highlighted or not, are other strategies for varying task difficulty.

SUMMARY

1. When neurogenic speech disturbances other than dysarthrias and AOS represent the only or primary impairment of communication or when they represent a major source of disability, their treatment may be appropriate and necessary. However, little is known about the treatment of such speech production deficits.
2. Because NS can be associated with drug effects, particularly anticonvulsants and psychotropic drugs, modifications of drug regimens may help to reduce dysfluencies. Behavioral treatment of NS usually should be deferred until after any pending, related neurosurgery. The literature

suggests that neurogenic dysfluencies may be modified by rate-reduction strategies that are effective for modifying rate in people with dysarthria or AOS. Training in the self-monitoring of dysfluencies has reduced dysfluencies in some aphasic patients. Traditional approaches for managing developmental stuttering, as well as biofeedback and relaxation treatment, represent other possible treatment strategies for NS.

3. Little is known about the treatment of palilalia, but approaches that are appropriate for hypokinetic dysarthria and NS may be applicable to its management in some cases. Palilalic patients with PD may improve with drug management.
4. Echolalia and other speech abnormalities associated with primary cognitive and affective disturbances are generally not approached by attempts to modify the motor aspects of speech production. Hypophonia associated with frontal lobe–limbic system pathology may, in some cases, benefit from vocal exercise to increase loudness, similar to that used for some patients with hypokinetic dysarthria. Behavioral efforts to improve loudness and phonation may be most appropriate when the degree of speech attenuation is disproportionate to other cognitive or affective deficits.
5. Deficits in verbal expression associated with aphasia reflect the underlying language disturbance and therefore are not appropriately managed by focusing on motor aspects of speech production. Dysfluencies associated with aphasia may require direct intervention.
6. Little is known about the effectiveness of management of pseudoforeign accent. Because of its association with aphasia and AOS, however, therapy for those disorders may improve the accent. Techniques for improving prosody, stress, rhythm, and naturalness that are appropriate for managing dysarthria and AOS may be of value, as may be some techniques for reducing foreign accent in non–neurologically impaired speakers.
7. Data regarding the management of aprosodia in patients with right hemisphere lesions are limited. Counseling about the nature of the deficit may help patients and their significant others, as may some actively taught strategies for expressing or clarifying emotional feelings when they are inadequately conveyed by prosody. Techniques used in managing pro-sodic impairments in dysarthric and apraxic patients may be of value. A small number of studies suggest that treatment hierarchies involving prosodic imitation or cognitive-linguistic strategies can result in improved expressive prosody.

References

1. Ackerman H, Ziegler W, Oertel W: Palilalia as a symptom of L-DOPA induced hyperkinesia, J Neurol Neurosurg Psychiatry 52:805, 1989.

2. Alexander MP: Chronic akinetic mutism after mesencephalic-diencephalic infarction: remediated with dopaminergic medications, Neurorehabil Neural Repair 15:151, 2001.

3. Anderson JM et al: Developmental stuttering and Parkinson's disease: the effects of levodopa treatment, J Neurol Neurosurg Psychiatry 66:776, 1999.

4. Anderson JM et al: Treatment of expressive aprosodia associated with right hemisphere injury, J Int Neuropsychol Soc 5:157, 1999.

5. Andy OJ, Bhatnagar SC: Stuttering acquired from subcortical pathologies and its alleviation from thalamic stimulation, Brain Lang 42:385, 1992.

6. Bar KJ, Hager F, Sauer H: Olanzapine- and clozapine-induced stuttering: a case series, Pharmacopsychiatry 37:131, 2004.

7. Baratz R, Mesulam M: Adult onset stuttering treated with anticonvulsants, Arch Neurol 38:132, 1981.

8. Berthier ML et al: Foreign accent syndrome: behavioral and anatomic findings in recovered and non-recovered patients, Aphasiology 5:129, 1991.

9. Bhatnagar S, Andy OJ: Alleviation of acquired stuttering with human centromedian thalamic stimulation, J Neurol Neurosurg Psychiatry 52:1182, 1989.

10. Boller F, Albert M, Denes F: Palilalia, Br J Disord Commun 10:92, 1975.

10a. Brady JP: Drug-induced stuttering: a review of the literature, J Clin Psychopharmacol 18:50, 1998.

11. Brookshire RH: Introduction to neurogenic communication disorders, ed 6, St Louis, 2003, Mosby.

12. Canter G: Observations on neurogenic stuttering: a contribution to differential diagnosis, Br J Disord Commun 6:139, 1971.

13. Chapey R: Language intervention strategies in aphasia and related disorders, ed 4, Philadelphia, 2001, Lippincott Williams & Wilkins.

14. Davis GA: Aphasiology: disorders and clinical practice, Needham Heights, Mass, 2000, Allyn & Bacon.

15. Donnan GA: Stuttering as a manifestation of stroke, Med J Aust 1:44, 1979.

16. Downie AW, Low JM, Lindsay DD: Speech disorders in parkinsonism: use of delayed auditory feedback in selected cases, J Neurol Neurosurg Psychiatry 44:852, 1981.

17. Duggal HS et al: Clozapine-induced stuttering and seizures, Am J Psychiatry 159:315, 2002.

18. Fleet WS, Heilman KM: Acquired stuttering from a right hemisphere lesion in a right-hander, Neurology 35:1343, 1985.

19. Giacino JT: Disorders of consciousness: differential diagnosis and neuropathologic features, Semin Neurol 17:105, 1997.

20. Goberman AM, Blomgren M: Parkinsonian speech dysfluencies: effects of L-dopa-related fluctuations, J Fluency Disord 28:55, 2003.

21. Helm NA: Management of palilalia with a pacing board, J Speech Hear Disord 44:350, 1979.

22. Helm NA, Butler RB: Transcutaneous nerve stimulation in acquired speech disorder, Lancet 3:1177, 1977.

23. Helm-Estabrooks N: Stuttering associated with acquired neurological disorders. In Curlee RF, editor: Stuttering and related disorders of fluency, New York, 1993, Thieme.

24. Helm-Estabrooks N: Diagnosis and management of neurogenic stuttering in adults. In St Louis KO, editor: The atypical stutterer: principles and practices of rehabilitation, New York, 1986, Academic Press.

25. LaPointe LL: Progressive echolalia and echopraxic: what could it be? what could it be? In Helm-Estabrooks N, Aten JL, editors: Difficult diagnoses in adult communication disorders, Boston, 1989, College-Hill Press.

26. Market KE et al: Acquired stuttering: descriptive data and treatment outcome, J Fluency Disord 15:21, 1990.

27. Marshall RC, Starch SA: Behavioral treatment of acquired stuttering, Aust J Commun Disord 12:245, 1969.

28. McClean MD, McLean A: Case report of stuttering acquired in association with phenytoin use for post–head-injury seizures, J Fluency Disord 10:241, 1985.

29. Meyers SC, Hall NE, Aram DM: Fluency and language recovery in a child with a left hemisphere lesion, J Fluency Disord 15:159, 1990.

30. Mueller U, Von Cramon DY: The therapeutic potential of bromocriptine in neuropsychological rehabilitation of patients with acquired brain damage, Prog Neuropsychopharmacol Biol Psychiatry 18:1103, 1994.

31. Myers PS: Right hemisphere damage: disorders of communication and cognition, San Diego, 1999, Singular Publishing Group.

32. Myers PS: Communication disorders associated with right hemisphere brain damage. In Chapey R, editor: Language intervention strategies in adult aphasia, ed 3, Baltimore, 1994, Williams & Wilkins.

33. Peach RK: Acquired neurogenic stuttering, Grand Rounds Commun Disord 9:177, 1984.

34. Rentschler GJ, Driver LE, Callaway EA: The onset of stuttering following drug overdose, J Fluency Disord 9:265, 1984.

35. Robin DA, Klouda GV, Hug LN: Neurogenic disorders of prosody. In Vogel D, Cannito MP, editors: Treating disordered speech motor control, Austin, Tex, 1991, Pro-Ed.

36. Rosenbek JC: Stuttering secondary to nervous system damage. In Curlee RF, Perkins WH, editors: Nature and treatment of stuttering: new directions, San Diego, 1984, College-Hill.

37. Rosenbek JC, LaPointe LL, Wertz RT: Aphasia: a clinical approach. Boston, 1989, College-Hill.

38. Rosenbek J et al: Stuttering following brain damage, Brain Lang 6:82, 1978.

38a. Rosenbek JC et al: Novel treatments for expressive aprosodia: a phase I investigation of cognitive linguistic and imitative interventions, J Int Neuropsychol Soc 10:786, 2004.

39. Ross ED, Stewart RM: Akinetic mutism from hypothalamic damage: successful treatment with dopamine agonists, Neurology 31:1435, 1981.

40. Rousey CG, Arjunan KN, Rousey CL: Successful treatment of stuttering following closed head injury, J Fluency Disord 11:257, 1986.

41. Sandyk R: Speech impairment in Parkinson's disease is improved by transcranial application of electromagnetic fields, Int J Neurosci 92:63, 1997.

42. Sapir S, Aronson AE: Aphonia after closed head injury: aetiologic considerations, Br J Disord Commun 20:289, 1985.

43. *Schreiber S, Pick CG: Paroxetine for secondary stuttering: further interaction of serotonin and dopamine, J Nerv Ment Dis 185:465, 1997.*

44. *Serra-Mestres J, Shapleske J, Tym E: Treatment of palilalia with trazodone, Am J Psychiatry 153:580, 1996.*

45. *Stringer AY: Treatment of motor aprosodia with pitch biofeedback and expression modeling, Brain Inj 10:583, 1996.*

46. *Supprian T, Retz W, Deckert J: Clozapine-induced stuttering: epileptic brain activity? Am J Psychiatry 156:1663, 1999.*

47. *Whitney JL, Goldstein H: Using self-monitoring to reduce dysfluencies in speakers with mild aphasia, J Speech Hear Disord 54:576, 1989.*

Managing Acquired Psychogenic and Related Nonorganic Speech Disorders

"The therapist must show a considerable knowledge of neurological and psychiatric aspects of the patient's illness to maintain credibility and obtain the patient's cooperation with treatment."

(Ron,[20] discussing therapy for somatization and conversion disorders)

CHAPTER OUTLINE

I. General principles and guidelines
A. Many people with psychogenic speech disorders can be managed effectively by speech pathologists
B. Prognosis for recovery is usually good
C. Symptoms and explanations must be addressed
D. A patient's belief that the problem is organic must be addressed
E. Treatment often should be attempted within the diagnostic session
F. Clinician attitude and manner of relating to the patient are crucial
G. The future must be discussed
H. When symptomatic therapy succeeds, the patient should have an explanation for it
I. Not everyone wants to be helped, is ready to be helped, or can be helped

II. General treatment techniques
A. The sequence of assessment and management
B. The psychosocial history
C. Addressing beliefs about organicity
D. Symptomatic therapy
E. Addressing the nature of the problem and its improvement
F. Addressing the future

III. Symptomatic treatment for specific psychogenic speech disorders
A. Psychogenic voice disorders
B. Psychogenic stuttering
C. Other psychogenic speech disorders

IV. Summary

Psychogenic and related nonorganic speech disorders (psychogenic/nonorganic speech disorders) can be disabling and handicapping because of the barriers they introduce to communicative interaction and because of the psychologic difficulties they represent. Their diagnosis—discussed in Chapters 14 and 15—is essential to setting the direction of treatment and is usually derived from the medical and psychosocial history and from careful assessment of the speech disturbance.

People with changes in speech due to major depression, schizophrenia, and other serious psychiatric disturbances generally are not referred for speech evaluation or treatment. In such cases the speech abnormality is usually neither a presenting complaint nor a direct focus of treatment. In contrast, changes in speech that reflect a conversion disorder or response to life stresses may be a presenting complaint and the focus of concerted medical efforts at diagnosis and management. Gratifyingly, a significant proportion of people with these latter types of speech disturbances seem responsive to treatment provided by the speech pathologist. Such positive outcomes obviously benefit the affected person, and they can be satisfying to the clinicians who provide treatment.

This chapter emphasizes general principles, guidelines, and techniques for managing psychogenic/nonorganic speech disorders. Many of them are derived from the literature on voice disorders, because treatment of psychogenic voice disorders is more fully developed and refined than is treatment of other psychogenic speech disorders, and because psychogenic voice disorders probably represent the largest subcategory of psychogenic/nonorganic speech disturbances seen in speech pathology practices.* Because there do not appear to be clear

---

*For example, psychogenic voice disorders represented 80% of the psychogenic speech disorders in the Mayo Clinic cases reviewed in Chapter 14.

differences in the histories and psychosocial dynamics among people with different types of psychogenic/nonorganic speech disorders, and because their various speech symptoms seem to respond equally well to similar techniques, the general principles and techniques discussed in the next section form the foundation for treating all psychogenic/nonorganic speech disorders. Following this discussion, management of several specific types of psychogenic speech disturbances are addressed.

▨ GENERAL PRINCIPLES AND GUIDELINES

The personality traits of individuals afflicted by psychogenic/nonorganic speech disorders, the life events that help to trigger and maintain the disorders, the specific characteristics of the abnormal speech, and the degree to which additional influential organic and psychologic variables are at work are too heterogeneous to permit simple prescriptive treatment. In this section, general principles and guidelines that seem important to management are addressed. They help to set the clinician's attitude about management, and they highlight the major issues that must be addressed in decision making and management activities.

Many People with Psychogenic Speech Disorders Can Be Managed Effectively by Speech Pathologists

There is an odd and persistent belief among some clinicians that psychogenic speech disorders are not within their scope of practice or, if they are, that the clinician's role is to treat the symptoms while avoiding the psychosocial history and its relationship to the speech disorder. The psychosocial issues, and perhaps even symptom management, are seen as the responsibility of the psychiatrist or psychologist, because they are, after all, experts in problems of "the mind." This belief is analogous to arguing that motor speech disorders (MSDs) should not be managed by speech pathologists, because neurologists are the experts in problems of "the brain." These arguments ignore the expertise of speech clinicians in the diagnosis and management of neurogenic and psychogenic speech disorders and their ability to determine when consultation from other medical subspecialties should be pursued—along with, or instead of, speech therapy—for optimal patient care.

One source of concern about managing the symptoms of conversion disorder speech abnormalities without psychiatric treatment is that the underlying psychologic disorder will simply generate a different symptom if the speech symptom is removed. Few psychiatrists today subscribe to this view, and there are many reported cases in which speech symptom resolution is not associated with adverse effects or the subsequent appearance of different conversion symptoms.[2,21] Aronson also suggested that premature referral to psychiatry may guarantee failure to improve speech, because the speech symptom is often dissociated from awareness on the part of the patient of any emotional problem; thus referral may be rejected by the patient. In addition, symptom removal often requires explicit attention to modifying symptoms, something most psychiatrists are not trained to do.[17] Patients are more likely to be receptive to psychiatric referral after speech has improved, because the etiology has then been established as nonorganic and, when appropriate, because the possible links between the speech problem and psychologic issues have been discussed in the course of speech therapy.

Psychiatric referral is neither invariably necessary nor appropriate following successful speech treatment. Psychogenic speech disorders can occur as a way of handling acute emotional distress or stress in people who are otherwise psychologically healthy. In some cases the experienced speech clinician and the patient may conclude that further intervention is unnecessary.* This receives some support from psychiatrists who note that psychoanalysis is not appropriate for the majority of patients with conversion disorders[19,30] and that treatment and remission of conversion symptoms can occur in various ways, including through behavioral management and "brief supportive therapy."[†14,27] Thus the speech pathologist has an important diagnostic and management role to play. In many cases, the role is a central one.

Prognosis for Recovery Is Usually Good

The prospect for recovery, especially with treatment, is often good, even when neurologic disease is present. In general, for example, patients with conversion disorders tend to improve over the course of weeks or months, and spontaneous remission may be the rule rather than the exception.[27,30] The prognosis for recovery from a conversion disorder is especially

---

*For example, Aronson, Peterson, and Litin[4] reported that none of the 27 patients they studied with conversion aphonia or dysphonia had serious psychopathology warranting immediate psychiatric help.

†Baker and Silver[5] found that patients with "hysterical paraplegia," originally thought to have paraplegia from physical trauma, responded rapidly to treatment. The most successful management was "a firm diagnosis; a confident prediction of improvement; sympathy; interest; and common sense."

good when the patient is young, symptoms are of recent onset and are not intermittent, there is an identifiable precipitating stressful event, premorbid health is good, there is an absence of serious psychopathology, and the patient has some insight into the connection between negative life events and his or her symptoms.[7,14,16,20,27,28] Prognosis becomes complicated when these conditions are not met, especially when severe psychopathology is present.

Conversion aphonias and dysphonias, as well as other nonorganic speech disturbances, may normalize in minutes or over several therapy sessions in a high proportion of patients.[1,2,8,17,26] However, although the relapse rate in some studies is low,[1] a significant minority may not do well.[17] Sustained recovery is more of a problem for patients in whom increased musculoskeletal tension represents their lifelong pattern of responding to stress or if they remain clinically anxious and depressed; although normal voice may be achieved during symptomatic therapy, the improvement may be short-lived unless ongoing anxiety and depression or the habitual pattern of responding to stress can be changed.[22] The same may be true for patients with conversion disorder if the underlying cause is still active and the patient remains unwilling or unable to acknowledge or deal with it more directly; in such cases, psychotherapy or time may be necessary instead of, or before, symptomatic speech therapy. Case[10] also suggests that people with psychogenic voice problems that are situation specific (e.g., only at work) are unlikely to respond to symptomatic treatment and may be in need of psychotherapy. Overall, "prognosis for improvement with speech therapy is excellent for conversion disorders, good for anxiety-induced speech disorders, and guarded for depression-related speech disorders."[23]

A good prognosis is not precluded by the presence of neurologic disease. For example, rapid improvement of acquired psychogenic stuttering and aphonias/dysphonias has been reported in people with various neurologic diseases, some with cooccurring neurogenic speech or language disorders.*[6,9,24,25,29]

---

*The literature may lead to an overestimate of the "true" proportion of cases that recover from psychogenic speech disorders in response to speech therapy. This is because it is much more likely that positive rather than negative treatment results are reported, especially for conditions in which the best external criterion for establishing the accuracy of diagnosis is a rapid positive response to symptomatic treatment. Put another way, cases that do not respond to symptomatic treatment may not be reported as treatment failures because the lack of positive response may produce doubt about whether the disorder is psychogenic in the first place, especially when neurologic disease is present.

To summarize, based on general impressions about recovery from conversion disorders and frequent reports of effective treatment of psychogenic speech disorders, the prognosis for recovery generally can be considered good. Clinicians are thus justified in bringing a positive, optimistic attitude to their management of people with these speech disorders.

Symptoms and Explanations Must Be Addressed

Effective management requires that the clinician be prepared to address symptoms, as well as the psychologic explanations for them, although neither is always necessary or possible. For example, speech may normalize in some patients as they reveal their psychosocial history and "discover" the psychologic trigger for their symptoms. Others respond to symptomatic treatment without ever identifying plausible explanatory factors. Nonetheless, these two components of management must be kept in mind by the clinician during diagnostic and any subsequent treatment sessions.

Underlying explanations for the speech disorder may be addressed at various levels. The most basic is during the psychosocial history, in which potential causal mechanisms may be brought to light. This can be accomplished by reviewing the events surrounding the onset of the speech disorder from both physical and psychologic perspectives. Patients' responses help set the sequence of subsequent events—for example, whether to move quickly to symptomatic management or to delve immediately into psychosocial issues.

Following symptomatic treatment—especially if it is successful—the relationship between the speech symptoms and their emotional causes can be addressed. Techniques for doing this are discussed in the next section. *It is essential to remember that the psychosocial history and its relationship to the speech problem are crucial for both diagnosis and treatment.*[3]

A Patient's Belief That the Problem Is Organic Must Be Addressed

People with psychogenic speech disorders often believe their problem has an organic basis. This belief may stem from the inaccessibility to them of the psychologic dynamics that have produced the speech problem, and it is often reinforced by multiple medical tests and treatments that are directed at possible neurologic or other organic causes. Rather than dispelling fears of organic disease, negative medical evaluations sometimes generate uncertainty and increase anxiety about the possible seriousness of the condition; this may be particularly true for patients who are afraid of contracting a disease to which they have been exposed or that has affected someone close to them. Unfortunately, acceptance of the nonorganic basis for their symptoms is rarely dispelled by professionals who dismiss them by saying "the problem is all in your head" without having explored the psychosocial history and without further explanation. This kind of confrontation rarely works and often promotes an adversarial relationship or patient withdrawal.[11,16,20,27,30]

Even when a specific cause cannot be found, the nonorganic basis for the speech problem should be addressed. The degree to which this is done directly or indirectly will vary as a function of the evidence for a specific causal mechanism, the patient's willingness to discuss psychologic issues, and the clinician's degree of certainty about the nonorganic etiology. In some cases, discussion of this issue should occur before any attempt at symptomatic therapy. In others, discussion should be deferred until after speech has improved. Often, the idea of nonorganic causes is introduced briefly before symptoms are managed and then in more detail after improvement has occurred. The gradual unfolding of these issues is nearly always more effective than telling the patient abruptly that his or her problem has no organic basis. It is generally counterproductive and destructive to a therapeutic alliance to directly challenge a patient's strong belief that there is a physical cause for his or her problem.[20,31]

The process of developing acceptance of the problem as nonorganic is not synonymous with identifying it as psychogenic and discovering its exact psychodynamics. This may happen in some cases, but *the primary goal is to have the patient accept that there are no organic barriers that preclude the possibility of speech improvement and maintenance of improvement once it has occurred.* For many patients, the triggering events are no longer active and may have been forgotten or become inaccessible to them (these patients are particularly "ready" to improve). Many readily accept an explanation that the cause is not clear but that there are no "active" organic explanations for the problem. This may be particularly effective for patients whose speech problems developed at the time of a physical injury or organic illness that subsequently resolved. By accepting that organic barriers to normal speech are not currently present, the way is paved for symptomatic therapy, improvement, and maintenance of normal speech.

Treatment Often Should Be Attempted within the Diagnostic Session

When the clinician is reasonably certain that the etiology is nonorganic and that the speech disorder should be treated symptomatically, treatment should be attempted immediately if possible. This is important, because the majority of people can be helped considerably or completely within the diagnostic session or within one or two subsequent therapy sessions.[2,8,26] This assertive approach can accomplish several things: (1) if treatment results in significant improvement, the diagnosis of the disorder as nonorganic will be confirmed; (2) the confirmed diagnosis may alter or modify previously planned medical and psychiatric evaluations; (3) the patient is likely to accept that the problem is not organic and may be receptive to addressing the psychologic causes for the disorder; (4) many patients will be pleased (although often perplexed) at the rapid return of their speech and be in a position to resume their lives in a more normal way, especially if the underlying psychologic causes are no longer active; and (5) patient and medical resources and costs will be saved.

Clinician Attitude and Manner of Relating to the Patient Are Crucial

In 1922 Henry Head said, "No one is a greater failure than the medical officer who wishes all hysterics could be shot at dawn. On the other hand, the firm diplomatist with subtle and demonstrable reasons why the patient can stand, walk, or feel often produces miraculous cures."[15] This reference to the attitude of some clinicians toward people with conversion disorders, if not literally true, captures what people with physical manifestations of nonorganic problems feel from people who dismiss them as having "nothing wrong" or a problem that is "all in your head." Such pronouncements, especially in the absence of any exploration of the psychosocial history, or when unaccompanied by supportive recommendations, are rarely accepted by the patient and usually do not put an end to his or her search for organic explanations. At best, such attitudes reflect ignorance, discomfort, or impatience in dealing with psychologic issues or a belief that problems that are psychologic in origin are not legitimate problems. They may also reflect insensitivity or a lack of respect for the effects that stress, anxiety, and conflict can exert on people's lives. The basic attitude with which to approach people with physical deficits caused by nonorganic disturbances is to acknowledge to them that the problem is indeed genuine and disabling, despite the absence of a detectable organic explanation.[11,28,31]

Clinician attitudes are crucial to management, and the attitudes should be clear to the patient. There can be no prescription for the style in which these attitudes are expressed, because style is a highly personal trait, but it is important that the following attitudes and beliefs be conveyed:

1. *Respect* for patients' concern about the possible organic cause of their problem and acknowledgment that their symptoms and the frustrations and limitations imposed by them are legitimate. For example, much can be done to develop a therapeutic alliance with a patient by responding to his or her story that "All the doctors say there's nothing wrong with me" with "That seems a foolish thing to say. You can't talk normally—of course there's something wrong!"

2. *Reassurance and optimism* about the negative findings of medical workups. Reviewing with seriousness the results of general and subspecialty medical workups and concluding that an absence of an organic explanation is encouraging rather than worrisome helps to set the stage for effective symptomatic treatment and discussion of possible nonorganic explanations.

3. *Support and approval* for the patient's desire and ability to improve. Some patients are indifferent to an invitation to work to improve their speech, or make excuses about why they are unable to do so; they usually do not respond to symptomatic treatment or discussion of psychologic issues. Many others state that they want to improve and are willing to work to do it when asked directly if that is their desire. An explicit invitation to work hard to improve speech places responsibility with the patient to play an active role in therapy, puts the patient in a position to take credit for his or her improvement, and begins to establish a capacity to do well in the future, independent of reliance on formal symptomatic therapy.

4. *Empathy and compassion* for the ordinary or extraordinary psychologic burdens the patient has been under, when he or she is willing to reveal and discuss them. Assuming the patient is "ready" to improve, the manner in which psychologic issues are discussed is crucial. It has much to do with kindness, an attitude that respects the reality and seriousness of the problem despite the lack of organic explanation, and one that involves as much as possible the patient's participation in the process of exploration of underlying psychologic issues.

5. *Assertiveness and confidence* that symptomatic therapy can be effective. The literature indicates that "suggestion" is a common denominator in successful treatment of conversion disorders,[5,17,27,28] meaning that it is important to convey a belief that the symptoms will remit; it is also reasonable to suggest that speech problems often can improve *rapidly*. Because symptomatic therapy involves trial and error techniques, it must be conducted with an air of confidence that each technique has the capacity to be effective. As treatment progresses, it is also important that the clinician immediately acknowledge changes in speech and enlist the patient's recognition of those changes.

6. *Honesty.* The patient should be told directly when the clinician does not understand completely the reasons for the speech problem or why he or she has or has not improved, but the uncertainty should be conveyed with confidence. This can be done with prefaces like "We don't always understand how these things develop" or "I don't know for certain why or how this problem developed, but it does seem that there's no physical barrier present that is in the way of your speech improving." Often, after symptomatic therapy has resulted in a return to normal speech, the patient asks what caused the problem or why it improved so rapidly. This then allows the clinician to say, "I'm not sure, let's explore that." This represents an ideal opportunity to discuss psychosocial issues.

7. *Pleasure and respect* for the patient's efforts and progress during symptomatic therapy and, when appropriate, his or her courage in confronting the psychologic issues tied to the symptoms. This opens the door to discussing the future.

The Future Must Be Discussed

When symptomatic therapy results in significant improvement or a return of normal speech, it is nonetheless important to discuss the future. If emotional issues that triggered the speech disturbance are no longer active or are resolving, discussion of the relationship between them and the speech disorder may establish that psychiatric referral or further symptomatic treatment are unnecessary. The experienced clinician usually develops a sense about whether psychiatric referral is necessary.[2] It is essential to involve the patient in this decision and also to review other ways available to him or her for dealing with similar psychologic burdens in the future. Reassurance that the speech problem may never recur can usually be given, but the patient should be urged to contact the clinician if the problem returns; in many cases, a routine follow-up appointment may reassure the patient that help is still available.

Whether or not speech has improved, if major ongoing psychologic issues are present, discussion about the need for psychiatric or psychologic referral should be pursued. Patients with somatization disorders frequently reject such referrals,[17] as do those who deny the presence of psychologic factors or their relevance to their current physical symptoms. Patients who have revealed the presence of such issues and have confronted their impact and importance are usually willing to accept such referral.

When Symptomatic Therapy Succeeds, the Patient Should Have an Explanation for It

Tied to discussion of the future is the fact that *most patients need an explanation for their recovery,* if not an explanation for the cause of the problem. Explanations vary greatly, and *it is not essential that patients have insight into the cause of their symptoms for them to maintain improvement.*[20] Explanations depend on the degree to which causal mechanisms have been discovered, whether the patient has insight into them, the patient's social and cultural beliefs and customs, and so on. It is nearly always important to explore what significant others, colleagues at work, and others have thought about the patient's problem and what they are likely to think about its resolution. Patients frequently ask how they can explain their improvement to others, partly as a way of admitting they do not understand it well themselves, but also as a way of saying they need a strategy for "saving face."

There is a fairly pervasive attitude in our society that psychologic difficulties, particularly those that produce unusual physical symptoms (e.g., aphonia, stuttering-like behavior), are a sign of personal weakness or intrinsic instability. These attitudes may be reinforced when symptoms resolve rapidly. As a result, saving face is important to patients' future ability to cope in their social environment and, perhaps, to their ability to maintain their gains. Without an adequate explanation, the patient may be unable or unwilling to maintain normal speech because of the possible psychosocial penalties for doing so. It is thus important to develop plausible explanations with the patient that they understand and that will be acceptable to those they know who will desire or demand an explanation. There is no formula for such explanations, but they should be structured to support the legitimacy of the symptoms, the inability of the patient to improve in the past, and the patient's active participation in resolving the speech problem. The understanding of these issues is usually optimized if it is developed in a negotiated way between clinician and patient, using a shared, common language.*[31]

Not Everyone Wants To Be Helped, Is Ready To Be Helped, or Can Be Helped

Contraindications to pursuing symptomatic therapy are relatively uncommon among patients referred for speech evaluation in rehabilitation and multidisciplinary medical practices. There are, however, some circumstances in which symptomatic therapy should not be pursued or is unlikely to be successful.

Some patients who are referred for evaluation do not come with a desire to be helped. Some will assertively or angrily state that they think such assessment is nonsensical because the problem is certainly due to some threatening organic disease. They may reject any attempt to address their psychosocial history and any effort to modify their speech symptoms, even when approached with empathy and confidence that symptomatic therapy may help them. These patients generally are not candidates for symptomatic therapy. If the experienced clinician is certain of this, symptomatic efforts should be aborted early. The best that can be done is to document the reasons for concluding that the speech disorder is nonorganic.

Some patients initially do not resist examination but may become threatened by inquiries about psychologic issues or the prospect that symptomatic therapy might resolve their speech symptom. They may give numerous excuses why they cannot participate in treatment, such as lack of time or other pending medical tests, or they may display severe pain in response to touch or manipulation of speech structures by the clinician. They may become hostile or angry at attempts to discuss emotional issues or work on speech symptoms. Many of these patients are not ready to be helped by symptomatic therapy.

Some patients have nonorganic speech disturbances that are present transiently and unpredictably or are situation specific (e.g., present only during or after an encounter with an estranged spouse). Symptomatic therapy is unlikely to be successful with such patients, and it can be impossible if speech is normal during speech evaluation. Assessment during an episode of speech difficulty may be of value to establish the nonorganic nature of the problem and to see if speech improvement can be achieved with symptomatic therapy, but the gains are unlikely to be

---

*Tucker and colleagues[31] point out that the concept of stress as a contributor to symptoms is less stigmatizing than depression or anxiety. Many patients who resist admitting to depression will admit to considerable stress and show an interest in reducing its effects on their lives.

lasting if psychologic issues are not dealt with. These patients should be referred for psychiatric assessment.[10]

Sometimes a patient is oblivious to or denies the presence of speech abnormality, despite floridly abnormal speech. Others reveal ongoing events or residual effects of prior psychologically traumatic events that are so profoundly disturbing that symptomatic therapy would be inconsequential or even risky if it provided a mechanism for further repressing or denying the trauma. Symptomatic therapy in these cases should be deferred until psychiatric evaluation has established if it is appropriate or necessary.

GENERAL TREATMENT TECHNIQUES

A number of treatment techniques were implied in the preceding discussion. They, as well as additional techniques, are discussed here to provide a sense of how to approach management. Treatment within the diagnostic session is emphasized, but the techniques discussed here can be applied over a number of sessions.

The emphasis on single-session treatment is not intended to imply that nonorganic speech disorders are always effectively treated in one or a few sessions, nor that people with such disorders might not require more time in order to achieve a return to normal speech. It is not entirely clear why some patients respond rapidly to symptomatic therapy while others require treatment and recovery over time, although it seems that gradual improvement is more often the course for people with more serious psychiatric difficulties, some requiring inpatient psychiatric care. For others, it may be that the need to save face requires that they recover in a manner that more closely resembles that which occurs in response to organic disease.

The Sequence of Assessment and Management

The speech evaluation and subsequent management are ideally conducted following all medical evaluations that are directly relevant to establishing the nature of the speech disorder. For most patients, this means that speech assessment should follow ear, nose, and throat or neurologic examinations, or both. Preceding medical examinations allow the clinician to review those findings, reassure the patient that there is no apparent organic explanation for his or her speech problem, and introduce the notion that there are no physical barriers to improving speech.

It is often effective to ask patients to review what they have been told by examining physicians because their interpretation of the meaning of such findings can then be reinforced or reinterpreted for them by the clinician. For example, in response to the patient's comment that "they said that everything looks normal," the clinician may say, "That's good news, isn't it?" In response to "Just like everyone else, they can't find the reason for this; one doctor told me there's absolutely nothing wrong with me," the clinician might say, "Well, there's obviously something wrong, because you're not talking very well, but the fact that there's nothing physically threatening going on is encouraging, isn't it?"

Patients for whom medical examinations have not yet been conducted are more likely to maintain a belief that their problem is organic and thus be less willing to accept the clinician's conclusion that it probably is not organic. In fact, the clinician may require such information to be confident that the problem is nonorganic. In such cases it may be best to defer symptomatic treatment until after medical assessments are complete, although some patients do respond well to symptomatic treatment before such assessments. When they do, it may nonetheless be important to complete medical assessments even after resolution of the speech problem, especially if it is apparent that the patient may still harbor fears of organic disease.

When there is evidence of neurologic or other organic disease, but the speech disorder is wholly or partly nonorganic, the clinician must then use medical assessment results as a basis for addressing the relationship between the organic findings and the speech disorder. It is necessary to establish that, in spite of organic factors, there are no major barriers to improving those aspects of the speech problem that cannot be explained by organic disease. This is obviously more difficult to convey, but it can be accomplished (e.g., "Despite the fact that you have multiple sclerosis, it's unlikely that MS would affect speech in this way. Even though it might have played some role in triggering your speech problem, I think it's possible that right now it won't prevent you from making significant improvements in your speech").

The Psychosocial History

The psychosocial history can be obtained while reviewing the history of the current illness. The facts of the history determine the direction and sequence of inquiry. The interview may begin with a review of the circumstances surrounding the onset of the speech problem. Was onset associated with an obvious illness, physically traumatic event, surgery, or a suspected or confirmed neurologic event? Was the speech problem immediately apparent, or was there a delay between the physical event and onset of speech difficulty? If so, what was going on at or shortly before the time the speech problem began? How has the speech problem changed and what conditions make it better or worse? Has it ever remitted, even for short periods of time? Answers to these questions help determine the degree to which there is an association of the speech problem with actual or perceived organic illness, as well as the degree to which the patient is convinced the problem is organic.

When the physical facts of the problem have been reviewed, and especially when there is no evidence of a possible organic cause, the patient can be asked about the facts of his or her job, family situation, and social life. This can be followed by asking how things have been going and were going in each of those areas when the speech problem began. The patient may not have been asked such questions before, despite numerous medical consultations. For some, this inquiry will be welcome, whereas for others it will be perceived as inappropriate or threatening. It is generally the case, however, that patients rarely reveal information about their personal lives without being asked, especially when they fail to see a connection between nonorganic factors and their physical symptoms.

Some patients reveal potentially significant psychosocial problems, but many deny any difficulties and insist that life is happy and stable. If they nonetheless seem receptive to inquiries about these issues, it is often appropriate to ask directly what stresses, conflicts, or pressures they are under or were under when their speech problem began. Sometimes etiologically significant psychosocial problems are immediately revealed in response to questions like "What was going on that might have been stressful to you at the time your speech problem began?" "Were you or are you been having any difficulties at home or at work?" Sometimes this leads to immediate discussion of the possible connection between the speech problem and psychologic factors, occasionally producing catharsis and resolution of the speech problem. More often the clinician will simply tuck the information away for later discussion.

Patients sometimes respond aggressively, angrily, or sarcastically to inquiries about their psychosocial history. Statements like "You think I'm crazy (just like everybody else), don't you?" can be responded to with something like "Not at all. It's just important to understand all of the things that can influence problems like this, and we know that stress is sometimes important," "No, but what is it that other people have said about that?" or "What do you think about that?" The patient's belief about the possibility of psychologic explanations will determine the extent to which discussion of such issues should be pursued at the time. If there is resistance or denial, it is usually best to proceed to speech assessment and symptomatic treatment. It should be kept in mind,

however, that patients who are resistant to the notion of possible social and psychologic *causes* of their symptoms are nonetheless often willing to discuss the social and psychologic *consequences* of them.[20] Such discussion can open the door to later discussion of psychologic causes and consequences.

When patients do reveal evidence of psychologically significant events, they may ask if the clinician sees a connection between them and the speech disorder. It is helpful to ask the patient what he or she thinks in this regard. If the answer demonstrates recognition of a possible causal relationship, the clinician should support and perhaps elaborate upon the explanation, acknowledging that psychologic issues can affect physical symptoms, and that this can occur in people without serious psychiatric difficulty who are under great stress, conflict, and so on. At the same time, it is often important to acknowledge that such problems are often complex and difficult to understand.

It is not essential that the clinician explicitly explore the connection between the psychosocial history and the speech disorder during history taking. This sometimes happens in a natural way, but often it does not. What is important is to gather some initial facts that contribute to hypotheses about causal mechanisms, the patient's beliefs about the disturbance, his or her willingness to discuss psychologic issues, and his or her capacity for insight. The actual drawing together of the psychosocial data and speech symptoms will often be deferred until after or during symptomatic treatment.

Addressing Beliefs about Organicity

The medical and psychosocial history should establish the degree to which the patient believes the problem has an organic basis. It is often valuable to ask directly, "What do you believe is the cause of this problem?" when it is not readily apparent or when the clinician is ready to address the issue. When there are no readily apparent possible physical explanations, it is valid to state that "right now it's difficult to know just what has caused this problem," and after the basic speech mechanism examination is complete to indicate that "at this point I don't see or hear anything that should prevent your speech from improving. It may be that something (the cold, the surgery, the physical trauma, the stroke) happened when this problem began that prevented you from speaking normally, but right now there's no evidence that that's still active or that it should prevent improvement in your speech." At this point the notion of symptomatic treatment can be introduced. Further discussion of the organicity of the problem can be deferred until after an assertive attempt at symptomatic treatment is complete.

Symptomatic Therapy

Symptomatic treatment should be introduced with the notion that a concerted effort to improve speech can result in significant and, often, rapid improvement. This can be followed by an explicit invitation to the patient ("Should we give it a try?") and a confident, pleased response when the patient accepts.

The direction of symptomatic efforts is determined by the specific abnormal speech characteristics. Several general techniques are frequently applicable. They include the following:

1. Identify for the patient the behaviors that represent the disorder (e.g., tight, effortful voice; whispering; facial grimacing; neck extension; eye blinking; speaking only one syllable per breath group; general muscle tension; sound repetitions; slow speech rate; consistent articulatory substitutions). Often these characteristics reflect excessive or misdirected muscular efforts.

2. After the behaviors are identified, it is appropriate to convey that they reflect a well-intentioned effort to speak that is actually physically exhausting and acting as a barrier to more normal speech ("You're working so hard to talk that you're unable to speak naturally"). The patient can then be told that an attempt will be made to redirect or reduce the amount of effort required to speak.

3. Have the patient do something with speech that will approximate a normal response. This may range from a grunt to a sigh to a prolonged sound to a single syllable. It should be reinforced if adequate and modified if accompanied by struggle or abnormal quality. It often helps to have the patient do something different, even if not normal, from what he or she has been doing habitually. For example, if the patient is grimacing, point out the behavior and have him or her do something else instead (e.g., open eyes widely). Any change should be reinforced. The patient should be told to listen to and feel the difference from his or her habitual response and then prompted to repeat the new response. When consistent, the response should be shaped toward normal or to a lengthier normal response (e.g., moving from a vowel to a syllable or word).

   Patients sometimes express or display signs of fatigue, exhaustion, or discomfort during these efforts. They should be reinforced for working hard, praised for each small gain, and told that speaking may become easier than it has been within a short time. It may help to tell them that the first steps are the hardest and that success often builds momentum, with progress becoming rapid after the initial period of hard work. Failed techniques should be accompanied by explanations that it is often necessary to try several things, each of which might work but some more adequately than others. The clinician should not let the patient's physical discomfort inhibit assertive efforts to work for change. The patient should have a sense that the clinician is willing to commit considerable physical effort of his or her own to work for change.

4. Talk to the patient about what is going on during symptomatic efforts. Statements such as "You've been trying hard to speak well, but your efforts have not been quite in the right direction. It's as if a train has been knocked off track (perhaps by your cold, accident, etc.). You've been trying by yourself to get it back on track but haven't quite known how. What we're doing here is putting you back on the track in a way that will make it easier to do what you're trying so hard to do" can motivate continued effort and begin to address possible causal mechanisms at the same time.

5. *Physical contact may be important to symptomatic therapy.* Laryngeal manipulation and massage is an effective way of reducing musculoskeletal tension and modifying voice in psychogenic voice disorders. The physical benefits of relieving musculoskeletal tension are clearly significant for many patients, but the physical contact between clinician and patient also may have considerable psychologic value by "bonding" them together in the therapeutic effort and providing evidence that something physical is being done to induce change. Physical contact may be important for the management of other psychogenic speech disorders as well, both for its value in identifying points of excessive musculoskeletal tension (e.g., the face, jaw, eyes, hands) and for its psychologic value. Touch may thus be invaluable as both a physical and psychologic tool. It is important that it is be used naturally and confidently.

6. As speech begins to improve and the clinician senses that symptomatic treatment will be successful, it is appropriate to accelerate enthusiasm about the patient's progress. Gradual withdrawal of physical manipulation or touch can take place, with increased expectations that the patient modify speech without physical assistance.

7. When speech has normalized or improved noticeably, the patient can be asked to read a paragraph and get the "feel" for his or her improved speech. The clinician can interrupt to ask some general questions; the patient's improved speech during such responses should be pointed out. Some patients pass these transition points rapidly. Others may need to proceed much more gradually. It is crucial that the clinician repeatedly let the patient know that each step of improvement reflects a capacity for normal speech and that it is his or her efforts that are determining the outcome.

As normalization takes place, many patients begin to ask "What can I do to keep my speech like this or get it back if I lose it again?" The clinician can indicate that it is likely that gains will be maintained without any special help now that the patient has regained the feel for normal speech.

Addressing the Nature of the Problem and Its Improvement

How the nature of the problem is addressed is highly dependent on the degree to which the clinician understands the problem. If the patient has good insight into causal stresses and if there is a logical link between them and the speech problem, a frank discussion of the role of stress, anxiety, or conflict in the production of physical symptoms may be accepted and understood. For patients with a clear history of an organic trigger for the problem, an explanation may be more difficult. It may include the notion that a physical event was initially responsible for triggering the speech abnormality, but that when the organic event was no longer active the speech problem persisted, either because the patient developed faulty habits that he or she could not overcome or because there were psychologic issues at work that expressed themselves in speech abnormalities.

It is often important at this point to address the possible role of ongoing stress and anxiety, because it bears on the patient's sense of security about whether the improvement will last and whether psychosocial issues need to be dealt with more directly. It often is also valuable to have significant others join the patient and clinician.* This is an opportunity to

establish that the improved speech can be maintained with familiar people. In many cases it is also appropriate to review with the patient and significant others the dynamics of the problem and its resolution. This is particularly valuable for patients who may have difficulty explaining these things to others on their own.

Addressing the Future

When speech assessment and subsequent symptomatic therapy are complete, the future should be addressed. In general, discussion should address (1) the likelihood that speech will remain normal or return to normal, (2) the need to address directly the psychologic issues, if any, that were or are related to the speech problem, and (3) how to explain the problem and its resolution to others. There are multiple permutations of these issues that may need to be addressed. The following scenarios provide some examples:

1. When symptomatic therapy results in a return of normal speech that is maintained with ease, the clinician should establish how the patient feels he or she will do in the future relative to speech. Many believe that speech will remain normal without future symptomatic help. In most instances, this will be correct. If triggering or maintaining psychogenic factors have been identified by the patient, if their role in the speech problem is understood, and if the factors seem no longer to be active, it helps to review the sequence of events from onset to symptom resolution and discuss how the patient thinks he or she will deal with similar issues in the future. Addressing directly whether the patient feels a need for professional counseling regarding his or her manner of dealing with stress or conflict or the specific events that triggered the speech problem is important, not necessarily because this will lead to an immediate decision to pursue psychiatric help, but at least to establish if such counseling may be of benefit in the future.

   It is often valuable to discuss concerns about how to explain the problem and its resolution to others and others' likely response to such explanations. If significant others are available, the clinician often should assist in this explanation. At the least, the patient should leave with a plan for talking with others about his or her speech problem and its resolution and for dealing with similar psychosocial stresses and conflicts in the future.

2. When symptomatic therapy results in a return of normal speech that the patient is main-

---

*It is the author's bias, admittedly not held by all clinicians, that the initial history, examination, and treatment of most adults with confirmed or possible neurologic or nonorganic speech disorders should be conducted between the clinician and patient alone, regardless of the severity of deficits. It is a way to acknowledge the patient's independence, privacy, and competence and permits interaction and assessment of the patient's abilities and disabilities free of possible assistance, interference, or inhibition by others.

taining with ease, but psychosocial factors that could be related to the problem have not been identified, the future is less certain. This situation occurs quite frequently. The clinician may be left to speculate about the significance of what is known from the history or to conclude that the reasons for the problem are uncertain, but that it is clear there are no physical barriers to maintaining normal speech. Reviewing the general role of stress and conflict in producing speech disorders may help some patients be more attuned to the effects of psychosocial factors in the future, although this will not necessarily be the outcome for people whose basic insight into their feelings is superficial.

3. When symptomatic therapy fails to produce any change in speech, but the clinician believes that continuing therapy will be beneficial because of the patient's motivation to improve, then further sessions should be scheduled. When underlying psychologic explanations for the problem have not been identified, it is also valuable to ask the patient to review in the interim the stresses and conflicts with which he or she is currently dealing, especially those that were also active at the time the speech problem began. This review should be discussed during the next session.

4. When the patient has failed to improve, but salient psychosocial issues have been identified, the need to pursue psychiatric or psychologic evaluation and counseling should be addressed. Sometimes the issues are volatile, pervasive, and profound and sometimes previously have not been apparent to the patient. Sometimes the patient has been aware of them but has minimized their importance until it has become apparent that they are affecting his or her physical well being. These patients often accept a referral for counseling. Symptomatic therapy can be conducted concurrently with psychiatric counseling, but sometimes it should be deferred until counseling is under way and it is clear that speech is not improving. For some, a multidisciplinary approach to management (e.g., psychiatry, pain management, speech pathology, physical therapy) is most appropriate and effective.[17]

5. When symptomatic therapy has not succeeded, when psychologic difficulties are denied, and when the patient insists on the organicity of his or her problem, it is unlikely that a referral for psychiatric consultation will be accepted. Nonetheless, if the clinician is confident that the speech problem is not organic, he or she can explain to the patient that nonorganic factors may be at work and that discussing their psychologic history with a specialist would be of value to leaving no stone unturned in efforts to get to the bottom of the problem. Many of these patients are unlikely to respond to further symptomatic therapy unless they express an acceptance of the possibility that causal organic (or nonorganic) factors are no longer active and that it may be possible to resolve the problem symptomatically.

◼ SYMPTOMATIC TREATMENT FOR SPECIFIC PSYCHOGENIC SPEECH DISORDERS

The general principles, guidelines, and techniques that have just been discussed probably apply equally well to the broad range of symptoms that characterize psychogenic/nonorganic speech disorders. Differences in management probably vary more as a function of patients' past and current psychosocial and medical status and their insight, readiness, and manner of responding during evaluation and treatment than to differences in abnormal speech characteristics. The differences that do exist in management among these speech disorders seem to lie mostly in some of the symptomatic techniques that are used. In the remainder of this chapter some techniques that are successful during symptomatic treatment for different types of psychogenic/nonorganic speech symptoms are reviewed. The review, although neither exhaustive nor prescriptive, will hopefully convey the theme that characterizes symptomatic treatment.

Psychogenic Voice Disorders

Psychogenic voice disorders are usually characterized by aphonia, hoarseness, or spasmodic dysphonia. The theme that runs through the manner of voice production in these patients is one of *excessive musculoskeletal tension* or *vocal hyperfunction*.[2] The goal of treatment is to reduce that tension because then the voice usually returns to normal. When the tension is not released psychologically or when psychologic tension is no longer the factor that is maintaining the voice disorder, symptomatic reduction of musculoskeletal tension can be effective. A general outline of steps that are useful in accomplishing this follows*:

1. People suspected of having a psychogenic voice disorder should be examined for laryngeal musculoskeletal tension. This is most readily detected by placing the thumb and

---

*A more detailed description of this approach to treating psychogenic voice disorders can be found in Aronson,[2] Case,[10] and Stemple.[26]

index or middle finger in the thyrohyoid space and determining if that space is narrower than normal (Figure 20-1) or if the patient experiences discomfort or pain with digital pressure or gentle kneading in the area. Normal speakers and people without excessive musculoskeletal tension feel pressure but not discomfort or pain. Many patients with psychogenic voice disorders will respond with pain or discomfort. Even when they do not, the steps that follow often are successful.

2. The patient can be told that his or her discomfort reflects excessive musculoskeletal tension and that the tension is a significant contributor to his or her abnormal voice. If psychosocial explanations have already been uncovered, it helps to indicate that muscular tension represents a response to those factors. If not, it usually suffices to indicate that the tension does not represent an irreversible or uncontrollable muscular abnormality or that the tension represents the patient's great but misdirected physical effort to achieve a normal voice.

3. With gentle kneading of the laryngeal muscles, the height of the larynx in the neck

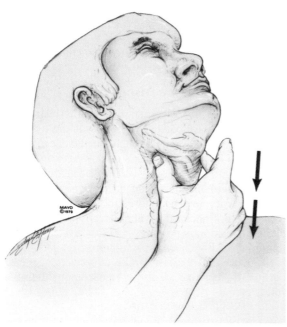

FIGURE 20-1 Placement of fingers in the thyrohyoid space for examination of musculoskeletal tension and for maneuvering the larynx to a lower position in the neck during symptomatic therapy. (From Aronson AE: *Clinical voice disorders,* New York, 1990, Thieme. With permission.)

should lower (the thyrohyoid space should become less narrow) and the laryngeal cartilages should become looser. Patients sometimes protest because of the discomfort, but they should be reassured that this is temporary and necessary to relax muscles.

4. During efforts to reduce musculoskeletal tension, the patient should be asked to produce some lax vowels, a nasal /m/, or a gentle oral or nasal "uh huh." This is often done while manually lowering the thyroid cartilage (see Figure 20-1). Aphonic patients may be asked to clear the throat, grunt, cough gently, or briefly hum and then attempt to prolong the act into a short vowel. The clinician should provide immediate feedback about positive changes in the quality of such productions, because patients are not always aware of them. The clinician should tell the patient that these traces of normal voice establish the capacity for normal phonation and that there is no barrier present to prevent further improvement. When voice is reliably achieved, the patient should attempt to produce the improved voice without physical assistance from the clinician.

The goal of these efforts is to elicit even a brief trace of improved or normal voice so that it may be shaped toward normal quality or extended to lengthier utterances. These efforts sometimes succeed rapidly, but they may take an extended period of time that is physically demanding of both clinician and patient. Much of the efforts are trial and error and require the clinician to take advantage of accidental or unplanned voice improvements; the clinician should use whatever works during this step and drop whatever fails.[2]

5. Once a brief but relatively normal voice can be achieved reliably, the patient should be asked to prolong a vowel or /m/ or to reflexively answer some yes-no questions with an appropriately inflected oral or nasal "uh huh" or "uh." Voiced phrases such as "one Monday morning" may then be attempted. Manual lowering of the larynx may continue or be reintroduced at this point, with a goal of fading it as soon as possible. The patient should be asked to feel as well as listen to his or her voice and to note how much easier it is to produce voice under these conditions than with the degree of tension that had been exhibited earlier.

6. Patients who can produce short phrases or count with the improved voice should be asked to read a paragraph. They should be stopped and assisted by verbal instruction or

manual assistance in regaining normal voice if they slip back to their previous pattern. They can then be asked to "play with" the voice, as if reading to entertain. When successful, they should then be engaged in casual conversation that may begin with basic biographic and factual information, proceed to narratives, and finally to a discussion of their feelings about their improved voice, explanations for the improvement and causes for the problem, prognosis, the future relative to their voice and psychosocial issues, and so on. In most cases the improved voice will be maintained without effort and may improve further during conversation. This should be pointed out so that patients recognize their control over the voice. Some patients will comment about how much easier it is to speak, whereas others will note that it feels odd or that the neck is sore from laryngeal manipulation. They can be reassured that any soreness will not persist.

The rate of improvement in response to this kind of symptomatic therapy varies. If the problem was due to musculoskeletal tension alone, if it was not present for long, or if underlying psychologic triggers are no longer active, normal voice is sometimes achieved in minutes. Stemple[26] suggests that the average time frame for achieving normal voice is 30 to 45 minutes, but some patients may require a few sessions.[2,8] Most who benefit go through various stages of dysphonia as improvement occurs, rather than making a sudden jump from baseline to normal voice.

Regarding efficacy, Aronson[2] notes that "the majority of patients can be helped considerably, if not completely, within that time [a single session]. Patients whose voices fail to improve . . . may not be ready to relinquish the abnormal voice because of musculoskeletal tension secondary to conversion reaction." Similarly, Boone[8] indicates that symptomatic therapy is usually effective in restoring normal voice and that the normal voice usually remains.

The presence of neurologic disease does not preclude the effectiveness of symptomatic therapy. Sapir and Aronson[25] reported two cases with aphonia and evidence of associated laryngeal musculoskeletal tension following closed head injury whose voices returned to normal in one or two sessions of symptomatic therapy. Similarly, Sapir and Aronson[24] discussed a patient with a psychogenic strained voice plus a unilateral upper motor neuron dysarthria from stroke. They also examined a patient with a severely breathy voice exceeding that expected for a postsurgical vocal fold paralysis. Both patients' voices improved rapidly with symptomatic treatment. They also discussed two additional patients, one with

organic voice tremor and hoarseness and another with myasthenia gravis and a strained dysphonia, whose voices improved markedly during discussion of psychosocial concerns and fears they had about physical illness. These cases highlight the role of psychologic mechanisms in some dysphonias that develop in people with organic illness, as well as the responsiveness of at least some of these patients to methods that are effective for those with psychogenic voice disorders but no organic illness.

Chewing therapy, progressive relaxation, and biofeedback approaches are other symptomatic treatments that can be used.[2,10,23] Some patients also may respond to methods of psychiatry that are sometimes effective for treating conversion and anxiety-induced disorders, such as counseling, minor tranquilizers, hypnosis, and sodium amobarbital (Amytal) interview. Some have spontaneous remission of their symptoms.[23,27,30]

Psychogenic Stuttering

The speech characteristics of psychogenic stuttering (PS) are highly variable but usually include sound/syllable/word repetitions, prolongations, hesitations, and blocking that are frequently accompanied by secondary struggle behavior such as facial grimacing. These and other characteristics were discussed in Chapter 14.

Relatively little is known about the management of PS. The literature contains few reports that focus on its management, but the general principles, guidelines, and techniques that have already been discussed are probably applicable. The symptomatic management of PS can be quite effective, possibly as often and as rapidly as it is for psychogenic voice disorders.

Similar to psychogenic voice disorders, the dysfluencies of PS are *often associated with excessive musculoskeletal tension in speech and sometimes nonspeech muscles.* Therefore an important and sometimes crucial goal of symptomatic therapy is to reduce musculoskeletal tension, because then fluency often normalizes. Because of this, many of the techniques that were described for reducing musculoskeletal tension in people with psychogenic voice disorders can be applied to people with PS. In fact, in some people with PS the focus of tension reduction may also be on the larynx, in which case the exact same techniques may be applied. The following steps summarize some techniques that seem to be effective in the symptomatic treatment of PS.

1. People suspected of having PS should be observed for evidence of excessive musculoskeletal tension in speech and nonspeech muscles. When phonation is perceived as effortful, the larynx may be examined in the

same way described for psychogenic voice disorders. The jaw, face, and eyes also should be observed for evidence of exaggerated movement or excessive contraction. Excessive neck flexion or extension may occur during speech, as may secondary movements or muscle tightness in the shoulders, torso, arms, or legs. If multiple loci of increased tension are apparent, those structures that can be manipulated by the clinician should be identified; they may become the initial focus of symptom reduction.

2. The patient often can be told that his or her dysfluencies at least partially reflect excessive musculoskeletal tension generated by his or her efforts to speak. The patient can also be told that this effort is actually preventing normal speech, that it does not represent an irreversible or uncontrollable abnormality, and that it can be brought under control.

3. The clinician should select a high-frequency and high-amplitude abnormal behavior for modification, preferably one associated with tension in muscles that can be touched or manipulated. The muscle tension during speech should be pointed out to the patient (e.g., neck extension, lower face retraction, eye closing, arm movements). The patient should then be asked to identify the behavior when it occurs, with reinforcement provided for accurate identification. If laryngeal muscle tension is chosen, the steps for treating psychogenic voice disorders can then be followed.

4. The patient should be asked to speak without abnormal movement or excessive tension in the selected structure (e.g., without excessive lower face retraction, eye closing, or neck extension). It may be necessary to begin with the production of single sounds, such as vowel prolongation. It may help for the clinician to touch the structure of focus during these initial attempts in order to focus attention and provide a source of feedback. Patients may benefit from being told to do something different than what they have been doing, even if it is not part of normal motor behavior. For example, a patient who abnormally retracts the lips when speaking may be told to open the eyes widely instead; these alternative behaviors (that probably serve as distracters) usually can be faded quickly once the target behavior changes.

5. When a sound can be prolonged without excessive muscle tension, the patient should produce some single words, with reinforcement for doing so without tension in the target structure and without dysfluencies. Adopting a slow, prolonged rate may help patients whose dysfluencies are characterized by hesitation and repetition. The patient should be reminded frequently about his or her success in reducing muscle tension and modifying dysfluencies. Sentence repetition and reading then can be pursued using similar strategies.

Some patients who have difficulty reducing dysfluencies benefit from learning to be dysfluent in a different way. For example, if PS is characterized by repetitions, the patient may be asked instead to prolong all syllables rather than repeat; if he or she hesitates before initiating each word or phrase, the patient can be told to "never stop" by using continuous voicing and not pausing at phrase boundaries. Once the pattern of baseline dysfluencies has been altered, these alternative abnormalities usually can be faded quickly.

6. When excessive tension, abnormal movements, and dysfluencies arising from a single structure have been modified, it frequently is the case that all musculoskeletal tension and dysfluencies begin to decrease. This should be pointed out to the patient. When this does not occur, the remaining abnormalities should be attacked with the same strategies. Any return of musculoskeletal tension or dysfluencies should be pointed out immediately and modified.

7. As dysfluencies are reduced, the patient may maintain a slow rate with flattened prosody. If so, he or she should be asked to "play with" speech during reading, as if to entertain. When successful, the patient should then engage in conversation. Most patients who have moved rapidly to this point continue to improve during conversation.

Like psychogenic voice disorders, rate of improvement varies, with many patients dramatically improving in less than an hour and others requiring several sessions. Most go through a gradual reduction of dysfluency, rather than making a sudden jump from their baseline behavior to fluency.

A number of clinical reports provide support for the efficacy of behavioral management of PS in people without, as well as those with, neurologic disease. As discussed in Chapter 14, Baumgartner and Duffy's[6] retrospective study of 49 cases with PS in the absence of neurologic disease established that among the patients in the group who were treated symptomatically with methods similar to those just described, 48% improved to normal in one or two sessions, often including during the diagnostic evaluation; another 29% improved nearly to normal; and 19% showed some improvement. Similarly, in their review of 20 patients with PS who did have evidence of neurologic disease, of the 55% of the cases who were treated, 45% improved to normal in one or two sessions, often including during the diagnostic evaluation; another 18% improved nearly to normal; and 18% showed some improvement. Thus symptomatic treatment was quite successful, sometimes dramatically so, and success was often achieved rapidly, even in people with neurologic disease.*

Several case studies also illustrate the duration, specific techniques, and efficacy of symptomatic treatment. Mahr and Leith[18] discussed four cases of adult-onset PS associated with probable conversion disorder. One person improved to normal after 9 months of twice-weekly sessions that focused on careful articulation and slow production of speech. Another improved within minutes when instructed to reduce rate and articulate clearly. Another whose PS began during the process of divorce improved when instructed to speak slowly and finally normalized when the person accepted the marriage's termination. A fourth individual failed to improve after $2\frac{1}{2}$ years of symptomatic therapy three times a week.

Duffy[13] detailed a case of PS without neurologic disease in which speech became normal during a diagnostic session that addressed contributing psychosocial issues and symptomatic treatment. The report also noted the importance of interdisciplinary contributions to management. That is, follow-up psychiatric evaluation and completion of comprehensive neurologic and medical examinations were essential to the overall management of the patient's psychologic difficulties.

Roth, Aronson, and Davis[21] summarized in detail 12 cases of PS without neurologic disease (most of whom were included in Baumgartner and Duffy's[6] retrospective study). Eleven of the 12 cases

improved, 5 in response to symptomatic speech therapy, 1 during group psychotherapy, 1 during a discussion of events surrounding the onset of the problem, and 4 spontaneously. Symptomatic treatment included "traditional techniques" such as easy onset of voicing, light touch articulation, or bouncing during blocking or struggle.

Brookshire[9] reported a case in which stuttering was considered at least partially psychogenic in origin, even though it began several months after a stroke. The patient did not improve significantly during 21 sessions of a commercially available relaxation program but responded dramatically within a single session to a behavior modification program that focused on decreasing muscle tension that preceded dysfluencies. It was concluded that placing contingencies on behaviors that precede dysfluent speech could produce dramatic and durable effects. The patient remained fluent during 8 years of follow-up.

Two additional case reports suggest that PS can respond favorably to techniques that often modify developmental stuttering. Tippett and Siebens[29] summarized speech therapy for a man with anoxic encephalopathy, weakness and spasticity, depression, and pseudoseizures (psychogenic seizures). His stuttering began to improve during an initial treatment session that emphasized rhythmic speaking techniques, became normally fluent without rhythmic speaking during 2 weeks of therapy, and was maintained at 3-month follow-up. Deal[12] reported on a patient whose dysfluencies began after a suicide attempt. He became increasingly fluent over the course of approximately 7 weeks in a treatment program that initially used delayed auditory feedback; he concurrently participated in group psychotherapy. Fluency was normal at follow-up 2 months later.

Other Psychogenic Speech Disorders

As noted in Chapter 14, psychogenic speech disorders can express themselves in ways that are less conventional than disturbances of voice or fluency. If the Mayo Clinic experience is an accurate reflection of the frequency with which such problems are encountered in speech pathology practices, however, they represent less than 10% of psychogenic speech disorders (see Table 14-1). These unusual problems most often reflect abnormalities in articulation, resonance, and prosody. The literature on their symptomatic management by speech pathologists is nearly nonexistent. The following guidelines for the management of these problems seem reasonable and have been effective for some patients in the author's clinical practice.

---

*These success rates may not be representative of those for the population with PS. They apply only to patients treated in a large tertiary care center, and there may be features of such patients that could make effective treatment outcome rates higher or lower for them than for the population as a whole. More important, perhaps, is the fact that only about half of the patients in Baumgartner and Duffy's review were treated; the reasons for not pursuing treatment in untreated cases were highly diverse or unclear but sometimes due to patient resistance to treatment or to the clinician's belief that treatment was inappropriate or unlikely to be effective at that time. The rates of treatment success are, nonetheless, impressive.

1. Psychogenic articulation, resonance, and prosodic disturbances probably reflect psychodynamic mechanisms like those that lead to psychogenic voice and fluency disorders. Thus the different symptoms probably represent different routes of expression that are determined by factors such as somatic compliance, secondary gain, notions about and experiences with illness and speech disorders, and, possibly, differences in the symbolic meaning of various symptoms. If this is true, then the general principles, guidelines, and techniques for management that have already been discussed should apply to people with these unusual symptoms. Differences in management, therefore, are mostly related to specific symptomatic techniques.

2. When psychogenic articulation, resonance, or prosodic disorders are accompanied by excessive musculoskeletal tension, the reduction of such tension should be undertaken in a manner similar to that described for psychogenic voice and stuttering problems. However, *musculoskeletal tension may not be a primary feature of these disorders.*

3. Psychogenic articulation disorders often seem characterized by substitution or distortion of specific sounds (e.g., w/r, w/l, all sounds produced with lingual retraction) rather than general imprecision. In this case, it seems reasonable to employ "traditional" articulation therapy techniques for their modification.

4. Psychogenic hypernasality, particularly when somatic compliance and conversion reaction mechanisms seem to be at work, may respond to "traditional" approaches to modifying articulation and resonance in people with organic velopharyngeal insufficiency.

5. Psychogenic prosodic disturbances can be quite variable. Because they may be accompanied by abnormalities in fluency, articulation, and even resonance, it may be best to focus on modification of fluency, articulation, or resonance because they are more easily localized to specific muscles and structures, making it simpler to focus symptomatic efforts. When the prosodic disturbance resembles that of a foreign accent, techniques for modifying foreign accent or neurogenic pseudoforeign accent (see Chapter 19) may be appropriate. When the prosodic disturbance conveys an impression of infantile speech or abnormally high pitch, "developmental" articulation errors that may be more modifiable than the abnormal prosodic pattern often accompany it. Similarly, people with psychogenic stuttering sometimes also have infantile speech characteristics; modifying the dysfluencies often results in a simultaneous spontaneous resolution of the infantile pattern of articulation and prosody.

When an infantile speech pattern is accompanied by prominent infantile affective behavior, the patient often denies speech difficulty and is incapable of interacting as an adult. It is not likely that he or she will respond to symptomatic efforts to modify this speech pattern, at least without concurrent psychiatric treatment.

6. People with psychogenic (conversion) mutism are quite similar in personality traits and histories to those with conversion aphonia and dysphonias[4] and may exhibit other psychogenic voice or fluency problems as they emerge from their mute state.[2] In general, they seem to respond well to symptomatic treatment techniques that are effective for people with psychogenic aphonia and dysphonia, including the physical techniques that are effective in reducing musculoskeletal tension.

SUMMARY

1. People with psychogenic/nonorganic speech disorders that are associated with conversion disorder or responses to life stresses often respond to treatment provided by a speech pathologist. Symptom resolution with speech therapy can be achieved for some patients before psychiatric evaluation, and psychiatric referral is not always necessary. The prognosis for recovery from psychogenic speech disorders is generally good.

2. Management usually requires that speech symptoms, as well as the explanations for their existence, be addressed with the patient. In many cases, treatment should be initiated within the diagnostic session.

3. The clinician's attitude and manner of interacting with the patient are crucial to management. Empathy, compassion, respect, honesty, confidence, and assertiveness are as important to competent, effective, and caring treatment for people with psychogenic speech disorders as they are to the management of MSDs.

4. When symptomatic therapy is successful, it is usually important to address the mechanisms that may explain the improvement, as well as the possible need for psychiatric referral.

5. Not all people with psychogenic speech disorders wish or are ready to be helped, and not all can be helped by speech therapy.

6. Therapy is best conducted following completion of all relevant medical evaluations.

7. The psychosocial history is crucial to both diagnosis and management. Symptomatic treatment usually involves the identification of abnormal behaviors and the gradual behavioral shaping of more normal speech responses with continuous explanation and reinforcement for change. Physical contact may be important to the success of symptomatic therapy.

8. Symptomatic therapy for psychogenic voice disorders (including mutism) and psychogenic stuttering often involves efforts to reduce excessive musculoskeletal tension and the gradual shaping of normal phonation and fluency. A high proportion of patients with psychogenic voice disorders and stuttering respond well to symptomatic therapy, many of them during the diagnostic encounter or within one or two treatment sessions.

9. Little is known about the symptomatic treatment of infrequently occurring psychogenic disorders of articulation, resonance, and prosody, but it is likely that the principles, guidelines, and techniques that seem important to managing psychogenic voice and stuttering disorders are applicable to them. The need to reduce musculoskeletal tension may not be as pervasive in patients with them, however, and symptomatic therapy may employ traditional techniques for modifying articulation, resonance, and prosody.

References

1. Andersson K, Schaléen L: Etiology and treatment of psychogenic voice disorder: results of a follow-up study of thirty patients, J Voice 12:96, 1998.

2. Aronson AE: Clinical voice disorders, New York, 1990a, Thieme.

3. Aronson AE: Importance of the psychosocial interview in the diagnosis and treatment of "functional" voice disorders, J Voice 4:287, 1990b.

4. Aronson AE, Peterson HW, Litin EM: Psychiatric symptomatology in functional dysphonia and aphonia, J Speech Hear Disord 31:115, 1966.

5. Baker JHE, Silver JR: Hysterical paraplegia, J Neurol Neurosurg Psychiatry 50:375, 1987.

6. Baumgartner J, Duffy JR: Psychogenic stuttering in adults with and without neurologic disease, J Med Speech-Lang Pathol 5:75, 1997.

7. Binzer M, Andersen PM, Kullgren G: Clinical characteristics of patients with motor disability due to conversion disorder: a prospective control group study, J Neurol Neurosurg Psychiatry 63:83, 1997.

8. Boone DR: The voice and voice therapy, Englewood Cliffs, NJ, 1977, Prentice-Hall.

9. Brookshire RH: A dramatic response to behavior modification by a patient with rapid onset of dysfluent speech. In Helm-Estabrooks N, Aten JL, editors: Difficult diagnoses in communication disorders, Boston, 1989, College-Hill Press.

10. Case JL: Clinical management of voice disorders, ed 2, Austin, Tex, 1991, Pro-Ed.

11. Chabolla DR et al: Psychogenic nonepileptic seizures, Mayo Clin Proc 71:493, 1996.

12. Deal JL: Sudden onset of stuttering: a case report, J Speech Hear Disord 47:301, 1982.

13. Duffy JR: A puzzling case of adult onset stuttering. In Helm-Estabrooks N, Aten JL, editors: Difficult diagnoses in communication disorders, Boston, 1989, College-Hill Press.

14. Ford CV, Folks DG: Conversion disorders: an overview, Psychosomatics 26:371, 1985.

15. Head H: An address on the diagnosis of hysteria, BMJ 1:827, 1922.

16. Lazare A: Current concepts in psychiatry: conversion symptoms, N Engl J Med 305:745, 1981.

17. Mahr G: Psychogenic communication disorders. In Johnson AF, Jacobson BH, editors: Medical speech-language pathology: a practitioner's guide, New York, 1998, Thieme.

18. Mahr G, Leith W: Psychogenic stuttering of adult onset, J Speech Hear Res 35:283, 1992.

19. Nemiah JC: Psychoneurotic disorders. In Nicholi AM, editor: The new Harvard guide to psychiatry, Cambridge, Mass, 1988, Belknap Press of Harvard University.

20. Ron MA: Somatization and conversion disorders. In Fogel BS, Schiffer RB, editors: Neuropsychiatry, Philadelphia, 1996, Williams & Wilkins.

21. Roth CR, Aronson AE, Davis LJ: Clinical studies in psychogenic stuttering of adult onset, J Speech Hear Disord 54:634, 1989.

22. Roy N, Bless DM, Heisey D: Personality and voice disorders: a superfactor trait analysis, J Speech Lang Hear Res 43:749, 2000.

23. Sapir S, Aronson AE: The relationship between psychopathology and speech and language disorders in neurologic patients, J Speech Hear Disord 55:503, 1990.

24. Sapir S, Aronson AE: Coexisting psychogenic and neurogenic dysphonia: a source of diagnostic confusion, Br J Disord Commun 22:73, 1987.

25. Sapir S, Aronson AE: Aphonia after closed head injury: aetiologic considerations, Br J Disord Commun 20:289, 1985.

26. Stemple JC: Voice therapy: clinical studies, St Louis, 1993, Mosby.

27. Stoudemire GA: Somatoform disorders, factitious disorders, and malingering. In Talbott JA, Hales RE, Yudofsky SC, editors: Textbook of psychiatry, Washington, DC, 1988, American Psychiatric Press.

28. Teitelbaum ML, McHugh PR: Psychiatric conditions presenting as neurologic disease. In Johnson RT, editor: Current therapy in neurologic disease, ed 3, Philadelphia, 1990, BC Decker.

29. Tippett DC, Siebens AA: Distinguishing psychogenic from neurogenic dysfluency when neurologic and psychologic factors coexist, J Fluency Disord 16:3, 1991.

30. Tomb DA: Psychiatry for the house officer, Baltimore, 1981, Williams & Wilkins.

31. Tucker GJ: Dealing with patients who have medically unexplained symptoms, Continuum 3:25, 1997.

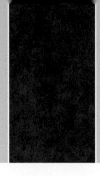

Index

A

Abdominal muscles
  and respiration, 84-85
  role in forced exhalation, 43
Abdominal trussing, 467
Abducens nerves
  anatomic origin and function of, 22t
Abductor spasmodic dysphonia, 244
Abscess formation
  with CNS inflammatory diseases, 33
Abulia
  definition and features of
    and mutism, 343-344
  distinguishing characteristics of
    versus other speech disturbances, 426t,
      428-429
  due to vascular disturbances, 26t
Accessory muscles
  of respiration, 43
Accessory nerves
  anatomic origin and function of, 22t
  bones associated with, 19f
  description of, 43
  diagram illustrating, 25f, 40f
  lesions
    associated with flaccid dysarthrias, 127
  and UMN innervation, 48t
Accuracy
  of speech, 72-73
Acetylcholine
  actions of, 30f
  definition of, 29
  functions of, 53
  imbalance with dopamine
    and Parkinson's disease, 191
  implicated in myasthenia gravis, 24-25
  as part of neurochemical system, 24
Acoustic analyses
  of motor speech disorders, 10
  of vocal fold activity, 84
Acoustic nerves
  anatomical diagram of, 25f
  control circuit influences on, 62
Acoustic neuroma
  causing facial paralysis, 121
Acquired communication disorders
  distribution of, 4f
Acquired immunodeficiency syndrome (AIDS)
  causing chorea, 224
  causing flaccid dysarthrias, 114-115
  causing parkinsonism, 192
  types of dysarthrias caused by
    and differential diagnoses, 414t
Acquired neurogenic mutism
  akinetic, 343-344
  and anarthria, 336-338
  and apraxia of speech, 336t, 341-342
  and biopercular syndrome, 336t, 339-340
  case studies, 346-349
  and cerebellar mutism, 336t, 340-341
  of cerebellar origin, 340-341
  definition and overview of, 335-336
  following corpus callosotomy, 345
  forms of, 335, 336t
  and locked-in syndrome, 336t, 338-339
  motor speech disorders associated with
    localization and clinical features of, 336t
  and speech arrest, 345
  with supplemental motor area damage, 61

Acquired neurologic communication disorders
  distribution of, 8f
Acquired psychogenic speech disorders
  case studies, 397-405
  definition and overview of, 381-382
  distinguishing between neurogenic, 426t,
    428-429, 430t
  etiologies of
    conversion disorders, 383-385
    depression, 382-383
    schizophrenia, 383
    stress and reactions to stress, 385
    volitional disorders, 386
  examination of, 387-388
  management of
    general principles and guidelines, 536-541
    general treatment techniques, 541-545
    symptomatic treatment of specific, 545-550
  other nonorganic disorders associated with
    articulation disorders, 395
    infantile speech, 396
    psychogenic mutism, 396
    resonance and prosodic disorders, 396
  speech characteristics, 389-396
    with depression and manic-depression, 389
    dysfluencies, 394b
    with psychogenic stuttering, 392-395
    with psychogenic voice disorders, 390-392
    with schizophrenia, 389-390
Action myoclonus (AM)
  characteristics of, 237-238
  definition of, 220
Action tremors
  definition of, 221
  examining motor speech, 72
"Acute"
  descriptive of disease development, 33
Adductor spasmodic dysphonia, 243-244, 469-
  470, 491-493
Aerodynamic measures
  to study motor speech disorders, 10
Affective disorders
  associated with CNS lesions, 360b, 361
  management of, 529
  causing mutism, 333, 336t, 342-343
Afferent fibers
  in direct activation pathway, 47-48
  within sensory system, 27
  types of, 30
Afferent nerves
  within visceral system, 24
Afferent pathways
  in sensory system, 36
Aging
  changes of speech with, 7
  and depression, 383
  and unilateral upper motor neuron (UUMN)
    dysarthria, 264
  as variable at onset of MSDs, 12
Airway compromise
  with vagus nerve damage, 126
Akinesia
  with bradykinesia, 188-189
  examples of, 189t
Akinetic mutism
  definition and features of, 26t, 343-344
  distinguishing among mutism forms
    and differential diagnosis, 424t, 425
  due to vascular disturbances, 26t

Alcohol
  withdrawal from
    causing chorea, 223
    causing temporary parkinsonism, 192
Alcoholism
  causing ataxic dysarthria, 168-169
Alexia without agraphia
  due to vascular disturbances, 26t
Alpha motor neurons
  movement and origins of, 37
Alphabet board supplementation, 482
Alternate motion rates (AMRs)
  with apraxia of speech, 318b, 319-320,
    322b
  characteristics of, 89, 90b
  defects with UUMN dysarthria, 263b, 264t
  definition of, 92
  examples of, 165
  illustrating ataxic dysarthria, 173f
  of jaws, 79, 80f, 81
  slow rates of
    with ataxic dysarthria, 173f, 177
  statistics
    for normal adults, 93t
  tracings
    with hypokinetic dysarthria, 195f
    of speech, 154f
Alzheimer's disease
  associated with primary progressive aphasia,
    311
  and depression, 383
  and echolalia, 359, 360b
  neurofibrillary degeneration with, 31
  neurofibrillary tangles in, 33
  causing palilalia, 258b, 359
  possibly leading to mutism, 338
  and speech disorders, 25
  types of dysarthrias caused by
    and differential diagnoses, 413t
Amantadine
  for Parkinson's disease, 191
Amino acids
  as part of neurochemical system, 24
Amphetamines
  causing dyskinesias, 222
Amyloid
  and dementia, 31
Amyotrophic lateral sclerosis (ALS)
  associated with mixed dysarthria, 276-277,
    281t, 285-289
  associated with primary progressive aphasia,
    311, 314b
  as degenerative disease, 12
  causing flaccid dysarthrias, 111-112
  leading to mutism, 337t, 338
  Mayo Clinic dysarthria studies on, 89
  physiologic and acoustic characteristics of,
    286-289
  speech impairment statistics with, 7
  types of dysarthrias caused by
    differential diagnoses of, 413t
Anarthria
  definition and clinical characteristics of,
    336-337
  differential diagnoses of, 423, 424t
  distinguishing among mutism forms
    and differential diagnosis, 423, 424t
  due to vascular disturbances, 26t-27t
  and mutism, 336-338

Anatomic levels
  and differential diagnoses, 411-419
  relationships between nervous system, 21t
    and motor speech disorders, 21t
Anatomic malformations
  and differential diagnoses, 412, 413t-414t,
    415
  distribution and types of, 4f
  causing flaccid dysarthria, 112b
Aneurysms
  definition of, 35
  types of dysarthrias caused by
    and differential diagnoses, 413t
Annulospiral endings, 38
Anoxia
  types of dysarthrias caused by
    and differential diagnoses, 413t
Anoxic encephalopathy, 238, 338
Anterior cerebral arteries
  anatomical location of, 24f, 25f
  function of, 23
Anterior communicating arteries
  anatomical location of, 24f, 25f
  function of, 22
Anterior fossae
  anatomical relationships with
    and motor speech disorders, 21t
  definition of, 18
  illustration of, 19f
Anterior limb
  of internal capsule, 47-48
Anterior lobes
  definition and location of, 54, 55
Anterior spinal arteries
  anatomical diagram of, 25f
Anterocollis, 221
Anticholinergic drugs
  for PD resting tremor
Anticonvulsants
  causing ataxic dysarthria, 169
Antiemetic medications
  leading to parkinsonism, 191-192
Antipsychotic drugs
  affecting neurotransmitter balance
    and causing hyperkinetic dysarthria,
    222-223
  leading to parkinsonism, 191-192
  orofacial dyskinesias due to, 220
Aortic arch
  blood vessels rising from, 23
Apallic state
  and mutism, 336t, 343
Aphasia
  versus apraxia of speech, 312
  distinguishing among dysfluencies associated
    with, 425t, 426-428
  distinguishing among mutism forms
    and differential diagnosis, 424t, 425
  distinguishing from apraxia of speech,
    421-423, 422t
  distinguishing from dysarthria, 421, 422t
  distribution statistics, 8f
  due to vascular disturbances, 26t
  language-related, 362-363
  management of, 529
  causing mutism, 333, 336t
  with sensorimotor impairment, 422
  signs of, 59
  study of, 4
  types of, 4f
Aphasic phonologic impairments, 312
Aphaxia of speech (AOS)
  differential diagnosis of
    as function of etiologies, 413t-414t
Aphemia, 312
Aphonia
  inertial, 392
  motor system disorders associated with
    summary to aid differential diagnosis, 417,
    418t
  with vagus nerve lesions, 126
Apneustic breathing, 44
Apneustic center, 44f
Appendicular ataxia, 167-168

Apraxia of phonation
  with apraxia of speech, 320, 322b
Apraxia of speech (AOS)
  acoustic and physiologic findings with
    articulation, 322b, 323-324
    fluency, 322b, 323-324
    nonspeech motor control, 322b
    prosody, 320, 322b, 323-324
    and speech rate, 321-323, 322b
    stress, 322b, 323-324
    summary of, 322b
    variability, 322b, 324
    and voice onset time (VOT), 321, 322b
  anatomical relationships associated with, 21t
  anatomy and functions
    and motor speech programming, 308-310
  behavioral management
    approaches, 514-521
    baseline data and motor learning, 511-512
    principles and guidelines, 510-514
  case studies, 325-330
  characteristics of, 310, 320b
  clinical findings with, 316-325
  with corticobasal degeneration (CBD), 292-
    293
  definition and overview of, 307-308
  definition of, 5-6
  and depression, 383
  and disrupted auditory feedback, 317
  distinctions among dysfluencies associated
    with, 425t, 426
  distinguishing among mutism forms
    and differential diagnosis, 424-425
  distinguishing from aphasia, 421-423, 422t
  distinguishing from dysarthrias
    anatomic and vascular distribution, 419
    etiologies, 413t-414t, 419
    oral mechanism finding, 416t, 419-420
    speech characteristics, 418t, 420-421
  distribution statistics, 8f
  due to dominant hemisphere abnormalities,
    64, 311, 314b
  due to vascular disturbances, 26t
  etiologies of, 311-312, 314-316
    degenerative diseases, 311-312, 314
    pie chart illustrating distribution of, 314t
    stroke, 311, 314-315, 314f
    surgical trauma, 311-312, 314-315, 314b
    tumors and trauma, 311-312, 314-315,
    314b
    vascular diseases, 311, 314-315, 314f
  general perspectives concerning
    management goals and guidelines, 508
    treatment focus and duration, 508-509
  lesion loci and vascular source
    and differential diagnoses, 411, 412t
  localization and neuromotor basis of, 13t
  management approaches to
    behavioral management, 510-518
    medical interventions, 509
    prosthetics, 509-510
  mutism with
    localization and clinical features of, 333,
    336t, 341-342
  published tests for diagnosing, 94, 96
  rate and prosodic characteristics with, 318b,
    319
  and sequential motion rates (SMRs), 93
  speech pathology, 312-313
  symptoms of, 315-316
  tasks for assessing, 95b
  terms that designate, 312b
Aprosodia
  acoustic findings, 368-369
  assessing prosodic production, 365-366
  definition of, 365
  distinctions among other speech disturbances
    aiding differential diagnosis, 426t, 428-429
  management of, 530
  nonspeech characteristics, 369-370
  symptoms of, 367b
Aqueduct of Sylvius
  within cerebrospinal fluid system (CSF), 23
  description and illustration of, 21, 22f

Arachnoid
  description of, 19
  diagram illustrating, 20f
Arachnoid villi, 20f, 21f
  absorbing cerebrospinal fluid, 23
Arcuate
  degeneration of, 168
Arnold-Chiari malformations
  causing flaccid dysarthria, 114
  types of dysarthrias caused by
    and differential diagnoses, 414t, 415
Arteries
  inferior view of, 25f
  supplying the brain, 24f
Arteriovenous malformations (AVMs)
  causing ataxic dysarthria, 168
  definition of, 35
Articulation
  abnormalities
    with hypokinetic dysarthria, 203-205, 206t-
    207t
  acoustic and physiologic findings
    with traumatic brain injuries (TBIs), 294t
  affected by chorea, 229
  affected by cranial nerve damage, 119t-120t
  affected by dystonia, 232
  affected by spinal nerves, 43
  with apraxia of speech (AOS)
    acoustic and physiologic findings with,
    322b, 323-324
  characteristics
    with amyotrophic lateral sclerosis (ALS),
    287t
    with apraxia of speech, 318b, 319, 320
    with ataxic dysarthria, 179t
    with hypokinetic dysarthria, 187
    with spasmodic dysphonia, 244t
  defects
    with UUMN dysarthria, 263b, 264t, 265t,
    266
  impairments
    with spastic dysarthria, 155-156
  imprecise
    with hypoglossal nerve lesions, 128, 129f
  levels affected by ataxic dysarthria, 163
  Mayo Clinic rating scale for, 89, 90b
  with palatopharyngolaryngeal myoclonus,
    237t
  psychogenic disorders of, 395
  with spasmodic torticollis, 235t
  strength training, 477-479
  and supplemental motor areas, 61
  treatment approaches to improve
    for different dysarthria types, 486t
  undershooting
    with hypokinetic dysarthria, 196, 203
Articulatory disorders
  ataxic dysarthria as, 172
Articulatory groping
  motor system disorders associated with
    summary to aid differential diagnosis, 417,
    418t
Articulatory inaccuracy
  with ataxic dysarthria, 173, 175t
Articulatory muscles
  innervating for speech, 3
Articulatory speech valves, 71-72
Articulatory-resonatory incompetence
  with chorea, 229
  with spastic dysarthria, 151
Aryepiglottic folds, 42
Arytenoid adduction surgery, 469
Arytenoid cartilage, 42
Ascending aorta, 24f
Assessment of Intelligibility in Dysarthric
    Speakers (AIDS), 98
Association fiber tracts, 30
Associations
  structure and function of nervous system, 28t
Astrocytes
  as part of blood-brain barrier, 31
  scars formed by, 32
  structure and function of nervous system, 28t
Astrocytomas, 33

Astrocytosis, 32
Astrogliosis, 32
Asymmetric cortical degeneration syndromes, 311, 314b
Ataxia
   due to vascular disturbances, 26t
   and movement, 165
   with vitamin E deficiency, 168
Ataxia telangiectasia, 167-168
Ataxic breathing
   definition of, 44
Ataxic dysarthria, 163-184
   acoustic and physiologic findings, 175-177, 179t
   as articulatory and prosodic disorder, 172
   associated with parkinsonism, 169
   case studies, 180-183
   and cerebellar control circuit damage, 163-183
   and cerebellar disease, 164
   clinical findings with, 171-175
      nonspeech oral mechanism, 171-172
   definition of, 163
   deviant speech characteristics with, 172-175, 173, 175t
   differential diagnosis of
      as function of etiologies, 413t-414t
   due to cerebellar lesions, 57
   due to vascular disturbances, 26t-27t
   etiologies of
      degenerative diseases, 166-168, 170
      distribution pie chart, 166f
      neoplastic diseases, 166f, 168-169, 170
      other causes, 166f, 169-170, 171
      toxic/metabolic conditions, 166f, 169
      trauma, 166f, 169, 170
      vascular diseases, 166f, 168, 170
   lesion loci and vascular source
      and differential diagnoses, 411, 412t
   localization and neuromotor basis of, 13t
   Mayo Clinic dysarthria studies on, 89
   and mixed dysarthria, 283-284
   neuromuscular deficits with, 172, 173t
   slowness of speech with, 173f, 177
   speaker-oriented treatments, 486t-487t, 488
   speech characteristics with, 163, 172, 176t
      summary of, 417, 418t
   subtypes of, 175
   summary of etiologies, 166f, 167b, 170
   summary of oral mechanism findings, 415, 416t
   summary of speech characteristics with, 417, 418t
Ataxic gait, 165
Ataxic hemiparesis
   description of, 258
Ataxic-like dysarthria
   with amyotrophic lateral sclerosis, 286
Atherosclerotic plaque
   description of, 35
   and strokes, 35
Athetosis
   affecting speech steadiness, 72
   description of, 220-221, 232-233
   rate, rhythm, and substrate of, 219t
Atrophy
   definition of muscle, 32
   with flaccid dysarthrias, 110
   with masticatory nucleus lesions, 41
   of muscles with innervation loss, 38
   summary of dysarthrias associated with, 416t
   types of dysarthrias caused by
      and differential diagnoses, 413t
Attention deficits
   due to vascular disturbances, 26t
   with Huntington's disease, 223-224
Attenuation of speech, 360b, 361
Atypical parkinsonian disorders, 191
Audible inspiration
   with flaccid dysarthrias, 133
   motor system disorders associated with
      summary to aid differential diagnosis, 417, 418t

Audible nasal emission
   with vagus nerve lesions, 126
Auditory feedback
   disrupted with apraxia of speech, 317
Auditory nerves
   bones associated with, 19f
Auditory-perceptual assessments
   of speech disorders, 9
Augmentative and alternative communication (AAC), 441, 443-444
Autism
   and echolalia, 359, 360b
Autoimmune diseases;See also acquired immunodeficiency syndrome (AIDS)
   and mixed dysarthria, 280-281, 281t
Autologous fat
   injections, 470
Automatic movements
   affected by flaccid dysarthrias, 110-111
Axonal reactions
   process of, 31
Axons
   function of, 28-29
   illustration of, 29f
   problems and flaccid dysarthria, 109
   of Purkinje cells, 55
   regeneration of, 31
   shearing of
      with diffuse axonal injury, 34

B

Babinski reflex, 144, 257, 310, 317t
Bacillar arteries
   anatomical relationships with
      and motor speech disorders, 21t
   definition and function of, 23
   diagram illustrating, 24f, 25f
   inferior view of, 25f
Bacteria
   clumps of
      and strokes, 35
Balance
   nerves associated with, 22t
Ballism
   rate, rhythm, and substrate of, 219t
Ballismus
   definition of, 220
Balloon cells, 31
Basal ganglia
   anatomical relationships with
      and motor speech disorders, 21t
   components of, 187-188
   diagram illustrating, 48f
   diseases
      clinical signs of hypokinetic dysarthria with, 194-198
   diseases of, 53
   dopaminergic/ cholinergic overactivity in
      and dystonia, 221
   and hyperkinetic dysarthria, 217-244
   influencing gamma motor neurons, 38
   lesions
      and depression, 383
      and parkinsonism, 191
      causing spastic dysarthria, 147b, 148
   location of, 187-188
   motor system involvement in, 27-28
   as neural area of programming, 60
   role in motor speech programming, 310
Basal ganglia control circuits
   associated with hyperkinetic dysarthria
      action myoclonus, 237-238
      athetosis, 232-233
      cervical dystonia, 233-235
      chorea, 227-230
      dystonia, 228t, 230-232, 233f, 234t, 242t
      organic voice tremors, 239-240, 241f, 242t
      palatopharyngolaryngeal myoclonus, 235-237
      spasmodic dysphonia (SD), 240-244
      spasmodic torticollis, 233-235
      Tourette's syndrome/tics, 238-239

Basal ganglia control circuits—cont'd
   associated with hypokinetic dysarthria
      anatomy and basic functions of, 187-188
      clinical characteristics of disorders of, 188-190
      components of, 188
      functions of, 188
      and parkinsonism, 188-189
   diagram illustrating, 53f
   effects of damage to, 54
   function of, 53-54
   important role of, 54
   lesions, 54
   location and course of, 52-53
   role in speech programming and control, 62
   and speech motor system, 52-54
Behavioral compensation method
   description of, 442-443
Behavioral management
   of apraxia of speech, 510-518
      biofeedback, 517-518
      integral stimulation, 515
      melodic intonation therapy (MIT), 516-517
      other, 518-521
      PROMPT, 516
      sound production, 515-516
   of dysarthrias
      speaker-oriented treatments
         articulation, 476-479
         overview of, 465-466
         phonation, 469-472
         prosody, 483-484
         rate, 479-483
         resonance, 472-476
         respiration, 466-469
   of motor speech disorders (MSDs)
      baseline data, 448
      basic principles of, 445-452
      communication -oriented approaches, 443
      evidence-based practice, 455-456
      goals of, 440
      medical and speech diagnoses, 446-447
      motor learning principles, 449-453
      motor reorganization, 446
      and neural adaptation, 445-446
      organizing sessions, 453-454
      speech-oriented approaches, 442-443
      treatment efficacy, 454-456
      treatment timing, 447-448
   speaker-oriented treatments
      of specific dysarthrias
         ataxic dysarthria, 486t-487t, 488
         flaccid dysarthria, 485, 486t-487t
         hyperkinetic dysarthria, 486t-487t, 488-491
         hypokinetic dysarthria, 486t-487t, 488-491
         mixed dysarthria, 486t-487t, 493
         spastic dysarthria, 485, 486t-487t, 488
         UUMN dysarthria, 486t-487t, 493
      summary of, 486t
      types of
         and techniques of, 486t
Bell's palsy
   causing facial paralysis, 121
   causing flaccid dysarthria, 112b, 115
Benztropine
   for Parkinson's disease, 191
Binswanger's disease, 146
Biofeedback
   and behavioral management of AOS, 517-518
   to improve articulation, 478-479
   to improve respiration, 468-469
   in motor learning, 450-451
   prostheses that provide, 441
Biopercular syndrome
   definition and clinical characteristics of, 339-340
Bite blocks, 476-477
Blepharospasms
   description of, 221
   rate, rhythm, and substrate of, 219t
Blood clots
   nonneoplastic characteristics of, 34
   and strokes, 35

Blood-brain barrier
  definition of, 31
Blurred speech
  with hypokinetic dysarthria, 194, 197
  motor system disorders associated with
    summary to aid differential diagnosis, 417,
      418t
Bones
  of the skull
    diagram illustrating, 18f
    function of, 18-19
Bony boundaries
  of skull and spinal column, 18-19
Botox, 440-441, 470-471, 476, 491-492
Botulinum toxins, 440-441, 470-471, 476, 491-
  492
Botulism
  description of, 113
  types of dysarthrias caused by
    and differential diagnoses, 413t, 415
Brachium pontis
  anatomical diagram of, 25f
Bradykinesia
  definition of, 188-189
  examples of, 189t
  affecting speed of muscle activation, 490
Brain;See also traumatic brain injuries (TBIs)
  arteries that supply, 24f
  diagram illustrating, 18f
  and motor speech processes
    summary of, 64-66
  as a nonstatic organ, 445
  traumatic brain injuries (TBIs)
    causing ataxic dysarthria, 169, 170
    and depression, 383
    description and types of, 34
    and differential diagnoses, 412, 413t-414t
    dysarthria with, 12
    causing hypokinetic dysarthria, 189b, 192
    and mixed dysarthria, 280, 281t, 293-295
    causing mixed dysarthria, 294t
    causing spastic dysarthria, 147b, 147f, 148
  traumatic injuries to
    causing ataxic dysarthria, 169, 170
  vascular system supply to, 26t
Brainstem
  anatomical relationships with
    and motor speech disorders, 21t
  description and illustration of, 21, 22f
  diffuse axonal injury in, 34
  lesions of, 51
  sensory systems of, 27
  strokes
    causing flaccid dysarthria, 113-114
    causing spastic dysarthria, 145, 147b, 147f
    and UUMN dysarthria, 257-258
  tumors
    leading to mutism, 337
    within visceral system, 24
Breathiness
  with amyotrophic lateral sclerosis (ALS),
    285t, 289
  with flaccid dysarthrias, 133
  with hypokinetic dysarthria, 196
  motor system disorders associated with
    summary to aid differential diagnosis, 417,
      418t
  with spastic dysarthria, 151, 152t
  transient, 229
  with vagus nerve lesions, 126
Breathing;See respiration
Broca's aphasia, 313, 363
Broca's area, 46t, 61, 309
Brodmann's area, 45-46
Bromocriptine
  for Parkinson's disease, 191
Bulbar muscles
  Wilson disease affect on, 293
Bulbar palsy
  description of, 131-132
  Mayo Clinic dysarthria studies on, 89
  progressive
    description of, 112
Bupropion, 192

C
Carbamazepine
  causing ataxic dysarthria, 169
Carbidopalevodopa
  for treatment of Parkinson's disease, 191
Carbon disulfide
  causing parkinsonism, 192
Carbon monoxide poisoning
  and echolalia, 359, 360b
  types of dysarthrias caused by
    and differential diagnoses, 413t
Carcinomatosis
  causing facial paralysis, 121
Cardiac arrest anoxia
  types of dysarthrias caused by
    and differential diagnoses, 413t
Carotid arterial system
  anatomical relationships with
    and motor speech disorders, 21t
Carotid arteries
  inferior view of, 25f
Carotid endarterectomy, 115-116
Carotid system
  blood entering brain through, 23
  vascular supply regions of
    and motor speech disorders (MSDs), 26t
Caudate nucleus
  anatomical diagram of, 25f
  associated with basal ganglia, 188
  definition of, 52
  diagram illustrating, 53f
  function and damage to, 53-54
  lacunar strokes in
    and UUMN dysarthria, 257-258
Cavities
  causing speech disorders, 6
Cell bodies
  function of, 28-29
  illustration of, 29f
Central chromatolysis, 31
Central nervous system (CNS);See also nervous
    system
  bony boundaries of, 18-19, 20f, 21-23
  covering layers of, 19, 20f
  damage and mutism, 335
  function of cerebrospinal fluid in, 23
  and motor speech programmer, 308-310
  nerves versus tracts, 30
  pathways of, 27-28
  and reflex testing, 86-87
  regulating speech motor programs, 3
  structural elements of, 28t
  tuberculosis
    types of dysarthrias caused by, 414t
Central pontine myelinolysis
  and mixed dysarthria, 280, 282b
  causing parkinsonism, 192
  types of dysarthrias caused by
    and differential diagnoses, 413t
Central programs, 60
Central sulcus, 45-46
Centrum semiovale
  diffuse axonal injury in, 34
Cerebellar control circuits
  anatomical diagram of, 56f
  anatomy and functions of, 163-164
  components of, 54, 55f
  damage to
    causing ataxic dysarthria, 163
  definition of, 54
  location and course of, 54-55
  role in speech programming and control, 62
Cerebellar degeneration
  types of dysarthrias caused by
    and differential diagnoses, 413t
Cerebellar hemispheres
  definition and location of, 54, 55f
  importance in speech, 55
  and movement, 164
Cerebellar mutism
  definition and clinical characteristics of, 340-341
  and mutism, 336t, 340-341
Cerebellar tremors
  definition of, 221

Cerebellopontine angle meningioma
  causing facial paralysis, 121
Cerebellum
  anatomical diagram of, 25f
  anatomical relationships with
    and motor speech disorders, 21t
  anatomy of, 54, 55f
  associated with timing and movement, 164
  and ataxic dysarthria, 163-183
  degeneration
    types of dysarthrias caused by, 413t
  description and illustration of, 21, 22f
  dysfunction in, 163-184
  influencing gamma motor neurons, 38
  lesions
    and ataxia, 165-166
  Mayo Clinic dysarthria studies on, 89
  localization of speech within, 164-165
  major anatomic subdivisions of, 54, 55
  metastatic brain tumors in, 168-169
  motor system involvement in, 27-28
  as neural area of programming, 60
  neurons of, 55, 56f
  role in speech, 56-57
  and speech muscles, 57
Cerebral arteries
  anatomical diagram of, 25f
  anatomical relationships with
    and motor speech disorders, 21t
  strokes and UUMN dysarthria, 257-258
Cerebral autosomal dominant arteriopathy
    with subcortical infarcts
    and leukoencephalopathy (CADASIL), 146
Cerebral cortex
  diagram illustrating, 20f
  and speech, 188-190
Cerebral edema
  in stroke patients, 35
Cerebral hemispheres, 21f
Cerebral hemorrhages
  description of, 35
Cerebral hypoxia
  and parkinsonism, 191
Cerebral palsy
  athetosis with, 220-221, 232-233
  as congenital disorder, 12
Cerebrospinal fluid
  description of, 19
Cerebrospinal fluid system (CSF)
  description and function of, 23
  illustration of, 21f
Cerebrovascular accident;See also strokes
  neurologic description of, 34
Cerebrovascular diseases;See also strokes
    stroke
    description of neurology of, 34
Cervical dystonia
  description and illustration of, 233-235
Cervical plexus, 43
Cervical vertebrae, 22
Channelopathies, 224
Cheeks
  sustained postures, 76, 78f
Chemicals
  causing parkinsonism, 192
  toxicity
    types of dysarthrias caused by, 413t
Chewing
  difficulties
    with unilateral upper motor neuron
      (UUMN) dysarthria, 261
  hypoglossal nerve role in, 43
  questioning patient concerning, 75
Cheyne-Stokes respiration
  definition of, 44
Choking
  questioning patient concerning, 75
Chorea
  affecting speech steadiness, 72, 228-230
  definition of, 220
  description and illustration of, 227-228
  deviant speech characteristics with, 228-230
  drugs or toxins that cause, 222-223
  with Huntington's disease, 223-224

Chorea—cont'd
　neuromuscular deficits associated with, 228t
　rate, rhythm, and substrate characteristics of, 219t
Chorea gravidarum, 220, 224
　types of dysarthrias caused by
　　and differential diagnoses, 414t
Choreiform movements
　with chorea, 227
Choreoathetosis, 168, 221
　Mayo Clinic dysarthria studies on, 89
Choroid plexus of lateral ventricle, 21f
Choroid plexuses, 23
Choroidal arteries
　anatomical diagram of, 25f
"Chronic"
　descriptive of disease development, 33
Chronic demyelinating polyneuritis
　definition of, 114
　types of dysarthrias caused by
　　and differential diagnoses, 414t
Chronic disorders
　description and examples of, 12
Chronic spasms, 221
Cingulate gyrus, 63
Circle of Willis
　anatomical location of, 24f
　definition and function of, 23
Cleft lip
　causing speech disorders, 6
Cleft palate
　causing speech disorders, 6
Clonic spasms
　description of, 221
Clonus
　definition of, 144
Closed head injuries (CHIs)
　causing apraxia of speech, 314-315
　definition of, 34
　causing flaccid dysarthria, 112b
　leading to mutism, 337-338
　causing palilalia, 258b, 359
　types of dysarthrias caused by
　　and differential diagnoses, 413t
Clusters
　of deviant speech
　　among bulbar palsy patients, 132-133
　　definition of
　　　89
CNS lymphoma, 114-115
CNS tuberculosis
　types of dysarthrias caused by
　　and differential diagnoses, 414t
Coarticulation
　definition of, 61
　patterns, 324
Cobulbar tracts
　function of, 143-144
Cocaine
　causing dyskinesias, 222
Cochleovestibular nerves
　anatomic origin and function of, 22t
Cognitive disturbances
　affecting speech, 63
　associated with CNS lesions, 360b, 361
　with ataxic dysarthria, 171
　due to vascular disturbances, 26t
　management of, 439, 529
　with mixed dysarthria, 282b, 285
　and mutism, 333, 335, 336t, 342-343
Cognitive system
　and neuron activity, 29-30
Cognitive-affect disorders
　distinguishing among mutism forms
　　and differential diagnosis, 424t, 425, 427-428
Cognitive-language disorders
　"other" as defined by Mayo Clinic
　　distribution statistics, 8f
Cognitive-linguistic disorders
　Mayo clinic definition of "other"
　　distribution and types of, 4f
Cognitive-linguistic processes
　definition of, 3

Cogwheel rigidity
　definition of, 188
Collagen
　injections, 470
Collet-Sicard syndrome
　associated with flaccid dysarthria, 114
Coma
　due to vascular disturbances, 26t-27t
　and mutism, 3443
Coma vigil
　and mutism, 343
Commissural
　structure and function of nervous system, 28t
Commissural fiber tracts, 30
Commissurotomy
　mutism with, 336t
Communication
　among neurons and muscles, 29
　augmentative and alternative, 441
　basic processes of, 3
　behavioral management to improve, 442-443
　disorders
　　acquired neurologic, 8f
　maximizing effectiveness of
　　as management's primary goal, 436-437
　motivation and needs, 438
　treatment oriented toward
　　interaction strategies, 496-498
　　listener strategies, 495-496
　　speaker strategies, 494-495
　　summary of, 494t
Communicative efficiency ratio, 98
Comprehensibility
　definition of, 96
　rating scale
　　for motor speech disorders, 97t
Conceptualization
　deficits in, 59
　definition of, 58
Conceptual-programming level
　five stages of
　　conceptualization, 58-59
　　feedback, 58t, 64
　　linguistic planning, 59
　　motor planning and programming, 58t, 59-64
　　performance, 58t, 64
　and speech
　　definition of, 57
　　key components of, 57-58
Concussion
　definition and course of, 34
Conduction aphasia, 313
Confirmatory signs
　definition and types of, 73
　reflexes as, 86-88
Congenital disorders
　description and examples of, 12
Connective tissue
　in CNS and PNS, 31
　structure and function of nervous system, 28t
Consciousness system
　components of, 25, 27
Consonants
　imprecise
　　with ataxic dysarthria, 173
　and vowels
　　with apraxia of speech, 321-322
Consonant-vowel (CV) syllables, 92
Consonant-vowel-consonant (CVC) syllables, 94
Contextual speech
　testing of, 93
Continuous positive airway pressure (CPAP), 475
Contralateral hemianesthesia
　due to vascular disturbances, 26t
Contralateral hemiplegia
　due to vascular disturbances, 26t
Contralateral lower extremity weakness
　due to vascular disturbances, 26t
Contrastive stress tasks, 484
Contrecoup injuries, 34
Control circuits
　diagram illustrating, 37f
　function of, 52

Contusions, 34
Conversion aphonia
　voice abnormalities with, 390-391
Conversion disorders
　affecting speech, 7
　characteristics and course of, 384
　definition of, 383
　and distinguishing neurogenic versus psychogenic
　　aiding differential diagnosis, 426t, 428-429
　causing psychogenic speech disorders, 383-385
　relationship to neurologic diseases, 383-385
Conversion dysphonia, 391
Coprolalia
　motor system disorders associated with
　　summary to aid differential diagnosis, 417, 418t
　with Tourette's syndrome, 238-239
Corona radiata
　diagram illustrating, 47f
　lesions
　　causing spastic dysarthria, 147b, 148
Corpora quadrigemina
　description and illustration of, 21, 22f
Corpus callosotomy
　mutism following, 345
Corpus callosum
　diffuse axonal injury in, 34
Cortex
　lesions
　　causing spastic dysarthria, 147b, 148
　localization of components of, 61
　and plasticity, 445
　role in speech, 56-57
　strokes
　　and UUMN dysarthria, 257-258
Cortical
　component of basal ganglia control circuit, 188
Cortical degeneration
　and mixed dysarthria, 279, 281t, 292-293
Cortical motor areas
　illustration of, 47f
Cortical sensory defects
　due to vascular disturbances, 26t
Cortical-cerebellar pathways
　important for speech control, 55-56
Corticobasal degeneration (CBD)
　and apraxia of speech, 311
　and echolalia, 359, 360b
　mixed dysarthria with, 292-293
　with Parkinson's disease, 191
　types of dysarthrias caused by
　　and differential diagnoses, 413t
Corticobulbar fibers, 30
　in genu, 48
Corticobulbar tracts
　diagram illustrating, 50f
　in direct activation pathway, 45
　location of, 46t
Corticonigral degeneration
　associated with primary progressive aphasia, 311
Corticoreticular fibers
　in genu, 48
Corticoreticular tracts
　definition of, 50
　diagram illustrating, 50f
Corticorubral fibers, 30
Corticorubral tracts
　definition of, 50, 51
　diagram illustrating, 50f
Corticospinal tracts
　diagram illustrating, 50f
　in direct activation pathway, 45
　function of, 143-144
Coughing
　observing patient during, 84
　questioning patient concerning, 75
　to test for nonverbal oral apraxia, 88
Counseling
　as part of behavioral management, 444

Coup
  injuries, 34
  sharpness of, 84
Coup de glotte, 84
Cranial nerves
  anatomical relationships with
    and motor speech disorders, 21t
  bones associated with, 19f
  connections of, 30
  distribution causing flaccid dysarthrias, 132t
  functions and locations of, 22t
  lesions
    associated with flaccid dysarthrias, 116-131
    and Bulbar palsy, 131
    summary of speech defects with, 119t-120t
  motor nuclei of, 27-28
  origins of, 21, 22f
  in peripheral nervous system (PNS), 23
  primary speech, 38-45
    accessory nerves, 43
    diagram illustrating, 40f
    facial nerves, 41
    glossopharyngeal nerves, 41-42
    hypoglossal nerves, 43
    trigeminal nerves, 39-41
    vagus nerves, 42
  within sensory system, 27
  and UMN innervation
    associated with speech, 48t
Cranial neuropathies
  definition of, 111
Creutzfeldt-Jacob disease (CJD)
  apraxia of speech with, 311
  leading to cerebellar dysfunction, 169
  and parkinsonism, 192
  possibly leading to mutism, 338
  types of dysarthrias caused by
    and differential diagnoses, 414t
Cricothyroid muscles, 42
Crying
  limbic system role in, 63
  with spastic dysarthria, 149-150
  with unilateral upper motor neuron (UUMN)
    dysarthria, 261
Cryptococcal meningitis, 114-115
Cyanide
  causing parkinsonism, 192
Cytosine arabinoside
  causing ataxic dysarthria, 169
Cytotoxic
  edema, 35

D

Decerebrate posturing
  definition of, 51
Decision making
  about prosthetics, 441-442
Decomposition
  of movement, 165
Decorticate posturing
  definition of, 51
Deep brain stimulation (DBS)
  to treat hypokinetic dysarthria, 488-489
Definitions
  basic speech pathology, 5-7
Degenerative diseases
  causing ataxic dysarthria, 166-168, 170
  characteristics of
    and progression, 33
    for various neurologic disease etiologies,
      32t
  description and examples of, 12
  and differential diagnoses, 412, 413t-414t
  causing flaccid dysarthria, 111, 112b
  and hyperkinetic dysarthria, 222f, 223-224
  and hypokinetic dysarthria, 189b, 190-191
  and mixed dysarthria, 276-279, 281t, 282b
  causing spastic dysarthria, 146
Degenerative neurologic diseases
  causing apraxia of speech, 311-312, 314-315
  apraxia of speech as manifestation of, 312
Delayed auditory feedback (DAF)
  to aid rate reduction, 480, 481f
  prostheses that provide, 441

Dementia
  associated with parkinsonism, 169
  and echolalia, 359, 360b
  with Huntington's disease, 223-224
  with lacunar state, 146
  with neurofibrillary degeneration, 31
  causing palilalia, 258b, 359
  with Parkinson's disease, 190-191
Dementia pugilistica, 169, 192
Demyelinating diseases
  description of, 32
  and differential diagnoses, 412, 413t-414t,
    415
  causing flaccid dysarthria, 112b, 114
Dendrites
  function of, 28-29
  illustration of, 29f
Dentate nuclei, 55, 56f
Depression
  affecting speech, 7
  definition of, 382-383
  and differential diagnoses, 411
  distinguishing neurogenic *versus* psychogenic
    aiding differential diagnosis, 426t, 428-
      429, 430t
  with Huntington's disease, 223-224
  with Parkinson's disease, 190-191
  psychogenic mutism with, 396
  speech characteristics with, 387
  symptoms of, 383
Descending aorta, 24f
Deterioration
  motor system disorders associated with
    summary to aid differential diagnosis, 417,
      418t
Development
  of neurologic diseases
    descriptive terminology of, 32t, 33
Diadochokinetic rates, 92, 93t
Diagnoses;*See also* differential diagnoses
  defining, 73-74
  of motor speech disorders (MSDs), 69-70
  patient awareness of, 75
  and prognoses
    of motor speech disorders (MSDs), 437-438
  speech
    related to management, 446-447
  terminology, 73
Diagnostic labels, 411
Dialysis encephalopathy
  types of dysarthrias caused by
    and differential diagnoses, 413t
Diaphragm
  myoclonic movement of
    with palatopharyngolaryngeal myoclonus,
      237t
  and speech, 43, 84-85
Diaschisis
  definition of, 32
Differential diagnoses
  case study, 431
  definition of process, 409
  distinguishing among speech disorders
    apraxia of speech *versus* dysarthrias,
      419-421
    dysarthrias *versus* apraxia of speech,
      411-419
    motor speech disorders *versus* aphasia,
      421-423
    motor speech disorders *versus* other
      disorders, 425-429
    neurogenic *versus* psychogenic, 429-430
  general guidelines for speech-related, 409-
    411
  process of, 69-70
"Diffuse"
  as descriptive of localization, 33
Diffuse axonal injuries, 34
Diffuse frontal lobe white matter lesions
  associated with parkinsonism, 191
Diffuse Lewy body disease, 191
Digastric muscles, 39
Diphtheria
  and chorea, 224

Diplophonia
  motor system disorders associated with
    summary to aid differential diagnosis, 417,
      418t
  with vagus nerve damage, 126
Direct activation pathways
  anatomy and basic functions of, 143-144
  damage to
    and spastic dysarthria, 144t
  diagram illustrating, 37f, 47f
  effects of damage to, 49
  function of, 49
  versus indirect activation pathway, 45t
  major cortical components of
    diagram illustrating, 46t
  nature of, 144
  and speech
    cortical components of, 45-47
    importance of, 45
    motor cortex, 46-47
    tracts, 47-48
  UMN innervation
    nerves associated with, 48t
  of upper motor neuron (UUMN) system
    clinical features of, 257b
    definition of, 256
Direct motor system;*See* direct activation
    pathways
Discrete movements, 144
Disease
  clinical localization of, 18
Disinhibited vocalization, 360b, 361
Disrupted auditory feedback, 317
Distal muscle atrophy, 168
Distorted vowels
  with chorea, 229
  motor system disorders associated with
    summary to aid differential diagnosis, 417,
      418t
  with spastic dysarthria, 151
Distribution pie chart
  and hyperkinetic dysarthria, 222f
Dominant hemisphere perisylvian cortex, 59
Dopamine
  antagonist drugs
    leading to parkinsonism, 191-192
  depletion
    and hypokinetic dysarthria, 187-188
  depletors, 192
  functions of, 53
  implicated in Parkinson's disease, 24-25
Dopamine-blocking agents
  tardive dyskinesia (TD) associated with, 222
Dopaminergic agonists
  for Parkinson's disease management, 191,
    440-441
Dorsal nerve roots
  attaching nerves to spinal cord, 22
Dorsal respiratory neurons, 44
Dorsal root ganglia
  within sensory system, 27
Drills
  intelligibility, 479
  speaking, 449-450
Drooling
  with chorea, 227
  with hypokinetic dysarthria, 193-194
  questioning patient concerning, 75
  with spastic dysarthria, 149
  summary of dysarthrias associated with, 416t
  with unilateral upper motor neuron (UUMN)
    dysarthria, 261, 263b, 264t
  with Wilson disease, 293
Drug abuse
  types of dysarthrias caused by
    and differential diagnoses, 413t
Drug toxicity
  causing flaccid dysarthria, 112b
  types of dysarthrias caused by
    and differential diagnoses, 413t
Drugs
  causing hyperkinetic dysarthria, 222-223
  inducing mutism, 336t
  to manage phonation, 471

Drugs—cont'd
  and managing motor speech disorders, 440-441
  and mutism, 346
  and stuttering, 356
  therapy
    for different dysarthria types, 488t
    for hypokinetic dysarthria, 489-490
  toxicity, 112b, 413t
  withdrawal from
    and tardive dyskinesia (TD), 222
    causing toxic tremors, 221
Duchenne's muscular dystrophy, 113
Dura mater
  layers of
    description and diagram illustrating, 19, 20f
Dysarthria
  action myoclonus (AM), 237-238
  and anarthria, 336-337
  anatomical relationships associated with, 21t
  anatomy and vascular distribution, 411, 412t
  versus apraxia of speech, 320
  with apraxia of speech, 315
  of athetosis, 232-233
  basic definition of, 5
  caused by dopamine-blocking agents, 222
  communication-oriented treatment of
    interaction strategies, 496-498
    listener strategies, 495-496
    speaker strategies, 494-495
  deviant speech dimensions, 103-104
  different types of
    treatment approaches to improve, 486t-487t
  distinctions among dysfluencies associated with, 425t, 426
  distinctive speech characteristics of, 89, 90b
  distinguishing among, 91
    and differential diagnosis, 411-419
  distinguishing from aphasia, 421, 422t
  distinguishing from apraxia of speech
    anatomic and vascular distribution, 419
    etiologies, 413t-414t, 419
    oral mechanism finding, 416t, 419-420
    speech characteristics, 418t, 420-421
  distribution statistics, 8f
  flaccid
    acoustic and physiologic findings with, 134t
    case reviews of, 135-139
    clinical characteristics of, 110-111
    clusters of abnormal speech with, 133t
    cranial nerves associated with, 118-127
    definition and overview of, 109
    deviant speech, 133t
    deviant speech clusters with, 132-133
    differential diagnosis of, 413t-414t
    distinctive speech characteristics with, 417, 418t
    distribution of cranial nerves causing, 132t
    due to vascular disturbances, 26t-27t
    etiologies of, 111-115, 116t
    lesion loci and vascular source, 411, 412t
    localization and neuromotor basis of, 13t
    Mayo Clinic dysarthria studies on, 89
    and mixed dysarthria, 283-284
    mutism with, 336t, 337
    neurochemical systems indicated in, 24-25
    neuromuscular deficits associated with, 116t
    speaker-oriented treatments, 485, 486t-487t
    subtypes of, 109
    summary of oral mechanism findings, 415, 416t
    terminology, 111
  with Huntington's disease, 223-224
  hyperkinetic
    action myoclonus, 237-238
    anatomical relationships associated with, 21t
    athetosis, 232-233
    and basal ganglia control circuit diseases and involuntary movements of speech, 217-221

Dysarthria—cont'd
  hyperkinetic—cont'd
    case studies of, 245-249
    cervical dystonia, 233-235
    chorea, 227-230
    definition and overview of, 217-218
    diagnosis and frequency of, 218
    differential diagnosis of
      as function of etiologies, 413t-414t
    distinctive speech characteristics with
      summary of, 417-418, 418t
    due to vascular disturbances, 26t
    dystonia, 228t, 230-232, 233f, 234t
    etiologies of, 221-224
    lesion loci and vascular source, 411, 412t
    localization and neuromotor basis of, 13t
    Mayo Clinic dysarthria studies on, 89
    and mixed dysarthria, 283-284
    mutism with, 336t
    neurochemical systems indicated in, 24-25
    neuromuscular deficits associated with, 228t
    organic vocal tremors, 239-240, 241f, 242t
    palatopharyngolaryngeal myoclonus, 235-237
    patient perceptions and complaints, 226-227
    spasmodic dysphonia (SD), 240-244
    spasmodic torticollis, 233-235
    speaker-oriented treatments, 486t-487t, 488-491
    summary of oral mechanism findings, 415, 416t
    symptoms of, 226-244
    Tourette's syndrome/tics, 238-239
  hypokinetic, 187-211
    acoustic and physiologic findings of, 198-205, 206t-207t
    anatomical relationships associated with, 21t
    and basal ganglia control circuits, 187-188, 188-190
    blurred speech with, 194
    case studies of, 207-211
    clinical signs of, 194-198
    definition of, 187
    dementia pugilistica leading to, 192
    deviant speech characteristics with, 195-197
    differential diagnosis of, 413t-414t
    distinctions among other speech disturbances, 426t, 428-429
    distinctive speech characteristics with, 417, 418t
    due to vascular disturbances, 26t
    etiologies of, 189b, 190-192, 193f
    "fused" speech with, 205
    lesion loci and vascular source, 411, 412t
    localization and neuromotor basis of, 13t
    masked facial expression with, 189, 190f
    Mayo Clinic dysarthria studies on, 89, 189, 190f
    and mixed dysarthria, 283-284
    mutism with, 336t
    neurochemical systems indicated in, 24-25
    neuromuscular deficits associated with, 195t
    and neurotransmitter depletion, 187
    patient's perceptions of, 193-194
    primary speech characteristics with, 198t
    respiration abnormalities with, 198-199, 206t
    with rigidity, 54
    speaker-oriented treatments, 486t-487t, 488-491
    summary of oral mechanism findings, 415, 416t
    surgery interventions for, 488-489
  with lacunar state, 146
  mixed
    amyotrophic lateral sclerosis (ALS), 276-277, 281t, 282b, 285-289
    from autoimmune diseases, 280-281, 281t, 282b

Dysarthria—cont'd
  mixed—cont'd
    case studies, 296-301
    characteristics of, 284-285
    cortical degeneration, 279, 281t, 282b, 292-293
    definition and overview of, 275-276
    from degenerative diseases, 276-279, 281t, 282b
    description of, 275-276
    deviant speech characteristics with, 285t
    etiologies of, 276-281, 282-295, 282b
    Friedreich's ataxia, 278, 281t, 282b, 290
    from infectious diseases, 280-281, 281t, 282b
    localization and neuromotor basis of, 13t
    Mayo Clinic dysarthria studies on, 89
    from motor neuron diseases, 276-277, 281t, 282b
    multiple sclerosis, 277, 281t, 282b, 289-290
    multiple system atrophy, 278, 281t, 282b, 291-292
    progressive supranuclear palsy (PSP), 278, 281t, 282b, 290, 291
    severity of, 284-285
    speaker-oriented treatments, 486t-487t, 493
    speech pathology, 281-295, 282b
    summary of etiologies, 281t, 282b
    from toxic/metabolic conditions
      central pontine myelinolysis, 280, 282b
      hepatocerebral degeneration, 279, 282b
      hypoxic encephalopathy, 279-280, 282b
      Wilson's disease (WD), 279-280, 282b
    from traumatic brain injuries (TBIs), 280, 281t, 282b, 293-295
    types and mixtures of, 283-284
    from vascular disorders, 280, 282b
  causing mutism, 333
  from posterior lobe lesions, 57
  published tests for diagnosing, 94
  spastic
    acoustic and physiologic findings, 152, 153t, 154f, 155-157
    anatomical relationships associated with, 21t
    with bilateral lesions, 52
    case reviews of, 158-161
    clinical characteristics of, 144-145
    clusters of abnormal speech with, 151t, 152
    definition and overview of, 49, 143
    deviant speech characteristics with, 150-151
    diagnosing, 70
    differential diagnosis of, 413t-414t
    from direct/indirect activation pathway damage, 143-144
    distinctive speech characteristics with, 417, 418t
    distribution of causes, 146-148
    etiologies of, 145-146
    lesion loci and vascular source, 411, 412t
    localization and neuromotor basis of, 13t
    Mayo Clinic dysarthria studies on, 89
    and mixed dysarthria, 283-284
    mutism with, 336t, 337
    neuromuscular deficits with, 150t
    patient perceptions and complaints, 148-149
    versus spastic paralysis, 145
    speaker-oriented treatments, 485, 486t-487t, 488
    summary of acoustic and physiologic findings, 153t, 155-157
    summary of oral mechanism findings, 415, 416t
    tracings illustrating, 154f
    and upper motor neuron (UMN) disease, 143
  speaker-oriented treatment of
    articulation, 476-479
    overview of, 465-466
    phonation, 469-472

Dysarthria—cont'd
  speaker-oriented treatment of—cont'd
    prosody, 483-484
    rate, 479-483
    resonance, 472-476
    respiration, 466-469
  for specific dysarthria types, 484-485,
      486t-487t, 488-493
  with traumatic brain injuries (TBIs), 12
  types of, 13t
  unilateral upper motor neuron (UUMN)
      system
    acoustic and physiologic findings, 265-266
    anatomy and functions of, 256-257
    case studies of, 268-270
    clinical characteristics of, 261-265
    clinical features of lesions of, 257, 259-260
    definition and overview of, 255-256
    distinctiveness of, 267-268
    etiologies of, 257-258, 259f, 259t, 260
    patient perceptions and complaints, 261
    severity of, 261
    speech characteristics of, 261-265
Dysarthria clumsy hand syndrome
  description of, 258
Dysdiadochokinesia, 165
Dysfluencies
  definition of, 197
  distinctions among, 425t
  versus "nonfluent," 362
  with stuttering, 394b
Dyskinesia
  affecting speech steadiness, 72
  definition of, 219
  rate, rhythm, and substrate characteristics of, 219t
Dysmetria
  definition of, 165
Dysmetric jaw
  summary of dysarthrias associated with, 416t
Dysphagia
  with Huntington's disease, 223-224
  with lacunar state, 146
  with spastic dysarthria, 149
  summary of dysarthrias associated with, 416t
  with Wilson disease, 293
Dysphasia
  signs of, 59
Dysphonia
  conversion, 391
  inertial, 392
Dysprosody, 366
Dyssynergia, 165
Dystonia, 168
  affecting speech steadiness, 72
  description of, 221
  distinguishing speech characteristics with,
      234t
  drugs or toxins that cause, 222-223
  Mayo Clinic dysarthria studies on, 89
  movements with
    waxing and waning, 228, 229f
  neuromuscular deficits associated with, 228t
  rate, rhythm, and substrate of, 219t
  speech characteristics with, 230-232
Dystonia musculorum deformans
  clinical features of, 224
  types of dysarthrias caused by
      and differential diagnoses, 413t

E
"Ear clicks"
  with palatopharyngolaryngeal myoclonus,
      236, 237t
Echolalia
  anatomic correlates, 360
  definition and clinical characteristics of, 359,
      360b
  distinctions among dysfluencies associated
      with, 425t, 427
  etiologies of, 359-360
  management of, 528
  motor system disorders associated with
    summary to aid differential diagnosis, 417,
        418t

Echolalia—cont'd
  with progressive supranuclear palsy (PSP),
      291, 292
  with Tourette's syndrome, 239
Edema
  nonneoplastic characteristics of, 34
Effectors
  within visceral system, 24
Efferent connections
  of cortex
    in motor system, 27-28
Efferent fibers
  in direct activation pathway, 47-48
  types of, 30
Efferent nerves
  within visceral system, 24
Efferent pathways
  in motor system, 36
Efficacy
  determining AOS management, 521
  treatment, 454-456
Efficiency
  definition of, 96, 443
  rating scale
    for motor speech disorders, 97t
Effort closure technique, 472
Elderly;See aging
Electroglottography, 84
Electromagnetic articulography, 517
Electromyography
  to study motor speech disorders, 10
Emboli
  and stroke, 35
Emboliform nuclei, 55, 56f
Embolism
  description of, 35
Emotional disorders
  affecting speech, 63
Emotional prosody, 366
Emotions
  difficulty controlling
    with spastic dysarthria, 149
  limbic system role in sensations of, 63
  and psychogenic speech disorders, 381-396
Emphatic stress, 366
Encephalitis
  and chorea, 220
  location of, 33
  types of dysarthrias caused by
      and differential diagnoses, 414t
End organs
  peripheral, 30
Engrams
  definition of, 60
Ependymal cells
  function in nervous system, 31
  structure and function of nervous system,
      28t
Epidural space
  description of, 19
  diagram illustrating, 20f
Epiglottis
  nerve sensations of, 42
Epilepsy
  and depression, 383
  myoclonic, 220
Episodic ataxia, 168
Equal stress
  motor system disorders associated with
    summary to aid differential diagnosis, 417,
        418t
Essential tremors
  definition of, 221
  rate, rhythm, and substrate of, 219t
Essential voice tremors
  description and waveforms illustrating, 239-
      240, 241f
  distinguishing speech characteristics of,
      242t
Eustachian tube
  and glossopharyngeal nerve, 41
  myoclonic "ear clicks"
    with palatopharyngolaryngeal myoclonus,
        237t

Evidence-based practice (EBP)
  description of principles of, 455-456
  guidelines, 463
Evolution
  characteristics of neurologic diseases, 32t
  of neurologic diseases
    descriptive terminology of, 33
"Exacerbating-remitting"
  descriptive of disease evolution, 33
  disorders
    description and examples of, 12
Examinations
  and forming differential diagnoses,
      409-410
  four parts of
    history, 74-75
    intelligibility, comprehensibility and
        efficiency, 96-99
    nonspeech analysis, 76, 77f-78f, 79, 80f,
        81, 82f, 83-88
    perceptual speech characteristics, 88-96
  general guidelines for
    confirmatory signs, 73
    diagnoses, 73-74
    history, 71
    salient features of, 71-73
  observations
    summary of, 430
  volitional versus automatic nonspeech, 88
Excess loudness variation
  motor system disorders associated with
    summary to aid differential diagnosis, 417,
        418t
Excess stress
  with chorea, 229-230
  motor system disorders associated with
    summary to aid differential diagnosis, 417,
        418t
  with progressive supranuclear palsy (PSP),
      291
Excessive rebound
  and impaired check, 165
Exercises
  to improve articulation, 478
Expiration
  MSDs associated with forced
    summary to aid differential diagnosis, 417,
        418t
Explosive loudness
  with ataxic dysarthria, 173, 174-175
External auditory meatus
  diagram illustrating, 18f
External laryngeal nerves, 42
External occipital protuberance, 18f
External respiration, 43
Extracellular space
  fluid collecting in, 35
Extracerebral hemorrhages, 35
Extracranial lesions
  of vagus nerve, 123
Extradural hemorrhages, 35
Extrafusal muscle fibers, 37
Extramedullary lesions
  of vagus nerve, 123
Extrapyramidal tract;See indirect activation
      pathway
Eyeballs
  myoclonic movement of
    with palatopharyngolaryngeal myoclonus,
        237t
Eyes
  blinking
    reduced
      with hypokinetic dysarthria, 194
      summary of dysarthrias associated with,
          416t
    and twitching with Tourette's syndrome,
        238-239
  fixed gaze
    with depression, 383
  movement of
    nerves associated with, 22t
  nystagmus, 57
  vascular supply to, 26t

F

Face
  abnormalities
    with hyperkinetic dysarthria, 225t, 226
  anatomical relationships with
    and motor speech disorders, 21t
  dyskinesia waveforms, 234f
  involuntary movements of
    with dystonia, 232, 233f, 234f
    summary of dysarthrias associated with,
      416t
  masked
    with hypokinetic dysarthria, 194
    summary of dysarthrias associated with,
      416t
  motor cortex neurons associated with, 46
  movement
    nerves associated with, 22t
    observing during, 76, 78f
  normal appearance of, 76-77
    at rest
      analysis of, 76
      illustration of, 77f
    during sustained postures, 76, 77f
  trigeminal nerve sensory role in, 39
  tumors
    causing facial paralysis, 121
Facial asymmetry, 41
Facial expressions
  with depression, 383
  and facial nerve, 41
Facial grimacing
  with adductor spasmodic dysphonia, 243,
    244t
  with psychogenic stuttering, 394b
  summary of dysarthrias associated with, 416t
  with Tourette's syndrome, 238-239
  with vagus nerve lesions, 126
Facial myokymia
  description of, 122
  rate, rhythm, and substrate of, 219t
  summary of dysarthrias associated with, 416t
Facial nerves
  anatomic origin and function of, 22t
  anatomical diagram of, 25f
  bones associated with, 19f
  description of
    and speech, 41
    lesions, 41
      associated with flaccid dysarthrias, 118,
        121-122
    and UMN innervation, 48t
Facial paralysis
  causes of, 121
Facial weakness
  with apraxia of speech, 316, 317t
  with flaccid dysarthria, 118f
  with unilateral upper motor neuron (UUMN)
    dysarthria, 257, 262, 267
Facilitatory
  nature of direct activation pathways, 144
Factitious disorders, 386
Falls
  and traumatic brain injury, 34
  with truncal ataxia, 57
Falx cerebri
  anatomical relationships with
    and motor speech disorders, 21t
  layers of
    description and diagram illustrating, 19,
      20f
Familial basal ganglia calcification
  types of dysarthrias caused by
    and differential diagnoses, 413t
Familial tremors
  definition of, 221
Fasciculations
  definition of, 38, 111
  with flaccid dysarthrias, 110-111
  with hypoglossal nerve lesions, 128, 129f
  with LMN lesions, 41
  rate, rhythm, and substrate of, 219t
  summary of dysarthrias associated with, 416t
  of tongue, 81

Fascioscapulohumeral
  definition of, 113
Fast Fourier transformation (FFT), 288
Fastigial nuclei, 55, 56f
Fatigue;See also weakness
  assessing patient, 93-94
  and speech
    with hypokinetic dysarthria, 193-194, 204
    motor learning techniques, 454
Feedback
  components and disorders associated with,
    58t
  within conceptual-programming level, 64
  instrumental, 450-451
  and motor learning, 450-451
Festination
  with parkinsonism, 189t, 190
Fiber tracts
  through cerebellum, 55
Fibrillations
  definition of, 111
  with flaccid dysarthrias, 110-111
  of muscles with innervation loss, 38
Final common pathways (FCPs)
  alpha motor neurons and extrafusal fibers, 37
  common terminology, 111
  of cranial nerves, 21, 22t
  diagram illustrating, 37f
  effects of damage, 38-39
  and flaccid dysarthrias
    causes of, 109-110
  function and structure of, 36t
  gamma motor neurons and intrafusal fibers,
    37-38
  influences upon, 38
  nerve and muscle interactions, 36-37
  and speech, 38-45
    accessory nerves, 43
    facial nerves, 41
    glossopharyngeal nerves, 41-42
    hypoglossal nerves, 43
    spinal nerves, 43-45
    trigeminal nerves, 39-41
    vagus nerves, 42
  and speech muscle strength, 71
Fisher syndrome, 169-170
Fissure of Rolando, 46t
Flaccid
  definition of, 109
Flaccid dysarthria
  acoustic and physiologic findings with, 134t
  case reviews of, 135-139
  clinical characteristics of, 110-111
  clusters of abnormal speech with, 133t
  cranial nerves associated with
    accessory nerves, 127
    facial nerves, 118, 120-122
    glossopharyngeal nerves, 122-123
    hypoglossal nerves, 127-130
    multiple nerves, 131-132
    trigeminal nerves, 116-117
    vagus nerves, 123-124
  definition and overview of, 109
  deviant speech, 133t
  deviant speech clusters with, 132-133
  differential diagnosis of
    as function of etiologies, 413t-414t
  distinctive speech characteristics with
    summary of, 417, 418t
  distribution of cranial nerves causing, 132t
  due to vascular disturbances, 26t-27t
  etiologies of, 111-115
    distribution of, 115b, 116t
  localization and neuromotor basis of, 13t,
    411, 412t
  Mayo Clinic dysarthria studies on, 89
  and mixed dysarthria, 283-284
  mutism with
    localization and clinical features of, 336t,
      337
  neurochemical systems indicated in, 24-25
  neuromuscular deficits associated with, 116t
  speaker-oriented treatments, 485, 486t-487t
  subtypes of, 109

Flaccid dysarthria—cont'd
  summary of oral mechanism findings, 415, 416t
  terminology, 111
Flaccid facial deplegia;See biopercular
  syndrome
Flexible fiberoptic laryngoscope, 84
Flocculonodular lobes
  definition and location of, 54, 55, 56f
  lesions
    associated with truncal ataxia, 57
Flocculus
  definition and location of, 54, 55
Fluency
  with apraxia of speech (AOS)
    acoustic and physiologic findings with,
      322b, 323-324
  characteristics with apraxia of speech, 318b,
    319
"Flutter"
  with amyotrophic lateral sclerosis, 286
  of the cheeks
    with nerve lesions, 122
  with hypokinetic dysarthria, 197
"Focal"
  as descriptive of localization, 32
  inflammatory diseases, 33
Focal cortical atrophy syndromes, 311
Focal dystonia
  of jaw, tongue, or face
    sensory tricks, 482
Focal mouth dystonia, 221
Foix-Chavany-Marie syndrome;See biopercular
  syndrome
Foramen lacerum
  cranial nerves associated with, 19f
  view from above, 19f
Foramen magnum
  accessory nerves through, 43
  cranial nerves associated with, 19f
  nerves associated with, 19f, 20f, 22
  view from above, 19f
Foramen of Luschka
  within cerebrospinal fluid system (CSF), 23
Foramen of Magendie, 21f
  within cerebrospinal fluid system (CSF), 23
Foramen of Monro, 21f
  within cerebrospinal fluid system (CSF), 23
Foramen ovale, 40
  cranial nerves associated with, 19f
  view from above, 19f
Foramen rotundum, 40
  cranial nerves associated with, 19f
  view from above, 19f
Foramen spinosum
  cranial nerves associated with, 19f
  view from above, 19f
Foramina
  definition of, 18
  illustration of, 19f
Foreign accent syndrome, 354t, 363-365, 529-
  530
Formant trajectories, 322b, 324
Fractures
  causing speech disorders, 6
"Freezing"
  with bradykinesia, 188-189
  with hypokinetic dysarthria, 197
Frenchay Dysarthria Assessment (FDA), 99
Friedreich's ataxia
  associated with mixed dysarthria, 278, 281t,
    290
  causing ataxic dysarthria, 167
  types of dysarthrias caused by
    and differential diagnoses, 413t
Frontal bones
  diagram illustrating, 18f
Frontal lobe premotor cortex
  component of basal ganglia control circuit, 188
Frontal lobes
  anatomical diagram of, 25f
  diagram illustrating tracts in, 50f
  motor system involvement in, 27-28
  tumors
    causing apraxia of speech, 314-315

Frontolimbic system
  and mutism, 336t
  as neural area of programming, 60
Fundamental frequency
  measurement of speech
    with apraxia of speech, 323
    with hypokinetic dysarthria, 199-200

G

Gag reflexes
  definition of, 86
  examining soft palate during, 83f
  motor neurons that mediate, 41
  questioning patient concerning, 75
  with spastic dysarthria, 150
  summary of dysarthrias associated with, 416t
Gait
  apraxia
    due to vascular disturbances, 26t
  ataxic, 57, 165, 169
  disturbances with truncal ataxia, 57
Gait apraxia
  due to vascular disturbances, 26t
Gait ataxia
  and anterior lobe lesions, 57
Gamma loops
  components of, 38
  description and illustration of, 38, 39f
  and reticular formation, 50-51
Gamma motor neurons
  definition of, 37-38
  reticulospinal tract termination on, 50-51
  role of, 38
Gamma motor system
  and stretch reflex, 38, 39f
Gamma-aminobutyric acid (GABA)
  functions of, 53
Ganglia
  within visceral system, 24
Gasserian ganglia, 39-40
Gegenhalten, 344
Genders
  speech variances between, 7
Generalized motor programs, 60
Genu
  definition of, 48
Gilles de la Tourette's syndrome (TS)
  definition of, 220
Glial cells
  function of, 28t
  types of, 30-31
Gliosis, 32
Globose nuclei, 55, 56f
Globus pallidus
  anatomical diagram of, 25f
  associated with basal ganglia, 188
  definition of, 52
  diagram illustrating, 53f
  function and damage to, 53-54
Glossopharyngeal breathing, 468
Glossopharyngeal nerves
  anatomic origin and function of, 22t
  anatomical diagram of, 25f
  bones associated with, 19f
  damage and lesions of, 41
  and gag reflex, 86
  lesions
    associated with flaccid dysarthrias, 122-123
    and speech
      description of, 41
    and UMN innervation, 48t
Glossopharyngeal neuralgia, 42, 122
Glottal coup, 84
Golgi tendon organs, 41
Grandfather passage, 104
Groaning
  with amyotrophic lateral sclerosis (ALS), 285t, 289
  with progressive supranuclear palsy (PSP), 291
Groping
  motor system disorders associated with
    summary to aid differential diagnosis, 417, 418t

Group therapy
  for motor learning, 454
Grunting
  with adductor spasmodic dysphonia, 243, 244t
  with Tourette's syndrome, 238-239
Guillain-Barre syndrome
  definition of, 114
  demyelination with, 32
  causing facial paralysis, 121
  causing flaccid dysarthria, 112b
  leading to cerebellar dysfunction, 169-170
  leading to mutism, 337
  types of dysarthrias caused by
    and differential diagnoses, 414t
Guillain-Mollaret triangle, 219t, 220, 236
Gums
  trigeminal nerve sensory role in, 39

H

Handicaps, 438
Hard palate;See also palate
  trigeminal nerve sensory role in, 39
Harshness
  motor system disorders associated with
    summary to aid differential diagnosis, 417, 418t
  with phonatory-prosodic insufficiency, 173-174
Head
  involuntary movements of
    summary of dysarthrias associated with, 416t
  movement of
    and accessory nerves, 43
  tremors
    summary of dysarthrias associated with, 416t
Health care system
  and motor speech disorder management, 439
Hearing
  loss
    and speech, 6
    nerves associated with, 22t
  within sensory system, 27
Heart
  transplant drugs
    and mutism, 346
Heat stroke
  leading to cerebellar dysfunction, 169
Heavy metals
  exposure
    causing parkinsonism, 192
  types of dysarthrias caused by
    and differential diagnoses, 413t
Hematomas
  nonneoplastic characteristics of, 34
  from trauma, 34
Hemianopsia
  due to vascular disturbances, 26t
Hemifacial spasms, 221
  description of, 121-122
  rate, rhythm, and substrate of, 219t
Hemiplegia
  due to vascular disturbances, 26t-27t
Hemispheres
  anatomical relationships with
    and motor speech disorders, 21t
Hemorrhagic infarcts, 35
Hemorrhagic leukoencephalitis, 146
Hemorrhagic strokes
  types of dysarthrias caused by
    and differential diagnoses, 413t
Hepatic encephalopathy
  types of dysarthrias caused by
    and differential diagnoses, 414t
Hepatocerebral degeneration
  and mixed dysarthria, 279, 282b
  types of dysarthrias caused by
    and differential diagnoses, 414t
Herbicides
  and Parkinson's disease, 190
Hereditary ataxia, 166-167

Hereditary cerebellar disease
  types of dysarthrias caused by
    and differential diagnoses, 413t
Hereditary cerebral calcinosis
  types of dysarthrias caused by
    and differential diagnoses, 413t
Hereditary degenerative CNS disease
  types of dysarthrias caused by
    and differential diagnoses, 413t
Hereditary spinocerebellar ataxia (SCAs), 167
Herpes zoster
  description of, 114
  causing facial paralysis, 121
  types of dysarthrias caused by
    and differential diagnoses, 414t, 415
Hiccups
  causes of, 85
  due to vascular disturbances, 26t-27t
  as form of myoclonus, 220
History
  basic data gathering, 74
  diagnosis and prognosis, 75-76
  examining a patient's, 71
  introduction and goal setting, 74
  onset and course, 75
  taking psychogenic, 387
Hoarseness
  with hypokinetic dysarthria, 196, 197
  with progressive supranuclear palsy (PSP), 291
  with vagus nerve lesions, 126
Homeostasis
  within visceral system, 24
Homonymous hemianopsia
  due to vascular disturbances, 26t
Human immunodeficiency virus (HIV)
  causing flaccid dysarthrias, 114-115
Humming
  with progressive supranuclear palsy (PSP), 291
Hunger
  limbic system role in sensations of, 63
Huntington's chorea, 220, 223-224, 225
  types of dysarthrias caused by
    and differential diagnoses, 413t
Huntington's disease
  associated with parkinsonism, 192
  and depression, 383
  deviant speech characteristics with, 228-229
  possibly leading to mutism, 338
  symptoms and progression of, 223-224
Hydrocephalus
  types of dysarthrias caused by
    and differential diagnoses, 414t
Hyoid elevation
  nerves associated with, 22t
Hyperactive gag
  summary of dysarthrias associated with, 416t
Hyperkinesia
  definition of, 54, 219
  with dopamine hyperactivity, 54
  causing speech unsteadiness, 72
Hyperkinetic dysarthria
  acoustic and physiologic findings
    action myoclonus, 237-238
    athetosis, 232-233
    cervical dystonia, 233-235
    chorea, 227-230
    dystonia, 228t, 230-232, 233f, 234t
    organic voice tremors, 239-240, 241f, 242t
    palatopharyngolaryngeal myoclonus, 235-237
    spasmodic dysphonia (SD), 240-244
    spasmodic torticollis, 233-235
    Tourette's syndrome/tics, 238-239
  action myoclonus (AM)
    characteristics of, 237-238
  anatomical relationships associated with, 21t
  and basal ganglia control circuit diseases
    and involuntary movements of speech, 217-221
  case studies of, 245-249

Hyperkinetic dysarthria—cont'd
  categories of abnormal movement with, 219t
  clinical characteristics of
    athetosis, 219t, 220-221, 223b
    ballismus, 219t, 220, 223b
    chorea, 219t, 220, 223b
    dyskinesias, 219-220
    dystonia, 219t, 221, 223b
    myoclonus, 219t, 220, 223b
    spasms, 219t, 221, 223b
    tics, 219t, 220, 223b
    tremors, 219t, 221, 223b
  definition and overview of, 217-218
  diagnosis and frequency of, 218
  differential diagnosis of
    as function of etiologies, 413t-414t
  distinctive speech characteristics with
    summary of, 417-418, 418t
  due to vascular disturbances, 26t
  with dystonia
    distinguishing speech characteristics with,
      234t
  etiologies of, 221-224
    and basal ganglia control circuits, 218-221
    degenerative diseases, 222f, 223-224
    distribution pie chart, 222f
    infectious diseases, 222f, 223b, 224
    neoplastic diseases, 222f, 223b, 224
    other, 224
    toxic-metabolic conditions, 222-223
    vascular diseases, 222f, 223b, 224
  lesion loci and vascular source
    and differential diagnoses, 411, 412t
  localization and neuromotor basis of, 13t
  Mayo Clinic dysarthria studies on, 89
  and mixed dysarthria, 283-284
  mutism with
    localization and clinical features of, 336t
  neurochemical systems indicated in, 24-25
  neuromuscular deficits associated with, 228t
  organic vocal tremors, 239-240, 241f, 242t
  patient perceptions and complaints, 226-227
  speaker-oriented treatments, 486t-487t, 488-
    491
  summary of oral mechanism findings, 415,
    416t
  symptoms of, 226-244
  with Tourette's syndrome, 238-239
Hypernasality
  with adductor spasmodic dysphonia, 243,
    244t
  with amyotrophic lateral sclerosis (ALS),
    285t, 286-289
  with chorea, 229
  with flaccid dysarthrias, 133
  motor system disorders associated with
    summary to aid differential diagnosis, 417,
      418t
  with progressive supranuclear palsy (PSP),
    291
  with spastic dysarthria, 151
  with vagus nerve lesions, 126
  with Wilson disease, 293t
Hyperreflexia
  with lacunar state, 146
Hypertension
  and lacunar infarcts, 145-146
Hypervigilance, 392
Hypoactive gag
  summary of dysarthrias associated with, 416t
Hypoglossal canal
  cranial nerves associated with, 19f
  view from above, 19f
Hypoglossal foramen, 43
Hypoglossal nerves
  anatomic origin and function of, 22t
  anatomical diagram of, 25f
  bones associated with, 19f
  function of, 43
  lesions
    associated with flaccid dysarthrias, 127-
      130
  location of, 40f
  and UMN innervation, 48t

Hypoglossal nucleus
  damage to, 43
  and taste and tactile information, 43
Hypokinesia
  with bradykinesia, 188-189
  definition of, 54
  examples of, 189t
Hypokinetic dysarthria
  acoustic and physiologic findings of, 198-
    205, 206t-207t
    articulation, 203-205
    phonation, 199-202
    resonance, 202-203
    respiration, 198-199
    sensory and perceptual deficits, 205, 206t-
      207t
    stress and pause, 205
  anatomical relationships associated with, 21t
  and basal ganglia control circuits
    anatomy and basic functions of, 187-188
    clinical characteristics of, 188-190
  blurred speech with, 194
  case studies of, 207-211
  clinical signs of, 194-198
  definition of, 187
  dementia pugilistica leading to, 192
  deviant speech characteristics with, 195-197
  differential diagnosis of
    as function of etiologies, 413t-414t
  distinctions among other speech disturbances
    aiding differential diagnosis, 426t,
      428-429
  distinctive speech characteristics with
    summary of, 417, 418t
  due to vascular disturbances, 26t
  etiologies of, 189b, 190-192, 193f
    degenerative diseases, 189b, 190-191
    distribution of, 192, 193f
    infectious conditions, 189b, 192
    toxic/metabolic diseases, 189b, 191-192
    trauma, 189b, 192
    vascular diseases, 189b, 191
  "fused" speech with, 205
  lesion loci and vascular source
    and differential diagnoses, 411, 412t
  localization and neuromotor basis of, 13t
  masked facial expression with, 189, 190f
  Mayo Clinic dysarthria studies on, 89
  Mayo Clinic pie chart
    on etiologies of, 189b, 193f
  and mixed dysarthria, 283-284
  mutism with
    localization and clinical features of, 336t
  neurochemical systems indicated in, 24-25
  neuromuscular deficits associated with, 195t
  and neurotransmitter depletion, 187
  patient's perceptions of, 193-194
  primary speech characteristics with, 198t
  respiration abnormalities with, 198-199,
    206t
  with rigidity, 54
  speaker-oriented treatments, 486t-487t, 488-
    491
  summary of oral mechanism findings, 415,
    416t
  surgery interventions for, 488-489
Hyponasality
  with ataxic dysarthria, 175
Hypoparathyroidism
  causing parkinsonism, 192
Hypothalamic nuclei, 63
Hypothalamus, 24
Hypothyroidism
  causing ataxic dysarthria, 169
  types of dysarthrias caused by
    and differential diagnoses, 414t
Hypotonia
  definition of, 165
  with flaccid dysarthrias, 110
  from posterior lobe lesions, 57
  summary of dysarthrias associated with,
    416t
Hypoxia
  in response to trauma, 34

Hypoxic encephalopathy
  and mixed dysarthria, 279-280, 282b
  types of dysarthrias caused by
    and differential diagnoses, 413t,
      414t
Hysterical neurosis, 384

I
Iatrogenic voice disorders, 391
Ictal speech arrests, 345
Idiopathic
  definition of, 115
Idiopathic disorders
  distribution and types of, 4f
Idiopathic torsion dystonia
  clinical features of, 224
Immobility
  with bradykinesia, 188-189
Immunosuppressive agents
  and mutism, 346
Impaired check
  and excessive rebound, 165
Imprecise articulation
  with chorea, 229
  with hypoglossal nerve lesions, 128,
    129f
Imprecise consonants
  with hypokinetic dysarthria, 196t, 197
  with spastic dysarthria, 151
"Improving"
  descriptive of disease evolution, 33
  disorders
    description and examples of, 12
Inappropriate silences
  with chorea, 229-230
  with hypokinetic dysarthria, 196-198
  motor system disorders associated with
    summary to aid differential diagnosis, 417,
      418t
Inborn errors
  of metabolism
    types of dysarthrias caused by, 414t
Inclusion bodies
  definition of, 31
Incontinence
  associated with parkinsonism, 169
  due to vascular disturbances, 26t
  with lacunar state, 146
Incoordination
  from posterior lobe lesions, 57
Increased rate
  motor system disorders associated with
    summary to aid differential diagnosis, 417,
      418t
Indirect activation pathways
  basal ganglia associated with, 188
  damage to
    and spastic dysarthria, 144t
  description and function of, 144
  versus direct activation pathway, 45t
  influencing gamma motor neurons, 38
  lesions, 51-52
  major cortical components of
    diagram illustrating, 46t
  and speech
    cortical components and tracts, 49-50
    destination of, 51
    effects of damage to, 51-52
    motor function roles in, 50-51
  UMN innervation
    nerves associated with, 48t
  of upper motor neuron (UUMN) system
    clinical features of, 257b
    definition of, 256
Indirect motor system;See indirect activation
    pathways
Inertial aphonia, 392
Inertial dysphonia, 392
Infantile speech
  psychogenic disorders of, 395-396
Infarcts
  hemorrhagic, 35
  ischemic, 35
  neurologic description of, 34

Infectious disorders
   associated with mixed dysarthria, 280-281, 281t
   and differential diagnoses, 412, 413t-414t
   causing flaccid dysarthria, 112b
   and hyperkinetic dysarthria, 222f, 223b, 224
   with hypokinetic dysarthria, 189b, 192
Infectious encephalopathy
   types of dysarthrias caused by
      and differential diagnoses, 414t
Infectious processes
   causing flaccid dysarthrias, 113
Inferior cerebellar peduncle, 42, 55
Inferior colliculi
   description and illustration of, 21, 22f
Inferior ganglia, 41, 42
Inferior olive, 42, 56f
Inferior pharyngeal constrictors, 42
Inflammatory diseases
   characteristics of
      and progression, 33
      for various neurologic disease etiologies, 32t
   and differential diagnoses, 412, 413t-414t
   causing spastic dysarthria, 146
Inflammatory polyradiculoneuropathy
   causing facial paralysis, 121
Information
   gathered during history-taking process, 73-75
Inhalation
   speaking on
      with spinal nerve lesions, 131
      with vagus nerve lesions, 126
   spinal nerve role in, 43
Inhalation speaking
   motor system disorders associated with
      summary to aid differential diagnosis, 417, 418t
Inhalatory stridor
   definition of, 84, 126
Inhibitory movements
   and indirect activation pathway, 144
Inion
   diagram illustrating, 18f
Injuries
   motor reorganization after, 445-446
Innervation
   loss and atrophy, 38
Innervation ratio
   definition of, 37
Inspiration
   MSDs associated with forced
      summary to aid differential diagnosis, 417, 418t
Instrumental biofeedback, 478-479
Instrumental feedback, 450-451
Instrumental methods
   of studying motor speech disorders, 9-10
Instrumentation
   for acoustic analysis, 10
Insula
   anatomical diagram of, 25f
   location in direct activation pathway, 47f
   role in motor speech programming, 310
   role in speech, 61-62
Integral stimulation
   and behavioral management of AOS, 515
Intelligibility
   assessment of, 96-97
   behavioral management to improve, 442
   definition of, 96
   drills, 479
   with hyperkinetic dysarthria, 226
   prostheses to treat abnormal, 441
   rating scale
      for motor speech disorders, 97t
   reduction
      with ataxic dysarthria, 171
   reduction of
      with mixed dysarthria, 284-285
   reduction with hypokinetic dysarthria, 193
   with spastic dysarthria, 147b, 148
   tests that measure, 98-99
Intensity
   measurement of speech
      with hypokinetic dysarthria, 199-200

Intention tremors, 165
   from posterior lobe lesions, 57
Intermittent hyponasality, 175
Internal acoustic meatus
   cranial nerves associated with, 19f
   view from above, 19f
Internal auditory arteries
   anatomical diagram of, 25f
Internal auditory meatus
   motor fibers through, 41
Internal capsule
   anatomical diagram of, 25f
   diagram illustrating, 48f, 53f
   in direct activation pathway, 47f
   lacunar strokes in
      and UUMN dysarthria, 257-258
   lesions
      causing spastic dysarthria, 147b, 148
   three major divisions of, 47-48
Internal carotid arteries
   anatomical location of, 24f
   definition and function of, 23
   sympathetic nerves, 19f
Internal laryngeal nerves
   function of, 42
Internal regulation system
   function and description of, 24
Internal respiration, 43
Interword intervals, 322-323
Intracerebral hemorrhages, 35
Intracranial arteritis
   types of dysarthrias caused by
      and differential diagnoses, 413t
Intracranial venous sinuses
   layers of
      description and diagram illustrating, 19, 20f
Intrafusal muscle fibers
   innervation of
      by gamma motor neurons, 38
Intramedullary lesions
   of vagus nerve, 123
Intraoral pressure
   Mayo Clinic rating scale for, 89, 90b
Intraparenchymal hemorrhages, 35
Involuntary movements
   abnormal
      with chorea, 227-228
      definition of, 218-219
      with hyperkinetic dysarthria, 226-227
   drugs that cause, 222-223
   of speech
      and hyperkinetic dysarthria, 217-218
   causing speech unsteadiness, 72
   summary of dysarthrias associated with, 416t
   with Tourette's syndrome, 238-239
Involuntary vocalizations
   description of, 361-362
   with progressive supranuclear palsy (PSP), 291
Iowa Oral Performance Instrument (IOPI), 83
Ipsilateral ataxia
   due to vascular disturbances, 26t-27t
Ipsilateral blindness
   due to vascular disturbances, 26t
Ipsilateral cerebellar ataxia
   due to vascular disturbances, 26t-27t
Irregular articulatory breakdowns
   with ataxic dysarthria, 173, 174, 175t
   with chorea, 229
Ischemia
   causes of, 34
   definition of, 31
   neuronal reactions to, 31
   in response to trauma, 34
Ischemic infarcts
   percentage of strokes, 35
Isochrony, 178

J
Jaw
   abnormal movements of
      with adductor spasmodic dysphonia, 243, 244t
      with hyperkinetic dysarthria, 225t, 226
      with tardive dyskinesia, 220

Jaw—cont'd
   alternate motion rates (AMRs), 79, 80f, 81
   appearance of
      at rest, 79, 80
      during sustained posture, 79, 80f
   dyskinesia waveforms, 234f
   dysmetric
      summary of dysarthrias associated with, 416t
   groping movements of
      with apraxia of speech, 320, 322b
   involuntary movements of
      with dystonia, 232, 233f, 234f
      summary of dysarthrias associated with, 416t
   and jaw jerk reflex, 86-87
   motor cortex neurons associated with, 46
   movements of
      and basal ganglia control circuit malfunctions, 188
      nerves associated with, 22t
      reduced with biopercular syndrome, 339-340
      and trigeminal nerve, 40-41
   myoclonic movement of
      with palatopharyngolaryngeal myoclonus, 237t
   tremulousness
      with hypokinetic dysarthria, 194, 197, 204
      summary of dysarthrias associated with, 416t
   trigeminal nerve sensory role in, 39
Jaw jerk reflexes
   description and illustration of, 86-87
   with spastic dysarthria, 144, 150
   summary of dysarthrias associated with, 416t
"Jitters"
   and voice quality
      with Parkinson's disease, 201
Jugular foramen
   accessory nerves through, 43
   cranial nerves associated with, 19f
   glossopharyngeal nerve through, 41
   syndrome, 124
   vagus nerve through, 42
   view from above, 19f

K
Kennedy's disease
   description of, 112-113
   types of dysarthrias caused by
      and differential diagnoses, 413t
Kinematics measures
   to study motor speech disorders, 10
Kinesthetic senses
   and normal speech development, 6
Kinetic tremors, 165
Knee-pat test, 165

L
Lability of affect
   with spastic dysarthria, 149-150
Lacerations, 34
Lacrimal glands
   facial nerve innervation of, 41
Lacrimation
   nerves associated with, 22t
Lacunar infarcts
   definition of, 145-146
   with unilateral upper motor neuron (UUMN) dysarthria, 258
Lacunar state
   definition of, 146
Lacunar syndromes
   with unilateral upper motor neuron (UUMN) dysarthria, 258
Lacunes
   definition of, 145-146
   with unilateral upper motor neuron (UUMN) dysarthria, 258
Lambert-Eaton syndrome
   myasthenic, 113
   types of dysarthrias caused by
      and differential diagnoses, 414t

Language
  deficits
    with apraxia of speech, 316, 317t
Laryngeal framework surgery, 469-471
Laryngeal hyperkinesia
  symptoms of, 227
Laryngeal speech valves, 71-72
Laryngeal surgeries
  and phonation, 469-471
Laryngectomy
  causing speech disorders, 6
Laryngoresponders, 390
Larynx
  abnormalities
    with hyperkinetic dysarthria, 225t, 226
  acoustic and physiologic findings
    with traumatic brain injuries (TBIs),
      294t
  characteristics
    with amyotrophic lateral sclerosis (ALS),
      287t
    with unilateral upper motor neuron
      (UUMN) dysarthria, 265-266, 265t
  lesions of, 84
  motor cortex neurons associated with, 46
  myoclonic movements
    with palatopharyngolaryngeal myoclonus,
      236, 237t
  nerve sensations of, 42
  nerves associated with, 22t
  problems with ataxic dysarthria, 175-177,
    179f
  structure, airflow and movement
    with Parkinson's disease, 201-202, 206t
  vagus nerve innervation of, 42
Laughter
  limbic system role in, 63
  with unilateral upper motor neuron (UUMN)
    dysarthria, 261
Learning
  limbic system role in sensations of, 63
Lee Silverman Voice Treatment (LSVT), 472,
  490-491
Left hemisphere
  description and illustration of, 21
  dominant in linguistic planning, 59
  lesions
    and depression, 383
    speech disorders associated with, 362-363,
      363-365
  tumors
    causing apraxia of speech, 314b
Lenticulostriate arteries
  anatomical diagram of, 25f
Lentiform nucleus
  associated with basal ganglia, 188
  definition of, 52
  diagram illustrating, 53f
  function and damage to, 53-54
Leptomeninges
  absorbing cerebrospinal fluid, 23
  description of, 19
  giving rise to meningiomas, 33
Lesions
  anatomic levels and vascular distribution
    and differential diagnoses, 411, 412t
  associated with apraxia of speech, 314-315
  associated with motor speech disorders, 12
  location of
    and differential diagnoses, 411, 412t
  nerve
    causing flaccid dysarthrias, 116-131
  sites of UMN system, 259-260
  unilateral upper motor neuron (UUMN)
    dysarthria, 257
Leukodystrophies
  affecting myelin, 32
Leukoencephalitis
  definition of, 146
Leukoencephalopathy
  types of dysarthrias caused by
    and differential diagnoses, 413t
Levator veli palatini, 43
Levodopa
  causing hyperkinetic dysarthria, 222

Lewy body disease
  types of dysarthrias caused by
    and differential diagnoses, 413t
Lexical stress, 366
Life stress
  and distinguishing neurogenic versus
    psychogenic
    aiding differential diagnosis, 426t, 428-429
Limb apraxia
  definition of, 310
  due to vascular disturbances, 26t
Limb ataxia
  from posterior lobe lesions, 57
Limb motor deficits
  management of, 439
Limbic lobes, 24
Limbic system
  and aprosodia, 365-370
  important role of
    in pain, smell and taste sensations, 62
  lesions
    and depression, 383
    and mutism, 344
  and mutism, 336t
Limbs
  movement deficits
    associated with apraxia of speech, 316,
      317t
Lingual dyskinesia, 233f
Linguistic planning
  description of, 59
  left hemisphere role in, 59
Linguistic units, 59
Lips
  abnormal movement of
    with adductor spasmodic dysphonia, 243,
      244t
  abnormal movements of
    with tardive dyskinesia, 220
  dyskinesia waveforms, 234f
  dysmetric
    summary of dysarthrias associated with,
      416t
  groping movements of
    with apraxia of speech, 320, 322b
  involuntary movements of
    with dystonia, 232, 233f, 234f
    summary of dysarthrias associated with,
      416t
  movements
    reduced with biopercular syndrome, 339-
      340
  myoclonic movement of
    with palatopharyngolaryngeal myoclonus,
      237t
  at rest, 76, 77f
  smacking with Tourette's syndrome,
    238-239
  sustained postures, 76, 77f
  tremulousness of
    with hypokinetic dysarthria, 194, 197, 204-
      205, 206t-207t
    summary of dysarthrias associated with,
      416t
Lithium
  causing ataxic dysarthria, 169
Liver
  disorders of
    causing parkinsonism, 192
  failure
    types of dysarthrias caused by, 414t
  transplant drugs
    and apraxia of speech, 311, 315
    and mutism, 346
Lobes
  anatomical relationships with
    and motor speech disorders, 21t
Localization
  characteristics of neurologic diseases, 32t
  and distinctions among dysfluencies
    associated with different speech disorders,
      425t
  of neurologic diseases
    definition of, 32-33
  stage of conceptualization, 59

"Locked-in" syndrome
  definition and clinical characteristics of, 338-
    339
  due to vascular disturbances, 26t-27t
  and mutism, 336t, 338-339
Locus ceruleus
  nerve cell loss
    with Parkinson's disease, 191
Long-term average spectrum (LTAS), 200
Loudness
  Mayo Clinic rating scale for, 89, 90b
  reduced
    with vagus nerve lesions, 126
Low pitch
  motor system disorders associated with
    summary to aid differential diagnosis, 417,
      418t
Lower face nerves
  and UMN innervation, 48t
Lower motor neuron (LMN) system;See also
    final common pathways (FCPs)
  alpha motor neurons and extrafusal fibers,
    37
  effects of damage, 38-39
  function and structure of, 36t
  gamma motor neurons and intrafusal fibers,
    37-38
  influences upon, 38
  nerve and muscle interactions, 36-37
  and speech, 38-45
    accessory nerves, 43
    facial nerves, 41
    glossopharyngeal nerves, 41-42
    hypoglossal nerves, 43
    spinal nerves, 43-45
    trigeminal nerves, 39-41
    vagus nerves, 42
  and speech muscle strength, 71
  versus upper motor neuron (UMN) system,
    45t
Lumbar vertebrae, 22
Lyme disease
  causing facial paralysis, 121

M

Macrophages
  function of, 31
Major longitudinal systems
  cerebrospinal fluid system within, 21f, 23
  of nervous system, 23-28
Malingering, 386
Malnutrition
  severe
    associated with cerebellar dysfunction, 169
Management
  approaches and issues
    augmented communication, 443-444
    behavioral management, 442-443, 445-454
    counseling and support, 444
    duration of treatment, 439-440
    factors influencing decisions, 437-439
    focus on treatment, 439
    medical interventions, 440-441
    prosthetics, 441-442
  of speaker-oriented dysarthria treatments
    articulation, 476-479
    overview of, 465-466
    phonation, 469-472
    prosody, 483-484
    rate, 479-483
    resonance, 472-476
    respiration, 466-469
  of specific dysarthria types
    ataxic dysarthria, 486t-487t, 488
    flaccid dysarthria, 485, 486t-487t
    hyperkinetic dysarthria, 486t-487t, 488-491
    hypokinetic dysarthria, 486t-487t, 488-491
    mixed dysarthria, 486t-487t, 493
    spastic dysarthria, 485, 486t-487t, 488
    UUMN dysarthria, 486t-487t, 493
Mandible
  diagram illustrating, 18f
Manic-depression
  definition of, 382-383
  speech characteristics with, 387

Manometers
  description and illustration of, 85-86
Masked facies
  definition of
    with parkinsonism, 189-190
  description of
    with hypokinetic dysarthria, 194
  illustration of expression, 190f
  summary of dysarthrias associated with, 416t
Masseter muscles, 41
Mastication
  nerves of, 40-41
  trigeminal nerve sensory role in, 39
Masticatory nucleus lesions, 41
Mastoid process
  diagram illustrating, 18f
Maxilla
  diagram illustrating, 18f
  trigeminal nerve branches from, 39
Maxillary reflexes, 86-87
Maxillary sinus
  trigeminal nerve branches from, 39
Maximum phonation time (MPT)
  measuring with hypokinetic dysarthria, 201
Maximum vowel prolongation, 91t
Mayo Clinic
  on ataxic dysarthria, 166f, 167f
  classifying acquired communication
    disorders, 4f
  classifying acquired neurologic disorders, 8f
  classifying motor speech disorders (MSDs),
    14f
  on deviant speech characteristics
    in dysarthrias, 103-104
  dysarthria studies, 89, 103-104
  on flaccid dysarthrias etiologies, 112b
  on hyperkinetic dysarthria
    etiologies of, 222f, 223b
  on mixed dysarthria, 89
  on speech pathology diagnosis
    of hypokinetic dysarthria, 192-194
  on unilateral upper motor neuron (UUMN)
    dysarthria
    etiologies of, 259
Mechanisms
  and distinctions among dysfluencies
    associated with different speech disorders,
      425t
  oral
    distinguishing among motor speech
      disorders, 416t
Medial longitudinal fasciculus, 51
Medial medullary syndrome, 114
Medial striate arteries
  anatomical diagram of, 25f
Medialization laryngoplasty, 469-471
Medical interventions
  for apraxia of speech (AOS), 509
  description of motor speech disorder, 440-441
  and diagnosis, 446
  for different dysarthria types, 488t
Medications;See also drugs
  and managing motor speech disorders, 440-
    441
  therapy
    for different dysarthria types, 488t
Medulla
  anatomical relationships with
    and motor speech disorders, 21t
  description and illustration of, 21, 22f
  diagram illustrating tracts in, 50f
  lesions
    causing spastic dysarthria, 147b, 148
Meige's syndrome, 224, 243
Melodic intonation therapy (MIT)
  and behavioral management of AOS,
    516-517
Memory
  deficits
    due to vascular disturbances, 26t
  limbic system role in sensations of, 63
Meninges
  anatomical relationships with
    and motor speech disorders, 21t

Meninges—cont'd
  layers of
    description and diagram illustrating, 19,
      20f
Meningitis
  causing facial paralysis, 121
  causing flaccid dysarthria, 112b
  location of, 33
  types of dysarthrias caused by
    and differential diagnoses, 414t
Mental illness;See also psychogenic speech
      disorders
  affecting speech, 7
  and echolalia, 359, 360b
Mesencephalic nucleus, 41
Metabolic conditions
  astrocyte reaction to, 32
  causing ataxic dysarthria, 166f, 169
  characteristics of
    and progression, 33
    for various neurologic disease etiologies,
      32t
  and differential diagnoses, 412, 413t-414t
  and hyperkinetic dysarthria, 222-223
  with hypokinetic dysarthria, 189b, 191-192
Metastasizing
  definition of, 33
Metathetic articulatory errors
  motor system disorders associated with
    summary to aid differential diagnosis, 417,
      418t
Methanol
  causing parkinsonism, 192
Metronomes, 441
Microglia
  structure and function of nervous system, 28t
  transformation of, 31
Micrographia
  with parkinsonism, 190
Midbrain
  anatomical relationships with
    and motor speech disorders, 21t
  description and illustration of, 21, 22f
  diagram illustrating tracts in, 50f
Middle cerebellar peduncles, 55
  degeneration of, 168
Middle cerebral arteries
  anatomical diagram of, 25f
  anatomical location of, 24f, 25f
  function of, 23
Middle fossae
  anatomical relationships with
    and motor speech disorders, 21t
  definition of, 18
  illustration of, 19f
Mixed dysarthria
  amyotrophic lateral sclerosis (ALS), 276-277,
    281t, 282b, 285-289
  from autoimmune diseases, 280-281, 281t,
    282b
  case studies, 296-301
  characteristics of, 284-285
  cortical degeneration, 279, 281t, 282b, 292-
    293
  definition and overview of, 275-276
  from degenerative diseases, 276-279, 281t,
    282b
  description of, 275-276
  deviant speech characteristics with, 285t
  etiologies of, 276-281, 282-295, 282b
  Friedreich's ataxia, 278, 281t, 282b, 290
  from infectious diseases, 280-281, 281t, 282b
  localization and neuromotor basis of, 13t
  Mayo Clinic dysarthria studies on, 89
  from motor neuron diseases, 276-277, 281t,
    282b
  multiple sclerosis, 277, 281t, 282b, 289-290
  multiple system atrophy, 278, 281t, 282b,
    291-292
  progressive supranuclear palsy (PSP), 278,
    281t, 282b, 290, 291
  severity of, 284-285
  speaker-oriented treatments, 486t-487t, 493
  speech pathology, 281-295, 282b

Mixed dysarthria—cont'd
  summary of etiologies, 281t, 282b
  from toxic/metabolic conditions
    central pontine myelinolysis, 280, 282b
    hepatocerebral degeneration, 279, 282b
    hypoxic encephalopathy, 279-280, 282b
    Wilson's disease (WD), 279-280, 282b
  from traumatic brain injuries (TBIs), 280,
    281t, 282b, 293-295
  types and mixtures of, 283-284
  from vascular disorders, 280, 282b
Modified tongue-anchor test, 84
Monoamines
  as part of neurochemical system, 24
Monoloudness
  with amyotrophic lateral sclerosis (ALS),
    285t, 289
  with hypokinetic dysarthria, 196t, 197
  motor system disorders associated with
    summary to aid differential diagnosis, 417,
      418t
  with phonatory-prosodic insufficiency, 173-
    174
  with spastic dysarthria, 151
Mononeuritis
  definition of, 33
Mononeuropathy
  definition of, 111
Mononucleosis
  causing facial paralysis, 121
Monopitch
  with amyotrophic lateral sclerosis (ALS),
    285t, 289
  with chorea, 229-230
  with hypokinetic dysarthria, 196t, 197
  motor system disorders associated with
    summary to aid differential diagnosis, 417,
      418t
  with phonatory-prosodic insufficiency, 173-
    174
  with progressive supranuclear palsy (PSP),
    291
  with spastic dysarthria, 151
Motor control
  in Parkinson's disease patients, 201
  and sensations, 62
  and Tourette's syndrome, 238-239
Motor cortex
  characteristics of, 46-47
  injuries
    motor reorganization after, 445-446
  as neural area of programming, 60
Motor end plates
  diagram illustrating, 30f
Motor equivalence
  definition of, 60
Motor fibers
  diagram illustrating, 30f
  innervating facial expressions, 41
Motor impersistence
  definition of, 92
Motor learning
  principles of, 449-453
Motor neuron diseases
  definition of, 111-112
  causing mixed dysarthria, 276-277, 281t
  types of dysarthrias caused by
    and differential diagnoses, 413t
Motor plasticity, 445
Motor reorganization, 445-446
Motor speech disorders (MSDs)
  anatomical relationships and, 21t
  basic definition of, 6
  behavioral management of
    baseline data, 448
    basic principles of, 445-452
    communication -oriented approaches, 443
    evidence-based practice, 455-456
    goals of, 440
    medical and speech diagnoses, 446-447
    motor learning principles, 449-453
    motor reorganization, 446
    and neural adaptation, 445-446
    organizing sessions, 453-454

Motor speech disorders (MSDs)—cont'd
  behavioral management of—cont'd
    speech-oriented approaches, 442-443
    treatment efficacy, 454-456
    treatment timing, 447-448
  categorizing and characterizing, 11-14
  and cerebellar control circuit damage, 163-
    183
  course of
    during neurologic disease progression, 33
  and cranial nerve lesions, 119t-120t
  defining, understanding and categorizing, 3-
    15
  differential diagnoses of, 409-431
  distinctions among
    and anatomic and vascular levels, 411,
      412t
  distinguishing from aphasia, 421, 422t
  distribution and types of, 4f
  examination procedures, 69-100, 71-74
    confirmatory signs, 73
    description of, 69-70
    diagnosis, 73-74
    diagnosis process, 70
    history, 71
    neurologic localization, 70
    procedures, 74-99
    purpose of, 69-70
    salient features, 71-73
    severity, 70
  flaccid dysarthrias, 109-140
  hierarchies of symptoms, 477
  hyperkinetic dysarthria
    deviant speech characteristics of, 228-244
    and involuntary movements of speech,
      217-218
  hyperkinetic dysarthria subtypes
    action myoclonus, 237-238
    athetosis, 232-233
    cervical dystonia, 233-235
    chorea, 227-230
    dystonia, 228t, 230-232, 233f, 234t
    organic voice tremors, 239-240, 241f, 242t
    palatopharyngolaryngeal myoclonus, 235-
      237
    spasmodic dysphonia (SD), 240-244
    spasmodic torticollis, 233-235
    Tourette's syndrome/tics, 238-239
  hypokinetic dysarthria, 187-211
    acoustic and physiologic findings of, 198-
      205, 206t-207t
    anatomical relationships associated with,
      21t
    and basal ganglia control circuits, 187-188,
      188-190
    blurred speech with, 194
    case studies of, 207-211
    clinical signs of, 194-198
    definition of, 187
    dementia pugilistica leading to, 192
    deviant speech characteristics with, 195-
      197
    differential diagnosis of, 413t-414t
    distinctions among other speech
      disturbances, 426t, 428-429
    distinctive speech characteristics with, 417,
      418t
    due to vascular disturbances, 26t
    etiologies of, 189b, 190-192, 193f
    "fused" speech with, 205
    lesion loci and vascular source, 411, 412t
    localization and neuromotor basis of, 13t
    masked facial expression with, 189, 190f
    Mayo Clinic dysarthria studies on, 89, 189,
      190f
    and mixed dysarthria, 283-284
    mutism with, 336t
    neurochemical systems indicated in, 24-25
    neuromuscular deficits associated with, 195t
    and neurotransmitter depletion, 187
    patient's perceptions of, 193-194
    primary speech characteristics with, 198t
    respiration abnormalities with, 198-199,
      206t

Motor speech disorders (MSDs)—cont'd
  hypokinetic dysarthria—cont'd
    with rigidity, 54
    speaker-oriented treatments, 486t-487t,
      488-491
    summary of oral mechanism findings, 415,
      416t
    surgery interventions for, 488-489
  intelligibility, comprehensibility, and
    efficiency, 96-97
  know etiologies for
    aiding differential diagnoses, 412, 413t-
      414t, 415
  major types of, 13t
  management approaches
    augmented communication, 443-444
    behavioral management, 442-443, 445-454
    counseling and support, 444
    medical interventions, 440-441
    prosthetics, 441-442
  management issues
    duration of treatment, 439-440
    factors influencing decisions, 437-439
    focus on treatment, 439
  medical diagnoses and prognoses, 437-438
  methods of studying
    acoustic, 10
    instrumental, 9-10
    perceptual, 9
    physiologic, 10
    visual imaging, 10-11
  mixed dysarthria
    amyotrophic lateral sclerosis (ALS), 276-
      277, 281t, 282b, 285-289
    from autoimmune diseases, 280-281, 281t,
      282b
    case studies, 296-301
    cortical degeneration, 279, 281t, 292-293
    definition and overview of, 275-276
    from degenerative diseases, 276-279, 281t,
      282b
    description of, 275-276
    etiologies of, 276-281, 282-295, 282b
    Friedreich's ataxia, 278, 281t, 282b, 290
    from infectious diseases, 280-281, 281t,
      282b
    localization and neuromotor basis of, 13t
    Mayo Clinic dysarthria studies on, 89
    from motor neuron diseases, 276-277,
      281t, 282b
    multiple sclerosis, 277, 281t, 282b, 289-
      290
    multiple system atrophy, 278, 281t, 282b,
      291-292
    progressive supranuclear palsy (PSP), 278,
      281t, 282b, 290, 291
    speech pathology, 281-295
    from toxic/metabolic conditions, 279-280,
      281t, 282b
    from traumatic brain injuries (TBIs), 280,
      281t, 282b, 293-295
    from vascular disorders, 280, 282b
  and mutism, 336t
    anarthria, 336-338
    apraxia of speech, 336t, 341-342
    biopercular syndrome, 336t, 339-340
    cerebellar mutism, 336t, 340-341
    locked-in syndrome, 336t, 338-339
    types of, 336t
  neurologic bases and pathologies of, 17-66
  neurologic basis for
    differential diagnoses and localization of, 4
    management of, 5
    prevalence of, 4-5
  nonorganic speech disorders
    management of
      general principles and guidelines, 536-541
    prevalence and distribution of, 7-8
  psychogenic speech disorders
    management of
      general principles and guidelines, 536-541
      general treatment techniques, 541-545
      symptomatic treatment of specific, 545-
        550

Motor speech disorders (MSDs)—cont'd
  rating deviant characteristics of, 89, 90b, 103-
    104
  relevant functional and anatomic divisions of,
    36t
  resource information related to, 461-462
  salient neuromuscular features of, 71-73
  sensorimotor characteristics of, 6
  summary of oral mechanism findings, 415,
    416t
  taking patient history, 73-75
  unilateral upper motor neuron (UUMN)
      dysarthria
    acoustic and physiologic findings, 265-266
    anatomy and functions of, 256-257
    case studies of, 268-270
    clinical characteristics of, 261-265
    clinical features of lesions, 257, 259-260
    definition and overview of, 255-256
    distinctiveness of, 267-268
    etiologies of, 257-258, 259f, 259t, 260
    patient perceptions and complaints, 261
    severity of, 261
    speech characteristics of, 261-265
  variables of
    age at onset, 12
    course of disease, 12
    neurologic diagnosis, 12
    pathophysiology, 13
    perceptual characteristics, 13
    severity, 13
    site of lesion, 12
    speech components involved, 13
  and vascular brain supply, 26t, 27t
  vascular diseases causing, 34-35
Motor speech planning
  assessment of, 94
  definition of, 3
  different disorders involving, 313
  dominant hemisphere damage affecting, 64
  elements of, 60
  introduction to, 307
  versus motor programming, 60
  and programming
    of speech, 59-64
Motor speech processes
  definition of, 3
  summary of, 64-66
Motor speech programmer
  anatomy and functions of, 308-310
  definition of, 308
  diagram illustrating, 37f
  network, 309-310
Motor speech programming
  assessing capacity of, 94, 95b
  definition of, 3
  different disorders involving, 313
  discussion of, 59-60
  dominant hemisphere damage affecting, 64
  elements of, 60
  introduction to, 307
  versus motor planning, 60
  as sensorimotor process, 316, 317t
Motor strip, 45-46
Motor system
  components of, 27-28
  and conceptual-programming, 57-59
  damage and mutism, 335
  function of, 27
  functional and anatomic divisions of
    basal ganglia control circuit, 36t, 52-54
    cerebellar control circuit, 36t, 54-57
    control circuits, 36t, 52
    direct activation pathway, 36t, 45-49
    final common pathway, 36-45
    indirect activation pathway, 36t, 49-52
  and neuron activity, 29-30
  relationships among divisions of, 37f
  of speech
    description of, 35-36
    functions of, 35, 36t
Motor units
  components of
    associated with flaccid dysarthrias, 110t

Motor units—cont'd
  definition of, 37
  diagram illustrating, 30f, 39f
  effects of damage to, 38
  and neural adaptation, 445
Motor vehicle accidents
  and traumatic brain injury, 34
Mouth
  abnormal movements of
    with adductor spasmodic dysphonia, 243, 244t
    with tardive dyskinesia, 220
  movements
    nerves associated with, 22t
  sustained postures, 76, 78f
  trigeminal nerve sensory role in, 39
  xerostomia, 81
Movements
  abnormal
    with amyotrophic lateral sclerosis (ALS),
      285-289
    with Tourette's syndrome, 238-239
    and basal ganglia control circuit
      malfunctions, 188
    categories of abnormal
      rate and rhythm characteristics of, 219t
    impairments
      with hypokinetic dysarthria, 193-194
    and indirect activation pathway, 144
    involuntary
      summary of dysarthrias associated with,
        416t
    and motor speech programming, 308-310
    rate of
      slowed by spastic dysarthria, 155-156
    reduced with biopercular syndrome, 339-340
    slowness of
      and spastic paralysis, 144t, 145
    and speech, 62-63
Moyamoya disease, 146
Multifocal
  as descriptive of localization, 33
Multifocal leukoencephalopathy
  types of dysarthrias caused by
    and differential diagnoses, 414t
Multiple motor tics
  summary of dysarthrias associated with, 416t
Multiple sclerosis (MS)
  associated with mixed dysarthria, 277, 281t,
    289-290
  demyelination with, 32
  and depression, 383
  as exacerbating-remitting disease, 12
  leading to mutism, 337t, 338
  causing palilalia, 258b, 359
  types of dysarthrias caused by
    and differential diagnoses, 414t
Multiple system atrophy (MSA)
  associated with mixed dysarthria, 278, 281t,
    291-292
  with ataxic dysarthria, 168
  with Parkinson's disease, 191
  types of dysarthrias caused by
    and differential diagnoses, 413t
Munchausen's syndrome
  as factitious disorder, 386
Muscle diseases
  and differential diagnoses, 412, 413t-414t
  causing flaccid dysarthria, 112b, 113
  types of dysarthrias caused by
    and differential diagnoses, 414t, 415
Muscle fibers
  diagram illustrating, 30f
  and stretch reflex, 38, 39f
Muscle spindles
  innervation of
    by gamma motor neurons, 38
Muscle tone
  and basal ganglia, 53
  basal ganglia control circuit regulating, 188
  exercises
    to improve articulation, 478
  and gamma motor neurons, 38, 39f, 51
  hypotonia
    with flaccid dysarthrias, 110

Muscle tone—cont'd
  and indirect activation pathway, 144
  reduction with neurologic disease, 72
Muscles
  atrophy with flaccid dysarthrias, 110
  bulbar
    Wilson disease affect on, 293
  drugs that treat disorders of, 440-441
  innervating for speech, 3
  of mastication, 39
  motor system involvement in, 27-28
  and neural adaptation, 445
  palatoglossus, 42
  of speech
    and flaccid dysarthrias, 109
  strength
    of speech, 71
  strength training for oral, 452-453
  and stretch reflex, 38, 39f
  trigeminal nerve sensory role in, 39
Muscular dystrophy
  causing flaccid dysarthria, 112b
  types of dysarthrias caused by
    and differential diagnoses, 414t
Musculoskeletal activities
  in speech, 3
Musculoskeletal defects
  causing speech disorders, 6
Musculoskeletal tension disorders
  voice abnormalities with, 390
Mutism
  akinetic, 343-344
  and anarthria, 336-338
  and apraxia of speech, 336t, 341-342
  and biopercular syndrome, 336t, 339-340
  case studies, 346-349
  and cerebellar mutism, 336t, 340-341
  of cerebellar origin, 340-341
  definition and overview of, 335-336
  distinguishing among forms of
    akinetic mutism, 424t, 425
    anarthria, 423, 424t
    aphasia, 424t, 425
    apraxia of speech, 424-425
    cognitive-affect disorders, 424t, 425
  following corpus callosotomy, 345
  forms of, 335, 336t, 424t
  and locked-in syndrome, 336t, 338-339
  motor speech disorders associated with
    localization and clinical features of, 336t
  and speech arrest, 345
  with supplemental motor area damage, 61
Myasthenia gravis (MG)
  drugs that treat, 440-441
  causing flaccid dysarthria, 111, 112b, 115f
  with multiple cranial nerve lesions, 131-132
  ptosis as sign of, 113
  types of dysarthrias caused by
    and differential diagnoses, 414t
Mycoplasma pneumoniae
  causing parkinsonism, 192
Myelin
  diseases which affect, 32
  formation of, 30-31
Myelin sheaths
  regeneration of, 31
Myelinated nerve fibers
  relevant to speech motor and sensory functions, 30
Myelitis
  definition of, 111
Myelopathy
  definition of, 111
Mylohyoid, 39
Myoclonic epilepsy, 220
  types of dysarthrias caused by
    and differential diagnoses, 414t
Myoclonic vowel prolongation
  motor system disorders associated with
    summary to aid differential diagnosis, 417,
      418t
Myoclonus
  definition of, 220
  rate, rhythm, and substrate characteristics of,
    219t

Myoclonus—cont'd
  summary of dysarthrias associated with, 416t
  toxins that cause, 223
Myopathy
  definition of, 111
  causing flaccid dysarthria, 112b
  types of dysarthrias caused by
    and differential diagnoses, 414t
Myositis
  definition of, 111
Myotonic dystrophy
  causing flaccid dysarthria, 112b
  types of dysarthrias caused by
    and differential diagnoses, 414t
Myotonic muscular dystrophy
  definition of, 113
Myxedema
  leading to ataxic dysarthria, 169

N
Nasal bones
  diagram illustrating, 18f
Nasal cavity
  diagram illustrating, 18f
Nasal emission
  motor system disorders associated with
    summary to aid differential diagnosis, 417,
      418t
Nasal regurgitation
  summary of dysarthrias associated with, 416t
Nasopharyngeal obturator, 441
Naturalness, 483-484
  treatment approaches to improve
    for different dysarthria types, 486t
Nausea
  due to vascular disturbances, 26t-27t
Neck
  breathing, 468
  injuries
    causing flaccid dysarthria, 112b
  movement
    nerves associated with, 22t
  trauma
    types of dysarthrias caused by, 413t
Neocerebellum, 54, 55f
Neoplastic diseases
  causing ataxic dysarthria, 166f, 168-169, 170
  characteristics of
    and progression, 33-34
  for various neurologic disease etiologies, 32t
  and differential diagnoses, 412, 413t-414t
  and hyperkinetic dysarthria, 222f, 223b, 224
Nerve cells;See neurons
Nerve fibers
  collecting to form nerves, 30
Nerve roots
  attaching nerves to spinal cord, 22
Nerve tracts
  damage to, 31
Nerves
  components of, 30-31
  composition of, 30
  diagram illustrating, 30f
Nervous system
  anatomical relationships at levels of, 21t
  astrocytes, 31
  bony boundaries of, 18-19
  characteristics of, 19, 21t
  and conceptual programming, 57
  connective tissue, 31
  and diagnoses, 70
  disorders and speech, 3-5
  ependymal cells, 31
  glial cells, 30-31
  importance of understanding, 4
  major anatomic levels of, 19, 20f, 21-23
  microglia, 31
  and motor speech disorders, 21t
  and motor speech processes
    summary of, 64-66
  nerve cells responding
    to neurologic disease, 31
  neurons, 28-29
  normal reflexes with, 86

Nervous system—cont'd
  recovery of, 445-446
  reflexes and learning, 62-63
  structural elements of, 28t
  tracts and pathways, 29-30
  tumors, 33-34
  vascular components of, 23, 24f
Nervous system diseases;*See also* neurologic
      diseases
  localizing and course of, 32-33
Neural adaptation
  definition of, 445
Neuritis
  definition of, 111
Neuroanatomy
  as foundation
    for motor speech disorder diagnosis and
        management, 17
  summary of, 64-66
Neurochemical systems
  components of, 24
  and motor speech disorders, 24-25
Neurocognitive activities
  in speech, 3
Neurocytomas, 33
Neurofibrillary degeneration
  definition of, 31
Neurofibrillary tangles
  in Alzheimer's disease, 33
Neurogenic mutism
  akinetic, 343-344
  and anarthria, 336-338
  and apraxia of speech, 336t, 341-342
  and biopercular syndrome, 336t, 339-340
  case studies, 346-349
  and cerebellar mutism, 336t, 340-341
  of cerebellar origin, 340-341
  definition and overview of, 335-336
  distinguishing among forms of
    akinetic mutism, 424t, 425
    anarthria, 423, 424t
    aphasia, 424t, 425
    apraxia of speech, 424-425
    cognitive-affect disorders, 424t, 425
  following corpus callosotomy, 345
  forms of, 335, 336t
  and locked-in syndrome, 336t, 338-339
  motor speech disorders associated with
    localization and clinical features of,
        336t
  and speech arrest, 345
  with supplemental motor area damage, 61
Neurogenic speech disorders
  aphasia, 354t, 362-363
  aprosodia, 354t, 365-370
  case studies, 371-375
  cognitive/affective, 354t, 360-362
  distinguishing between psychogenic, 426t,
      428-429, 430t
  dysarthrias
    management of
      communication-oriented treatment of,
          494-498, 496-498
  echolalia, 354t, 359-360
  foreign accent syndrome, 354t, 363-365
  management of other, 525-530
  neurogenic stuttering, 354-358, 364t
  "other" as defined by Mayo Clinic
      distribution statistics, 8f
  palilalia, 354t, 358-359
Neurogenic stuttering
  anatomic correlates, 357
  with apraxia of speech, 316
  behavioral management
    rate reduction strategies, 527
    self-monitoring, 527
  definition and clinical characteristics of,
      354-355
  distinctions among dysfluencies associated
      with, 425t, 426
  etiologies of, 355-357
  management of
    behavioral management, 526-527
    medical management, 526

Neurogenic stuttering—cont'd
  nature of the problem, 357-358
  with progressive supranuclear palsy (PSP),
      291
  terminology, 392
  varieties of, 356
Neuroleptic medications
  affecting neurotransmitter balance
    and causing hyperkinetic dysarthria, 222-
        223
  leading to parkinsonism, 191-192
Neurologic diagnosis
  broad categories of, 12
Neurologic diseases;*See also* nervous system
      diseases
  broad etiologic categories
    degenerative diseases, 33
    inflammatory diseases, 33
    neoplastic diseases, 33-34
    toxic-metabolic diseases, 33
    traumatic diseases, 34
    vascular diseases, 34-35
  characteristics for various etiologies of, 32t
  and conversion disorders, 384
  and depression, 383
  localization, development and evolution of,
      32t
  localization of
    definition of, 32-33
    and motor speech processes
      summary of, 64-66
    nerve cells responding to, 31
  and speech changes, 3-5
  causing speech unsteadiness, 72
Neurologic speech disorders
  apraxia of speech
    and motor speech planning/programming,
        307-308
  definitions of
    apraxia of speech, 5-6
    dysarthria, 5
    Mayo clinic definition of "other"
        distribution and types of, 4f
    other cognitive and linguistic, 6
Neuromuscular activities
  in speech, 3
Neuromuscular deficits
  associated with hyperkinetic dysarthria
    and chorea and dystonia, 228t
Neuromuscular execution
  definition of, 3
Neuromuscular junctions
  diseases
    description and signs of, 113
    and differential diagnoses, 412, 413t-414t
  diseases of, 111
  problems and flaccid dysarthria, 109
Neuronal neoplasms, 33
Neurons
  combined activities of, 30
  damaged, 31-32
  description and components of, 28-29
  diagram illustrating, 29f
  regeneration of, 31-32
  structure and function of nervous system,
      28t
Neuropathology
  summary of, 64-66
Neuropathy
  definition of, 111
  causing flaccid dysarthria, 112b
Neuropeptides
  as part of neurochemical system, 24
Neurophysiology
  as foundation
    for motor speech disorder diagnosis and
        management, 17
  summary of, 64-66
Neurosyphilis, 114-115
Neurotransmitters
  acetylcholine, 29, 30f
  and basal ganglia, 53
  depletion
    with hypokinetic dysarthria, 187-188

Neurotransmitters—cont'd
  drugs that affect balance of, 222-223
  imbalances
    causing basal ganglia control circuit
        malfunctions, 188
Nigrostriatal degeneration
  with Parkinson's disease, 191
Nigrostriatal tracts, 53
Nodes of Ranvier
  description of, 31
  diagram illustrating, 30f
Nodose ganglia, 42
Nodules, 55f
Noncranial bones
  anatomical relationships with
    and motor speech disorders, 21t
Nonhemorrhagic strokes
  causing ataxic dysarthria, 170
  types of dysarthrias caused by
    and differential diagnoses, 413t
Nonorganic disorders
  affecting speech, 7
Nonorganic speech disorders
  case studies, 397-405
  definition and overview of, 381-382
  distinguishing between neurogenic, 426t,
      428-429, 430t
  etiologies of
    conversion disorders, 383-385
    depression, 382-383
    schizophrenia, 383
    stress and reactions to stress, 385
    volitional disorders, 386
  examination of, 387-388
  management of
    general principles and guidelines, 536-541
    general treatment techniques, 541-545
    symptomatic treatment of specific, 545-550
  other nonorganic disorders associated with
    articulation disorders, 395
    infantile speech, 396
    psychogenic mutism, 396
    resonance and prosodic disorders, 396
  speech characteristics, 389-396
    with depression and manic-depression, 389
    dysfluencies, 394b
    with psychogenic stuttering, 392-395
    with psychogenic voice disorders, 390-392
    with schizophrenia, 389-390
  statistical distributions of, 386t
Nonspeech motor control
  with apraxia of speech (AOS)
    acoustic and physiologic findings with,
        322b
Nonspinal bones
  anatomical relationships with
    and motor speech disorders, 21t
Nonverbal oral apraxia (NVOA)
  with apraxia of speech, 316, 317t
  assessment of, 88
  corticobasal degeneration (CBD), 311
  definition and characteristics of, 316, 317t
  summary of dysarthrias associated with,
      416t
Normal pressure hydrocephalus (NPH)
  associated with parkinsonism
    and hypokinetic dysarthria, 169
  ataxic dysarthria from, 169
Nose
  trigeminal nerve sensory role in, 39
Nuclei
  problems and flaccid dysarthria, 109
Nucleus ambiguus, 41, 42, 43
Nystagmus
  definition of, 165
  due to flocculonodular lesions, 57
  due to vascular disturbances, 26t-27t

O

Obscene gestures
  with Tourette's syndrome, 238-239
Obstructive hydrocephalus
  associated with parkinsonism
    and hypokinetic dysarthria, 169

Occipital bones
    diagram illustrating, 18f
Occipital lobes
    sensory systems of, 27
Ocular dysmetria
    definition of, 165
Oculomotor deficits
    due to vascular disturbances, 26t-27t
Oculomotor nerves
    anatomic origin and function of, 22t
Oculomotor palsy
    due to vascular disturbances, 26t
Oculopharyngeal muscular dystrophy, 113
Older adults;See aging
Olfactory nerves
    anatomic origin and function of, 22t
    role in speech, 63
Oligodendroglia cells
    forming myelin, 30-31
    structure and function of nervous system, 28t
Olivary nuclei
    degeneration of, 168
Olivopontocerebellar ataxia, 167
Olivopontocerebellar atrophy (OPCA)
    definition of, 168
    with Parkinson's disease, 191
    types of dysarthrias caused by
        and differential diagnoses, 413t
On-off effects
    definition of, 191
Opercular syndrome;See biopercular syndrome
Ophthalmic arteries
    anatomical relationships with
        and motor speech disorders, 21t
Optic atrophy
    due to vascular disturbances, 26t
Optic nerves
    anatomic origin and function of, 22t
    anatomical diagram of, 25f
Optic tract
    vascular supply to, 26t
Optimal breath group, 467
Oral secretions
    and glossopharyngeal nerve, 42
Oral verbal apraxia, 312
Orbit
    vascular supply to, 26t
Orbital cavity
    diagram illustrating, 18f
Organic vocal tremors
    description and waveforms illustrating, 239-240, 241f
    distinguishing speech characteristics of, 242t
Organic voice
    rate, rhythm, and substrate of, 219t
Oro-buccalingual dyskinesia, 220
Orofacial dyskinesias
    definition of, 219
    and dystonia, 221
Orofacial dystonia, 221
Orofacial mobility
    reduced with biopercular syndrome, 339-340
Orofacial tremors
    with spasmodic dysphonia, 243
Oromandibular-lingual dystonia
    illustration of patient with, 231f
Oromotor reflex testing, 86
Otitis media
    causing facial paralysis, 121

P

Pacing boards, 441, 481-482
Pain
    limbic system role in sensations of, 63
    nerve fibers, 40
    transmission through trigeminal nerves, 39
Palatal lift prosthesis, 441, 473, 474f, 493
Palatal myoclonus, 220
    due to vascular disturbances, 26t-27t
Palatal tremors, 220
Palatal weakness
    unilateral
        summary of dysarthrias associated with, 416t

Palate
    abnormal movements of
        with adductor spasmodic dysphonia, 243, 244t
        with hyperkinetic dysarthria, 225t, 226
    and gag reflex, 86
    involuntary movements of
        summary of dysarthrias associated with, 416t
    motor cortex neurons associated with, 46
    movements
        reduced with biopercular syndrome, 339-340
    nerves associated with, 22t
    weakness
        with hypoglossal nerve lesions, 128, 129f
Palatoglossus muscles, 42, 43
Palatopharyngolaryngeal myoclonus (PM)
    definition of, 220
    description and illustration of, 235-236
    effects on speech, 237
    hyperkinetic dysarthria of
        distinguishing speech characteristics of, 237t
        rate, rhythm, and substrate characteristics of, 219t
Palilalia
    causes and anatomic correlates, 359
    clinical characteristics of, 358-359
    distinctions among dysfluencies associated with, 425t, 427
    management of, 528
    motor system disorders associated with
        summary to aid differential diagnosis, 417, 418t
    with progressive supranuclear palsy (PSP), 291, 292
    with Tourette's syndrome, 238-239
Pallidotomy
    to treat hypokinetic dysarthria, 488-489
Palmomental reflexes
    description of, 87-88
    with spastic dysarthria, 144, 150
Paralysis
    with masticatory nucleus lesions, 41
Paraneoplastic cerebellar degeneration, 169
Paraneoplastic syndrome
    types of dysarthrias caused by
        and differential diagnoses, 413t
Paraplegia
    due to vascular disturbances, 26t
Paratonia, 344
Parenchyma, 31
Paresis
    with masticatory nucleus lesions, 41
    and nerve damage, 38
Parietal bones
    diagram illustrating, 18f
Parietal lobes
    sensory systems of, 27
    somatosensory cortex, 309-310
Parkinsonism
    akathisia with, 220
    and basal ganglia control circuit
        malfunctions, 188-189
    common nonspeech signs of, 189t
    defining clinical signs of
        versus Parkinson's disease, 191
    dementia pugilistica leading to, 192
    Mayo Clinic dysarthria studies on, 89
    causing palilalia, 258b, 359
    respiration abnormalities with, 198-199, 206t
    types of dysarthrias caused by
        and differential diagnoses, 413t
Parkinson-plus syndromes, 191
Parkinson's disease (PD)
    akathisia with, 220
    associated with hypokinetic dysarthria, 187
    deep brain stimulation (DBS) to treat, 488-489
    and depression, 383
    diagnosing, 70
    facial masking with, 54
    and fundamental frequency, 199-200

Parkinson's disease (PD)—cont'd
    and inclusion bodies, 31
    causing palilalia, 258b, 359
    versus parkinsonism, 191
    possibly leading to mutism, 338
    respiration abnormalities with, 198-199, 206t
    speech impairment statistics with, 7
    statistics concerning, 190-191
    types of dysarthrias caused by
        and differential diagnoses, 413t
Parotid tumors
    causing facial paralysis, 121
Paroxysmal ataxia, 168
Paroxysmal ataxic dysarthria (PAD), 168
Paroxysmal dystonic choreoathetosis, 224
Paroxysmal exercise-induced dystonia, 224
Paroxysmal kinesigenic choreoathetosis, 224
Pathologic crying
    with spastic dysarthria, 149-150
    with unilateral upper motor neuron (UUMN)
        dysarthria, 261
Pathologic laughing
    with spastic dysarthria, 149-150
    with unilateral upper motor neuron (UUMN)
        dysarthria, 261
Pathologic oral reflexes
    description of, 86
    in UMN disease, 144
Pathophysiology
    as variable in motor speech disorders, 13
Pathways
    definition of nerve fiber, 30
    structure and function of nervous system, 28t
Pause
    abnormalities
        with hypokinetic dysarthria, 205
    time, 480
Pendulousness
    definition of, 165
Penetrating head injuries
    definition of, 34
    types of dysarthrias caused by
        and differential diagnoses, 413t
Perceptual analysis
    of motor speech disorders
        clinical salience of, 11
    of speech characteristics, 88-96
        distinctive dysarthria, 89-90
        Mayo Clinic dysarthria studies, 88-90
        published tests, 94, 96
        tasks for, 91-94
        styles used for, 90-91
Perceptual methods
    of classifying speech disorders, 13
    of studying motor speech disorders, 9
Percussion myotonia
    definition of, 113
Performance
    components and disorders associated with, 58t
    within conceptual-programming level, 64
Pergolide
    for Parkinson's disease, 191
Peripheral end organs, 30
Peripheral nerves
    anatomical relationships with
        and motor speech disorders, 21t
    diagram illustrating, 30f
    within sensory system, 27
Peripheral nervous system (PNS);See also
        nervous system
    cranial and spinal nerves in, 21, 22t, 23
    damage and mutism, 335
    major structures of, 30
    nerves versus tracts, 30
    and reflex testing, 86-87
    regulating speech motor programs, 3
Peripheral neuropathy
    definition of, 111
Peripheral receptor organs
    within sensory system, 27
Persistent vegetative state
    mutism with, 336t, 343

Personality
and psychogenic speech disorders, 381-396
Pesticides
and Parkinson's disease, 190
Petrosal ganglia, 41
Pharyngeal branch
of vagus nerve, 42
Pharyngeal movement
nerves associated with, 22t
Pharyngeal plexus
formation of, 42
Pharyngeal reflexes, 86
Pharynx
abnormal movement of
with adductor spasmodic dysphonia, 243,
244t
contractions
with palatopharyngolaryngeal myoclonus,
236, 237t
examining at rest, 83f
and glossopharyngeal nerve, 41
movement of
nerves associated with, 22t
vagus nerve innervation of, 42
Phasic movements
definition of, 71
Phenytoin
causing ataxic dysarthria, 169
causing dyskinesias, 222
Phonation
affected by chorea, 228-229
affected by dystonia, 231
behavioral management of, 472
characteristics
with spasmodic dysphonia, 244t
defects with UUMN dysarthria, 263b, 264t
effect of vagus nerve damage on, 42
examining soft palate during, 83f
with hypokinetic dysarthria, 199-202, 206t
with palatopharyngolaryngeal myoclonus,
237t
prosthetic management of, 471-472
quantifying, 84
with spasmodic torticollis, 235t
summary of cranial lesion effects on, 119t-120t
and supplemental motor areas, 61
treatment approaches to improve
for different dysarthria types, 486t
and vowel prolongation, 91
Phonatory incompetence
with flaccid dysarthrias, 133
Phonatory instability
with ataxic dysarthria, 176-177
Phonatory muscles
innervating for speech, 3
Phonatory stenosis
with hyperkinetic dysarthria, 229
with spastic dysarthria, 151, 152t
Phonatory-prosodic insufficiency
with ataxic dysarthria, 173-174
with flaccid dysarthrias, 133
Phonatory-respiratory instability
with ataxic dysarthria, 176-177
Phonemes
and motor speech programmer, 309
motor system disorders associated with
repeated
summary to aid differential diagnosis, 417,
418t
repeating
with hypokinetic dysarthria, 197
Phonosurgery, 469-471
Phrases
short
with spastic dysarthria, 151
Phrenic nerves, 43
Physiologic analysis
of motor speech disorders, 10
Physiologic tremors
causes of, 72
definition of, 221
Pia mater
layers of
description and diagram illustrating, 19, 20f

Pick's disease
description of, 191
and echolalia, 359, 360b
and inclusion bodies, 31
types of dysarthrias caused by
and differential diagnoses, 413t
Pin-rolling movements
with parkinsonism, 188
Pitch
low or breaking
with spastic dysarthria, 151, 152t
Mayo Clinic rating scale for, 89, 90b
reduced
with vagus nerve lesions, 126
tracings illustrating, 154f
Pitch breaks
motor system disorders associated with
summary to aid differential diagnosis, 417,
418t
Plasticity
and cortex, 445
and neural adaptation, 445
Pleasure
limbic system role in sensations of, 63
Plexopathy
definition of, 111
Pneumotaxic center, 44
Polio
definition of, 114
causing flaccid dysarthria, 112b
types of dysarthrias caused by
and differential diagnoses, 414t
Poliomyelitis
definition of, 114
Polymyositis, 113
types of dysarthrias caused by
and differential diagnoses, 414t
Polyneuritis
definition of, 33
Polyneuropathy
definition of, 111
Pons
anatomical relationships with
and motor speech disorders, 21t
description and illustration of, 21, 22f
lacunar strokes in
and UUMN dysarthria, 257-258
lesions
causing spastic dysarthria, 147b,
148
Pontine
degeneration of, 168
Pontine branch
anatomical diagram of, 25f
Pontine nuclei, 55, 56f
Ponto-medullary respiratory oscillator, 44
Positive Babinski's sign
definition of, 144
Positron emission tomography (PET)
to study neuronal cell deaths, 32
Postanoxic myoclonus, 220
Postencephalitic parkinsonism, 192
Posterior cerebral arteries
anatomical diagram of, 25f
definition and function of, 23
diagram illustrating, 24f, 25f
Posterior communicating arteries
anatomical diagram of, 25f
Posterior fossae
anatomical relationships with
and motor speech disorders, 21t
definition of, 18
description and structures of, 21-22
illustration and structures of, 19f
locational diagram of, 20f, 21-22
Posterior limb
of internal capsule, 47-48
Posterior lobes
definition and location of, 54, 55
Post-polio syndrome, 114
Postsynaptic membranes
diagram illustrating, 30f
Postural adjustments
and speech, 467

Postural instability
deep brain stimulation (DBS) to treat,
488-489
Postural tremors
definition of, 221
examining for motor speech, 72
Posture
abnormalities
examples of, 189t
adjustments, 467
affected by hypokinetic dysarthria, 188-189
examining patient's, 85
and indirect activation pathway, 144
with spasmodic torticollis, 235f
stooped
with depression, 383
sustained
summary of dysarthrias associated with,
416t
Pramipexole
for Parkinson's disease, 191
Precentral gyrus, 45-46
Prefrontal syndrome, 344
Premotor cortex
diagram illustrating, 46t
function of, 61
Preprogrammed movement sequences, 60
Preprogramming
description of, 60
Pressure consonants
with vagus nerve lesions, 126
Presynaptic membranes
diagram illustrating, 30f
Primary generalized dystonia, 221
clinical features of, 224
types of dysarthrias caused by
and differential diagnoses, 413t
Primary language cortex, 46t
Primary lateral sclerosis (PLS)
causing flaccid dysarthria, 112b
causing spastic dysarthria, 146
types of dysarthrias caused by
and differential diagnoses, 413t
Primary motor cortex
anatomic diagram illustrating, 46f
description of, 45
Primary progressive aphasia (PPA)
with corticobasal degeneration, 292
definition and features of, 311, 314b
types of dysarthrias caused by
and differential diagnoses, 413t
Primary sensory cortex, 46t, 47
Primidone
causing ataxic dysarthria, 169
Primitive reflexes, 86
Prognoses
patient awareness of, 75
for recovery from psychogenic speech
disorders, 536
"Progressive"
descriptive of disease evolution, 33
Progressive bulbar palsy
description of, 112
types of dysarthrias caused by
and differential diagnoses, 413t
Progressive disorders
description and examples of, 12
Progressive multifocal leukoencephalopathy,
338
Progressive pseudobulbar palsy, 146
Progressive supranuclear palsy (PSP)
associated with mixed dysarthria, 278, 281t,
290-291
associated with primary progressive aphasia,
311
and echolalia, 359, 360b
leading to mutism, 337t, 338
causing palilalia, 258b, 359
types of dysarthrias caused by
and differential diagnoses, 413t
Projection fiber tracts, 30
Projections
structure and function of nervous system,
28t

Prolonged intervals
    motor system disorders associated with
        summary to aid differential diagnosis, 417,
            418t
Prolonged phonemes
    with chorea, 229-230
    motor system disorders associated with
        summary to aid differential diagnosis, 417,
            418t
Prompts for restructuring oral muscular
        phonetic targets (PROMPT)
    and behavioral management of AOS, 516
Proprioceptive senses
    and normal speech development, 6
Prosodic disturbances
    ataxic dysarthria as, 172
    with chorea, 229
Prosodic excess
    with ataxic dysarthria, 173-174, 175t
    with chorea, 229-230
    with spastic dysarthrias, 151
Prosodic insufficiency
    with chorea, 229-230
    with hypokinetic dysarthria, 196t, 197
    with Wilson disease, 293t
Prosodic production
    assessment of, 365-366
Prosody
    acoustic and physiologic findings
        with traumatic brain injuries (TBIs), 294t
    affected by chorea, 229-230
    affected by cranial nerve damage, 119t-120t
    affected by dystonia, 232
    with apraxia of speech (AOS)
        acoustic and physiologic findings with,
            320, 322b, 323-324
    characteristics of
        with amyotrophic lateral sclerosis (ALS),
            287t
        with hypokinetic dysarthria, 187
        with spasmodic dysphonia, 244t
    with chorea, 229
    impairments
        with ataxic dysarthria, 173t, 177, 179t
        with spastic dysarthria, 155-156
    levels affected by ataxic dysarthria, 163
    Mayo Clinic rating scale for, 89, 90b
    with palatopharyngolaryngeal myoclonus,
            237t
    prostheses to treat abnormal, 441
    psychogenic disorders of, 395-396
    with spasmodic torticollis, 235t
    treatment approaches to improve
        for different dysarthria types, 486t
Prosthetic devices
    for apraxia of speech (AOS), 509-510
    for different dysarthria types, 488t
    management of
        description of motor speech disorder,
            440-441
    postural support with, 467
"Pseudo smile"
    with Wilson disease, 293
Pseudobulbar affect
    with lacunar state, 146
    with spastic dysarthria, 149-150
    summary of dysarthrias associated with, 416t
Pseudobulbar crying
    with unilateral upper motor neuron (UUMN)
            dysarthria, 261
Pseudobulbar laughter
    with unilateral upper motor neuron (UUMN)
            dysarthria, 261
Pseudobulbar palsy
    deviant speech with, 151-152
    Mayo Clinic dysarthria studies on, 89
    with spastic dysarthria, 149, 155
Pseudoforeign accents, 354t, 363-365
    management of, 529-530
Psychiatric diseases;See also psychogenic
            speech disorders
    causing psychogenic speech disorders, 382-
            386
    speech changes caused by, 4

Psychogenic mutism
    definition of, 396
Psychogenic spasmodic dysphonia
    voice abnormalities with, 391
Psychogenic speech disorders
    case studies, 397-405
    definition and overview of, 381-382
    distinguishing between neurogenic, 426t,
            428-429, 430t
    distribution and types of, 4f
    etiologies of
        conversion disorders, 383-385
        depression, 382-383
        schizophrenia, 383
        stress and reactions to stress, 385
        volitional disorders, 386
    examination of, 387-388
    management of
        general principles and guidelines, 536-541
        general treatment techniques, 541-545
        symptomatic treatment of specific, 545-550
    other nonorganic disorders associated with
        articulation disorders, 395
        infantile speech, 396
        psychogenic mutism, 396
        resonance and prosodic disorders, 396
    principles to remember concerning, 382
    and speech changes, 7
    speech characteristics, 389-396
        with depression and manic-depression, 389
        dysfluencies, 394b
        with psychogenic stuttering, 392-395
        with psychogenic voice disorders, 390-392
        with schizophrenia, 389-390
    speech pathology issues, 386-396
    statistical distributions of, 386t
Psychogenic stuttering
    characteristics of, 392-395
    definition of, 392
    statistics concerning, 393t
    symptomatic treatment of, 545-547
    terminology, 392
Psychogenic voice disorders
    description of, 390
    symptomatic treatment of, 545-547
Psychologic factors;See also psychogenic
            speech disorders
    and differential diagnoses, 411
Psychomotor retardation
    with depression, 383
Psychosomatic disorders, 385
Ptosis
    due to vascular disturbances, 26t-27t
    as sign of myasthenia gravis, 113
"Punch-drunk" encephalopathy, 169
Pupil constriction
    nerves associated with, 22t
Pure dysarthria
    description of, 258
Pure motor hemiparesis
    description of, 258
Purines
    as part of neurochemical system, 24
Purkinje cells, 169
    definition of, 55
Purposeful activity, 448-449
Putamen
    anatomical diagram of, 25f
    associated with basal ganglia, 188
    definition of, 52
    diagram illustrating, 53f
    function and damage to, 53-54
    lacunar strokes in
        and UUMN dysarthria, 257-258
Pyramidal tract;See direct activation pathway

Q

Quadriplegia
    due to vascular disturbances, 26t-27t

R

Radiation necrosis
    types of dysarthrias caused by
        and differential diagnoses, 414t

Radiation therapy
    causing flaccid dysarthria, 112b, 115
Radiculopathy
    definition of, 111
Rage
    limbic system role in sensations of, 63
Ramsay-Hunt syndrome, 114
Range
    of speech, 72
Range of movement
    and articulation defects
        with hypokinetic dysarthria, 203-205,
            206t-207t
    and basal ganglia control circuit
        malfunctions, 188
    of jaw and lips
        during speech AMRs, 92-93
    reduction of
        conditions associated with, 73
        with hypokinetic dysarthria, 187, 194,
            195
    restricted with dopamine deficiency, 54
    and rigidity
        with parkinsonism, 188-189, 194
    and spastic paralysis, 144t, 145
Rate
    acoustic and physiologic findings
        with traumatic brain injuries (TBIs),
            294t
    characteristics
        with amyotrophic lateral sclerosis (ALS),
            287t
    MSDs associated with increased
        summary to aid differential diagnosis, 417,
            418t
    nonprosthetic reduction strategies, 482
    and prosody
        characteristics with apraxia of speech,
            318b, 319
        defects with UUMN dysarthria, 263b, 264t,
            265t
    prostheses to treat abnormal, 441
    treatment approaches to improve
        for different dysarthria types, 486t
Receptors
    within visceral system, 24
Recurrent laryngeal branch
    of vagus nerve, 42
Red nucleus
    definition of, 51
    diagram illustrating, 50f
    location of, 56f
Reduced loudness
    motor system disorders associated with
        summary to aid differential diagnosis, 417,
            418t
Reduced stress
    with hypokinetic dysarthria, 196t, 197
    motor system disorders associated with
        summary to aid differential diagnosis, 417,
            418t
Referential tasks, 484
Reflexes
    and central nervous system, 27-28
    as confirmatory clues, 86-88
    damaged by flaccid dysarthria, 110
    and indirect activation pathway, 144
    and sensory-motor and alpha motor neurons,
            38
    and speech, 62-63
Reflexive movements
    affected by flaccid dysarthrias, 110-111
Relaxation
    to improve articulation, 478
Release phenomena, 86
Renshaw cells
    innervation of, 37
Repetitive transcranial magnetic stimulation
            (rTMS), 345
Reserpine, 192
Resonance
    affect of spinal nerves on, 43
    affected by chorea, 229
    affected by cranial nerve damage, 119t-120t

Resonance—cont'd
    affected by dystonia, 231-232
    characteristics
        with spasmodic dysphonia, 244t
    defects with UUMN dysarthria, 263b, 264t
    hypokinetic dysarthria's effect on, 202-203,
        206t
    Mayo Clinic rating scale for, 89, 90b
    with palatopharyngolaryngeal myoclonus,
        237t
    psychogenic disorders of, 395-396
    treatment approaches to improve
        for different dysarthria types, 486t
Resonatory incompetence
    with chorea, 229
Resonatory muscles
    innervating for speech, 3
Resources
    related to motor speech disorders (MSDs),
        461-462
Respiration
    affected by chorea, 228
    affected by dystonia, 231
    characteristics
        with amyotrophic lateral sclerosis (ALS),
            287t
        with palatopharyngolaryngeal myoclonus,
            237t
        problems with ataxic dysarthria, 175-177,
            179f
        rapid or shallow, 85
        with spasmodic dysphonia, 244t
        with spasmodic torticollis, 235t
        with spastic dysarthria, 152, 155
        with unilateral upper motor neuron
            (UUMN) dysarthria, 265-266, 265t
    difficulties
        with traumatic brain injuries (TBIs), 294t
    examining patient, 84-86
    with hypokinetic dysarthria, 198-199, 206t
    Mayo Clinic rating scale for, 89, 90b
    nerves associated with, 43-44
    neurons associated with
        diagram illustrating, 44f
    treatment approaches to improve
        for different dysarthria types, 486t
Respiratory muscles
    abnormalities
        with hyperkinetic dysarthria, 225t, 226
    affected by cranial nerve lesions, 119t-120t
    innervating for speech, 3
Restiform body
    anatomical diagram of, 25f
Resting tremors
    definition of, 221
    examining for motor speech, 72
    examples of, 189t
    with parkinsonism, 188
Reticular activating system (RAS), 343
Reticular formation, 21
    definition of, 50
    diagram illustrating, 50f, 53f
    role in speech, 64
    in visceral system, 24
Reticulospinal tract
    diagram illustrating, 50f
Retrocollis, 221
Rhythm
    abnormalities with ataxic dysarthria, 173f, 177
    and supplemental motor areas, 61
Rhythmic cueing, 482-483
Right hemisphere
    and aprosodia, 365-370
    description and illustration of, 21
    influence on speech, 64
    lesions
        and depression, 383
Rigid oral laryngoscope, 84
Rigidity
    causing articulation defects
        with hypokinetic dysarthria, 203-205, 206t-
            207t
    with dopamine deficiency, 54
    examples of, 189t

Rigidity—cont'd
    with hypokinetic dysarthria, 188-189
    with parkinsonism, 188
Rolandic fissure, 45-46
Rolandic operculum
    causing mutism, 339-340
Romberg test, 165
Rooting reflexes, 87
Ropinirole
    for Parkinson's disease, 191
Rubella
    leading to cerebellar dysfunction, 169
Rubrospinal tract, 51
    diagram illustrating, 50f

S

Salient neuromuscular features
    accuracy-73, 72
    associated with diagnoses, 71-73
    range, 72
    speed, 71-72
    steadiness, 72
    strength, 71
    tone, 72
Salivation
    nerves associated with, 22t
Saltatory conduction
    diagram illustrating, 29f, 30f
    process of, 31
Sarcoidosis
    definition of, 114
    causing facial paralysis, 121
    types of dysarthrias caused by
        and differential diagnoses, 414t
"Scanning" speech, 173, 178, 289-290
Scavenger cells
    function of, 31
Schizophrenia
    affecting speech, 7
    and distinguishing neurogenic versus
        psychogenic
            aiding differential diagnosis, 426t, 428-429
    and echolalia, 359, 360b
    psychogenic mutism with, 396
    causing psychogenic speech disorders, 383
    speech characteristics with, 389
    tardive dyskinesia (TD) in patients with, 222
Schwann cells
    forming myelin, 30-31
    giving rise to schwannomas, 33
    structure and function of nervous system, 28t
Seizure disorders
    and mutism, 336t, 345
    types of dysarthrias caused by
        and differential diagnoses, 414t
Selegiline
    for Parkinson's disease, 191
Semilunar ganglia, 39-40
Senile plaques, 31
Sensorimotor commands
    for planning and programming speech, 308
Sensorimotor disorders
    with apraxia of speech, 422
    characterizing, 6
    Tourette's syndrome, 238-239
Sensorimotor programs
    controlled by motor speech
        programming/planning, 316, 317t
    functions of, 3
Sensory ataxia, 170
Sensory cortex
    within sensory system, 27
Sensory dysarthria, 118
Sensory functions
    loss of, 168
    and Tourette's syndrome, 238-239
    of trigeminal nerves, 39-41
Sensory motor integration
    and basal ganglia control circuit
        malfunctions, 188
    and Tourette's syndrome, 238-239
Sensory processes
    and speech, 6
    in speech motor control, 62

Sensory system
    components of, 27
    diagram illustrating, 37f
    and neuron activity, 29-30
    role of
        in speech programming, 62
Sensory tics, 239-239
Sensory tricks
    to correct abnormal involuntary movements,
        227
    to inhibit dystonic movements, 230
    for jaw, tongue, or face focal dystonia, 482
    with spasmodic torticollis, 235t
    summary of dysarthrias associated with,
        416t
Sentence intelligibility test (SIT), 98-99
Sequential motion rates (SMRs)
    with apraxia of speech, 318b, 319-320,
        322b
    definition of, 93
    with motor impersistence, 92
    motor system disorders associated with
        summary to aid differential diagnosis, 417,
            418t
    statistics for normal adults, 93t
"Severity"
    of motor speech disorders (MSDs), 70
Sex
    limbic system role in sensations of, 63
"Shimmer"
    and voice quality
        with Parkinson's disease, 201
Short phrases
    motor system disorders associated with
        summary to aid differential diagnosis, 417,
            418t
Short rushes of speech
    motor system disorders associated with
        summary to aid differential diagnosis, 417,
            418t
Shoulders
    movements of
        nerves associated with, 22t
        with spasmodic dysphonia, 243, 244t
    shrugging of
        and accessory nerves, 43
Shy-Drager syndrome
    mixed dysarthria with, 292
    with Parkinson's disease, 191
    types of dysarthrias caused by
        and differential diagnoses, 413t
Silences
    inappropriate
        with hypokinetic dysarthria, 196-198
    and pauses
        with Parkinson's disease, 205, 206t-207t
Silent articulatory movements
    with adductor spasmodic dysphonia, 243,
        244t
Sinemet
    for treatment of Parkinson's disease, 191
Singultus, 85, 220
Skeleton
    anatomical relationships with
        and motor speech disorders, 21t
Skilled movements, 144
Skull
    anatomical relationships with
        and motor speech disorders, 21t
    diagram illustrating bones of, 18f
    fractures
        causing flaccid dysarthria, 112b
        types of dysarthrias caused by, 413t
    function of, 18-19
    and major nervous system levels, 19, 20f, 21-
        23
Skull base tumors
    causing flaccid dysarthria, 115
Sleep disorders
    and dysarthria, 5
Slow or irregular AMRs
    motor system disorders associated with
        summary to aid differential diagnosis, 417,
            418t

Slow rate, 394b
  motor system disorders associated with
    summary to aid differential diagnosis, 417, 418t
    with progressive supranuclear palsy (PSP), 291
Slurred speech
  with ataxic dysarthria, 171
  with unilateral upper motor neuron (UUMN) dysarthria, 261, 264b, 264t
Smell
  limbic system role in sensations of, 63
  nerves associated with, 22t
Smiling
  observing facial appearance when, 76, 77f
Snout reflexes
  description of, 87
  with spastic dysarthria, 144, 150
  summary of dysarthrias associated with, 416t
Soft palate
  beating-like elevation of
    with palatopharyngolaryngeal myoclonus, 236, 237t
  examining at rest, 83f
  vagus nerve innervation of, 42
  vagus nerve lesion effects on, 124t
Somatic compliance, 385
Somatization disorders
  causing psychogenic speech disorders, 385
Somatosensory cortex
  and motor speech programming, 309-310
  role in speech, 61-62
Somnolence
  due to vascular disturbances, 26t-27t
Sound production
  and behavioral management of AOS, 515-516
Spasmodic dysphonia (SD)
  description and causes of, 240-244
  distinguishing speech characteristics with, 243, 244t
  psychogenic
    voice abnormalities with, 391
  rate, rhythm, and substrate of, 219t
Spasmodic torticollis (ST)
  associated with spasmodic dysphonia, 243
  description and illustration of, 233-235
  distinguishing speech characteristics with, 235t
  patient posture with, 235f
  rate, rhythm, and substrate of, 219t
Spasms
  description of, 221
  rate, rhythm, and substrate of, 219t
Spastic dysarthria
  acoustic and physiologic findings, 152, 153t, 154f, 155-157
  anatomical relationships associated with, 21t
  with bilateral lesions
    of direct/indirect activation pathways, 52
  case reviews of, 158-161
  clinical characteristics of, 144-145
  clusters of abnormal speech with, 151t, 152
  definition and overview of, 49, 143
  deviant speech characteristics with, 150-151
  diagnosing, 70
  differential diagnosis of
    as function of etiologies, 413t-414t
  from direct/indirect activation pathway damage, 143-144
  distinctive speech characteristics with
    summary of, 417, 418t
  distribution of causes, 146-148
  etiologies of, 145-146
    degenerative disease, 146
    inflammatory disease, 146
    vascular disorders, 145-146
  lesion loci and vascular source
    and differential diagnoses, 411, 412t
  localization and neuromotor basis of, 13t
  Mayo Clinic dysarthria studies on, 89
  and mixed dysarthria, 283-284
  mutism with
    localization and clinical features of, 336t, 337

Spastic dysarthria—cont'd
  neuromuscular deficits with, 150t
  patient perceptions and complaints, 148-149
  versus spastic paralysis, 145
  speaker-oriented treatments, 485, 486t-487t, 488
  summary of acoustic and physiologic findings, 153t, 155-157
  summary of oral mechanism findings, 415, 416t
  tracings illustrating, 154f
  and upper motor neuron (UMN) disease, 143
Spastic paralysis
  clinical characteristics of, 144-145
  versus spastic dysarthria, 145
Spasticity
  causes of, 51
  definition of, 143
  effects on speech, 52
  and muscle tone, 144
  with spastic dysarthria, 150-151
  and spastic paralysis, 144t, 145
Spatial dyscoordination, 324
Spatial summation, 37
Speaker-oriented treatments
  of dysarthrias
    articulation, 476-479
    overview of, 465-466
    phonation, 469-472
    prosody, 483-484
    rate, 479-483
    resonance, 472-476
    respiration, 466-469
  for specific dysarthria types
    ataxic dysarthria, 486t-487t, 488
    flaccid dysarthria, 485, 486t-487t
    hyperkinetic dysarthria, 486t-487t, 488-491
    hypokinetic dysarthria, 486t-487t, 488-491
    mixed dysarthria, 486t-487t, 493
    spastic dysarthria, 485, 486t-487t, 488
    UUMN dysarthria, 486t-487t, 493
  summary of, 486t
  types of
    and techniques of, 486t
Speaking
  drills, 449-450
Spectatoring, 392
Speech
  abnormal
    diagnostic variables, 69-70
  abnormalities with rhythm
    with ataxic dysarthria, 173f, 177, 179t
  and apraxia of speech
    symptoms, 315-316
  auditory-perceptual attributes of, 9
  and basal ganglia control circuit, 53-54
  blurred with hypokinetic dysarthria, 194
  characteristics
    and distinctions among dysfluencies, 425t
  cognitive and linguistic disorders, 6
  complaints with UUMN dysarthria, 261
  conceptual-programming level, 57-59
  cranial nerves affect on, 119t-120t
  defects
    with amyotrophic lateral sclerosis, 285-286
    with chorea, 228
    with dystonia, 230-232
    with psychogenic speech disorders, 388-389
    with UUMN dysarthria, 263b, 264t
  definition of, 3
  deviant characteristics
    with mixed dysarthria, 285
  deviant dimensions of, 152t
  difficulties with apraxia of speech, 317-321
  and direct activation pathway
    cortical components of, 45-47
    importance of, 45
    motor cortex, 46-47
    tracts, 47-48
  effect of basal ganglia control circuit on, 188-190
  effect of palatopharyngolaryngeal myoclonus on, 237

Speech—cont'd
  examinations, 69-100, 409-410
    diagnoses, 73-74, 409-430
    four parts of, 74-99
    guidelines for, 71-74
    during nonspeech activities, 76-88
    procedures, 74-99
    purpose of, 69-70
  functional and anatomic divisions of
    basal ganglia control circuit, 36t, 52-54
    cerebellar control circuit, 36t, 54-57
    control circuits, 36t, 52
    direct activation pathway, 36t, 45-49
    final common pathway, 36-45
    indirect activation pathway, 36t, 49-52
  indirect activation pathway
    cortical components and tracts, 49-50
    destination of, 51
    effects of damage to, 51-52
    motor function roles in, 50-51
  linguistic units, 59
  localization of
    within cerebellum, 164-165
  management of, 435-456
  measurements of
    fundamental frequency and intensity, 199-200
  methods of studying, 9-11
  motor system
    description of, 35-36
  neurological breakdown of, 3-5
  neurology of, 3
  normal variations in, 7
  patient perceptions
    with hypokinetic dysarthria, 193-194
  planning and programming, 59-64
  primary distinguishing characteristics
    with hypokinetic dysarthria, 198t
  production of
    conceptual-programming levels, 58-64
  rates of
    impairments with hypokinetic dysarthria, 194-197
  rating deviant characteristics, 89, 90b
  right hemisphere influences on, 64
  role of cerebellar control circuit in, 56-57
  with spasmodic dysphonia (SD), 243, 244t
  study of normal, 3
  summary of examinations, 85-86
  tasks for assessment of, 91
Speech apraxia, 312
Speech arrests
  and mutism, 345
  with seizures
    mutism with, 336t
Speech disorders
  causes of
    and basal ganglia control circuit lesions, 54
    and genu lesions, 48
  motor
    basic definition of, 6
    defining and categorizing, 3-15
  neurologic
    distribution of, 4f
  nonneurologic, 6-7
  other neurogenic
    aphasia, 362-363
    aprosodia, 365-370
    cognitive/affective, 360-362
    echolalia, 359-360
    foreign accent syndrome, 363-365
    neurogenic stuttering, 354-358
    "other" as defined by Mayo Clinic, 8f
    palilalia, 358-359
  psychogenic
    case studies, 397-405
    definition and overview of, 381-382
    distinguishing between neurogenic, 426t, 428-429, 430t
    distribution and types of, 4f
    etiologies of
      conversion disorders, 383-385
      depression, 382-383
      schizophrenia, 383

Speech disorders—cont'd
    etiologies of—cont'd
        stress and reactions to stress, 385
        volitional disorders, 386
    examination of, 387-388
    other nonorganic disorders associated with
        articulation disorders, 395
        infantile speech, 396
        psychogenic mutism, 396
        resonance and prosodic disorders, 396
    and speech changes, 7
    speech characteristics, 389-396
        with depression and manic-depression,
            389
        dysfluencies, 394b
        with psychogenic stuttering, 392-395
        with psychogenic voice disorders, 390-
            392
        with schizophrenia, 389-390
    psychogenic versus neurogenic, 429-430
Speech motor control
    definition of, 57
Speech motor system
    control circuits, 52
    final common pathway (FCP), 38-45
        accessory nerves, 43
        facial nerves, 41
        glossopharyngeal nerves, 41-42
        hypoglossal nerves, 43
        spinal nerves, 43-45
        trigeminal nerves, 39-41
        vagus nerves, 42
    relationships among divisions of, 37f
Speech pathology
    and mixed dysarthria, 281-295
Speech rate
    with apraxia of speech (AOS)
        acoustic and physiologic findings with,
            321-323, 322b
    and articulation defects
        with hypokinetic dysarthria, 203-205, 206t-
            207t
Speech sensorimotor system
    five stages of
        conceptualization, 58-59
        feedback, 58t, 64
        linguistic planning, 59
        motor planning and programming, 58t, 59-
            64
        performance, 58t, 64
Speech valves, 71
Speed
    of speech, 71-72
Sphenoid bones
    diagram illustrating, 18f
Sphincteric contractions, 86
Spinal accessory nerves;See accessory nerves
    bones associated with, 19f
Spinal arteries
    anatomical relationships with
        and motor speech disorders, 21t
Spinal column
    bony boundaries of, 18-19
    and major nervous system levels, 19, 20f,
        21-23
Spinal cord
    anatomical relationships with
        and motor speech disorders, 21t
    anatomy of, 19f, 20f, 22
    diagram illustrating, 20f, 50f
    injuries
        causing flaccid dysarthrias, 130
Spinal meninges
    anatomical relationships with
        and motor speech disorders, 21t
Spinal muscle atrophies
    description of, 112
    types of dysarthrias caused by
        and differential diagnoses, 413t
Spinal nerves
    affecting voice resonance and articulation,
        43
    anatomical relationships with
        and motor speech disorders, 21t

Spinal nerves—cont'd
    attached to spinal column, 22
    connections of, 30
    lesions
        associated with flaccid dysarthrias, 130-131
    motor nuclei of, 27-28
    in peripheral nervous system (PNS), 23
    within sensory system, 27
Spinal tract
    of trigeminal nerve, 40
Spinocerebellar ataxia, 167, 192
    types of dysarthrias caused by
        and differential diagnoses, 413t
Spirantization
    with apraxia of speech, 322b, 324
    causing articulation defects
        with hypokinetic dysarthria, 203-205, 206t-
            207t
    with hypokinetic dysarthria, 196, 203
Sports injuries
    and traumatic brain injury, 34
Stabilization
    of stroke victims, 34-35
"Staging"
    of management, 444
Stapedius muscles
    and facial nerve, 41
Stapedius reflex
    nerves associated with, 22t
Static encephalopathy
    as congenital disorder, 12
Static tremors
    with parkinsonism, 188
"Stationary"
    descriptive of disease evolution, 33
    disorders
        description and examples of, 12
Status epilepticus
    and echolalia, 359, 360b
Steadiness
    of speech, 72
Sternocleidomastoid muscles, 43
Straight sinus
    diagram illustrating, 20f, 21f
Strained-strangled quality
    motor system disorders associated with
        summary to aid differential diagnosis, 417,
            418t
Strength
    of muscles affecting speech, 71
    of speech
        motor learning techniques, 451-453
Strength training
    to improve articulation, 477-479
Stress
    abnormalities
        with hypokinetic dysarthria, 205
    with apraxia of speech (AOS)
        acoustic and physiologic findings with,
            322b, 323-324
    and distinguishing neurogenic versus
            psychogenic
        aiding differential diagnosis, 426t, 428-429
    causing psychogenic speech disorders, 385
    reduced
        with spastic dysarthria, 151
Stress testing
    for speech assessment, 93-94
Stretch reflex
    diagram illustrating, 39f
    and gamma motor neurons, 38, 39f
Stretching
    to improve articulation, 478
Striated muscles
    and motor cortex, 46-47
    motor system involvement in, 27-28
Striatonigral degeneration
    types of dysarthrias caused by
        and differential diagnoses, 413t
Striatum
    components of, 187-188
    definition of, 52
    diagram illustrating, 53f
    function and damage to, 53-54

Stridor
    motor system disorders associated with
        summary to aid differential diagnosis, 417,
            418t
Strokes
    causing akinetic mutism, 343-344
    causing ataxic dysarthria, 168
    causing biopercular syndrome, 339-340
    and depression, 383
    and diagnosing UUMN dysarthria, 267-268
    and echolalia, 359, 360b
    causing flaccid dysarthria, 112b
    hyperkinetic dysarthria from, 224
    "improving" speech following, 12
    leading to mutism, 337t, 338
    and mixed dysarthrias, 280, 281t, 282b
    as most common cause of AOS, 311-312,
        314-315
    neurologic description of, 34
    causing palilalia, 258b, 359
    causing spastic dysarthria, 145, 147b, 147f,
        155
    speech impairment statistics with, 7
    types of dysarthrias caused by
        and differential diagnoses, 413t
    causing unilateral upper motor neuron
        (UUMN) damage, 257-258
Struggle behavior, 394b
Stuttering
    anatomic correlates, 357
    with apraxia of speech, 316
    characteristics of, 392-395
    definition and clinical characteristics of, 354-
        355
    definition of, 392
    etiologies of, 355-357
    nature of the problem, 357-358
    neurogenic
        anatomic correlates, 357
        with apraxia of speech, 316
        definition and clinical characteristics of,
            354-355
        etiologies of, 355-357
        nature of the problem, 357-358
        with progressive supranuclear palsy (PSP),
            291
        varieties of, 356
    with progressive supranuclear palsy (PSP),
        291
    statistics concerning, 393t
    symptomatic treatment of, 545-547
    terminology, 392
    varieties of, 356
Stylopharyngeus muscles, 41
"Subacute"
    descriptive of disease development, 33
Subacute spongiform encephalopathy, 311
Subarachnoid hemorrhages, 35
Subarachnoid space
    anatomical relationships with
        and motor speech disorders, 21t
    within cerebrospinal fluid system (CSF), 23
    description of, 19
    diagram illustrating, 20f, 21f
Subclavian arteries, 24f
Subcortical arteriosclerotic encephalopathy,
    146
Subcortical infarcts, 146, 258
Subdural hematomas, 34
Subdural hemorrhages, 35
Subdural space
    description of, 19
    diagram illustrating, 20f
Sublingual glands
    facial nerve innervation of, 41
Submandibular glands
    facial nerve innervation of, 41
Substantia nigra
    associated with basal ganglia, 188
    definition of, 52
    diagram illustrating, 53f
    function and damage to, 53-54
    nerve cell loss
        with Parkinson's disease, 191

Subthalamic nuclei
    associated with basal ganglia, 188
    definition of, 52
    diagram illustrating, 53f
    function and damage to, 53-54
Sucking reflexes
    due to vascular disturbances, 26t
    hypoglossal nerve role in, 43
    with spastic dysarthria, 144, 150
    summary of dysarthrias associated with,
        416t
    testing for, 87
Superior cerebellar arteries
    anatomical diagram of, 25f
Superior cerebellar peduncle, 55
Superior colliculi
    description and illustration of, 21, 22f
Superior laryngeal nerve branches
    of vagus nerve, 42
Superior sagittal sinus
    diagram illustrating, 20f, 21f
Supplemental motor areas (SMAs)
    function of, 61
    as neural area of programming, 60
Supplementary motor area, 46
Supporting cells;See glial cells
Supramarginal gyrus, 46t
    role in speech, 61-62
Supratentorial levels
    anatomical relationships with
        and motor speech disorders, 21t
    locational diagram of, 20f
    of nervous system, 18-19, 19, 21t
Surgeries
    causing flaccid dysarthria, 112b
    for hypokinetic dysarthria, 488-489
    interventions
        for different dysarthria types, 488t
    laryngeal, 469-471
    trauma
        causing apraxia of speech, 311-312, 314-
            315
    types of dysarthrias caused by
        and differential diagnoses, 413t
    types of dysarthrias caused by
        and differential diagnoses, 413t
Surgical interventions
    for different dysarthria types, 488t
Surgical trauma
    causing apraxia of speech, 311-312, 314-315
    types of dysarthrias caused by
        and differential diagnoses, 413t
Swallowing
    difficulties
        with chorea, 227
        with hypokinetic dysarthria, 193-194
        with spastic dysarthria, 149
        with unilateral upper motor neuron
            (UUMN) dysarthria, 261
    and glossopharyngeal nerve, 41-42
    hypoglossal nerve role in, 43
    questioning patient concerning, 75
Sydenham's chorea, 220, 224
    types of dysarthrias caused by
        and differential diagnoses, 414t
Symptomatic therapy
    for psychogenic speech disorders, 543-550
Synapses
    definition and illustration of, 29
Synaptic cleft
    definition and illustration of, 29
    diagram illustrating, 30f
Synaptic vesicles
    definition and illustration of, 29
Synkinesis
    definition and appearance of, 118f, 121
    rate, rhythm, and substrate of, 219t
    summary of dysarthrias associated with,
        416t
Syphilis
    causing facial paralysis, 121
    causing parkinsonism, 192
    types of dysarthrias caused by
        and differential diagnoses, 414t

Syringobulbia
    definition of, 114
    causing flaccid dysarthria, 112b
    types of dysarthrias caused by
        and differential diagnoses, 414t, 415
Syringomyelia
    definition of, 114
    causing flaccid dysarthria, 112b
    types of dysarthrias caused by
        and differential diagnoses, 414t, 415
Systemic lupus erythematosus
    and chorea, 224

T

Tactile senses
    and normal speech development, 6
    transmission through trigeminal nerves, 39
Tardive dyskinesia (TD)
    description and causes of, 220
    in schizophrenic patients, 222
Taste
    deficits
        due to vascular disturbances, 26t-27t
        facial nerve innervation of, 41
        limbic system role in sensations of, 63
        nerves associated with, 22t
Teeth
    poor care of
        causing speech disorders, 6
    trigeminal nerve sensory role in, 39
Teflon
    injections, 470
Tegmentum
    definition of, 21
Telegraphic syntax, 394b
Telescoping
    with ataxic dysarthria, 173, 174, 175t
    motor system disorders associated with
        summary to aid differential diagnosis, 417,
            418t
Temperature
    nerve fibers, 40
Temporal bones
    diagram illustrating, 18f
Temporal dyscoordination, 324
Temporal dysregulation
    with ataxic dysarthria, 173f, 177
Temporal lobes
    anatomical diagram of, 25f
    within limbic system, 63
    sensory systems of, 27
Temporal summation, 37
Temporalis muscles, 41
Temporomandibular joint
    trigeminal nerve sensory role in, 39
Tensilon test, 113
Tensor tympani, 39
Tensor veli palatini, 39, 236
Tentorium cerebelli
    anatomical relationships with
        and motor speech disorders, 21t
    layers of
        description and diagram illustrating, 19, 20f
Terminal tremors
    with ataxic dysarthria, 165
    definition of, 221
    examining for motor speech, 72
Terminology
    basic speech pathology definitions, 5-7
Tetrabenazine, 192
Thalamic nuclei, 63
Thalamic system
    lesions
        and depression, 383
Thalamocortical connections
    within sensory system, 27
Thalamocortical fibers, 30
Thalamocortical radiation, 47
Thalamotomy
    causing palilalia, 258b, 359
    to treat hypokinetic dysarthria, 488-489
Thalamus
    anatomical relationships with
        and motor speech disorders, 21t

Thalamus—cont'd
    component of basal ganglia control circuit,
        188
    diagram illustrating, 48f
    illustration of, 53f
    influences on speech, 64
    lacunar strokes in
        and UUMN dysarthria, 257-258
    within sensory system, 27
Thalamus-ventral nuclei, 56f
Thermal senses
    transmission through trigeminal nerves, 39
Thirst
    limbic system role in sensations of, 63
Thoracic vertebrae, 22
Thrombosis
    definition of, 35
Thrombotic strokes, 35
Tic douloureux, 117
Tics
    definition of, 220, 238-239
    multiple motor
        summary of dysarthrias associated with,
            416t
    rate, rhythm, and substrate characteristics of,
        219t
    vocal characteristics of, 239
Titubation
    definition of, 165
Tongue
    abnormal movements of
        with adductor spasmodic dysphonia, 243,
            244t
        with amyotrophic lateral sclerosis (ALS),
            287
        with hyperkinetic dysarthria, 225t, 226
        with tardive dyskinesia, 220
    appearance at rest, 81
    atrophy
        with hypoglossal nerve lesions, 128, 129f
    dyskinesia waveforms, 234f
    dysmetria
        summary of dysarthrias associated with,
            416t
    and gag reflex, 86
    and glossopharyngeal nerve, 41
    groping movements of
        with apraxia of speech, 320, 322b
    and hypoglossal nerve, 43
    involuntary movements of
        with dystonia, 232, 233f, 234f
        summary of dysarthrias associated with,
            416t
    motor cortex neurons associated with, 46
    movements
        reduced with biopercular syndrome, 339-
            340
    movements and sensations
        nerves associated with, 22t
    myoclonic movement of
        with palatopharyngolaryngeal myoclonus,
            237t
    nerve sensations of, 42
    palatoglossus muscles of, 42
    during sustained postures, 81, 82f, 83
    tremulousness of
        with hypokinetic dysarthria, 194, 197
        summary of dysarthrias associated with, 416t
Tonic spasms
    description of, 221
Torticollis
    summary of dysarthrias associated with, 416t
Tourette's syndrome (TS)
    definition of, 220, 238-239
    distinguishing speech characteristics of, 239t
    and echolalia, 359, 360b
    causing palilalia, 258b, 359
    types of dysarthrias caused by
        and differential diagnoses, 414t
Toxic conditions
    causing ataxic dysarthria, 166f, 169
    characteristics of
        and progression, 33
        for various neurologic disease etiologies, 32t

Toxic conditions—cont'd
    and differential diagnoses, 412, 413t-414t
    and hyperkinetic dysarthria, 222-223
    with hypokinetic dysarthria, 189b, 191-192
    causing mixed dysarthria
        central pontine myelinolysis, 280
        hepatocerebral degeneration, 279
        hypoxic encephalopathy, 279-280
        Wilson's disease (WD), 279-280
Toxic tremors
    causes for, 221
Toxins
    and mutism, 346
Tracts
    definition of nerve fiber, 30
    indirect activation pathway, 49-50
    structure and function of nervous system, 28t
Tractus solitarius, 41, 42
Transcortical motor aphasia, 342, 360
"Transient"
    descriptive of disease evolution, 33
Transient breathiness, 229
Transient ischemic attacks (TIAs);See also
        strokes
    description of, 35
Transient mutism, 340
Trapezius muscles, 43
Trauma; See also traumatic brain injuries (TBIs)
    causing apraxia of speech, 311-312, 314-315
    causing ataxic dysarthria, 166f, 169, 170
    characteristics of
        for various neurologic disease etiologies,
            32t
    and differential diagnoses, 412, 413t-414t
    causing flaccid dysarthria, 111, 112b
    causing hypokinetic dysarthria, 189b, 192
    types of dysarthrias caused by
        and differential diagnoses, 413t
Traumatic brain injuries (TBIs)
    acoustic and physiologic findings
        with mixed dysarthria, 294t
    causing ataxic dysarthria, 169, 170
    and depression, 383
    description and types of, 34
    and differential diagnoses, 412, 413t-414t
    dysarthria with, 12
    causing hypokinetic dysarthria, 189b, 192
    and mixed dysarthria, 280, 281t, 293-295
    causing spastic dysarthria, 147b, 147f, 148
Traumatic injuries
    description of, 34
Treatment;See management
Tremors
    with amyotrophic lateral sclerosis, 286
    and articulation defects
        with hypokinetic dysarthria, 203-205, 206t-
            207t
    deep brain stimulation (DBS) to treat, 488-
        489
    due to vascular disturbances, 26t
    essential voice, 239-240, 241f, 242t
    measuring voice
        with hypokinetic dysarthria, 200-201
    with parkinsonism
        description of, 188
    and speech unsteadiness, 72
    summary of dysarthrias associated with, 416t
    toxins that cause, 222-223
    types and descriptions of, 221
Tremulousness
    with hypokinetic dysarthria, 196
    of jaw, lips and tongue
        with hypokinetic dysarthria, 194, 197
    summary of dysarthrias associated with, 416t
    during sustained facial postures, 76
Tricyclic antidepressants
    causing dyskinesias, 222
Trigeminal ganglia, 39-40
Trigeminal nerves
    anatomic origin and function of, 22t
    anatomical diagram of, 25f
    branches of, 39-41
    lesions
        associated with flaccid dysarthrias, 116-118

Trigeminal nerves—cont'd
    maxillary and mandibular divisions of, 19f
    role in speech production, 39-41
    sensory functions of, 39
    and UMN innervation, 48t
Trigeminal neuralgia
    description of, 117
Trigeminothalamic tracts, 40
Trihexyphenidyl
    for Parkinson's disease, 191
Trochlear nerves
    anatomic origin and function of, 22t
Truncal ataxia, 167-168
    definition of, 57
Trussing, 467
Tuberculosis
    leading to cerebellar dysfunction, 169
    causing parkinsonism, 192
    types of dysarthrias caused by
        and differential diagnoses, 414t
Tumors
    causing apraxia of speech, 311-312, 314-315
    causing ataxic dysarthria, 168-169
    of basal ganglia
        causing chorea and dystonia, 224
    causing facial paralysis, 121
    causing flaccid dysarthria, 112b
    metastasizing, 33
    neoplastic, 33-34
    causing spastic dysarthria, 147f, 148
    and strokes, 35

U

Undetermined dysarthria
    localization and neuromotor basis of, 13t
Unilateral blindness
    due to vascular disturbances, 26t
Unilateral palatal weakness
    summary of dysarthrias associated with, 416t
Unilateral sensory loss
    due to vascular disturbances, 26t
Unilateral upper motor neuron (UUMN) system
    anatomical relationships associated with, 21t
    deviant speech characteristics with, 263b,
        264t
    diagnosis of, 267-268
    differential diagnosis of
        as function of etiologies, 413t-414t
    diseases of
        differential diagnosis of, 426t, 428-429
    dysarthria
        acoustic and physiologic findings, 265-266
        anatomy and functions of, 256-257
        case studies of, 268-270
        cerebral hemisphere lesions, 52
        clinical characteristics of, 261-265
        clinical features of lesions of, 257,
            259-260
        definition and overview of, 255-256
        distinctiveness of, 267-268
        etiologies of, 257-258, 259f, 259t, 260
        localization and neuromotor basis of, 13t,
            14
        patient perceptions and complaints, 261
        severity of, 261
        speaker-oriented treatments, 486t-487t, 493
        speech characteristics of, 261-265
        symptoms of, 49
    including direct and indirect pathways, 256-
        257
    lesion loci and vascular source
        and differential diagnoses, 411, 412t
    pathways
        lacunar strokes in, 257-258
    spasticity with, 264
    summary of oral mechanism findings with,
        416t
Upper constrictor muscles
    of pharynx, 41
Upper face nerves
    and UMN innervation, 48t
Upper motor neuron (UMN) lesions
    definition of, 144
    and spastic paralysis, 144-145

Upper motor neuron (UMN) system
    anatomy and basic functions, 256-257
    clarification and distinctions of, 45
    corticospinal and corticobulbar tracts, 45
    cranial nerves of innervation
        related to speech, 48t
    direct and indirect activation pathways of,
        256-257
    disease
        and spastic dysarthria, 143
    dysarthria
        with direct activation pathway lesions, 49
        due to vascular disturbances, 26t
    lesions of, 52
    versus lower motor neuron (LMN) system,
        45t
Uvula, 43

V

Vagus nerves
    anatomic origin and function of, 22t
    anatomical diagram of, 25f
    bones associated with, 19f
    branches of, 42
    damage to, 42
    description of, 42
    effects of lesions
        unilateral and bilateral, 125f
    and gag reflex, 86
    innervating palate, pharynx and larynx, 42
    lesions
        associated with flaccid dysarthrias, 123-
            124
        effects of, 123, 124t
    and UMN innervation, 48t
Valium
    causing ataxic dysarthria, 169
Valproic acid
    causing ataxic dysarthria, 169
Variability
    with apraxia of speech (AOS)
        acoustic and physiologic findings with,
            322b
Variable rate
    motor system disorders associated with
        summary to aid differential diagnosis, 417,
            418t
Vascular disorders
    associated with mixed dysarthria, 280, 281t,
        282b
    causing ataxic dysarthria, 166f, 168, 170
    as cause of neurologic disease, 34-35
    characteristics of
        for various neurologic disease etiologies,
            32t
    and differential diagnoses, 412, 413t-414t
    causing flaccid dysarthria, 112b
    and hyperkinetic dysarthria, 222f, 223b, 224
    with hypokinetic dysarthria, 189b, 191
    causing spastic dysarthria, 145, 147b, 147f
    causing unilateral upper motor neuron
        (UUMN) dysarthria, 257-259
Vascular parkinsonism, 191
Vascular supply
    and differential diagnoses, 411, 412t
Vascular system
    anatomical diagram of, 24f, 25f
    anatomical relationships with
        and motor speech disorders, 21t
    definition and function of, 23
    supply to brain, 26t
Vasogenic edema, 35
Vegetative state
    and mutism, 343
Velopharyngeal inadequacy, 472-476
Velopharyngeal speech valves, 71-72
Velopharynx
    acoustic and physiologic findings
        with traumatic brain injuries (TBIs), 294t
    characteristics
        with amyotrophic lateral sclerosis (ALS),
            287t
        with unilateral upper motor neuron
            (UUMN) dysarthria, 265t, 266

Velopharynx—cont'd
  hypokinetic dysarthria's effect on, 202-203,
    206t
  during movement, 83f, 84
  at rest, 83-84
  with spastic dysarthria, 155
Ventral nerve roots
  attaching nerves to spinal cord, 22
Ventral respiratory neurons, 44
Ventricles
  anatomical relationships with
    and motor speech disorders, 21t
  within cerebrospinal fluid system (CSF),
    23
  locational diagram of, 21f
Ventricular system
  anatomical relationships with
    and motor speech disorders, 21t
  within cerebrospinal fluid system (CSF),
    23
  diagram illustrating, 22f
Verbal apraxia, 312
Vermis
  definition and location of, 54, 55f
  description and illustration of, 21
Vertebral arteries
  anatomical diagram of, 25f
  anatomical relationships with
    and motor speech disorders, 21t
  definition and function of, 23
  diagram illustrating, 24f, 25f
  inferior view of, 25f
Vertebral column
  anatomical relationships with
    and motor speech disorders, 21t
  description of, 22
Vertebrobasilar system
  anatomical relationships with
    and motor speech disorders, 21t
  blood entering brain through, 23
  vascular supply regions of
    and motor speech disorders (MSDs),
    26t-27t
Vertigo
  due to vascular disturbances, 26t-27t
Vestibular nuclei, 56f
  function of, 51
Vestibulospinal tract
  description of, 51
Videostroboscopy, 84
Viral infections
  astrocyte reaction to, 32
  and inclusion bodies, 31
Visceral system
  activities
    limbic system role in sensations of, 63
  function and description of, 24
  organs
    nerves associated with, 22t
Vision
  nerves associated with, 22t
  within sensory system, 27
Visual deficits
  due to vascular disturbances, 26t
Visual imaging methods
  of studying motor speech disorders, 10-11
Visuomotor tracking tasks, 325

Vitamin E
  deficiency with ataxia, 168
Vitamins
  deficiency
    associated with cerebellar dysfunction, 169
Vocal flutter
  with progressive supranuclear palsy (PSP),
    291
  with vagus nerve lesions, 126
Vocal fold paralysis
  with conversion aphonia
    voice abnormalities with, 390-391
Vocal fold weakness
  with conversion aphonia
    voice abnormalities with, 390-391
Vocal folds
  adduction and paresis, 84
  bowing
    with Parkinson's disease, 201-202, 206t
  nerve sensations of, 42
  paralyses
    causing flaccid dysarthria, 112b, 115
  for pitch
    innervation of, 42
  vagus nerve lesion effects on, 124t
  weakness of
    characteristics of, 126
    with unilateral upper motor neuron
      (UUMN) dysarthria, 262
Vocal tics
  with Tourette's syndrome, 238-239
Voice
  affect of spinal nerves on, 43
  characteristics
    with hypokinetic dysarthria, 187
    with spasmodic dysphonia, 244t
  distribution and types of, 4f
  measurements
    fundamental frequency and intensity, 199-
      200
  normal versus organic tremor, 241f
  quality
    Mayo Clinic rating scale for, 89, 90b
    with Parkinson's disease, 201
  tremors
    with hypokinetic dysarthria, 200-201
Voice amplifier, 441
Voice arrests
  motor system disorders associated with
    summary to aid differential diagnosis, 417,
      418t
Voice onset time (VOT)
  with apraxia of speech (AOS)
    acoustic and physiologic findings with,
      321, 322b
  with chorea, 229-230
Voice stoppages
  with hyperkinetic dysarthria, 229
  motor system disorders associated with
    summary to aid differential diagnosis, 417,
      418t
Voice tremors
  with cerebellar disease, 175
  motor system disorders associated with
    summary to aid differential diagnosis, 417,
      418t
  organic, 239-240, 241f, 242t

Volitional disorders
  versus automatic nonspeech, 88
  speech disorders from, 386
Voluntary movements
  affected by flaccid dysarthrias, 110-111
  and neuron activity, 29-30
Vomiting
  due to vascular disturbances, 26t-27t
Von-Hippel Lindau disease, 168
Vowel prolongation
  parameters of, 92
  for speech assessment, 91
Vowels
  and consonants
    with apraxia of speech, 321-322

W

Wada testing, 345
Wallenberg's lateral medullary syndrome
  associated with flaccid dysarthria, 114
Wallerian degeneration
  description of, 31
Water glass manometers, 85f
Weakness
  facial
    with apraxia of speech, 316, 317t
    with flaccid dysarthria, 110, 118f
    with unilateral upper motor neuron
      (UUMN) dysarthria, 257, 262, 267
  lower face
    summary of dysarthrias associated with,
      416t
  and nerve damage, 38
  and spastic paralysis, 144t, 145
  of speech
    motor learning techniques, 451-453
  of voice
    with hypokinetic dysarthria, 193-194
Wernicke's aphasia, 313, 325, 389
Whipple's disease
  causing parkinsonism, 192
White matter
  lacunar strokes in
    and UUMN dysarthria, 257-258
Wilson's disease (WD)
  deviant speech characteristics with, 293t
  disorders of
    causing parkinsonism, 192
  drugs that treat, 440-441
  mixed dysarthria with, 279-280, 282b,
    293
  types of dysarthrias caused by
    and differential diagnoses, 414t
  wing-beating tremors with, 221
Wing-beating tremors
  definition of, 221
Work intelligibility test, 99

X

Xerostomia, 81

Y

Yes-no reversals, 292

Z

Zygomatic arch
  diagram illustrating, 18f